T0175462

TENTH EDITION

Handbook of
Clinical Anesthesia
Procedures of the
Massachusetts
General Hospital

TENTH EDITION

Handbook of Clinical Anesthesia Procedures of the Massachusetts General Hospital

Senior Editor
Richard M. Pino, MD, PhD, FCCM

Associate Editors
Edward A. Bittner, MD, PhD, FCCM
Hovig V. Chitilian, MD
Wilton C. Levine, MD
Susan A. Vassallo, MD

Department of Anesthesia, Critical Care, and Pain Medicine
Harvard Medical School
Massachusetts General Hospital
Boston, Massachusetts

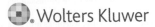. Wolters Kluwer

Philadelphia · Baltimore · New York · London
Buenos Aires · Hong Kong · Sydney · Tokyo

Acquisitions Editor: Keith Donnellan
Senior Development Editor: Ashley Fischer
Editorial Coordinator: Sean Hanrahan and Oliver Raj
Marketing Manager: Kirsten Watrud
Production Project Manager: Justin Wright
Design Coordinator: Stephen Druding
Manufacturing Coordinator: Beth Welsh
Prepress Vendor: TNQ Technologies

10th edition

Copyright © 2022 Wolters Kluwer.

Copyright © 2016 Wolters Kluwer. Copyright © 2010, 2007 Lippincott Williams & Wilkins, a Wolters Kluwer business. Copyright © 2002 Lippincott Williams & Wilkins. Copyright © 1998 Lippincott-Raven. Copyright © 1994 JB Lippincott. All rights reserved. This book is protected by copyright. No part of this book may be reproduced or transmitted in any form or by any means, including as photocopies or scanned-in or other electronic copies, or utilized by any information storage and retrieval system without written permission from the copyright owner, except for brief quotations embodied in critical articles and reviews. Materials appearing in this book prepared by individuals as part of their official duties as U.S. government employees are not covered by the above-mentioned copyright. To request permission, please contact Wolters Kluwer at Two Commerce Square, 2001 Market Street, Philadelphia, PA 19103, via email at permissions@lww.com, or via our website at shop.lww.com (products and services).

9 8 7 6 5 4 3 2 1

Printed in China

Library of Congress Cataloging-in-Publication Data

ISBN-13: 978-1-975154-40-0

Cataloging in Publication data available on request from publisher.

This work is provided "as is," and the publisher disclaims any and all warranties, express or implied, including any warranties as to accuracy, comprehensiveness, or currency of the content of this work.

This work is no substitute for individual patient assessment based upon healthcare professionals' examination of each patient and consideration of, among other things, age, weight, gender, current or prior medical conditions, medication history, laboratory data and other factors unique to the patient. The publisher does not provide medical advice or guidance and this work is merely a reference tool. Healthcare professionals, and not the publisher, are solely responsible for the use of this work including all medical judgments and for any resulting diagnosis and treatments.

Given continuous, rapid advances in medical science and health information, independent professional verification of medical diagnoses, indications, appropriate pharmaceutical selections and dosages, and treatment options should be made and healthcare professionals should consult a variety of sources. When prescribing medication, healthcare professionals are advised to consult the product information sheet (the manufacturer's package insert) accompanying each drug to verify, among other things, conditions of use, warnings and side effects and identify any changes in dosage schedule or contraindications, particularly if the medication to be administered is new, infrequently used or has a narrow therapeutic range. To the maximum extent permitted under applicable law, no responsibility is assumed by the publisher for any injury and/or damage to persons or property, as a matter of products liability, negligence law or otherwise, or from any reference to or use by any person of this work.

CCS0521

Mark Abraham, MD*
Department of Anesthesia, Critical Care and Pain Medicine
Massachusetts General Hospital
Boston, Massachusetts

Christopher M. Aiudi, MD, PharmD
Resident in Anesthesia
Department of Anesthesia, Critical Care, and Pain Medicine
Massachusetts General Hospital
Boston, Massachusetts

Daniel Ankeny, MD, PhD
Instructor in Anesthesia
Harvard Medical School
Department of Anesthesia, Critical Care and Pain Medicine
Massachusetts General Hospital
Boston, Massachusetts

Cliodhna Ashe, MD
Resident in Anesthesia
Department of Anesthesia, Critical Care and Pain Medicine
Massachusetts General Hospital
Boston, Massachusetts

Aditi Balakrishna, MD
Assistant Professor
Harvard Medical School
Department of Anesthesia, Critical Care, and Pain Medicine
Massachusetts General Hospital
Boston, Massachusetts

*Affiliation prior to publication.

Xiaodong Bao, MD, PhD
Assistant Professor of Anesthesia
Harvard Medical School
Department of Anesthesia, Critical Care and Pain Medicine
Massachusetts General Hospital
Boston, Massachusetts

Diana Barragan-Bradford, MD
Fellow in Critical Care
Department of Anesthesia, Critical Care and Pain Medicine
Massachusetts General Hospital
Boston, Massachusetts

William Benedetto, MD
Assistant Professor of Anesthesia
Harvard Medical School
Department of Anesthesia, Critical Care, and Pain Medicine
Massachusetts General Hospital
Boston, Massachusetts

Gloria Nadayil Berchmans, MD
Resident in Anesthesia
Department of Anesthesia, Critical Care, and Pain Medicine
Massachusetts General Hospital
Boston, Massachusetts

Sheri M. Berg, MD
Assistant Professor of Anesthesia
Harvard Medical School
Director of PACU
Department of Anesthesia, Critical Care and Pain Medicine
Massachusetts General Hospital
Boston, Massachusetts

Edward A. Bittner, MD, PhD, MSEd, FCCM
Associate Professor of Anesthesia
Harvard Medical School
Program Director, Critical Care-Anesthesiology Fellowship
Associate Director, Surgical Intensive Care Unit
Department of Anesthesia, Critical Care and Pain Medicine
Massachusetts General Hospital
Boston, Massachusetts

Juan M. Cotte Cabarcas, MD
Resident in Anesthesia
Department of Anesthesia, Critical Care and Pain Medicine
Massachussets General Hospital
Boston, Massachusetts

Shika Card, MD, MA
Resident in Anesthesia
Department of Anesthesia, Critical Care and Pain Medicine
Massachusetts General Hospital
Boston, Massachusetts

Andrew N. Chalupka, MD
Assistant Professor of Anesthesia
Senior Associate Consultant
Department of Anesthesiology and Perioperative Medicine
Mayo Clinic
Rochester, Minnesota

Marvin G. Chang, MD, PhD
Instructor of Anesthesia
Harvard Medical School
Assistant Program Director, Critical Care Anesthesiology Fellowship
Department of Anesthesia, Critical Care and Pain Medicine
Massachusetts General Hospital
Boston, Massachusetts

Frances K. W. Chen, MD
Resident in Anesthesia
Department of Anesthesia, Critical Care, and Pain Medicine
Massachusetts General Hospital
Boston, Massachusetts

Jenny Zhao Cheng, MD
Resident in Anesthesia
Department of Anesthesia, Critical Care and Pain Medicine
Massachusetts General Hospital
Boston, Massachusetts

Hovig V. Chitilian, MD
Assistant Professor of Anesthesia
Harvard Medical School
Department of Anesthesia, Critical Care and Pain Medicine
Neurosurgical, Vascular, and Thoracic Division Chief
Massachusetts General Hospital
Boston, Massachusetts

Kate Cohen, MD
Instructor of Anesthesia
Department of Anesthesia, Critical Care and Pain Medicine
Harvard Medical School
Massachusetts General Hospital
Boston, Massachusetts

Devan Cote, MD
Resident in Anesthesia
Department of Anesthesia, Critical Care, and Pain Medicine
Massachusetts General Hospital
Boston, Massachusetts

Jennifer Cottral, MD
Instructor of Anesthesia
Harvard Medical School
Department of Anesthesia, Critical Care, and Pain Medicine
Massachusetts General Hospital
Boston, Massachusetts

Stephanie L. Counihan, MSN, CRNA
Staff Nurse Anesthetist
Massachusetts General Hospital
Department of Anesthesia, Critical Care, and Pain Medicine
Boston, Massachusetts

Jerome Crowley, MD, MPH*
Instructor of Anesthesia
Harvard Medical School
Department of Anesthesia, Critical Care and Pain Medicine
Massachusetts General Hospital
Boston, Massachusetts

Adam A. Dalia, MD, MBA, FASE
Assistant Professor of Anesthesia
Harvard Medical School
Division of Cardiac Anesthesia
Department of Anesthesiology, Critical Care and Pain Medicine
Massachusetts General Hospital
Boston, Massachusetts

Michelle Dyrholm, DO
Resident in Anesthesia
Department of Anesthesia, Critical Care and Pain Medicine
Massachusetts General Hospital
Boston, Massachusetts

Affiliation prior to publication.

Dan Ellis, MD
Instructor of Anesthesia
Harvard Medical School
Department of Anesthesia, Critical Care and Pain Medicine
Massachusetts General Hospital
Boston, Massachusetts

Michael R. Fettiplace, MD, PhD
Resident
Department of Anesthesia, Critical Care and Pain Medicine
Massachusetts General Hospital
Boston, Massachusetts

Gregory H. Foos, MD
Resident in Anesthesia
Department of Anesthesia, Critical Care and Pain Medicine
Massachusetts General Hospital
Boston, Massachusetts

Hilary Gallin, MD
Resident in Anesthesia
Department of Anesthesia, Critical Care and Pain Medicine
Massachusetts General Hospital
Boston, Massachusetts

Erica L. Gee, MD
Resident in Anesthesia
Department of Anesthesia, Critical Care and Pain Medicine
Massachusetts General Hospital
Boston, Massachusetts

Philipp Gerner, MD
Resident in Anesthesia
Department of Anesthesia, Critical Care and Pain Medicine
Massachusetts General Hospital
Boston, Massachusetts

Gregory E. Ginsburg, MD
Assistant Professor of Anesthesia
Harvard Medical School
Department of Anesthesia, Critical Care, and Pain Medicine
Massachusetts General Hospital
Boston, Massachusetts

Paul D. Guillod, MD
Resident in Anesthesia
Department of Anesthesia, Critical Care, and Pain Medicine
Massachusetts General Hospital
Boston, Massachusetts

Casey Hamilton, MD
Resident in Anesthesia
Department of Anesthesia, Critical Care and Pain Medicine
Massachusetts General Hospital
Boston, Massachusetts

David Hao, MD
Resident in Anesthesia
Department of Anesthesia, Critical Care, and Pain Medicine
Massachusetts General Hospital
Boston, Massachusetts

Evan Hodell, MD
Resident in Anesthesia
Department of Anesthesia, Critical Care, and Pain Medicine
Massachusetts General Hospital
Boston, Massachusetts

Ryan J. Horvath, MD, PhD
Instructor of Anesthesia
Harvard Medical School
Department of Anesthesia, Critical Care, and Pain Medicine
Massachusetts General Hospital
Boston, Massachusetts

Omar Hyder, MD, MS
Instructor of Anesthesia
Harvard Medical School
Department of Anesthesia, Critical Care, and Pain Medicine
Massachusetts General Hospital
Boston, Massachusetts

Oluwaseun Johnson-Akeju, MD, MMSc
Anesthetist in Chief
Department of Anesthesia, Critical Care and Pain Medicine
Massachusetts General Hospital
Boston, Massachusetts

Alexander S. Kuo, MS, MD
Assistant Professor
Harvard Medical School
Department of Anesthesia, Critical Care and Pain Medicine
Massachusetts General Hospital
Boston, Massachusetts

Jean Kwo, MD
Assistant Professor in Anesthesia
Harvard Medical School
Department of Anesthesia, Critical Care, and Pain Medicine
Massachusetts General Hospital
Boston, Massachusetts

Maximilian Frank Lang, MD
Resident in Anesthesia
Department of Anesthesia, Critical Care and Pain Medicine
Massachusetts General Hospital
Boston, Massachusetts

Stephanie Lankford, CRNA
Certified Registered Nurse Anesthetist
Department of Anesthesia, Critical Care, and Pain Medicine
Massachusetts General Hospital
Boston, Massachusetts

Thomas J. Lavin, DO
Resident in Anesthesia
Department of Anesthesia, Critical Care, and Pain Medicine
Massachusetts General Hospital
Boston, Massachusetts

Johanna Lee, MD
Resident in Anesthesia
Department of Anesthesia, Critical Care and Pain Medicine
Massachusetts General Hospital
Boston, Massachusetts

Wilton C. Levine, MD
Assistant Professor of Anesthesia
Harvard Medical School
Medical Director Perioperative Services
Department of Anesthesia, Critical Care and Pain Medicine
Massachusetts General Hospital
Boston, Massachusetts

Jason M. Lewis, MD
Instructor of Anesthesia
Harvard Medical School
Director
Clinical Operations
Department of Anesthesia, Critical Care and Pain Medicine
Massachusetts General Hospital
Boston, Massachusetts

Rupeng Li, MD, PhD
Resident in Anesthesia
Department of Anesthesia, Critical Care and Pain Medicine
Massachusetts General Hospital
Boston, Massachusetts

Lucy T. Li, MD
Resident in Anesthesia
Department of Anesthesia, Critical Care and Pain Medicine
Massachusetts General Hospital
Boston, Massachusetts

James Taylor Lloyd, MD
Instructor of Anesthesia
Harvard Medical School
Department of Anesthesia, Critical Care and Pain Medicine
Massachusetts General Hospital
Boston, Massachusetts

Ying Hui Low, MD
Instructor of Anesthesia
Harvard Medical School
Department of Anesthesia, Critical Care and Pain Medicine
Massachusetts General Hospital, Harvard Medical School
Boston, Massachusetts

Christopher J. Mariani, MD, PhD
Resident in Anesthesia
Department of Anesthesiology, Critical Care, and Pain Medicine
Massachusetts General Hospital
Boston, Massachusetts

John Marota, MD, PhD
Associate Professor
Harvard Medical School
Department of Anesthesia, Critical Care and Pain Medicine
Massachusetts General Hospital
Boston, Massachusetts

Lukas H. Matern, MD
Resident in Anesthesia
Department of Anesthesia, Critical Care and Pain Medicine
Massachusetts General Hospital
Boston, Massachusetts

Joseph L. McDowell, MD
Instructor of Anesthesia
Harvard Medical School
Department of Anesthesia, Critical Care and Pain Medicine
Massachusetts General Hospital
Boston, Massachusetts

Rebecca D. Minehart, MD, MSHPEd
Assistant Professor of Anesthesia
Harvard Medical School
Department of Anesthesia, Critical Care and Pain Medicine
Massachusetts General Hospital
Boston, Massachusetts

Ilan Mizrahi, MD
Instructor of Anesthesia
Harvard Medical School
Department of Anesthesia, Critical Care, and Pain Medicine
Massachusetts General Hospital
Boston, Massachusetts

Miguel A. Patino Montoya, MD
Resident in Anesthesia
Department of Anesthesia, Critical Care and Pain Medicine
Massachusetts General Hospital
Boston, Massachusetts

Jeremi Mountjoy, MD
Instructor of Anesthesia
Harvard Medical School
Department of Anesthesia, Critical Care and Pain Medicine
Massachusetts General Hospital
Boston, Massachusetts

Eleanor M. Mullen, MSN, CRNA
Staff CRNA
Department of Anesthesia, Critical Care, and Pain Medicine
Harvard Medical School
Massachusetts General Hospital
Boston, Massachusetts

Alexander Nagrebetsky, MD, MSc
Assistant Professor of Anesthesia
Harvard Medical School
Department of Anesthesia, Critical Care and Pain Medicine
Massachusetts General Hospital
Boston, Massachusetts

John H. Nichols, MD
Instructor of Anesthesia
Harvard Medical School
Department of Anesthesia, Critical Care, and Pain Medicine
Massachusetts General Hospital
Boston, Massachusetts

Raissa Quezado da Nobrega, MD
Resident in Anesthesia
Department of Anesthesia, Critical Care and Pain Medicine
Massachusetts General Hospital
Boston, Massachusetts

Peter O. Ochieng, MD
Resident in Anesthesia
Department of Anesthesia, Critical Care, and Pain Medicine
Massachusetts General Hospital
Boston, Massachusetts

Riccardo Pinciroli, MD
Instructor
Harvard Medical School
Research Staff
Department of Anesthesia, Critical Care, and Pain Medicine
Massachusetts General Hospital
Boston, Massachusetts

Richard M. Pino, MD, PhD, FCCM*
Associate Professor of Anesthesia
Harvard Medical School
Division Chief, Critical Care
Department of Anesthesia, Critical Care and Pain Medicine
Massachusetts General Hospital
Boston, Massachusetts

*Affiliation prior to publication.

Triffin J. Psyhojos, MD
Instructor of Anesthesia
Harvard Medical School
Department of Anesthesia, Critical Care, and Pain Medicine
Massachusetts General Hospital
Boston, Massachusetts

Jason Zhensheng Qu, MD
Assistant Professor of Anesthesia
Harvard Medical School
Department of Anesthesia, Critical Care and Pain Medicine,
Massachusetts General Hospital
Boston, Massachusetts

Katarina Ruscic, MD, PhD
Instructor of Anesthesia
Harvard Medical School
Department of Anesthesia, Critical Care and Pain Medicine
Massachusetts General Hospital
Boston, Massachusetts

A. Sassan Sabouri, MD
Assistant Professor of Anesthesia
Harvard Medical School
Department of Anesthesia, Critical Care and Pain Medicine
Massachusetts General Hospital
Boston, Massachusetts

Kyan C. Safavi, MD, MBA
Assistant Professor of Anesthesia
Harvard Medical School
Department of Anesthesia, Critical Care and Pain Medicine
Massachusetts General Hospital
Boston, Massachusetts

Aubrey Samost-Williams, MD, MS
Instructor of Anesthesia
Harvard Medical School
Department of Anesthesia, Critical Care and Pain Medicine
Massachusetts General Hospital
Boston, Massachusetts

Kendrick Shaw, MD, PhD
Instructor of Anesthesia
Harvard Medical School
Department of Anesthesia, Pain, and Critical Care Medicine
Massachusetts General Hospital
Boston, Massachussetts

Jamie L. Sparling, MD
Instructor of Anesthesia
Harvard Medical School
Department of Anesthesia, Critical Care and Pain Medicine
Massachusetts General Hospital
Boston, Massachusetts

Peter Stefanovich, MD
Assistant Professor of Anesthesia
Harvard Medical School
Department of Anesthesia, Critical Care and Pain Medicine
Massachusetts General Hospital
Boston, Massachusetts

Rachel Steinhorn, MD
Cardiovascular Fellow
Harvard Medical School
Department of Anesthesia, Critical Care and Pain Medicine
Massachusetts General Hospital
Boston, Massachusetts

Matthew W. Vanneman, MD
Instructor of Anesthesia
Harvard Medical School
Department of Anesthesia, Critical Care and Pain Medicine
Massachusetts General Hospital
Boston, Massachusetts

Susan A. Vassallo, MD
Associate Professor of Anesthesia
Harvard Medical School
Department of Anesthesia, Critical Care and Pain Medicine
Massachusetts General Hospital
Boston, Massachusetts

Rafael Vazquez, MD
Assistant Professor of Anesthesia
Harvard Medical School
Department of Anesthesia, Critical Care, and Pain Medicine
Massachusetts General Hospital
Boston, Massachusetts

Elisa C. Walsh, MD
Resident in Anesthesia
Department of Anesthesia, Critical Care and Pain Medicine
Massachusetts General Hospital
Boston, Massachusetts

Jeanine P. Wiener-Kronish, MD
Distinguished Professor
Henry Isaiah Dorr Professor of Anesthetics and Anesthesia
Harvard Medical School
Emeritus Chair
Department of Anesthesia, Critical Care and Pain Medicine
Massachusetts General Hospital
Boston, Massachusetts

Shauna Williams, CRNA
Staff CRNA
Department of Anesthesia, Critical Care and Pain Medicine
Massachusetts General Hospital
Boston, Massachusetts

Samuel Wood, MD
Resident in Anesthesia
Department of Anesthesia, Critical Care, and Pain Medicine
Massachusetts General Hospital
Boston, Massachusetts

Jared R. B. Wortzman, MD*
Instructor of Anesthesia
Harvard Medical School
Department of Anesthesia, Critical Care and Pain Medicine
Massachusetts General Hospital
Boston, Massachusetts

Nancy M. Wu, MD
Assistant in Anesthesia
Harvard Medical School
Department of Anesthesia, Critical Care and Pain Medicine
Massachusetts General Hospital
Boston, Massachusetts

Luca Zazzeron, MD
Resident in Anesthesia
Department of Anesthesia, Critical Care and Pain Medicine
Massachusetts General Hospital
Boston, Massachusetts

*Affiliation prior to publication.

PREFACE

Dr. Richard Kitz, as the Anesthetist-in-Chief at Massachusetts General Hospital, had a vision for a "manual of anesthetic practice that was written primarily by recent house staff" that was "intended to be the foundation of practical knowledge for the inexperienced or incompletely trained anesthetist." The goal was to have each chapter written by a resident mentored by a faculty member. Although Dick is no longer with us, the legacy that he started in the 1970's continues today with the 10th edition of *Clinical Anesthesia Procedures of the Massachusetts General Hospital.* These chapters have been passed on from generation to generation with updating to meet the needs of our ever-changing specialty.

This 10th edition has several new features. Each senior author of the previous edition was given a choice to write a new chapter with the hope that new authors would significantly update each chapter as needed rather than just making minor edits of previous ones. Several of the chapters now have online links to videos and graphics. Anesthesia at MGH is conducted as a care team of residents, CRNAs, fellows, and staff anesthesiologists. Several of the chapters in this edition are now coauthored by a CRNA who has expertise of the subject matter. Finally, this edition was written almost entirely during the COVID-19 pandemic. During this time, all of the authors were administering to the needs of incredibly sick patients with respiratory and multisystem organ failure.

The Tenth edition continues to focus on clinical fundamentals that are required for the safe administration of anesthesia and perioperative care. Each chapter reflects the current clinical practice at MGH that is the foundation of our residency and fellowship programs. It is designed to be an easily accessible and accurate source of information for practicing anesthesiologists, CRNAs, anesthesia assistants, learners in anesthesia and other disciplines, medical students, and healthcare professionals interested in perioperative care. The information should be augmented with consultation of other in-depth published works and online sources.

I wish to gratefully acknowledge the many past editors of, and contributors to, the previous editions of this handbook. I have enjoyed working with Sean Hanrahan, Ashley Fischer, Oliver Raj, and Keith Donnellan at Wolters Kluwer. My executive assistant, Amanda Bourgeois, has been indispensable throughout the planning and organization of this book, communicating with the publishing staff, and "gently reminding" my colleagues to submit the chapters on time.

During the writing of this book and the COVID-19 pandemic, the support of our families was essential for maintaining some semblance of normalcy. Thanks to my wife, Patti, and son, Daniel, for their continued love and support.

I have been privileged to work with my mentors and friends, Hassan Ali, MD, and Jeanine Wiener-Kronish, MD. Thirty years ago, I purchased the third edition of *Clinical Anesthesia Procedures of the Massachusetts General Hospital* during an anesthesia elective with Mack Thomas, MD, at LSUMC in New Orleans. I am forever grateful for his teaching, enthusiasm that inspired me to become an anesthesiologist and critical care physician, and his continued friendship.

Richard M. Pino, MD, PhD, FCCM

CONTENTS

Evaluating the Patient Before Anesthesia

Michelle Dyrholm and Kate Cohen

I. INTRODUCTION

The clinic model for anesthesiologists' preoperative evaluation of patients is evolving. Historically, prior to the day of surgery, a patient was evaluated in person at an office. The visit established rapport and allowed the anesthesiologist to become familiar with the patient's surgical illness, identify and medically optimize comorbidities, develop a perioperative management strategy, and obtain informed consent. Due to patient and hospital factors, this approach is being modified. Telemedicine consults are burgeoning as a cost- and time-saving method of accomplishing the same preoperative evaluation. Electronic consults, or eConsults, are also being used as a direct pathway of communication between the anesthesiologist and other patient providers. The anesthesiologist gathers clinical information through fragmented healthcare systems and synthesizes an overall clinical picture to determine optimization and complete workup prior to surgery. Physical examination and consent forms are completed on the day of surgery. Some centers with known low-risk patients and low-risk procedures defer the entire evaluation to the day of surgery. Regardless of the model of preoperative evaluation, the basic tenants remain the same.

II. HISTORY

Relevant information is obtained through chart review followed by corroboration with the patient interview. When the medical record is not available, a history is obtained from the patient and supplemented by the patient's other physicians.

- **A. History of presenting illness.** The anesthesiologist should review the symptoms of the present surgical illness, presumptive diagnosis, initial treatment, and diagnostic studies.
- **B. Medications.** The provider should establish the current dosing and schedules of all the patient's medications. Antihypertensive, antianginal, antiarrhythmic, anticoagulant, anticonvulsant, and specific endocrine (eg, insulin and hypoglycemics) medications are especially important. Deciding to continue medication during the preoperative period depends on the severity of the underlying illness, potential consequences of discontinuing treatment, half-life of the medication, and likelihood of deleterious interactions with anesthetic agents. As a general rule, most medications may be continued up through the time of surgery (see Section VI).

C. **Allergies and drug reactions.** True allergic reactions are relatively uncommon. Adverse reactions to perioperative medications are common, however, and may be reported by the patient. Therefore, it is important to obtain a careful description of the exact nature of the reaction.

1. **True allergic reactions.** IgE-mediated reactions and anaphylaxis can be presumed based upon characteristic symptoms that occurred within a narrow timeframe after exposure to an allergen. Multiple organ systems can be affected, and common symptoms include pruritic rash, urticaria, angioedema, bronchospasm, shortness of breath, wheezing, hypotension, persistent vomiting, and intestinal cramping.

2. **Antibiotic allergy.** Allergies to antibiotics, especially to sulfonamides, penicillins, and cephalosporin derivatives, are the most common drug allergies. While skin testing can help determine true penicillin allergy, 90% to 99% of patients with self-reported allergy have a negative skin test. Therefore, it should not be used as the sole predictor. In patients with a penicillin allergy, the major determinant of immunological reaction to a cephalosporin is the similarity between the side chain of first-generation drug rather than the β-lactam structure that they share. There is a 0.5% to 3% cross reactivity to first- and second-generation cephalosporins. Some institutions implement a test dose procedure prior to administering a therapeutic dose and monitor for adverse reaction. However, anaphylaxis is not dose dependent. For patients with a penicillin allergy, there is a threefold increased coincidental risk of reaction to even an unrelated drug. That is, they are more likely to react to any medication.

3. **Soybean oil and/or egg yolk allergy.** Propofol is commonly formulated as an emulsion containing soybean oil, egg lecithin, and glycerol which has created concerns regarding its use in patients with a history of associated food allergies. Egg allergies are predominantly to the ovalbumin protein found in the egg white, rather than the lecithin in the egg yolk. Similarly, soy allergy is typically to the soy protein rather than the soy oil. Current data suggest low likelihood of adverse reaction to propofol in these patients.

4. **Inhalational agent or succinylcholine "allergy."** A history of allergy to "anesthesia," inhalational agents, or succinylcholine, in the patient or any close relative, may represent a history of malignant hyperthermia (Chapter 17) or atypical plasma cholinesterase.

5. **Local anesthetic allergy.** Allergy to ester-type local anesthetics can be anaphylactic (see Chapter 19), while allergy to the amide-type local anesthetics is exceedingly rare. Tachycardia or palpitations associated with perivascular injection of local anesthetic mixed with epinephrine may be reported as an occurrence during regional anesthetics. A history of local anesthetic systemic toxicity (LAST) can uncover relevant neurological or cardiac sequelae and inform patient preferences but is unlikely to recur.

6. **Shellfish or seafood allergy.** Patients with an allergy to shellfish, seafood, or topical antiseptic containing iodine are not at increased risk of adverse reaction to iodinated intravenous contrast. However, patients with a prior documented reaction to contrast are at risk if exposed to the same agent. It is important to note that there is no allergy cross reactivity between different classes of contrast, and alternate contrasts can typically be safely administered.

7. **Latex allergy or hypersensitivity reactions.** Latex allergy must be ascertained preoperatively to allow for preparation of a latex-free operating

room. Additionally, banana, avocado, chestnut, kiwi, or papaya allergy should be elicited as 30% to 50% of individuals with these allergies have cross-reactive allergies to latex. Other risk factors for latex allergy include repeated exposure to latex (eg, healthcare workers or patients with multiple prior surgeries), atopy, and certain medical disorders, such as spina bifida. If these risk factors exist, and no prior skin or serologic tests have been conducted, it may be warranted to treat the patient as latex allergic.

D. Anesthetic history. It is crucial to question the patient about their prior experience with anesthesia. Common descriptions of anesthetic problems include postoperative nausea and vomiting (PONV), sore throat, neuropathy, difficult intubation, and prolonged emergence. Reviewing previous anesthetic records can shed light on other patient-specific considerations.

1. **Response to medications.** Patient response to sedative, analgesic, and anesthetic agents varies widely among individuals. Cognitive changes, such as memory loss, delirium, or dullness, are frequently described in elderly patients and can be minimized by avoiding burst suppression, anticholinergic drugs, and benzodiazepines. Intraoperative awareness may be reported. Describing to the patient the experience of sedation versus general anesthesia may clarify a prior experience and provide reassurance. Those with true recall may require higher doses of hypnotic medication, modified electroencephalographic (EEG) assessment, and other mechanisms of confirming depth of anesthesia.

2. **Vascular access and invasive monitoring.** Determining the need for ultrasound-guided IV placement or central access can help to avoid repeated attempts in a patient who is a "difficult stick." In morbidly obese patients, noninvasive blood pressure (BP) monitoring may be impossible due to the conical shape of the upper extremity and an arterial line may be required.

3. **Airway management.** Determine past ease of mask ventilation, view obtained on direct laryngoscopy, size and type of laryngoscope blade and endotracheal tube, and depth of endotracheal tube insertion. A prior history of a difficult intubation is the primary predictor of a difficult airway.

4. **Perianesthetic complications.** Review prior records for complications such as adverse drug reactions, dental injury, protracted PONV, hemodynamic instability, respiratory compromise, postoperative myocardial infarction (MI), unanticipated admission to an intensive care unit (ICU), prolonged emergence, or need for reintubation.

5. **Opioid requirements.** Opioid administration perioperately can lend insight into future requirements and the need for alternative pain management strategies such as neuraxial anesthetics, peripheral nerve blocks, and multimodal pharmacology.

E. Family history. A history of adverse anesthetic outcomes in family members should be assessed with open-ended questions, such as "Has anyone in your family experienced unusual or serious reactions to anesthesia?" Additionally, patients should be specifically asked about a family history of malignant hyperthermia.

F. Social history and habits

1. **Smoking.** The perioperative period is a powerful time to provide counseling and support smoking cessation in patients and is associated with a higher rate of success. Smoking cessation reduces postoperative complications, and evidence suggests that abstinence should be encouraged regardless of surgical interval timing. A history of exercise

intolerance or the presence of a productive cough or hemoptysis may indicate the need for further evaluation.

2. **Drug and alcohol use.** Although self-reporting of drug and alcohol intake typically underestimates use, it is a helpful start to define the type of drugs used, routes of administration, frequency, and timing of most recent use. Stimulant abuse may lead to palpitations, angina, and lowered thresholds for serious arrhythmias and seizures. Marijuana use can cause airway hyperreactivity and significantly increase the requirements of propofol and analgesics. Acute alcohol intoxication decreases anesthetic requirement and predisposes to hypothermia and hypoglycemia. Alcohol withdrawal may precipitate severe hypertension (HTN), tremors, delirium, and seizures and may markedly increase anesthetic and analgesic requirements. Risk of intraoperative awareness is also increased with chronic opioid or benzodiazepine use.

III. REVIEW OF SYSTEMS
The purpose of review of systems (ROS) is to elicit symptoms of occult disease and to determine the stability of current disease. Coexisting illnesses should be evaluated by an organ-systems approach with an emphasis on recent changes in symptoms, signs, and treatment (see Chapters 3-7). A minimum ROS should seek to elicit the following information:

A. **Cardiovascular.**

1. **Coronary artery disease.** Preexisting coronary artery disease (CAD) may predispose the patient to spontaneous myocardial ischemia, demand ischemia, or ventricular dysfunction. Angina, dyspnea on exertion (DOE), paroxysmal nocturnal dyspnea, and reduced exercise capacity can help characterize the severity of disease.

2. **Pacemakers (permanent pacemaker, PPM) and implanted cardioverter-defibrillators (ICD).** ICDs should be interrogated within 6 months of surgery, PPMs within 12 months, and cardiac resynchronization therapy (CRT) devices within 3 to 6 months. The decision to deactivate functions of an ICD or change a PPM to asynchronous mode via transcutaneous magnet placement should be made based on the likelihood of electrocautery interference (ie, distance from the generator) causing unwanted shocks or failure to pace.

3. **HTN.** Baseline blood pressure ranges should be established, and the perioperative goal should be to maintain pressures within 10% to 20% of the baseline. Poorly controlled HTN is frequently associated with marked preoperative HTN and labile intraoperative pressures. If the planned surgical position is prone or beach chair, the procedure may be delayed for BP optimization so the risk of blindness and stroke is minimized.

4. **DOE.** DOE is an important sign that can be caused by myriad underlying etiologies, including physical deconditioning, obesity, or cardiopulmonary pathology. If the DOE is acute or acute-on-chronic, the patient should be evaluated and referred for appropriate testing to determine etiology and treatment.

5. **Exercise capacity.** Assessment of functional capacity helps in risk stratification for predicting a perioperative cardiac event. Functional capacity is quantified in terms of metabolic equivalents of task (METs) rated on a scale of poor (<4 METs) to excellent (≥10). A METs of moderate (≥4) or greater, such as the ability to climb two flights of stairs, is associated with reduced perioperative morbidity and mortality for those having noncardiac surgery.

B. Respiratory.
1. **Upper respiratory infection (URI).** URI can predispose patients to bronchospasm and laryngospasm during induction and emergence from general anesthesia. In severe cases, this can lead to inability to oxygenate and ventilate. Therefore, the patient with active signs and symptoms of a URI (productive cough, rhinorrhea, sore throat, fever) should have elective procedures postponed for 4 to 6 weeks after recovery.
2. **Asthma.** Reactive airway disease may result in acute bronchospasm in the perioperative period. Specific questions about previous asthma-related hospitalizations, intubations, emergency room visits, and medication requirement (specifically, steroid use) can help delineate the severity of asthma.
3. **Obstructive sleep apnea (OSA).** Symptoms of OSA should be elicited as they may herald difficulty with bag-mask ventilation or episodes of perioperative hypoxia/hypercarbia. The STOP-BANG criteria helps rate the likelihood of having OSA. Long-standing and untreated OSA can lead to pulmonary HTN, and a transthoracic echocardiogram (TTE) can be used to confirm severity.
C. Neurological. Anesthetic agents may exacerbate underlying neurological disorders. It is important to evaluate the patient's current neurological state and for history of seizure disorder, stroke, amyotrophic lateral sclerosis (ALS), multiple sclerosis, myasthenia gravis, Lambert-Eaton syndrome, Parkinson disease (presence of deep brain stimulator), and cerebral palsy, among others. Baseline neurological deficits should be documented with precision to allow for accurate postoperative comparison and intervention. Neuromuscular blockade should be carefully considered prior to administration, as it may result in prolonged weakness or lethal hyperkalemia.
D. Renal. Renal disease can be categorized according to severity, etiology, and acuity. All types affect perioperative management. Hemodialysis for end-stage renal disease (ESRD) should be performed 24 hours prior to surgical procedure to optimize electrolyte imbalances and volume status. Evaluation of creatinine, glomerular filtration rate (GFR), anemia, and electrolyte abnormalities are imperative. Nonsteroidal anti-inflammatory drug (NSAID) use should be avoided, and cisatracurium is often a preferred neuromuscular blockade agent.
E. Endocrine.
1. **Diabetes mellitus.** Diabetes is a risk factor for cardiovascular disease, nephropathy, neuropathy, and gastroparesis. The patient with autonomic nervous system dysfunction may have silent myocardial ischemia and endovascular disease. Endotracheal intubation may prove difficult secondary to arthritis of the temporomandibular joints and cervical spine as a result of glycosylation of synovium. Home blood glucose measurements, hemoglobin A1c level, and symptomatic swings in blood glucose may elucidate whether the diabetes is well controlled.
2. **Thyroid disease.** Thyroid storm can lead to an intraoperative emergency and occurs in patients with thyrotoxicosis secondary to Graves disease and as well in those with untreated disease. Severe hypothyroidism can lead to slow metabolism of medication, hypothermia, and prolonged emergence from anesthesia.
F. Gastrointestinal.
1. **Gastroesophageal reflux disease (GERD).** Symptoms of reflux with or without hiatal hernia increase the risk of pulmonary aspiration and

may alter the anesthetic plan. An awake intubation or rapid sequence induction may be indicated. The patient should be asked specifically about chest pain/burning sensation, globus sensation, sour taste in the mouth after meals, frank regurgitation of food, or unexplained cough.

2. **Dysphagia/odynophagia.** Those with a subjective feelings of difficulty swallowing or pain with swallowing may have stricture, mass, or a motility syndrome. They are poor candidates for transesophageal echocardiogram (TEE) and may require coordination of care to have an esophagogastroduodenoscopy (EGD) preoperatively in the presence of severe cardiac disease.

3. **Motion sickness or PONV history.** A history of motion sickness and/or PONV increases the risk for PONV. Other factors associated with increased PONV risk include, but are not limited to, history of vertigo, female gender, nonsmoking status, gynecologic and laparoscopic procedures, strabismus surgery, and the need for large doses of perioperative or postoperative opioids. A different anesthetic technique, such as total intravenous anesthesia, may be warranted in the patient with multiple risk factors.

G. **Musculoskeletal.** A history of radiation to the head or neck may increase the risk of distorted airway anatomy, reduce range of motion, and alter intubation technique. Rheumatoid arthritis and Down syndrome are associated with atlantoaxial instability, and ankylosing spondylitis may significantly reduce cervical spine range of motion. The patient should also be questioned about scoliosis when neuraxial anesthesia is being considered as well as joint pain for purposes of intraoperative positioning.

H. **Obstetric/gynecologic.** Possibility of pregnancy and timing of last menses should be elicited in women of childbearing age as some medication may be teratogenic. Elective surgery should be postponed until the postpartum period. Maternal arterial pressures are directly proportional to uteroplacental perfusion, so sustained hypotension could result in fetal distress. For 2 weeks following nonobstetric surgery, the parturient is also at risk of preterm labor.

I. **Hematologic.** A history of easy bruising, bleeding diathesis, heavy menses, or unprovoked blood clots warrant further questioning and workup. Idiopathic thrombocytopenia, von Willebrand disease, thalassemia, hemophilia, sickle cell disease, and inherited thrombophilias add a layer of complexity to peripheral nerve blocks, neuraxial anesthetics, planning for surgical blood loss, and need for anticoagulation postoperatively.

IV. THE PHYSICAL EXAMINATION

The physical examination should be thorough, but focused. Special attention is directed toward evaluation of the airway, heart, lungs, and neurologic status. Assessment of the block site is warranted before a regional anesthetic.

A. **Vital signs.**

1. **Blood pressure.** If the patient has aortic arch disease, blood pressure measurement should be taken in both arms. Noninvasive blood pressure measurements should be avoided on an extremity with an arteriovenous fistula. While there is controversial evidence for causing lymphedema with a blood pressure cuff after axillary lymph node dissection or radiation, it is reasonable to avoid the limb for patient preference and assuaging anxiety. Arterial lines should, however, be avoided

on the side of breast cancer surgery to reduce the risk of cellulitis causing lymphedema.

2. **Pulse.** Resting heart rate should be noted for rhythm and rate.
3. **Respiratory rate.** Respirations should be observed for rate, depth, effort, and pattern.
4. **Oxygen saturation.** Etiology of a saturation less than 93% should be investigated.

B. **Height and weight.** Height and weight measurement are necessary for determining drug dosages, fluid requirements, adequate urine output, and ventilator settings. Ideal body weight (IBW) should be calculated using the formula:
1. Males: IBW (kg) = 50 + 2.3 kg for each inch over 5 ft
2. Females: IBW (kg) = 45.5 + 2.3 kg for each inch over 5 ft

C. **Head and neck.** During the basic preoperative examination, the anesthesiologist should evaluate the following:
1. **Maximal mouth opening.**
2. **Ability to prognath.** Upper lip bite test.
3. **Mallampati classification** (see Chapter 13).
4. **Thyromental distance.** Thyromental distance is the distance between the tip of the chin and the thyroid notch. Approximately three fingerbreadths distance is considered normal.
5. **Dentition.** Evaluate teeth for those loose, chipped, or missing. Crowns, bridges, dentures, braces, retainers, and other dental appliances should be noted.
6. **Facial hair.** A large beard or mustache may be taped with Tegaderm or shaved so as not to interfere with achieving a seal for bag-mask ventilation.
7. **Cervical spine.** Evaluate range of motion in flexion, extension, and rotation of the cervical spine.
8. **Superficial neck.** Check for tracheal deviation, cervical masses, and jugular venous distention. The presence of a carotid bruit is nonspecific but may suggest a need for evaluating carotid stenosis.
9. **Neck circumference.** A neck circumference measurement of 17 inches for men and 16 inches for women are associated with OSA and obstruction during bag-mask ventilation.

D. **Precordium.** Auscultation of the heart may reveal murmurs, S3, S4, or a pericardial rub.

E. **Lungs.** Auscultate for wheezing, rhonchi, or rales, which should be correlated with observations regarding the ease of breathing and the use of accessory muscles of respiration.

F. **Abdomen.** Any evidence of abdominal distention, masses, or ascites should be noted as these may predispose the patient to regurgitation or ventilatory compromise.

G. **Extremities.** Evaluate for muscle wasting and weakness, distal perfusion, clubbing, cyanosis, edema, and the presence of any cutaneous infections (especially over sites of planned vascular cannulation or regional nerve block). Ecchymosis or unexplained injury, especially in children, women, and elderly patients, can be an indication of an abusive relationship.

H. **Back.** Note any deformity, scoliosis, bruising, rash, cellulitis, or skin condition that could lead to difficulty in patient positioning or performance of neuraxial analgesia.

I. **Neurologic examination.** Document mental status, cranial nerve function, cognition, and peripheral sensorimotor function.

V. LABORATORY STUDIES

Routine laboratory screening tests are generally not indicated. Tests should be selected based on the patient's medical condition and the proposed surgical procedure.

A. Hematologic studies. Hematologic studies are indicated if there are concerns regarding significant preexisting anemia, perioperative blood loss, or coagulopathy.

1. **Recent hematocrit/hemoglobin level.** There is no universally accepted minimum hematocrit before anesthesia. The etiology and duration of anemia should be ascertained.

2. **Platelet studies.** By history, platelet function can be assessed by easy bruising, petechiae, excessive bleeding from gums or minor cuts, and family history. Repeat complete blood count (CBC), smear, evaluation of liver function, autoimmune disease, and infectious etiology should be considered. A hematology consultation for etiology evaluation such as TTP, ITP, HIT, vWD, or malignancy may be pursued.

3. **Coagulation studies.** Coagulation studies may be ordered to assess level of pharmacological anticoagulation, readiness for nerve block or neuraxial anesthesia after discontinuation of anticoagulant, synthetic liver function, and clinically relevant nutritional deficiency. Coagulation status of the patient on low-molecular-weight heparin may be monitored through measurement of anti–factor Xa levels.

4. **Blood type/antibody screen.** Type and screen should be obtained if anticipating a significant intraoperative blood loss or if the patient has alloantibodies that are challenging to crossmatch.

B. Serum chemistry. A metabolic panel should be ordered in patients with risk factors for renal or hepatic disease that would affect their serum electrolytes, ability to metabolize drugs, and impact their response to fluid. It is also indicated for patients taking diuretics, digoxin, steroids, or aminoglycoside antibiotics.

1. **Hypokalemia.** Low potassium levels are common in the patient receiving diuretics and are usually readily corrected by preoperative oral potassium supplementation. Mild hypokalemia (2.8-3.5 mEq/L) should not preclude elective surgery. Rapid correction with intravenous potassium may lead to dysrhythmias and cardiac arrest.

2. **Hyperkalemia.** Elevated potassium is often seen in the patient with end-stage renal disease. Mild elevations in serum potassium among those with already elevated baselines is well tolerated. Treatment of hyperkalemia is warranted if concentrations exceed 6 mEq/L or if electrocardiogram (ECG) changes occur, such as peaked T waves, prolonged PR interval, P wave flattening, or widened QRS.

3. **Hyponatremia.** Serum sodium levels <135 mEq/L are an independent negative prognostic indicator for perioperative outcomes. Even mild hyponatremia in healthy patients undergoing nonemergent surgery is associated with an increased incidence of 30 day mortality, coronary events, pneumonia, wound infections, and hospital length of stay. The severity of hyponatremia corresponds to worse outcomes. Low serum sodium should be considered a surrogate marker for medical comorbidities, and perhaps not itself the cause of poor outcomes. The etiology should be determined, and if possible, severe abnormalities should be corrected preoperatively.

C. ECG. The most recent ACC/AHA guidelines for patients undergoing noncardiac surgery state that a preoperative ECG is not beneficial in asymptomatic patients undergoing low-risk procedures. Preoperative ECG may be reasonable for patients with known severe arrhythmia, cerebrovascular disease, peripheral arterial disease, or structural or coronary heart disease undergoing greater than a low-risk surgical intervention. An ECG should not be done for the sole indication of advanced patient age.

D. Chest radiography. A chest x-ray (CXR) should be obtained in the patient with signs or symptoms of acute or unstable chronic cardiopulmonary disease.

E. Pulmonary function tests. Pulmonary function tests (PFTs) are used to evaluate the severity of lung disease. They have a recognized role in the evaluation of patients undergoing lung resection surgery; however, they have not been shown to be predictive of postoperative pulmonary complications in surgeries other than lung resection (see Chapters 4 and 27).

VI. PREOPERATIVE MEDICAL OPTIMIZATION

Preexisting medical conditions should be controlled or stabilized before surgery. Many of the complications associated with these conditions may be prevented by thoughtful administration of standard medications.

A. HTN. Untreated HTN can cause end-organ damage. Acute treatment of chronic HTN may be indicated in the patient with systolic blood pressures greater than 20% of their baseline. If HTN persists despite treatment or if the blood pressure is greater than 180/110 mm Hg, elective surgery should be postponed until the blood pressure is better controlled. Angiotensin-converting enzyme inhibitors and angiotensin receptor blocking agents may cause refractory vasoplegia and should be held the night before or on the day of surgery. β-blockers, calcium channel blockers, and clonidine may be continued perioperatively.

B. Coronary artery disease. In patients with a recent history of percutaneous coronary intervention or coronary artery bypass grafting on dual anti-platelet therapy (DAPT), careful consideration must be given to medication management and timing of surgical procedure. See the 2016 ACC/AHA Guideline Focused Update on Duration of DAPT Therapy in Patients With Coronary Artery Disease for comprehensive guidelines. Chapter 3 further outlines the stepwise approach to preoperative evaluation in patients with CAD.

Individuals on long-term β-blocker therapy should continue their medication in the perioperative period. Postoperative dose modification in the setting of bradycardia or hypotension is appropriate. Current literature does not support initiating prophylactic β-blockade immediately prior to or on the day of surgery, as this has been associated with increased all-cause mortality. Detailed recommendations for perioperative beta-blocker administration is further outlined in the 2014 AHA/ACC Guideline on Perioperative Cardiovascular Evaluation and Management of Patients Undergoing Noncardiac Surgery.

With regard to aspirin, new evidence reveals that the risks may outweigh the benefits for primary prevention. Guidelines at MGH state that aspirin (81-325 mg) be continued up to and including the day of surgery, **except in the case of** intracranial neurosurgical procedures, intramedullary spine surgery, surgery of the middle ear or posterior eye, and possibly prostate surgery. Complete reversal of aspirin effects requires 7 to 10 days for new platelet synthesis. Discontinuing aspirin in a patient receiving aspirin for secondary prophylaxis necessitates an explicit discussion with the patient's primary care physician, cardiologist, or vascular physician. The decision should weight the cardiovascular risks of stopping aspirin versus the risk of bleeding from the surgery.

C. **Anticoagulation therapy.** Depending on the indication for the anticoagulation, a patient on warfarin may need to be bridged with low-molecular-weight heparin or unfractionated heparin regimens prior to surgery. This decision should be made with the surgeon and physician prescribing the anticoagulation.

D. **NSAIDs.** The modest inhibition of platelet function caused by NSAIDs does not increase bleeding risk nor does it increase the risk of hematoma associated with spinal or epidural anesthesia. Celecoxib does not affect platelet function and therefore may be continued perioperatively in those who take it chronically. Some surgeons still hesitate to continue NSAIDs given data suggesting deleterious effects on bone healing. Given the oppositional literature, a discussion with the surgeon regarding NSAID use is justified. As part of expedited recovery after surgery (ERAS) protocols, NSAIDs are often given as part of a preoperative cocktail. Caution should be taken with patients who have severe coronary disease, peptic ulcer disease, HTN, renal disease, and asthma.

E. **Opioid tolerance.** Usual doses of opioids should be continued in the perioperative period to avoid withdrawal. Multimodal analgesia and regional anesthetics should be pursued as determined by patients and surgical factors. A patient taking methadone should continue maintenance dosing through the day of surgery. A patient taking Suboxone should have a plan formulated by their prescribing physician, surgeon, and anesthesiologist. Guidelines at MGH recommend patients on Suboxone ≤8 mg/d (4 mg BID) continue their baseline regimen throughout the perioperative period. Higher daily dosage may require preoperative titration to optimize surgical pain management. For inpatient procedures, an Addictions Consult Team should be consulted to assist in the postoperative titration of Suboxone.

F. **Asthma.** A patient with moderate to severe asthma may require treatment with albuterol or ipratropium via metered dose inhaler immediately prior to airway instrumentation. A wheezing patient should be referred to a pulmonologist or internist for optimization and symptom control before surgery. All asthma medications—inhaled and oral—should be continued perioperatively.

G. **Diabetes mellitus.** A diabetic patient may present with hyperglycemia or hypoglycemia. A blood glucose level should be obtained by finger stick preoperatively and abnormal levels addressed (see Chapter 7). Severe and acute hyperglycemia can lead to a hyperosmolar state that can result in impaired enzyme function, diabetic ketoacidosis, or a hyperosmolar hyperglycemic nonketotic state. Oral hypoglycemic agents and short-acting insulin should all be held on the day of surgery. Basal insulin should be continued, albeit many recommend a reduction of 20% to 50%, and blood glucose levels closely monitored.

H. **High aspiration risk.** Guidelines to reduce the risk of pulmonary aspiration have been published by the ASA and include preoperative assessment risk factors, nil per os (NPO) status, and pharmacological agent recommendations. These precautions should be implemented for patients at high risk of aspiration, like those with a hiatal hernia, difficult airway, ileus, obesity, poorly controlled diabetes, depressed sensorium, pregnancy, and acute trauma. The following medications can be administered to decrease gastric acid and/or decrease gastric volume: **H_2 antagonists** such as cimetidine, famotidine, and ranitidine reduce the volume and acidity of gastric secretions. Cimetidine inhibits the CYP P450 system and prolongs the elimination of many drugs, including theophylline, diazepam, propranolol, and lidocaine, potentially increasing the toxicity of these agents. Ranitidine has recently been withdrawn from the market due to FDA concerns over contamination. **Proton-pump inhibitors** are highly effective in reducing acid production but do not work quickly enough to be used in the immediate preoperative period; the greatest benefit is seen in patients on long term therapy. **Nonparticulate antacids**, such as sodium citrate and citric acid (Bicitra) raise gastric pH. **Metoclopramide** enhances gastric emptying by increasing lower esophageal sphincter tone and simultaneously relaxing the pylorus. As with all dopamine antagonists, it may produce dystonia or other extrapyramidal effects. Metoclopramide is contraindicated in suspected bowel obstruction due to increased risk of perforation.

I. **Other medications.** In general, anticonvulsants, antiarrhythmics, steroids, and hormonal supplements may be continued through the perioperative period. Vitamins and herbal supplements should be discontinued a minimum of 7 days prior to surgery.

VII. ANESTHETIC ASSESSMENT AND PLAN

A. **ASA physical status class.** ASA class provides an overall impression of the severity of the patient's illness. The six physical classes are described in **Table 1.1.**

B. **Airway management.** Plan for a natural airway or placement of either a laryngeal mask airway (LMA) or endotracheal tube should take into consideration the patient's current airway examination, past airway management, aspiration risk, and the planned procedure, including positioning and estimated duration.

C. **Monitoring.** The healthy patient undergoing minimally invasive surgery needs only the standard ASA monitors. However, if the patient has significant cardiovascular disease, pulmonary disease, or is at risk for blood loss, invasive monitoring such as a central line and arterial line should be considered for the granularity of hemodynamic status and assessing blood gases and cell counts frequently.

D. **Anesthetic options.** Numerous methods are available for providing anesthesia, analgesia, and hemodynamic stability for any given type of surgery. General anesthesia, regional anesthesia, and combinations thereof should be reviewed and considered.

VIII. PATIENT DISCUSSION

The perioperative period is emotionally stressful for patients who frequently have fears about surgery, anesthesia, diagnoses, complications, and mortality. The anesthesiologist can alleviate much of this stress with a thoughtful discussion. Moreover, the anesthesiologist should explain the events of the perioperative period and give instruction and information on the following:

A. **Perioperative procedures.** Explanation of the procedures that will occur prior to induction—placement of intravenous, arterial, or epidural catheters, placement of routine monitors, preoxygenation, cricoid pressure—with reassurance that supplemental sedation and analgesia will be provided as necessary.

B. **Perioperative medication use.** If a necessary medication was forgotten on the morning of surgery, it should be given by the anesthesiologist. Preoperative oral medications, such as acetaminophen, gabapentin, and celebrex, are commonly seen in patients getting multimodal pain control (see Section VI).

C. **Preoperative fasting.** Specific instructions about fasting should be addressed. See **Table 1.2.**

TABLE 1.1	ASA Physical Status Classification System	
ASA PS Classification	**Definition**	**Adult Examples, Including, But Not Limited to**
ASA I	A normal healthy patient	Healthy, nonsmoking, no or minimal alcohol use
ASA II	A patient with mild systemic disease	Mild diseases only without substantive functional limitations. Examples include (but not limited to): current smoker, social alcohol drinker, pregnancy, obesity (30 < BMI < 40), well-controlled DM/HTN, mild lung disease
ASA III	A patient with severe systemic disease	Substantive functional limitations; one or more moderate to severe diseases. Examples include (but not limited to): poorly controlled DM or HTN, COPD, morbid obesity (BMI ≥ 40), active hepatitis, alcohol dependence or abuse, implanted pacemaker, moderate reduction of ejection fraction, ESRD undergoing regularly scheduled dialysis, premature infant PCA < 60 wk, history (>3 mo) of MI, CVA, TIA, or CAD/stents.
ASA IV	A patient with severe systemic disease that is a constant threat to life	Examples include (but not limited to): recent (<3 mo) MI, CVA, TIA, or CAD/stents, ongoing cardiac ischemia or severe valve dysfunction, severe reduction of ejection fraction, sepsis, DIC, ARD or ESRD not undergoing regularly scheduled dialysis
ASA V	A moribund patient who is not expected to survive without the operation	Examples include (but not limited to): ruptured abdominal/thoracic aneurysm, massive trauma, intracranial bleed with mass effect, ischemic bowel in the face of significant cardiac pathology or multiple organ/system dysfunction
ASA VI	A declared brain-dead patient whose organs are being removed for donor purposes	

ARD, acute respiratory distress; ASA, American Society of Anesthesiologists; BMI, body mass index; CAD, coronary artery disease; COPD, chronic obstructive pulmonary disease; CVA, cerebrovascular accident; DIC, disseminated intravascular coagulation; DM, diabetes mellitus; ESRD, end-stage renal disease; HTN, hypertension; MI, myocardial infarction; PCA, postconceptual age; TIA, transient ischemic attack. The addition of "E" denotes Emergency surgery: (An emergency is defined as existing when delay in treatment of the patient would lead to a significant increase in the threat to life or body part). Excerpted from *ASA Physical Status Classification System, 2019 of the American Society of Anesthesiologists.* A copy of the full text can be obtained from ASA, 1061 American Lane Schaumburg, IL 60173-4973 or online at www.asahq.org

D. Postoperative recovery. Explain the intended plan for postoperative recovery in the postanesthesia care unit or ICU.

E. Pain control. Detail the plan for perioperative pain control.

F. Autologous blood donation. Autologous donation may be considered in the stable patient scheduled for surgery in which blood transfusion is likely.

TABLE 1.2	ASA Practice Guidelines for Preoperative Fasting	
Ingested Material		**Minimum Fasting Period**[a]
Clear liquids		2 h
Breast milk		4 h
Infant formula, nonhuman milk, light meals		6 h
Full meal		8 h

ASA, American Society of Anesthesiologists.
[a]Healthy patients, elective cases.

IX. INFORMED CONSENT

Informed consent involves discussing the anesthetic plan, alternatives, and potential complications. The patient must demonstrate decision-making capacity; that is, understanding, appreciation, reasoning, and choice. Consent must be voluntary, free from coercion. Descriptions should be made in layman's terms and conducted in the patient's native language, using a trained medical interpreter when appropriate. Children should not be used as interpreters, although adult family members may serve as interpreters if the patient signs a waiver of disclosure stating they choose to waive access to a hospital-appointed translator.

A. **Explanation of general anesthesia.** Many aspects of anesthetic management are outside the realm of common experience and must be explicitly defined. Examples of this include endotracheal intubation, mechanical ventilation, invasive hemodynamic monitoring, regional anesthesia techniques, blood product transfusion, and postoperative ICU care.

B. **Alternatives.** Alternatives to the suggested management plan should be presented as they may become necessary if the planned procedure fails or if there is a change in clinical circumstances.

C. **Risks.** Risks associated with anesthesia-related procedures should be disclosed in a manner that the average person would find helpful in making a decision. The best case/worst case communication tool is useful to guide this discussion. Offering the most likely situation is clarifying for patients as well. The discussion should also include complications that occur with a relatively high frequency and those that are just remote risks.

1. **Regional anesthesia.** The risks of regional and neuraxial anesthesia include infection, local bleeding, nerve injury, headache, drug reaction, and possible failure to provide adequate anesthesia. Certain regional anesthetic techniques may carry more specific risks, for example, pneumothorax after an infraclavicular nerve block, and should be weighed against the associated benefits specific to the patient. General anesthesia and its attendant risks should also be discussed as it could become necessary.

2. **General anesthesia.** The risks of airway instrumentation include sore throat, hoarseness, and dental injury. The anesthetic agents may cause nausea and vomiting or produce an allergic reaction. The possibility of intraoperative awareness, pulmonary or cardiac injury, stroke, postoperative visual loss, postoperative cognitive dysfunction, postoperative intubation, ICU admission, or death should be discussed when appropriate.

3. **Blood transfusion.** The risks associated with blood transfusion are fever, hemolytic reactions, and infection. Currently, the risk of transmission

of the hepatitis B virus is ~1 in 360,000, whereas the risk of transmission of the human immunodeficiency and hepatitis C viruses is ~1 in 1,500,000 units transfused.

4. **Vascular cannulation**. The risks of intravenous catheters include injury of peripheral nerves, tendons, blood vessels, and site infection causing a phlebitis or cellulitis. Hemothorax, pneumothorax, and central line bloodstream infection are risks associated with central venous access.

D. **Extenuating circumstances**. Anesthetic procedures may proceed without informed consent in emergency situations as consent is assumed under dire circumstances.

X. DAY OF SURGERY PREMEDICATION

A. **Sedatives and analgesics**. The goal for administering sedatives and analgesics before surgery is to allay the patient's anxiety, to decrease pain during administration of regional anesthesia or preoperative line placement, and to facilitate smooth induction of anesthesia. The dose of sedatives and analgesics should be reduced or withheld for the elderly, debilitated, or acutely intoxicated patient. The dose should also be decreased in a patient with upper airway obstruction, central apnea, neurologic deterioration, or severe pulmonary disease.

1. **Benzodiazepines**.
   a. **Midazolam**. Midazolam, 1 to 3 mg intravenously or intramuscularly, is a short-acting benzodiazepine that provides excellent anterograde amnesia and anxiolysis. It plays a role in preventing PONV. It is known to cause delirium in the elderly and to be synergistic with opioids in causing respiratory depression.
   b. **Lorazepam**. Lorazepam, 1 to 2 mg orally or intravenously, may cause more prolonged amnesia and postoperative sedation than midazolam.

2. **Opioids**. Opioids may be given preoperatively to a patient who has, or is anticipated to have, significant pain or to a patient who is opioid dependent. The opioid-dependent patient should receive sufficient premedication to overcome tolerance and to prevent perioperative withdrawal. Intravenous fentanyl is ideally dosed at least 2 to 5 minutes prior to airway instrumentation so that its effect blunts the reaction from laryngoscopy.

B. **Anticholinergics**. Anticholinergics are not frequently used for premedication. Glycopyrrolate, 0.2 to 0.4 mg intravenously for adults and 10 to 20 μg/kg for pediatric patients, may be given in conjunction with ketamine as an antisialagogue. Occasionally, this antisialagogue effect is desirable during oral surgery, bronchoscopy, fiberoptic intubation, or to treat secretions related to recent smoking cessation.

C. **Antiemetics**. Antiemetics may be given prior to induction or intraoperatively to prevent PONV (see Chapter 37). Adequate prophylaxis includes the use of at least two antiemetics with differing mechanisms of action (see **Table 1.3**).

D. **Aspiration risk-mitigating agents**. Aspiration risk-mitigating agents may be warranted on the day of surgery in the at-risk patient (see Section VI.H).

XI. DELAYING SURGICAL PROCEDURES

Occasionally, it is in the best interest of the patient to delay elective surgical procedures for further medical evaluation and optimization. Some conditions can significantly increase morbidity and mortality if not appropriately evaluated and treated.

A. **Recent myocardial infarction**. If the patient has had a recent MI that was managed medically, then elective noncardiac surgery should be delayed

	Antiemetic Agents		
Antiemetic Agent	**Mechanism of Action**	**Side Effects**	**Dose**
Ondansetron	Serotonin (5-HT$_3$) receptor antagonist	Dizziness, headache, and QTc prolongation	4 mg intravenously
Droperidol[a]	Dopamine (D$_2$) receptor antagonist	Dystonia, prolonged QTc, and decreased seizure threshold	0.5-1.25 mg intravenously
Haloperidol	D$_2$ receptor antagonist	Dystonia, prolonged QTc, and decreased seizure threshold	1 mg intravenously
Dexamethasone	Unknown	Anal/vulvar pruritus and hyperglycemia	4 mg intravenously
Metoclopramide	Dopamine receptor antagonist	GI upset with abdominal cramping and dystonia	10 mg intravenously
Promethazine	Antihistamine	Sedation and decreased seizure threshold	6.25 mg intravenously
Scopolamine	Anticholinergic	Dry mouth, blurred vision, confusion, and urinary retention	1.5 mg transdermally

Table 1.3

[a]The Food and Drug Administration requires 2 to 3 h of electrocardiogram (ECG) monitoring following administration given the risk of QTc prolongation and torsades de pointes.

for 60 days. If the patient underwent percutaneous coronary intervention, surgery should be delayed in accordance with antiplatelet therapy recommendations. See Chapter 3 for further details.

B. **New dysrhythmia.** New-onset atrial fibrillation, atrial flutter, supraventricular tachycardia, sustained ventricular tachycardia, and second-degree, type II, or third-degree heart block must be evaluated with an ECG, rhythm strip, electrolyte replenishment, and a cardiology consultation. Surgery should be postponed until workup and treatment are complete and stability is established.

C. **Coagulopathy.** Coagulopathies can predispose the patient to massive intraoperative blood loss. As such, surgery should be postponed until all possible etiologies have been thoroughly investigated and treated.

D. **Hypoxia.** If hypoxia is of unclear etiology, surgery should be postponed until the cause is investigated and the patient optimized. VQ mismatch, dead space, shunt, decreased fraction of inspired oxygen (FIO$_2$), and inadequate respiratory rate/effort should be considered. Workup should begin with a physical examination and evaluation of vital signs. Diagnostic studies such as a CXR, computed tomography (CT) scan, or arterial blood gas may be ordered as needed.

E. **New cardiovascular symptoms.** Unstable angina and new shortness of breath or DOE are concerning symptoms. Surgery should be postponed until they can be fully evaluated by an appropriate specialist. New ECG changes, especially those indicative of silent MI, such as bifascicular block or new Q waves, must be evaluated prior to elective procedures.

F. **New murmurs.** New heart murmurs may be indicative of a change in valvular pathology and should be evaluated by an echocardiography and/or cardiologist before proceeding with elective surgery.

XII. ETHICAL CONSIDERATIONS IN PATIENT CARE

A highly valued ethical principle that guides patient care in the United States is the concept of **patient autonomy.** Adult patients with decision-making capacity can and may choose to accept or refuse life-sustaining medical therapies in accordance with their own morals and beliefs. Respect for patient autonomy is demonstrated in the physician's ethical responsibility of attaining informed consent and including the patient in the medical decision-making process whenever possible.

A. **Advance directive.** Also referred to as a **living will**, is a legal document written by a patient which outlines instructions for medical care should the patient become unable to communicate their wishes in the future. It often designates a surrogate decision maker.

B. A **healthcare proxy** or **durable power of attorney for health care** is a designated surrogate who has legal charge to execute the patient's wishes should they become unable to do so. If a representative has not been designated by the patient, the next of kin may become the de facto surrogate.

C. **Physician orders for life-sustaining treatment (POLST).** Patients who have been diagnosed with a serious, life-limiting medical condition can create an advanced set of **portable medical orders** which are signed by their healthcare provider and placed in their medical record.

D. **The pediatric patient** deserves special consideration when ethical issues are confronted. Legally, such decisions are deferred to the parents. Ethically, the child may participate in these decisions depending on their developmental level and decision-making capacity.

E. **Religious/personal beliefs.** Certain personal beliefs and desires may warrant special consideration prior to surgery. The Jehovah's Witness patient undergoing elective surgery should have a clear plan that is understood and agreed to by the patient and the entire surgical team; specifically, their consent or refusal to use blood subfractions or contiguous autotransfusion should be documented. The same considerations apply to the patient with a preexisting DNI/DNR order where further discussion should guide suspending those directives versus proceeding with goal-directed resuscitation.

F. **Ethical issues for the anesthetist.** The ethical and moral beliefs of the anesthetist must be taken into consideration for elective procedures. It is within the right of the individual to refuse to participate in the care of, for example, a therapeutic abortion, or a patient who is DNR. Additionally, physicians are not bound to provide care that they deem futile. Involving palliative care physicians in patient and family meetings is often critical to determining a patient's thought process and highlighting their ultimate goals.

Suggested Readings

American Society of Anesthesiologists. Ethical Guidelines for the Anesthesia Care of Patients with Do-Not-Resuscitate Orders or Other Directives that Limit Treatment. Approved October 17, 2001, reaffirmed October 17, 2018.

Baron TH, Kamath PS, McBane RD. Management of antithrombotic therapy in patients undergoing invasive procedures. *N Engl J Med.* 2013;368:2113-2124.

Bittl JA, Baber U, Bradley SM, Wijeysundera DN. Duration of dual antiplatelet therapy: a systematic review for the 2016 ACC/AHA guideline focused update on duration of dual antiplatelet therapy in patients with coronary artery disease. A report of the American College of Cardiology/American Heart Association Task Force on clinical practice guidelines. *J Am Coll Cardiol.* 2016;68:1116-1139.

Blumenthal K, Peter J, Trubiano J, Phillips E. Antibiotic allergy. *Lancet.* 2019;393(10167):183-198.

Blumenthal KG, Shenoy ES, Varughese CA, Hurwitz S, Hooper DC, Banerji A. Impact of a clinical guideline for prescribing antibiotics to inpatients reporting penicillin or cephalosporin allergy. *Ann Allergy Asthma Immunol.* 2015;115(4):294-300.e2. doi:10.1016/j.anai.2015.05.011

Crossley GH, Poole JE, Rozner MA, et al. The Heart Rhythm Society (HRS)/American Society of Anesthesiologists (ASA) Expert Consensus Statement on the perioperative management of patients with implantable defibrillators, pacemakers and arrhythmia monitors: facilities and patient management. *Heart Rhythm.* 2011;8:1114-1154.

Douketis JD, Spyropoulos AC, Spencer FA, et al. Perioperative management of antithrombotic therapy: antithrombotic therapy and prevention of thrombosis, 9th ed. American College of Chest Physicians evidence-based clinical practice guidelines. *Chest.* 2012;141(2 suppl):e326S-e350S.

Fihn SD, Gardin JM, Abrams J, et al. 2012 ACCF/AHA/AATS/PCNA/SCAI/STS guideline for the diagnosis and management of patients with stable ischemic heart disease: a report of the American College of Cardiology Foundation/American Heart Association Task Force on practice guidelines, and the American College of Physicians, American Association for Thoracic Surgery, Preventive Cardiovascular Nurses Association, Society for Cardiovascular Angiography and Interventions, and Society of Thoracic Surgeons. *Circulation.* 2012;126:e354.

Fleisher LA, Fleischmann KE, Auerbach AD, et al. 2014 ACC/AHA guideline on perioperative cardiovascular evaluation and management of patients undergoing noncardiac surgery: executive summary. A report of the American College of Cardiology/American Heart Association Task Force on practice guidelines. *Circulation.* 2014;130:1-141.

Kristensen SD, Knuuti J, Saraste A, et al. 2014 ESC/ESA guidelines on non-cardiac surgery: cardiovascular assessment and management the joint task force on non-cardiac surgery. Cardiovascular assessment and management of the European Society of Cardiology (ESC) and the European Society of Anaesthesiology (ESA). *Eur Heart J.* 2014;35(35):2383-2431.

MGH Guidelines for perioperative aspirin administration. Consensus Statement from the Departments of Anesthesia, Medicine, Cardiology, and Surgery. 12/2011.

Piccolo R, Windecker S. Low-dose aspirin to reduce the risk for myocardial infarction among patients with coronary stents undergoing noncardiac surgery. *Ann Intern Med.* 2018;168(4):289-290.

Practice advisory for preanesthesia evaluation. An updated report by the American Society of Anesthesiologists Task Force on preanesthesia evaluation. *Anesthesiology.* 2012;116:522-538.

Practice advisory for the perioperative management of patients with cardiac implantable electronic devices: pacemakers and implantable cardioverter–defibrillators 2020. An updated report by the American Society of Anesthesiologists Task Force on perioperative management of patients with cardiac implantable electronic devices. *Anesthesiology.* 2020;132:225-252.

Practice guidelines for the perioperative management of patients with obstructive sleep apnea. An updated report by the American Society of Anesthesiologists Task Force on perioperative management of patients with obstructive sleep apnea. *Anesthesiology.* 2014;120:268-286.

Practice guidelines for preoperative fasting and the use of pharmacologic agents to reduce the risk of pulmonary aspiration: application to healthy patients undergoing elective procedures. An updated report by the American Society of Anesthesiologists Task Force on preoperative fasting and the use of pharmacologic agents to reduce the risk of pulmonary aspiration. *Anesthesiology.* 2017;126(3):376-393.

Prins KW, Neill JM, Tyler JO, et al. Effects of beta-blocker withdrawal in acute decompensated heart failure: a systematic review and meta-analysis. *JACC Heart Fail.* 2015;3:647-653.

Ridker P. Should aspirin Be used for primary prevention in the post-statin era? *N Engl J Med.* 2018;379(16):1572-1574.

Stern T, Cifu AS. Perioperative beta-blocker therapy. *J Am Med Assoc.* 2015;313(24):2486-2487.

Updated by the Committee on Standards and Practice Parameters, Apfelbaum JL, Hagberg CA, Caplan RA, et al. The previous update was developed by the American Society of Anesthesiologists Task Force on Difficult Airway Management; Caplan RA, Benumof JL, Berry FA, et al. Practice guidelines for management of the difficult airway: an updated report by the American Society of Anesthesiologists Task Force on Management of the Difficult Airway. *Anesthesiology.* 2013;118:251-270.

Wijeysundera DN, Duncan D, Nkonde-Price C, et al. Perioperative beta blockade in noncardiac surgery: a systematic review for the 2014 ACC/AHA guideline on perioperative cardiovascular evaluation and management of patients undergoing noncardiac surgery. A report of the American College of Cardiology/American Heart Association Task Force on practice guidelines. *J Am Coll Cardiol.* 2014;64:2406.

Zhang Y, et al. MGH Guidelines for Perioperative Management of Patients on Opioid Therapy. 01/2018.

2 Basics of Echocardiography

Thomas J. Lavin and Alexander S. Kuo

Echocardiography is the use of ultrasound to image the heart and associated structures. It allows real-time assessment of the cardiac structure, cardiac function, and hemodynamic parameters. There are two primary modalities of echocardiography, transthoracic (TTE) and transesophageal (TEE).

I. TRANSTHORACIC IMAGE ACQUISITION

A. During a TTE, the ultrasound probe is applied to the chest or upper abdomen. TTE imaging can be more technically difficult to obtain because of intervening structures such as the chest wall, ribs, or lung. A review of the comprehensive TTE examination is beyond the scope of this chapter, but the basic views will be discussed.

B. Basic TTE views

1. Parasternal window
    a. Long axis (LAX)
        i. Position the transducer in the second, third, or fourth intercostal space at the left parasternal border with the marker oriented toward the right shoulder (**Figure 2.1**).
        ii. Place the mitral valve and aortic valve in the center of the image (**Figure 2.2**).
    b. Right ventricular (RV) inflow
        i. Obtain the parasternal LAX view.
        ii. Tilt the face of the transducer inferiorly and medially until only the RV can be visualized (**Figure 2.3**).
    c. Short axis (SAX)
        i. Aortic valve and great vessels.
            a. Position the transducer in the second, third, or fourth intercostal space at the left parasternal border with the marker oriented toward the left shoulder. If you are in the parasternal LAX view, the SAX can be obtained by rotating the probe 90° counterclockwise (**Figure 2.4**).
            b. Tilt the transducer to ensure that the aortic valve is in the center of the image (**Figure 2.5**).
        ii. Basal
            a. Obtain the parasternal SAX view.
            b. Tilt the transducer to ensure that the left ventricle (LV) is in the center of the image.
            c. Tilt the transducer slightly inferiorly and laterally toward the LV apex from the aortic valve SAX until both mitral valve leaflets are appreciated (**Figure 2.6**).
            d. Consider changing rib interspace to make the LV appear rounder in shape and the RV crescent-shaped.

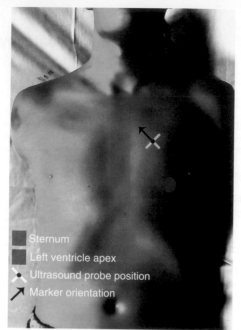

FIGURE 2.1 Parasternal long-axis transthoracic echocardiogram probe position.

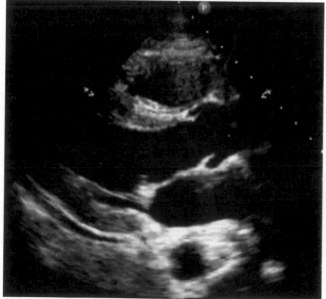

FIGURE 2.2 Parasternal long-axis transthoracic echocardiographic image.

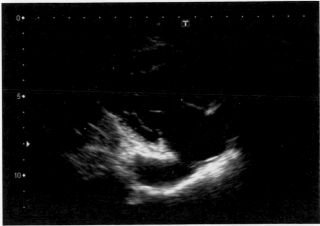

FIGURE 2.3 Right ventricular inflow transthoracic echocardiographic image.

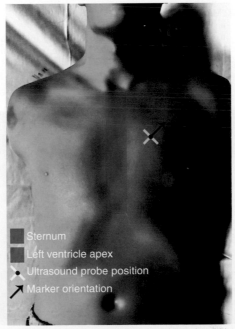

FIGURE 2.4 Parasternal short-axis aortic valve and great vessels probe position.

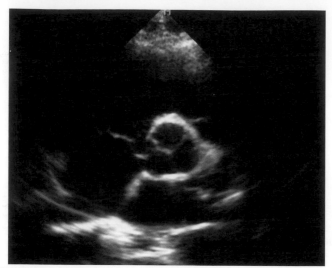

FIGURE 2.5 Parasternal short-axis aortic valve and great vessels transthoracic echocardiographic image.

    iii. Midpapillary
        a. Obtain the parasternal basal view.
        b. Tilt or slide the transducer slightly inferiorly and laterally toward the LV apex until both the papillary muscles can be visualized attaching to the LV wall (**Figure 2.7**).

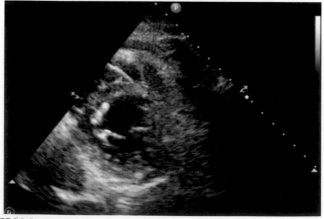

FIGURE 2.6 Parasternal short-axis basal transthoracic echocardiographic image.

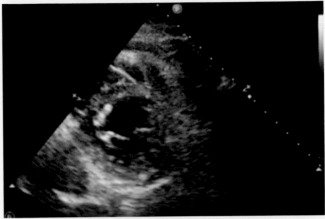

FIGURE 2.7 Parasternal short-axis midpapillary transthoracic echocardiographic image.

       iv. Apical
         a. Obtain the parasternal midpapillary view.
         b. Tilt or slide the transducer slightly inferiorly and laterally towards the LV apex until no papillary muscles can be visualized (**Figure 2.8**).
    2. Apical window
       a. Four-chamber
         i. Position the transducer in the fourth or fifth intercostal space between the anterior and midaxillary lines, along the point of maximal pulsation (apex) with the marker pointing toward the left axilla (**Figure 2.9**).
         ii. Move the probe laterally so the interventricular septum is in the center of the image and vertical (**Figure 2.10**).

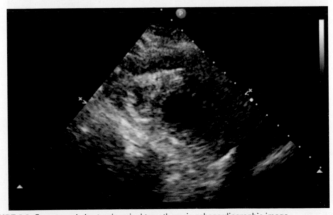

FIGURE 2.8 Parasternal short-axis apical transthoracic echocardiographic image.

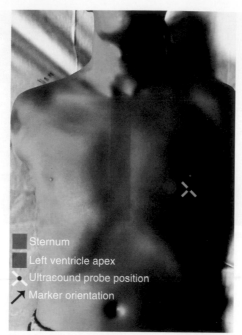

FIGURE 2.9 Apical four-chamber probe position.

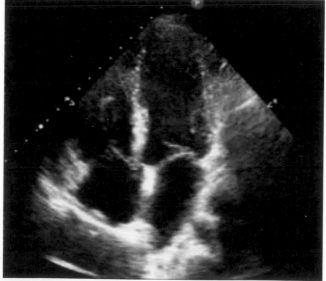

FIGURE 2.10 Apical four-chamber transthoracic echocardiographic image.

      iii. If atria cannot be appreciated, tilt the probe face anteriorly.

      iv. If ventricles appear too spherical, move the transducer inferiorly, down one rib interspace.

  b. Five-chamber

      i. Obtain the apical four-chamber view.

      ii. Tilt the transducer face anteriorly along the chest wall to visualize the aortic valve and left ventricle outflow tract (LVOT) in the center of the image (**Figure 2.11**).

      iii. Consider moving the transducer superiorly, up a rib interspace, or more laterally to align the LVOT.

  c. LAX/three-chamber

      i. Obtain the apical four-chamber view.

      ii. Rotate the transducer 100 to 140° counterclockwise pointing toward the right shoulder so the aortic valve and LVOT are visualized (**Figure 2.12**).

      iii. Place the left atria and ventricle in the center of the image by sliding the transducer more laterally (**Figure 2.13**).

3. Subcostal window

  a. Four-chamber

      i. Position the transducer in the subxiphoid region of the abdomen, at a flat angle parallel to the skin surface, with the index marker directed toward the left flank (**Figures 2.14** and **2.15**).

      ii. Consider moving the probe slightly right of the patient's midline to utilize the liver as an echogenic window.

  b. SAX

      i. Obtain the subcostal four-chamber view.

      ii. Rotate the transducer 90° counterclockwise so the index marker is oriented toward the patient's head (**Figure 2.16**).

      iii. Slide the probe so that the left ventricle is in the center of the image (**Figure 2.17**).

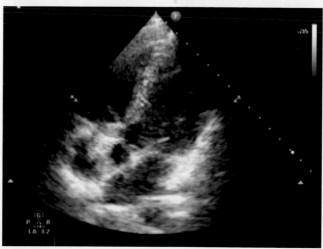

FIGURE 2.11 Apical 5-chamber transthoracic echocardiographic image.

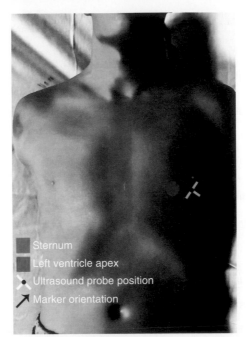

Sternum
Left ventricle apex
Ultrasound probe position
Marker orientation

FIGURE 2.12 Apical long-axis (three-chamber) probe position.

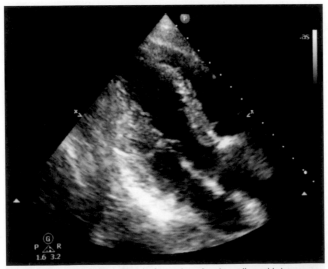

FIGURE 2.13 Apical long-axis (three-chamber) transthoracic echocardiographic image.

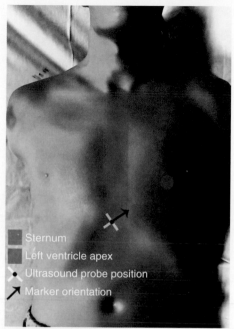

Sternum
Left ventricle apex
Ultrasound probe position
Marker orientation

FIGURE 2.14 Subcostal four-chamber probe position.

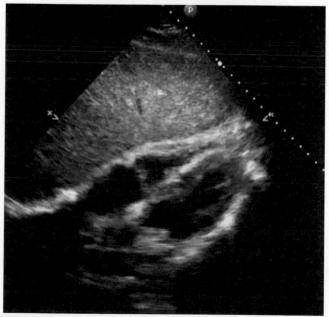

FIGURE 2.15 Subcostal four-chamber transthoracic echocardiographic image.

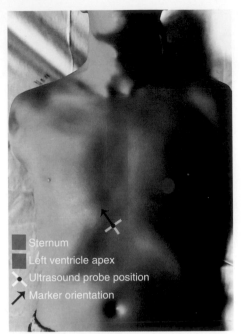

FIGURE 2.16 Subcostal short-axis probe position.

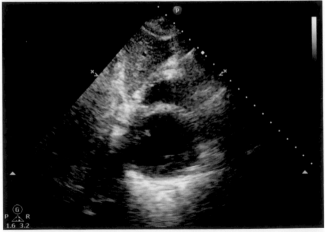

FIGURE 2.17 Subcostal short-axis transthoracic echocardiographic image.

    iv. Rotate the probe to make the left ventricle appear round in shape, trying to optimize the view of the two papillary muscles without any mitral valve.

  c. Inferior vena cava (IVC)

    i. Obtain the subcostal four-chamber view.

    ii. Rotate the transducer 90° counterclockwise so the index marker is oriented toward the patient's head, while keeping the right atrium in the center of the image (**Figure 2.18**).

    iii. Visualize the junction of the IVC and right atrium by tilting the probe face inferiorly (**Figure 2.19**).

    iv. Attempt to make the IVC appear more horizontal and appreciate hepatic veins draining into IVC.

    v. Ensure that the IVC is nonpulsatile (aorta is pulsatile).

II. TRANSESOPHAGEAL IMAGE ACQUISITION

A. In TEE, the ultrasound probe is inserted in the mouth and is advanced down the esophagus and then into the stomach. TEE can more consistently obtain higher resolution images than TTE because the esophagus is adjacent to the posterior heart, without any intervening structures of the ribs and lung. However, image alignment may be more difficult because the probe is confined to the esophagus. A review of the comprehensive TEE examination is beyond the scope of this chapter, but basic views will be discussed.

B. TEE complications

TEE is an invasive procedure, and a topical or general anesthetic is often required. It is associated with a minor complication rate of

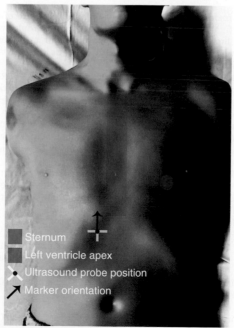

FIGURE 2.18 Subcostal inferior vena cava probe position.

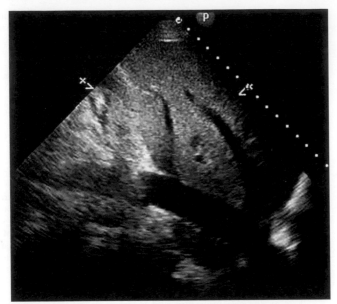

FIGURE 2.19 Subcostal inferior vena cava transthoracic echocardiographic image.

approximately 1% and a major complication rate of approximately 0.1%. Minor complications include lip or oropharyngeal trauma, self-limited dysphagia, or dyspepsia. Major complications include esophageal perforation and gastric injury or bleeding.

C. TEE probe manipulation

1. **Advancement or withdrawal:** Pulling the probe in and out of the esophagus moves the image plane superiorly and inferiorly in the body.

2. Rotation left or right: **Rotation** of the probe to move the imaging plane left or right.

3. **Omniplane:** Rotation of the ultrasound imaging plane allows changing from transverse orientation at 0° through sagittal orientation at 90°. This is performed electronically in modern TEE probes with button controls.

4. **Flexion of probe tip:** This is performed by rotating the wheel controls on the probe. The larger wheel allows anteflexion and retroflexion. The smaller wheel allows flexion left and right of the probe tip.

D. Basic TEE views

1. Midesophageal window

   a. Four-chamber

      i. Insert the probe approximately 20 cm, so that the transducer is behind the left atrium, and deep enough so no part of the aortic valve or LVOT can be seen (**Figure 2.20**).

      ii. Ensure that the probe omniplane is set between 0° and 10°.

   b. Five-chamber

      i. Obtain the four-chamber view.

      ii. Withdraw the probe until the LVOT can be seen (**Figure 2.21**).

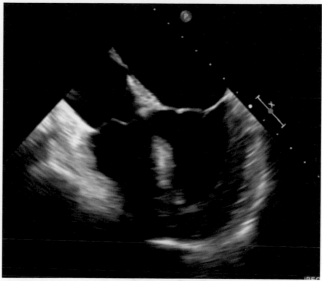

FIGURE 2.20 Midesophageal four-chamber transesophageal echocardiographic image.

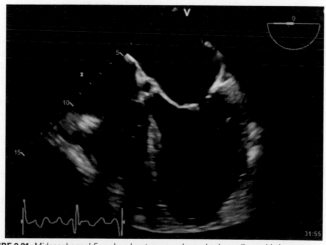

FIGURE 2.21 Midesophageal five-chamber transesophageal echocardiographic image.

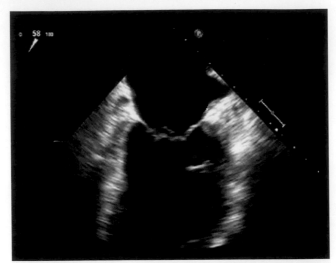

FIGURE 2.22 Midesophageal midcommissure transesophageal echocardiographic image.

   c. Midcommissural view
      i. Obtain the four-chamber view.
      ii. Place the mitral valve in the center of the image and omniplane to 45° to 60° so that the right atrium and right ventricle disappear.
      iii. Rotate the probe so the tip of the anterior mitral leaflet is seen in the middle of the screen, with the posterior mitral leaflet on both sides of the anterior leaflet tip (**Figure 2.22**).
   d. Two-chamber view
      i. Obtain the midcommissural view
      ii. Place the mitral valve in the center of the image and omniplane to 80° to 100° so that the right atrium and right ventricle disappear and the left atrial appendage appears (**Figure 2.23**).
   e. LAX view
      i. Obtain the two-chamber view.
      ii. Place the mitral valve in the center of the image and omniplane to 120° to 130° so that the aortic valve and LVOT are visualized in the LAX (**Figure 2.24**).
      iii. Adjust the depth to ensure that the entire LV remains in view.
   f. Right ventricular inflow-outflow
      i. Obtain the five-chamber view.
      ii. Omniplane to 30° to 45° and place the aortic valve in the center of the image to make the 3 cusps symmetric.
      iii. Advance the probe deeper to visualize the LVOT; retract the probe to visualize the coronary ostia (**Figure 2.25**).
   g. Bicaval
      i. Obtain the two-chamber view at approximately 90° omniplane.
      ii. Turn the entire probe to the right.
      iii. Adjust the omniplane angle or degree of rotation to simultaneously image the superior and inferior vena cava (**Figure 2.26**).

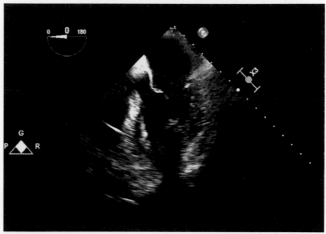

FIGURE 2.23 Midesophageal two-chamber transesophageal echocardiographic image.

2. Transgastric window
   a. SAX
      i. Advance the probe until stomach rugae or the liver becomes visible.
      ii. Anteflex to contact the stomach wall and inferior aspect of the heart.
      iii. Ensure that the omniplane is set to 0°.
      iv. Turn the probe to the left or right in order to center the LV.
      v. Slightly advance or withdraw the probe or adjust flexion until both papillary muscles appear (**Figure 2.27**).

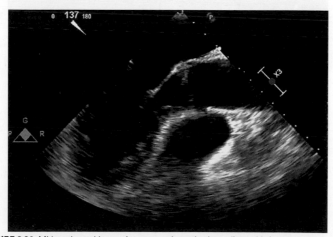

FIGURE 2.24 Midesophageal long-axis transesophageal echocardiographic image.

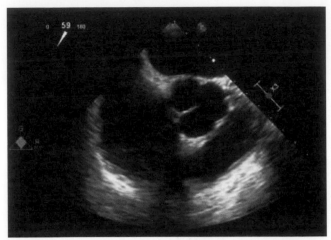

FIGURE 2.25 Midesophageal right ventricular inflow-outflow transesophageal echocardiographic image.

    b. Two-chamber
        i. Obtain the transgastric SAX view.
        ii. Omniplane to approximately 90°.
        iii. Anteflex until the LV is horizontal (**Figure 2.28**).
    c. LAX
        i. Obtain the transgastric two-chamber view.
        ii. Omniplane to 110° to 120°.

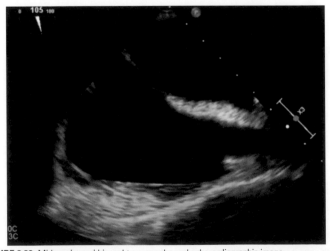

FIGURE 2.26 Midesophageal bicaval transesophageal echocardiographic image.

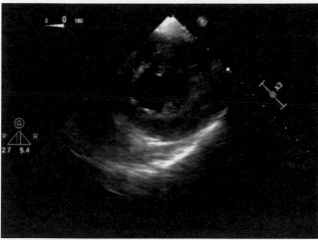

FIGURE 2.27 Transgastric short-axis transesophageal echocardiographic image.

        iii. Consider slightly turning probe to the right.

        iv. Adjust the depth of the probe so that the aortic valve is near the center of the image (**Figure 2.29**).

    d. RV inflow

        i. Obtain the transgastric SAX view.

        ii. Turn the probe to the right to put the right ventricle in the center of the image.

        iii. Omniplane to approximately 90°.

        iv. Anteflex until the RV is horizontal (**Figure 2.30**).

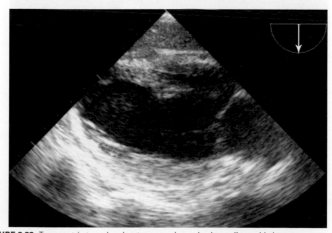

FIGURE 2.28 Transgastric two-chamber transesophageal echocardiographic image.

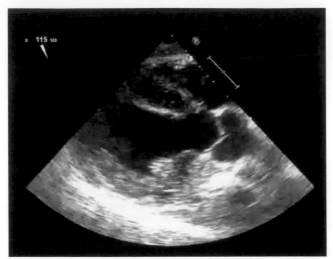

FIGURE 2.29 Transgastric long-axis transesophageal echocardiographic image.

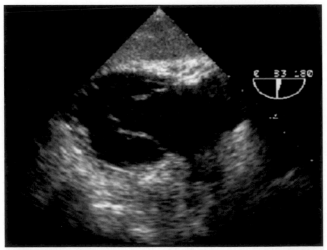

FIGURE 2.30 Transgastric right ventricular inflow transesophageal echocardiographic image.

    e. Deep transgastric LAX
       i. Obtain the transgastric SAX view and advance the probe.
      ii. Anteflex and slowly withdraw the probe until the LVOT is seen
         (**Figure 2.31**).

III. ECHOCARDIOGRAPHIC ASSESSMENT

A. Focused cardiac ultrasound versus comprehensive echocardiography:

Ultrasonography has been clinically used since the mid-20th century; however, ultrasound devices have evolved from expensive, largely cumbersome machines to affordable, handheld instruments over the recent years. As a result, there has been increasing use of echocardiography by noncardiologists to supplement the physical examination and other physiologic monitors in order to rapidly rule out or diagnose numerous pathologies in an unstable patient. The American Society of Echocardiography defines focused cardiac ultrasound (FoCUS) as a technique to supplement physical examination to recognize explicit ultrasonic signs that represent a narrow list of potential diagnoses in a specific clinical setting. The remainder of this chapter will address FoCUS assessment.

B. Left ventricular assessment

1. Assessment of left ventricular function can be conducted from a number of views including parasternal LAX, parasternal SAX, apical four-chamber, and subcostal views. The assessment of the left ventricle should begin with an evaluation of the architecture of the chamber, noting whether it is dilated or hypertrophied. Subsequently, the systolic function of the left ventricle, both globally and regionally, should be assessed. LV assessment is a basic skill that can be rapidly obtained with training and practice. Research has shown that medical students and junior resident physicians were able to improve clinical diagnosis with only a two-hour bedside ultrasound tutorial.

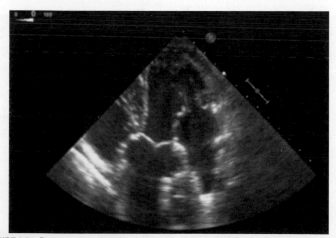

FIGURE 2.31 Deep transgastric long-axis transesophageal echocardiographic image.

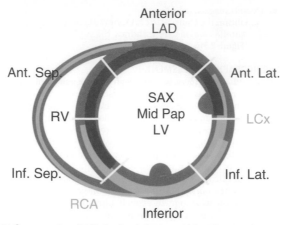

FIGURE 2.32 Coronary artery distribution in relation to ventricle wall segments.

2. The parasternal SAX is particularly useful for appreciating gross regional wall motion abnormalities corresponding to the coronary circulation. Typically, the left anterior descending artery perfuses the anterior portion of the left ventricle; the circumflex artery perfuses the lateral portion of the left ventricle; and the right coronary artery perfuses the inferior portion of the ventricle (**Figures 2.32** and **2.33**). Accurate and specific evaluation of wall motion abnormalities requires a significant amount of expertise and experience that transcends the purpose of a focused examination.

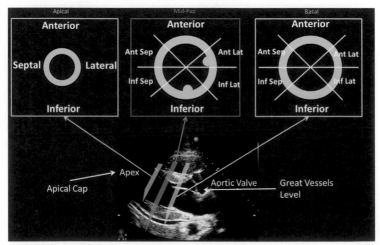

FIGURE 2.33 Standard left ventricular myocardial segmentation for tomography.

3. **Visual LV assessment:** As individuals practice and become more familiar with imaging the left ventricle, they will be able to quickly and objectively appreciate left ventricular function without having to make measurements. Clinicians should determine whether an ejection fraction is grossly normal or abnormal and whether the walls of the left ventricle are moving and thickening symmetrically or asymmetrically. The parasternal SAX view, at the midpapillary level, is typically the easiest view for appreciating global LV function. The American Society of Echocardiography evaluates wall motion of the segments by examining endocardium thickening and inward radial motion. The grading system ranges from normal or grade I, hypokinetic or grade II, akinetic or grade III, and, finally, dyskinetic or grade IV (**Table 2.1**). It is important to evaluate each segment for both parameters during examination, and in order to do so, it may be useful to visually cover the segments not being evaluated since a pathologic segment that does not thicken may still seem to move due to the inward motion of adjacent walls.

4. **Fractional shortening** is a one-dimensional method for evaluating LV function. It is measured by using an M-mode tracing in the parasternal LAX or SAX view. In the parasternal LAX view, the M-mode line should be perpendicular to the left ventricle and just beyond the tips of the mitral valve leaflets. In the parasternal SAX view, the M-mode line should be obtained through the center of the left ventricle at the midpapillary level. After obtaining each image, one can determine end-diastolic and end-systolic diameters and determine the fraction of shortening percentage by dividing their difference by the end-diastolic diameter. Normal fractional shortening is greater than 30%, whereas a fractional shortening less than 15% is consistent with severe hypokinesis. To approximate ejection fraction from this measurement, one can multiply the fractional shortening percentage by two; however, this technique can be very inaccurate, especially in the setting of regional wall motion abnormalities.

5. **Fractional area change (FAC)** is a two-dimensional (2D) technique that relies on the parasternal SAX view at the midpapillary level, comparing the traced area at end diastole and end systole. To calculate the area change, one would divide the difference between the end-diastolic area and end-systolic area by the end-diastolic area. Normal FAC is greater than 35%.

TABLE 2.1	Standard Grading System for Left Ventricle Wall Motion	
Qualitative Descriptor	**Systolic thickening and motion**	**Clinical Implication**
1. Normal/Hyperkinetic	Thickens and shortens	Normal
2. Hypokinetic	Reduced thickening and shortening	Ischemia or dysfunction
3. Akinetic	Does not thicken or shorten	Myocardial scar, infarction, hibernating
4. Dyskinetic	Thins or elongates	Aneurysm

Derived from Lang RM, Badano LP, Mor-Avi V, et al. Recommendations for cardiac chamber quantification by echocardiography in adults: an update from the American Society of Echocardiography and the European Association of Cardiovascular Imaging. *J Am Soc Echocardiogr.* 2015;28(1):1-39.e14.

6. E-point septal separation (EPSS) is another method for evaluating left ventricle function. It is determined by measuring the narrowest distance during early diastole between the anterior leaflet of the mitral valve and the interventricular septum in the parasternal LAX view, utilizing an M-mode beam through both structures. A distance greater than 7 mm is a marker for left ventricular ejection fraction less than 30%.

C. Right ventricular assessment

1. The right ventricle can be assessed from a number of different views; however, due to its irregular crescent shape, no single view can offer a comprehensive assessment. The four-chamber view allows good assessment of the free wall and septal motion, but only in a single plane. The SAX allows assessment of the midventricle, while the RV inflow-outflow allows assessment of basal function only.

2. Interventricular septal morphology:

   a. It is important to evaluate the shape of the interventricular septum when evaluating the right ventricle since the geometry of this anatomic structure significantly contributes to right ventricular pressure and function. Normally, the left ventricle is round while the right ventricle is crescent shaped when examining the structures in the parasternal SAX view. During right ventricular overload, the interventricular septum flattens causing the left ventricle to become "D" shaped. Ultimately, this change in shape will impair left ventricular filling and the cardiac output (CO).

   b. Volume overload: The interventricular septum will flatten during diastole if the right ventricle is volume overloaded with restoration of normal shape during systole. Circumstances that would cause the right ventricle to experience volume overload include tricuspid regurgitation and left-to-right shunts such as atrial or ventricular septal defects.

   c. Pressure overload: The interventricular septum will flatten during systole and restore normal shape during diastole if the right ventricle is pressure overloaded. Pathologic conditions that would increase pressure over include pulmonary hypertension.

   d. If the right ventricle experiences both pressure and volume overload, the interventricular septum will be flattened throughout the entire duration of the cardiac cycle.

3. Right ventricular systolic function:

   a. FAC: It is determined in the same manner as for the left ventricle. The apical four-chamber view is most useful for measuring right ventricle FAC. An operator will trace the endocardium to the tricuspid annulus and compare the area between end diastole and end systole before dividing by end-diastolic area. Normally, right ventricle FAC is >35%.

   b. TAPSE: Tricuspid annular plane systolic excursion (TAPSE) is the distance the lateral annulus travels toward the apex during systole. In the apical four-chamber view, an M-mode beam is placed through the interventricular septum and lateral wall tricuspid annulus to measure the systolic excursion of the right ventricle in a longitudinal plane. Normal TAPSE is >1.6 cm; however, the major limitation of this measurement is that it only evaluates the free wall of the right ventricle, neglecting the contributions of the interventricular septum and right ventricular outflow tract.

4. **Right ventricular wall thickness:** Wall thickness is useful for evaluating the presence of right ventricular hypertrophy, which can result from pulmonary hypertension or chronic right ventricular volume overload. RV lateral wall thickness is best measured by TTE using the subcostal four-chamber. Using M-mode, the measurement is made at end diastole at the level of the tip of the anterior tricuspid valve leaflet. The right ventricular wall is normally less than 5 mm thick.

5. **Right ventricular dilation:** Right ventricular size is best evaluated in the apical four-chamber view. During end diastole, one measures the diameter right above the tricuspid annulus at the base of the right ventricle. The normal value is less than 4.2 cm. Generally speaking, the normal RV is no more than two-thirds the size of the left ventricle in an apical four-chamber view. If the RV makes up the apex or is larger than the LV, then the RV is most likely significantly enlarged.

D. **IVC**

1. The IVC can be readily assessed by surface ultrasound. The patient should be supine for measurements. The vena cava is a tubular structure that runs cephalad to caudad. Imaging is performed from the subcostal window to the right of midline in the sagittal plane to obtain LAX view of the IVC. The morphology of the IVC can provide insight into the filling pressures of the heart and provide supportive data for diagnoses such as tamponade, hypovolemia, or heart failure.

2. **IVC diameter and central venous pressure (CVP)**
   a. In spontaneously breathing patients, IVC diameter correlates to CVP.
      i. If the IVC diameter is less than 2.1 cm AND collapses more than 50% with sniff, this indicates filling pressures are normal, CVP < 5 mm Hg.
      ii. If the IVC diameter is greater than 2.1 cm AND collapses less 50% with sniff, this indicates elevated filling pressures, CVP > 15 mm Hg.
      iii. Other conditions are indeterminate, and filling pressures may be intermediate, CVP 5 to 10 mm Hg.

3. **IVC for fluid responsiveness:** In intubated patients without any spontaneous effort, variations in CVP diameter can be used to predict fluid responsiveness. Please see the section below on Hemodynamic Measurements and Fluid Responsiveness.

IV. **HEMODYNAMIC MEASUREMENTS AND FLUID RESPONSIVENESS**

1. The difference in pressure between chambers can be assessed by measuring the velocity of fluid flow between the two chambers. This relationship is given by simplified Bernoulli equation.

2. **Simplified Bernoulli equation (Figure 2.34):**

$$P_2 - P_1 \left(mm\,Hg\right) = 4V^2 \left(m/s\right)$$

where $P_1 - P_2$ is the difference in pressure between the two chambers in mm Hg and V is the velocity of the fluid flow jet between the chambers in meters per second. A common usage of this equation is in the measurement of right ventricular systolic pressure (RVSP).

3. **RVSP measurement:** The tricuspid regurgitant jet is measured in the apical four-chamber or parasternal RV-inflow view using continuous wave Doppler. The peak velocity is then inserted in the simplified Bernoulli equation. CVP is then added to the calculated pressure gradient, since the

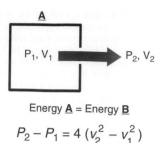

Energy **A** = Energy **B**

$$P_2 - P_1 = 4\left(v_2^2 - v_1^2\right)$$

FIGURE 2.34 Bernoulli equation for calculating transvalvular gradients.

calculated pressure difference is between the RV and the right atrium and not the absolute pressure.

$$RVSP = 4V_{\text{tricuspid regurg.}}^2 + CVP$$

If the fluid is starting with a significant initial velocity, a slightly more accurate modified Bernoulli equation must be used to account for this. An example of this would be measurement of the aortic stenosis with high cardiac output since the LVOT would have significant velocity. Modified Bernoulli equation:

$$P_2 - P_1\left(mm\,Hg\right) = 4\left(V_2^2 - V_1^2\right)\left(m/s\right)$$

1. Although ultrasound cannot measure flow directly, velocity can be measured and integrated over time, velocity time integral (VTI), to determine distance travelled. Multiplying the VTI by the cross-sectional area of the structure through which the velocity is measured yields the rate of flow. A common application of this approach is the measurement of stroke volume and cardiac output.

2. **Stroke volume measurement:** This is performed by measuring first measuring the LVOT diameter in the parasternal LAX view. Assuming the LVOT is a circle, the area can be calculated, $LVOT_{area}$. Then the flow in the LVOT from the apical five-chamber view using pulse wave Doppler. From the pulse wave Doppler waveform, the area under the curve of ejection is then measure to obtain the VTI. This VTI is then multiplied by $LVOT_{area}$ to give the stroke volume (SV). The SV can then be multiplied by the heart rate (HR) to give the cardiac output.

$$LVOT_{area} = \left(\pi/4\right) \times \left(LVOT_{diameter}\right)^2$$
$$\text{Stroke volume} = LVOT_{area} \times VTI_{LVOT}$$
$$\text{Cardiac output} = SV \times HR$$

a. **SVV:** In order to calculate SVV, an apical five-chamber view is obtained to determine the blood flow through the LVOT using pulse wave Doppler. Placing the marker through the LVOT will produce a series of VTIs, and SVV is calculated by subtracting the maximum velocity by the minimum velocity divided by the average of the two velocities. Changes > 12% correlate with a likelihood of fluid responsiveness;

however, this technique has only been validated for patients in sinus rhythm who are mechanically ventilated with neuromuscular blockade and receiving a tidal volume of 8 mL/kg.

$$SVV = \frac{SV_{Max} - SV_{Min}}{SV_{average}}$$

b. **IVC diameter variation** is measured in a manner similar to the static assessment of IVC diameter. In the subcostal IVC LAX view, the M-mode beam is sited approximately 1 to 2 cm proximal to the cavoatrial junction and used to measure the change in maximum diameter (at the end of positive pressure inspiration) and minimum diameter (at the end of positive pressure expiration). A value greater than 12% after calculating the difference between the maximum and minimum diameters divided by the mean of each has been shown to predict fluid responsiveness to an 8 mL/kg intravenous (IV) volume bolus (**Table 2.2**). Although this technique has only been validated in mechanically ventilated patients, IVC diameter variation does not require sinus rhythm, unlike SVV.

c. **PLR** test is a reversible preload challenge that translocates approximately 300 mL of blood from the lower extremities by changing a semirecumbent positioned patient into a supine position with leg elevation. The maximal cardiac response to PLR occurs within 2 minutes of the positioning change. Similar to conventional SVV, a sonographer will calculate the LVOT velocity in the apical five-chamber view, both before and after the maneuver. An increase in the velocity by 10% to 15% corresponds with likelihood of fluid responsiveness. A meta-analysis of studies of PLR found the diagnostic value of this technique to be excellent. A particular advantage of this approach is the lack of requirement for mechanical ventilation, sinus rhythm, or normal pulmonary compliance.

d. **Fluid challenge:** A final method is to measure CO before administration of an IV fluid bolus and then measure the CO after. If the cardiac output does not increase with the fluid challenge, the patient is presumed not to be fluid responsive and no further IV fluids are administered until there has been a change in physiologic state. Measurement of CO using echocardiography is describe the above in the section on "*Flow Measurement.*"

TABLE 2.2	Inferior Vena Cava Diameter correlation to Central Venous Pressure	
IVC Diameter	**Collapse With Sniff**	**Approximate CVP**
Less than 2.1 cm AND	Greater than 50%	Normal, 0-5 mm Hg
Greater than 2.1 cm AND	Less than 50%	Elevated, >15 mm Hg
Does not meet both conditions above		Indeterminate or intermediate

CVP, central venous pressure; IVC, inferior vena cava.
Derived from Lang RM, Badano LP, Mor-Avi V, et al. Recommendations for cardiac chamber quantification by echocardiography in adults: an update from the American Society of Echocardiography and the European Association of Cardiovascular Imaging. *J Am Soc Echocardiogr.* 2015;28(1):1-39.e14.

A. Doppler ultrasound

1. Ultrasound cannot directly measure pressures or blood flow, but using Doppler measurements, velocity can be assessed and pressure and flows can be inferred. This is a powerful tool that allows for quantitative hemodynamic measurements. It is important to recognize that Doppler can only measure velocity along the direction of the ultrasound beam. Thus, measurement accuracy is dependent on angle and is most accurate when the angle of the transducer beam is less than 20° to the direction of blood flow. There are three main modes of Doppler used: continuous wave, pulse wave, and color.

2. **Continuous wave Doppler** continuously transmits and receives Doppler signals. This allows measurement of the highest velocity of blood flow along the path of the beam and is useful for assessing regurgitant jets or the flow through a stenotic aortic valve. However, it does not allow the position of the velocity measurement to be known.

3. **Pulse wave Doppler** allows velocity measurements at a specific location. However, due to the Nyquist limit, the maximum measurable velocity is limited by aliasing. Thus, only lower velocities flows can be measured, such as ventricular ejection or mitral inflow.

4. **Color Doppler** allows visualization of flow overlaid on the 2D image. Like pulse wave, it is also limited to accurate measurement of lower velocities. It is a very useful tool to qualitatively evaluate flow patterns.

B. Pressure gradient assessment

A. Flow measurements

A. Fluid responsiveness

1. The concept of fluid responsiveness is central to optimizing fluid therapy. Fluid overload has been associated with prolonged duration of mechanical ventilation, in addition to increased overall morbidity and mortality; thus, fluids should only be administered to patients who are fluid responsive. The use of echocardiography for fluid responsiveness remains a controversial topic.

2. Fluid responsiveness is defined by a 10% to 15% increase in stroke volume after receiving a 500 mL fluid bolus over 10 to 15 minutes. Conceptually, administering additional fluid will only increase stroke volume if it increases stressed blood volume and if both ventricles are volume responsive and functioning on the ascending portion of the Frank-Starling curve. It is important to consider that a heart with impaired systolic function can respond to an increase in fluid; however, the overall response will be relatively reduced.

3. **Static echocardiograph parameters:** Overall, static parameters are poor predictors of volume responsiveness, but they do correlate with values such as central venous and pulmonary capillary wedge pressure.

4. **Left ventricular end-diastolic area (LVEDA)** is best measured in the parasternal SAX view at the midpapillary level and has been shown to more accurately reflect left ventricle preload relative to pulmonary capillary wedge pressure. A publication reviewing fluid responsiveness in intensive care unit (ICU) patients included two studies that found patients more likely to respond to a fluid bolus if they had lower LVEDAs relative to individuals who would not respond; however, these two studies relied on TEE rather than TTE. Overall, LVEDA < 10 cm^2 has been associated with severe hypovolemia, and conversely, >20 cm^2 has been associated with volume overload.

5. **Left ventricular end-systolic area (LVESA)** is measured at the midpapillary level in the parasternal SAX views. Particular attention should be paid to the positioning of the papillary muscles. The classical teaching is

that contact between opposing papillary muscles at the end of systole ("kissing papillary muscles") is indicative of severe hypovolemia. There are various other factors that can also cause a small LVESA, including distributive shock, hyperdynamic left ventricle contractility, right ventricular failure, acute mitral regurgitation, or cardiac tamponade to name a few.

6. IVC diameter: Please see the section above on IVC assessment.

7. **Dynamic echocardiographic parameters** are more evidence supported indices for determining fluid responsiveness relative to static tests. Some examples of dynamic parameters of fluid responsiveness are stroke volume variation (SVV), IVC variation, passive leg raise (PLR) testing, and fluid challenge.

V. CONCLUSION

Driven by progressive advances in ultrasound technology, the use of echocardiography and FoCUS by noncardiologists is rapidly expanding. This allows the clinician at the bedside to rapidly and repeatedly evaluate a patient. It supplements physical examination and obviates the potential risk involved in waiting for, or transporting an unstable patient for, additional forms of diagnostic testing. A focused bedside ultrasound examination does not replace the role of a comprehensive echocardiographic examination and care must be taken to practice within the limitations of one's own expertise. Consultation of an expert echocardiographer is recommended when there is any question or complex diagnosis. However, point of care cardiac ultrasound is a powerful new tool for the bedside clinician, and the applications will continue to develop in the future.

Suggested Readings

Beigel R, Cercek B, Luo H, Siegal RJ. Noninvasive evaluation of right atrial pressure. *J Am Soc Echocardiogr*. 2013;26(9):1033-1042.

Cherpanath TG, Hirsch A, Geerts BF, et al. Predicting fluid responsiveness by passive leg raising: a systematic review and meta-analysis of 23 clinical trials. *Crit Care Med*. 2016;44(5):981-991. doi:10.1097/CCM.0000000000001556

Cherpanath TG, Geerts BF, Lagrand WK, Schultz MJ, Groeneveld AB. Basic concepts of fluid responsiveness. *Neth Heart J*. 2013;21(12):530-536.

Feissel M, Michard F, Faller JP, Teboul JL. The respiratory variation in inferior vena cava diameter as a guide to fluid therapy. *Intensive Care Med*. 2004;30:1834-1837. doi:10.1007//s00134-004-2233-5

Feissel M, Michard F, Mangin I, Ruyer O, Faller JP, Teboul JL. Respiratory changes in aortic blood velocity as an indicator of fluid responsiveness in ventilated patients with septic shock. *Chest*. 2001;119(3):867-873.

Goldberg BB, Goodman GA, Clearfield HR. Evaluation of Ascites by ultrasound. *Radiology*. 1970;96:15-22.

Kristensen JK, Buemann B, Kuhl E. Ultrasonic scanning in the diagnosis of splenic haematomas. *Acta Chir Scand*. 1971;137:653-657.

Labovitz AJ, Noble VE, Bierig M, et al. Focused cardiac ultrasound in the emergent setting: a consensus statement of the American Society of Echocardiography and American College of Emergency Physicians. *J Am Soc Echocardiogr*. 2010;23:1225-1230.

Lang RM, Badano LP, Mor-Avi V, et al. Recommendations for cardiac chamber quantification by echocardiography in adults: an update from the American Society of Echocardiography and the European Association of Cardiovascular Imaging. *J Am Soc Echocardiogr*. 2015;28(1):1-39.e14.

McKaigney CJ, Krantz MJ, La Rocque CL, Hurst ND, Buchanan MS, Kendall JL. E-point septal separation: a bedside tool for emergency physician assessment of left ventricular ejection fraction. *Am J Emerg Med*. 2014;32(6):493-497.

Monnet X, Marik PE, Teboul JL. Prediction of fluid responsiveness: an update. *Ann Intensive Care*. 2016;6(1):111.

Michard F, Teboul JL. Predicting fluid responsiveness in ICU patients: a critical analysis of the evidence. *Chest.* 2002;121(6):2000-2008.

Panoulas VF, Daigeler AL, Malaweera ASN, et al. Pocket-size hand-held cardiac ultrasound as an adjunct to clinical examination in the hands of medical students and junior doctors. *Eur Heart J Cardiovasc Imaging.* 2013;14(4):323-330. doi:10.1093/ehjci/jes140

Spencer KT, Kimura BJ, Korcarz CE, Pellikka PA, Rahko PS, Siegel RJ. Focused cardiac ultrasound: recommendations from the American Society of Echocardiography. *J Am Soc Echocardiogr.* 2013;26:567-581.

Wetterslev M, Haase N, Johansen RR, Perner A. Predicting fluid responsiveness with transthoracic echocardiography is not yet evidence based. *Acta Anaesthegiol Scan.* 2013;57(6):692-697. doi:10.1111/aas.12045

Wojciech M, Dyla A, Zawada T. Utility of transthoracic echocardiography (TTE) in assessing fluid responsiveness in critically ill patients—a challenge for the bedside sonographer. *Med Ultrason.* 2016;18(4):508-514. doi:10.11152/mu-880

3 Specific Considerations With Cardiac Disease

Adam A. Dalia and Casey Hamilton

I. GENERAL CONSIDERATIONS

An estimated one in three Americans has one or more types of cardiovascular disease (CVD). Mortality data show that one of every three deaths in the United States is secondary to CVD.

II. CORONARY ANATOMY

The coronary arteries perfuse the myocardium. The left and right coronary arteries originate from the coronary sinuses distal to the aortic valve. The left main coronary artery (LMCA) branches into the left anterior descending artery (LAD) and the left circumflex artery (LCX) to supply most of the left ventricle (LV), interventricular septum (IVS), and the left atrium (LA). The right coronary artery (RCA) supplies the right atrium (RA) and ventricle (RV), as well as portions of the IVS, including the sinoatrial (SA) and atrioventricular (AV) nodes (**Figure 3.1**). In approximately 70% of the population, the posterior descending artery (PDA) is supplied by the RCA. This circulation is described as "right dominant." The remainder of the population is either "left dominant," with the PDA emerging from the LCX (10% of the population), or "codominant," with the PDA receiving contributions from both the LCX and RCA (20% of population).

III. PREOPERATIVE CARDIOVASCULAR EVALUATION FOR NONCARDIAC SURGERY

The American College of Cardiology and the American Heart Association (ACC/AHA) have developed joint guidelines for the preoperative cardiovascular evaluation and management of patients undergoing noncardiac surgery. The initial evaluation consists of the patient's history, focused physical examination, and routine laboratory investigation. Based on the patient's history, cardiac risk factors, functional status, and the nature of the surgical procedure, the ACC/AHA guidelines provide a stepwise approach for identifying patients who may benefit from further cardiovascular testing (**Figure 3.2**).

A. Initial screening

1. The need for **emergency surgery** preempts further cardiac workup. The ACC/AHA guidelines define an emergency procedure as one that must be started within 6 hours. As there is little to no time, the patient must proceed often with no or very limited clinical preoperative evaluation. Emergent surgery should proceed with appropriate patient monitoring and management strategies based on the patient's clinical risk factors for coronary artery disease (CAD). Bedside focused cardiac ultrasound (FoCUS) via transthoracic echocardiography can be performed to rule out life-threatening cardiac conditions such as tamponade, aortic dissection, or myocardial infarction (MI) to help with perioperative management in the emergent setting.

2. If the **surgery is not emergent**, determine whether the patient has an acute coronary syndrome (ACS). An ACS is an unstable angina or an MI. The patient may present with chest pain, shortness of breath,

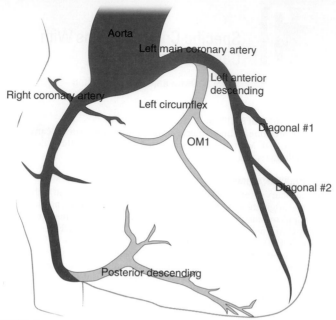

FIGURE 3.1 Coronary anatomy.

diaphoresis, or nausea. The electrocardiogram (ECG) may show ST segment depressions or elevations. If the patient has an ACS, the surgical procedure should be postponed and the patient should immediately undergo cardiac evaluation and guideline-directed medical therapy (GDMT). If the patient does not have an ACS, then proceed with an assessment of the patient's postoperative risk for a major adverse cardiac event (MACE).

B. Risk of MACE. The patient's risk of MACE should be determined based on clinical characteristics and the surgical procedure. Clinical risk factors for MACE include a history of heart failure, CAD, cerebrovascular disease, diabetes, and chronic kidney disease. Validated risk prediction tools, such as the Revised Cardiac Risk Index (RCRI) and the American College of Surgeons National Surgical Quality Improvement Program (ACS NSQIP) Surgical Risk Calculator (riskcalculator.facs.org), can be used to help predict the risk of perioperative MACE.

1. If the patient has a **low risk of MACE** (<1%), then **no further testing** is needed and the patient may **proceed to surgery.**

2. If the patient has an **elevated risk of MACE** (≥1%), then the **functional capacity** should be determined. **Functional capacity** can be expressed as metabolic equivalents (METs). A single MET represents oxygen consumption at rest. If the patient has moderate or excellent functional capacity without cardiac symptoms, then the patient may proceed to surgery without further evaluation. **Moderate or excellent functional capacity** is defined as an **exercise capacity greater than or equal to 4 METs.** Activities that correspond to moderate functional capacity include

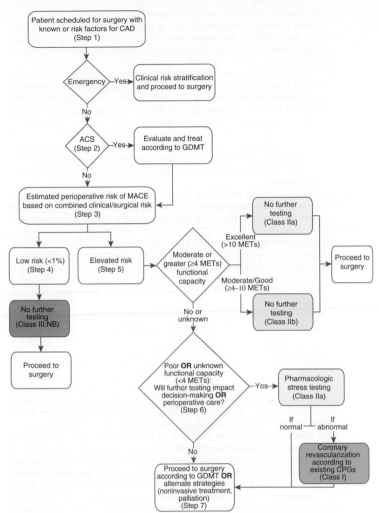

FIGURE 3.2 Stepwise approach to perioperative cardiac assessment for CAD from the latest ACC/AHA guidelines. Colors correspond to classes of recommendations. ACC/AHA, American College of Cardiology and American Heart Association; ACS, acute coronary syndrome; CAD, coronary artery disease; CPGs, clinical practice guidelines; GDMT, guideline-directed medical therapy; MACE, major adverse cardiac event; METs, metabolic equivalents. (Reprinted from Fleisher LA, Fleischmann KE, Auerbach AD, et al. 2014 ACC/AHA guideline on perioperative cardiovascular evaluation and management of patients undergoing noncardiac surgery: a report of the American College of Cardiology/American Heart Association Task Force on practice guidelines. *J Am Coll Cardiol.* 2014;64(22):e77-e137. Copyright © 2014 American College of Cardiology Foundation and the American Heart Association, Inc. With permission.)

climbing two flights of stairs, walking on level ground at 4 mph, running a short distance, scrubbing floors, or playing a game of golf without a cart. The ability to participate in strenuous sports such as swimming, singles tennis, or football generally corresponds to excellent functional capacity.

3. If the patient has poor or unknown functional capacity, then further testing may be needed if the results will change a patient's management. **Poor functional capacity** is defined as an **exercise capacity less than 4 METs**. Examples include the inability to walk more than two blocks on level ground without stopping due to symptoms and activity limited to eating, dressing, and walking indoors. Further testing may include exercise or pharmacologic stress testing. If abnormal, coronary angiography may be considered. The patient can then proceed to surgery with GDMT. Testing may not be necessary if the results will not alter patient management.

C. **Supplemental cardiac evaluation.** Supplemental cardiac evaluation should be performed when indicated to measure functional capacity, identify the presence of cardiac dysfunction, and provide an estimate of the perioperative cardiac risk.

1. **Preoperative resting 12-lead ECG** should be considered for patients with known coronary heart disease, significant arrhythmia, peripheral arterial disease, cerebrovascular disease, or other structural heart diseases, except for those undergoing low-risk surgery. Routine preoperative ECG is not indicated for asymptomatic patients undergoing low-risk surgery.

2. **Rest echocardiography** may be used to evaluate ventricular function in patients with history of heart failure or dyspnea of unknown origin. It is also useful to assess valvular pathology in patients with a history of valvular disease or a newly identified heart murmur.

3. **Stress testing** is recommended for patients with elevated risk of MACE and poor or unknown functional capacity if outcome will change management. Patients who have an elevated risk of MACE and moderate to good (4-10 METs) functional capacity may proceed to surgery without stress testing. Routine screening with stress testing is not useful for patients undergoing low-risk noncardiac surgery.

   a. **Exercise stress testing** provides an objective measure of functional capacity. It is the preferred modality in patients who are capable of achieving adequate workloads. Sensitivity and specificity for multivessel CAD are 81% and 66%, respectively. Exercise stress tests are highly predictive when ST segment changes are characteristic of ischemia (>2 mm, sustained into recovery, and/or associated with hypotension). The risk of perioperative cardiac events is increased significantly in patients who have abnormal exercise ECGs at low workloads. Radionuclide imaging or echocardiography can be combined with exercise stress testing for patients whose baseline ECGs render interpretation invalid.

   b. **Pharmacologic stress testing** can be conducted with either an agent that increases myocardial oxygen demand (dobutamine) or dilates coronary arteries and causes coronary steal from diseased vessels (dipyridamole or adenosine). Pharmacologic stress tests are suitable for patients who are unable to exercise. Dobutamine stress testing is typically combined with echocardiography to detect wall motion abnormalities brought about by the increased myocardial workload. Dipyridamole or adenosine stress tests are typically combined with radionuclide imaging to detect areas of myocardium that are at risk. Pharmacologic vasodilation has the risk of a false-negative test in patients with multivessel CAD where all vessels are already maximally vasodilated. In both cases, perioperative cardiac risk is directly proportional to the extent of myocardium that is found to be at risk on imaging.

4. **Cardiac catheterization** is considered the "gold standard" for evaluating CAD. Information obtained includes coronary anatomy with visualization of direction and distribution of flow, hemodynamics, and overall function of the heart. Routine preoperative coronary angiography is not recommended. Revascularization before noncardiac surgery is recommended in circumstances in which revascularization is indicated according to existing clinical practice guidelines.

5. **Noninvasive imaging** including cardiac MRI (CMR) and coronary computed tomography angiogram (CCTA) have emerged as reasonable options for preoperative cardiac evaluation. CMR is usually reserved for patients after first-line imaging (echocardiography) is either inconclusive or indeterminant; it is generally reserved for patients with complex disease. Contraindications to CMR include the presence of implants or cardiovascular implantable electronic devices (CIEDs) that are not MRI safe. CCTA can be utilized to rule out obstructive CAD in low- to medium-risk patients, but it is not advised for high-risk patients; coronary catheterization remains the gold standard for high-risk patients. Contraindications to cardiac CTA include renal failure or allergy to contrast.

6. **Cardiac consultation** may be helpful in determining which tests will be useful and in interpreting the results. The consultant can help optimize the patient's preoperative medical therapy and provide follow-up in the postoperative period. Such follow-up is crucial with the initiation of new drug therapies and often for patients with pacemakers and implantable cardioverter-defibrillator (ICD) devices (see Section XI).

D. Indications for preoperative coronary revascularization with either **coronary artery bypass grafting** or **percutaneous coronary intervention (PCI)** are in general the same as in the nonoperative setting. Surgery, in and of itself, is not an indication for coronary revascularization, regardless of extent of vessel disease or left ventricular dysfunction.

IV. PREANESTHETIC CONSIDERATIONS

A. Patients are likely to be anxious. Reassurance during the preoperative visit has been shown to be useful in decreasing anxiety. **Anxiolytics** may blunt rises in sympathetic tone and may be invaluable.

B. **Cardiac medications** are usually continued perioperatively. Possible exceptions include angiotensin-converting enzyme inhibitors (due to proposed prolonged vasodilation), sustained-release or long-acting medications, and diuretics.

1. **β-blockers.** While the evidence for initiating β-blockers in the perioperative period is mixed, there is a consensus that patients already taking β-blockers should continue them in the perioperative period. Initiating β-blocker therapy in the perioperative period has been associated with an increased incidence of MACEs such as nonfatal stroke and MI. In patients with moderate to high risk of perioperative myocardial ischemia or with three or more Revised Cardiac Risk Index (RCRI) risk factors (eg, diabetes mellitus, HF, CAD, renal insufficiency, cerebrovascular accident), it may be reasonable to start β-blockers before surgery. When possible, β-blockers should be started days to weeks

before elective surgery and titrated cautiously. **They should not be started on the day of surgery**; starting β-blockers within 1 day or less of surgery increases the risk of stroke, death, hypotension, and bradycardia.

2. **Statins.** Patients taking statins should continue to receive statins perioperatively. Preoperative initiation of statin therapy is reasonable in patients undergoing vascular surgery as well as in patients with standard clinical indications for statin therapy who are undergoing elevated-risk procedures.

3. **Aspirin.** The efficacy of aspirin for the secondary prevention of MI in patients with ischemic heart disease has been well documented. Data on the risk of discontinuing antiplatelet therapy in patients with coronary stents have strongly suggested continuing aspirin in the perioperative period. The data on continuing aspirin in patients undergoing elective noncardiac, noncarotid surgery who have not had previous coronary stenting, however, are controversial. Some publications recommend that aspirin should not be stopped routinely in the perioperative period at all, while a recent systematic review and metanalysis suggests that aspirin has no significant effect on overall survival, cardiovascular mortality, or arterial ischemic events, while reducing venous thromboembolic events at the expense of increased risk of major bleeding.

C. **Timing of elective surgery in the setting of previous PCI** presents a special challenge. Management decisions should be made in consultation with the patient's cardiologist and surgeon.

1. **Balloon angioplasty without stent placement.** The ACC/AHA recommend that elective noncardiac surgery should be **delayed 14 days** after balloon angioplasty. Aspirin therapy should be continued in the perioperative period.

2. **Bare-metal coronary stents (BMS).** Current recommendations are to **delay elective noncardiac surgery for 30 days** following PCI with BMS. This time period allows for the completion of thienopyridine therapy and the endothelialization of the stent. The risk of ischemic events is greatest within 30 days of PCI, significantly lower at 30 to 90 days, and lowest after 90 days. Aspirin therapy should be continued perioperatively.

3. **Drug-eluting stents (DES).** Thrombosis of DES can occur months after placement and is often related to the omission of dual antiplatelet therapy (DAPT) perioperatively. The current consensus recommendation is to **defer elective surgery for at least 3 months, and optimally 6 months**, following placement. Aspirin therapy should be continued perioperatively. Elective noncardiac surgery after DES implantation **may be considered after 3 to 6 months** if the risk of further delay is greater than the expected risks of ischemia and stent thrombosis.

4. Should a noncardiac surgical procedure be required within the time frame recommended for DAPT following PCI, consider continuing the therapy throughout the perioperative period. If bleeding risk necessitates the discontinuation of thienopyridine therapy, continue aspirin therapy and restart thienopyridines as soon as possible.

D. **Supplemental oxygen** should be provided to all patients who have a significant risk of ischemia.

E. **Monitoring** is discussed in Chapter 15.

F. **Anesthetic technique.** There are no convincing data to support the superiority of one particular anesthetic technique over another in the management of patients at risk for perioperative cardiac events; the anesthetic technique should be decided upon based on patient and surgical factors. The use of MAC, local, or neuraxial combination can be more hemodynamically stable compared to general anesthesia but presents challenges with regard to anticoagulation status, level of consciousness, and pain control (tachycardia and hypertension). For major open abdominal aortic surgery, it has been shown that epidural anesthesia with general anesthesia improved pain control while reducing postoperative respiratory failure and MI; however, there was no observed difference in mortality.

V. ISCHEMIC HEART DISEASE

CAD afflicts an estimated 30% of patients undergoing surgery in the United States. CAD increases in prevalence with age. Other risk factors include hypercholesterolemia, male gender, hypertension, cigarette smoking, diabetes mellitus, obesity, and family history of premature development of ischemic heart disease. CAD is a risk factor for perioperative cardiac complications, including MI, unstable angina, congestive heart failure (CHF), and serious dysrhythmias.

A. Pathophysiology. Myocardial ischemia occurs when oxygen demand exceeds oxygen delivery.

B. Supply. The myocardium is supplied via coronary arteries. Myocardial oxygen supply depends on coronary artery diameter, LV diastolic pressure, aortic diastolic pressure, and arterial oxygen content.

  1. **Coronary blood flow** is dependent on the aortic root-to-downstream coronary pressure gradient. Most **coronary blood flow occurs during diastole**. Coronary artery blood flow in normal individuals is controlled primarily through local mediators. The coronary arteries of patients with significant CAD may be maximally dilated at rest.

  2. **Heart rate** is inversely proportional to the length of diastole. Faster heart rates decrease the duration of maximal coronary perfusion.

  3. **Blood oxygen** content is determined by hemoglobin concentration, oxygen saturation, and dissolved oxygen content. Increasing inspired oxygen fraction and/or hemoglobin concentration increases blood oxygen content.

C. Demand. Myocardial oxygen consumption (MVO_2) is increased by increases in ventricular wall tension and heart rate (velocity of shortening) and, to a lesser degree, contractility.

  1. **Ventricular wall tension** is modeled by Laplace law: wall tension is directly proportional to the ventricular transmural pressure and the ventricular radius and inversely proportional to the ventricular wall thickness. Changes in these parameters affect oxygen demand.

  2. **Heart rate.** Tachycardia is well tolerated in normal hearts. Atherosclerotic coronary arteries may not adequately dilate to meet increased demands of faster heart rates.

  3. **Contractility** increases with the increased chronotropy, myocardial stretch, calcium, and catecholamines. Increasing contractility increases oxygen consumption.

D. Supply and demand balance. Atherosclerosis is the most common etiology for supply-demand imbalances. Conditions such as aortic stenosis, systemic hypertension, and hypertrophic cardiomyopathy, which are characterized by marked ventricular hypertrophy and high intraventricular pressures, may also increase MVO_2. These conditions may create imbalances, even in the setting of normal coronary arteries. The goal of treatment is to improve the myocardial oxygen supply-demand balance.

  1. **Increase supply**
     a. **Increase coronary perfusion pressure** with the administration of volume or α-adrenergic agonists to increase aortic root diastolic pressure.

    b. **Increase coronary blood flow** with nitrates to dilate coronary arteries.

    c. **Increase oxygen content** by raising hemoglobin concentration or oxygen partial pressure.

2. **Decrease demand**

    a. **Decrease heart rate** either directly with β-adrenergic antagonists or indirectly by treating underlying causes of tachycardia (eg, pain, anxiety).

    b. **Decrease ventricular size** (decrease wall tension) by decreasing preload with nitrates, calcium channel antagonists, or diuretics. Occasionally, increasing inotropy may decrease demand by decreasing ventricular size and wall tension.

    c. **Decreasing contractility** may decrease MVO_2 if ventricular size and wall tension do not increase excessively. Calcium channel blockers and volatile anesthetics decrease contractility.

    d. **Intra-aortic balloon counter pulsation** increases coronary perfusion pressure by augmenting diastolic pressure. It also reduces resistance to LV ejection, thereby reducing LV size and wall tension.

VI. VALVULAR HEART DISEASE

A. Aortic stenosis

1. **The etiology** is usually progressive calcification and narrowing of a tricuspid or bicuspid valve. Severity is defined by valve area and mean gradient (mild, greater than 1.5 cm² or less than 25 mm Hg; moderate, between 1.0 and 1.5 cm² or between 25 and 40 mm Hg; and severe, less than 1.0 cm² or greater than 40 mm Hg, respectively).

2. **Symptoms** of angina, syncope, or heart failure develop late in the disease process. In the absence of surgical intervention, the average survival is 2 to 3 years following the onset of symptoms.

3. **Pathophysiology.** The **ventricle** becomes **hypertrophied** and stiff in response to the increased pressure load. Coordinated atrial contraction becomes critical to maintaining adequate ventricular filling and stroke volume. The ventricle is susceptible to ischemia due to increased muscle mass and decreased coronary perfusion in the setting of increased intraventricular pressure.

4. **Anesthetic considerations.** Aortic stenosis is the only valvular lesion associated with an increased risk of perioperative ischemia, MI, and death.

    a. **Normal sinus rhythm** and adequate **volume status** should be maintained.

    b. **Avoid systemic hypotension.** Hypotension should be treated immediately and aggressively with an α-agonist such as phenylephrine to maintain adequate coronary perfusion pressure.

    c. **Avoid tachycardia.** Tachycardia results in increased oxygen demand along with a shorter period of diastole leading to decreased coronary perfusion and reduced cardiac output. Severe bradycardia can lead to reduced cardiac output and should be avoided as well. **Cardiac pacing** capabilities should be considered to treat severe bradycardia. Supraventricular tachydysrhythmias should be treated aggressively with direct current cardioversion.

    d. **Nitrates** and **peripheral vasodilators** should be administered with extreme caution.

    e. The **treatment of ischemia** in these patients is directed at increasing oxygen delivery by raising coronary perfusion pressure and decreasing oxygen consumption (by increasing blood pressure and lowering heart rate).

B. Aortic regurgitation
1. **Etiologies** include rheumatic heart disease, endocarditis, trauma, collagen vascular diseases, and processes that dilate the aortic root (eg, aneurysm, Marfan syndrome, and syphilis).
2. **Pathophysiology**
   a. Acute aortic regurgitation may cause sudden LV volume overload with increased LV end-diastolic pressure and pulmonary capillary occlusion pressure. Manifestations include decreased cardiac output, CHF, tachycardia, and vasoconstriction.
   b. Chronic aortic regurgitation leads to LV dilation and eccentric hypertrophy. Symptoms may be minimal until late in the disease process when left-sided heart failure occurs.
3. **Anesthetic considerations**
   a. Maintain a **normal to slightly increased heart rate** to minimize regurgitation and maintain aortic diastolic and coronary artery perfusion pressure.
   b. Maintain adequate volume status.
   c. **Improve forward flow** and decrease LV end-diastolic pressure and ventricular wall tension with vasodilators.
   d. Avoid peripheral arterial vasoconstrictors, which may worsen regurgitation.
   e. Consider pacing. These patients have an increased incidence of conduction abnormalities.
   f. Intra-aortic balloon counter pulsation is generally **contraindicated** in the setting of aortic regurgitation.

C. Mitral stenosis
1. **The etiology** is almost always rheumatic.
2. **Pathophysiology**
   a. Increased left atrial pressure and volume overload increase left atrial size and may cause **atrial fibrillation** and **pulmonary edema.**
   b. **Elevated left atrial pressure** increases pulmonary venous pressure and pulmonary vascular resistance. In turn, right ventricular pressure is increased for a given cardiac output. Chronic pulmonary hypertension produces pulmonary vascular remodeling. **Pulmonary hypertension** may lead to tricuspid regurgitation, RV failure, and decreased cardiac output.
3. **Anesthetic considerations**
   a. **Avoid tachycardia.** Tachycardia is poorly tolerated because of decreased diastolic filling time leading to decreased cardiac output and increases in left atrial pressure. Control ventricular response pharmacologically or consider cardioversion for patients with atrial fibrillation. Continue digoxin, calcium channel blockers, and β-adrenergic blockers perioperatively.
   b. **Avoid pulmonary hypertension.** Hypoxia, hypercarbia, acidosis, atelectasis, and sympathomimetics increase pulmonary vascular resistance. Oxygen, hypocarbia, alkalosis, nitrates, prostaglandin E_1, and inhaled nitric oxide decrease pulmonary vascular resistance.
   c. **Hypotension** may indicate RV failure. Inotropes and agents that decrease pulmonary hypertension may be useful (eg, dobutamine, milrinone, nitrates, prostaglandin E_1, and inhaled nitric oxide).
   d. **Pulmonary artery catheter** may assist in the perioperative evaluation of volume status, intracardiac pressures, and cardiac output.
   e. **Premedication** should be adequate to prevent anxiety and tachycardia. Exercise caution in patients with hypotension, pulmonary hypertension, or low cardiac output.

D. Mitral regurgitation

1. **Etiologies** include mitral valve prolapse, ischemic heart disease, endocarditis, and post-MI papillary muscle rupture.

2. **Pathophysiology.** Mitral regurgitation allows blood to be ejected into the LA during systole. The amount of regurgitant flow depends on the ventricular-atrial pressure gradient, size of the mitral orifice, and duration of systole.

   a. **Acute mitral regurgitation** usually occurs in the setting of MI. Acute volume overload of the left side of the heart leads to LV dysfunction with increased ventricular wall tension.

   b. **Chronic mitral regurgitation** causes gradual left atrial and LV overload and dilation with compensatory eccentric hypertrophy.

   c. **Measurement of ejection fraction** does not accurately reflect forward flow, because the incompetent valve permits immediate bidirectional ejection with systole.

3. **Anesthetic considerations**

   a. **Relative tachycardia** is desirable to decrease ventricular filling time and ventricular volume.

   b. **Afterload reduction** is beneficial. Increased systemic vascular resistance will increase regurgitation.

   c. **Maintain preload**.

VII. CONGESTIVE HEART FAILURE

Heart failure results from impairment of ventricular systolic or diastolic function. Heart failure manifests as dyspnea, fatigue, decreased exercise tolerance, and pulmonary or peripheral edema. Heart failure can be classified into two categories: (1) heart failure with reduced ejection fraction (HFrEF) that is associated with variable degrees of LV enlargement and depressed ventricular ejection and (2) heart failure with preserved ejection fraction (HFpEF) in which diastolic dysfunction is pronounced.

A. Etiologies include ischemic cardiomyopathy; hypertension; valvular heart disease; endocrine and metabolic causes such as diabetes, thyroid disease, and acromegaly; toxic cardiomyopathies due to alcohol, cocaine, or chemotherapy; nutritional causes such as carnitine deficiency; infective causes such as viral myocarditis, human immunodeficiency virus (HIV) infection, and Chagas disease; iron overload states; amyloidosis; sarcoidosis; and catecholamine-induced takotsubo.

B. Pathophysiology of heart failure is the culmination of progressive changes in myocyte architecture that result in changes in ventricular shape, chamber size, ventricular wall thickness, and stiffness that lead to reduced myocardial function and cardiac output.

C. Anesthetic considerations. Hemodynamic goals aim to preserve cardiac output and minimize myocardial work. Medical management should be optimized preoperatively.

1. **Maintain preload but with caution.** Patients with impaired LV function depend on preload to maintain cardiac output; however, they are at risk of pulmonary edema with fluid overload.

2. **Avoid tachycardia** to minimize myocardial work and preserve ventricular filling during diastole.

3. **Aggressively treat arrhythmias** as they may lead to reduction in cardiac output. In a failing ventricle, left ventricular end-diastolic volume (LVEDV) is heavily dependent on atrial contraction. The absence of coordinated atrial contractions (such as in atrial fibrillation) can lead to significant compromise of ventricular preload.

4. **Preserve contractility.** Patients with heart failure may rely on increased sympathetic tone to maintain cardiac output. As a result, they may become profoundly hypotensive following induction or even after analgesic or anxiolytic therapy. Inotropic support may be required.

5. **Afterload reduction** is favorable as it reduces myocardial work. If vasopressors are needed, they should be used with caution.

D. **Anesthetic considerations for durable left ventricular assist devices (LVADs)**
Approximately 20% to 30% of patients with durable LVADs will present for noncardiac surgery. The two most commonly implanted LVADs are the HeartMate 3 (Abbott, Abbott Park, IL) and the HeartWare HVAD (Medtronic, Dublin, Ireland). These are both considered continuous centrifugal flow assist devices and are FDA approved for bridge to transplant or destination therapy that is a final intervention for patients who are poor heart transplant candidates. Hemodynamic goals should focus on maintaining adequate preload and preserved afterload. Patients with LVADs may not be good candidates for regional techniques due to anticoagulation but should be considered for local or MAC techniques when indicated.

1. **Preoperative considerations**
   a. Perform a **system controller history review** and contact the institutional or patient's **LVAD care team.** The team can help in interpretation of any alarms or faults the device may have as well as any previous interventions required.
   b. Review pertinent laboratory studies and physical examination to assess for other sequelae of end-stage heart failure (progression of kidney or liver disease).
   c. Discuss any current home **inotropic** medications, **anticoagulation**, and/or presence of **CIEDs.** Most LVAD patients will have had a CIED placed prior to LVAD implantation due to their reduced EF and risk for sudden cardiac death.

2. **Intraoperative considerations**
   a. **Ensure reliable AC power and/or backup battery power** for the LVAD
   b. Monitor with standard ASA monitors, and consider the use of an invasive arterial line if unable to obtain NIBP or if clinically indicated. A pulmonary artery catheter for monitoring pulmonary artery pressure and central venous pressure should be considered depending on procedure type and patient status. We can also consider the use of cerebral oximetry for monitoring of cerebral perfusion. Transesophageal echocardiography is not mandatory but should be available to assist in troubleshooting hemodynamic events.
   c. Induction of anesthesia should be focused on adequate preoxygenation, **avoidance of significant reductions in afterload, maintaining heart rate** and **rhythm**, and optimizing fluid balance.
   d. Patient can be positioned in the usual fashion including prone and lateral as long as close attention is paid to the driveline of the LVAD.
   e. Administer surgical site infection prophylaxis with antibiotics in the usual fashion; however, close attention should be paid to proper sterile technique around the driveline site.
   f. Target **mean arterial pressure goals 65 to 80 mm Hg**, to be maintained with either **volume resuscitation or afterload support** (vasopressin preferred due to reduced effect on PVR). If continued hemodynamic instability is observed, consider increasing LVAD pump speed.

g. **Maintenance of right ventricular function** and **reducing pulmonary artery pressure** is crucial. Preventing hypoxia, hypercarbia, acidosis, and immediate correction of arrhythmias is imperative. For additional reduction in pulmonary artery pressure, consider the use of pulmonary vasodilators such as inhaled epoprostenol, nitric oxide, or milrinone.

h. If mechanically ventilating, strategy is aimed at mitigating hypoxia and hypercarbia with an **avoidance of excessive positive end-expiratory pressure (PEEP)** or high tidal volumes, which can result in a hemodynamically significant reduction in preload.

i. Intraoperative challenges specific to LVAD patients include

1. **Suction events**

    a. Occurs when the **IVS is shifted** toward the inflow cannula located in the LV leading to **obstruction of the inflow cannula** and hypotension, arrythmias, and pump flow reductions. This can result from hypovolemia, increased PVR, and/or increased LVAD pump speeds. Treatment depends on the etiology but can include fluid bolus or transfusion, vasopressor therapy (phenylephrine or vasopressin bolus), and lowering LVAD pump speed.

2. **Power failure**

    a. This can occur when there is a disconnection of the driveline from the system controller or when the system is unplugged from AC power with inadequate backup battery. The best way to avoid this is to secure alternative AC power sources and ensuring backup batteries are charged.

3. **LVAD pump thrombosis**

    a. This critical event rarely occurs intraoperatively but can lead to **complete pump failure and hemodynamic collapse.** This occurs when thrombus forms inside the LVAD pump due to inadequate anticoagulation, acute increases in afterload, or dramatic reductions in pump speeds. Signs of pump thrombosis include sudden increases in pump power without resultant increases in pump flow and speed. Treatment usually involves replacement of the LVAD.

3. **Postoperative considerations**

    a. Recovery of LVAD patients can be performed in the postanesthesia care unit (PACU) but may require intensive care unit (ICU)–level care depending on the intraoperative course.

    b. Attention should be paid to any preoperative programming changes of a patient's CIED; it is advised to reverse these changes in the postoperative period prior to discharge.

    c. Reinitiate anticoagulation therapy in coordination with the surgical team.

VIII. HYPERTROPHIC CARDIOMYOPATHY

Hypertrophic cardiomyopathy is a cardiac disorder characterized by **asymmetric LV hypertrophy and impaired relaxation in diastole.** Although most patients with hypertrophic cardiomyopathy do not have an increased LV outflow tract gradient at rest, many of them develop **dynamic outflow tract obstruction** with decreased filling and increased contractility. Under these conditions, as flow accelerates through the narrowed LV outflow tract, it creates drag, which pulls the anterior leaflet of the mitral valve toward the septum. This systolic anterior motion (SAM) of the anterior mitral leaflet leads to further outflow obstruction and mitral regurgitation.

A. **Anesthetic considerations.** Factors that **worsen the outflow obstruction** include decreased arterial pressure, decreased intraventricular volume, increased contractility, and increased heart rate.

1. **Maintain normal volume status.**
2. **Avoid tachycardia.** Continue β-adrenergic and calcium channel blocker therapy for heart rate control.
3. **Maintain normal sinus rhythm.** Consider cardioversion for supraventricular tachycardia.
4. **Avoid hypotension.** Correct vasodilation with α-adrenergic agonists to avoid tachycardia and marked changes in contractility. Use nitrates and peripheral dilators with extreme caution.
5. **Use inotropes with caution.** Increased inotropy may exacerbate the outflow obstruction.

IX. CONGENITAL HEART DISEASE

With improvement in the survival of congenital heart disease (CHD) patients, anesthesiologists are encountering them with greater frequency as adults in noncardiac surgical settings. Depending on the underlying lesion, an adult with a history of CHD (ACHD) may have an **uncorrected** lesion or may have undergone a **reparative** or **palliative** procedure in the past. As the medical and surgical management of these conditions continues to evolve, different patients with the same original congenital defect may present having undergone significantly different procedures and, as a result, may differ in their anatomy and physiology. Transferring patient care to institutions with extensive experience in managing these disorders should be considered.

A. **General considerations**

1. A thorough understanding of the patient's **cardiac anatomy, physiology, and functional status** along with the **physiologic stresses** associated with the surgical procedure is essential.
2. **Myocardial dysfunction** may be present as a long-term consequence of the physiology of the original lesion or the subsequent reparative or palliative procedure. It may also be a consequence of chronic hypoxemia.
3. **Dysrhythmias** are common and may be due to the pathophysiology of the cardiovascular defect or scarring from prior surgery. Intra-atrial reentrant tachycardia and ventricular tachycardia are commonly encountered in this patient population.
4. **Cyanotic patients** are often polycythemic and at risk for stroke and thrombosis. Intravenous hydration is important. Hemodilution may be considered in the instance of a preoperative hematocrit greater than 60%. **Abnormal hemostasis**, usually mild in severity, has been noted in patients with cyanotic CHD.
5. **Systemic air emboli** are a constant danger in the presence of bidirectional or right-to-left shunts. Intravenous lines must be purged of air bubbles, and air filters should be used.
6. **Infective endocarditis prophylaxis.** Some CHD patients require antibiotic prophylaxis for infective endocarditis with certain procedures. See Chapter 8.
7. A complete discussion of the specific lesions common in ACHD patients is beyond the scope of this chapter. For a more thorough treatment of the subject, please refer to the Suggested Readings.

X. CARDIAC TRANSPLANT PATIENT

Globally, more than 5500 cardiac transplants are performed each year. The 1-year survival rate is approximately 84%, and the 3-year survival rate is approximately 78%. These patients are increasingly encountered in the noncardiac surgical setting.

A. Physiology of the transplanted heart

1. Sympathetic reinnervation may occur over time. Parasympathetic reinnervation is not thought to occur; however, bradycardia related to the administration of neostigmine has been reported.

2. Transplanted hearts exhibit accelerated graft atherosclerosis and are at increased risk for myocardial ischemia.

3. **Hemodynamics of the transplanted heart**

   a. Cardiac impulse formation and conduction are normal, although the resting heart rate is increased.

   b. The Frank-Starling mechanism remains intact. Transplanted hearts respond normally to circulating catecholamines.

   c. Autoregulation of coronary blood flow is intact.

   d. Due to autonomic denervation, the transplanted heart meets the demand for increased cardiac output initially by increasing stroke volume and subsequently by increasing heart rate in response to circulating catecholamines.

4. **Drug effects**

   a. Drugs that act via the autonomic system (eg, atropine and digoxin) are ineffective.

   b. Direct-acting agents are effective. Isoproterenol, dopamine, or epinephrine may be used to increase heart rate. Norepinephrine or phenylephrine may be used to increase blood pressure. Response to ephedrine is blunted.

   c. β-adrenergic receptors are intact and may be present in increased density.

   d. Traditional teaching dictates that anticholinesterases have no effect on the rate of a denervated heart; however, over time, other receptor-related mechanisms may take over and allow anticholinesterases to exert bradycardic effect. A muscarinic antagonist should always be coadministered to block the cardiac and other muscarinic side effects.

B. Anesthetic considerations

1. The patient's activity level and **exercise capacity** should be determined. A cardiology consultant may provide data concerning cardiac function and anatomy as measured by echocardiography and catheterization.

2. Underlying **CAD may be asymptomatic**. Evidence of ischemia may include a history of dyspnea, signs of reduced cardiac function, and dysrhythmias.

3. A baseline 12-lead ECG should be obtained and may demonstrate multiple P waves and right bundle branch block.

4. To assess the effect of immunosuppression and concomitant drug therapy, baseline laboratory studies should include complete blood count, serum electrolytes, blood urea nitrogen, serum creatinine, glucose, and liver function tests.

5. Strict aseptic technique is required for all interventions (eg, intravenous access), because the patient may be receiving long-term immunosuppression.

6. **Monitoring.** Invasive monitoring is used when indicated by the patient's cardiopulmonary status and the surgical procedure. The right internal jugular vein is often the access site for repetitive endocardial biopsies and may need to be reserved for this purpose.

7. **Anesthesia**

   a. General, regional, and spinal anesthesia have been administered to cardiac transplant patients. Selection of a specific anesthetic technique should be guided by considerations other than the patient's history of cardiac transplantation.

b. **Hemodynamic goals**
   i. Maintain preload.
   ii. Avoid sudden vasodilation. Initial compensatory changes in cardiac output depend on the Frank-Starling mechanism because of the delayed heart rate response.
   iii. If sudden hypotension occurs, administer volume and direct-acting vasopressors such as phenylephrine and norepinephrine.

XI. CARDIAC IMPLANTABLE ELECTRONIC DEVICES: PACEMAKERS AND IMPLANTABLE CARDIOVERTER-DEFIBRILLATORS

A. CIEDs

1. Increasing numbers of patients with permanent pacemaker (PPM) and ICD devices are undergoing noncardiac surgery. Familiarity with the indications, functions, and perioperative management of these devices is essential.

2. PPMs are utilized in a variety of conditions where the patient's native conduction is compromised or inadequate, including from structural or ischemic heart disease, infiltrative diseases, and postprocedural alterations in conduction pathways, among many others.

3. ICDs have significantly improved the mortality of patients at high risk for sudden cardiac death. The four key ICD functions are **antitachycardia pacing** (ATP), **cardioversion**, **defibrillation**, and **backup pacing.** The conventional ICD is implanted in the upper chest and is connected to one or two defibrillating transvenous leads that also have sensing and pacing capabilities.

4. Current PPM and ICD devices include traditional subcutaneous generators with transvenous leads that have single or dual chamber sensing and pacing and possibly antitachycardia therapies (ie, cardioversion-defibrillation, antitachycardia pacing), as well as newer technologies including leadless pacemakers and subcutaneous ICDs (see below).

5. **Indications for PPM**
   a. Symptomatic bradycardia.
   b. Third-degree (complete) AV block.
   c. Type II, second-degree AV block.
   d. Cardiac resynchronization therapy. Biventricular pacing to synchronize RV and LV depolarization in patients with symptomatic HFrEF (left ventricular ejection fraction [LVEF] ≤ 35%) with sinus rhythm and interventricular conduction abnormality (left bundle branch block [LBBB], QRS ≥ 150 ms).

6. **Indications for ICD**
   a. **Primary prevention** in patients at high risk for sudden cardiac death (LVEF ≤ 35%, at risk for ventricular tachyarrhythmias).
   b. **Secondary prevention** in patients with prior sudden cardiac death or unstable ventricular arrhythmias.

B. Pacemaker nomenclature

1. A standard five-letter code is used to describe pacemaker settings and function. The first letter designates the **chamber paced** (O, none; A, atrium; V, ventricle; D, dual [both atrium and ventricle]).

2. The second letter describes the **chamber sensed** (O, none; A, atrium; V, ventricle; D, dual).

3. The third letter describes the **pacemaker's response** to sensed events (O, none; I, inhibition of pacemaker output; T, triggering of pacemaker output; D, dual response: spontaneous atrial and ventricular activity inhibit atrial and ventricular pacing and atrial activity triggers a ventricular response).

4. The fourth letter indicates the presence or absence of **rate modulation** (O, no rate modulation; R, rate modulation present).

5. The fifth letter specifies the presence and type of multisite **pacing** (O, none; A, more than one stimulation site in either atrium, stimulation sites in each atrium, or a combination of the two; V, more than one stimulation site in either ventricle, stimulation sites in each ventricle, or a combination of the two; D, any combination of A and V).

6. For example, a **VVI** pacemaker will sense and pace the ventricle yet will be inhibited and will not fire if an R wave is detected. A **DDD** pacemaker senses and paces both the atrium and ventricle. A VVIRV pacemaker has ventricular inhibitory pacing with rate modulation and multisite ventricular pacing. This mode is often used in patients with heart failure, chronic atrial fibrillation, or intraventricular conduction delay. A **DDDRD** pacemaker has dual-chamber pacing with rate modulation and multisite pacing in both the atrium (or atria) and ventricle(s).

C. **Considerations for magnet application to CIEDs**

1. **Applying a magnet to most pacemakers** (excluding leadless pacemakers) will cause them to function in an **asynchronous mode** (eg, VOO), which may be desirable in the pacing-dependent patient undergoing a procedure with possible electromagnetic interference (EMI). However, **the magnet response of a pacemaker is most reliably determined by device interrogation.** Typically, normal pacemaker function is restored upon removal of the magnet. Use of a magnet during surgical procedures is necessary only if a patient that has not undergone preoperative interrogation and reprogramming is pacing dependent and inhibition of pacemaker output is noted coincident with EMI. If used, the magnet should be placed directly over the pacemaker. It is best to tape the magnet in place to avoid inadvertent dislodgment. **Magnet application should be used with caution**, as asynchronous pacing has the potential to cause unstable arrhythmias through the R-on-T phenomenon if ventricular pacing output occurs during the relative refractory period of cardiomyocyte repolarization.

2. All ICDs are exquisitely sensitive to EMI associated with electrocautery above the level of the umbilicus. EMI can be interpreted by an ICD as ventricular fibrillation leading to **inappropriate shocks.** Inappropriate shocks can be difficult to detect in an anesthetized and paralyzed patient and can lead to battery depletion.

3. Most ICDs are designed to **suspend antitachycardia therapies in response to a magnet** application and resume function upon removal of the magnet. Some models of St. Jude and Boston Scientific ICDs can be programmed to ignore magnet application. Furthermore, some older models of Boston Scientific ICDs may be programmed to suspend function with magnet application but require magnet removal and reapplication to resume function. It is **best to have ICD function interrogated preoperatively** to determine its settings and response to magnet application.

4. **Indiscriminate use of magnets for ICDs is best avoided.** It is preferable to reprogram and disable antitachycardia therapies while taking steps to prepare for prompt treatment of any unstable arrhythmia as described below. Also, magnet application to ICDs **does not change pacing to an asynchronous mode**, and pacing-dependent patients should have the device reprogrammed to an asynchronous mode if indicated.

D. **Leadless pacemakers**

1. CIED technology is rapidly evolving, and there is currently only one leadless pacemaker system available (Medtronic Micra). It comprises of a small generator with contained sensing and pacing electrodes, which is **implanted (and removed) directly into the RV** via a femoral transcatheter approach. The battery life is approximately 8-12 years.

2. This system **eliminates the need for transvenous leads** and subcutaneous pockets, reducing risks of infection and lead-related problems, which can lead to perforation, venous occlusion, tricuspid regurgitation, oversensing, and infection. Major risks of the device itself include perforation, dislodgement and embolization, and tamponade.

3. The leadless system is designed predominantly for bradyarrhythmias with functional pacing modes of VVI-R, VVI, and VOO. It has a baseline/reset mode of VVI at 65 bpm and is MRI conditional when set in "SureScan" mode (VOO/OVO setting).

4. There are currently no consensus societal guidelines on the perioperative management of such devices, but the same general principles for other CIEDs described below should apply, with the following unique considerations:

    a. The Medtronic Micra leadless system does not have a Hall sensor; thus, it **cannot detect the presence of a magnet** and will not switch to an asynchronous mode if a magnet is applied. It **requires the use of the leadless programmer to change the settings** of the device.

    b. Therefore, consultation with a specialist with the knowledge, equipment, and ability to interrogate the device and reprogram to an appropriate setting for the given clinical circumstance is necessary. There is some evidence to suggest that given its location and sensitivity, electrocautery may not be detected by the Micra device and thus would not need perioperative reprograming.

5. Wireless ultrasound endocardial pacing, a system which involves a subcutaneous generator and endocardial receiver used with a traditional CIED, is another system which may be seen more in noncardiac surgery patients.

E. Subcutaneous ICDs (S-ICDs)

1. New devices that include a subcutaneous generator implanted in the left lateral chest with a tunneled parasternal lead are available for patients with indications for an ICD who have inadequate vascular access, very high risk of infection, or for very young people with a long life-expectancy. These devices avoid the complications associated with transvenous leads. S-ICDs have a battery life of approximately 7 years, can withstand external cardiopulmonary resuscitation (CPR), and can be implanted under monitored anesthesia care.

2. Limitations include the absence of bradycardia pacing, antitachycardia pacing, or cardiac resynchronization therapies. Unlike traditional ICDs, the S-ICD does not contain any permanent pacemaker functions except a 30-second backup pacing function immediately following a shock (VVI at 50 bpm). The generator is larger than traditional ICDs and delivers a higher energy shock of 80 J. It is susceptible to the same oversensing problems from EMI as traditional ICDs, which could lead to inappropriate shocks.

3. Currently available S-ICDs respond to external magnet application by temporarily suspending shock therapy while the magnet is applied, with resumption of the permanent settings on removal of the magnet. However, the lateral location of the device and off-centered placement of the magnet may make magnet application more challenging than traditional anteriorly located ICD generators.

F. Preoperative evaluation and preparation

1. Determine if a CIED is present by conducting a focused history and physical examination and reviewing any available imaging or cardiology reports.

2. Determine the **type, manufacturer, primary indication, and if the patient is pacing dependent** (eg, prior AV nodal ablation, no spontaneous ventricular activity noted on prior interrogation, or concerning history such as syncope related to symptomatic bradycardia).

3. Determine the **current device settings** and **status** (ie, properly functioning generator, leads if present, and battery life) by patient history, electrophysiology records, and ECG. Device interrogation is the only reliable method for determining the settings and battery function of the device.

4. If the information is not readily available, the manufacturer and model number may be obtained from a radiograph of the generator. The manufacturer of the device must be identified in order to be able to program the pacemaker, as each manufacturer has a unique programming device. Determine whether rate modulation is active. Also, determine the response of the device to a magnet.

5. Determine if EMI is likely (sources include monopolar electrosurgery or radiofrequency ablation superior to the umbilicus, transcutaneous electrical nerve stimulation, lithotripsy, magnetic resonance, radiofrequency identification devices, and electroconvulsive therapy).

   a. If EMI is likely, reprogram to asynchronous pacing in patients who are pacing dependent, and suspend any antitachycardia therapies if an ICD is present. Rate-responsive mode should also be disabled to prevent inappropriate tachycardia.

   b. Continuously monitor patient and ensure that temporary backup pacing and/or defibrillating methods are immediately available

G. **Intraoperative management**

1. Modern pacemakers are extremely resistant to EMI. If interference does occur, the pacemaker output may be inappropriately inhibited or the pacemaker may be reset to a committed pacing mode (ie, DOO or VOO).

2. **Resetting of pacemakers** by EMI will produce asynchronous pacing that can be noted on the ECG.

3. Intraoperative exposure of the device to EMI can be reduced by placing the current return pad (**"grounding pad"**) in a location on the patient such that the **current path** from the electrocautery or radiofrequency ablation catheter **does not pass near the pulse generator or leads.** Other measures include the use of **short, intermittent, irregular bursts** at the lowest possible energy level and the use of a **bipolar electrocautery** system or an **ultrasonic (harmonic) scalpel.** During lithotripsy, the beam should not be focused near the generator.

4. **Monitor heart rate** during EMI with a pulse oximeter, arterial line, precordial or esophageal stethoscope, or a finger on the pulse.

5. For procedures or diagnostic **tests involving MRI**, it is essential to **follow institutional protocols**, and in the event that an external defibrillator, device programmer, or any other MRI unsafe equipment is necessary, the **patient should be removed from the MRI area prior to use of these devices.**

6. Prior to any MRI scan in patients with MRI conditional devices, the device should be interrogated as described above, antitachycardia therapies should be suspended, and asynchronous pacing should be activated in pacing-dependent patients.

7. **Avoid using radiofrequency identification devices** in close proximity to CIEDs, and ensure continuous monitoring for signs of EMI to allow for prompt discontinuation if interference is noted.

8. For **electroconvulsive therapy (ECT)**, take the same considerations as above including suspending antitachycardia therapies and switching to an asynchronous mode in pacing-dependent patients, while being prepared to promptly manage any sinus tachycardia or ventricular arrhythmias that can be associated with ECT.

9. **Postoperative evaluation of pacemaker function** is recommended by most manufacturers if electrocautery is used or if settings are changed perioperatively.

H. **Temporary perioperative pacing and cardioversion-defibrillation options**

1. **Transcutaneous.** External pacing and cardioversion-defibrillation can be performed via large pads placed on the anterior and posterior thorax. This is an easy and inexpensive method of ventricular pacing and antitachycardia therapy. Avoid placing pads directly over subcutaneous generators.

2. **Transvenous**

   a. A temporary pacing electrode can be inserted via a central vein into the heart.

   b. Various pulmonary artery catheters that have pacing options exist (see Chapter 15).

3. **Transesophageal.** The LA can be paced with a pacing probe placed in the esophagus. Transesophageal pacing requires intact AV nodal conduction.

I. **Emergency external cardioversion or defibrillation**

1. If unstable arrhythmias occur and a magnet is being used to disable antitachycardia therapies of an ICD, immediate steps should be to terminate the source of EMI and remove the magnet from the ICD, which should resume antitachycardia therapies usually within 10 seconds.

2. If after removal of the magnet there is not prompt restoration of antitachycardia therapies with appropriate response to any arrhythmia, or if the antitachycardia therapies were suspended by device interrogation preoperatively, advanced cardiac life support (ACLS) guidelines including external defibrillation should be followed.

   a. If possible, avoid placing pads directly over the generator to minimize current flow through the generator and the leads.

   b. Use the clinically appropriate energy level regardless of the presence of a CIED.

   c. Any device should be immediately interrogated after external cardioversion/ defibrillation, as device reset or malfunction is possible after external electrical therapy.

J. **Postoperative management**

1. Ongoing monitoring of rate and rhythm with electrocardiogram and pulse oximetry should continue in the immediate postoperative period.

2. If the device was reprogrammed periprocedurally, ensure that backup pacing and cardioversion-defibrillation methods are readily available if indicated until permanent settings are restored.

3. Have the device interrogated immediately if there is any concern for inappropriate or unreliable device settings or function (eg, emergency surgery without thorough preoperative evaluation, concern for disabled rather than suspended antitachycardia therapy from magnet application in an older device, observed or suspected shocks from device intraoperatively, or any concern for malfunction from EMI, physical disruption, or large fluid shifts).

Suggested Readings

Al-Khatib SM, Stevenson WG, Ackerman MJ, et al. 2017 AHA/ACC/HRS guideline for management of patients with ventricular arrhythmias and the prevention of sudden cardiac death: A report of the American College of Cardiology/American Heart Association Task Force on clinical practice guidelines and the Heart Rhythm Society. *Circulation.* 2018;138:e272-e391.

American Society of Anesthesiologists. Practice advisory for the perioperative management of patients with cardiac implantable electronic devices: Pacemakers and implantable cardioverter-defibrillators. *Anesthesiology.* 2020;132:225-252.

Baehner T, Ellerkmann RK. Anesthesia in adults with congenital heart disease. *Curr Opin Anaesthesiol.* 2017;30:418.

Blasco LM, Parameshwar J, Vuylsteke A. Anaesthesia for noncardiac surgery in the heart transplant recipient. *Curr Opin Anaesthesiol.* 2009;22:109-113.

Cronin B, Essandoh MK. Update on cardiovascular implantable electronic devices for anesthesiologists. *J Cardiothorac Vasc Anesth.* 2018;32:1871-1884.

Dalia AA, Cronin B, Stone ME, et al. Anesthetic management of patients with continuous-flow left ventricular assist devices undergoing noncardiac surgery: an update for anesthesiologists. *J Cardiothorac Vasc Anesth.* 2018;32(2):1001-1012.

Devereaux PJ, Yang H, Yusuf S, et al. Effects of extended-release metoprolol succinate in patients undergoing non-cardiac surgery (POISE trial): a randomised controlled trial. *Lancet.* 2008;371:1839-1847.

Devereaux PJ, Mrkobrada M, Sessler D, et al. Aspirin in patients undergoing noncardiac surgery. *N Engl J Med.* 2014;370:1494-1503.

Epstein AE, DiMarco JP, Ellenbogen KA, et al. 2012 ACCF/AHA/HRS focused update incorporated into the ACCF/AHA/HRS 2008 guidelines for device-based therapy of cardiac rhythm abnormalities: a report of the American College of Cardiology Foundation/American Heart Association Task Force on Practice Guidelines and the Heart Rhythm Society. *J Am Coll Cardiol.* 2013;61:e6-e75.

Fleisher LA, Fleischmann KE, Auerbach AD, et al. 2014 ACC/AHA guideline on perioperative cardiovascular evaluation and management of patients undergoing noncardiac surgery: a report of the American College of Cardiology/American Heart Association Task Force on practice guidelines. *J Am Coll Cardiol.* 2014;64(22):e77-e137.

Hawn MT, Graham LA, Richman JR, et al. The incidence and timing of noncardiac surgery after cardiac stent implantation. *J Am Coll Surg.* 2012;214:658.

Hindler K, Shaw AD, Samuels J, et al. Improved postoperative outcomes associated with preoperative statin therapy. *Anesthesiology.* 2006;105:1260-1272.

Kertai MD. Preoperative coronary revascularization in high-risk patients undergoing vascular surgery: a core review. *Anesth Analg.* 2008;106:751-758.

Levine GN, Bates ER, Bittl JA, et al. 2016 ACC/AHA guideline focused update on duration of dual antiplatelet therapy in patients with coronary artery disease: a report of the American College of Cardiology/American Heart Association Task Force on Clinical Practice Guidelines. *J Am Coll Cardiol.* 2016;68:1082-1115.

Mahmoud KD, Sanon S, Habermann EB, et al. Perioperative cardiovascular risk of prior coronary stent implantation among patients undergoing noncardiac surgery. *J Am Coll Cardiol.* 2016;67:1038.

Nishimura RA, Otto CM, Bonow RO, et al. 2017 AHA/ACC focused update of the 2014 AHA/ACC guideline for the management of patients with valvular heart disease: a report of the American College of Cardiology/American Heart Association Task Force on Clinical Practice Guidelines. *Circulation.* 2017;135(25):e1159-e1195.

Reddy VY, Exner DV, Cantillon DJ, et al. Percutaneous implantation of an entirely intracardiac leadless pacemaker. *N Engl J Med.* 2015;373(12):1125-1135.

Stout KK, Daniels CJ, Aboulhosn JA, et al. 2018 AHA/ACC guideline for the management of adults with congenital heart disease: a report of the American College of Cardiology/American Heart Association Task Force on Clinical Practice Guidelines. *J Am Coll Cardiol.* 2019;73:e81-e192.

Wijeysundera DN, Duncan D, Nkonde-price C, et al. Perioperative beta blockade in noncardiac surgery. A systematic review for the 2014 ACC/AHA guideline on perioperative cardiovascular evaluation and management of patients undergoing noncardiac surgery: a report of the American College of Cardiology/American Heart Association Task Force on Practice Guidelines. *Circulation.* 2014;130(24):2246-2264.

Wolff G, Navarese EP, Brockmeyer M, et al. Perioperative aspirin therapy in non-cardiac surgery: a systematic review and meta-analysis of randomized controlled trials. *Int J Cardiol.* 2018;258:59-67.

4 Specific Considerations With Pulmonary Disease

Riccardo Pinciroli, Jeanine P. Wiener-Kronish and Rachel Steinhorn

I. OVERVIEW

The focus of this chapter is on the physiology of "normal" lungs for patients undergoing anesthetic procedures. In addition, important concepts for the care of patients with obesity, asthma, chronic obstructive pulmonary disease (COPD), or acute respiratory distress syndrome (ARDS) are described.

II. PULMONARY FUNCTION

General anesthesia (GA) alters pulmonary function through direct impact on the lungs and indirect action on associated systems.

A. Pulmonary mechanics

1. **Minute ventilation and alveolar ventilation** decrease under both volatile inhaled anesthetics and the most common intravenous (IV) induction agents. Volatile anesthetics reduce tidal volumes (Vt) while increasing respiratory rate, leading to a relatively preserved minute ventilation, but a greater proportion of dead space ventilation versus alveolar ventilation. Both propofol and barbiturates cause a decrease in Vt and respiratory rates, reducing minute ventilation. Agents that have less impact on muscle tone, such as ketamine, etomidate, and dexmedetomidine, cause less reduction in lung volumes.

2. **Functional residual capacity** (FRC) decreases irrespective of the anesthetic agent used. Moving from an upright to a supine position decreases FRC (normally ~3L) by 0.8 to 1L as the diaphragm is displaced cephalad by pressure from the abdominal contents. Elevating the patient's head by 30° significantly increases FRC compared to the supine position, which can be an important consideration in patients with increased intraabdominal pressure, such as pregnancy or obesity. The relaxation in muscle tone caused by induction of GA decreases FRC by another 0.4 to 0.5 L, as the diaphragm is further displaced upward, and the intercostal muscles relax.

   GA induces atelectasis and worsens ventilation perfusion (V/Q) mismatch. Once FRC decreases to the patient's closing capacity, small airways collapse. Closing capacity increases with age and obstructive lung disease, making the risk of atelectasis greater in these patient populations. The addition of positive end-expiratory pressure (PEEP) can increase FRC and decrease atelectasis. Atelectasis occurs primarily in dependent portions of the lung and to a greater extent when spontaneous ventilation is permitted compared to controlled ventilation with sufficient PEEP.

B. Gas exchange

Shunt and dead space both increase during GA, impairing oxygenation and CO_2 elimination. Pulmonary blood flow is primarily distributed by the effect of gravity, and this distribution shifts as the patient moves from the upright to supine or a lateral decubitus position for surgery. These shifts in perfusion are not accompanied by compensatory changes in ventilation, leading to V/Q mismatch. As minute ventilation decreases during a GA, anatomical dead space remains unchanged, but alveolar dead space increases. Atelectasis increases shunt.

C. Respiratory reflexes

1. A rise in $Paco_2$ is the primary factor that promotes an increase in ventilation. Both volatile inhaled and IV anesthetics cause a dose-dependent blunting of the ventilatory response to hypercapnia and the apneic threshold by decreasing the sensitivity of chemoreceptors at the carotid and aortic bodies to a reduction in Pao_2.

2. Volatile anesthetics cause a dose-dependent decrease in hypoxic pulmonary vasoconstriction, while IV anesthetics have minimal effect on it. Some antihypertensive infusions such as sodium nitroprusside, nitroglycerin, and nicardipine worsen shunt from nonselective pulmonary vasodilation.

3. Volatile anesthetics are bronchodilators that reduce airway resistance in a dose-dependent fashion and can be useful in patients with reactive airway disease. The pungent volatile agents desflurane and isoflurane can increase airway irritability, breath-holding, and coughing; they should not be used for inhaled inductions due to the risk of laryngospasm or bronchospasm.

4. Propofol and barbiturates decrease upper airway reflexes during induction, which reduces reaction to the stimulation of laryngoscopy but increases the risk of micro- and macroaspiration. Relaxed oropharyngeal muscle tone displaces the tongue posteriorly and increases obstruction.

D. Ciliary function. Volatile anesthetics and nitrous oxide reduce ciliary beat frequency, slowing the rate of mucous clearance from the airways, and decrease surfactant production. GA is often administered with nonhumidified gasses delivered at high flow rates, which dries secretions and can damage the respiratory epithelium. Intubation and laryngeal mask airways bypass the nasopharynx that would typically warm and humidify inspired air. An increased quantity of thickened secretions places the patient at higher risk of airway obstruction and pulmonary infection.

E. Surgical site considerations. Abdominal, thoracic, and spine surgeries can restrict the ability to cough and breathe deeply due to splinting from pain. This places the patient at risk for persistent postoperative atelectasis and poor secretion clearance, impairing gas exchange and increasing the risk for a postobstructive pneumonia. Incentive spirometry is frequently utilized postoperatively in an attempt to reduce perioperative pulmonary complications, but there are limited data supporting its efficacy and no standard protocol to optimize its use.

III. ASTHMA

A. Background. Asthma is a chronic inflammatory disease characterized by bronchial hyperresponsiveness and remodeling. It affects more than 300 million people worldwide. The affected population is heterogeneous, with multiple inciting etiologies, but with a common endotype involving eosinophilic inflammation associated with Th2 response that usually responds to inhaled steroids. One endotype, a neutrophilic inflammatory asthma (T2-low asthma) is, however, very poorly responsive to routine asthma treatment.

B. Perioperative considerations

1. A very common trigger for asthma exacerbation is infection with human rhinovirus, with peak infections occurring in the fall and spring months. Other viruses associated with exacerbations and hospitalizations include influenza, respiratory syncytial virus, coronaviruses,

human metapneumoviruses, parainfluenza viruses, adenoviruses, and bocaviruses. Given the high potential for postoperative complications, an elective procedure should be rescheduled if a patient has an exacerbation/infection with a viral illness. The most severe asthmatics can often be recognized by their treatment regimens. These regimens include anti-IgE (omalizumab) utilized in patients with persistent asthma on high-dose inhaled corticosteroids (ICS), anti-IL-5 (mepolizumab and reslizumab) for persistent eosinophilic asthma, and treatment with ICS in combination with long-acting beta-agonists. Leukotriene antagonists are inferior to ICS in terms of lowering exacerbation rates.

2. Bronchospasm develops in about 9% of asthmatics in the perioperative period and most often occurs in patients who have asthma, COPD, smoking-related diseases, or bronchitis. All patients with respiratory disease should be maintained on their home medications.

a. Ketamine has bronchodilating properties.

b. Dexmedetomidine does not.

IV. CHRONIC OBSTRUCTIVE PULMONARY DISEASE

COPD is a leading cause of death worldwide and is associated with exposure to tobacco, biomass, and pollution. The major symptoms of COPD include dyspnea, cough, and or/sputum production. Exacerbations and rates of decline in respiratory mechanics are variable, reflecting the heterogenous nature of this syndrome that is influenced by genetics and environmental issues. The longterm prognosis of patients with COPD is usually assessed when these patients are hospitalized with "exacerbations" or a need for increased medications. Variables associated with poor prognosis include older age, lower body mass index (BMI), more and frequent exacerbations, and poor quality of life.

Perioperative Considerations

1. Patients should utilize their inhalers on the day of the operation and should be in optimal condition in terms of their baseline lung function. Right heart function should be evaluated prior to the operation, and right heart failure and pulmonary hypertension should be treated since it is a significant risk factor for any procedure.

2. Lung protective ventilation using Vt of 6 to 8 mL/kg based on predicted body weight (PBW) should be utilized intraoperatively to limit the risk of lung trauma (volutrauma). Many of these patients have intrinsic auto-PEEP (iPEEP), which is a failure to collapse alveoli at end exhalation. This will require a ventilator setting that allows a longer duration for exhalation. PEEP should be used judiciously; some suggest using PEEP levels to match or be just below auto-PEEP levels. If the patient is hypercapnic at baseline, the hypercapnia should be maintained during and after the operation/procedure. The patient may need supplemental oxygen after the operation, and high flow nasal cannula (HFNC) may be beneficial to decrease the work of breathing. Patients may require noninvasive mechanical ventilation postoperatively. Narcotics should be used judiciously in patients with hypercapnia.

V. OBESITY

Obesity is defined as the abnormal accumulation of excessive fat, leading to risks for a patient's health. The ratio of weight to the square of height, known as BMI, is a widely used anthropometric measurement, with 30 kg/m^2 being the typical threshold for the definition of obesity. Severe, or class III, obesity is defined as a BMI of 40 kg/m^2 or higher. Morbid obesity (BMI 40-49.9 kg/m^2) and super morbid obesity (BMI $\geq$ 50 kg/m^2) are often associated with multisystem disease.

Obesity leads to a complex series of alterations, including—but not limited to—airway and lung physiology.

A. Respiratory pathophysiology

1. Respiratory alterations in obesity are linked to the presence of excess visceral fat pushing against the diaphragm and displacing it cranially.

2. Respiratory pathophysiology of the obese patient is characterized by
   a. elevated pleural pressure
   b. reduced expiratory reserve volume (ERV)
   c. atelectasis
   d. air trapping and iPEEP
   e. V/Q mismatch and shunting.

3. Obese patients chronically live in a tenuous balance of altered respiratory mechanics that predispose them to respiratory failure. Due to chronic reduction of ERV, tidal breathing occurs typically at low lung volumes. Under such conditions, distal airways tend to narrow (possibly closed) during expiration, predisposing to air trapping. However, even in morbidly obese patients, in standard conditions and if positioned upright, the overall distribution of ventilation remains homogeneous. Oxygen saturation is also preserved with significant reductions of ERV. Increased elastic recoil of the lung may help to maintain expiratory flow in the setting of the low lung volume, thereby preventing air trapping. A change to the supine position proves challenging for many, otherwise stable, obese individuals, likely due to the disruption of such a fragile homeostasis.

4. The net result of these pathophysiologic changes is an increased susceptibility of obese patients to the development of perioperative pulmonary complications.

B. Preoperative evaluation

1. Given the increased risk for complications in patients with central compared to peripheral obesity, consider measuring the waist circumference, and not limiting risk considerations to the BMI value only.

2. Screen patients for the presence of obstructive sleep apnea (OSA), as it is prevalent and
   a. often underdiagnosed in the obese population. Patients with OSA who use continuous positive airway pressure (CPAP) at home should continue this therapy during the perioperative period. **Always consider that the obese patient may have sleep-disordered breathing** (Chapter 1).

3. Airway examination and history of previous airway management are important to evaluate risk of difficult intubation and/or mask ventilation.

4. Thorough pulmonary assessment is important to assess risk for perioperative complications. This includes the following:
   a. Baseline Spo_2 with arterial blood gas analysis if Spo_2 <95% on room air.
   b. Preoperative spirometry testing as needed to exclude baseline obstructive disease.
   c. Evaluation for signs of airway hyperresponsiveness (eg, wheezing), chronic respiratory acidosis, or hypoxia.

C. Intraoperative issues

1. **Airway.** A comprehensive airway strategy with backup plans is important, given rapid oxygen desaturation with induction of anesthesia and potential difficulty with mask ventilation and intubation.
   a. Maximal denitrogenation with 100% Fio_2 administration is essential. Obesity results in a reduced apneic time before developing

desaturation compared to nonobese patients. Low lung volumes and reabsorption atelectasis cause rapid desaturations and limit the time to perform laryngoscopy and intubation before critical desaturation develops.

b. CPAP or bilevel positive airway pressure (BiPAP) may improve oxygenation by maintain lung volumes during induction in selected high-risk patients.

c. Ramped positioning may be beneficial for intubation. It consists of 25° head-up position of the torso, which can be visualized with an imaginary horizontal line connecting the auditory meatus with the sternal notch.

D. Maintenance of anesthesia

1. Pharmacology. Obesity has significant effects on the metabolism and pharmacokinetic profiles of most anesthetic agents. Although bolus dose recommendations based on actual or total body weight (TBW) are valid in normal-weight patients, large doses based on TBW in morbidly obese patients can be dangerous.

a. The use of intraoperative depth of anesthesia monitoring is recommended, particularly when total intravenous anesthesia is administered.

b. Assessment of neuromuscular blockade by train-of-four monitoring is essential to maintain an adequate depth of paralysis and to ensure the complete reversal prior to emergence.

c. Due to its low fat-blood solubility coefficient, several studies have reported more rapid emergence and recovery with the inhalation of **desflurane**, compared with sevoflurane, isoflurane, or the use of propofol.

d. Limit, ideally spare, long-acting opioids.

E. Mechanical ventilation

1. Under GA and complete paralysis, there is a decrease in respiratory system compliance. The dominant contribution to such alteration comes from the lung, while the elastic properties of the chest wall are less relevant.

2. The abdominal load is associated with elevated pleural pressure. Negative end-expiratory transpulmonary pressure is not uncommon in obese patients, even while undergoing mechanical positive pressure ventilation. Atelectasis and hypoxemia can be readily apparent consequences. Consequently, higher levels of PEEP may be required in obese patients compared to nonobese patients.

3. Initial ventilator settings:

a. Pressure- or volume-controlled modes can be used. However, pressure control will result in hypoventilation if Vt are not achieved due to elevated pressure resulting from increased chest wall mass.

b. Vt: 6 mL/kg PBW (4-8 mL/kg PBW).

c. Inspiratory time: 0.6 to 1.0 seconds.

d. Setting of PEEP should be to optimize plateau and driving pressures as well as lung compliance. PEEP setting during anesthesia in obese patients is currently debated. In the case of a stable patient with no major pulmonary comorbidity, an initial PEEP of 6 to 8 cmH_2O should suffice. Recruitment maneuvers can be used judiciously during anesthesia (ideally delivered by a stepwise increase/decrease in PEEP targeting a plateau pressure >40 but <55 cmH_2O) to improve oxygenation and restore homogeneous ventilation.

   e. Adjust F_{IO_2}, ideally below 0.5, to maintain SpO_2 >92, minimizing hyperoxia.

     1. Injurious ventilation may predispose even healthy lungs to ventilator-induced lung injury. In order to guarantee protective ventilation, the following should be pursued:

       a. Plateau pressure <28 cmH_2O.

       b. Driving pressure (plateau − [PEEP + PEEPi]) <15 cmH_2O. Driving pressure should not increase when PEEP is increased.

     2. Flow-volume loops on the ventilator can be used to identify signs of airflow limitation.

     3. Esophageal manometry may be considered in very-high-risk patients to select optimal PEEP.

     4. Electrical impedance tomography (EIT) is a noninvasive radiation-free monitoring technique that provides images based on the electrical conductivity of the contents of the chest. Due to the susceptibility to lung collapse and airway closure in obese patients EIT may be a useful tool for the titration of intraoperative PEEP.

F. Effect of surgical procedure

   1. Pneumoperitoneum during laparoscopy leads to an increase in respiratory system elastance, from effects on the chest wall. Lung compliance is mostly unaltered. However, the effects of obesity and pneumoperitoneum on respiratory mechanics are often concomitant (eg, bariatric surgery), with a synergistically detrimental effect for the patient.

   2. Trendelenburg position. The head-down position at 15° or more is often required for laparoscopic surgery. Trendelenburg positioning results in displacement of the diaphragm toward the thoracic cavity due to the effects of gravity, which may be detrimental to the respiratory mechanics of obese patients. End-expiratory lung volume further decreases as a result of Trendelenburg positioning, and a higher airway opening pressure is required to avoid airway closure. iPEEP might also increase, ultimately leading to difficult ventilation, altered gas exchange, and, potentially, ventilator-induced lung injury.

   3. Emergence. Considerations prior to extubation include the type of surgery that was performed (abdominal and thoracic surgery are increased risk for pulmonary complications), the state of the baseline pulmonary function, the volume status of the patient, and confirmation that neuromuscular blockade has been completely reversed. Extubation directly to CPAP or BiPAP may be beneficial in obese patients. Patients should be closely monitored after extubation and narcotics administered sparingly given the increased risk for postoperative respiratory depression.

VI. ACUTE RESPIRATORY DISTRESS SYNDROME

   A. Background: ARDS is a life-threatening condition of hypoxemic respiratory failure with reduced lung compliance secondary to diffuse alveolar damage. Alveoli are flooded with a protein-rich exudate, leading to multifocal, bilateral pulmonary consolidation. A myriad of direct and indirect conditions predispose patients to ARDS (**Table 4.1**). Ten percent of ICU patients and 23% of mechanically ventilated patients have ARDS, and the syndrome is likely underdiagnosed in most ICUs. ARDS remains primarily a clinical diagnosis, and its severity is typically graded as mild, moderate, or severe according to the Berlin criteria (**Table 4.2**).

TABLE 4.1	Direct and Indirect Conditions That Place Patients at Risk of Developing ARDS

Conditions Precipitating ARDS

Direct	Indirect
• Pneumonia (bacterial, viral, mycobacterial, fungal, parasitic) • Aspiration pneumonitis • Pulmonary contusion • Inhalational injury • Near drowning	• Nonthoracic trauma • Pancreatitis • Burns • Transfusion-associated lung injury • Hematopoietic stem cell transplant • Cardiopulmonary bypass • Reperfusion injury after lung transplant or embolectomy • Medications (chemotherapy, amiodarone, radiation) • *Immunologic response to viruses (COVID-19)

ARDS, acute respiratory distress syndrome.

B. Preoperative considerations. Patients with trauma, pancreatitis, or sepsis may require urgent or emergent surgery before pulmonary function can be optimized. Many patients with ARDS benefit from higher levels of PEEP to improve oxygenation and decrease atelectrauma. Care should be taken when transferring between transport ventilators and ICU/operating room (OR) ventilators to avoid the loss of PEEP, which can precipitate atelectasis.

C. Intraoperative considerations

   1. Preoxygenation with noninvasive positive pressure intubation can reduce atelectasis. Apneic oxygenation with HFNC or nasal cannula during intubation may increase the safe apneic time and reduce hypoxia.

TABLE 4.2	Clinical Diagnosis and Severity Grading Criteria for ARDS

The Berlin Criteria

Timing	New/worsening respiratory symptoms within 1 wk of a known clinical insult		
Chest imaging	Bilateral opacities (not fully explained by effusions, lobar/lung collapse, nodules)		
Origin of edema	Hypoxemic respiratory failure not explained by cardiac failure or volume overload		
	Mild	**Moderate**	**Severe**
Oxygenation	$200 < P{:}F < 300$ PEEP or CPAP > 5 cmH$_2$O	$100 < P{:}F < 200$ PEEP > 5 cmH$_2$O	$P{:}F < 100$ PEEP > 5 cmH$_2$O

ARDS, acute respiratory distress syndrome; CPAP, continuous positive airway pressure; PEEP, positive end-expiratory pressure.

2. **Lung protective ventilation** should be prioritized. The ARDS net protocol established guidelines for mechanical ventilation in patients with ARDS in the ICU and can be extrapolated to the operative setting.

   a. Vt of 6 to 8 mL/kg based on PBW rather than actual weight should be used to minimize ventilator-induced lung injury and volutrauma. Vt as low as 4 mL/kg may be tolerated to maintain lung-protective pressures, provided gas exchange remains adequate.

   b. Respiratory rate with goal <35 breaths/min to maintain adequate minute ventilation with low Vt.

   c. FIO_2 should be minimized to keep SpO_2 90% to 95%. Hyperoxia can cause increased oxidative stress with sequelae of endothelial inflammation, mitochondrial dysfunction, and direct lung injury.

   d. Plateau pressure should be maintained <30 cmH$_2$O.

   e. PEEP should be adjusted to minimize atelectasis. Patients with moderate to severe ARDS may require high PEEP (12-15 cmH$_2$O) to maximize alveolar recruitment. Overdistention with increased PEEP even with lung-protective plateau pressures can lead to hypotension and the need for vasoactive drugs or fluid resuscitation.

   f. Driving pressure (Pplat-PEEP) should be limited to <15 cmH$_2$O.

   g. Ventilator mode. No definitive evidence suggests benefit of volume control versus pressure control ventilation for patients with ARDS. Important metrics for lung protection such as plateau pressure and pulmonary compliance are more easily measured with volume control settings.

3. Failure to achieve goals of lung protective ventilation despite adequate depth of anesthesia is an indication for paralysis if not required for the surgical procedure.

   A **recruitment maneuver** is a transient increase in transpulmonary pressure applied to reaerate the collapsed alveoli. Recruitment maneuvers followed by decremental PEEP titration to the best pulmonary compliance are frequently used for patients with ARDS in the ICU, but there is equivocal evidence that these strategies improve mortality or liberation from the ventilator. If a recruitment maneuver is to be performed, it should be approached in a stepwise fashion.

4. **Fluid management.** Excessive fluid administration in patients with ARDS can worsen pulmonary edema and may be associated with increased mortality. Transfusion of blood products can also precipitate or worsen ARDS. A conservative fluid strategy and transfusion threshold (Hgb <7 g/dL) should be adopted. Avoiding excessive fluid administration is particularly challenging in clinical conditions associated with ARDS including trauma, sepsis, and pancreatitis since adequate tissue perfusion needs to be maintained.

D. **Postoperative considerations.** Patients with ARDS often require postoperative mechanical ventilation and ICU care. If patients receive neuromuscular blockade intraoperatively, particular care should be taken to ensure complete reversal if extubation is planned. Adoption of opioid-sparing analgesic approach can reduce risk of postoperative respiratory depression. If you plan to extubate the patient, consider positioning the patient in reverse trendelenburg to optimize pulmonary mechanics. Extubation to noninvasive positive pressure ventilation or HFNC may reduce the risk of postoperative respiratory failure and reintubation in these high-risk patients.

E. Other pulmonary conditions

1. **Pulmonary contusion** occurs in two-thirds of blunt thoracic trauma cases that present emergently to the OR. Imaging findings of pulmonary contusion may lag behind the clinical manifestations. Bedside lung ultrasound can be used to evaluate evolving pulmonary injury more rapidly than imaging modalities such as CT or CXR with a high sensitivity and specificity. Disruption of the alveolar capillary endothelium leads to intraparenchymal and alveolar hemorrhage and edema, increasing the shunt fraction. The inflammatory response provoked often leads to ARDS. Splinting due to pain associated with rib fractures or pleuritic pain results in more atelectasis. Opioid-sparing analgesia with neuraxial techniques such as epidural or paravertebral catheters can decrease atelectasis.

2. **Pneumonia** can result in inflammation and endothelial leak that result in impaired gas exchange. It can precipitate severe hypotension when combined with the decrease in systemic vascular resistance caused by IV and volatile anesthetic agents.

Suggested Readings

Agusti A, Bel E, Thomas M, et al. Treatable traits: toward precision medicine of chronic airway diseases. *Eur Respir J.* 2016;47(2). 410-419. doi:10.1183/13993003.01359-201

Amato MB, Meade MO, Slutsky AS, et al. Driving pressure and survival in the acute respiratory distress syndrome. *N Engl J Med.* 2015;372(8):747-755.

ARDS Definition Task Force; Ranieri VM, Rubenfeld GD, Thompson BT, et al. Acute respiratory distress syndrome: the Berlin definition. *J Am Med Assoc.* 2012;307(23):2526-2533.

Barrot L, Asfar P, Mauny F, et al. Liberal or conservative oxygen therapy for adult respiratory distress syndrome. *N Engl J Med.* 2020;382:999-1008.

Casthely PA, Lear S, Cottrell JE, Lear E. Intrapulmonary shunting during induced hypotension. *Anesth Analg.* 1982;61:231-235.

Castillo JR, Peters SP, Busse WW. Asthma exacerbations: pathogenesis, prevention and treatment. *J Allergy Clin Immunol Pract.* 2017;5:918-927.

Del Sorbo L, Goligher EC, McAuley DF, et al. Mechanical ventilation in adults with acute respiratory distress syndrome. Summary of the experimental evidence for the clinical practice guideline. *Ann Am Thorac Soc.* 2017;14(suppl 4):S261-S270.

Eltorai AEM, Szabo AL, Antoci V, et al. Clinical effectiveness of incentive spirometry for the prevention of postoperative pulmonary complications. *Respir Care.* 2018;63(3):347-352.

Evgenov OV, Liang Y, Jiange Y, Blair JL. Pulmonary pharmacology and inhaled anesthetics. In: Gropper M, Eriksson L, Fleisher L, Wiener-Kronish J, Cohen N, eds. *Millers Anesthesia.* 9th ed. Elsevier; 2020:541.

Futier E, Constantin JM, Pelosi P, et al. Noninvasive ventilation and alveolar recruitment maneuver improve respiratory function during and after intubation of morbidly obese patients: a randomized controlled study. *Anesthesiology.* 2011;114:1354-1363.

Gattinoni L, Cressoni M, Brazzi L. Fluids in ARDS. *Curr Opin Crit Care.* 2014;20:373-377.

Gleason JM, Christian BR, Barton ED. Nasal cannula apneic oxygenation prevents desaturation during endotracheal intubation: an integrative literature review. *West J Emerg Med.* 2018;19(2):403-411.

Goligher EC, Tomlinson G, Hajage D, et al. Extracorporeal membrane oxygenation for adult respiratory distress syndrome and posterior probability of mortality benefit in a post hoc Bayesian analysis of a randomized clinical trial. *J Am Med Assoc.* 2018;320(21):2251-2259.

Hignett R, Fernando R, McGlennan A, et al. A randomized crossover study to determine the effect of a 30° head-up versus a supine position on the functional residual capacity of term parturients. *Anesth Analg.* 2011;113:1098-1102.

LaGrew JE, Olsen KR, Frantz A. Volatile anesthetic for treatment of respiratory failure from status asthmaticus requiring extracorporeal membrane oxygenation. *BMJ Case Rep.* 2020;13:e231507. doi:10.1136/bcr-2019-231507

Lipson DA, Crim C, Criner GJ, et al. Reduction in all-cause mortality with fluticasone furoate/umeclidinium/vilanterol in COPD patients. *Am J Respir Crit Care Med.* 2020;201:1508-1516.

Lumb AB. Pre-operative respiratory optimization: an expert review. *Anaesthesia*. 2019;74(suppl 1):43-48.

Lumb AB, Slinger P. Hypoxic pulmonary vasoconstriction: physiology and anesthetic implications. *Anesthesiology*. 2015;122:932-946.

National Heart, Lung, and Blood Institute PETAL Clinical Trials Network; Moss M, Huang DT, Brower RJ, et al. Early neuromuscular blockade in the acute respiratory distress syndrome. *N Engl J Med*. 2019;380(21):1997-2008.

Pandit JJ. Effect of low dose inhaled anaesthetic agents on the ventilatory response to carbon dioxide in humans: a quantitative review. *Anaesthesia*. 2005;60:461-469.

Robba C, Ball L, Pelosi P. Between hypoxia or hyperoxia: not perfect but more physiologic. *J Thorac Dis*. 2018;10(suppl 17):S2052-S2054.

Rothen HU, Sporre B, Engberg G, Wegenius G, Hedenstierna G. Airway closure, atelectasis and gas exchange during general anaesthesia. *Br J Anaesth*. 1998;81:681-686.

Saraswat V. Effects of anaesthesia techniques and drugs on pulmonary function. *Indian J Anaesth*. 2015;59(9):557-564.

Satoh D, Kurosawa S, Kirino W, et al. Impact of changes of positive end-expiratory pressure on functional residual capacity at low tidal volume ventilation during general anesthesia. *J Anesth*. 2012;26:664-669.

Soldati G, Testa A, Silva FR, Carbone L, Portale G, Silveri NG. Chest ultrasonography in lung contusion. *Chest*. 2006;130(2):533.

Specjalski K, Niedoszytko M. MicroRNAs: future biomarkers and targets of therapy in asthma? *Curr Opin Pulm Med*. 2020;26:285-292.

Vogelmeier CF, Roman-Rodriguez M, Singh D, Han MK, Rodriguez-Roisin R, Ferguson GT. Goals of COPD treatment: focus on symptoms and exacerbations. *Respir Med*. 2020;166:105938.

Vuyk J, Sitsen E, Reekers M. Intraveous anesthetics. In: Gropper M, Eriksson L, Fleisher L, Wiener-Kronish J, Cohen N, eds. *Millers Anesthesia*. 9th ed. Elsevier; 2020:664.

Writing Group for the Alveolar Recruitment for Acute Respiratory Distress Syndrome Trial (ART) Investigators; Cavalcanti AB, Suzumura ÉA, Laranjeira LN, et al. Effect of lung recruitment and titrated positive end-expiratory pressure (PEEP) vs low PEEP on mortality in patients with acute respiratory distress syndrome: a randomized clinical trial. *J Am Med Assoc*. 2017;318(14):1335-1345. doi:10.1001/jama.2017.14171

Zhan Q, Sun B, Liang L, et al. Early use of noninvasive positive pressure ventilation for acute lung injury: a multicenter randomized controlled trial. *Crit Care Med*. 2012;40:455-460.

Specific Considerations With Renal Disease

Katarina Ruscic and Cliodhna Ashe

I. GENERAL CONSIDERATIONS

Approximately 15% of the population has renal disease, with a trend towards increasing prevalence with age. Perioperative renal dysfunction complicates patient management and results in increased morbidity and mortality. Aside from optimizing intravascular volume status, there is no definite consensus on prophylaxis for the development of acute kidney injury (AKI).

II. PHYSIOLOGY

The kidneys regulate intravascular volume, osmolality, acid-base and electrolyte balance, produce hormones, and excrete the end products of metabolism and drugs.

A. Fluid regulation

1. The kidney plays an important role in fluid regulation via neurohumoral interactions as outlined below.

   a. **Renin-angiotensin-aldosterone system** (RAAS). The juxtaglomerular apparatus of the kidney secretes **renin** in response to renal hypoperfusion, decreased sodium chloride delivery to the distal nephron, and increased sympathetic activity. Renin cleaves angiotensinogen to form angiotensin I, which is then converted to angiotensin II by angiotensin-converting enzyme (ACE) in the lung and other tissues.

   b. **Angiotensin II** produces arteriolar vasoconstriction and stimulates aldosterone release.

   c. **Aldosterone** is a mineralocorticoid released by the adrenal cortex in response to angiotensin II, increased potassium levels, decreased sodium content, and adrenocorticotropic hormone. Aldosterone acts on the distal tubules to increase reabsorption of sodium in exchange for potassium and protons.

   d. **Antidiuretic hormone (ADH)**, also known as arginine vasopressin (AVP), is released by the posterior pituitary gland in response to increased osmolality, decreased extracellular volume, positive pressure ventilation, and surgical stimuli, including pain. ADH increases the permeability of the collecting duct to water through insertion of aquaporin water channels. Thus, ADH conserves water and concentrates urine.

   e. **Atrial natriuretic peptide** is a hormone released from the atrial myocytes during atrial stretch and contributes to a natruretic response largely by decreasing RAAS activity. The resultant increase in renal sodium and water excretion decreases blood volume.

   f. **Kinins** are converted from kininogens by kallikreins and are regulated by salt intake, renin release, and hormone levels. They cause vasodilatation and natriuresis.

B. Electrolyte balance

1. **Disorders of sodium homeostasis**

   a. **Hyponatremia:** Plasma sodium concentration less than 134 mEq/L.

1. **Clinical features** vary with the degree of hyponatremia and the rapidity of onset. Symptoms generally do not appear until the sodium concentration falls below 125 mEq/L.
   a. **Moderate hyponatremia or gradual onset:** Confusion, muscle cramps, lethargy, anorexia, and nausea.
   b. **Severe hyponatremia or rapid onset:** Seizures and coma.
2. **Treatment:** Generally, acute normalization of the serum [Na⁺] is not necessary unless the patient has severe symptoms. **Correct no more than 8 mEq/L/d** until 120 mEq/L is reached to prevent complications from rapid correction (eg, osmotic demyelination syndrome [formerly central pontine myelinolysis] and seizures). At this point, the patient should be out of danger, and the [Na⁺] should be normalized slowly over a period of days. Treatment depends on the volume status of the patient. In some cases, desmopressin can be preemptively coadministered to slow the rate of [Na⁺] rise, preventing unintended overcorrection.
   a. **Hypervolemic hyponatremia** due to renal failure, congestive heart failure, cirrhosis, pregnancy, transurethral resection of prostate/hysteroscopy syndrome, or nephrotic syndrome is treated by sodium and water restriction and possibly with diuresis.
   b. **Hypovolemic hyponatremia** from renal losses (diuretics, especially thiazides, renal tubular acidosis with bicarbonaturia, salt wasting nephropathy, mineralocorticoid deficiencies), gastrointestinal losses (vomiting, bowel obstruction, bowel preparations), or sweating is treated with normal saline. Renal versus nonrenal etiology can be determined by the urine sodium (>20 mmol/L if renal loss, or appropriately low if extra-renal). For severe hypovolemic hyponatremia, the [Na⁺] may be partially corrected over 6 to 8 hours with 3.5% hypertonic saline. Hypertonic saline is dangerous in volume-expanded salt-retaining states such as congestive heart failure.
   c. **Normovolemic hyponatremia** from the syndrome of inappropriate ADH (most common cause of SIADH is malignancy), hypothyroidism, drugs that impair renal water excretion, or water intoxication is treated by fluid restriction.
   d. **Pseudohyponatremia** from hyperglycemia (uncontrolled diabetes mellitus), hyperlipidemia, or hyperproteinemia (multiple myeloma) should be ruled out to avoid mistreatment. Corrected [Na⁺] = measured [Na⁺] + (glucose − 100) × 0.024, where Na is in milliequivalents per liter and glucose is in milligrams per deciliter.
b. **Hypernatremia:** Plasma sodium concentration greater than 144 mEq/L. It is usually caused by impairment of thirst or the ability to obtain water. In inpatients, it can be seen after aggressive use of loop diuretics for several days.
   1. **Clinical features** vary with the degree of hypernatremia and rapidity of onset, ranging from tremulousness, weakness, irritability, and mental confusion to seizures and coma.
   2. **Treatment** depends on determining the volume status of the patient, treating the underlying cause, and correcting the potential water deficit. Rapid correction can induce cerebral edema (with the feared complication of uncal herniation),

seizures, permanent neurologic damage, and death. Plasma [Na⁺] should be corrected at a **maximum rate of 0.5 mEq/L/h.** The water deficit, if present, can be calculated as follows:

$$\text{Volume to be replaced}\left(L\right) = \left(0.6 \times \text{body weight}\left(kg\right)\right)$$

$$\times \left[\left(\left[Na^{+}\right] - 140\right)\bigg/140\right]$$

a. **Hypervolemic hypernatremia** occurs secondary to Na⁺ overload from mineralocorticoid excess, dialysis with hypertonic solutions, or treatment with hypertonic saline or sodium bicarbonate ($NaHCO_3$). The excess total body Na⁺ (ie, volume) may be removed by dialysis or with diuretic therapy, and the blood [Na⁺] is gently decreased with intravenous isotonic water such as 5% dextrose (D5W).

b. **Hypovolemic hypernatremia** occurs secondary to water loss exceeding Na⁺ loss (eg, diarrhea, vomiting, heat injury, and diuresis) or inadequate water intake (eg, impaired thirst mechanism and altered mental status). If **hemodynamic instability or evidence of hypoperfusion** is present, replenish volume with lactated Ringer solution (which has [Na⁺] 130 mEq/L). **After volume replenishment,** the remaining free water deficit can be replaced gently with D5W to decrease the [Na⁺].

c. **Normovolemic hypernatremia** is typically the result of diabetes insipidus (central or nephrogenic). Other causes include increased mineralocorticoid (primary hyperaldosteronism), increased glucocorticoid, or ectopic ACTH. Therapy consists of treating the underlying etiology, correcting the free water deficit with D5W, and exogenous vasopressin in central diabetes insipidus.

2. **Disorders of potassium homeostasis**
   a. **Hypokalemia:** Plasma [K⁺] less than 3.5 mEq/L.
      1. Serum [K⁺] is a poor index of **total body potassium** stores as 98% of body potassium is located intracellularly. Thus, large total K⁺ deficits must be present or a significant proportion of K⁺ must have shifted intracellularly before seeing a decrease in serum [K⁺].
      2. **Etiologies**
         a. **Total body K⁺ deficit** due to [K⁺] losses:
            i. **Gastrointestinal tract** (eg, vomiting, diarrhea, fistula, nasogastric suctioning, chronic malnutrition, or obstructed ileal loops).
            ii. **Kidney** (eg, diuretics, some antibiotics, mineralocorticoid and glucocorticoid excess, and some types of renal tubular acidosis). Magnesium depletion increases renal K⁺ loss.
         b. **Shifts in distribution** of K⁺ (extracellular to intracellular):
            i. Alkalosis (H⁺ shifts to the extracellular fluid and K⁺ moves intracellularly). Thus, rapid correction of acidosis, by hyperventilation or $NaHCO_3$ administration, may produce undesirable hypokalemia.
            ii. Insulin therapy.
            iii. Beta-agonists.

3. **Clinical features** rarely appear unless [K⁺] is less than 3 mEq/L or the rate of decrease is rapid.
   a. **Signs** include weakness, augmentation of neuromuscular block, ileus, and disturbances of cardiac contractility.
   b. Hypokalemia **increases excitability** and predisposes the patient to **arrhythmias.** Electrocardiographic (ECG) changes include flattened T waves, U waves, increased PR and QT intervals, ST segment depression, and atrial and ventricular dysrhythmias.
   c. Serum [K⁺] less than 2.0 mEq/L is associated with vasoconstriction and rhabdomyolysis.
4. **Treatment.** Rapid replacement of K⁺ may cause more problems than hypokalemia. There is some evidence that there is no need to correct chronic hypokalemia ([K⁺] ≥ 2.5 mEq/L) before induction of anesthesia.

b. **Hyperkalemia:** Plasma [K⁺] > 5.5 mEq/L.
   1. **Etiologies**
      a. **Decreased excretion** (eg, renal failure and hypoaldosteronism).
      b. **Increased production/extracellular shift** (eg, acidosis, catabolic stress, ischemia, rhabdomyolysis, tumor lysis syndrome, administration of blood, gastrointestinal [GI] bleeding). Acidosis increases the serum [K⁺] by 0.6 mEq (with wide variability) for every 0.1 unit decrease in the pH.
      c. **Drugs:** succinylcholine, nonsteroidal anti-inflammatory drugs (NSAIDs), ACE inhibitor (ACEI), angiotensin receptor blocker (ARB), potassium-sparing diuretics, heparin, and β-blockers.
      d. **Pseudohyperkalemia** from a hemolyzed specimen, erythrocytosis, or thrombocytosis.
   2. **Clinical features** are more likely with acute changes.
      a. **Signs and symptoms** include muscle weakness, paresthesias, and cardiac conduction abnormalities, which become dangerous with levels >6.5 mEq/L. Bradycardia, ventricular fibrillation, and cardiac arrest may result.
      b. Hyperkalemia suppresses electrical conduction. **ECG findings** include peaked T waves, ST segment depression, prolonged PR interval, loss of the P wave, diminished R-wave amplitude, QRS widening, prolongation of the QT interval, and appearance of a sine wave ("preterminal" rhythm).
   3. **Treatment** depends on the nature of ECG changes and serum levels.
      a. **Rapidly acting therapies in the setting of clinical symptoms:**
         i. Slow IV administration of 0.5 to 1.0 g of **calcium chloride** stabilizes the membrane of cardiac myocytes. The dose may be repeated in 5 minutes if changes persist.
         ii. **Insulin** shifts K⁺ intracellularly. Ten units regular insulin is given IV simultaneously with 25 g of glucose IV (one 50-mL ampule of a 50% solution) over 5 minutes. Check the glucose level 30 minutes later to avoid hypoglycemia.
         iii. **Hyperventilation and NaHCO₃** administration shifts K⁺ intracellularly. Between 50 and 100 mEq of NaHCO₃ may be given IV over 5 minutes, with a repeated dose in 10 to 15 minutes.
      b. **Definitive treatment**
         i. Diagnose and treat the underlying etiology.
         ii. Potassium elimination (decrease total body potassium).
         iii. Diuretics (loop and thiazide) waste potassium in the urine. Depending on the volume status of the patient, concomitant fluid resuscitation may be required.

        iv. Cation exchange resins (sodium polystyrene sulfonate [Kayexalate], 20-50 g with sorbitol) given orally or rectally will remove K^+ through the intestinal route.

        v. Serum $[K^+]$ can also be lowered by dialysis (ideally intermittent hemodialysis with high blood and dialysis flow rates, low $[K^+]$ and [high HCO_3^-] dialysate).

C. Extrarenal regulatory and metabolic functions

1. **Erythropoietin** is produced by the kidney to stimulate red blood cell production. Treatment of patients with exogenous recombinant erythropoietin can combat the anemia due to chronic kidney disease (CKD).

2. **Vitamin D** is converted to its most active form, 1,25-dihydroxycholecalciferol, by the kidney.

3. **Parathyroid hormone** acts on the kidney to conserve calcium, waste phosphate, and increase formation of 1,25-dihydroxycholecalciferol.

4. **Metabolization of protein hormones**, eg, insulin, accounting for the generally decreased insulin requirements as renal failure progresses.

III. RENAL FAILURE

A. Acute kidney injury (AKI)

1. **Epidemiology.** Estimated to occur in 12% of hospital admissions and 50% or greater of intensive care unit (ICU) patients. Risk increases with age. Perioperative acute kidney injury is common, accounting for 30% to 40% of all in-hospital cases of AKI. Development of postoperative AKI is associated independently with increased morbidity and mortality.

2. **Etiology**

    a. **Traditional categorization** is by the anatomical groups of prerenal, intrarenal, and postrenal.

       1. **Prerenal.** Due to decreased circulating blood volume (hypovolemia) or a perceived decrease in circulating volume (decreased cardiac output or hypotension). Early correction of the underlying cause usually results in rapid reversal of renal dysfunction, but continued renal hypoperfusion may result in intrinsic renal damage.

       2. **Intrarenal.** The most common cause is ATN due to ischemia. Other intrarenal causes include toxins, acute glomerulonephritis, and interstitial nephritis.

       3. **Postrenal.** Obstructive lesions result in disrupted emptying and can be caused by renal calculi, neurogenic bladder, prostatic disease, or an encroaching tumor. Unilateral obstruction rarely causes AKI.

    b. **Modern description** favors describing specific syndromes (eg, hepatorenal, cardiorenal, nephrotoxic, sepsis-associated AKI) that do not always fit the traditional classification scheme, since each has a unique treatment.

       1. **Cardiorenal syndrome:** Inflammation and neurohormonal activation affect blood flow autoregulation, impairing compensation for the abnormal kidney perfusion pressure caused by low cardiac output and/or renal vein congestion.

       2. **Hepatorenal syndrome:** Hepatic dysfunction causes systemic vasodilation, triggering a high level of activation of the RAAS and subsequent renal dysfunction. Portal hypertension-induced splanchnic vasodilation seems to play a central role. Profound oliguria and sodium retention result.

3. **Classification:** There are three widely used classification systems for AKI (**Table 5.1**):

   a. The **RIFLE** criteria classifies three levels of kidney injury (*r*isk, *i*njury, or *f*ailure) and two outcomes (*l*oss and *e*nd-stage renal disease [ESRD]) based upon (1) the increase in serum creatinine over 7 days or (2) a decrease in urine output (UOP).

   b. The **AKIN** criteria modifies the RIFLE criteria by including absolute increases in serum creatinine and limiting the period of injury to a 48-hour window.

   c. The **Kidney Disease: Improving Global Outcomes (KDIGO)** criteria fuse the RIFLE and AKIN criteria.

4. **Diagnosis:** History and physical examination, in particular assessing the patient's volume status, to determine etiology. Pertinent laboratory tests should include urinalysis, serum creatinine level and fractional excretion of sodium (FE_{Na}), or fractional excretion of urea (FE_{Urea}) if the patient has been exposed to diuretics. Imaging studies can help rule out obstruction (**Table 5.2**).

TABLE 5.1	Criteria for Acute Kidney Injury		
	RIFLE	**AKIN**	**KDIGO**
Diagnostic criteria		Increase in SCr of ≥0.3 mg/dL or ≥50% within 48 h OR UOP <0.5 mL/kg/h for >6 h	Increase in SCr of ≥0.3 mg/dL within 48 h or ≥50% within 7 d OR UOP <0.5 mL/kg/h for >6 h
Staging Criteria			
Risk (RIFLE) AKIN/KDIGO **stage 1**	Increase in SCr to ×1.5 baseline OR UOP <0.5 mL/kg/h for 6-12 h	Increase in SCr of ≥0.3 mg/dL or to 150%-200% baseline OR UOP <0.5 mL/kg/h for 6-12 h	Increase in SCr of ≥0.3 mg/dL or ×1.5-1.9 baseline OR UOP <0.5 mL/kg/h for 6-12 h
Injury (RIFLE) AKIN/KDIGO **stage 2**	Increase in SCr of ×2 baseline OR UOP <0.5 mL/kg/h for 12-24 h	Increase in SCr to 200%-300% baseline OR UOP <0.5 mL/kg/h for 12-24 h	Increase in SCr to ×2.0-2.9 baseline OR UOP <0.5 mL/kg/h for 12-24 h
Failure (RIFLE) AKIN/KDIGO **stage 3**	Increase in SCr to ×3 baseline OR Increase in SCr by 0.5 mg/dL to >4.0 mg/dL OR UOP <0.3 mL/kg/h for <24 h or anuria for >12 h OR Initiation of RRT	Increase in SCr to >300% baseline OR SCr ≥4.0 mL/dL with an acute increase of >0.5 mg/dL OR UOP of <0.3 mL/kg/h for >24 h or anuria for >12 h OR Initiation of RRT	Increase in SCr to ≥3.0 times baseline OR Increase in SCr to ≥4.0 mg/dL OR Urine output of <0.3 mL/kg/h for ≥24 h or anuria for >12 h OR Initiation of RRT

	Criteria for Acute Kidney Injury (Continued)		
	RIFLE	**AKIN**	**KDIGO**
Loss (RIFLE)	Need for RRT >4 wk		
End-stage (RIFLE)	Need for RRT >3 mo		

AKIN, Acute Kidney Injury Network; ESRD, end-stage renal disease; KDIGO, Kidney Disease: Improving Global Outcomes; RIFLE, risk, injury, failure, loss, ESRD; SCr, serum creatinine.
Derived from Palevsky PM. Definition of acute kidney injury. In: Curhan GC, ed. *UpToDate*. UpToDate. Accessed June 2020. https://www.uptodate.com/contents/definition-and-staging-criteria-of-acute-kidney-injury-in-adults

5. **Clinical features.** Depending on the severity, the condition may be silent. It can present with hypervolemia due to an impaired ability to excrete water and sodium with resultant hypertension, cardiac arrhythmia, pulmonary edema, and peripheral edema. In the setting of cardiac failure, volume overload can precipitate cardiogenic shock (sometimes referred to as falling off the Starling curve). Uremia can affect cognitive function and platelet efficacy. Urinary tract obstruction might present with pain. Inability to concentrate the urine can present with hypovolemia. AKI also can cause electrolyte derangements, impaired excretion of drugs and toxins, and potential progression to CKD. Two-thirds of cases of AKI resolve within 7 days, cases that do not resolve are associated with 47% hospital mortality.

6. **Prevention.** Mainly based on tradition and extrapolation from animal models. A modest goal is to keep UOP greater than 0.5 mL/kg/h and to avoid hypovolemia, hypoxia, renovascular constriction, and maintenance of renal vasodilation and renal tubular blood flow along with attenuation of renal ischemic reperfusion injury. N-acetylcysteine (NAC) and bicarbonate do not provide benefit beyond fluid hydration.

7. **Management**
   a. **Medications** Although medications such as diuretics, dopamine, and fenoldopam can increase UOP, treat hypertension, and manage electrolyte, fluid, and acid-base disturbances, they have not been proven to prevent or treat AKI.
   b. **Optimization:** Remove toxic drugs, renally dose medications, and favor medications that do not require renal clearance. Avoid hydroxyethyl starch, especially in septic shock. Normal saline has a higher risk for composite death, dialysis, and renal dysfunction compared with more physiological solutions (eg, lactated Ringer's). Order imaging with contrast only if essential. Control inflammation, correct anemia (hemoglobin >7 g/dL), optimize cardiac output, and correct volume status. This may require invasive hemodynamic monitoring.

	Urine and Serum Diagnostic Indexes		
	Prerenal	**Renal**	**Postrenal**
FE_{Na}	<1%	>2%	>2%
FE_{Urea}	<35%	>50%	>50%
Serum (BUN)/creatinine	>20	10	10

BUN, blood urea nitrogen; FE_{Na}, fractional excretion of sodium.

If adequately intravascularly replete, vasopressors may be needed to maintain mean arterial pressure (MAP) >65 mm Hg.

c. **Specific syndromes:** In addition to the above optimization, address the underlying condition.

d. **Renal replacement therapy (RRT):** Incidence of patients with postoperative AKI requiring renal replacement therapy varies depending on the underlying surgical operation (eg, coronary artery bypass grafting 1.1% vs general surgery 0.6%). Indications for RRT in AKI and CKD include hyperkalemia, acidosis, volume overload, and uremic complications (pericarditis, tamponade, and encephalopathy). Best timing for RRT initiation remains controversial.

   1. **Hemodialysis** uses an artificial semipermeable membrane that separates the patient's blood from the dialysate and allows the exchange of solutes by **diffusion** along a gradient. Vascular access (via central venous catheters or a surgically created arteriovenous fistula) and systemic or regional anticoagulation are often required. Hemodialysis typically is performed three times a week, and serum electrolyte and volume abnormalities are corrected by adjusting the dialysis bath fluid. Blood samples taken immediately after dialysis will be inaccurate, because redistribution of fluid and electrolytes takes approximately **6 hours**. Complications include arteriovenous fistula infection or thrombosis, dialysis disequilibrium or dementia, hypotension, pericarditis, and hypoxemia.

   2. **Ultrafiltration** and **hemofiltration** allow for the removal of volume with minimal removal of waste products. These techniques are useful in volume-overloaded patients. As with standard hemodialysis, anticoagulation is usually required.

      a. **Ultrafiltration** uses hemodialysis equipment to create a hydrostatic driving force across the membrane without a dialysate on the opposing side. Thus, an ultrafiltrate of serum is removed, and this volume is not replaced. If large volumes of fluid are removed rapidly, hypotension may ensue.

      b. **Hemofiltration** uses the same principle as ultrafiltration; however, replacement fluid is given to the patient either before or after the membrane filter and solutes/electrolytes are removed by convection. Volume shifts are minimized so that patients can tolerate longer periods of continuous filtration.

   3. **Continuous renal replacement therapy (CRRT)** refers to any continuous mode of extracorporeal solute or fluid removal. Slower blood flow rates with CRRT improve hemodynamic stability compared with regular hemodialysis.

TABLE 5.3	National Kidney Foundation Classification of CKD		
Stage	**Description**	**GFR**	**US Prevalence (%)**
I	Normal	≥90	3.3
II	Mild	60-89	3.0
III	Moderate	30-59	4.3
IV	Severe	15-29	0.2
V	Failure	<15	0.1

B. **CKD** is defined by kidney damage manifested as abnormalities in the composition of blood or urine, abnormalities in imaging tests, or a glomerular filtration rate (GFR) < 60 mL/min/1.73 m^2 for ≥3 months.

1. **Epidemiology.** CKD affects 15% of adults (**Table 5.3**).

2. **Etiology.** Common causes include diabetes mellitus (single largest cause of ESRD in the United States), hypertension, glomerulonephropathies, tubulointerstitial disease, renovascular disease, polycystic kidney disease, and obesity.

3. **Clinical features**

   a. **Hypervolemia and hypertension,** sometimes resulting in congestive heart failure and edema.

   b. **Accelerated atherosclerosis** and **hypertriglyceridemia,** which may increase the risk of coronary artery disease.

   c. **Uremic pericarditis and pericardial effusions,** which may cause cardiac tamponade.

   d. **Hyperkalemia, hypermagnesemia,** and **hyponatremia** may occur.

   e. **Hypocalcemia** and **hyperphosphatemia** due to elevated parathyroid hormone, resulting in renal osteodystrophy.

   f. **Metabolic acidosis** due to retained sulfates and phosphates and an inability to excrete products of metabolism.

   g. **Chronic anemia** secondary to decreased erythropoietin production and decreased red blood cell survival.

   h. **Platelet dysfunction,** secondary to uremia, which can be temporarily treated with desmopressin acetate.

   i. **Gastrointestinal dysfunction** is common as a result of accumulated urea that may result in inflammation of the entire GI tract. Increased gastric volume, acid production, and delayed gastric emptying result in an increased risk of regurgitation and aspiration during anesthesia.

   j. Increased **susceptibility to infection** due to leukocyte and immune dysfunction from uremia, malnutrition, and inflammatory reaction to dialysis.

   k. **Central nervous system changes** range from mild changes in mentation to severe encephalopathy and coma. Peripheral and autonomic neuropathies are common.

   l. **Glucose intolerance.**

4. **Management.** When needed, approximately 85% of patients receive hemodialysis and 15% receive peritoneal dialysis. Transplantation is the preferred method of treatment for most patients with ESRD.

   a. **Hemodialysis** (see Section III.A.7.d).

   b. **Peritoneal dialysis** uses the capillaries of the peritoneum as a semipermeable exchange membrane with the dialysate infused into the peritoneal cavity via an indwelling peritoneal catheter. Advantages over hemodialysis include less hypotension or disequilibrium and no need for heparin treatment. However, peritoneal dialysis is less efficient and limited in catabolic states compared with hemodialysis. Complications include infection, hyperglycemia from the dextran in the dialysate, and increased protein loss into the dialysate.

IV. ANESTHETIC MANAGEMENT

A. **Preoperative assessment.** The etiology of renal disease should be elucidated (eg, diabetes mellitus, hypertension). Elective surgery should be postponed in the setting of an acute, unoptimized disease process (eg, new type 1 hepatorenal syndrome). The degree of residual renal function is best estimated by creatinine clearance (see Section IV.A.3.b). A thorough, systems-based history and physical should be performed (see Chapter 1).

1. **History**
   a. **Signs and symptoms** can be varied depending on the cause of renal failure but may include polyuria, polydipsia, dysuria, edema, dyspnea, arrhythmia, and mental status changes.
   b. **Relevant medications** should be detailed: diuretics, antihypertensives, potassium supplements, digitalis, and nephrotoxic agents (NSAIDs, aminoglycosides, exposure to heavy metals, and recent radiographic dye).
   c. **Schedule of hemodialysis** should be noted for coordination with procedures. Dry weight should be confirmed.
2. **Physical examination**
   a. Patients should be thoroughly examined for the stigmata of renal failure as described in Section III.B.3.
   b. **Arteriovenous fistula** should be evaluated for patency (by the presence of a thrill or bruit). Intravenous access and blood pressure determinations should be performed on the opposite limb to preserve the fistula.
   c. **Avoid inserting peripherally inserted central venous catheters** in patients with CKD given the risk of upper-extremity venous thrombosis and central venous stenosis, which impairs future RRT vascular access.
   d. For **central lines** in CKD, if clinically appropriate, choose smaller-bore catheters to preserve the veins. Internal jugular vein sites rather than subclavian veins are also less prone to thrombose or permanently damage vessels.
3. **Laboratory studies**
   a. **Serum creatinine (SCr)** is normally 0.6 to 1.2 mg/dL but is affected by the patient's skeletal muscle mass and activity level. SCr concentration is inversely proportional to GFR; thus, a doubling of SCr generally corresponds to a 50% reduction in GFR. In pregnancy, physiologic increase in GFR and expansion of extracellular fluid volume mean normal SCr is 0.4 to 0.8 mg/dL (thus SCr of 1.0 mg/dL in pregnancy may mean renal failure, the etiology of which must be investigated).
   b. **Creatinine clearance** is used to estimate GFR and provides the best estimate of renal reserve. It is normally 80 to 120 mL/min. A gross estimate of creatinine clearance can be calculated by: $\{[140\text{-age (years)}] \times \text{weight (kg)}\}/[72 \times \text{serum creatinine (mg/dL)}]$. Multiply by 0.85 for women. Ideal body weight should be used in obesity. This formula is invalid with gross renal insufficiency or changing renal function. Medications such as trimethoprim, H_2 receptor antagonists, and salicylates block the secretion of creatinine and may elevate serum creatinine and decrease creatinine clearance.
   c. **Blood urea nitrogen** is an insensitive measure of GFR because it is influenced by volume status, cardiac output, diet, and body habitus. The ratio of blood urea nitrogen to creatinine is normally 10 to 20:1; disproportionate elevation of the blood urea nitrogen may reflect hypovolemia, low cardiac output, gastrointestinal bleeding, or steroid use.
   d. **Electrolytes:** Serum Na^+, K^+, Cl^-, and HCO_3^- concentrations will usually be normal until renal failure is advanced. Careful consideration of the risk and benefit of proceeding with elective surgery should be made if $[Na^+]$ is less than 131 or greater than 150 mEq/L, or if $[K^+]$ is less than 2.5 or greater than 5.9 mEq/L, because these abnormalities may exacerbate arrhythmias and compromise cardiac function. Serum Ca^{2+}, PO_4^-, and Mg^{2+} concentrations are altered in renal failure.

   e. Urinalysis provides a qualitative assessment of general renal function.

     1. Findings suggestive of renal disease include abnormal pH, proteinuria, pyuria, hematuria, and casts.

     2. The kidney's ability to concentrate urine is often lost before other changes become apparent. A specific gravity of 1.018 or greater after an overnight fast suggests that concentrating ability is intact. However, radiographic dye and osmotic agents will elevate specific gravity and invalidate this test.

   f. Urine electrolytes, osmolality, urine creatinine, and urine urea can help determine volume status and concentrating ability and are used to help differentiate between prerenal and intrarenal diseases (see **Table 5.2**).

   g. Hematologic studies should assess anemia and coagulation abnormalities.

   h. ECG may reveal myocardial ischemia or infarction, pericarditis, and the effects of electrolyte abnormalities (see Section II.B).

   i. Imaging may show evidence of fluid overload, pericardial effusion, infection, uremic pneumonitis, or cardiomegaly.

4. Risk assessment for postoperative renal dysfunction

   a. Patient factors:

     1. Demographics: age >65 years, male gender, higher ASA score, ICU patient

     2. Acute Pathology: sepsis, trauma, abdominal hypertension

     3. Comorbidities: CKD, obesity, hypertension, diabetes mellitus, vascular disease, liver disease, cardiac dysfunction

   b. Potential nephrotoxins

     1. NSAIDs: associated with increased risk of perioperative AKI in patients with underlying risk factors (age, higher burden of comorbidity). Consider avoiding or dose-reducing.

     2. ARB/ACEI: Angiotensin II increases efferent arteriolar vasoconstriction to maintain glomerular filtration pressure. However, in patients taking ACEI or ARB, this compensatory mechanism may be decreased, which could cause a decrease in renal perfusion pressure and urine production. Consider stopping these on the day of surgery.

     3. Antibiotics: aminoglycosides, multitherapy versus monotherapy.

     4. Contrast media: These cause a decrease in O_2 supply by causing intrarenal vasoconstriction, decreased medullary blood supply, and an increase in O_2 demand. The osmotic load increases work to the medullary nephrons.

   c. High-risk surgery: renal artery surgery, thoracic and abdominal aortic surgery, nonrenal organ transplantation, surgery with large blood loss, and prolonged (>3 hours) cardiopulmonary bypass.

5. Preoperative optimization

   a. Patients on hemodialysis should be dialyzed before surgery, allowing time between dialysis and surgery to permit equilibration of fluids and electrolytes. Blood samples taken immediately after hemodialysis may be inaccurate owing to redistribution of fluid and electrolytes. Equilibration may take up to 6 hours.

   b. If the patient is on CRRT, the decision to continue intraoperatively must be based on the underlying reason for the CRRT, the duration of the procedure, and the type of procedure. Most patients will be able to tolerate discontinuation of CRRT before surgery and reinstitution afterward.

    c. It may be prudent to postpone major elective vascular surgery for a few days after contrast media exposure. In addition, pretreatment with isotonic crystalloid for **volume expansion**, NAC, or **sodium bicarbonate infusion** (SBI) before radiographic contrast administration may prevent contrast-induced (CI) nephropathy in patients at increased risk of **CI-AKI**.

        1. **Volume expansion** with crystalloid has been shown to be beneficial. There is no clear consensus on optimal rate or duration of infusion.

        2. **NAC** 20% (200 mg/mL) 1200 mg is given orally every 12 hours, on the day before and on the day of contrast administration, for a total of 2 days. There are conflicting data regarding the effectiveness of NAC in preventing CI-nephropathy.

        3. **SBI** of 150 mEq/L of sodium bicarbonate (three ampules of 50 mEq sodium bicarbonate in 1 L of D5W or free water) is administered at 3 mL/kg/h for 1 hour before contrast administration, followed by an infusion of 1 mL/kg/h for 6 hours after the procedure. Most likely the benefit is from crystalloid volume expansion rather than the bicarbonate component.

B. Intraoperative management. There are limited data comparing general and regional anesthesia in terms of renal protection; currently, there is no beneficial effect of one anesthetic technique over the other. When regional anesthesia is considered, coexisting neuropathies should be determined (and documented) and the coagulation profile checked for coagulopathies.

    1. **Premedication** should be administered carefully because patients with renal failure may have an increased sensitivity to central nervous system depressants especially if significant uremia is present (see Section VI.A.1).

    2. The dose of **induction agents** may need to be reduced and their rate of administration slowed to avoid hypotension (see Section VI.A.2). Serum potassium should be checked before administration of succinylcholine.

    3. Many anesthetics cause peripheral vasodilation and myocardial depression necessitating the use of **vasopressors**. Current clinical data are insufficient to recommend one vasoactive agent as superior to another in preventing AKI. Appropriate use of vasoactive agents can improve kidney perfusion and should not be withheld from the patient in distributive shock owing to concern over kidney perfusion.

    4. Adequate **hemodynamic management**, in particular maintenance of adequate MAP, is vital in ensuring adequate renal perfusion pressure. Data suggest intraoperative hypotension is associated with postoperative AKI. Maintain at least MAP >65 mm Hg. There is evidence that targeting an individualized systolic blood pressure (SBP) within 10% of the patient's baseline SBP decreases postoperative organ dysfunction.

    5. Surgical stimulation results in an increase in circulating catecholamines, catabolic hormones, and cytokines that increase ADH, resulting in sodium/water retention, potassium loss, and decreased UOP. Narcotics also increase ADH release, which may further reduce UOP (see Section VI.A.3).

    6. **Positioning** should be done carefully. Patients with CKD are prone to fractures secondary to renal osteodystrophy.

7. **Hyperglycemia and glycemic variability** may increase the risk of postoperative AKI; thus, intraoperative glucose monitoring in high-risk patients may be of benefit.

8. **Ventilation** with excessive positive-pressure ventilation can impair venous return by reducing preload, causing a resultant reduction in renal perfusion pressure. Avoidance of hypoxia, hypercarbia, and ventilator-induced lung injury through the use of lung protective ventilation may help reduce inflammatory AKI risk factors. Determine optimal PEEP by oxygenation and compliance.

9. **Fluid management** should take into account maintenance fluid requirements, evaporative/insensible losses (eg, open abdominal procedures with losses up to 10 mL/kg/h), extravasation/third-space losses of fluids, and intravascular/blood loss.

   a. Fluid replacement should proceed cautiously with balanced crystalloids. Liberal versus restrictive perioperative fluid management is a much debated topic. A goal-directed, patient-specific approach is recommended.

   b. Large volumes of 0.9% sodium chloride administration may result in a hyperchloremic metabolic acidosis. Data suggests that lactated Ringer's solution is associated with less metabolic acidosis and hyperkalemia, especially in patients undergoing renal transplant surgery.

   c. For more extensive procedures, arterial line waveform analysis, bedside point-of-care ultrasound, central venous pressure, or pulmonary artery catheter may help guide fluid management (see Chapter 3).

   d. **Urine output** in patients who are neither oliguric nor anuric can be a helpful marker of adequate resuscitation with goal 0.5 mL/kg/h (although this should be adjusted for the individual case and patient).

10. **Rhabdomyolysis** is skeletal muscle breakdown with release of nephrotoxic breakdown products, such as myoglobin. It may result from suboptimal positioning, compartment syndrome, tourniquet use, prolonged procedures, hypotension, neuroleptic malignant syndrome, and malignant hyperthermia. High BMI is an additional risk factor. Diagnose with serum creatinine kinase >5000 U/L. Treat the underlying source and concomitant electrolyte abnormalities, and give generous volumes of crystalloid fluids (classically NS, although recent data suggest LR is equivalent).

11. **Hematologic disturbances** are common in CKD, including anemia, leukocyte dysfunction, and coagulopathy. Accordingly, these patients are at an increased risk for intraoperative bleeding. Interventions to reduce bleeding include:

    a. **Recombinant erythropoietin** corrects anemia, normalizes starting hemoglobin, and may restore platelet function.

    b. **DDAVP** improves platelet function by stimulating release of von Willebrand-Factor VIII complex from the endothelium into the plasma where it binds and activates platelets. Effects are seen 1 to 2 hours post infusion and last approximately 6 to 12 hours.

    c. **Cryoprecipitate** contains von Willebrand-Factor VIII complex, which corrects prolonged bleeding in about 50% of cases. However, there is a risk of bloodborne infection.

d. Conjugated estrogens may reduce bleeding and have a longer duration of action than DDAVP.

e. Heparin-free or low-dose heparin hemodialysis.

12. Specific considerations for renal transplantation: Recipients have ESRD and generally have hypertension and/or diabetes mellitus, are at increased risk for cardiac disease, and may have disturbances in electrolytes, acid-base balance, platelet function, and volume status. Specific considerations:

   a. IV access may be limited, and placement in extremities with fistulas or shunts should be avoided. The benefits of additional invasive monitors (central venous or arterial lines) should be weighed against the risks of catheter-related infections in functionally immunosuppressed patients.

   b. Patients may have delayed gastric emptying from diabetes, uremic neuropathy, and preoperative opioids, so a rapid sequence induction may be indicated. Succinylcholine is safe to use in ESRD, provided serum potassium is normal as the increase in plasma potassium is no greater than in the general population. If a rapid sequence induction is not indicated, either a benzylisoquinolinium or aminosteroid may be used (see Pharmacology and Renal Failure).

   c. Graft function depends on adequate intravascular volume before and after vascular anastomosis to maintain perfusion to the transplanted kidney. Crystalloid, and albumin are useful volume expanders. If pharmacologic support is necessary, inotropes may be preferable to α-agonists, but data are limited.

   d. Most patients receive immunosuppressants to prevent graft rejection, including induction therapy with anti-thymocyte globulin that can induce an anaphylactic reaction.

C. Postoperative management

   1. Postoperative fluid management:

   a. Repletion should take into account effusions, drainage tube losses, and mobilization of third-space fluid back into the vascular compartment.

   b. Replacement fluid should consist of balanced crystalloids and dextrose until the patient is able to take adequate fluid orally.

   c. Postoperative oliguria can be a normal physiological response to pain and surgical trauma. Remembering this can avoid over-zealous fluid administration that may be harmful.

   2. Hypertension is a common postoperative problem and is aggravated by fluid overload. For those not on dialysis, diuretics and short-acting antihypertensives are effective. For those on dialysis, postoperative dialysis may be required.

V. PHARMACOLOGY AND THE KIDNEY

   A. Pharmacological interventions for renal protection in the perioperative period
   At present, no convincing evidence indicates that any of these measures are of benefit.

   1. Diuretics are used to facilitate management of fluid balance and manage electrolyte and acid-base disturbances (**Table 5.4**). However, the KDIGO guidelines 2012 recommend against use of diuretics specifically to prevent or treat AKI, except in management of volume overload.

T A B L E 5.4	Diuretics			
	Primary Site of Action	Primary Effect	Side Effects	Comments
Nonosmotic				
Loop (furosemide, etarynic acid, and bumetanide)	Thick ascending loop of Henle and Na^+/K^+/Cl^- symporter	Moderate to severe natriuresis and chloruresis	Hypokalemia, alkalosis, and volume contraction	Interferes with both urinary concentration and dilution
Thiazides (chlorothiazide, and metolazone)	Distal tubules and Na^+/Cl^- symporter	Mild to moderate natriuresis	Hyponatremia, hypokalemia, alkalosis, and volume contraction	Interferes with urinary dilution and tends to be ineffective in renal failure and CHF
Carbonic anhydrase inhibitors (acetazolamide)	Proximal tubule and carbonic anhydrase	Mild natriuresis	Hyperchloremia, hypokalemia, and metabolic acidosis	Used primarily for ophthalmology; self-limiting renal effect
Potassium sparing (spironolactone, triamterene, and amiloride)	Collecting duct and ENaC channel or aldosterone receptor	Mild to moderate natriuresis	Hyperkalemia	Used in conjunction with K^+ losing diuretics or in hyperaldosterone states
Osmotic				
Mannitol	Proximal tubule, descending loop of Henle and collecting duct	Moderate to severe diuresis	Early: vasodilation and volume expansion; Late: hyperosmolality and volume contraction	Draws intracellular fluid into intravascular space

CHF, congestive heart failure.

There is no evidence that use of diuretic therapy reduce severity or mortality in AKI. In fact, it may precipitate AKI.

2. **Dopamine** dilates renal arterioles, increases renal blood flow, and augments natriuresis and the GFR. Low-dose dopamine (0.5-3 µg/kg/min) has been proposed to prevent and treat AKI, but efficacy has never been demonstrated.

3. **Fenoldopam** is a specific dopamine-1 receptor agonist. Emerging data suggest possible protective effects in AKI; larger studies are needed. It is found to be ineffective for prevention of CI-AKI.

4. **Natriuretic peptides:** There are currently no definitive trials to support use of ANP, BNP, or nesiritide.

B. **Anesthetic effects on the kidney.** Patients with normal kidney function experience transient postanesthetic alterations in renal function. These alterations may occur despite insignificant changes in blood pressure and cardiac output, suggesting that changes in intrarenal distribution of blood flow are responsible. With brief exposures to anesthesia, the observed changes in renal function are reversible (renal blood flow and GFR return to baseline within a few hours). With extensive surgery and prolonged anesthesia, impaired ability to excrete a water load or concentrate urine may last for several days.

1. All inhalational agents and many induction agents cause myocardial depression, hypotension, and a mild to moderate increase in renal vascular resistance, leading to a decreased renal blood flow and GFR.

2. Compensatory catecholamine secretion causes redistribution of renal cortical blood flow.

3. ADH release increases with the onset of surgical stimulation. Hydration before the induction of anesthesia attenuates the rise in ADH produced by painful stimuli.

4. Spinal and epidural anesthesia produce decreases in renal blood flow, GFR, and UOP.

5. There are **concerns regarding adverse renal effects** of some fluorinated volatile agents, in particular sevoflurane. Strong bases in CO_2 absorbents can theoretically accumulate at low fresh gas flow (FGF), degrading sevoflurane to the nephrotoxic by-product, Compound A. However, current data show that renal effects of low-flow (≤1 L/min) sevoflurane are no different from low-flow isoflurane. Package insert in the United States currently recommends sevoflurane exposure should not exceed 2 MAC hours at flow rates of 1 to 2 L/min and that FGF <1 L/min is not recommended.

6. There are data to suggest volatile anesthetics exert cardioprotective properties during cardiac surgery. This is largely attributed to anesthetic preconditioning.

7. The VAPOR-1 trial suggests possible longer-term benefits in recipients receiving sevoflurane (vs propofol) during renal transplantation, with lower acute rejection rate after 2 years.

VI. PHARMACOLOGY AND RENAL FAILURE

Many common anesthetic drugs may be affected by renal dysfunction owing to changes in:

- Volume of distribution and electrolytes.
- **pH** (resulting in a higher percentage of nonionized drug).
- **Decreased serum protein concentration** resulting in increased bioavailability of protein-bound drugs, impaired biotransformation, and decreased rates of excretion (**Table 5.5**).
- **Loading doses** do not need to be altered significantly in CKD as the duration of action of drugs administered by bolus is **determined by redistribution,** not elimination. With repeated dosing or long-term infusion, the duration of action is dependent on elimination, and maintenance doses of drugs with significant renal excretion should be reduced.

A. **Lipid-soluble drugs** generally are poorly ionized and must undergo metabolism by the liver to water-soluble forms before elimination by the kidney. With few exceptions, the metabolites have little biological activity.

1. **Benzodiazepines** are metabolized in the liver to both active and inactive compounds, which are then eliminated by the kidney. Benzodiazepines are 90% to 95% protein bound. Great care must be taken in using diazepam because of its long half-life and its active metabolites. Accumulation of benzodiazepines and their metabolites may occur in severe renal failure. Benzodiazepines are not appreciably removed by dialysis.

TABLE 5.5	Pharmacologic Considerations for Perioperative Drugs Used in Patients With Chronic Renal Insufficiency	
Drug Class	**Pharmacokinetics**	**Considerations**
Volatile anesthetics	Pulmonary metabolism	Sevoflurane produces compound A, a potentially nephrotoxic metabolite.
Lipid Soluble		
Barbiturates	Free fraction of induction dose is almost doubled in patients with CKD.	Exaggerated hypotension and other clinical effects in CKD. Need to reduce induction dose.
Benzodiazepines	Increased free fraction in CKD	Potentiates clinical effects in CKD. Active metabolites accumulate with repeated dosing.
Propofol	Rapid, extensive hepatic metabolism. Pharmacokinetics unchanged in CKD	CKD does not alter clinical effects.
Etomidate	Increased free fraction in CKD	CKD does not alter clinical effects.
Ketamine	Redistribution and hepatic metabolism largely responsible for termination of anesthetic effects. Minimal change in free fraction in CKD	CKD does not alter clinical effects.
Opioids	Metabolized in liver	May have increased and prolonged effect in CKD. Active metabolites may prolong action with chronic administration: Morphine-6-glucoronide (morphine) has potent analgesic and sedative effects. Normeperidine (meperidine) has neurotoxic effects. Hydromorphone-3-glucoronide (hydromorphone) can cause cognitive dysfunction and myoclonus. Fentanyl has no active metabolite.
Ionized Drugs		
Muscle relaxants	Standard dose of succinylcholine increases serum K^+ by 0.5-0.8 mEq/L in CKD. Many nonpolarizing NMBs result in prolonged effects due to reliance on renal excretion	Succinylcholine is not contraindicated in CKD if serum K^+ is not elevated. Cisatracurium, mivacurium, and rocuronium are preferable in CKD.

(*continued*)

	Pharmacologic Considerations for Perioperative Drugs Used in Patients With Chronic Renal Insufficiency (Continued)

Drug Class	Pharmacokinetics	Considerations
Cholinesterase inhibitors	Decreased elimination in CKD, and half-life is prolonged	Half-life prolongation is similar or greater than the duration of blockade from long-acting NMB so recurarization is rarely seen.
Digoxin	Excreted in urine	Increased risk of toxicity in CKD.
Vasoactive Drugs		
Catecholamines		Catecholamines with α-adrenergic effects constrict renal vasculature and may reduce renal blood flow
Sodium nitroprusside	Metabolized by the kidney and excreted as thiocyanate	Toxicity from thiocyanate accumulation is more likely in CKD
Antibiotics		
Penicillin, cephalosporins, aminoglycosides, and vancomycin	Predominately dependent on renal elimination	Loading dose is unchanged, but maintenance doses need adjustment.

2. **Barbiturates, etomidate, and propofol** are highly protein bound, and in hypoalbuminemic patients, a much greater proportion will be available to reach the receptor sites. Acidosis and changes in the blood-brain barrier will further reduce induction requirements. Lower initial doses are recommended in renal failure.

3. **Opioids** are metabolized in the liver but may have a more intense and prolonged effect in patients with renal failure, particularly in hypoalbuminemic patients in whom protein binding will be reduced. Active metabolites of morphine and meperidine may prolong their actions, and accumulation of normeperidine may cause seizures. The pharmacokinetics of fentanyl, sufentanil, alfentanil, and remifentanil are unchanged in renal failure.

B. **Ionized drugs.** Drugs that are highly ionized at physiologic pH tend to be eliminated unchanged by the kidney, and their duration of action may be prolonged by renal dysfunction.

1. **Depolarizing neuromuscular blockers (NMBs).** Succinylcholine can be used safely in ESRD provided the potassium concentration is <5.5 mmol/L and repeated doses are avoided. An increase of ~0.5 mmol/L in serum potassium is observed both in ESRD and in healthy subjects.

2. **Nondepolarizing NMBs.** Traditionally, benzylisoquinolinium muscle relaxants (such as cisatracurium) are preferable in ESRD given their organ-independent metabolism. However, their metabolism is pH dependent, and acidosis in ESRD may prolong their effects. Rocuronium (an aminosteroid NMB) is excreted primarily in bile, and ~33% is excreted in urine resulting in prolonged action in renal failure. However, use of sugammadex in ESRD is becoming more

prevalent. Sugammadex is a modified gamma-cyclodexrin that binds to and encapsulates aminosteroid neuromuscular blocking agents. It is excreted unchanged in urine. Its efficacy as a reversal agent appears to be independent of excretion of the cyclodextrin-NMB complex and no evidence of recurarization has been reported in studies. In ESRD, excretion of the cyclodextrin-NMB complex is prolonged. No known adverse side effects of delayed excretion are known; however, more study in this area is warranted. Reassuringly, the cyclodextrin-NMB complex can be removed by dialysis.

3. **Cholinesterase inhibitors.** With impaired renal function, elimination of the reversal drugs is decreased and their half-lives are prolonged.

4. **Digoxin** is excreted in the urine, and patients with renal failure are at increased risk of digitalis toxicity.

VII. FUTURE CONSIDERATIONS FOR IDENTIFICATION OF PATIENTS AT RISK OF PERIOPERATIVE AKI

Neither SCr nor urine output are direct markers of kidney injury. In addition, both are delayed and insensitive biomarkers affected by many variables. A number of novel potential biomarkers have been identified that show promise, including kidney injury molecule 1 (KIM-1), interleukin 18, liver-type fatty acid-binding protein (L-FABP), **tissue inhibitor of metalloproteinase-2 (TIMP-2), insulin-like growth factor binding protein 7 (IGRBP7), and neutrophil gelatinase-associated lipocalin (NGAL).** Only TIMP-2 × IGRBP7 has entered routine clinical practice. These show great potential in identifying AKI early in which timely intervention may change the course and progression of the disease. With regards to intraoperative diagnostic technologies, research is ongoing into development of real-time GFR monitoring using novel fluorescent GFR tracer agents.

Suggested Readings

Abuelo JG. Normotensive ischemic acute renal failure. *N Engl J Med.* 2007;357:797-805.

Bito H, Ikeuchi Y, Ikeda K. Effects of low-flow sevoflurane anesthesia on renal function: comparison with high-flow sevoflurane anesthesia and low-flow isoflurane anesthesia. *Anesthesiology.* 1997;86(6):1231-1237.

Bugaj JE, Dorshow RB. Pre-clinical toxicity evaluation of MB-102, a novel fluorescent tracer agent for real-time measurement of glomerular filtration rate. *Regul Toxicol Pharmacol.* 2015;72(1):26-38.

Cammu G, Van Vlem B, van den Heuvel M, et al. Dialysability of sugammadex and its complex with rocuronium in intensive care patients with severe renal impairment. *Br J Anaesth.* 2012;109(3):382-390.

Colson P, Ryckwaert F, Coriat P. Renin angiotensin system antagonists and anesthesia. *Anesth Analg.* 1999;89:1143-1155.

Craig RG, Hunter JM. Recent developments in the perioperative management of adult patients with chronic kidney disease. *Br J Anaesth.* 2008;101:296-310.

Craig RG, Hunter JM. Recent developments in the perioperative management of adult patients with chronic kidney disease. *Br J Anaesth.* 2008;101(3):296-310.

Futier E, Lefrant JY, Guinot PG, et al. Effect of individualized vs standard blood pressure management strategies on postoperative organ dysfunction among high-risk patients undergoing major surgery: a randomized clinical trial. *J Am Med Assoc.* 2017;318(14):1346-1357.

Hirsch IA, Tomlinson DL, Slogoff S, Keats AS. The overstated risk of preoperative hypokalemia. *Anesth Analg.* 1988;67(2):131-136.

Khwaja A. KDIGO clinical practice guidelines for acute kidney injury. *Nephron Clin Pract.* 2012;120(4):c179-c184.

Kunst G, Klein AA. Peri-operative anaesthetic myocardial preconditioning and protection – cellular mechanisms and clinical relevance in cardiac anaesthesia. *Anaesthesia.* 2015;70(4):467-482.

Massoth C, Zarbock A, Meersch M. Risk stratification for targeted AKI prevention after surgery: biomarkers and bundled interventions. *Semin Nephrol.* 2019;39(5):454-461.

Mazze RI, Jamison RL. Low-flow (1 l/min) sevoflurane: is it safe? *Anesthesiology.* 1997;86(6):1225-1227.

McKinlay J, Tyson E, Forni LG. Renal complications of anaesthesia. *Anaesthesia.* 2018;73(suppl 1):85-94.

Merten GJ, Burgess P, Gray LV. Prevention of contrast induced nephropathy with sodium bicarbonate. *J Am Med Assoc.* 2004;291:2328-2334.

Nieuwenhuijs-Moeke GJ, Nieuwenhuijs VB, Seelen MAJ, et al. Propofol-based anaesthesia versus sevoflurane-based anaesthesia for living donor kidney transplantation: results of the VAPOR-1 randomized controlled trial. *Br J Anaesth.* 2017;118(5):720-732.

Ong Sio LCL, Dela Cruz RGC, Bautista AF. Sevoflurane and renal function: a meta-analysis of randomized trials. *Med Gas Res.* 2017;7(3):186-193.

Pépin MN, Bouchard J, Legault L, Ethier J. Diagnostic performance of fractional excretion of urea and fractional excretion of sodium in the evaluations of patients with acute kidney injury with or without diuretic treatment. *Am J Kidney Dis.* 2007;50(4):566-573.

Petroni KC, Cohen NH. Continuous renal replacement therapy: anesthetic implications. *Anesth Analg.* 2002;94:1288-1297.

Ronco C, Bellomo R, Kellum JA. Acute kidney injury. *Lancet.* 2019;394(10212):1949-1964.

Schmid S, Jungwirth B. Anaesthesia for renal transplant surgery: an update. *Eur J Anaesthesiol.* 2013;29:552-558.

Sear JW. Kidney dysfunction in the postoperative period. *Br J Anaesth.* 2005;95:20-32.

Sladen RN. Renal physiology. In: Miller R, ed. *Anesthesiology.* 7th ed. Churchill Livingstone; 2010:441-476.

Staals LM, Snoeck MM, Driessen JJ, Flockton EA, Heeringa M, Hunter JM. Multicentre, parallel-group, comparative trial evaluating the efficacy and safety of sugammadex in patients with end-stage renal failure or normal renal function. *Br J Anaesth.* 2008;101(4):492-497. doi:10.1093/bja/aen216

Sterns RH. Disorders of plasma sodium – causes, consequences, and correction. *N Engl J Med.* 2015;372(1):55-65.

Suneja M, Kumar AB. Obesity and perioperative acute kidney injury: a focused review. *J Crit Care.* 2014;29:694.e1-694.e6.

Thakar CV. Perioperative acute kidney injury. *Adv Chronic Kidney Dis.* 2013;20:67-75.

Thapa S, Brull SJ. Succinylcholine-induced hyperkalemia in patients with renal failure: an old question revisited. *Anesth Analg.* 2000;91(1):237-241. doi:10.1097/00000539-200007000-00044

Wagener G, Brentjens TE. Anesthetic concerns in patients presenting with renal failure. *Anesthesiol Clin.* 2010;28:39-54.

Weldon BC, Monk TG. The patient at risk for acute renal failure. *Anesthesiol Clin North Am.* 2000;18(4):705-737.

Wong KC, Schafer PG, Schultz JR. Hypokalemia and anesthetic. *Anesth Analg.* 1993;77(6):1238-1260. Published correction appears in *Anesth Analg.* 1994;78(5):1035.

Zarbock A, Koyner JL, Hoste EAJ, Kellum JA. Update on perioperative acute kidney injury. *Anesth Analg.* 2018;127(5):1236-1245.

6 Specific Considerations With Liver Disease

Mark Abraham and Jerome Crowley

I. HEPATIC ANATOMY

A. Liver structure

1. The anatomic unit of the liver is **lobule.** The lobule is composed of hexagonal plates of hepatocytes and portal triads (terminal portal vein, hepatic artery, and bile duct branch) surrounding a central hepatic vein.

2. Hepatocytes are classified by their position in relation to their portal triad. Those closest to the triad are labeled **Zone 1 cells (periportal).** These cells receive the most oxygen and nutrients and are responsible for most nitrogen metabolism, oxidation, and gluconeogenesis. **Zone 2** is a transitional area. **Zone 3 hepatocytes (pericentral)** are the farthest from the triad and are at the greatest risk for ischemic injury.

B. Hepatic blood supply. The liver comprises only 2% of the total body mass, but it receives 20% to 25% of the cardiac output.

1. The **hepatic artery** supplies 25% of the total liver blood flow and 50% of the liver's oxygen requirement.

2. The **portal vein** drains the stomach, spleen, pancreas, and intestine. It supplies 75% of the hepatic blood flow and 50% of hepatic oxygen.

3. **Total hepatic blood flow** depends greatly on venous return from the preportal organs. Flow in the hepatic artery is regulated by sympathetic tone and local adenosine concentration and is inversely related to portal vein flow (PVF). A reduction in PVF will lead to an increased adenosine concentration in the liver, which causes local arteriole dilation and an increase in hepatic artery flow. Total hepatic blood flow may be reduced in diseases causing increased hepatic vascular resistance (eg, cirrhosis, infiltrative disease as in metastatic liver disease, and Budd-Chiari syndrome).

II. HEPATIC FUNCTION

A. Synthesis and storage

1. **Proteins.** The normal adult liver produces 12 to 15 g of protein per day including the following:

   a. **Albumin** is manufactured exclusively in the liver and has a half-life of approximately 20 days. It comprises 50% of all circulating plasma proteins and is the most important drug-binding protein, especially for organic acids such as penicillins and barbiturates. Albumin contributes to oncotic pressure and also serves as a carrier protein for bilirubin and hormones.

   b. α_1**-acid glycoprotein** is an "acute phase reactant" and is responsible for binding basic drugs such as amide local anesthetics, propranolol, and opioids.

   c. **Pseudocholinesterase** is responsible for the degradation of succinylcholine, mivacurium, and ester-type local anesthetics. In the presence of severely depressed hepatocellular function or a genetically mediated enzyme deficiency, decreased plasma levels may cause profound clinical effects.

    d. All proteinaceous **clotting factors** are produced in the liver with the exception of factor VIII, which is produced in the vascular endothelium. Synthesis of factors II (prothrombin), VII, IX, and X as well as proteins C, S, and Z is vitamin K dependent; deficiency of vitamin K or disturbances of liver function may lead to deficiencies of clotting factors and excess bleeding. Factor VII has the shortest half-life (4-6 hours) and therefore declines at nearly the same rate as protein C (9 hours). Because factor VII is located in the extrinsic pathway, which is assessed by the prothrombin time (PT), this early decline in the factor VII activity prolongs the PT even though other pathways have not yet been affected. Factors II, IX, and X have half-lives of approximately 60 hours, 24 hours, and 36 hours, respectively. Consequently, it takes 4 to 6 days before their activities are at a minimum level, and an antithrombotic effect is achieved that correlates with the international normalized ratio (INR).

2. Carbohydrates. The liver is actively involved in the homeostatic regulation of plasma glucose levels **(glycogen synthesis** and **gluconeogenesis).** The normal liver can store enough glycogen to provide glucose during a fast of 12 to 24 hours. After that time, glucose is derived by gluconeogenesis from amino acids, glycerol, and lactate.

3. Lipids. Most of the body's lipoproteins, as well as cholesterol and phospholipids, are formed in the liver.

4. Heme and bile

    a. The liver is the primary erythropoietic organ of the fetus and continues to be a major site of hematopoiesis until approximately 2 months of age. In healthy adults, the liver is responsible for 20% of heme production. Abnormalities in **heme synthesis** can result in porphyria.

    b. The liver forms approximately 800 mL of bile per day. **Bile** salts are detergents that aid in absorbing, transporting, and excreting lipids. Bile also carries metabolic waste products and drug metabolites to the intestine from the liver. As an emulsifier, bile facilitates fat absorption by the small intestine. Failure to produce or release bile causes jaundice and an inability to absorb fat and fat-soluble vitamins (A, D, E, and K) and can result in steatorrhea, vitamin deficiencies, and coagulopathy.

B. Degradation

1. Proteins. The liver is the major site of protein degradation where amino acids are broken down through a process that generates urea for the elimination of ammonia. Patients with liver disease may lack the ability to form urea, resulting in rapidly rising plasma ammonia levels and hepatic encephalopathy.

2. Steroid hormones. Cholesterol is degraded principally by the liver, and its by-products serve as substrates for the production of bile salts, steroid hormones, and cell membranes. The liver also serves as the major site of steroid hormone degradation, and **hepatic failure results in steroid excess.** Elevations of serum aldosterone and cortisol result in increased resorption of sodium and water, and loss of potassium in the urine, contributing to the edema, ascites, and electrolyte abnormalities frequently seen with liver disease. Decreased metabolism of estrogens and impaired conversion to androgens causes other clinical stigmata of liver disease including spider angiomata, gynecomastia, palmar erythema, and testicular atrophy.

3. **Heme and bile.** Bilirubin that is bound to albumin is delivered to hepatocytes where it then undergoes conjugation with glucuronic acid, which makes it water soluble. These products are excreted within the bile and are eliminated via the feces or urine.

C. **Drug metabolism**

1. The liver has a dual blood supply, receiving blood from the hepatic artery and the portal veins. The hepatic extraction ratio (HER) is a measure of the efficiency of the liver in removing drugs from hepatic inflow. It is defined as the fraction of a drug concentration flowing into the liver that is removed through hepatic elimination and metabolism. High-extraction drugs are absorbed from the gut and delivered to the liver, where they may be metabolized before reaching the systemic circulation (first-pass metabolism). Drugs with a high extraction ratio and significant first-pass metabolism have low oral bioavailability.

2. **Hepatic clearance** = HER × hepatic blood flow rate. Some drugs are extensively metabolized by the liver and have an HER of close to 1.0 (propofol). In these cases, hepatic metabolism depends predominantly on hepatic blood flow, and moderate changes in hepatic function have little effect on clearance. Other drugs have an HER of less than 1.0, and clearance depends on both hepatic function and changes in hepatic blood flow.

3. **Protein binding.** The degree of protein binding depends on the specific drug's affinity for protein binding and the protein concentration. Decreased concentrations of plasma proteins, as often seen in liver disease, will result in a greater proportion of unbound drug. Only free, unbound drug is pharmacologically active and is available for conversion to a less active form. A decrease in plasma proteins may therefore affect the potency and/or elimination of a drug.

4. **Volume of distribution** is often increased in patients with liver disease, and **portal-systemic shunting** permits orally administered drugs to bypass the liver, reducing the first-pass effect. Both can alter drug effects and metabolism.

5. **Enzyme induction/cytochrome p450** enzymes are produced in the liver and are responsible for much drug metabolism. Certain drugs such as barbiturates, ethanol, and phenytoin induce cytochrome p450 enzymes. Induction of cytochrome p450 increases tolerance to a drug's effect and tolerance to other drugs that are also metabolized by the cytochrome p450 system.

6. Two steps are involved in **hepatic drug elimination:**

   a. **Phase I** reactions change a compound's structure via oxidation, reduction, or hydrolysis (primarily via cytochrome p450 enzymes). The products of this phase may be metabolically active. Drugs that have a high affinity for the p450 complex (eg, ciprofloxacin) may decrease the metabolism of concurrently administered drugs.

   b. **Phase II** reactions may or may not follow Phase I reactions and are enzymatically enhanced conjugations with glucuronide, sulfate, taurine, or glycine. These conjugations increase the water solubility of the metabolite for excretion via urine.

III. **METABOLISM OF ANESTHETICS**

A. **Intravenous anesthetics**

1. **Induction agents**

   a. **Propofol** is metabolized by the liver (HER ~ 1) to water-soluble compounds that are excreted by the kidneys. Extrahepatic metabolism of propofol also contributes to total propofol clearance. Termination of action of propofol is largely due to redistribution, so propofol is a reasonable anesthetic in patients with liver disease.

b. **Barbiturates** have a duration of action that is determined by redistribution and hepatic metabolism and may have prolonged effects in patients with liver disease. Hypoalbuminemia, as seen in patients with altered liver function, may reduce protein binding and increases the free active fraction of these drugs. Therefore, barbiturates must be titrated carefully in patients with liver disease.

c. **Ketamine** is metabolized by the hepatic microsomal enzyme system to norketamine, which has approximately 30% of the activity of the parent drug. Ketamine has an HER of approximately 1.

d. **Etomidate** is metabolized by the liver through ester hydrolysis to inactive metabolites. Similar to ketamine, etomidate has a high HER, so clearance is affected by conditions that reduce hepatic blood flow. Recovery from an initial induction dose is primarily due to rapid redistribution. Etomidate may be considered in acute liver failure in order to maintain cerebral perfusion pressure.

2. **Benzodiazepines and opioids** are metabolized primarily by the liver and have significantly increased half-lives in patients with liver disease. Additionally, they have increased potency in cases of hypoalbuminemia as these drugs, which are usually protein bound, are now free in the plasma resulting in higher drug levels. This issue may confound the clinical picture of hepatic encephalopathy and should be titrated carefully. Remifentanil may be an appropriate choice as its clearance is not affected by liver dysfunction.

3. **Neuromuscular blocking agents.** Patients with liver disease often demonstrate **resistance to nondepolarizing neuromuscular blockers**, probably because of increased volume of distribution or increased neuromuscular receptors. However, a slower elimination time may decrease the requirement for maintenance dosing.

a. **Intermediate-acting neuromuscular blocking drugs, vecuronium** and **rocuronium**, are highly dependent on hepatobiliary excretion and metabolism (both are excreted, 50% unchanged, in the bile). This translates to a decreased clearance and a prolonged effect in patients with liver disease. Vecuronium undergoes hepatic metabolism to several compounds, one of which is 3-desacetylvecuronium that has 50% of vecuronium's neuromuscular blocker activity. **Cisatracurium** and atracurium are degraded via Hofmann elimination and are unaffected by liver disease.

b. Succinylcholine and mivacurium (not available in the United States) are completely metabolized in the plasma by pseudocholinesterase. Cholinesterase production may be depressed in severe liver disease, and its duration may be prolonged in patients with hepatic dysfunction.

IV. LIVER DISEASE

A. **Liver disease** is classified by time course and severity.

1. **Parenchymal**

a. **Acute hepatocellular injury** has many etiologies, including viral infection (hepatitis A, B, C, D, and E; Epstein-Barr virus; cytomegalovirus; herpes simplex virus; ECHO virus; and coxsackievirus), acute shock, congestion from heart failure, drugs, chemicals and poisons (including alcohol, halothane, phenytoin, propylthiouracil, isoniazid, tetracycline, and acetaminophen), and inborn errors of metabolism (eg, Wilson disease and α_1-antitrypsin deficiency).

  b. **Chronic parenchymal disease** may be associated with varying degrees of functional impairment. **Cirrhosis** may result from many insults, including chronic active hepatitis, alcoholism, hemochromatosis, primary biliary cirrhosis, and congenital disorders. End-stage hepatic fibrosis causes significant resistance to portal blood flow, leading to portal hypertension and esophageal varices. Further complications from the combination of portal hypertension and decreased hepatic function include ascites, coagulopathy, gastrointestinal bleeding, and encephalopathy.

2. **Cholestasis** occurs most frequently in cholelithiasis and acute or chronic cholecystitis. Primary biliary cirrhosis and primary sclerosing cholangitis also begin as cholestatic diseases, ultimately leading to parenchymal damage and liver failure. **Hyperbilirubinemia** is an important marker for hepatobiliary disease. **Unconjugated hyperbilirubinemia** is due to excess bilirubin production (eg, massive transfusion, absorption of large hematomas, or hemolysis) or impaired uptake of unconjugated bilirubin by the hepatocyte (eg, Gilbert syndrome). **Conjugated hyperbilirubinemia** generally occurs with hepatocellular disease (eg, alcoholic or viral hepatitis and cirrhosis), disease of the small bile ducts (eg, primary biliary cirrhosis and Dubin-Johnson syndrome), or obstruction of the extrahepatic bile ducts (eg, pancreatic carcinoma, cholangiocarcinoma, and gallstones).

B. **Manifestations of liver disease**

1. **Central nervous system.** Hepatic dysfunction can lead to **encephalopathy.** Although the exact pathogenesis is unclear, impaired neurotransmission, presence of intrinsic γ-aminobutyric acid-ergic substances, and altered cerebral metabolism may be involved in its pathogenesis. **Ammonia levels** are often elevated in encephalopathic patients but do not correlate with the severity or outcome of encephalopathy. Signs may vary from sleep disturbances to the presence of asterixis or coma. Patients with severe acute liver failure often present with a rapidly progressive encephalopathy complicated by **cerebral edema.** Elevated intracranial pressure must be aggressively managed to prevent cerebral ischemia. Extreme hyponatremia or its overly aggressive treatment may lead to fatal osmotic demyelination syndrome (also called **central pontine myelinolysis).** Changes in mental status and increased sensitivity to sedatives mandate caution in dosing premedications.

2. **Cardiovascular system**

   a. Patients with advanced liver disease exhibit a **hyperdynamic circulatory state** with an elevated **cardiac output**, resting tachycardia, and **decreased systemic vascular resistance.** Elevated levels of nitric oxide, glucagon, and prostaglandins are thought to be responsible for the arteriolar vasodilation. **Arteriovenous shunts**, such as spider angiomata in the skin, can be present in almost all vascular beds. Severe liver disease can lead to portopulmonary hypertension, which can result in right ventricular dysfunction and hemodynamic collapse on induction of anesthesia.

   b. Patients with advanced liver failure also have a reduced effective intravascular volume due to vasodilation and portosystemic shunting. In addition, hypoalbuminemia, increased levels of aldosterone, and inappropriate secretion of antidiuretic hormone all lead to **increased total body fluid volume** that worsens ascites and edema/anasarca.

c. **Alcoholic cardiomyopathy (ACM)** should always be considered in patients with a history of alcohol abuse. ACM is characterized by an increase in myocardial mass, dilation of the ventricles, and wall thinning. Changes in ventricular function may depend on the stage of the disease, in that asymptomatic ACM is associated with diastolic dysfunction, whereas systolic dysfunction is a common finding in symptomatic ACM patients characterized by a dilated left ventricle, normal or reduced left ventricular wall thickness, and increased left ventricular mass.

3. **Respiratory system**
    a. **Airway protection** is a major concern in patients with liver disease. Patients with the typical stigmata of advanced disease have ascites (increased abdominal pressure—causing a reduction in functional residual capacity) and encephalopathy (altered mental status), which can affect their ability to protect their airway and should be considered at increased risk for aspiration. In addition, there is an increased risk of aspiration due to delayed gastric emptying. Definitive airway protection with rapid sequence induction and intubation is frequently advisable when general anesthesia is required.
    b. **Chronic hypoxemia** results from many causes. Massive ascites and pleural effusions lead to atelectasis and restrictive lung physiology. Diminished hypoxic pulmonary vasoconstriction results in ventilation perfusion mismatch; intrapulmonary shunting can be significant (10%-40%). Pulmonary hypertension can coexist with portal hypertension and can produce right-sided heart failure. The hepatopulmonary syndrome is a triad of liver disease, increased alveolar-arterial oxygen gradient, and intrapulmonary vascular dilatations. The syndrome of platypnea-orthodeoxia may be seen (postural hypoxemia and dyspnea induced by upright posture) as the presence of a hyperdynamic circulation, and low pulmonary resistance results in the rapid transit of blood through the lungs and potentiates the transit of deoxygenated blood to the systemic circulation. Because of gravity, shifting of blood to the dilated precapillary beds of the lung bases results in an increased hypoxemic dyspnea when the patient is in the upright position. The platypnea-orthodeoxia may not always be apparent as anatomic effects on respiration from pleural effusions and ascites may worsen breathing in the supine position. If the patient is symptomatic, arterial blood gas analysis may be necessary to determine the degree of hypoxia.

4. **Gastrointestinal system**
    a. The increased pressure in the portal system due to increased volume of blood through these vessels or increased resistance (scarring, fibrosis) to portal blood flow results in **portal hypertension**, splenomegaly, and splanchnic venous congestion. This increases collateral circulation, which is manifested as hemorrhoids, esophageal varices, and dilated abdominal wall veins (caput medusae). **Ascites** is due to splanchnic venous congestions coupled with hypoalbuminemia and decreased oncotic pressure. Ascites may increase the risk of abdominal wound dehiscence, abdominal wall herniation, and respiratory compromise. Ascites can be managed with diuretics, with careful attention to electrolytes and renal function. If a large volume of ascites is uncontrolled prior to surgery, paracentesis may be advisable. Replacement of ascites with albumin, colloids, or blood products is advisable to reduce the risk of hepatorenal syndrome (HRS).

    b. **Variceal bleeding** can progress rapidly to hemorrhagic shock. After volume resuscitation, treatment consists of vasopressin, somatostatin, β-adrenergic blockade, sclerotherapy, or endoscopic ligation.

5. **Renal system**
    a. Intravascular volume depletion may produce **prerenal azotemia.** The blood urea nitrogen level may be deceptively low because of the liver's inability to synthesize urea from ammonia.
    b. **Water and electrolyte balance** is complicated by frequent use of diuretics. Metabolic alkalosis, hypokalemia, and hyponatremia (despite total body sodium overload) are common in patients with hepatic disease. Hyponatremia may lead to seizures and worsening of hepatic encephalopathy; caution should be used when treating hyponatremia as rapid correction may lead to central pontine myelinosis. Correction of hyponatremia is typically done with fluid restriction and discontinuation of diuretics.
    c. **HRS** is characterized by increased renal vascular resistance, oliguria, and renal failure in the presence of hepatic failure. The sequelae include decreased renal blood flow, sodium retention, and increased sensitivity to nonsteroidal anti-inflammatory medications. The diagnosis is one of exclusion and is based on clinical criteria. Two subtypes of HRS are defined. Type 1 is at least a twofold increase in serum creatinine (to greater than 2.5 mg/dL) in a period of less than 2 weeks, It is often associated with significant oliguria. Type 2 is less severe and usually represents a resistance to diuretics. Normal renal function may return after liver transplantation or if liver failure resolves. Maintenance of normal intravascular volume and renal perfusion pressure is important to preserve renal function in cirrhotic patients.

6. **Coagulopathy** is caused by several factors.
    a. **Synthesis of clotting factors** (II, VII, IX, and X) as well as that of endogenous anticoagulants (proteins C, S, and Z) is impaired in liver failure.
    b. **Cholestasis** causes impaired absorption of fat and fat-soluble vitamins (A, D, E, and K). **Vitamin K,** produced in the intestinal mucosa, is an important cofactor in the synthesis of clotting factors II, VII, IX, and X.
    c. **Thrombocytopenia** secondary to hypersplenism, alcohol-induced bone marrow failure, and consumption is frequently seen.
    d. **Preoperative correction of clotting abnormalities** with fresh frozen plasma (FFP) or vitamin K should be performed as necessary. In emergency situations, vitamin K should be avoided due to its prolonged time of onset (approximately 8 hours). In these situations, FFP can be administered, and cryoprecipitate, DDAVP (1-desamino-8-d-arginine vasopressin), factor VIIa, and platelets should be considered for refractory situations. Regional anesthesia may not be appropriate in the setting of liver failure or anticipated liver failure. The potential for postoperative coagulopathy should be taken into account before placing an epidural. Invasive monitoring can help evaluate and guide volume status. The importance of adequate venous access for intraoperative infusion of crystalloid, colloid, blood products, and vasoactive drugs should not be underestimated.

7. **Nutritional deficiency,** as manifested by the forms of protein–energy malnutrition marasmus and kwashiorkor, can be part of liver disease, especially in alcoholics. Nutritional deficiency is a risk factor for increased

morbidity and mortality postoperatively and should be treated with supplementation high in carbohydrate/lipid content and low in amino acid content to prevent worsening of hepatic encephalopathy. Nutritional supplementation is especially important in alcoholics and should include vitamin B$_1$ supplementation. If surgery is not urgent, nutritional status should be optimized preoperatively. Due to the low risk of intravenous thiamine, it should be administered before any dextrose in patients presented with any concern for nutritional deficiency.

8. **Glycemic control** depends heavily on the liver. **Hypoglycemia** may occur in end-stage hepatic insufficiency, during the anhepatic phase of liver transplantation, or in liver failure that may accompany an episode of severe circulatory shock. Close monitoring of blood glucose levels should be performed frequently, and glucose-containing solutions should be administered as necessary. Severe hepatic insufficiency leads to diminished **glycogen** stores, requiring gluconeogenesis to maintain normoglycemia. **Gluconeogenesis** is also impaired in severe liver disease and alcoholism.

V. SURGICAL RISK IN PATIENTS WITH LIVER DISEASE
A. Mortality
1. Reported mortality rates in patients with cirrhosis undergoing various elective noncardiac and nontransplant surgical procedures range from **6%** to **27%** (in comparison with 1.1% for noncirrhotic patients). Wide range of mortality is related to **severity of the disease, type of surgery, patient demographics, and expertise of the surgical, anesthetic, and ICU teams.**
B. Risk assessment
1. Preoperative risk assessment can help predict survival and may reduce perioperative morbidity and mortality.
2. The **Child-Turcotte-Pugh (CTP)** classification was designed to evaluate the risk of surgical portosystemic shunt procedures and was subsequently found to predict long-term survival in patients with cirrhosis. This risk stratification system includes **ascites, bilirubin level, albumin level, nutritional status, encephalopathy, and PT (Table 6.1).** CTP is considered to be the best prognostic indicator for overall mortality.

TABLE 6.1	Modified Child-Pugh Score		
	Points		
Parameter	1	2	3
Albumin (g/dL)	>3.5	2.8-3.5	<2.8
Bilirubin (mg/dL)[a]	<2.0	2.0-3.0	>3.0
Ascites	Absent	Slight	Moderate
Encephalopathy	Absent	Grades I and II	Grades III and IV
PT prolongation (s)	<4.0	4.0-6.0	>6.0

Class A, 5-6 points; class B, 7-9 points; class C, 10-15 points.
PT, prothrombin time.
[a]For primary biliary cirrhosis: 1 point for bilirubin <4.0 mg/dL, 2 points for bilirubin 4-10 mg/dL, and 3 points for bilirubin more than 10 mg/dL.

3. Other predictors of perioperative risk include **type of surgery**, presence of **sepsis, reoperation**, and **elective versus emergent** surgery. Procedures involving a laparotomy (greater reduction in hepatic arterial blood flow) or other intra-abdominal incisions (open cholecystectomy, gastric surgery, and colectomies), cardiac surgery, or those associated with increased blood loss have particularly high mortality rates.

4. The **model for end-stage liver disease (MELD)** is a prognostic scoring system originally designed for predicting 3-month mortality following transjugular intrahepatic portosystemic shunt (TIPS) insertion. It was subsequently found to be useful for predicting mortality of patients on the liver transplantation waiting list. The score is calculated based on a patient's serum bilirubin, serum creatinine, and INR (**Table 6.2**). A newer refinement to the MELD scoring system, MELD-sodium (MELD-Na), has been shown to be better at predicting overall 1 year mortality compared to both CTP and MELD scores.

C. **Preoperative assessment**
   1. Routine screening of liver function with lab tests has not proven to be useful when applied to a general surgical population.
   2. A careful **history** and **physical examination** are the best screening tools in the preoperative period. Symptoms of concern include a history of jaundice, pruritus, malaise, and anorexia. Exposure to drugs, alcohol, and other toxins should be considered. Physical examination may reveal stigmata of liver disease such as hepatosplenomegaly, ascites, peripheral edema, spider angiomata, testicular atrophy, caput medusae, hemorrhoids, asterixis, gynecomastia, and temporal wasting. In addition, frequency of paracentesis, date of last paracentesis, hospitalizations for decompensation, and any history of a TIPS should be identified preoperatively.

TABLE 6.2	MELD Score and MELD-Na

MELD = 3.78[Ln Serum Bilirubin (mg/dL)] + 11.2[Ln INR] + 9.57[Ln Serum Creatinine (mg/dL)] + 6.43
MELD-Na = MELD − Na − (0.025 × MELD × (140 − Na)) + 140

In interpreting the MELD score in hospitalized patients, the 3-month mortality is:
- 40 or more—100% mortality
- 30-39—83% mortality
- 20-29—76% mortality
- 10-19—27% mortality
- <10—4% mortality

In interpreting the MELD-Na score in hospitalized patients, the 3-month mortality is:
- 32 or more—65%-66% mortality
- 27-31—27%-32% mortality
- 23-26—14%-15% mortality
- 21-22—7-10% mortality
- 17-20—3-4% mortality
- <17—less than 2% mortality

The maximum score given for MELD is 40. All values higher than 40 are given a score of 40. If the patient has been dialyzed twice within the last 7 d, then the value for serum creatinine used should be 4.0. Any value <1 is given a value of 1 (ie, if bilirubin is 0.8, a value of 1.0 is used).
INR, international normalized ratio; MELD, model for end-stage liver disease; MELD-Na, MELD-sodium.

3. **Liver imaging** is essential to characterize extent of injury. CT and MRI are preferable modalities to evaluate liver architecture, vasculature, presence of hepatocellular carcinoma, and portal hypertension. Ultrasound with Doppler may be used if there is a contraindication to CT or MRI.

4. Any history of **gastrointestinal bleeding** needs to be investigated and recent results of esophagogastroduodenoscopy are necessary, particularly for major operations.

5. **Identify comorbid conditions.** Presence of cardiac disease, chronic kidney disease, and diabetes are common in patients with liver disease and may affect anesthetic management.

6. **Laboratory tests** should be considered for the patient in whom liver disease is suspected (complete blood count, basic metabolic panel, bilirubin, transaminases, alkaline phosphatase, albumin, total protein, PT, and hepatitis serologies). In addition to liver synthetic function, progressive liver disease is also associated with renal dysfunction and recent relevant laboratory results should be checked.

7. **ECG, chest radiograph, and evaluation of the myocardial function** should be considered when indicated based on age, disease severity, and duration. If significant limitation of exercise is present, transthoracic echocardiography should be considered to identify coexisting cardiac disease as well as potential portopulmonary syndrome (right ventricular systolic pressure) and hepatopulmonary syndrome (evidence of extracardiac shunts on contrast echocardiography).

8. **Duration** and severity of liver disease have general prognostic implications, and **percutaneous liver biopsy** may be indicated to establish a diagnosis before elective surgery.

D. Every effort should be made to **correct abnormalities before surgery**, including coagulopathies, poorly controlled ascites, volume and electrolyte imbalances, renal dysfunction, encephalopathy, thrombocytopenia, and inadequate nutritional status.

VI. ANESTHESIA IN PATIENTS WITH LIVER DISEASE

A. Planning the anesthetic must take into account the surgical procedure, type and severity of liver disease, and alterations to hepatic blood flow due to anesthetics. Meticulous attention must be paid to **maintaining adequate hepatic perfusion** and oxygen delivery. Both **general and regional anesthesia** techniques can decrease total hepatic blood flow. Episodes of perioperative hepatic ischemia (due to surgical manipulation or anesthetics) can exacerbate preexisting liver disease. Hypotension, hemorrhage, and vasopressors can compromise hepatic oxygenation delivery, resulting in increased postoperative hepatic dysfunction. Surgical traction and patient positioning can compromise hepatic blood flow. Positive-pressure ventilation and positive end-expiratory pressure may cause deleterious effects in hepatic venous pressure, resulting in decreased cardiac output and total hepatic blood flow. **Hyperventilation** should be avoided because hypocarbia can independently reduce hepatic blood flow.

B. Many factors must be considered when choosing an anesthetic agent in the setting of liver failure such as drug distribution and metabolism, protein binding, and often concurrent renal insufficiency. Benzodiazepines should be avoided to avoid oversedation. **Propofol is the preferred induction agent** because of its redistribution, but can cause hypotension and vasodilation that may reduce hepatic perfusion. Maintenance with volatile agents is preferred because they are mainly eliminated via the respiratory system. Older halogenated compounds are absorbed more readily because of their lipophilicity and require more hepatic metabolism than newer agents such as **sevoflurane and desflurane. Processed EEG monitoring** should be considered as duration of action of various agents may be affected to altered liver metabolism and renal impairment.

C. Neuromuscular blockade consideration is important given the different metabolism of various drugs noted earlier. Cisatracurium and atracurium are safe as they undergo Hoffman elimination. Considerations for renal dysfunction when must be assessed when using vecuronium and rocuronium. Mean time of recovery of TOF (train-of-four) ratio >0.9 in patients with liver dysfunction is not significantly different compared to patients with normal liver function with use of sugammadex reversal for rocuronium. Due to reduction of pseudocholinesterases, the action of succinylcholine may be prolonged in patients with liver disease. Patients with cirrhosis may exhibit a significantly elevated cardiac output, which will shorten the onset time of neuromuscular blockade agents; however, this is variable and should not change decision-making around choice of agents for rapid sequence intubation.

D. Caution must be exercised when **regional anesthesia** is considered in a patient with liver disease. Coagulopathy and thrombocytopenia put these patients at a higher risk for epidural bleeding and hematoma formation. However, in a patient with well-compensated liver disease and a reasonably normal coagulation profile and platelet count, regional anesthesia may be appropriate and may even be beneficial, but this must be considered on a case-by-case basis. Particularly with epidural placement, postoperative transfusion of FFP or administration of vitamin K may be necessary to remove the epidural catheter, and this risk should be discussed with the surgical team. Additionally, there is also a theoretical concern of hypotension with epidural anesthesia; more recent studies have demonstrated no difference in postoperative fluid administration, vasopressor support, and end-organ dysfunction with use of epidural anesthesia in liver resection.

E. Analgesia in patients with liver disease can be challenging due to altered drug metabolism and alterations in mental status. **Acetaminophen is deemed safe**; however, the dose must be reduced in patients with chronic liver disease. (Total daily dose less than 2000 mg is considered safe.) **Nonsteroidal anti-inflammatory drugs (NSAIDs) should be avoided** due to increased risk of renal injury and gastrointestinal bleeding. Additionally, NSAIDs may exacerbate coagulopathies associated with liver disease. **Long-acting opiates should be avoided** if possible. Measured doses of shorter-acting opiates such as fentanyl are tolerated in cirrhotic patients. Opioid-induced constipation may exacerbate encephalopathy in patients with liver disease. Coadministration of laxatives is imperative.

F. Sufficient **venous access** is of paramount importance, especially in surgery involving the liver parenchyma. **Large-bore peripheral intravenous cannulas** are inserted before or after the induction of anesthesia for major surgery (often 14 gauge or larger). In patients with insufficient peripheral access, **large-bore central venous catheters** (ie, 8.5F single-lumen or 12F double-lumen catheters) may be inserted. Universal precautions are mandatory given the high risk of infection in this patient population.

G. Invasive monitoring is also an important component of anesthetic planning. An **arterial catheter** facilitates blood sampling for monitoring serial blood gases, glucose, and electrolytes and is needed for measuring arterial blood pressure. It is considered routine in major surgery for patients with end-stage liver disease. **Central venous catheterization** is indicated for pressure monitoring and rapid drug administration into the central circulation. **Pulmonary artery catheters** may help guide fluid and vasopressor therapy in some patients. Skillful line placement is important in coagulopathic patients. Ultrasonographic visualization of the vein before or during cannulation will reduce the incidence of carotid arterial puncture and the number of needle passes needed to cannulate the jugular vein.

H. Transesophageal echocardiography (TEE) may be safely performed if clinically indicated in patients with liver disease with a low risk of bleeding provided that any varicies are grade II or better. Risk/benefit of a TEE must certainly be considered in this patient population but may be beneficial in patients who are at a high likelihood of hemodynamic deterioration (such as liver transplant or emergent surgery in a cirrhotic patient).

I. A low threshold for performing a **rapid sequence induction** should exist for these patients given their elevated intra-abdominal pressure and increased risk of aspiration.

J. Other physiologic variables that should be taken into consideration include urine output, body temperature, blood sugar levels, electrolyte disturbances, and coagulation status.

K. Proper **postoperative care** and the timing of **extubation** for patients presenting with severe comorbidities should also be considered.

L. **Surgical considerations for the anesthesiologist during procedures on the liver.** Excessive bleeding and transfusion requirements have been correlated with increased postoperative morbidity. Management must focus on the balance between reducing blood loss while maintaining adequate liver perfusion. Surgical techniques for hepatic resection and other procedures on the liver have been developed to decrease blood loss. **Total hepatic vascular exclusion** (TVE), the **Pringle maneuver** (PM), **low central venous pressure** (CVP) **anesthesia, and venovenous bypass** are four such techniques.

1. TVE consists of clamping the hepatic inflow vessels (portal vein and hepatic artery) to the liver as well as the outflow vessels (inferior vena cava and suprahepatic inferior vena cava). This can have profound deleterious effects on venous return and the hemodynamics of the patient. This also results in a significant amount of warm ischemic time to the liver and may increase postoperative hepatic dysfunction.

2. The PM consists of intermittent clamping of the hepatic inflow vessels (portal vein and hepatic artery) causing intermittent hepatic ischemia. There can be significant back bleeding through the hepatic veins and vena cava. A recent meta-analysis did not demonstrate a difference in blood loss using PM in patients undergoing liver resection; however, previous older studies have shown a reduction in blood loss. This difference is thought to be attributed to newer surgical techniques that limit blood loss without occluding the hepatic inflow vessels.

3. A low CVP (generally referred to as a CVP lower than 5 mm Hg) facilitates control of bleeding from hepatic veins and the inferior vena cava during parenchymal dissection. Low CVP anesthesia reduces the pressure gradient that promotes bleeding through inadvertent extrahepatic venous injuries as well as hepatic venous bleeding during parenchymal dissection. Low CVP anesthesia has been demonstrated to reduce blood loss; however, it has not been demonstrated to reduce postoperative morbidity. Caveats for CVP monitoring with liver resection include increased risk of AKI with hypoperfusion and limitations of CVP monitoring with structural cardiac disease and with surgical compression of the liver-associated hepatic inflow and outflow vessels.

4. Venovenous bypass consists of the placement of large-bore cannulas in the common femoral vein and potentially the portal vein to drain venous blood and then return the blood to the cannula in either the internal jugular or axillary vein. This allows for caval interruption of the liver during surgery for control of hemorrhage without a significant drop in preload. There is risk to placement of these cannulas, and this should only be performed by an experienced team but may allow for safer surgical manipulation particularly in patients with limited cardiac reserve. To date, no study has shown a benefit to this technique and clinical judgment, and surgical needs must be considered on a case-by-case basis.

M. **Enhanced Recovery after Surgery (ERAS) for liver resection** has been adopted in many respects as ERAS protocols have been shown to decrease morbidity and duration of postoperative admissions. In 2016, the ERAS society published guidelines for liver resection. Preoperative considerations specific for liver resection highlight ensuring adequate preoperative nutritional status and avoiding long-acting anxiolytics. The guidelines also recommend using abdominal wound catheters and intrathecal opioids instead of epidural anesthesia and maintaining low-CVP anesthesia with balanced crystalloids. Minimally invasive surgery is recommended when appropriate. Postoperative considerations are similar to other ERAS strategies with early oral intake, mobilization, and a strong recommendation for multimodal analgesia. While there is strong evidence for many of the ERAS recommendations for perioperative nutrition and early mobilizations, the data for some of the other recommendations are equivocal particularly for low CVP anesthesia and epidural analgesia as discussed above.

VII. POSTOPERATIVE LIVER DYSFUNCTION

Postoperative liver dysfunction after surgery and anesthesia is common and can range from mild enzyme elevations to fulminant hepatic failure. There are many etiologies for postoperative hepatic dysfunction.

A. **Surgical causes** include maneuvers that impair hepatic blood flow or obstruct the biliary system (clamped vessels, retraction, or direct injury). Postoperative elevations of hepatocellular enzymes or bilirubin also can be caused by increased bilirubin loads after massive transfusion, resorption of hematoma, or hemolysis. Overt hepatic failure can occur during or after shock of any etiology.

B. **Nonsurgical** causes of hepatic dysfunction include undiagnosed cases of preoperative viral hepatitis, alcoholism, and cholelithiasis. Drug therapy in the perioperative period must also be evaluated as a cause of jaundice.

C. **Halothane hepatitis** is clinically indistinguishable from viral hepatitis. The diagnosis is one of exclusion. The incidence is 1 in 6000 to 1 in 35,000 following single exposure to halothane and increases to about 1 in 3000 following multiple exposures. Halothane is not available in the United States, but it is still in many countries.

Suggested Readings

Agarwal V, Divatia JV. Enhanced recovery after surgery in liver resection: current concepts and controversies. *Korean J Anesthesiol.* 2019;72(2):119-129.

Bhangui P, Laurent A, Amathieu R, et al. Assessment of risk for non-hepatic surgery in cirrhotic patients. *J Hepatol.* 2012;57:874-884.

Child CG, Turcotte JG. Surgery and portal hypertension. *Major Probl Clin Surg.* 1964;1:1-85.

Dershwitz M, Hoke JF, Rosow CE, et al. Pharmacokinetics and pharmacodynamics of remifentanil in volunteer subjects with severe liver disease. *Anesthesiology.* 1996;84:812-820.

Diaz KE, Schiano TD. Evaluation and management of cirrhotic patients undergoing elective surgery. *Curr Gastroenterol Rep.* 2019;21(7):32.

Dundar HZ, Yilmazlar T. Management of hepatorenal syndrome. *World J Nephrol.* 2015;4(2):277-286.

Eid EA, Sheta SA, Mansour E. Low central venous pressure anesthesia in major hepatic resection. *Middle East J Anesthesiol.* 2005;18(2):367-377.

Hoteit MA, Ghazale AH, Bain AJ, et al. Model for end-stage liver disease score versus child score in predicting the outcome of surgical procedures in patients with cirrhosis. *World J Gastroenterol.* 2008;14(11):1774-1780.

Hughes MJ, Ventham NT, Harrison EM, Wigmore SJ. Central venous pressure and liver resection: a systematic review and meta analysis. *HPB (Oxford).* 2015;17(10):863-871.

Kamath PS. Clinical approach to the patient with abnormal liver test results. *Mayo Clin Proc.* 1996;71:1089-1095.

Kim WR, Biggins SW, Kremers WK, et al. Hyponatremia and mortality among patients on the liver-transplant waiting list. *N Engl J Med.* 2008;359(10):1018-1026.

Kim YK, Chin JH, Kang SJ, et al. Association between central venous pressure and blood loss during hepatic resection in 984 living donors. *Acta Anaesthesiol Scand.* 2009;53(5):601-606.

Lesurtel M, Lehmann K, de Rougemont O, Clavien P-A. Clamping techniques and protecting strategies in liver surgery. *HPB (Oxford).* 2009;11(4):290-295.

Li Z, Sun Y, Wu F, et al. Controlled low central venous pressure reduces blood loss and transfusion requirements in hepatectomy. *World J Gastroenterol.* 2014;20(1):303-309.

Liu E, Guha A, Dnleavy M, et al. Safety of transesophageal echocardiography in patients with esophageal varices. *J Am Soc Echocardiogr.* 2019;32(5):676-677.

Millwala F, Nguyen GC, Thuluvath PJ. Outcomes of patients with cirrhosis undergoing non-hepatic surgery: risk assessment and management. *World J Gastroenterol.* 2007;13(30):4056-4063.

Parks DA, Skinner KA, Gelman S, Maze E. Hepatic physiology. In: Miller RD, ed. *Anesthesia.* 5th ed. Churchill Livingstone; 2000:647-662.

Patel T. Surgery in the patient with liver disease. *Mayo Clin Proc.* 1999;74:593-599.

Picker O, Beck C, Pannen B. Liver protection in the perioperative setting. *Best Pract Res Clin Anaesthesiol.* 2008;22(1):209-224.

Ramzan MI, Somogyi AA, Walker JS, et al. Clinical pharmacokinetics of the non-depolarising muscle relaxants. *Clin Pharmacokinet.* 1981;6:25-60.

Scott VL, Dodson SF, Kang Y. The hepatopulmonary syndrome. *Surg Clin.* 1999;79:23-41.

Starczewska MH, Mon W, Shirley P. Anaesthesia in patients with liver disease. *Curr Opin Anaesthesiol.* 2017;30(3):392-398.

Villanueva C, Colomo A, Bosch A, et al. Transfusion strategies for acute upper gastrointestinal bleeding. *N Engl J Med.* 2013;368:11-21.

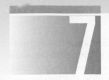

7 Specific Considerations With Endocrine Disease

Aubrey Samost-Williams and Jennifer Cottral

I. DIABETES MELLITUS

A. Diabetes mellitus (DM) is a chronic systemic disease characterized by an absolute or relative lack of insulin. As of 2020, approximately 10.5% of the US population has DM, 90% to 95% of which is DM type 2. DM is the most common endocrinopathy encountered in the perioperative period.

B. Types of DM

1. **DM type 1 (DM1)** is caused by autoimmune destruction of pancreatic β-cells resulting in an absolute insulin deficiency. Patients are usually diagnosed at a young age, not obese, and prone to ketoacidosis. Management is with insulin.

2. **DM type 2 (DM2)** is characterized by impaired insulin secretion and peripheral insulin resistance. Patients are typically diagnosed in adulthood and prone to hyperosmolar complications. Common comorbidities include hypertension (HTN), obesity, cerebrovascular disease, cardiovascular disease, and peripheral vascular disease. Common complications of DM2 include retinopathy, nephropathy, and neuropathy. With the increasing prevalence of childhood obesity, DM2 is now encountered in children and adolescents. Initial management is usually with diet and exercise. Oral hypoglycemic agents, insulin sensitizers, and/or insulin are added as needed.

3. **Gestational DM.** Between 6% and 9% of pregnancies are complicated by gestational DM. Parturients with gestational DM have a 3 to 7 times increased risk of developing DM2 within 5 to 10 years and a lifetime risk of up to 60%.

4. **Secondary DM** is due to other causes of absolute or relative insulin insufficiency. Insulin hyposecretion is seen with pancreatic destruction due to cystic fibrosis, pancreatitis, hemochromatosis, cancer, and after pancreatic surgery. Glucose intolerance may result from a glucagonoma or pheochromocytoma, thyrotoxicosis, acromegaly, or glucocorticoid excess.

C. Physiology of DM. Insulin is synthesized in pancreatic β-cells. Glucose, β-adrenergic agonists, arginine, and acetylcholine stimulate insulin secretion; α-adrenergic agonists and somatostatin inhibit insulin secretion. Insulin facilitates glucose and potassium transport across cell membranes, increases glycogen synthesis, and inhibits lipolysis. Peripheral tissues resist the effects of insulin during times of stress (eg, surgery, infection, cardiopulmonary bypass). Normally, low-level insulin production continues during fasting periods, preventing catabolism and ketoacidosis.

D. Obsolete terminology. The terms "juvenile-onset DM," "adult-onset DM," "insulin-treated DM," and "insulin-requiring DM" should be avoided. These terminologies fail to specify the actual type of DM and its implications. Instead use the terms listed above.

E. Outpatient therapy for DM
1. Oral hypoglycemic agents (Table 7.1)
a. Sulfonylureas (SFUs) increase pancreatic insulin release, thereby lowering blood glucose. There is an increased risk of hypoglycemia with these agents because circulating blood glucose levels do not influence the effect of SFUs. Glyburide and glimepiride, the two longest acting of the currently used SFUs, can induce hypoglycemia for more than 24 hours after administration. SFUs increase the effectiveness of thiazide diuretics, barbiturates, and anticoagulants by displacing these drugs from albumin.

TABLE 7.1	Noninsulin Agents Used to Treat DM		
Agent		**Onset (Hours)**	**Duration (Hours)**
Sulfonylurea	Tolbutamide[a]	≤0.25	6-12
	Tolazamide[a]	1	10-24
	Chlorpropamide[a]	1	60
	Glipizide (Glucotrol)	1	10-20
	Glipizide XL	1	20-24
	Gliclazide (glibenclamide)	1-2	12-24
	Glyburide (Micronase, Glynase, and Diabeta)	1	18-24
	Glimepiride (Amaryl)	1	24
α-Glucosidase inhibitor[b]	Acarbose (Precose)	Immediate	<0.3
	Miglitol (Glyset)	Immediate	<0.3
Biguanide[b]	Metformin (Glucophage, Glumetza, Riomet, and Fortamet)	1	8-12
Thiazolidinedione[b]	Pioglitazone (Actos)	1	24
	Rosiglitazone (Avandia)	1	24
Meglitinide	Repaglinide (Prandin)	1	3-4
D-Phenylalanine derivative	Nateglinide (Starlix)	1	4
GLP-1 receptor agonists[b,c]	Exenatide (Byetta)	<0.25	6-12
	Exenatide QW (Bydureon)[d]	2-4 wk[e]	
	Liraglutide (Victoza)[d]		24
	Albiglutide QW (Tanzeum)[d]		
	Dulaglutide (Trulicity)[d]		
	Lixisenatide (Lyxumia)		
Amylin analogue[b]	Pramlintide (Symlin)	<0.25	2-4

TABLE 7.1	Noninsulin Agents Used to Treat DM (Continued)		
Agent		**Onset (Hours)**	**Duration (Hours)**
DPP-IV inhibitor[b,g]	Sitagliptin (Januvia)	1	24
	Saxagliptin (Onglyza)	1-2	24
	Linagliptin (Tradjenta)[d]	1.5	
	Alogliptin (Nesina)[d]		
	Vildagliptin (Galvus)[d,f]		
Dopamine agonist	Bromocriptine Mesylate (Cycloset and Parlodel)	1	8-12
SGLT2 inhibitor	Canagliflozin (Invokana) Empagliflozin (Jardiance) Dapagliflozin (Farxiga) Ipragliflozin (Suglat)[f]	Within 24 (dose dependent)	24

[a]Historical agents that are no longer widely used.
[b]When used as the sole agent for treatment, hypoglycemia while fasting is unlikely.
[c]Glucagon-like peptide 1.
[d]Onset of action and/or duration of action are not reported.
[e]Steady state achieved by week 7.
[f]Currently not FDA approved.
[g]Dipeptidyl peptidase IV.

b. **Meglitinides and D-phenylalanine derivatives** act via a nonsulfony-lurea receptor pathway to rapidly increase insulin release from the pancreas. These drugs may also cause hypoglycemia but are more rapid and short acting than SFUs.

c. **Biguanides** decrease hepatic glucose production, inhibit intestinal glucose absorption, and increase peripheral glucose uptake and uti-lization. Metformin is the only currently marketed drug in this class and when used as monotherapy, is associated with a very low risk of hypoglycemia. Medical conditions leading to increased plasma metformin levels may predispose patients to lactic acidosis, such as renal dysfunction (reduced drug clearance), hepatic dysfunction (reduced lactate clearance), or heart failure. Diarrhea is a common side effect.

d. **Thiazolidinediones** increase insulin sensitivity and decrease hepatic glucose production. Side effects include weight gain, fluid retention leading to edema or heart failure, and upper respiratory tract infec-tion. Risk of hypoglycemia is low when used as monotherapy. As of 2020, rosiglitazone remains available in the United States despite an associated increased risk of heart attack, heart failure, and death.

e. **α-Glucosidase inhibitors** decrease the rise in postprandial glucose by preventing intestinal absorption of glucose. There is a low risk of hypoglycemia, and side effects include abdominal pain, flatulence, and diarrhea.

f. **Dipeptidyl peptidase IV (DPP-4) inhibitors** prevent the breakdown of endogenous glucagon-like peptide 1 (GLP-1), thereby enhancing insulin secretion and decreasing glucagon secretion in a glucose-dependent manner. They are not associated with significant gastrointestinal (GI) side effects, and there is a low risk of hypoglycemia. There is a potential increased risk of heart failure with some DPP-4 agents in susceptible patients.

g. **Dopamine (D2) agonists** improve glycemic control by increasing hypothalamic dopamine levels and decreasing excessive sympathetic tone within the central nervous system (CNS). This reduces fasting and postprandial glucose, triglyceride, and free fatty acid levels. Side effects include nausea, asthenia, constipation, and dizziness. Single-agent therapy is not associated with hypoglycemia.

h. **SGLT2 inhibitors** decrease renal glucose reabsorption by inhibiting sodium-glucose cotransporter 2 (SGLT2) in the nephron, which is responsible for more than 90% of renal glucose reabsorption. SGLT2 inhibitors do not usually cause hypoglycemia because they increase urinary excretion of glucose in a plasma glucose-dependent manner. Adverse effects include an increased risk of genitourinary infection, osmotic diuresis leading to volume depletion and orthostatic hypotension, euglycemic diabetic ketoacidosis, bone fractures, and lower limb amputations.

2. **Injectable agents**

   a. **Insulin (Table 7.2).** Rapid and short-acting insulins are given just before meals to prevent postprandial hyperglycemia. Intermediate and long-acting insulins are given 1 to 2 times a day to mimic basal insulin secretion needed to meet baseline metabolic requirements. Rapid and short-acting insulins can also be administered continuously via a subcutaneous pump. The liver and kidney metabolize insulin. As a result, renal insufficiency and hepatic impairment may produce clinically significant prolongation of insulin action and reduce insulin requirements. Adverse reactions associated with insulin analogues are vast, but the most relevant risk is severe hypoglycemia.

TABLE 7.2	Subcutaneous Insulin Preparations Used to Treat DM		
Class	**Agent**	**Onset (Hours)**	**Peak Effect (Hours)**	**Duration (Hours)**
Rapid Acting				
	Lispro (Humalog)	0.1-0.25	1-2	2-4
	Aspart (NovoLog)	0.1-0.25	1-2	2-4
	Glulisine (Apidra)	0.1-0.25	1-2	2-4
Short Acting				
	Regular (Humulin R, Novolin R)	0.5-1	2-4	6-10
Intermediate Acting				
	NPH	2-4	6-12	12-18
Long Acting				
	Glargine (Lantus)	1-3	No peak	20-24
	Detemir (Levemir)	1-3	No peak	20-24

When regular insulin is administered IV, the onset of action is immediate. The duration of action is ~1 h.

b. **Amylin analogues (Table 7.1)** suppress inappropriate postprandial glucagon secretion seen in DM (glucagon stimulates hepatic release of glucose) and reduce appetite by delaying gastric emptying. Amylin analogues do not cause hypoglycemia as monotherapy but may cause hypoglycemia when given concurrently with insulin. Common side effects include nausea and headache.

c. **GLP-1 analogues (Table 7.1)** enhance glucose-dependent insulin secretion, reduce inappropriate postprandial glucagon secretion seen in DM, and reduce appetite by delaying gastric emptying. Hypoglycemia is a risk only when GLP-1 analogues are taken with other agents known to cause hypoglycemia. The most common adverse events include nausea, vomiting, and diarrhea.

F. **Acute complications of diabetes.** Diabetic ketoacidosis (DKA) and hyperglycemic hyperosmolar syndrome (HHS) are the result of insulin deficiency, resistance to insulin during stress (eg, infection, surgery, myocardial infarction, intoxication [alcohol, cocaine], dehydration, and trauma), and/or medications.

1. **DKA** occurs primarily in DM1.

   a. **Pathophysiology of DKA** is related to an absolute low level of insulin leading to extracellular hyperglycemia and intracellular hypoglycemia. This shifts metabolism from glucose-based to ketogenic, leading to the uncontrolled production of ketone bodies and subsequent high anion gap metabolic acidosis. Extracellular hyperglycemia leads to fluid shifts, osmotic diuresis, and subsequent electrolyte abnormalities.

   b. **Clinical manifestations of DKA** include nausea, vomiting, abdominal pain, polyuria, polydipsia, weakness, renal failure, shock, deep rhythmic (Kussmaul) breathing with a fruity odor, and mental status changes. It is associated with depressed myocardial contractility, decreased vascular tone, high anion gap metabolic acidosis, electrolyte abnormalities, hyperglycemia, and hyperosmolarity. Patients are often profoundly hypovolemic owing to hyperglycemia-related osmotic diuresis, emesis, and reduced oral intake. Total body potassium (K^+) is depressed, but serum levels are spuriously normal or elevated because acidemia shifts K^+ out of cells via transcellular hydrogen (H^+)-K^+ exchange. Serum sodium (Na^+) concentrations may be spuriously low because hyperglycemia causes osmotic shifts of water from the intracellular to the extracellular space, leading to a relative dilutional hyponatremia. Hypophosphatemia and hypomagnesemia from osmotic diuresis are common.

   c. **Treatment of DKA** is based on the principles of volume replacement (fluid deficit in adult DKA averages 6-9 L), insulin therapy, correction of electrolyte abnormalities, identification and treatment of underlying stressors or precipitants, and supportive care. DKA management algorithms often vary by institution.

2. **HHS** is primarily a presentation of DM2.

   a. **Pathophysiology of HHS** is related to severe hyperglycemia owing to a relative insulin deficiency and increase in counterregulatory hormones (glucagon, catecholamines, cortisol) leading to osmotic diuresis and profound hypovolemia. Insulin levels are inadequate to prevent hyperglycemia but are sufficient to block ketogenesis and ketoacidosis.

   b. **Clinical manifestations of HHS** are often associated with serum glucose levels exceeding 600 mg/dL. They include electrolyte abnormalities,

CNS dysfunction (depressed sensorium, seizure, coma), blurred vision, neurologic deficits, weight loss, leg cramps, polydipsia, and polyuria. Mortality in HHS may be as high as 20%.

c. **Treatment of HHS** is similar to the treatment of DKA, with an emphasis on volume repletion, insulin therapy, correction of electrolyte abnormalities, and diagnosis and treatment of underlying precipitants. Intubation should be considered if there is a concern for lack of airway protection owing to altered mental status. Volume repletion is generally more aggressive in HHS owing to a higher fluid deficit (8-10 L in the average size adult), and initial target glucose level is higher than DKA (250-300 mg/dL in HHS, 200 mg/dL in DKA). The target glucose level in HHS is higher to prevent rapid correction of serum osmolality and subsequent cerebral edema.

G. **Anesthetic considerations in the patient with DM** focus on risk reduction, maintenance of euglycemia, avoidance or treatment of acute complications of DM, and prevention of perioperative complications related to chronic complications of DM.

1. **Perioperative glycemic targets.** Both hyperglycemia and hypoglycemia have been associated with increased morbidity and mortality in the preoperative period. However, the optimal target blood glucose range remains unclear and no consensus has been reached among affiliated professional societies. In addition, there is a growing body of evidence suggesting that the link between hyperglycemia and adverse outcomes in cardiac and noncardiac surgery may not be as strong in diabetic patients as compared with their nondiabetic counterparts. A consistent finding is that tighter glucose control leads to more frequent hypoglycemic events, which may be associated with increased morbidity and mortality. Most professional societies agree that treatment with insulin therapy should be initiated at blood glucose levels >180 mg/dL.

2. **Perioperative glycemic management** depends on anesthetic technique, duration and invasiveness of surgery, and anticipated time to resumption of oral intake.

   a. **Oral hypoglycemic agents** and insulin sensitizers that can cause hypoglycemia should be held the day of surgery.

      1. Amylin analogues and GLP-1 analogues, which cause delayed gastric emptying, should also be held in order to reduce the likelihood of postoperative nausea and vomiting.

      2. Metformin should be held from the day of surgery until normal postoperative renal function has been confirmed.

      3. Thiazolidinediones and DPP-IV inhibitors do not cause hypoglycemia and may be given the morning of surgery.

      4. α-Glucosidase inhibitors also do not produce hypoglycemia, but they are ineffective when patients are NPO (nothing by mouth). SGLT2 inhibitors should be continued if ambulatory surgery, and should be stopped the morning of any minor or major nonambulatory surgery.

   b. **Insulin**

      1. **Insulin-dependent DM2.**

         a. Insulin should be continued through the night before surgery. If the patient has a history of hypoglycemia, the dose should be reduced to half to two-thirds of the patient's customary dose.

         b. Patients should receive approximately half of their total normal morning dose of intermediate- or long-acting insulin in a subcutaneous dose. Rapid- and short-acting insulins should not be given.

    c. If glucose drops below 120 mg/dL, consider starting a glucose infusion. If glucose rises above 180 mg/dL consider starting insulin.

        i. IV insulin should be used if the patient is (1) expected to be hemodynamically unstable, (2) expected to have fluid shifts or temperature changes, (3) has an operative duration > 4 hours, (4) is critically ill, or (5) is poorly controlled at home. See **Table 7.3** for an example infusion regimen.

        ii. If the patient meets none of the above criteria, can consider subcutaneous insulin instead.

        iii. If insulin is started, check blood sugars at least every 2 hours. In addition, monitor potassium levels if using an insulin infusion.

  2. **DM1.** These patients must always receive insulin to prevent ketoacidosis, even in the setting of low or normal glucose levels. Simultaneous infusion of a glucose-containing solution may be necessary to prevent hypoglycemia.

    a. Perioperative insulin management for patients with DM1 receiving newer intensive regimens of three or more daily insulin injections should be discussed in advance with the physician responsible for managing the patient's diabetes.

    b. For the patient with an insulin pump, the following information should be obtained preoperatively: pump identification information, programmed settings information, insertion site,

---

TABLE 7.3   Guidelines for Routine Regular IV Insulin Infusion

If blood glucose (BG) >180: Start IV insulin bolus dose (blood sugar/40) units. Start IV insulin infusion (blood sugar/100) units/h. Check glucose at least hourly until stable and adjust infusion as appropriate. Then check glucose at least every 2 hours.

Adjustment of Regular Insulin Infusion Rate, units/hour

Blood Glucose (mg/dL)	Infusion change if BG has increased since last check	Infusion change if BG has decreased less than 30 mg/dL	Infusion change if BG has decreased more than 30 mg/dL
<70	Treat hypoglycemia with D50 boluses. Recheck and repeat as needed.		
71-109	Hold infusion and check blood sugars at least hourly. Restart infusion at half previous rate if BG >180 mg/dL.		
110-140	No change	Decrease rate by 0.5 U/h	Hold infusion
141-180	No change	No change	No change
181-210	Increase rate by 1 U/hr	Increase rate by 1 U/h	No change
211-240	Increase rate by 2 U/h	Increase rate by 2 U/h	No change
>241	Increase rate by 3 U/h	Increase rate by 3 U/h	No change

Guidelines assume the patient is fasting and not in DKA or HHS. Dosing must be individually titrated based on frequent blood glucose monitoring. D50 is a solution of dextrose, 50% (weight/volume) in water.
Adapted with permission from Duggan EW, Carlson K, Umpierrez GE. Perioperative hyperglycemia management: an update. *Anesthesiology*. 2017;126(3):547-560. Copyright © 2017 the American Society of Anesthesiologists, Inc.

blood sugar measurements, plans for correction dosing, pump failure plan, and diabetes provider contact information. **The anesthesia provider needs to know how to use the pump in case settings need to be changed intraoperatively.**

  i. The usual basal rates can be reduced by 10% to 20% while the patient is NPO to avoid hypoglycemia.
  ii. Only use if (1) the site does not interfere with the surgery, (2) there is no plan for MRI or other radiation, (3) the pump is out of the path of the electrocautery return circuit, and (4) there is minimal risk of needing defibrillation.
  iii. Blood glucose levels should be checked frequently with target glucose level of 120 to 180 mg/dL, which is typically more liberal than home management. This may require turning basal rate down to 80% of normal.

  c. **Fixed ratio insulin combinations** are prescribed for the outpatient management of some diabetics. In consultation with the physician managing the diabetes, these patients should be switched to preparations of individual insulins in the immediate preoperative period. An appropriately reduced dose (approximately 50%) of only the long-acting insulin can then be taken on the morning of surgery as described above.

3. **DKA, HHS, and metabolic abnormalities** should be treated before elective surgery and actively managed in the operating room if surgery cannot be postponed until the patient is medically stabilized.

4. **Vascular disease.** Diabetic patients have a strong predisposition to all types of vascular diseases. Macrovascular disease (coronary artery, cerebrovascular, and peripheral vascular) and microvascular disease (retinopathy, neuropathy, and nephropathy) occur more frequently, more extensively, and at an earlier age than in the general population. Insulin-dependent DM is a known independent risk factor for perioperative major adverse cardiac events. Diabetic patients with ischemic heart disease are more likely to be asymptomatic or have atypical anginal symptoms. Continuation of aspirin and β-blockade and a high index of suspicion for ischemic heart disease are mainstays of management. DM is the most common cause of chronic and end-stage renal disease. Avoid nephrotoxins and consider renal protective treatments in patients exposed to IV contrast.

5. **Neuropathy.** Diabetic autonomic neuropathy (DAN) can be present even in patients with well-controlled DM. It has widespread effects, including decreased lower esophageal sphincter tone, gastroesophageal reflux disease, gastroparesis, bladder atony, sexual dysfunction, orthostatic hypotension, and labile blood pressure. DAN is associated with an increased risk for silent myocardial ischemia, renal failure, stroke, obstructive sleep apnea (OSA), and overall mortality among patients with DM. Patients with DAN may be at higher risk for intraoperative hypothermia, be more susceptible to aspiration owing to higher residual gastric volumes, and be less able to compensate for the sympathectomy of neuraxial anesthesia. Signs of cardiac autonomic neuropathy include resting tachycardia, orthostatic hypotension, and decreased beat-to-beat variability with deep breathing. Peripheral neuropathies may cause pain and/or numbness. Patients with peripheral neuropathy may be more vulnerable to positioning injuries and should be padded carefully. Document neuropathies in the anesthesia preoperative evaluation and before initiating regional anesthesia.

6. **Airway management**
   a. DM has been associated with difficult laryngoscopy. Postulated mechanisms include obesity (excess pretracheal and occipital tissue, large neck circumference) and DM-related decrease in temporomandibular joint and cervical spine mobility. This may be predicted by signs of other joint stiffness, such as incomplete approximation of one or more digits when attempting to approximate palmar surfaces (prayer sign).
   b. Obesity, sleep apnea, and redundant pharyngeal tissue are common in patients with metabolic syndrome and DM2.
7. **Protamine.** Diabetic patients receiving NPH or NPL (Humalog mix) insulin are at increased risk for protamine reactions owing to the structural similarities between the drugs.

II. HYPOGLYCEMIA
A. **Etiologies** include excessive doses of insulin or oral hypoglycemic agents, particularly in the setting of decreased nutritional intake. Other causes of hypoglycemia include sepsis, liver failure, a spectrum of pancreatic diseases, some malignancies, hypopituitarism, adrenal insufficiency, and renal failure in patients who receive insulin (reduced insulin clearance).
B. **Signs and symptoms.** Adrenergic responses to hypoglycemia produce tachycardia, diaphoresis, palpitations, HTN, and tremulousness. Neuroglycopenia can result in irritability, headache, confusion, stupor, seizure, and coma. General anesthesia masks the signs and symptoms of hypoglycemia. Patients with long-standing DM and previous episodes of hypoglycemia often lose sympathetic responses to hypoglycemia, a condition termed hypoglycemic unawareness. Hypoglycemic unawareness is more common in patients with improved glucose control who experience more episodes of hypoglycemia. It is more common in DM1 than in DM2 and can be more severe in elderly patients.
C. **Anesthetic considerations** include providing a continuous glucose infusion and regularly checking blood glucose levels. Anticipate fluctuating glucose levels from surgical stress and infection and with insulinoma manipulation.

III. THYROID DISEASE
Thyroid disease is common in the US adult population, with a higher prevalence among women and with increasing age.
A. **Physiology.** Thyroid-stimulating hormone (TSH) from the anterior pituitary stimulates the thyroid gland to take up iodine and produce the hormones triiodothyronine (T_3) and L-thyroxine (T_4); 80% of serum T_3 is produced by the peripheral conversion from T_4, and T_3 is significantly more potent than T_4. Both forms of thyroid hormone are extensively (>99%) bound to plasma proteins and only the free (unbound) thyroid hormone is biologically active. T_3 and T_4 are major regulators of metabolic activity. They alter the speed of drug metabolism, biochemical reactions, total body oxygen consumption, and heat production.
B. **Evaluation and laboratory studies.** Serum TSH is currently the best initial screen for the determination of thyroid function in the ambulatory population. TSH levels rise in hypothyroidism and fall in hyperthyroidism. Evaluation of thyroid function is complex in sick patients since there are many other factors that influence thyroid function tests in otherwise euthyroid patients. As a result, thyroid function should only be assessed in sick patients if there is a strong suspicion of thyroid dysfunction and with the guidance of consulting endocrine services.

C. Thyrotoxicosis

1. **Etiologies** include Graves disease, toxic multinodular goiter, subacute thyroiditis (acute phase), toxic adenoma, TSH receptor stimulation by β-human chorionic gonadotropin overproduction (pituitary or placental tumors), ovarian tumors secreting thyroid hormone (struma ovarii), intake of excess iodine, and supratherapeutic doses of thyroid hormone.

2. **Symptoms** generally result from a hypermetabolic state and include nervousness, heat intolerance, fatigue, diarrhea, insomnia, increased perspiration, muscle weakness, tremors, irregular menses, and weight loss. Cardiovascular signs include an increase in cardiac output and pulse pressure, decrease in peripheral vascular resistance, dysrhythmias, palpitations, HTN, and high output heart failure in predisposed patients. Ophthalmic disease occurs only with Graves hyperthyroidism.

3. **Treatment** involves medical and surgical options. Two commonly used medications that inhibit thyroid hormone production include propylthiouracil (PTU) and methimazole. Symptoms may also be addressed with β-blockade. Thyroid gland ablation is another approach and can be achieved with surgery or radioactive iodine.

4. **Thyroid storm** is an endocrine emergency and a state of physiologic decompensation due to severe thyrotoxicosis. Precipitants include infection, surgery, trauma, cessation of antithyroid medications, excess iodine, iodinated IV contrast agents, and amiodarone. Thyroid storm may occur 6 to 18 hours postoperatively. Manifestations include diarrhea, vomiting, hyperpyrexia, hypovolemia, tachycardia, heart failure, shock, weakness, irritability, delirium, and coma. Thyroid storm may mimic malignant hyperthermia, neuroleptic malignant syndrome, sepsis, hemorrhage, pheochromocytoma crisis, or transfusion/drug reaction. The mortality rate of thyroid storm is greater than 20%.

5. **Treatment for thyroid storm** (**Table 7.4**) includes blocking thyroid hormone synthesis and release, blocking T_4 to T_3 conversion, suppressing the sympathetic response with β-adrenergic blockade, and supportive therapy (active cooling, meperidine to attenuate heat production from shivering, volume resuscitation, and electrolyte replacement). Steroids should be administered if there is any indication of adrenal insufficiency (including cardiovascular collapse). Iodine must be given at least 1 hour **after** initiation of treatment with PTU or methimazole to prevent iodine from being used as a substrate for thyroid hormone synthesis.

6. **Anesthetic considerations**.

   a. Patients should be euthyroid prior to surgery to avoid precipitating thyroid storm.

   b. Antithyroid drugs, pharmacologic iodine doses, and β-adrenergic antagonist medications should be continued through surgery.

   c. Strongly consider invasive hemodynamic monitoring.

   d. In an emergent situation, thyrotoxic patients can be prepared for surgery with high-dose IV β-blockers titrated until the heart rate is less than 100 beats/min. Glucocorticoids may also be considered because they inhibit the peripheral conversion of T_4 to T_3 and treat a potentially reduced adrenocortical reserve.

   e. Avoid sympathetic stimulation (pain, anxiety, ketamine, and local anesthetics with epinephrine). Consider generous sedative premedication unless there is concern for airway compromise.

TABLE 7.4	Treatment of Thyroid Storm

Block Sympathetic Response

Propranolol	1-2 mg IV (repeat as needed) or 40-80 mg orally every 6 h
Verapamil	5-10 mg IV (repeat as needed)
Esmolol	50-100 µg/kg/min IV

Block Thyroid Hormone Synthesis (Thionamides)

PTU	200 mg orally every 4-6 h
Methimazole	20 mg orally or per rectum every 4 h

Block Thyroid Hormone Release

Iopanoic acid[a]	500 mg orally every 12 h
Iodine (SSKI)[a]	100 mg orally every 12 h
Dexamethasone	2 mg orally every 6 h

Block T_4 to T_3 Conversion

Propranolol, PTU, and iopanoic acid

Steroids (hydrocortisone, 100 mg orally/IV every 8 h or dexamethasone, 2 mg orally/IV every 6 h)

Supportive Therapy

Fluids, cooling (with meperidine to block shivering), electrolyte replacement, antipyretics (no aspirin), treatment of precipitating illness and congestive heart failure, oxygen, nutrition, consider plasmapheresis and airway support

SSKI, saturated solution of peotassium iodide.
[a]Give iopanoic acid or SSKI > 1 h after PTU or methimazole to avoid hormone production surge.

    f. Regional anesthesia may be beneficial in thyrotoxic patients because it blocks sympathetic responses. The addition of epinephrine to the local anesthetic should be avoided owing to the risk of systemic uptake and worsening tachycardia and HTN. Thrombocytopenia sometimes occurs in thyrotoxicosis. Consider checking the platelet count before initiating regional anesthesia.

    g. Patients may be hypovolemic owing to HTN, diarrhea, and perspiration. Hypotension should be treated with vasoconstrictor agents and fluids. Anticipate brisk tachycardic response to anticholinergic drugs.

    h. Assure full eye protection, as proptotic eyes may not have complete lid closure.

    i. Drug metabolism and anesthetic requirements may be increased owing to thyrotoxicosis-related hypermetabolism.

    j. Large goiters may displace and compress the trachea, compromising the airway. Emergency tracheostomy may be difficult in patients with goiter.

D. Hypothyroidism

  1. Etiologies of hypothyroidism include congenital disorders, thyroid gland damage from surgery, radioiodine, or radiation, pituitary disease, autoimmune disease (eg, Hashimoto thyroiditis), iodine deficiency, drug therapy (lithium or amiodarone with preexisting chronic thyroiditis), and late-phase subacute thyroiditis. Hashimoto thyroiditis is the most common etiology in adults and can be associated with other autoimmune processes.

2. **Clinical features of hypothyroidism** that influence anesthetic care are characterized by a hypometabolic state and include hypoventilation from respiratory muscle weakness and impaired responsiveness to hypoxia and hypercarbia, altered mental status, facial edema with an enlarged tongue, anemia, coagulation and electrolyte abnormalities, ileus with delayed gastric emptying, reduced cardiac output due to decreased contractility and heart rate, pericardial effusion, reversible cardiomyopathy, conduction abnormalities, and diminished baroreceptor reflexes. Symptoms associated with other endocrine disorders may be a feature of hypothyroidism due to pituitary disease.

3. **Treatment of hypothyroidism.** Chronic treatment involves oral supplementation with oral thyroid hormone. T_4 is administered once daily and requires 7 to 10 days to have initial effects; 3 to 4 weeks of therapy are needed to achieve a stable state. T_3 is not routinely used as therapy because of its short half-life. IV thyroid hormone should be given with caution in patients with coronary artery disease because the increased metabolic state and oxygen consumption may induce myocardial ischemia.

4. **Myxedema coma** (profound hypothyroidism) is a clinical diagnosis. Surgery, drugs, trauma, and infection can be precipitants in a severely hypothyroid patient. It is defined by decreased mental status associated with decreased responsiveness to CO_2, heart failure, hypothermia, and exaggerated symptoms of hypothyroidism.

5. **Treatment of myxedema coma** is with IV T_3 and T_4, passive rewarming, intubation if airway protection is a concern, correction of electrolyte abnormalities, stress dose steroids if concomitant primary or secondary adrenal insufficiency is suspected, and management of hypotension, heart failure, effusions, and the precipitating cause(s). Active warming may cause hypotension in these patients who are hypovolemic with peripheral vasoconstriction.

6. **Anesthetic considerations.** Adverse surgical outcomes in patients with hypothyroidism are generally associated only with severe hypothyroidism.
   a. Securing the airway may be difficult because of an enlarged tongue, relaxed oropharyngeal tissues, goiter, and delayed gastric emptying.
   b. Patients may be prone to hypotension owing to hypovolemia, blunted baroreceptor reflexes, reduced myocardial contractility, and bradycardia.
   c. Patients may be susceptible to hypoventilation owing to respiratory muscle weakness and impaired responsiveness to hypoxia and hypercarbia.
   d. There may be an increased sensitivity to CNS-depressant and paralytic medications.
   e. Corticosteroid supplementation may be necessary.
   f. There is an increased likelihood of heart failure, hypothermia, hypoglycemia, hyponatremia, and delayed emergence.

IV. CALCIUM METABOLISM AND PARATHYROID DISEASE
   A. **Physiology.** Calcium is essential for neuromuscular excitability, cardiac automaticity, mitotic division, coagulation, muscle contraction, neurotransmitter and hormone secretion and action, and the activity of many enzymes. Parathyroid hormone (PTH) and vitamin D maintain the

extracellular calcium concentration within a narrow range. PTH increases intestinal calcium absorption, increases osteoclastic release of calcium and phosphorus from bone, decreases renal clearance of calcium, and enhances formation of 1,25-dihydroxyvitamin D by the kidney. Levels of ionized calcium and magnesium determine the secretion of PTH. Vitamin D augments the effects of PTH and is necessary for calcium absorption from the GI tract. Calcitonin from thyroid parafollicular cells lowers serum calcium in two ways: by inhibiting osteoclast activity and by inhibiting renal reabsorption of calcium and phosphorus.

B. **Calcium measurement.** Serum calcium is found in both bound (primarily to albumin) and unbound forms, and only ionized calcium is physiologically relevant. Hypoalbuminemia produces a decrease in total calcium, and serum calcium levels should be corrected accordingly (0.8 mg/dL calcium per 1 g/dL albumin below normal). Acidemia increases and alkalemia decreases ionized calcium levels owing to alterations in albumin binding.

C. **Hypercalcemia**

1. **Etiologies of hypercalcemia** include hyperparathyroidism, malignancy, immobilization, granulomatous diseases, vitamin D intoxication, familial hypocalciuric hypercalcemia, thyrotoxicosis, drugs (lithium, thiazides, calcium, vitamin A, theophylline), Paget disease, renal disease, and adrenal insufficiency. Primary hyperparathyroidism is usually due to a parathyroid adenoma and is characterized by hypercalcemia and hypophosphatemia with an elevated PTH. Hypercalcemia of malignancy can be due to tumor release of PTH-related protein (a protein that binds the same receptor as PTH) or osteolytic metastases resulting in direct bony destruction and calcium resorption.

2. **Clinical features of hypercalcemia** are summarized in **Table 7.5.** Mild hypercalcemia is usually asymptomatic. When total serum calcium (corrected for albumin level) is >13 mg/dL, there is an increased risk

TABLE 7.5 Hypercalcemia: Signs and Symptoms

Gastrointestinal	Osteopenia/osteoporosis
• Nausea/vomiting	Weakness/atrophy/fatigability
• Anorexia	Central nervous system
• Constipation	• Seizures
• Pancreatitis	• Disorientation/psychosis
• Peptic ulcers	• Memory loss
• Abdominal pain	• Sedation/lethargy/coma
Hemodynamic	• Anxiety/depression
• Dehydration	Renal
• HTN	• Polyuria
• ECG/conduction changes	• Nephrolithiasis
• Digitalis sensitivity	• Decreased renal blood flow
• Dysrhythmias	• Oliguric renal failure (late)
• Catecholamine resistance	
Hematologic	
• Anemia	
• Thrombosis	

of end-organ calcification, renal calculi, and nephrocalcinosis. A total serum calcium level of >14 to 15 mg/dL is considered an endocrine emergency, as patients may experience uremia, coma, cardiac arrest, or death.

3. **Treatment of hypercalcemia**

a. **Hydration** with IV normal saline to maintain a urine output of 100 to 150 mL/h is the initial treatment for hypercalcemia. In patients with symptoms of volume overload, diuretics may be added. The patient must be monitored for hypokalemia, hypomagnesemia, fluid overload, and diuresis-induced hypovolemia. In patients with renal or cardiac failure, dialysis should be considered. Goals should also include treatment of the underlying cause of hypercalcemia. Intensive care unit (ICU) care may be necessary.

b. **Bisphosphonates** decrease bone resorption and are the treatment of choice in severe or life-threatening hypercalcemia and in hypercalcemia of malignancy. The maximum effect occurs in 2 to 4 days making them less important in the acute setting. Side effects include renal insufficiency, fever, myalgias, uveitis, and osteonecrosis of the jaw. Lower bisphosphonate doses are used in patients with renal insufficiency.

c. **Calcitonin** will lower serum calcium concentrations by 1 to 2 mg/dL in 4 to 6 hours, but its effects are transient, so it is useful acutely but must be followed up with more definitive treatment.

d. **Gallium nitrate** inhibits bone resorption and is effective in hypercalcemia of malignancy, but its use is limited by nephrotoxicity and the need for continuous infusion over 5 days.

e. **Glucocorticoid therapy** is effective in some cases of multiple myeloma, vitamin D toxicity, and granulomatous diseases.

f. **Denosumab and cinacalcet** are alternative therapies for severe hypercalcemia resistant to other therapies.

4. **Anesthetic considerations.**

a. Hypercalcemia > 12 mg/dL warrants preoperative correction.

b. Intravascular volume and other electrolyte abnormalities should be normalized and monitored.

c. Hypercalcemia has an unpredictable effect on neuromuscular blockade, so relaxants should be carefully titrated. Muscular weakness due to hypercalcemia may worsen respiratory function. Avoid hypoventilation because acidosis increases ionized calcium levels.

d. Careful positioning is required because patients can be osteoporotic.

e. Patients with hypercalcemia are predisposed to digitalis toxicity and may have conduction abnormalities. Shortened QTc and high-grade AV block have been described.

D. **Hypocalcemia** is serum calcium < 8.5 mg/dL in the absence of hypoalbuminemia or acid/base abnormalities.

1. **Etiologies** include hypoparathyroidism, hypoalbuminemia, alkalemia, vitamin D deficiency, chronic kidney disease, hyperphosphatemia, drug effects (furosemide, antiepileptics), and pancreatitis. Hypoparathyroidism is commonly due to destruction of parathyroid glands (surgery, autoimmune diseases, irradiation, infiltrative diseases) and less commonly due to PTH underproduction (sepsis, severe burns). Severe hypomagnesemia (<1 mg/dL) can also lead to PTH underproduction and may cause PTH resistance. In the operating room, hypocalcemia can be seen in hyperventilation leading to a respiratory alkalosis, as well as massive transfusion when citrate (an anticoagulant

used in blood products) binds calcium. Because the liver metabolizes citrate, hypocalcemia is often seen during the anhepatic phase of liver transplantation.

2. **Clinical features.** Patients are usually asymptomatic until total calcium is less than 7.0 mg/dL or ionized calcium is less than 2.8 mg/dL (0.7 mmol/L) especially if the onset is insidious.

   a. **Chronic hypocalcemia** causes lethargy, muscle cramps, a prolonged QT interval, renal failure, cataracts, dementia, and personality changes.

   b. **Acute hypocalcemia** produces neuromuscular irritability with muscle cramps and hand, foot, and circumoral paresthesias. Patients may demonstrate facial nerve irritability to percussion (Chvostek sign) or carpal spasm with tourniquet ischemia for 3 minutes (Trousseau sign).

   c. **Severe hypocalcemia** results in stridor, laryngospasm, tetany, apnea, coagulopathy, hypotension with catecholamine resistance, psychosis/confusion, and seizures unresponsive to conventional therapy.

3. **Treatment**

   a. Severe or symptomatic hypocalcemia should be treated with IV calcium. Calcium formulations cause a chemical phlebitis; administer calcium centrally whenever possible. One gram of elemental calcium gluconate contains 93 mg of elemental calcium; 1 g of calcium chloride contains 273 mg of elemental calcium. For urgent therapy, 1 to 2 g of calcium gluconate or 1 g of calcium chloride may be given IV over 10 to 20 minutes. Dilution may be needed depending on the available preparation of calcium gluconate or chloride. During parenteral therapy, calcium levels, creatinine, electrocardiogram (ECG), and hemodynamic status must be monitored. Therapeutic goals are a total serum calcium level near 8 mg/dL or an ionized calcium near >1.1 mmol/L in the setting of normal acid/base status. Evaluate and correct abnormalities in serum phosphorus, potassium, and magnesium levels. Treat elevated phosphorus levels with oral phosphate binders; treat low magnesium levels (<1 mg/dL) with parenteral magnesium sulfate.

   b. Mild to moderate hypocalcemia may be managed with oral calcium and activated vitamin D analogue. Patients require elemental calcium at 1.5 to 3 g/d (3750-7500 mg of calcium carbonate) and 1, 25-dihydroxyvitamin D (calcitriol, 0.25-3.0 µg/d) in 4 to 6 divided doses.

   c. For chronic replacement, patients receive calcitriol or vitamin D (ergocalciferol 50,000 IU, 1-3 times/wk) in addition to calcium.

4. **Anesthetic considerations.**

   a. Severe hypocalcemia should be corrected preoperatively if time allows.

   b. Calcium formulations cause a chemical phlebitis, so use the largest and most reliable intravenous access available when administering supplemental calcium.

   c. Respiratory alkalosis may cause a decrease in ionized calcium with no change in total calcium; consider the underlying cause of a low ionized calcium before treating.

   d. Check for and correct hypomagnesemia to sustainably address hypocalcemia.

   e. Frequently check ionized calcium levels during massive transfusion, as the citrate in blood products will chelate calcium.

    f. Cardiovascular effects of hypocalcemia include hypotension with insensitivity to β-adrenergic agonists, a prolonged QT interval, atrioventricular block, and digitalis insensitivity.

E. Parathyroid surgery

  1. Anesthetic considerations and surgical complications in parathyroid surgery are similar to those for thyroid surgery.

    a. General anesthesia or regional techniques (deep and/or superficial cervical plexus blockade bilaterally) can be used.

    b. Surgeons may perform recurrent laryngeal monitoring intraoperatively, but keep in mind that this is not possible under sedation with regional anesthesia.

    c. To ensure the appropriate removal of parathyroid tissue, blood may be sent intraoperatively for PTH levels with a 50% reduction and normalization of PTH level predicting surgical success. The circulating half-life of PTH is just a few minutes.

V. ADRENAL CORTICAL DISEASE

  A. Physiology. The adrenal glands consist of two functionally distinct endocrine systems contained within a single organ: the adrenal cortex and the adrenal medulla. The adrenal cortex contains three zones, each of which secrete a different hormone: mineralocorticoids, glucocorticoids, and androgens. The adrenal medulla secretes catecholamines.

    1. Glucocorticoids. Cortisol is the principal hormone of this class. It is produced daily in a diurnal manner in response to adrenocorticotropic hormone (ACTH) from the anterior pituitary, and its production can be augmented by stress. Cortisol is required for converting norepinephrine to epinephrine in the adrenal medulla, although cortisol does not increase sympathetic nervous system activity. It has anti-inflammatory and immunosuppressive properties. Cortisol raises blood glucose levels by stimulating gluconeogenesis and promoting insulin resistance. It also has multiple effects on carbohydrate, protein, and fatty acid metabolism. Cortisol raises blood pressure by unclear mechanisms and studies suggest cortisol-induced HTN may be independent of its tendency to increase sodium retention.

    2. Mineralocorticoids. Aldosterone is the principle hormone of this class and the major regulator of extracellular fluid volume and potassium homeostasis. Its production is regulated by the renin-angiotensin system and blood K^+ concentration. Increased renin levels promote the conversion of angiotensinogen to angiotensin I. Angiotensin-converting enzyme (ACE) cleaves angiotensin I to generate angiotensin II. Angiotensin II then stimulates aldosterone secretion. Aldosterone causes reabsorption of Na^+ and excretion of K^+ and H^+ in the distal tubule of the nephron.

    3. Androgens. Abnormalities in androgen secretion are rarely pertinent to anesthetic management.

  B. Pharmacology. Synthetic steroids are available with different potencies and ratios of glucocorticoid to mineralocorticoid effect (**Table 7.6**).

  C. Primary hyperaldosteronism (Conn's syndrome)

    1. Etiologies include aldosterone-producing adrenal adenomas or aldosterone excess from bilateral adrenal hyperplasia.

    2. Clinical features include HTN, mild hypernatremia, hypokalemic metabolic alkalosis, hypokalemia-related muscle weakness, and increased incidence of metabolic syndrome.

TABLE 7.6	Glucocorticoid and Mineralocorticoid Hormones			
	Relative Potency			
Steroid	Glucocorticoid	Mineralocorticoid	Equivalent Dose (mg)	Duration (hours)
Short acting				8-12
Cortisol	1.0	1.0	20	
Cortisone	0.8	0.8	25	
Aldosterone	0.3	3000	–	
Intermediate acting				12-36
Prednisone	4.0	0.8	5	
Prednisolone	4.0	0.8	5	
Methylprednisolone	5.0	0.5	4	
Fludrocortisone	10.0	125	–	
Long acting				>24
Dexamethasone	25-40	0	0.75	

3. **Treatment.** The definitive treatment for aldosterone-producing adrenal adenomas is adrenalectomy. The standard treatment for bilateral adrenal hyperplasia is with an aldosterone receptor inhibitor, either spironolactone or eplerenone.

D. **Glucocorticoid excess (Cushing syndrome)**

1. **Etiologies** include exogenous steroid administration, excess pituitary ACTH secretion, ectopic ACTH secretion, and excess cortisol secretion.

2. **Clinical features** include truncal obesity, moon facies, gastroesophageal reflux disease, peptic ulcers, HTN, hypernatremia, hypervolemia, hyperglycemia, hypokalemia, red or purple cutaneous striae, poor wound healing, muscle wasting and weakness, osteopenia/porosis, hypercoagulability, mental status changes, emotional lability, aseptic osteonecrosis, pancreatitis, benign intracranial HTN, cataracts, and glaucoma.

3. **Anesthetic considerations.**

   a. Patients often exhibit HTN refractory to treatment.

   b. Hypervolemia can be reduced with diuretics, but potassium must be replaced.

   c. Monitor serum glucose levels and treat as needed.

   d. Osteoporosis makes careful positioning necessary.

   e. Patients may have unrecognized insulin resistance and coronary artery disease.

   f. Consider venous thrombosis prophylaxis given hypercoagulability.

   g. Glucocorticoid replacement should begin postoperatively for both unilateral and bilateral adrenalectomies. Mineralocorticoid replacement is necessary only after bilateral adrenalectomy.

   h. Excess ACTH secretion is treated by excision of the secreting tumor. Anesthesia for transsphenoidal pituitary surgery is discussed elsewhere.

E. **Adrenal cortical hypofunction** generally refers to a deficiency in adrenal secretion of mineralocorticoids, glucocorticoids, or both. Hypofunction may be due to dysfunction of the adrenal gland (primary), pituitary gland (secondary), or hypothalamus (tertiary).

1. **Etiologies** include idiopathic hypofunction, autoimmune destruction, surgical removal, radiation, infection, hemorrhage, drugs, granulomatous or metastatic infiltration, vasculitis, adrenal vein thrombosis, or loss of ACTH stimulation.

2. **Clinical features** depend on which adrenal cortical hormone is lacking and the time course of hormone deficiency.

   a. **Primary adrenal insufficiency (Addison's disease)** is associated with low cortisol and aldosterone levels resulting in hyponatremia, hyperkalemia, anemia, psychiatric changes, weakness, fatigue, weight loss, nausea/vomiting, abdominal pain, myalgias, arthralgias, postural hypotension, salt craving, and hyperpigmentation.

   b. **Secondary adrenal insufficiency** results in low cortisol levels and normal serum aldosterone because aldosterone production is independent of ACTH. Patients may have panhypopituitarism with symptoms of low TSH, growth hormone (GH), and/or gonadotropin levels. Exogenous steroid use is a common cause and may suppress the hypothalamic-pituitary-adrenal axis for up to 12 months after cessation of treatment.

   c. **Acute adrenal insufficiency** (adrenal crisis) primarily presents as shock and is a life-threatening emergency. Other clinical features include hypoglycemia, hyponatremia, hyperkalemia, metabolic acidosis, nausea/vomiting, abdominal pain, and mental status changes. The precipitant is usually a physiologic stressor (eg, surgery, trauma, infection), but it can also be due to inadequate daily doses of mineralocorticoid and/or glucocorticoid, a missed dose, or reduced drug absorption from vomiting or diarrhea.

3. **Treatment.** During times of stress, the glucocorticoid dose must be increased beyond basal dosing. Treatment of adrenal crisis includes identification and treatment of the precipitating event, volume resuscitation, infusion of dextrose 5% in isotonic fluid for hypoglycemia, electrolyte correction, hemodynamic support as necessary, and steroid replacement (hydrocortisone 100 mg IV followed by 50 mg IV every 6 hours or as a continuous infusion with a total daily dose of 200 mg; subsequent doses after 24 hours are based on clinical response). If hydrocortisone is not available, other parental glucocorticoids may be used in equivalent dosages. In primary adrenal insufficiency, daily fludrocortisone is required once the daily hydrocortisone dose is <50 mg.

4. **Anesthetic considerations.**

   a. Evaluate and treat hemodynamic and electrolyte derangements.

   b. Avoid etomidate in adrenal insufficiency because of the potential for further adrenal suppression.

   c. Patients with adrenal hypofunction may exhibit marked sensitivity to sedative, anesthetic, or vasodilator drugs. Titrate drug doses carefully to avoid cardiovascular depression.

   d. Perioperative steroid replacement is controversial and should be individualized. Any patient who has received more than a 14-day course of supraphysiologic steroid dosing in the past year may need glucocorticoid supplementation perioperatively.

   e. The following is one recommendation for perioperative IV hydrocortisone dosing:

F. Perioperative corticosteroid replacement depends on surgical invasiveness.

1. **Minor surgery** (eg, inguinal herniorrhaphy, minor urologic or gynecologic procedures, colonoscopy, oral or minor plastic surgery): usual daily dose + hydrocortisone 50 mg IV before incision + hydrocortisone 25 mg every 8 hours for 24 hours, followed by usually daily dose only.

2. **Moderate surgery** (eg, cholecystectomy, joint replacement, colon resection, hysterectomy, extremity revascularization): same dosing regimen as for minor surgery.

3. **Major surgery** (eg, trauma, labor and delivery, esophagectomy, major cardiac, vascular, or abdominal surgery), usual daily dose + hydrocortisone 100 mg before incision + hydrocortisone 50 mg every 8 hours or 200 mg in 24 hours by continuous infusion. Taper dose by half per day until usual daily dose is reached. Consider continuous infusion of 5% dextrose in 0.45% normal saline based on degree of hypoglycemia.

VI. ADRENAL MEDULLARY DISEASE

A. Physiology. Preganglionic fibers of the sympathetic nervous system stimulate release of catecholamines from the adrenal medulla.

B. Pheochromocytoma

1. **Epidemiology.** Pheochromocytomas are rare, functionally active neuroendocrine tumors of the adrenal medulla. They are typically unilateral adrenal tumors but can be bilateral, metastatic, or extra-adrenal. They are also associated with an array of familial syndromic disorders. Most tumors secrete epinephrine, norepinephrine, and dopamine. Secretion is independent of neurogenic control.

2. **Clinical features** are generally due to excess catecholamine release. The classic presentation includes palpitations, headache, and diaphoresis in an episodically hypertensive patient. Other symptoms include anxiety, flushing, tremor, orthostatic hypotension, hypovolemia, and weight loss. Plasma fractionated metanephrines or a 24-hour urine collection for catecholamines and their metabolites are the routine screening tests. Preoperative diagnosis is important, as intraoperative diagnosis is associated with a high mortality rate. Treatment is with surgical excision.

3. **Preoperative evaluation/preparation** is important because inadequate preparation has been shown to correlate with significant perioperative morbidity and mortality. The goal of preoperative management is to achieve adequate blood pressure control and assess for evidence of the cardiovascular consequences of excess catecholamines. Patients can develop catecholamine-induced cardiomyopathy acutely (takotsubo) or chronically (dilated or hypertrophic). Additional preoperative concerns include hypovolemia, intracranial hemorrhage, hyperglycemia, and nausea/vomiting. Comorbid endocrinopathies should be sought and treated.

   a. α-Receptor blockade is often started as an outpatient with oral phenoxybenzamine, a long-acting, irreversible α_1-adrenergic and α_2-adrenergic blocker, or a shorter-acting competitive α_1-blocker (prazosin, doxazosin). A calcium-channel blocker can be used as supplemental or alternative therapy, especially if the patient cannot tolerate α-blockers. Achieving adequate α-receptor blockade may require 7 to 14 days. Clinical end points suggesting adequate α-receptor blockade are known as the Roizen criteria and include: no blood pressure readings >160/90 mm Hg within 24 hours before surgery, postural hypotension (but standing blood pressure >80/45 mm Hg), no more than one premature ventricular contraction every 5 minutes, and an ECG that is free of ST-T changes for >1 week.

b. After adequate α-receptor blockade, patients without heart failure or renal dysfunction are encouraged to start a high-sodium diet and increased fluid intake for volume expansion. This is done to attenuate catecholamine-induced volume contraction and prevent significant intraoperative hypotension.

c. β-Blockade is instituted **after** the onset of adequate α-blockade to prevent unopposed vascular α-receptor stimulation and catastrophic hypertensive crisis. β-Blockade should be used with extreme caution in patients with catecholamine-induced cardiomyopathy. Selective or nonselective β-blockers can be used, with dosing titrated to a heart rate of 60 to 80 bpm.

d. α-Metyrosine can also be used for preoperative blood pressure management. It decreases circulating catecholamine levels by competitively inhibiting tyrosine hydroxylase, an enzyme important in the biosynthesis of norepinephrine. It is less tolerated because of its side-effect profile and is not typically administered as monotherapy.

4. Anesthetic considerations. The goal is to avoid triggering an adrenergic crisis, the most common precipitants being hypotension and sympathetic stimulation. Preoperative sedation may be helpful. Avoid sympathomimetic, vagolytic, or histamine-releasing drugs and anticipate the need to blunt sympathetic responses to induction, intubation, pneumoperitoneum, and surgical stimulation. A thoracic epidural is effective in ablating some sympathetic responses, but it does not prevent catecholamine surges and may cause hypotension.

a. Blood pressure should be measured directly. The need for additional invasive hemodynamic monitoring depends on the patient's medical status.

b. Magnesium has many intraoperative uses during pheochromocytoma resection. It has both antiarrhythmic and vasodilating properties owing to its ability to antagonize catecholamine receptors and function as a calcium channel blocker. It can be a useful adjunct but may potentiate the effects of nondepolarizing neuromuscular blocking agents.

c. Arrhythmias and hypertensive crisis may occur intraoperatively. Treatment options include IV boluses of vasodilators and β-blockers. Sodium nitroprusside, clevidipine, and nicardipine reduce both preload and afterload, whereas nitroglycerin predominantly reduces preload. Esmolol is a preferred β-blocking agent because of its rapid onset and short duration of action. Arrhythmias can be addressed with β-blockers and magnesium.

d. Once the tumor's venous supply is ligated, a sudden decrease in blood pressure may occur owing to the decrease in circulating catecholamine levels and residual α and β-blockade. Volume loading prior to tumor resection may attenuate this hypotension, and treatment with a direct-acting vasopressor is customary. Vasopressin may be particularly helpful because its pressor effect is catecholamine independent.

e. Glucose should be monitored perioperatively. Hyperglycemia is common preoperatively owing to suppression of insulin release by catecholamine-mediated α_2 receptor blockade. Hypoglycemia is seen after tumor resection owing to a surge in insulin in the absence of excess catecholamines.

    f. Endogenous catecholamine levels should return to normal shortly after tumor removal, but blood pressure may take much longer to normalize. ICU care may be required in the postoperative period. Patients undergoing bilateral adrenalectomy will require glucocorticoid and mineralocorticoid replacement therapy.

VII. PITUITARY DISEASE
A. Anterior pituitary gland

1. **Physiology.** The anterior pituitary regulates the thyroid and adrenal glands, the ovaries and testes, growth, and lactation by producing TSH, ACTH, follicle-stimulating hormone, luteinizing hormone, GH, and prolactin. A negative feedback system mediated by peripheral hormones tightly controls anterior pituitary secretion. Anterior pituitary adenomas may lead to hormone excess or hypopituitarism. Macroadenomas (>1 cm in diameter) can compress adjacent structures producing visual disturbances, seizures, or increased intracranial pressure.

2. **Anterior pituitary hyperfunction.** Pituitary adenoma is the most common cause of anterior pituitary hyperfunction. Prolactinomas generally do not affect anesthetic management. The hyperthyroidism of a TSH-secreting adenoma and the hyperadrenalism of an ACTH-secreting adenoma are treated as described above. The anatomic and physiologic changes seen with GH-secreting tumors warrant careful consideration.

3. **Clinical features.** GH stimulates bone, cartilage, and soft tissue growth leading to prognathism, subglottic narrowing of the trachea, and soft tissue overgrowth of the lips, tongue, epiglottis, and vocal cords. Connective tissue overgrowth can cause recurrent laryngeal nerve paralysis, carpal tunnel syndrome, and other peripheral neuropathies. These patients often develop glucose intolerance, arthritis, osteoporosis, OSA, HTN, cardiomyopathy generally manifesting as diastolic dysfunction, arrhythmias, and heart failure. They also have an increased incidence of valvular heart disease, coronary artery disease, and colon carcinoma. The primary treatment is surgical removal of the tumor. Medical management for persistent disease after surgery includes dopamine agonists (bromocriptine and cabergoline), somatostatin analogues (octreotide and lanreotide), GH receptor antagonists (pegvisomant), and radiation therapy. Excision of GH-secreting pituitary adenomas is often performed via the transsphenoidal approach.

4. **Anesthetic considerations.**

    a. Blood pressure should be measured directly. The need for additional invasive hemodynamic monitoring depends on the patient's medical status.

    b. Patients should be evaluated for other endocrinopathies and cardiac disease preoperatively.

    c. Patients with OSA are at high risk for airway obstruction.

    d. Conventional mask airways are often difficult to achieve, and endotracheal intubation can be challenging. Advanced airway and tracheostomy equipment should be available, and awake fiberoptic intubation should be considered. Small-diameter endotracheal tubes may be required.

    e. Serum glucose levels should be carefully monitored and muscle relaxants titrated using a peripheral nerve stimulator.

    f. Patients may be osteoporotic and have an increased susceptibility to peripheral neuropathies. Careful positioning is necessary.

5. Anterior pituitary hypofunction
  a. Etiologies. Pituitary adenoma is the most common cause of anterior pituitary hypofunction. Other causes of pituitary failure include trauma, radiation, pituitary apoplexy, tumors, infiltrative disease, and surgical hypophysectomy. Sheehan syndrome is a condition of pituitary failure in which hemorrhagic shock causes vasospasm and subsequent pituitary necrosis in postpartum women.
  b. Anesthetic considerations. Adrenal insufficiency develops over 4 to 14 days after destruction of the pituitary gland. Perioperative glucocorticoid supplementation may be necessary. Because the half-life of thyroid hormone is 7 to 10 days, symptomatic hypothyroidism does not occur until 3 to 4 weeks after pituitary surgery or apoplexy.

B. Posterior pituitary gland
  1. Physiology. The posterior pituitary is composed of the nerve terminals of neurons originating in the hypothalamus. Antidiuretic hormone (ADH; vasopressin) and oxytocin are stored in the posterior pituitary. ADH regulates plasma osmolarity and extracellular fluid volume by facilitating renal tubular resorption of free water. Intravascular hypovolemia, pain from trauma or surgery, nausea, and positive airway pressure stimulate ADH secretion. Oxytocin stimulates uterine contraction in labor and milk ejection in lactation.
  2. Diabetes insipidus (DI)
    a. Etiologies. DI results from insufficient ADH secretion by the posterior pituitary (central DI) or failure of the renal tubules to respond to ADH (nephrogenic DI). Causes of central DI include intracranial trauma, hypophysectomy, metastatic disease to the pituitary or hypothalamus, and infiltrative diseases. Causes of nephrogenic DI include hypokalemia, hypercalcemia, sickle cell anemia, chronic myeloma, obstructive uropathy, chronic renal insufficiency, and lithium therapy. Nephrogenic DI may be seen in the third trimester of pregnancy and may also be congenital.
    b. Clinical features include polydipsia and polyuria. The urine is inappropriately dilute, and serum osmolarity is high. Urine output is greater than 2 L/d.
    c. Anesthetic considerations. Mild DI (daily urinary volumes of 2-6 L in patients with an adequate thirst mechanism) does not require treatment. In patients who cannot drink, initial therapy should be with isotonic fluids (normal saline) to reverse shock. Once osmolality is less than 290 mOsm/kg, hypotonic fluids (half normal saline) are necessary. Careful monitoring and titration of urine output and plasma volume, sodium, and osmolarity are necessary.
    d. Central DI may be treated with the synthetic vasopressin analogue desmopressin (DDAVP) at 1 to 2 µg subcutaneously or IV every 12 hours as needed (or with an infusion intraoperatively). Side effects of DDAVP include hyponatremia, HTN, and coronary artery vasospasm.
    e. Nephrogenic DI is associated with failure of vasopressin to reduce urinary volume. Adequate oral or parenteral hydration must be assured. Chlorpropamide (an oral hypoglycemic) potentiates the effects of ADH on renal tubules and may be helpful. Inhibition of prostaglandin synthesis (by ibuprofen, indomethacin, or aspirin) or mild salt depletion with a thiazide diuretic may reduce urine volume.

3. **Syndrome of inappropriate antidiuretic hormone secretion (SIADH)** is persistent secretion of ADH in the absence of an osmotic stimulus.

   a. **SIADH** can be caused by malignancy, CNS disorders (stroke, trauma, infection, and tumor), pulmonary disorders (tuberculosis, pneumonia, positive-pressure ventilation, and chronic obstructive pulmonary disease), and many drugs (nicotine, amitriptyline, chlorpropamide, clofibrate, serotonin reuptake inhibitors, nonsteroidal anti-inflammatory drugs, haloperidol, amiodarone, ciprofloxacin, valproate, methotrexate, and some chemotherapies). Other etiologies include lupus, HIV, Guillain-Barré, hypothyroidism, Addison disease, heart failure, and cirrhosis. SIADH is associated with urine osmolality greater than serum osmolality (with a low serum osmolality), urine sodium greater than 20 mEq/L, and serum sodium less than 130 mEq/L. If serum sodium falls below 110 mEq/L, cerebral edema and seizures may result.

   b. **Treatment** includes addressing the underlying cause and fluid restriction (800-1000 mL daily) for the mild and/or asymptomatic hyponatremia of SIADH. Chronic hyponatremia is generally not treated unless it is associated with symptoms or the serum sodium is <120 mEq/L. Treatments include oral salt tablets or hypertonic saline for severe cases. Hyponatremia should be corrected no faster than 0.5 mEq/L/h because overly aggressive correction may produce central pontine myelinolysis, an irreversible neurologic disorder. Demeclocycline antagonizes the effects of ADH on renal tubules and may be helpful. Vasopressin receptor antagonists may also be helpful but are associated with a concerning safety profile.

VIII. CARCINOID

A. **Carcinoid tumors** (neuroendocrine tumors) typically arise anywhere along the GI tract, but they can also be seen in the lungs and elsewhere. Carcinoid tumors are capable of secreting substances that affect vascular, bronchial, and GI smooth muscle tone. Serotonin and histamine are the most commonly secreted hormones, but carcinoid tumors are capable of secreting up to 35 peptides and hormones. Stimuli for the release of these chemical mediators include catecholamines, histamine, hypotension, and tumor manipulation.

B. **Carcinoid syndrome** is seen in <5% of patients with carcinoid tumors. This syndrome develops when substances produced by the tumor reach the systemic circulation. Substances secreted from GI tumors are metabolized in the liver (preventing carcinoid syndrome) until the secretion overwhelms the liver's neutralizing ability, either because of the quantity produced or because of decreased liver activity from metastases. Tumors or metastases located outside the GI tract may produce the syndrome by direct release of mediators into the systemic circulation. Around 40% to 50% of small bowel and proximal colon carcinoids produce carcinoid syndrome.

C. **Clinical features** of carcinoid syndrome depend on which mediators a tumor releases. Common symptoms include flushing, bronchoconstriction, GI hypermotility, and hypoglycemia or hyperglycemia. Peripheral vasodilation and vasoconstriction can produce profound hypotension and HTN. Plaque-like deposits of fibrous tissue can deposit in the structures of the right side of the heart, resulting in tricuspid regurgitation and pulmonic stenosis. Left-sided valvular disease is unusual owing to inactivation of humoral substances by the lung.

D. Treatment is by surgical removal of the tumor. Liver metastases may be surgically resected or embolized. Medical treatment is used in preparation for surgery or embolization, in patients with unresectable disease, or in patients who are not surgical candidates. Octreotide is a long-acting somatostatin analogue and is the mainstay of medical treatment.

E. Anesthetic considerations

1. Hypovolemia, glucose abnormalities, and electrolyte disturbances should be treated preoperatively. Patients should be evaluated for valvular heart disease.

2. Octreotide should be given preoperatively to prevent the development of intraoperative carcinoid crisis. Both dosing and timing of preoperative treatment depend on the presence of symptoms and whether the patient is octreotide naive.

3. Preoperative sedation may be helpful to minimize mediator release due to anxiety.

4. Large blood loss should be expected as these tumors are vascular and there may be liver dysfunction or metastases. Invasive blood pressure monitoring should be used in anticipation of large blood pressure swings. Other invasive hemodynamic monitoring may help differentiate causes of hypotension in patients with carcinoid heart disease.

5. Triggers of mediator release should be avoided (hypotension, anxiety, pain, hypoxia, hypercarbia, tumor compression, drugs that cause histamine or catecholamine release, or sympathetic stimulation). Anticipate intraoperative mediator release; treat with octreotide boluses or infusion. Flushing is a warning sign of potential cardiovascular instability and should be treated with octreotide boluses.

6. Hypotension or HTN should be treated with octreotide, fluids, and direct-acting vasoconstrictors (phenylephrine, vasopressin) or vasodilators (nitrates) as needed. Conventional therapies for these conditions (β-agonists, epinephrine, and NTP) can stimulate mediator release and exacerbate symptoms.

7. Bronchospasm is less common but may be severe and should be treated with octreotide, antihistamines, and nebulized ipratropium.

8. Patients with carcinoid syndrome may have delayed awakening owing to excess serotonin. Postoperative ICU care may be appropriate, especially if an octreotide taper is required.

Suggested Readings

Bajwa SJS, Sehgal V. Anesthetic management of primary hyperparathyroidism: a role rarely noticed and appreciated so far. *Indian J Endocrinol Metab.* 2013;17(2):235-239.

Buchleitner AM, Martínez-Alonso M, Hernández M, Solà I, Mauricio D. Perioperative glycaemic control for diabetic patients undergoing surgery. *Cochrane Database Syst Rev.* 2012;(9):CD007315.

Domi R, Sula H, Kaci M, Paparisto S, Bodeci A, Xhemali A. Anesthetic considerations on adrenal gland surgery. *J Clin Med Res.* 2015;7(1):1-7.

Duggan EW, Carlson K, Umpierrez GE. Perioperative hyperglycemia management: an update. *Anesthesiology.* 2017;126:547-560.

Farling PA. Thyroid disease. *Br J Anaesth.* 2000;85:15-28.

Gerlach R, Tung A. Insulin for perioperative glucose control: settled science? *Anesthesiology.* 2017;127(5):899-900.

Gosmanov AR, Gosmanova EO, Dillard-Cannon E. Management of adult diabetic ketoacidosis. *Diabetes Metab Syndr Obes.* 2014;7:255-264.

Kaltsas G, Caplin M, Davies P, et al. ENETS consensus guidelines for the standards of care in neuroendocrine tumors: pre- and perioperative therapy in patients with neuroendocrine tumors. *Neuroendocrinology.* 2017;105(3):245-254.

Langley RW, Burch HB. Perioperative management of the thyrotoxic patient. *Endocrinol Metab Clin North Am.* 2003;32:519-534.

Liu MM, Reidy AB, Saatee S, Collard CD. Perioperative steroid management: approaches based on current evidence. *Anesthesiology.* 2017;127:166-172.

Mancuso K, Kaye AD, Boudreaux JP, et al. Carcinoid syndrome and perioperative anesthetic considerations. *J Clin Anesth.* 2011;23(4):329-341.

Naranjo J, Dodd S, Martin YN. Perioperative management of pheochromocytoma. *J Cardiothorac Vasc Anesth.* 2017;31(4):1427-1439.

Nemergut EC, Dumont AS, Barry UT, Laws ER. Perioperative management of patients undergoing transsphenoidal pituitary surgery. *Anesth Analg.* 2005;101(4):1170-1181.

Pasquel FJ, Umpierrez GE. Hyperosmolar hyperglycemic state: a historic review of the clinical presentation, diagnosis, and treatment. *Diabetes Care.* 2014;37(11):3124-3131.

Preiser JC, Provenzano B, Mongkolpun W, Halenarova K, Cnop M. Perioperative management of oral glucose-lowering drugs in the patient with type 2 diabetes. *Anesthesiology.* 2020;133:430-438. doi:10.1097/ALN.0000000000003237

Rushworth RL, Torpy DJ, Falhammar H. Adrenal crisis. *N Engl J Med.* 2019;381(9):852-861.

Stathatos N, Wartofsky L. Perioperative management of patients with hypothyroidism. *Endocrinol Metab Clin North Am.* 2003;32:503-518.

Infectious Diseases and Infection Control in Anesthesia

Diana Barragan-Bradford and Jamie L. Sparling

I. INTRODUCTION
A. The Centers for Disease Control and Prevention (CDC) estimates that in the United States, there are approximately 687,000 nosocomial infections per year, which cause or contribute to 72,000 deaths per year. In addition to the morbidity and mortality, these complications cost billions of dollars annually.

B. Infection control responsibilities of anesthetists
1. **Participate in infection control** to prevent transmission of infectious agents between patients and between patients and operating room (OR) personnel.
2. **Prevent or avoid infectious complications associated with anesthetic procedures** such as central venous catheter (CVC) insertion and epidural placement.
3. **Participate in prevention of surgical wound infections and antibiotic stewardship** with timely and appropriate perioperative antibiotic selection.

II. INFECTION CONTROL IN THE OR
A. Methods of infection spread
1. **Contact** with a colonized person, an actively infected person, a host, or a fomite is the most frequent route of transmission in the OR.
2. **Body fluids** (blood, urine, CSF) are a method of transmission that depends on access to a mucosal surface or a break in the integrity of the skin barrier.
3. **Droplet transmission** is the transfer of infectious particles via suspension in large fluid droplets such as those released during coughing or sneezing, which travel short distances (ie, 3-6 feet).
4. **Airborne transmission** is similar to droplet transmission with the exception that the particles are small enough to remain suspended in air and travel in air currents.

B. Standard or universal precautions constitute a minimum of acceptable guidelines that should be used for all patient populations regardless of infectious status.
1. **Hand hygiene** has consistently been shown to be the single most important method for preventing nosocomial infections. Basic hand hygiene requires that alcohol-based hand rub or hand washing with soap and water be used before and after any patient contact including any contact with equipment in the immediate vicinity of the patient.
2. **Personal protective equipment (PPE)** including gloves, gowns, masks, eye protection, and face shields should be readily available. Gloves should be used any time there is potential for contact with body fluids, and additional protective gear should be used when indicated based on precaution requirements.
3. **Appropriate OR attire** to prevent infectious spread includes clean scrubs that have not been worn outside of the OR, a cap or bouffant that covers all hair including beards, a mask, and either OR-dedicated closed

toed shoes or shoe covers over general use closed toed shoes. The use of cloth hats, compared with disposable bouffants, does not significantly impact surgical site infection (SSI) rates.

C. **Specific precautions** are necessary based on specific pathogens and their mode of transmission.

   1. **Contact precautions** are applied to patients with pathogens that can be transmitted by direct or indirect contact. The most frequently encountered organisms are methicillin-resistant *Staphylococcus aureus* (MRSA), vancomycin-resistant *Enterococcus* (VRE), extended-spectrum beta-lactamase enterobacteriaceae, multidrug-resistant organisms, and vancomycin-intermediate sensitivity or vancomycin-resistant *S. aureus*. In recent years, many hospitals have discontinued contact precautions for MRSA due to its high prevalence in the community; nevertheless, the CDC continues to recommend contact precautions for patients colonized or infected with MRSA. Routine screening via rectal (VRE) and nasal (MRSA) swabs has increased the identification of colonized patients, thus increasing the number of patients on contact precautions.

      a. **Gloves and gown** should be donned prior to entering and removed upon exiting the patient room.

      b. **Alcohol based hand cleanser or hand washing** should occur prior to gowning and gloving and immediately following gown and glove removal.

      c. During **transportation**, cover or contain the infected or colonized areas of the patient's body. Policies regarding wearing PPE during transport vary according to institution.

      d. **Medical records** should be kept outside of the patient room and transported in a plastic bag.

      e. **Removal of contact precautions** is hospital specific and organism specific. Typical standards include cessation of antibiotics for at least 48 hours, negative cultures from the infected site if applicable, and three negative cultures on different dates from the common site of colonization (MRSA, nasal; VRE, rectal).

   2. **Contact precautions plus** is for patients with known or suspected infection with spore-forming or alcohol-resistant organisms that can be transmitted by direct or indirect contact. The most frequently encountered is *Clostridium difficile*. In addition to standard contact precautions, hands must be washed with water and soap after glove and gown removal. These precautions may be discontinued after completion of an appropriate antibiotic course and resolution of symptoms.

   3. **Droplet precautions** are for patients with known or suspected infection with organisms that are transmissible via large respiratory droplets. The most frequently encountered organisms/diseases include meningococcal meningitis, *Mycoplasma pneumoniae*, and influenza.

      a. **Disposable surgical masks** should be worn by providers when within 3 feet of the patient and should be disposed of immediately after exiting the room. **Hand hygiene** should be completed after disposing of the mask.

      b. **Transportation** of the patient requires the patient to wear a surgical mask.

   4. **Airborne precautions** are for patients with known or suspected infection with organisms that may remain suspended in the air and be dispersed by air currents. The most frequently encountered organisms include pulmonary tuberculosis and varicella.

  a. **N95 respirators** should be worn whenever in the patient's room. These are specialized masks that require fit testing and training prior to use. For those who are unable to tolerate N95 respirators, **powered air-purifying respirators (PAPRs)** are an alternative.
  b. **Negative pressure** isolation rooms are required, and doors should remain closed.
  c. **Transportation** of the patient requires the patient to wear a surgical mask and those providing direct care to wear an N95 respirator.

D. **OR hygiene standards**
  1. **Bactericidal cleaning agents** should be used between all cases on the anesthesia machine, monitors, and workstation.
  2. **Clean workstation standards** at Massachusetts General Hospital mandate that any item that has touched the anesthesia machine tray will be discarded between cases to prevent cross contamination.
  3. **Sterilization of reusable equipment** between uses is necessary (eg, laryngoscopes, reusable laryngeal mask airways, bronchoscopes, reusable stylets). Alternatively, single-use, disposable laryngoscope blades and handles are available.
  4. **Bacterial contamination of the anesthesia machine** and the possibility of cross contamination between patients is a controversial topic. Available data have shown no significant difference in postoperative pulmonary infection rate between reusable circuits that are appropriately cleaned and disposable circuits. The high oxygen content, metallic ions, and the shifts in temperature and humidity present within the machine are bactericidal.
  5. **Air exchanges** in the OR should occur at a minimum of 15 times per hour, and the OR should be maintained at a positive pressure relative to surrounding areas with few exceptions (ie, airborne precaution patient).

E. **Avoid anesthesia-associated infectious complications**
  1. **Peripheral intravenous lines** should be placed after cleaning of the insertion site with an approved cleaning solution (at MGH, these include 70% isopropyl alcohol, povidone iodine, or 2% chlorhexidine/70% isopropyl alcohol) and covered with a transparent occlusive dressing. Additionally, access ports should be disinfected by using an appropriate disinfectant with friction prior to any access.
  2. **Strict sterile technique** including site cleaning, drapes, mask, and sterile gloves should be used for other invasive procedures including epidural placement, spinals, arterial lines, and peripheral nerve blocks.
  3. **CVCs** are a major source of potentially avoidable nosocomial infections. The most common sites of venous cannulation are the femoral, internal jugular, and subclavian veins. It was traditionally taught that femoral lines were the "dirtiest," and subclavian lines the "cleanest," but recent studies indicate that sterile technique in placement and daily assessment is more important than site choice. Central line–associated bloodstream infection (CLABSI) is a source of major morbidity and healthcare expenditure, but the adoption of prevention bundles has decreased the rate of CLABSI by 46% from 2008 to 2013. Causes include infection from skin flora at the site, contamination of infusions or catheter hubs, and seeding from distant sites. Emergency insertion, long duration in situ, use for total parenteral nutrition, and an increased number of lumens heighten the risk of CLABSI. The most common pathogens are bacteria including *Staphylococcus* and *Streptococcus* spp. as well as *Candida* spp.

a. **Protocols** for placement and daily care decrease CLABSI. Use of checklist and dedicated monitoring personnel during placement ensures strict sterile technique including full draping of the patient, aseptic technique (hand prep, site prep, sterile gown and gloves, mask), and appropriate dressing. Use of a daily care checklist ensures site skin integrity, maintenance of a transparent occlusive dressing, and ongoing evaluation for necessity of central access as well as appropriateness of removal. Routine replacement of CVC has not shown any clinical benefit.

b. **Diagnosis** of CLABSI is based on clinical manifestations, ranging from localized signs of infection to septic shock, combined with laboratory culture data. Blood, sputum, and urine cultures as well as wound cultures if applicable should be obtained prior to antibiotic initiation. If further clarity is required, simultaneous quantitative blood cultures, one from a peripheral site and one from the CVC, should be obtained. A 5- to 10-fold higher colony count on the culture from the CVC supports the diagnosis of CLABSI.

c. **Treatment** of CLABSI. The CVC should be removed and replaced at a new site. Changing the catheter over a guidewire should be avoided. Empiric antibiotic coverage is appropriate with narrowing of coverage as soon as Gram stain and culture data allow. Typical antibiotic courses for uncomplicated CLABSI are 7 to 14 days, but longer courses may be indicated for fungal infections and immunocompromised hosts.

4. **Aspiration pneumonia** is a potentially lethal infectious anesthetic complication as a result of aspiration of oropharyngeal or gastric contents that can occur at any point when the airway is not secured. Microaspiration can also occur around the endotracheal tube cuff and is shown to correlate with ventilator-associated pneumonia in the ICU.

   a. **Aspiration pneumonia** indicates an actual infectious etiology, while aspiration pneumonitis reflects a noninfectious chemical pneumonitis. Differentiation between the two can be challenging and as such, antibiotic therapy should not be reflexively initiated for all aspiration events.

   b. **Risk factors for aspiration** include emergency surgery, insufficient time spent NPO prior to induction, pregnancy, gastroparesis or other functional obstruction, bowel obstruction, and severe gastroesophageal reflux.

   c. **Risk factors for aspiration pneumonia** include large volume of aspiration, aspiration of low pH content matter, aspiration of particulate matter, immunocompromised status, and known colonization of secretions.

   d. **Treatment** of aspiration pneumonia should target the most frequent bacteria encountered: *S. aureus, Escherichia coli, Pseudomonas aeruginosa, Klebsiella pneumoniae*, and anaerobes. Broad-spectrum antibiotics may be indicated if pneumonitis has not improved in the first 48 hours. Narrowing of antibiotics should be accomplished as soon as possible based on respiratory Gram stain and culture. Steroids are no longer routinely administered for aspiration pneumonia, and therapeutic bronchoalveolar lavage should be avoided.

5. **Transfusion-related infections** have been minimized by using increasingly stringent testing protocols for all donated blood products. Use of appropriate transfusion thresholds can decrease the frequency and quantity of transfusion to additionally decrease related infection rates (**Table 8.1**).

TABLE 8.1	Transfusion-Related Infection Risk	
Transfusion-Related Infection		**Risk**
Bacterial infection (seen in platelet transfusion)		1 in 10,000
Parvovirus		1 in 35,000
Hepatitis C		1 in 150,000-400,000
Hepatitis B		1 in 200,000-500,000
Hepatitis A		1 in 1,000,000
HIV		1 in 1,500,000-2,000,000
Human T-lymphocytic virus 1 and 2		1 in 2,000,000-3,000,000
Syphilis		1 in 4,000,000

III. PERIOPERATIVE ANTIBIOTICS

A. Indications for administration of antibiotics in the OR
  1. **Continuation of ongoing treatment** for active infection
  2. **Prophylaxis against SSI**
  3. **Prophylaxis against endocarditis**

B. Principles of prophylaxis
  1. SSIs occur approximately 110,800 per year in the United States, according to the CDC. These SSIs result in increased hospital stays, increased ICU admissions, increased healthcare expenses, and, most importantly, an increase in mortality of up to 50%.
  2. **Surgical Care Improvement Project (SCIP)** is a national initiative to improve surgical outcomes. Antibiotic prophylaxis and stewardship are a major part of the measures.
      a. **SCIP-1:** Preoperative antibiotic dosed within 1 hour before incision time. Exceptions include vancomycin and fluoroquinolones, which require administration within 120 minutes of incision due to longer administration times. Of note, not all procedures warrant routine antibiotic prophylaxis.
      b. **SCIP-2:** Prophylactic antibiotic must be SCIP recommended. See **Table 8.2** for SCIP-recommended regimens.
      c. **SCIP-3:** Prophylactic antibiotics must be discontinued within 24 hours of the anesthetic end time (exception is 48 hours for cardiac surgery).
  3. Timing and administration
      a. As noted above, **antibiotic administration must occur within 60 to 120 minutes of incision** to allow appropriate blood and tissue levels. Care must be taken to ensure this, as administration may occur in an inpatient unit, in the preoperative area, in the emergency department, or in the OR. The institutional guidelines for the correct dose of antibiotics should be followed.
      b. **Repeated dosing** is indicated for surgeries of long duration, surgeries with large blood loss (>1500 mL), or large fluid replacement. Redosing is antibiotic specific. Cefazolin is the most frequently used perioperative antibiotic with a typical redosing schedule of every 4 hours intraoperatively.

TABLE 8.2	SCIP-Recommended Perioperative Prophylactic Antibiotics
Surgical Procedure/Site	**SCIP-Approved Antibiotics**
Coronary artery bypass grafting (CABG), other cardiac, or vascular	Cefazolin, cefuroxime, OR vancomycin[a] If β-lactam allergy: vancomycin[b] OR clindamycin
Hip/knee arthroplasty	Cefazolin, cefuroxime, OR vancomycin[a] If β-lactam allergy: vancomycin[b] OR clindamycin[b]
Colon	Cefotetan, cefoxitin, ampicillin/sulbactam, OR ertapenem[c] OR cefazolin OR cefuroxime *and* metronidazole If β-lactam allergy: clindamycin *and* aminoglycoside OR clindamycin *and* quinolone OR clindamycin *and* aztreonam OR metronidazole *and* aminoglycoside OR metronidazole *and* quinolone
Hysterectomy	Cefotetan, cefazolin, cefoxitin, cefuroxime, OR ampicillin/sulbactam If β-lactam allergy: clindamycin OR metronidazole

SCIP, Surgical Care Improvement Project.
[a]Justification for vancomycin is acceptable with provider documentation.
[b]When undergoing cardiac, orthopedic, and vascular surgery, if patient is allergic to β-lactam antibiotics, vancomycin or clindamycin is an acceptable substitute.
[c]Single dose only.

    c. Parenteral administration is standard. Slow intravenous push is appropriate for some antibiotics (eg, cefazolin), and prolonged infusions are required for others (eg, vancomycin, fluoroquinolones).

    d. Observation for **adverse reactions**.

        1. Antibiotics are the second leading cause of anaphylaxis in the OR.

        2. Agent-specific hypersensitivity reactions may be encountered (ie, red man syndrome with vancomycin).

    e. As noted above, antibiotics should be discontinued within 24 hours to prevent development of drug-resistant organisms.

C. Endocarditis prophylaxis. Patients with certain congenital and acquired cardiac conditions are at increased risk for infective endocarditis following specific surgical and dental procedures. In 2007, the American Heart Association significantly narrowed the list of both cardiac abnormalities and procedures for which endocarditis prophylaxis is indicated. The latest guidelines are reflected in the 2017 update and summarized below.

    1. Prophylaxis for high-risk patients only. High-risk patients include (1) prosthetic cardiac valves including transcatheter-implanted prostheses and homografts, (2) prosthetic material used in cardiac valve repair, (3) history of infectious endocarditis, (4) specific congenital heart diseases (CHDs): unrepaired cyanotic CHD including palliative shunts and conduits, or repaired CHD with residual shunts or valvular regurgitation at the site of or adjacent to the site of a prosthetic patch or prosthetic device, and (5) cardiac transplant recipients who develop valvulopathies. All other cardiac abnormalities do not need endocarditis prophylaxis.

    2. Prophylaxis for high-risk procedures only. High-risk procedures include (1) dental procedures that involve manipulation of gingival tissue, periapical region of the teeth, or perforation of the oral mucosa; (2) respiratory tract procedures only if there is incision or biopsy of respiratory mucosa; and (3) skin and musculoskeletal tissue procedures only if the site is infected. Specifically, gastrointestinal and genitourinary procedures including endoscopic retrograde cholangiopancreatography, cystoscopies, and ureteral stent placements, in the absence of active infection, are no longer considered high risk.

D. Surgical wound classification. Surgical wounds are classified based on risk of infection and help to guide antibiotic therapy.

   1. **Clean** wounds are uninfected; show no signs of inflammation; do not enter the respiratory, gastrointestinal, or genitourinary tracts; and are closed primarily. The biggest risk for postoperative infections is from skin-colonizing bacteria such as *Staphylococcus* and *Streptococcus* spp.

   2. **Clean-contaminated** wounds enter the respiratory, gastrointestinal, or genitourinary tracts without spillage of contents. Common pathogens are site dependent. Common respiratory pathogens include *Streptococcus pneumoniae*, *K. pneumoniae*, *S. aureus*, and *P. aeruginosa*. Common gastrointestinal pathogens include *E. coli*, *Proteus* spp., *Bacteroides* spp., and *Enterococcus* spp. Common genitourinary pathogens include *E. coli*, *Proteus* spp., *Klebsiella* spp., and *Staphylococcus saprophyticus*.

   3. **Contaminated** wounds include gross spillage of nonpurulent contents and those with breaks in sterile technique. Common pathogens are site dependent.

   4. **Dirty** wounds include gross spillage of purulent contents, existing infection or perforation, and organisms known to be present prior to the procedure. Again, common pathogens are site dependent.

E. Commonly encountered perioperative antibiotics

   1. **β-Lactams** include penicillins, carbapenems, monobactams, and cephalosporins. The common mechanism of action is inhibition of cell wall synthesis.

      a. **Cefazolin**, a first-generation cephalosporin, is the most commonly administered perioperative antibiotic as it provides coverage of most of the gram-positive and many of the gram-negative bacteria that are seen with clean wounds. **Cefoxitin** and **cefotetan**, second-generation cephalosporins, extended coverage of gram-negative bacteria and anaerobic bacteria making them appropriate selections for clean-contaminated and contaminated wounds. **Ceftriaxone** and **ceftazidime**, third generation cephalosporins, and **cefepime**, a fourth generation cephalosporin, extend coverage further over gram-negative bacteria making them appropriate selections for dirty wounds in particular.

      b. **Adverse reactions** include (1) hypersensitivity reactions from rash to anaphylaxis, (2) central nervous system toxicity (especially high-dose penicillin), (3) hematologic (platelet dysfunction with piperacillin or ticarcillin and impairment of clotting factor production with cefotetan), and (4) interstitial nephritis (especially with methicillin or nafcillin).

      c. **Penicillin and cephalosporin cross-reactivity:** among patients who report penicillin allergy, between 0% and 8.1 % will react if given a cephalosporin. The higher estimate is based upon old retrospective studies that have several limitations that may lead to an overestimation of cross-reactivity.

   2. **Clindamycin** inhibits protein synthesis at ribosomal subunits and is an appropriate alternative for β-lactam allergic patients. Coverage includes most gram-positive bacteria (including MRSA) as well as many anaerobes. **Adverse reactions** include (1) rash (anaphylaxis is rare), (2) hypotension with rapid administration, (3) gastrointestinal distress, (4) *C. difficile* colitis, and (5) potentiation of neuromuscular blockade.

3. **Vancomycin** inhibits cell wall synthesis at a different site than the β-lactams. It covers most gram-positive bacteria including MRSA but provides no coverage of gram-negative bacteria, making it an appropriate selection for β-lactam allergic patients and patients colonized or infected with MRSA. **Adverse reactions** include (1) red man syndrome and hypotension from histamine release with rapid administration, (2) hypersensitivity reactions, and (3) increased nephrotoxicity and ototoxicity when administered with other agents at risk for causing nephrotoxicity and ototoxicity.

4. **Aminoglycosides** include gentamicin, tobramycin, streptomycin, and amikacin. The mechanism of action is inhibition of protein synthesis at a ribosomal subunit different from clindamycin. Coverage includes grampositive and gram-negative aerobes and *Mycobacteria* spp. making them appropriate choices for combination therapy in wounds other than clean. **Adverse reactions** include (1) nephrotoxicity especially in patients with baseline renal impairment or other risk factors for renal impairment, (2) ototoxicity, and (3) potentiation of neuromuscular blockade.

5. **Fluoroquinolones** include ciprofloxacin, levofloxacin, and moxifloxacin. Mechanism of action is inhibition of bacterial DNA replication. Coverage includes extensive gram-negative bacteria, many grampositive bacteria, and atypical bacteria making them appropriate choices for combination therapy in wounds other than clean. **Adverse reactions** include (1) gastrointestinal distress, (2) hepatotoxicity, (3) central nervous system effects, especially in the elderly, and (4) variable QT prolongation.

6. **Metronidazole** inhibits nucleic acid synthesis. Coverage includes most anaerobic organisms making it appropriate for combination therapy in wounds other than clean. Adverse reactions include (1) gastrointestinal distress, (2) thrombophlebitis, (3) hypersensitivity reactions, (4) neurologic effects including peripheral neuropathy, and (5) disulfiramlike reaction when combined with alcohol.

IV. **PATHOGENIC ORGANISMS OF ANESTHETIC CONCERN**
The CDC (www.cdc.gov) has current reviews of common pathogens, including all reviewed here.

A. **Viruses**

1. **Human immunodeficiency virus (HIV)**

a. **Transmission.** HIV is transmitted through percutaneous or mucosal exposure to infected blood or body fluids via needlestick or other sharps injury, blood transfusion, sexual contact, and perinatally from infected mother to neonate.

b. **Occupationally acquired HIV.** Risk is low for occupationally acquired HIV in healthcare workers. Risk of seroconversion after percutaneous exposure to blood from an HIV-positive patient is 0.3%. Risk is increased with deep injury, visible patient blood on the injurious device, a needle that was within a vein or artery in the HIV-positive patient, patients with higher viral loads, and larger bore hollow needles.

c. **Postexposure prophylaxis (PEP).** In case of exposure, the Occupational Health Service of the institution should be contacted. Frequently updated guidelines are available for management of exposed healthcare workers on the CDC Web site (www.cdc.gov) and from the National Clinicians' PEP Hotline (888-448-4911). PEP must be initiated within 3 days of exposure making immediate reporting of exposure to occupational health of paramount importance. The decision to initiate PEP and the choice and duration of the PEP regimen are based on numerous factors including type of exposure, volume of exposure, and sensitivity of the virus to antiretroviral agents. PEP is not 100% effective, and follow-up testing is necessary.

2. **Hepatitis B virus (HBV)**

   a. **Transmission.** HBV is transmitted through percutaneous or mucosal exposure to infected blood or body fluids via needlestick or other sharps injury, blood transfusion, sexual contact, and perinatally from infected mother to neonate.

   b. **Occupationally acquired HBV.** Risk depends on immunization status of the healthcare provider, hepatitis B e antigen (HBeAg) status of the HBV-positive patient, and quantity of inoculate. Risk is increased in unimmunized healthcare workers (currently most hospitals and healthcare facilities require HBV vaccination and antibody titers prior to employment), source patients who are HBeAg positive, and when percutaneous exposure is via a hollow large-bore needle. Risk of clinical hepatitis from HBeAg-negative percutaneous exposure via needlestick is 1% to 6%, but is 22% to 31% with HBeAg-positive percutaneous exposure via needlestick. 90% of acute HBV hepatitis resolves without sequelae; however, 10% become chronically infected and are at risk for chronic hepatitis, cirrhosis, and hepatocellular carcinoma.

   c. **HBV vaccination.** Recombinant vaccination consisting of three vaccinations over 3 months is effective at least 90% of the time. As the nonresponder rate is 10%, verification of antibody titers should be completed for those who will be in contact with blood or bloody body fluids.

   d. **PEP.** Exposure to blood or body fluids from patients who are known to be hepatitis B surface antigen (HBsAg) positive or patients with unknown status who are high risk for HBV may require PEP. Immediate reporting of the event is of utmost importance. Vaccinated healthcare workers who have appropriate levels of hepatitis B surface antigen antibodies (HBsAb) (≥10 mIU/mL) require no treatment. Vaccinated healthcare workers who have low levels of HBsAb (<10 mIU/mL) and previously unvaccinated healthcare workers are treated with hepatitis B immunoglobulin (HBIg) and vaccination/revaccination.

3. **Hepatitis C virus (HCV)**

   a. **Transmission.** HCV is typically transmitted through large volume or repeated percutaneous exposure to blood, blood transfusion, perinatally from infected mother to neonate, and less commonly from sexual contact.

   b. **Occupationally acquired HCV.** HCV seroconversion from percutaneous exposure via needlestick or other sharps injury is approximately 1.8%. Of those infected with HCV, 80% become chronically infected and are at risk for chronic hepatitis, cirrhosis, and hepatocellular carcinoma.

   c. **PEP.** No PEP is currently recommended for HCV exposure. Close clinical and laboratory follow-up should continue to evaluate for necessity of treatment for chronic infection.

4. **Herpes simplex virus (HSV) I and II**

   a. **Transmission.** HSV is transmitted by direct contact between infected individuals, whether symptomatic or not, or infected secretions, mucosa, or damaged skin.

    b. Occupationally acquired HSV. Herpetic whitlow is HSV infection of the finger that can occur in the healthcare setting from contact with oral secretions of an infected individual. Symptoms include fever, painful and inflamed lesions, and localized lymphadenopathy. Persons with active herpetic whitlow can transmit HSV, so patient contact should be avoided.

5. Cytomegalovirus (CMV). CMV is a herpesvirus that in healthy patients is usually asymptomatic; however, it can be life threatening in immunocompromised patients and in utero. Transmission of CMV occurs via direct contact between a susceptible host (severely ill or immunocompromised) and infected source in the form of blood transfusion or organ transplantation. Infection can be acute or reactivation of a latent infection. To reduce this risk, CMV-negative immunosuppressed patients and CMV-negative pregnant patients should receive blood transfusions from CMV-negative donors if transfusion is required.

6. Varicella-zoster virus (VZV)

    a. Transmission. VZV (chicken pox and shingles) is transmitted via direct contact or airborne routes. Anesthetists can be exposed or expose others to VZV. Like CMV, VZV can be life threatening to immunocompromised patients and in utero.

    b. VZV vaccination. VZV vaccination is indicated for all nonimmune healthcare workers who may come into contact with high-risk patient populations. A history of chicken pox as a child and/or antibody titer may be required by healthcare facilities as preemployment screening.

7. Influenza virus

    a. Transmission. Influenza is transmitted via respiratory secretions in the droplet route. Anesthetists can acquire and spread influenza via their close involvement with respiratory secretions. Influenza is generally not life threatening in healthy individuals but may be life threatening in the immunocompromised, the chronically ill, and elderly patients.

    b. Influenza vaccination. Most healthcare facilities now require annual vaccinations for healthcare workers.

B. Bacteria

1. *Mycobacterium tuberculosis*

    a. Transmission of tuberculosis (TB). TB is transmitted via respiratory secretions via an airborne route. TB is often a latent or inactive disease that may be asymptomatic. Active TB most often occurs in immunocompromised and chronically ill patients.

    b. Occupational TB. Most healthcare facilities require annual testing of healthcare workers for TB via purified protein derivative skin testing. Recent seroconversion warrants treatment with a course of isoniazid. Additionally, healthcare workers need to be fitted and trained for N95 respirators; as above, healthcare workers who cannot tolerate an N95 respirator should use a PAPR.

2. Antibiotic-resistant bacteria are a growing problem in medicine. The rate of growth in antibiotic-resistant bacteria is currently outpacing the development of new antimicrobial drugs. Poor antibiotic stewardship, prolonged hospitalizations, presence of indwelling catheters, and prolonged mechanical ventilation have contributed to the increase in antibiotic-resistant bacteria. Anesthetists can help prevent the transmission of and slow the rate of growth of antibiotic-resistant bacteria with strict infection control policies and antibiotic stewardship.

C. Prion diseases
1. **Protein-containing infectious particles (prions)** cause diseases such as **Creutzfeldt-Jakob** and **kuru.** Transmission is from direct inoculation of infected material into a host, with most commonly reported transmission being from dura transplantation. Epidemiologic studies are limited due to the long incubation time and rarity of the disease. Although the occupational risk for healthcare workers is believed to be very low, following a surgical procedure of confirmed or suspected disease decontamination of equipment is per specific protocols.

D. Emerging infectious disease
1. In the last 2 decades, several new pathogens have emerged requiring a coordinated, worldwide response on the behalf of governments, public health, and healthcare organizations. In the midst of these outbreaks, little evidence is available to guide treatment early on, and guidelines will be fluid. Please refer to your local organization's guidelines to inform management approaches. Examples include:
   a. **Ebola:** Ebolavirus is a genus of five species from the filoviridae family. Several outbreaks have been reported since 1976, most recently the Zaire virus in 2014 to 2016. All species in the genus are highly virulent and transmissible by direct contact with infected blood, secretions, tissues, organs, and other bodily fluids from dead or living infected persons. Transmission via fomites contaminated with infected bodily fluids is also possible.
   b. **Novel coronaviruses (MERS, SARS, SARS-CoV-2):** Novel coronaviruses have been responsible for worldwide outbreaks of the Middle East respiratory syndrome (MERS, 2012), severe acute respiratory syndrome (SARS, 2003), and COVID 19 (caused by SARS-CoV-2, 2019). These viruses spread from an infected person's respiratory secretions via droplets and presumably aerosols but may also spread via fomites contaminated with infectious droplets. The occupational risk for healthcare workers is believed to be high, for which the use of proper protective equipment is mandatory when treating these patients.

V. OCCUPATIONAL EXPOSURE TO INFECTIOUS DISEASE
A. Prevention of exposure
1. Use **standard or universal precautions** as above.
2. **Observe needle safety.** The CDC estimated that 385,000 needlestick and other sharps-related injuries occur in healthcare workers each year. Many safety needle and needleless systems have been designed and should be used preferentially over standard needles. Needles should never be recapped, and needles should be discarded in a labeled sharps container immediately after use.

B. Management of exposure
1. **Wash exposed area.** Soap and water or sterile saline should be used to wash skin, and water or sterile saline should be used to flush mucous membranes. Specialized eye washing stations should be available.
2. **Immediate reporting of exposure** to occupational health or the emergency room (if after normal work hours) to ensure initiation of protocols for testing, PEP, and counseling.

VI. IMMUNOCOMPROMISED PATIENTS
A. Immunocompromised patients are at increased risk for community-acquired, nosocomial, and opportunistic infections. Immunocompromise can be due to malignancy, chemotherapy, HIV infection, corticosteroids,

severe malnutrition, and immunosuppressive therapy for solid organ and bone marrow transplant recipients or severe autoimmune disease.

1. **Elective surgery** should be delayed if possible, in the severely immunocompromised (ie, total neutrophil count < 500 cells/mm³).
2. Strict adherence to **sterile technique** is essential.
3. **Anesthetist with respiratory infections** should not be involved in the care of severely immunocompromised patients. If unavoidable, the provider should wear a surgical mask during any contact with the patient.
4. Patients may be on **neutropenic precautions** that include specific dietary and environmental restrictions as well as the wearing of masks during transport.
5. **Antibiotic prophylaxis** is used in various immunocompromised patients for prophylaxis against postoperative wound infection and for long-term prophylaxis against opportunistic infections. It is important to verify which immunosuppressant drugs a patient is taking as many may interact with common perioperative medications. Cyclosporine, in particular, is associated with metabolism alteration and toxicity when combined with various antibiotics.

Suggested Readings

Centers for Disease Control and Prevention. Updated U.S. Public Health Service guidelines for the management of occupational exposures to HBV, HCV, and HIV and recommendations for postexposure prophylaxis. Last Updated April 25, 2014. http://www.cdc.gov/mmwr/preview/mmwrhtml/rr5011a1.htm

Centers for Disease Control and Prevention. Workbook for designing, implementing, and evaluating a sharps injury prevention program. Last reviewed February 11, 2015. http://www.cdc.gov/sharpssafety/pdf/sharpsworkbook_2008.pdf

Harbarth S, Frankhauser C, Schrenzel J, et al. Universal screening for methicillin-resistant *Staphylococcus aureus* at hospital admission and nosocomial infection in surgical patients. *J Am Med Assoc.* 2008;299:1149-1157.

Jensen PA, Lambert LA, Iademarco MF, Ridzon R; Centers for Disease Control and Prevention. Guidelines for preventing the transmission of Mycobacterium tuberculosis in health care facilities. *MMWR Recomm Rep.* 2005;54(RR-17):1-141.

Kothari SN, Anderson MJ, Borgert AJ, Kallies KJ, Kowalski TJ. Bouffant vs skull cap and impact on surgical site infection: does operating room headwear really matter? *J Am Coll Surg.* 2018;227(2):198-202.

Loftus RW, Brown JR, Koff MD, et al. Multiple reservoirs contribute to intraoperative bacterial transmission. *Anesth Analg.* 2012;114:1236-1248.

Loftus RW, Koff MD, Burchman CC, et al. Transmission of pathogenic bacterial organisms in the anesthesia work area. *Anesthesiology.* 2008;109:399-407.

Mandell LA, Niederman MS. Aspiration pneumonia. *N Engl J Med.* 2019;380:651-663.

Nishimura RA, Otto CM, Bonow RO, et al. 2017 AHA/ACC focused update of the 2014 AHA/ACC guideline for the management of patients with valvular heart disease: a report of the American College of Cardiology/American Heart Association Task force on Clinical Practice Guidelines. *Circulation.* 2017;135(25):e1159-e1195.

Parienti JJ, Mongardon N, Megarbane B, et al. Intravascular complications of central venous catheterization by insertion site. *N Engl J Med.* 2015;373:1220-1229.

The Joint Commission. Specifications manual for national hospital inpatient quality measures. 2019. https://www.jointcommission.org/-/media/tjc/documents/measurement/specification-manuals/hiqr_specsman_july2019_v5_6.pdf

Safety in Anesthesia

Miguel A. Patino Montoya and Rebecca D. Minehart

I. OVERVIEW OF SAFETY IN ANESTHESIA

A. Anesthesiology has led the patient safety movement, and anesthesia-related adverse outcomes have drastically declined since the 1960s. Despite this decline, the risks of both general and regional anesthesia remain. Recent data suggest that anesthetic-related mortality is 0.5 to 1/100,000 in the developed world.

B. The World Health Organization (WHO) and the World Federation of Societies of Anesthesiologists (WFSA) developed the International Standards for a Safe Practice of Anesthesia. These standards are intended to guide individuals and organizations in maintaining and improving safety and quality in anesthesia care.

C. Adverse events are injuries resulting from medical care. Many systems and human factors errors can contribute to adverse events. Reason's "Swiss cheese model" of adverse event causation describes how, although many layers of defense lie between hazards and adverse events, there are gaps in each layer that, if aligned perfectly, can allow an event to occur.

D. Errors can occur despite a practitioner's expertise, experience, and good intention. In the perioperative arena, errors can result from the following:

1. Organizational influences including production pressure or improperly maintained equipment

2. Inadequate supervision, which includes the unavailability of attending anesthesiologists to immediately assist less experienced residents

3. Preconditions for unsafe acts include fatigued clinicians or improper communication practices

4. Specific individual acts

E. Preventing adverse events therefore relies on optimizing practitioners' understanding of the system and resources of their workplace, in addition to individual practice improvement. Strategies to create safer systems include the following:

1. Simplification

2. Standardization

3. Improving teamwork and communication

4. Developing an organizational culture that promotes **learning from past mistakes**

5. Building **resilient recovery systems**

F. **Resilience** is a critical system property advocating for maintaining safety. It can be defined as the adaptability or capacity to recover quickly from difficulties or unforeseen complications. Special interest has developed to move from an error-based approach in safety to a preventative approach. This means that resilient systems do not wait for errors to occur so they can be analyzed, but rather focus on prevention, ensuring best performances, and/or quick recovery during any circumstances.

II. STANDARDS FOR SAFE ANESTHESIA CARE

The International Standards for a Safe Practice can be grouped in different categories:

A. **Professional aspects**, such as anesthetists having high levels of knowledge and skills, professional training through formal accredited training institutions, adequate numbers of anesthesiologists to meet the needs of the surgical workforce, and quality assurance mechanisms to implement improvements in care

B. **Facilities and equipment**, which must allow for safe care, according to the environment (preoperative area, operating room [OR], and postanesthesia recovery area)

C. **Available medications and intravenous fluids**, such as basic hypnotics, anxiolytics, opioids and other nonopioid analgesics, local anesthetics, dextrose solutions, normal saline, Ringer lactate, resuscitative medications and concentrated oxygen, and magnesium

D. **Monitoring**, including visualizing respiration rate and quality (including breathing system bag movement) and assessing tissue oxygen and perfusion, auscultating breath and heart sounds, palpating pulse rate and quality, enabling audible signals and alarms at all times, and using continuous pulse oximetry, intermittent noninvasive blood pressure monitoring, and a carbon dioxide detector for patients undergoing intubation

E. **Conduct of anesthesia**, such as a single anesthetist per patient responsible also for transport, assessment and informed consent procedures, WHO Safe Surgical Checklist procedures, and appropriate postanesthetic care and pain management

III. TYPES OF ERRORS

Errors are acts of commission (doing something wrong) or omission (failing to do the right thing) leading to an undesirable outcome. Anesthesiologists should be aware of, and actively work to mitigate, common types of errors.

A. **Medication errors.** It is estimated that at least 5% of hospital patients experience an adverse drug event. The cost of preventable medication errors in US hospitals has been estimated at $16.4 billion annually.

1. **Examples of medication errors** include administration of an inappropriate dose, administration through an inappropriate route, administration at an inappropriate rate, and administration to the incorrect patient. Some specific examples are as follows:

   a. The rapid intravenous (IV) administration of undiluted dilantin or undiluted potassium can cause cardiovascular collapse or death.

   b. Neostigmine administered without a corresponding antimuscarinic drug can lead to severe bradycardia, asystole, and death.

   c. Inadvertent administration of a medication to which a patient has a known allergy.

2. **Strategies to decrease medication errors:**
   a. Have a thorough understanding of the pharmacokinetics, pharmacodynamics, and effects of each medication administered.
   b. Exercise extreme vigilance in drug administration. Double-check medications prior to administration and consider implementing the "Five Rights" checklist: right patient, right route, right dose, right time, and right drug prior to each administration.
   c. Have only **unit dosing** available in the patient care area. Unit dosing refers to packaging medications in quantities and concentrations that are safe and appropriate for administration without dilution.
   d. Involve clinical pharmacists in perioperative care. Pharmacists can provide assistance with drug dosing questions and help identify medication errors immediately.
   e. Perform careful medication reconciliation when transitioning care between the floor, ICU, and perioperative or procedural areas. Medical reconciliation is the process of reviewing a patient's complete medication regimen on both ends of care to avoid unintended inconsistencies.
   f. Avoid confusing and potentially hazardous abbreviations. The Joint Commission has issued a list of high-risk "do not use" abbreviations. https://www.jointcommission.org/resources/patient-safety-topics/patient-safety/
   g. Consider bar coding technology to decrease medication identification errors.

B. **Procedure errors**
   1. **Examples of procedure errors** include wrong-site surgery, retained instruments, and OR fires. Higher volumes of certain surgeries or procedures being performed by a single physician or institution have been associated with better outcomes.
   2. **Strategies to reduce procedure errors:**
      a. "Universal Protocols" should be implemented including signing site of surgery, using preprocedural time-outs, and using checklists.
      b. Intraoperative surgical instrument and sponge counts are used to prevent retained surgical instruments in the patient. If the instrument counts at the end of the procedure indicate that an instrument is missing, radiography of the operative field is conducted in the OR to determine whether the instrument is in the patient.
      c. Recognize and avoid the fire safety triangle: ignition source (electrocautery, lasers) plus fuel source (gauze, drapes, endotracheal tube) plus oxidizers (oxygen, nitrous oxide) equals fire.
      d. The positive volume-outcome relationship for procedures argues for simulation training and specialization. Robust competency training should take place for procedures such as vascular catheterization, advanced intubation techniques, and bedside ultrasound use.

C. **Cognitive errors** are not due to faulty knowledge but involve faulty thought processes and subconscious biases. Cognitive errors are important contributors to missed diagnoses and patient injury.
   1. **Table 9.1** lists 14 common cognitive errors.
   2. **Strategies to decrease cognitive errors:**
      a. Use **Bayesian reasoning** and **iterative hypothesis testing**. In Bayesian reasoning, the probability estimate for a hypothesis is updated as additional evidence is acquired. With iterative hypothesis testing, a list of differential diagnoses is modified and re-ranked as more information becomes available. Each piece of new information triggers a recalibration of the probability of various diagnoses.

TABLE 9.1	Cognitive Error Catalog	
Cognitive Error	**Definition**	**Illustration**
Anchoring	Focusing on one issue at the expense of understanding the whole situation	While troubleshooting an alarm on an infusion pump, you are unaware of sudden surgical bleeding and hypotension
Availability bias	Choosing a diagnosis because it is in the forefront of your mind due to an emotionally charged memory of a bad experience	Diagnosing simple bronchospasm as anaphylaxis because you once had a case of anaphylaxis that had a very poor outcome
Premature closure	Accepting a diagnosis prematurely, failure to consider reasonable differential of possibilities	Assuming that hypotension in a trauma patient is due to bleeding, and missing the pneumothorax
Feedback bias	Misinterpretation of no feedback as "positive" feedback	Belief that you have never had a case of unintentional awareness, because you have never received a complaint about it
Confirmation bias	Seeking or acknowledging only information that confirms the desired or suspected diagnosis	Repeatedly cycling an arterial pressure cuff, changing cuff sizes, and locations, because you "do not believe" the low reading
Framing effect	Subsequent thinking is swayed by leading aspects of initial presentation	After being told by a colleague, "this patient was extremely anxious preoperatively," you attribute postoperative agitation to her personality rather than low blood glucose
Commission bias	Tendency toward action rather than inaction. Performing unindicated maneuvers, deviating from protocol. May be due to overconfidence, desperation, or pressure from others	"Better safe than sorry" insertion of additional unnecessary invasive monitors or access; potentially resulting in a complication
Overconfidence bias	Inappropriate boldness, not recognizing the need for help, tendency to believe we are infallible	Delay in calling for help when you have trouble intubating, because you are sure you will eventually succeed
Omission bias	Hesitation to start emergency maneuvers for fear of being wrong or causing harm, tendency toward inaction	Delay in calling for chest tube placements when you suspect a pneumothorax, because you may be wrong and you will be responsible for that procedure
Sunk costs	Unwillingness to let go of a failing diagnosis or decision, especially if much time/resources have already been allocated. Ego may play a role	Having decided that a patient needs an awake fiberoptic intubation, refusing to consider alternative plans despite multiple unsuccessful attempts

TABLE 9.1	Cognitive Error Catalog (*continued*)	
Cognitive Error	**Definition**	**Illustration**
Visceral bias	Countertransference; our negative or positive feelings about a patient influencing our decisions	Not troubleshooting on epidural for a laboring patient, because she is "high maintenance" or a "complainer"
Zebra retreat	Rare diagnosis figures prominently among possibilities, but physician is hesitant to pursue it	Try to "explain away" hypercarbia when malignant hyperthermia should be considered
Unpacking principle	Failure to elicit all relevant information, especially during transfer of care	Omission of key test results, medical history, or surgical event
Psych-out error	Medical causes for behavioral problems are missed in favor of psychological diagnosis	Elderly patient in postanesthesia recovery area is combative—prescribing restraints instead of considering hypoxia

Reprinted from Stiegler MP, Neelankavil JP, Canales C, et al. Cognitive errors detected in anaesthesiology: a literature review and pilot study. *Br J Anaesth*. 2012;108(2):229-235. Copyright © 2012 Elsevier. With permission.

    b. Be aware of performance-shaping factors that may adversely affect anesthetists' diagnostic abilities: noise, illness, aging, and especially sleep deprivation and fatigue.

    c. Continually learn from experience: self-reflect, discuss with senior and peer clinicians, and participate in M&M conferences.

D. Human factors errors. Human factors engineering is the applied science of systems design. It is concerned with the interplay between people and their work environments. Pioneering studies of human factors in anesthesia were integral to the redesign of anesthesia equipment, significantly reducing the risk of injury or death in the OR. Experts in this field perform usability tests and heuristic analyses to identify error-prone devices or systems before they lead to harm.

E. Care transition and handoff errors

    1. Examples of handoff errors: The most common errors at the time of transitions and handoffs are medication errors and failure to follow up diagnostic results.

    2. Strategies to decrease handoff errors:

        a. Handoffs should occur at designated times and without distractions. The anesthetic record should indicate the time of the change.

        b. If possible, care transitions should be avoided during short procedures. They should be used carefully in complex cases.

        c. During a handoff, the following information should be clearly and accurately presented:

            1. Prior clinical details. The patient's diagnosis, surgical procedure, allergies, past medical and surgical history, relevant medications, and any pertinent laboratory values or studies.

            2. Intraoperative management. Status of the surgical procedure, airway assessment and management techniques, anesthetic plan, current vital signs with an explanation for any apparent abnormalities or trends, details of IV access and monitoring, blood loss and volume status assessment, status of the patient's blood bank sample plus blood product availability, anticipated need for additional intraoperative, and plan for postoperative recovery of the patient.

    3. Handoffs should also address likely clinical scenarios and contingency plans.

  d. A handoff checklist may be used to ensure that complete information is communicated to the next responsible clinician. For example, "I-PASS" (Illness severity, Patient summary, Action list, Situation awareness and contingency planning, and Synthesis by the receiver) is a common strategy for handoffs.

F. Teamwork and communication errors. The perioperative, procedural, and intensive care units are team environments. Teamwork enhances safety and may be essential for preventing or recovering from a critical situation.

  1. Strategies to enhance teamwork and decrease communication errors:

    a. Start each day with effective **introductions**, consider **briefings and check-ins** with team members, and end with **debriefings**.

    b. Well-functioning teams are characterized by appropriate authority gradients and hierarchies that allow for "**speaking up.**" "Authority gradients" refer to the established or perceived power hierarchy within a team, and how the distribution of power is balanced. Concentration of power in one person or in overbearing team leaders leads to a steep and inappropriate authority gradient if that leader does not actively solicit information from others in an inclusive manner. Expressing concerns, questioning, or even clarifying instructions would require considerable determination on the part of team members who perceive their input as devalued or frankly unwelcome. In contrast, **inclusive leadership**, where input from team members is invited and appreciated, is thought to allow for improved collaboration.

    c. Develop an **understanding of the responsibilities and functions** of the other team members. During a crisis, maintain awareness of the other team members' actions.

    d. Make requests and **delegate tasks** clearly and specifically by name. Delegate tasks to those who can best perform them, and encourage confirmation that team members can perform tasks designated.

    e. Utilize **closed-loop communication** to avoid misunderstandings. When one individual gives a message, the receiver should repeat the message back to ensure it was heard correctly. Always **confirm** that critical interventions have been made as planned.

    f. Always communicate any concerns early and clearly.

IV. GENERAL SAFETY STRATEGIES

A. Crisis resource management

  1. In the early 1990s, the concept of Anesthesia Crisis Resource Management was introduced by Dr David Gaba. It was adapted from the aviation industry and their Crew (originally "cockpit") Resource Management principles and has extended to other specialties and fields under the name of Crisis Resource Management (CRM). CRM is a strategy to optimally identify, organize, and apply resources to preserve safety and acceptable outcomes for patients. CRM key principles were designed for team members to focus their attention on elements that can improve patient safety. See **Table 9.2** for more details.

T A B L E 9.2	Crisis Resource Management (CRM) Principles

CRM Principle	Elaboration on Principle
Call early for help	Know your limitations and call for help when a difference can be made. Anticipate and call people with special skills if they may be needed.
Anticipate and plan	Plan for possible difficulties ahead and the unexpected. Use wisely the time during low workload periods to prepare.
Know your environment	Know where things are and how they work. Know the vulnerabilities and strengths of your environment.
Use all available information	Use different sources to gather data and integrate them to have better understanding of patients and situations. Cross check your information.
Allocate attention wisely	Minimize distractions. Do not fixate on a single variable. Alternate focusing on details and the big picture.
Mobilize resources	Think of resources (people or equipment) and activate them to help with the crisis. Do not struggle alone.
Use cognitive aids	Flexibility can be helpful, but also a source of errors. Cognitive aids can help minimize such errors. Know their formats, location, and content.
Communicate effectively	All team members must understand the situation (ie, have "shared situational awareness"). All requests must be clear and confirmed (directed, "closed loop").
Distribute the workload	Team leaders must distribute tasks according to team members' abilities. Reassess distribution and identify overload or failure in tasks.
Establish role clarity	Responsibilities must be clear to each member. Roles must be concordant to skill and training.
Designate leadership	Clear leadership must be established. The leader plans and communicates effectively.

Reprinted from Gaba DM, Fish KJ, Howard SK, et al. *Crisis Management in Anesthesiology*. 2nd ed. Saunders; 2015. Copyright © 2015 Elsevier. With permission.

2. A simple mnemonic "Name/Claim/Aim High" integrates key CRM principles (see **Figure 9.1**):
   a. Name: The clinical problem/crisis must be identified and called out loud, including when the diagnosis is unknown.
   b. Claim: A leader must be established, and other roles must be assigned (either leader- or self-designated; roles may change).
   c. Aim: The team is aimed with a brief list of interventions, including diagnostic questions to resolve.
3. Under this strategy, a "Pre-Name" phase includes knowing the environment, anticipating and planning, and calling early for help. The naming phase includes effective communication, anticipating and planning, and mobilizing resources. The Claiming phase is the most extensive, as it incorporates all the other principles except for those included in the pre-name phase. The term "event manager" is often used

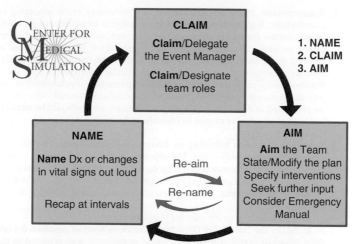

FIGURE 9.1 Name/Claim/Aim. This is an example of a tool to guide effective leadership, teamwork, and application of crisis resource management principles. (© Center for Medical Simulation, 2018.)

interchangeably with "team leader," as a means to facilitate "speaking up" by team members by flattening power hierarchy. Finally, the Aiming phase encompasses effective communication, mobilizing resources, using all available information, and using cognitive aids.

V. QUALITY ASSURANCE AND SAFETY IMPROVEMENT PROGRAMS

Institutional quality assurance programs should include a spectrum of activities aimed at maintaining and improving the quality of care and minimizing the risk of injury from anesthesia.

A. **Just culture.** Healthcare organizations should strive to create a **just culture.** A just culture is one that recognizes that even competent professionals make mistakes and that individual practitioners should not be held accountable for system failings over which they have no control. A just culture does not tolerate the conscious disregard of clear risks to patients: reckless behavior or gross misconduct. Personnel should always feel comfortable disclosing their own errors while maintaining professional accountability.

B. **Standards and guidelines.** Anesthesiologists should be aware of national and local safety policies and procedures. This includes policies for monitoring, response to adverse events, resuscitation protocols, perioperative testing protocols, and any special procedures or practices for the use of drugs, equipment, and supplies. The American Society of Anesthesiologists' standards and practice guidelines can be found at www.asahq.org.

C. **Safety training.** Anesthetists should obtain training in fire safety, electrical safety, OR evacuation, infection control procedures, and crisis management. They should also be certified in advanced cardiac life support and, under certain circumstances, pediatric advanced life support and advanced trauma life support. Simulation techniques should be used wherever practical to allow practice under controlled conditions.

D. **Documentation.** Many systems depend on voluntary error reporting by anesthetists. A safety report or quality assurance incident report should be completed for any unusual occurrence, unforeseen outcome, patient injury, or near miss, especially if follow-up action may be required to prevent recurrence. Incidents are reviewed by the departmental quality assurance committee, which receives additional information from those involved in the event and may suggest compensatory mechanisms as systematic factors are identified. Cases with special educational value should be presented at departmental case conferences. There should be ongoing analysis of all adverse events to identify and assess system problems and developing patterns.

E. **Guidelines for action following an adverse anesthesia event.** Despite best efforts, errors may still occur. **The objective** of these guidelines is to limit patient harm from errors when they do occur, to ensure the causes of the event are identified, and to help prevent recurrence.

1. **The anesthesiologist** involved in an adverse event should do the following:
   a. Continue to provide care for the patient.
   b. Notify the anesthesia OR administrator as soon as possible. If a resident or certified registered nurse anesthetist was involved in the event, he or she should notify the attending staff.
   c. Document events in the patient record. If appropriate, include serial numbers or lot numbers of equipment or medication that was involved.
   d. Do not alter the record.
   e. Stay involved with the follow-up care.
   f. Contact consultants as needed.
   g. Submit a follow-up report to the department quality assurance committee.
   h. Participate in apology and disclosure with the patient or patient's family.
   i. Obtain support as needed.

Suggested Readings

Agarwala AV, McCarty LK, Pian-Smith MC. Anesthesia quality and safety: advancing on a legacy of leadership. *Anesthesiology*. 2014;120(2):253-256.

American Society of Anesthesiologists. Accessed on May 21, 2020. https://www.asahq.org/standards-and-guidelines

Anesthesia Patient Safety Foundation. Accessed on May 21, 2020. www.asahq.org

Arriaga AF, Bader AM, Wong JM, et al. Simulation-based trial of surgical-crisis checklists. *N Engl J Med.* 2013;368:246-253.

Cooper JB, Gaba DM. A strategy for preventing anesthesia accidents. *Int Anesthesiol Clin.* 1989;27:148-152.

Cooper JB, Newbower RS, Kitz RJ. An analysis of major errors and equipment failures in anesthesia management: considerations for prevention and detection. *Anesthesiology*. 1984;60:34-42.

Gaba DM, Fish K, Howard S, Burden A. *Crisis Management in Anesthesiology.* 2nd ed. Saunders; 2015.

Gelb AW, Morris WW, Johnson W, et al. World Health Organization-World Federation of Societies of Anaesthesiologists (WHO-WFSA) International Standards for a Safe Practice of Anesthesia. *Anesth Analg.* 2018;126(6):2047-2055.

Guohua L, Warner M, Lang BH, et al. Epidemiology of anesthesia-related mortality in the United States, 1999-2005. *Anesthesiology.* 2009;110:759-765.

Institute for Safe Medication Practice. Accessed on May 21, 2020. www.ISMP.org

Kohn LT, Corrigan JM, Donaldson MS, eds. *To Err Is Human: Building a Safer Healthcare System.* National Academy Press; 1999.

Leape L, Berwick D, Clancy C, et al. Transforming healthcare: a safety imperative. *Qual Saf Health Care.* 2009;18:424-428.

Minehart RD, Foldy EG, Long JA, Weller JM. Challenging gender stereotypes and advancing inclusive leadership in the operating theatre. *Br J Anaesth.* 2020;124(3):e148-e154.

Østergaard D, Dieckmann P, Lippert A. Simulation and CRM. *Best Pract Res Clin Anaesthesiol.* 2011;25(2):239-249.

Oberfrank SM, Rall M, Dieckmann P, Kolbe M, Gaba DM. Chapter 6. Avoiding patient harm in anesthesia: human performance and patient safety. In: Gropper MA, Miller RD, eds. *Miller's Anesthesia.* 9th ed. Elsevier Churchill Livingstone; 2020:105-178e.

Shahian DM, McEachern K, Rossi L, Gino Chisari R, Mort E. Large-scale implementation of the I-PASS handover system at an academic medical centre. *BMJ Qual Saf.* 2017;26(9):760-770.

Smith AF, Plunkett E. People, systems and safety: resilience and excellence in healthcare practice. *Anaesthesia.* 2019;74(4):508-517.

Stiegler MP, Neelankavil JP, Canales C, et al. Cognitive errors detected in anaesthesiology: a literature review and pilot study. *Br J Anaesth.* 2012;108(2):229-235.

Watcher RM. *Understanding Patient Safety.* 2nd ed. McGraw Hill Medical Publishing; 2012.

The Anesthesia Machine

Samuel Wood and Jeremi Mountjoy

I. OVERVIEW

Over the past 2 decades, anesthesia machines have become increasingly more complex. These **anesthesia machines** present many challenges to anesthetists in terms of their increased complexity, changed layout and function, and integration of new technologies.

The basic function of the anesthesia machine is to prepare a gas mixture of known and variable composition, and then deliver that gas to the patient. The machine regulates a controlled flow of oxygen, nitrous oxide, and air, to which anesthetic vapors are added. These gases flow into a breathing system. The breathing system can provide positive pressure ventilation via a mechanical ventilator or manual bag ventilation, and also allow a patient to breathe the gases spontaneously. The breathing system incorporates means for warming and humidification of gases, and for removal of CO_2 from the exhaled gases. Anesthesia machines also provide a scavenger system to allow removal of waste gases from the immediate environment.

The anesthesia breathing system is unique among mechanical ventilators in that it is explicitly designed to allow patients to rebreathe exhaled gases, so that anesthetic agents can be conserved. To facilitate rebreathing, machine features are incorporated to ensure that the gas mixture delivered to the patient is safe. At a minimum, anesthesia machines incorporate an oxygen sensor, to measure the oxygen concentration in the gas mixture. Many anesthesia machines also incorporate a sophisticated gas analysis system, capable of measuring oxygen, carbon dioxide, and anesthetic agents. Anesthesia machines also comply with a complex set of standards, with built-in monitors and sensors used to survey the functioning of the ventilation system, and detect equipment malfunctions.

II. THE GAS DELIVERY SYSTEM (FIGURE 10.1)

A. Medical gas supply

1. **Pipeline gas system.** Wall outlets deliver oxygen, nitrous oxide, and air, from a central supply source, at a pressure of 50 to 55 pounds/in^2 (psi). These outlets and the supply hoses to the machine are diameter indexed and color coded by gas to safeguard against the administration of a hypoxic gas mixture. This schema is referred to as the Diameter Index Safety System.

2. **Gas cylinders.** Gas cylinders are used as backup sources when wall delivery fails or in locations where piped anesthesia gases are not available. Anesthesia machines use the size E cylinder. In a similar fashion to the gas supply hoses, cylinder colors are specific for each gas and pin indexed to prevent connection to the wrong regulator. This schema is referred to as the Pin Index Safety System.

    a. **A full cylinder of oxygen** (green, USA; white, international) has a pressure of 2000 to 2200 psi and contains the equivalent of 660 L of gas

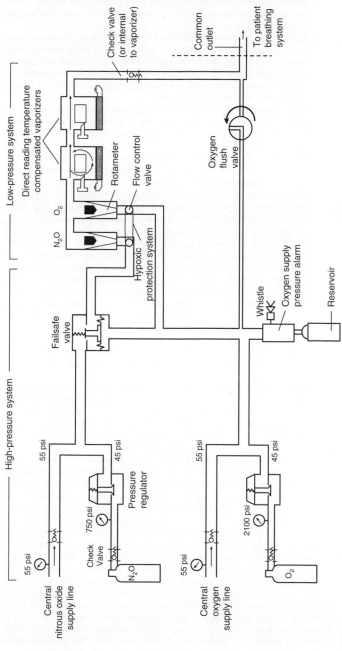

FIGURE 10.1 Schematic of an anesthesia machine. There are many variations in the design depending on vintage and manufacturer.

at atmospheric pressure and room temperature. The oxygen cylinder pressure decreases in direct proportion to the amount of oxygen remaining in the cylinder.

b. **A full cylinder of nitrous oxide** (blue) has a pressure of 745 psi and contains the equivalent of 1500 L of gas at atmospheric pressure and room temperature. The nitrous oxide in the full cylinder is primarily in the liquid phase; the cylinder pressure does not decrease until the liquid content is exhausted, at which time approximately one-fourth of the total volume of gas remains.

c. **Air cylinders** are present on some machines. A full cylinder (yellow, USA; black/white, international) has a pressure of 1800 psi and contains the equivalent of 630 L at atmospheric pressure and room temperature.

d. **Pressure regulators** reduce the high pressure from the cylinders to about 45 psi (just below pipeline pressure) so that, when cylinder gases are used, adjustments at the flow valves (rotameters) are not needed to compensate for the changing pressure that occurs as the cylinders empty. The regulators divide the machine into high-pressure (proximal to the regulator) and low-pressure (distal to the regulator) systems. It is important to keep the gas cylinder closed when relying on pipeline gas supply of the same gas. If both a cylinder and the pipeline are connected and open, gas should flow preferentially from the pipeline because its pressure is slightly higher than the regulated cylinder pressure. If the pipeline pressure fails or is less than the cylinder pressure, the cylinder will supply the gas until it is emptied. It is important to ensure that each anesthesia machine has a cylinder wrench to enable the user to open the cylinder valves when piped gases are not available.

B. **Flow control valves and flowmeters** control and measure gas flows.

1. On modern anesthesia machines, the flow control valves can be digital or mechanical. **Needle valves** control the flow of each gas, with the knob of the oxygen valve having a different shape, as a safety feature. Many newer machines have electronic controls. Typically the user specifies the gases to be mixed (ie, oxygen with air or nitrous oxide), then sets (1) the flow and (2) the percentage of oxygen. More advanced systems allow the user to specify the FiO_2 and concentration of anesthetic agent, and then manage the flows and the vaporizer electronically. These systems are not available in the US market at this time.

2. **Flowmeters.** The traditional flowmeter is a calibrated tapered glass tube in which a bobbin or a ball float is used to indicate the flow of gas. Flowmeters with a ball float should be read in the middle of the ball. Meters with a bobbin should be read at the top of the bobbin. Newer anesthesia machines have electronic flowmeter digital readouts. Gases are mixed sequentially after passing through their respective flowmeters. The oxygen is added last so that a leak occurring after the first gas is added will be less likely to result in delivery of a hypoxic gas mixture.

C. **Vaporizers.** Anesthesia machines are outfitted with one or more vaporizers calibrated to deliver a specific concentration of anesthetic agent measured as percent by volume. The vaporizers used in model anesthesia machines can be broadly classified into two groups: variable bypass vaporizer and measured flow vaporizers. Variable bypass vaporizers operate on the principle that a small proportion of the total gas mixture delivered to them is diverted into a vaporizing chamber, where it becomes fully saturated with anesthetic before it is added back to the main flow. The concentration of anesthetic delivered by the vaporizer is therefore proportional to the amount of gas passing through the vaporizing chamber. Many variable bypass vaporizers are strictly mechanical. They rely on precise calibration and mechanisms for temperature compensation. Additionally, the vaporizing chamber is enclosed in a thick metal case to enhance heat transfer and to provide a heat sink to prevent excessive cooling as the anesthetic evaporates. This style of vaporizer typically labels the amount of anesthetic delivered in units of percentage, but it is often a partial pressure of gas that is being delivered. As an example, a sevoflurane or isoflurane vaporizer set to 1% will deliver the same partial pressure of gas regardless of altitude, despite that partial pressure representing an increasing fraction of the total pressure. Some variable bypass vaporizers have electronic controls (eg, Aladin Cassettes from GE), which measure the concentration of anesthetic agent leaving the vaporizer and electronically adjust the bypass accordingly.

D. **Desflurane** is often administered using a measured flow vaporizer. This is to compensate for the unique physical properties of the agent. **Desflurane has a boiling point of about 23 °C.** If desflurane was allowed to reach its boiling point during delivery, the anesthetic agent would leave variable bypass vaporizer at an uncontrolled rate and enter the circuit in high concentration. (Note: this does not affect Aladin-type vaporizers.) Many, but not all, vaporizers address this problem by heating and pressurizing desflurane, thus preventing the transition from liquid to gas states in the vaporizer during administration. Heating also compensates for the anesthetic's relatively high vapor pressure and the extreme cooling that occurs when high concentrations are vaporized. A vapor pressure of approximately 2 atmospheres is created within the vaporizer regardless of ambient pressure. As a result, when desflurane is utilized at high altitude, the partial pressure of gas ultimately delivered to the patient is less than the amount delivered at sea level.

E. Vaporizers are calibrated for a specific anesthetic and several different proprietary filling systems exist to prevent inadvertent addition of an incorrect anesthetic to a vaporizer. These typically take the form of an adapter that will only attach to one type of anesthetic agent's bottle, and only fit into the corresponding vaporizer.

F. The **common gas outlet** is the port where gases exit the machine; it is connected to the breathing system via the fresh gas hose. Due to the integration of the breathing system with other components of modern anesthesia machines, the common gas outlet is usually not visible nor accessible to the user.

G. **Oxygen flush valve.** One hundred percent oxygen at 45 to 55 psi comes directly from the high-pressure system to the common gas outlet. Oxygen flow can be as high as 40 to 60 L/min. Caution should be taken when using this valve for intubated patients to prevent barotrauma. This warning does not apply to breathing systems with fresh gas isolation valves.

III. BREATHING SYSTEMS

The anesthesia breathing system is unique among ventilators in that it is specifically designed to allow patients to rebreathe exhaled gases. This allows for the conservation of anesthetic agent along with heat and moisture. While gases are rebreathed, they are also conditioned and mixed with the fresh gas flow, which changes their composition. Rebreathing is accomplished by a unidirectional circuit, controlled by at least two one-way valves called the circle system.

A. The **circle system** incorporates a carbon dioxide absorber and prevents rebreathing of exhaled carbon dioxide. The circle consists of an absorber, two one-way valves, a Y-piece adapter, a reservoir bag, and an adjustable pressure limiting (APL) "pop-off" valve (**Figure 10.2**).

1. The **carbon dioxide absorber.** Soda lime ($CaOH_2$ + NaOH + KOH + silica) or Baralyme ($Ba[OH]_2$ + $Ca[OH]_2$) contained in the absorber combines with carbon dioxide, forming $CaCO_2$ and liberating heat and moisture (H_2O). A pH-sensitive dye changes to blue-violet, indicating exhaustion of the absorbing capacity.

2. **One-way valves** ensure that exhaled gas is not rebreathed without passing through the carbon dioxide absorber.

3. The **Y-piece adapter** is used to connect the inspiratory and expiratory limbs of the circuit to the patient.

4. The **reservoir bag and APL valve** are located on the expiratory limb. The reservoir bag accumulates gas between inspirations. It is used to visualize spontaneous ventilation and to assist ventilation manually. Typically, a 3 L reservoir bag is used for adult patients; smaller bags may be appropriate for pediatric patients. The APL valve is used to control the pressure in the breathing system and allows excess gas to escape. The valve can be adjusted from fully open (for spontaneous ventilation, minimal peak pressure 1-3 cm H_2O) to fully closed (maximum pressure 75 cm H_2O or greater). Dangerously high pressures that may produce barotrauma and hemodynamic compromise can occur if the valve is left unattended in the fully or partially closed position.

IV. ANESTHESIA VENTILATORS

A. Anesthesia machines are equipped with mechanical ventilators that employ several different mechanisms to deliver gases to the patient. Conventional anesthesia machines are fitted with a mechanical ventilator that uses a **collapsible bellows. In these systems, a bellows is contained within a closed chamber.** The bellows is compressed when oxygen or air is directed into the chamber outside the bellows. Compressing the bellows causes the pressure in the breathing system to rise. Bellows ventilators come in two types: (1) ascending bellows that are attached to the bottom of their chamber and rise during exhalation, and (2) descending bellows that are attached to the top of their chamber and fall during exhalation. Draeger anesthesia machines typically use a piston to directly compress gas within the system, though one Draeger machine, the Perseus, uses a turbine fan to generate gas pressure within the system. Getinge anesthesia machines use a novel system where oxygen is metered directly into the breathing system to generate increased pressure. The oxygen is added to the system near the scavenger, and it is separated from the rest of the breathing system by a large dead space to prevent the composition of the inhaled gases from being affected. Although gas-driven ventilators can be safely driven with either oxygen or air, most often oxygen is chosen and is supplied by pipeline. Cylinder gases can be used to drive the ventilator in the event of pipeline failure. If the machine is set up to drive the ventilator using cylinder oxygen, mechanical ventilation should be discontinued in the event of pipeline failure to conserve oxygen in the cylinder.

B. **Ventilation modes.** Modern anesthesia machines feature versatile **microprocessor-controlled ventilators** that allow for sophisticated manipulation and monitoring of airway pressures and flow rates. Anesthesia machines are capable of multiple modes (such as pressure-regulated volume control, volume control, pressure control, pressure support, synchronized

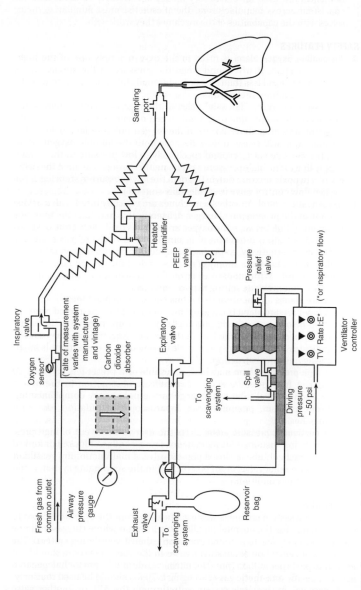

FIGURE 10.2 Representative circle breathing system with ventilator. The airway pressure gauge may sense on the patient side of the inspiratory valve. The PEEP (positive end expiratory pressure) valve may be integral to the ventilator. Other variations are possible depending on the manufacturer.

mandatory, and inverse ratio ventilation), thereby enabling the anesthetist to optimize ventilation, oxygenation, hemodynamics, and weaning. The nomenclature used for ventilatory modes is extremely variable, and not consistent across manufacturers. The anesthetist must familiarize themselves with the capabilities of the machines they work with.

V. SAFETY FEATURES
    A. An **audible oxygen alarm** is fitted in the oxygen supply line of the high-pressure system. It will sound when the pressure in the supply line is greater than 0 and less than 30 psi. Traditionally this was a reed or whistle, but is now commonly electronic.

    B. A pressure-operated **"fail-safe" valve** in the high-pressure system of the nitrous oxide supply line opens only when oxygen pressure in the high-pressure system is above 25 psi. If the oxygen pressure falls below that, nitrous oxide will cease to flow. Because both the audible oxygen alarm and the fail-safe valve respond specifically to low pressure in the oxygen supply line of the high-pressure system, neither protects against the delivery of a hypoxic mixture downstream in the low-pressure system (eg, if the oxygen flow control valve is accidentally shut off).

    C. **Oxygen ratio control.** Anesthesia machines are typically fitted with a device to control the proportion of oxygen delivered. This may take the form of a mechanical link between the oxygen and nitrous oxide flow control knobs that will not allow a fraction of inspired oxygen (FiO_2) of less than 25% to be set. Alternatively, some machines incorporate an oxygen ratio controller that cuts off the supply of nitrous oxide if the oxygen flow is below about 200 mL. With modern electron flow controls, this may simply be software that prevents setting hypoxic mixtures.

    D. **Pressure alarms** are incorporated into all anesthesia machines.

        1. A **low-pressure alarm** is triggered by a period of by a sustained pressure drop below atmospheric pressure. Low pressure may be caused by a disconnection or a large leak in the system. Negative pressure usually indicates a scavenging system malfunction or that the patient is inhaling against an obstruction.

        2. A **high-pressure alarm** may have a variable or a preset (eg, 65 cm H_2O) limit. A high-pressure alarm may indicate obstruction in the tubing or endotracheal tube or a change in the pulmonary compliance (eg, bronchospasm, pneumothorax, laparoscopic insufflation, or "light anesthesia").

        3. A **continuous pressure alarm** alerts the user in the event of high pressure being sustained for more than a few seconds. A blocked or kinked endotracheal tube, a closed pop-off valve, a malfunctioning ventilator pressure relief valve, or an obstruction in the scavenging system could create this condition.

VI. SCAVENGING
A scavenging system channels waste gases away from the operating room to a location outside the hospital building or a location where the gases can be discharged safely (eg, to a nonrecirculating exhaust ventilating system). The ambient concentration of anesthetic gases in the operating room should not exceed 25 parts per million (ppm) for nitrous oxide and 2 ppm for halogenated agents. Specific anesthetic gas-scavenging systems should be used routinely.

    Excess gas in the circle system exits through the APL or another valve during mechanical ventilation. Tubing carries these gases to a receiving system.

A. The **Receiving system** ensures that neither positive nor negative pressure builds at the patient end of the system. The system may be open or closed. An open system consists of a reservoir canister opened to atmosphere at one end. Suction usually is applied to the canister, exhausting the waste gas. A closed system consists of a reservoir bag with positive and negative pressure relief valves to maintain the pressure in the bag within an acceptable range.

B. **Disposal of gases from the receiving system** may be passive or active, although passive systems are inadequate for modern hospitals. A passive system consists of wide-bore tubing that carries gases directly to the exterior or into the exhaust ventilation ducts. Active systems typically employ waste anesthesia gas suction or general hospital suction but may also use fans, pumps, or Venturi systems.

VII. GAS ANALYSIS

Anesthesia machines must contain an oxygen sensor in the inspiratory limb of the circuit. The oxygen sensor prevents the delivery of hypoxic gas mixtures. These sensors are typically paramagnetic or galvanic.

Monitoring of expired CO_2 by waveform capnography and inspired/expired anesthetic gas concentrations are also standard of care. They are typically monitored by sidestream gas analysis. Gas analysis may be incorporated in the anesthesia machine itself, or monitored by a secondary device. When the gas analyzer is incorporated into the anesthesia machine, it is automatically turned on with the anesthesia machine; a stand-alone oxygen sensor may be omitted. Several methods are used to monitor concentrations of O_2, CO_2, and anesthetic gases in the breathing system. The oxygen analyzer is the most important monitor for detecting a hypoxic gas mixture. Capnometry, the measurement of CO_2, has many uses, including monitoring the adequacy of ventilation and detecting breathing system faults. Breath-to-breath monitoring of anesthetic concentrations provides tracking of anesthetic uptake and distribution. Most gas analyzers incorporate alarms. Among the techniques for measurement are the following:

A. **Infrared analysis** uses spectrophotometry and the Beer law (the concentration of a solution is proportional to its light absorption) to provide continuous measurement of the concentration of gas or anesthetic in a gas mixture. Gases that have two or more different atoms in the molecule absorb infrared radiation; thus, infrared analysis can be used to measure concentrations of CO_2, N_2O, and halogenated anesthetics but not O_2. Typically, some gas is withdrawn from the breathing system at a steady rate (50-300 mL/min) and passed into a small measurement chamber in the instrument. Pulses of infrared energy at a wavelength that is absorbed only by the gas of interest are beamed through the gas, and the difference in energy absorbed is used to determine the gas concentration. In some capnographs, a miniaturized measurement chamber and sensor are placed in the breathing system. In most infrared instruments, only one preselected volatile anesthetic can be measured at a time.

B. **Oxygen analyzers.** Continuous measurements of oxygen concentrations in a mixture of gases can be provided by galvanic, or paramagnetic analysis.

1. **Galvanic oxygen monitors** use an anode, cathode, and electrolyte material. This cell is similar to a battery that consumes oxygen.

2. **Paramagnetic analyzers.** These analyzers are based on the principle that oxygen is paramagnetic and therefore attracted to a magnetic field, whereas most other gases are weakly diamagnetic and therefore

repelled from a magnetic field. Modern miniaturized paramagnetic analyzers incorporate a rapidly oscillating magnetic chamber and are capable **of breath-to-breath analysis.** They are often combined with another gas analysis technique in an anesthetic agent monitor.

VIII. EMERGENCY EQUIPMENT

A. A **backup means of positive-pressure ventilation** (self-inflating bag) should be available for any anesthetic procedure. In many operating rooms, these bags can be found on the back of the anesthesia machine.

B. A **light source (eg, flashlight), which is not the laryngoscope,** should be available in case of power failure.

IX. ANESTHESIA MACHINE CHECKOUT RECOMMENDATIONS

Anesthesia machine function must be evaluated by a routine checkout, or a reasonable equivalent before administering anesthesia. Modern electronic anesthesia machines are able to perform most of this check automatically. A generic list of anesthetist-performed checks that should accompany the automatic check specified by your machines manufacturer are provided below:

A. **Emergency ventilation equipment.** Verify that backup ventilation equipment is available and functioning.

B. **Suction device.** Verify that a suction device is available and of adequate pressure remove airway fluids.

C. **High-pressure system**
   1. **Check oxygen cylinder supply.** Verify oxygen cylinder supply
   2. **Check central pipeline supplies.** Check if hoses are connected properly, and pipeline pressure gauges read approximately 50 psi.

D. **Low-pressure system**
   1. **Check initial status of low-pressure system.**
      a. Close flow control valves and turn vaporizers off.
      b. Check fill level and tighten vaporizers' filler caps.
   2. **Turn on the machine's master switch and all other necessary electrical equipment.**
   3. **Test flowmeters.** Adjust flow of all gases through their full range, checking for smooth operation of floats and undamaged flow tubes.

E. **Scavenging system.** Check and adjust the scavenging system.

F. **Breathing system**
   1. **Calibrate O_2 monitor (if present).** Verify that low O_2 alarm is enabled and functioning.
   2. **Check initial status of the breathing system.**
      a. Check that breathing circuit is complete, undamaged, and unobstructed.
      b. Verify that CO_2 absorbent is adequate.
   3. **Perform leak check of the breathing system (some or all portions of this section may be automated and/or require different values per manufacturer recommendation).**
      a. Set all flowmeters to 0 (or the minimum value).
      b. Close APL (pop-off) valve and occlude Y-piece.
      c. Pressurize breathing system to 30 cm H_2O with O_2 flush.
      d. Ensure that pressure remains fixed for at least 10 seconds.
      e. Open APL (pop-off) valve and ensure that pressure decreases.

G. **Manual and automatic ventilation systems.** Test ventilation systems and unidirectional valves.

H. **Monitors.** Check, calibrate, and/or set alarm limits of all monitors.

I. **Final position.** Check final status of the machine.
   1. Vaporizers off
   2. APL valve open
   3. Selector switch to "Bag"
   4. All flowmeters to 0
   5. Breathing system is now ready to use

Suggested Readings

Dorsch JA, Dorsch SE, eds. *A Practical Approach to Anesthesia Equipment.* Lippincott Williams & Wilkins; 2011.

Dorsch JA, Dorsch SE, eds. *Understanding Anesthesia Equipment.* 5th ed. Lippincott Williams & Wilkins; 2008.

Ehrenwerth J, Eisencraft J, Berry J, eds. *Anesthesia Equipment: Principles and Applications.* 2nd ed. Elsevier Saunders; 2013.

Olympio MA. Modern anesthesia machines offer new safety features. *Anesth Patient Saf Found Newsl.* 2003;18:17-32.

Sandberg WS, Urman RD, Ehrenfeld JM. *The MGH Textbook of Anesthesia Equipment.* Elsevier Saunders; 2011.

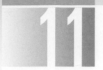

Administration of General Anesthesia

Luca Zazzeron and Kendrick Shaw

The primary goal of general anesthesia is to provide amnesia, hypnosis, analgesia, and immobility while surgical procedures are performed. In this chapter, we will review common indications for general anesthesia and considerations to be taken in the perioperative setting. We will summarize relevant aspects of intraoperative management of patients undergoing general anesthesia, including induction, airway management, and maintenance of general anesthesia. Finally, we will focus on side effects related to the administration of general anesthesia, both in the intraoperative and postoperative periods.

I. INDICATIONS

A. **Surgical procedure:** The most common factor determining whether a patient needs general anesthesia is the type of surgical procedure the patient needs. All procedures that require complete patient immobilization and muscle paralysis will require general anesthesia and mechanical ventilation. Common types of procedures that usually warrant general anesthesia are abdominal laparoscopic procedures and open chest (thoracic and cardiac surgery) or open abdominal procedures (hepatic, gastrointestinal, pancreatic, gynecologic, endocrinologic, urologic surgeries).

B. **Duration:** Another factor to be considered is the duration of the procedure. When the anticipated duration is long, even though the type of surgery itself would not require general anesthesia, general anesthesia may be preferred over conscious sedation to maintain patient comfort for the entire duration of the case.

C. **Patient's features:** The patient's characteristics and medical comorbidities also play a relevant role in the decision about anesthetic options. Whenever neuraxial anesthesia is contraindicated (such as in patients on anticoagulation or with bleeding disorders, sepsis, or severe aortic valve abnormalities), general anesthesia may be required for procedures that could otherwise be performed under neuraxial anesthesia. In patients with severe lung disease, pulmonary hypertension, or severe heart disease, regional techniques and sedation may be preferable. The patient's preference should always be considered, as many patients may refuse regional techniques and request general anesthesia or vice versa.

D. **Timing:** In some cases, when the procedure is emergent (eg, in cases of hemorrhagic shock, limb ischemia, or emergent C-sections for fetal distress), the fastest way to make the patient ready is by administering general anesthesia as compared to neuraxial or regional techniques which generally require more time.

II. PRE-OP EVALUATION AND PLANNING

A. **History:** In the perioperative period, a comprehensive evaluation of the patient's history and physical examination should be performed. Allergies, medications, and recent laboratory results should be reviewed. Relevant

T A B L E 11.1	ASA Practice Guidelines for Preoperative Fasting
Ingested Material	**Minimum Fasting Period**[a]
Clear liquids	2 h
Breast milk	4 h
Infant formula, nonhuman milk, light meals	6 h
Full meal	8 h

[a]Healthy patients, elective cases.

cardiac history should be collected and may affect choice of induction medications and cardiovascular monitoring. Evaluation of the timing of recent ingestion of liquids or solid food and any history of gastrointestinal disease such as gastroesophageal reflux is important and may guide in determining the preferable airway device (endotracheal tube [ETT] vs laryngeal mask airway [LMA]) when administering general anesthesia. Diabetic patients should have blood sugars checked before and during surgery to avoid hypoglycemia in the setting of NPO status (**Table 11.1**). The time of the last oral intake should be confirmed. The patient should be questioned about any individual or family history of difficulty with anesthesia, such as a difficult airway or malignant hyperthermia.

B. Physical examination: The airway examination and evaluation of prior general anesthetics and airway management is a critical portion of the physical examination. If a difficult airway is predicted, alternative intubating devices such as a video laryngoscope and/or a bronchoscope should be available in the operating room (OR) and an awake fiberoptic intubation should be considered.

C. Pain management: In the perioperative setting, although general anesthesia might be the primary anesthetic for the procedure, the need for regional anesthesia for postoperative pain control should be discussed with the surgical team. Regional nerve block or neuraxial anesthesia should be performed in a timely manner without delaying the surgical procedure. Other medications such as acetaminophen, gabapentin, and cox-2 inhibitors administered before the surgery can reduce the opioid requirement and improve pain control after surgery.

D. Intravenous (IV) access: Adequate IV access should be obtained before entering the OR. The size and the number of IV catheters placed vary with the procedure, anticipated blood loss, and the need for continuous drug infusions. In patients with significant cardiovascular disease or risk of brain ischemia, blood pressure should be closely monitored during induction and an arterial catheter should be placed preoperatively. If medications used for cardiovascular support (eg, epinephrine and norepinephrine) are likely to be used, a central venous catheter may be placed either before or after induction, depending on whether these are anticipated to be needed on induction or only as the surgical procedure progresses.

E. Anxiety medications: The preoperative period is one of high anxiety. Reassurance can be effective in mitigating anxiety in most patients. When deemed appropriate, a benzodiazepine (eg, diazepam and midazolam) with or without a small dose of an opioid (eg, fentanyl or morphine) may be administered, particularly when additional preoperative procedures such as epidural catheter or arterial line placement are planned. Patients complaining of pain on arrival in the OR may be given analgesics in incremental amounts to alleviate symptoms. Dosages are based on the patient's age, medical condition, and anticipated time of discharge. Appropriate monitoring should be used and resuscitative equipment available whenever benzodiazepines or opioids are administered IV.

F. **Drugs to neutralize gastric acid and decrease gastric volume:** H_2-antagonists, proton-pump inhibitors, nonparticulate antacids, and metoclopramide may be indicated when the patient is at increased risk of aspiration of gastric contents (ie, recent meal, trauma, bowel obstruction, pregnancy, history of gastric surgery, increased intra-abdominal pressure, difficult airway, or history of active reflux). When the risk of aspiration is high, such as when bowel obstruction is present, a nasogastric tube should be placed and the stomach emptied before induction of anesthesia, while promotility drugs should be avoided as they may increase retrograde peristalsis.

G. **Team huddle:** Except in emergent circumstances, specific airway, blood loss, or other surgical concerns should be discussed with other members of the care team before taking the patient to the OR (see WHO Surgical Safety Checklist). For the patient at high risk for life-threatening complications (eg, airway loss, nonperfusing arrhythmia, massive hemorrhage, or air embolus), specialized equipment and/or extra help should be immediately available, and preoperatively reviewing pertinent sections of an emergency manual is recommended.

III. INDUCTION OF ANESTHESIA

The induction of anesthesia consists in the administration of medications that produce unconsciousness and loss of reflexes and respiratory activity in a patient.

A. **Patient position:** During induction of anesthesia, the patient usually rests supine on the OR table. Maintaining a semirecumbent or reverse Trendelenburg position in obese patients or in patients with increased abdominal pressure (pregnancy) increases the functional residual capacity and decreases the risk of desaturation after induction. In some instances, such as when the procedure is to be performed in prone position or when the patient is experiencing significant pain with movement, the induction of anesthesia may be performed on the hospital bed or the stretcher and the patient moved to the OR table at a later time after induction. Regardless of whether the patient is to be induced on a stretcher or on the OR table, the anesthesiologist should make sure they have adequate physical access to the patient's airway before the induction of anesthesia.

B. **Monitoring:** During induction, patients should be monitored with electrocardiogram (ECG), noninvasive or invasive (when indicated) blood pressure monitoring, and continuous oxygen saturation monitoring.

C. **Preoxygenation:** Before induction, 100% oxygen should be administered using a nonrebreather mask or a sealed mask gently placed on the patient's face. Removing nitrogen from the lungs and replacing it with oxygen increases the time the patient can spend without ventilating before desaturation occurs (eg, from 2.8 minutes without preoxygenation to 9.9 minutes with preoxygenation in a healthy 70 kg male). End-tidal oxygen monitoring or end-tidal nitrogen monitoring can be used to assess the adequacy of preoxygenation: in most patients, an end-tidal oxygen concentration of 90% or an end-tidal nitrogen of less than 5% is achievable.

Most patients without respiratory disease will be able to reach an adequate level of preoxygenation after 3 minutes of normal breathing with 100% oxygen or after 8 vital capacity breaths of 100% oxygen.

D. **IV medications:** Most commonly, induction of anesthesia is obtained by injecting medications intravenously. A potent short-acting hypnotic agent is generally used to abolish consciousness. Common medications include propofol, etomidate, and ketamine. When muscle paralysis is required, succinylcholine or nondepolarizing neuromuscular blocking agents (NDNMBAs) such as rocuronium, vecuronium, or cisatracurium may be administered. Laryngoscopy is associated with strong sympathetic responses including hypertension and tachycardia; these can be attenuated by administration of opioids, lidocaine, or β-adrenergic blockers. IV lidocaine (ideally initially administered with a tourniquet above the injection site) is also used to minimize the pain at the site of IV injection of propofol and etomidate.

E. **Inhalational anesthetics:** When the maintenance of spontaneous ventilation due to a compromised airway is desired, or when an IV access cannot be obtained (eg, in pediatric patients), an inhalational anesthetic technique can be used. After preoxygenation, inhalational anesthetics are administered via a face mask at low concentration (0.5 times minimum alveolar concentration [MAC]) and then increased every three to four breaths until adequate depth of anesthesia is obtained for IV placement or airway manipulation. Alternatively, a "single vital capacity breath" inhalation induction can be achieved using a high concentration of a less pungent agent like halothane or sevoflurane.

F. **Other medications and routes of administration:** In uncooperative patients or young children, alternative induction agents and routes of administration include intramuscular injection of ketamine, rectal methohexital, oral transmucosal fentanyl, and oral midazolam.

IV. AIRWAY MANAGEMENT

After induction of general anesthesia, airway reflexes and respiratory drive are depressed. The airway should be secured, and mechanical ventilation should be provided to maintain oxygenation and remove CO_2. The most commonly used devices to secure the airway and provide ventilation are ETT and LMA.

A. **ETT placement:** If tracheal intubation is planned, a muscle relaxant may be given to facilitate laryngoscopy and intubation. Alternatively, remifentanil (4 μg/kg) can be used to effectively depress airway reflexes and facilitate intubation but frequently causes bradycardia and hypotension. Various techniques can be used to place the ETT. The most common technique is the direct laryngoscopy, which allows direct visualization of the glottis by means of a laryngoscope and insertion of the ETT in the trachea. When a difficult airway is predicted, a video laryngoscope can be used. Patients with difficult or unstable airways may be intubated safely before the induction of anesthesia by fiberoptic guidance under topical anesthesia and conscious sedation.

B. **LMA placement:** Laryngeal masks can be used to safely secure the airway and provide mechanical ventilation during general anesthesia. Typically, LMAs are used for short cases (<4 hours) as prolonged use is associated with increased risk of pharyngeal edema and necrosis. In patients with gastroesophageal reflux, LMAs are relatively contraindicated as they do not offer full protection of the airway against aspiration. Given the LMA is a supraglottic device and the trachea is not violated, neuromuscular blockade is generally not required.

V. MAINTENANCE OF ANESTHESIA

After induction of general anesthesia, maintaining the patient unconscious throughout the entire duration of the procedure is achieved by continuous administration of anesthetics. The depth of anesthesia should be continuously assessed and the dosage of anesthetics adjusted based on surgical stimulation and patient's features. Common reactions to surgical stimulation denoting insufficient depth of anesthesia include somatic responses such as movement, coughing, and changes of respiratory pattern or autonomic responses such as tachycardia, hypertension, mydriasis, sweating, or tearing. Patients with history of alcohol use disorder or on long-term use of sedatives and/or opioids may require larger doses of general anesthetic. Failure in providing adequate depth of anesthesia may result in intraoperative awareness, which occurs in 0.1% to 0.2% of general anesthetics and is more frequent in certain high-risk surgical populations (eg, trauma, cardiac surgery, and obstetrics). Factors that increase the risk of awareness include the use of muscle relaxants and anesthesia techniques such as nitrous oxide combined with opioid medications without other hypnotic agents. Intraoperative monitoring of the cortical electroencephalogram (eg, SedLine monitor or BIS) and auditory-evoked potentials may be useful for monitoring depth of anesthesia, especially for total IV anesthetics, but their utility is controversial when used with volatile anesthetics.

A. **Volatile agents:** Among others, potent inhaled anesthetics commonly used include sevoflurane, isoflurane, and desflurane. The concentration of the volatile anesthetic is titrated to patient movement (if muscle relaxants are not used), blood pressure (which decreases with increasing depth), and ventilation. The MAC is the concentration of a vapor in the lungs that is needed to prevent a motor response in 50% of subjects in response to a surgical stimulus. Maintaining total end-tidal drug concentrations above $0.7 \times$ MAC is associated with a low incidence of awareness. Typically, the use of volatile anesthetic with minimal opioid use allows maintenance of spontaneous ventilation. Nitrous oxide can be used in association with potent inhaled anesthetics or opioids (nitrous oxide-narcotic) to maintain general anesthesia. The use of nitrous oxide allows using a lower concentration of potent vapor anesthetic while maintaining adequate depth of anesthesia. If nitrous oxide is used, its concentration should be adjusted to ensure adequate oxygenation. High concentrations of nitrous oxide are contraindicated in patients with closed air-filled compartments such as pneumothorax, pneumocephalus, or bowel obstruction. In patients with vitamin B_{12} or folate deficiency or methionine synthase abnormalities, nitrous oxide can exacerbate hematologic or neurologic diseases.

B. **Total intravenous anesthesia (TIVA):** Maintenance of general anesthesia can be achieved by using a continuous infusion of a short-acting hypnotic drug (eg, propofol) with or without opioids (eg, remifentanil) or other adjunct medications such as lidocaine, ketamine, dexmedetomidine, and a muscle relaxant. A TIVA technique is particularly useful in situations where ventilation is frequently interrupted such as during surgical procedures on the lungs and the respiratory tree. TIVA is often preferred when neuromonitoring is performed such as during spine surgery and neurosurgery, as propofol causes a decrease in amplitude and prolongation of the evoked potential latencies which are less pronounced than the volatile anesthetics. TIVA is also the technique of choice in patients at high risk for postoperative nausea and vomiting (PONV).

C. **Balanced anesthesia:** Inhaled and IV anesthetic can be combined to maintain general anesthesia. A low concentration of a volatile or IV anesthetic (0.3–$0.5 \times$ MAC or ED_{50}) may be combined with nitrous oxide, opioids, and relaxant. Continuous ketamine, dexmedetomidine, magnesium, and lidocaine infusions can be combined with inhaled or IV anesthetics to reduce the need for intraoperative and postoperative opioids. Combining anesthetics reduces the need for and the potential toxicity of large doses of single agents but increases the risk of adverse drug interactions. General anesthesia can also be combined with a regional anesthetic technique (ie, peripheral or neuraxial nerve block). The required depth of general anesthesia is significantly reduced with blockade of painful surgical stimulation but still needs to be sufficient to ensure hypnosis.

VI. EMERGENCE AND EXTUBATION

To ensure timely wake up at the end of the procedures, anesthetic medications should be discontinued at an appropriate time based on medication half-life and pharmacodynamics. A common practice is to reduce the concentration of potent inhaled anesthetics and administer nitrous oxide. When using remifentanil, this should be slowly titrated in 30 minutes to avoid postoperative hyperalgesia. Before proceeding with emergence, adequate pain control should be ensured. Patients should be normothermic, hemodynamically stable, and with normal gas-exchange and metabolic status. Reversal of paralysis should be ensured using a quantitative assessment, such as a train-of-four with accelerometer, and muscle relaxant reversal should be administered when appropriate. In some instances, a deep extubation technique might be preferable. These situations include asthmatic patients at higher risk of bronchospasm during airway manipulation, patients at risk of bleeding due to cough and increased intrathoracic pressure (such as during neck or brain surgery), or patients with respiratory infectious disease.

VII. TRANSPORT AND DISPOSITION

Before leaving the OR, stable vital signs and adequate monitoring should be confirmed. Extubated patients should be able to breathe spontaneously without assistance and maintain stable oxygen saturation. Intubated patients should be connected to transport ventilators, and proper ventilation should be confirmed. All patients should be hemodynamically stable, and patients requiring vasopressors infusion should have proper hemodynamic monitoring during transport. Basic monitoring during transport includes a pulse oximeter, ECG, and noninvasive or invasive blood pressure monitoring. Emergency drugs and the equipment for emergent intubation should be available during transport of unstable patients. All patients who have received general anesthesia should be monitored in an appropriate postanesthesia care unit (PACU) or equivalent (eg, intensive care unit [ICU]) setting until they have recovered sufficiently to be discharged to a less closely monitored setting. During this time, oxygenation, ventilation, circulation, temperature, and level of consciousness should be monitored and treatment provided as needed.

VIII. INTRAOPERATIVE ADVERSE EFFECTS RELATED TO GENERAL ANESTHESIA AND MANAGEMENT

Medications that induce general anesthesia also cause blunting of many autoregulatory responses of the body. Various systems are affected by the administration of general anesthesia, including the cardiovascular system, the respiratory system, thermoregulation, and the motor/somatic system.

A. **Cardiovascular:** Anesthetic medications typically cause a reduction in systemic vascular resistance, with blunting of cardiovascular reflexes including reflex tachycardia and vasoconstriction in response to a reduced blood pressure or change in blood volume. Also, many anesthetic medications such as propofol and inhaled anesthetics reduce myocardial contractility. Together with the fact that many patients present with a reduced circulating blood volume due to NPO status, the administration of general anesthesia is often associated with the development of hypotension. Blood pressure and heart rate should be monitored carefully. Patients should be adequately fluid resuscitated. When appropriate, vasoconstricting drugs such as phenylephrine and vasopressin should be administered. In patients with underlying cardiac dysfunction, the administration of inotropic drugs such as norepinephrine or epinephrine might be necessary.

B. **Respiratory:** Patients under general anesthesia cannot protect their airway, and their respiratory drive is often depressed. Moreover, additional factors including peritoneal insufflation, open chest surgery, and patient positioning may significantly affect respiratory function during surgery. After securing the airway, assisted or controlled ventilation of the patient is provided. During assisted ventilation, the respiratory rate and pattern can help assess the depth of anesthesia and whether the patient requires more analgesics such as opioids. An assisted mode is typically preferred to minimize positive airway pressure when LMAs are used, as this will reduce the risk of inflating the stomach. When paralysis is required, controlled ventilation is necessary. Minute ventilation should be adjusted based on continuous monitoring of end-tidal CO_2 or the arterial partial pressure of CO_2 when available. During laparoscopic surgeries with CO_2 insufflation, minute ventilation should be increased due to CO_2 systemic absorption. In the OR while administering general anesthesia for surgery, a number of adverse airway events may occur, and continuous monitoring of airway pressure allows early detection and correction of many of these issues to ensure patient's safety. A decrease in airway pressure may signify a leak or a circuit disconnection. If such a decrease is seen, immediate and careful evaluation of the entire circuitry should be performed to identify and correct the issue. An increase in airway pressure may be a sign of an obstruction along the respiratory circuit from the ventilator to the alveoli. Common causes include ETT obstruction or movement, change in muscle relaxation, or surgical compression. Less frequently, this can be a sign of pneumothorax or increased airway resistance due to bronchospasm or mucus plug.

C. **Thermoregulation:** Hypothermia is the most common temperature derangement during general anesthesia and surgery. Volatile anesthetics, propofol, and opioids promote heat loss through vasodilation and heat redistribution from the core to the skin surface. Heat is then lost through various processes including radiation, conduction, convection, and evaporation, with radiation being the most significant mechanism and accounting for approximately 60% of total heat loss. Most general anesthetics also depress the hypothalamic thermoregulatory centers, resulting in impaired responses to changes in body temperature such as vasoconstriction and shivering. Current guidelines recommend continuous monitoring of central temperature, which can be achieved by means of disposable temperature probes. Common sites for temperature monitoring include the esophagus, nasopharynx, tympanic membrane, bladder, or mixed venous blood. The severity of hypothermia depends on many factors including the type of surgery, the area of the body exposed to the environment, room temperature, body mass index (BMI), age, and the temperature of fluids used for resuscitation.

The decrease in body temperature after administration of general anesthesia can be mitigated by warming the patient with warm forced air and blankets before induction. Strategies to treat hypothermia during surgery include adjusting the room temperature, reducing the uncovered areas of the body, applying warming devices on the patient's skin, and administering warm fluids.

D. **Motor/somatic:** During general anesthesia, movement, somatic perception, and proprioception are abolished. Patient positioning is important and pressure points padding should be used to reduce the risk of skin and soft-tissue damage.

IX. **POSTOPERATIVE ADVERSE EFFECTS RELATED TO GENERAL ANESTHESIA**

A. **Hypotension:** Persistent hypotension after general anesthesia is common, particularly in the elderly, in patients with underlying cardiovascular disease, and after long surgeries. Continuous infusion of vasopressor medications may be required to maintain adequate mean arterial pressure, while appropriate volume resuscitation should be ensured.

B. **PONV:** PONV are frequent side effects observed after general anesthesia. Risk factors for PONV include female gender, history of PONV, nonsmoking status, and younger age. Anesthesia-related factors include use of volatile anesthetic, duration of anesthesia, use of opioids, and nitrous oxide. Several drugs can be administered intraoperatively to reduce the risk of PONV. These include ondansetron, dexamethasone, haloperidol, and transdermal scopolamine. A propofol infusion can also be used to prevent or treat severe PONV. One medication can be used in patients at low risk, while up to three to four different medications should be administered to patients at high risk for PONV.

C. **Shivering:** Postanesthetic shivering is one of the leading causes of patients' discomfort after recovering from general anesthesia. The main mechanism is the anesthetic-mediated inhibition of thermoregulation. First-line treatment includes warming the patient. Pharmacologic interventions such as administration of meperidine, clonidine, ketamine, and tramadol are reserved for more severe cases.

D. **Complications related to muscle relaxant use:** Residual paralysis in the PACU has been documented in 5% to 50% of patients who underwent general anesthesia with muscle relaxant use. The frequency of this phenomenon depends on the type of neuromuscular blockade and whether reversal agents were administered, as well as the neuromonitoring system employed and the definition criteria. Residual paralysis is associated with increased risk of pulmonary complications due to weakness, atelectasis, and hypoventilation resulting in higher risk of pneumonia, hypoxemia, and respiratory failure. Quantitative neuromuscular blockade monitoring (eg, with a quantitative train-of-four stimulator) should be routinely used during general anesthesia whenever muscle relaxants are used. Before emergence and extubation, full reversal should be documented and reversal agents such as sugammadex or neostigmine should be administered when appropriate. Succinylcholine-induced postoperative myalgia is considered a minor side effect observed after succinylcholine-induced fasciculations; however, in some instances, it can be severe and interfere with return to activity. The most common intervention to decrease the incidence and severity of myalgia is pretreatment with a small dose of a nondepolarizing neuromuscular blocking agent prior to the administration of succinylcholine. Other methods include stretching exercises and supplementation of vitamin C.

E. **Upper airway complications:** Sore throat and hoarseness after general anesthesia are common and occur in up to 50% of the patients. More severe and rare complications due to airway manipulation and ETT or LMA placement include laceration of the pharyngeal mucosa, arytenoid dislocation, vocal cord injury, and recurrent laryngeal nerve injury. To minimize the risk of injury, airway devices that pass through the vocal cords should be gently inserted under vision (direct or using video techniques). Other complications related to laryngoscopy and LMA insertion include tooth damage or displacement, lip laceration, and injury to the frenulum. If voice changes persist, an otorhinolaryngologist should be consulted for further evaluation and management.

F. **Postoperative cognitive dysfunction (POCD) and delirium:** POCD is defined as a decline in patient's memory and learning after surgery. Up to 30% of patients experience short-term POCD, while 10% may have POCD persisting for up to 3 months. The incidence of POCD is affected by patient's factors (including age, level of education, and social support) and factors related to surgery and anesthesia (case complexity, duration, and type of anesthesia). Monitoring of depth of anesthesia and ensuring adequate brain perfusion, oxygenation, normoglycemia, and normothermia are critical in the intraoperative period. In the postoperative period, multimodal analgesia with an opioid-sparing strategy may be beneficial, particularly in elderly patients.

Suggested Readings

American Society of Anesthesiologists Committee. Practice guidelines for preoperative fasting and the use of pharmacologic agents to reduce the risk of pulmonary aspiration: application to healthy patients undergoing elective procedures. An updated report by the American Society of Anesthesiologists Committee on Standards and Practice Parameters. *Anesthesiology*. 2017;126(3):376-393.

Apfel CC, Korttila K, Abdalla M, et al. A factorial trial of six interventions for the prevention of postoperative nausea and vomiting. *N Engl J Med*. 2004;350(24):2441-2451.

Avidan MS, Jacobsohn E, Glick D, et al; BAG-RECALL Research Group. Prevention of intraoperative awareness in a high-risk surgical population. *N Engl J Med*. 2011;365:591-600.

Avidan MS, Zhang L, Burnside BA, et al. Anesthesia awareness and the bispectral index. *N Engl J Med*. 2008;358:1097-1108.

Cavallone LF, Vannucci A. Review article: extubation of the difficult airway and extubation failure. *Anesth Analg*. 2013;116(2):368-383.

Fleisher LA, Fleischmann KE, Auerbach AD, et al; American College of Cardiology; American Heart Association. 2014 ACC/AHA guideline on perioperative cardiovascular evaluation and management of patients undergoing noncardiac surgery: a report of the ACC/AHA Task Force on practice guidelines. *J Am Coll Cardiol*. 2014;64:e77-e137.

Kheterpal S, Vaughn MT, Dubovoy TZ, et al. Sugammadex versus neostigmine for reversal of neuromuscular blockade and postoperative pulmonary complications (STRONGER): a multicenter matched cohort analysis. *Anesthesiology*. 2020. 132(6):1371-1381.

Kotekar N, Shenkar A. Nagaraj R. Postoperative cognitive dysfunction – current preventive strategies. *Clin Interv Aging*. 2018;13:2267-2273.

Lewis SR, Pritchard MW, Fawcett LJ, Punjasawadwong Y. Bispectral index for improving intraoperative awareness and early postoperative recovery in adults. *Cochrane Database Syst Rev*. 2019;9:CD003843.

Myles PS, Leslie K, McNeil J, Forbes A, Chan MTV. Bispectral index monitoring to prevent awareness during anaesthesia: the B-Aware randomised controlled trial. *Lancet*. 2004;363:1757-1763.

Plaud B, Debaene B, Donati F, Marty J. Residual paralysis after emergence from anesthesia. *Anesthesiology*. 2010;112(4):1013-1022.

Stanski DR, Shafer SL. Monitoring depth of anesthesia. In: Miller RD, ed. *Anesthesia*. 6th ed. Churchill Livingstone; 2005:1227-1264.

Willenkin RL, Polk SL. Management of general anesthesia. In: Miller RD, ed. *Anesthesia*. 4th ed. Churchill Livingstone; 1994:1045-1056.

World Alliance for Patient Safety. *WHO Surgical Safety Checklist and Implementation Manual*. 2008. Accessed May, 2020. http://www.who.int/patientsafety/safesurgery/ss_checklist/en/

12 Intravenous and Inhalation Anesthetics

Juan M. Cotte Cabarcas and Gregory E. Ginsburg

I. PHARMACOLOGY OF INTRAVENOUS ANESTHETICS

Intravenous (IV) anesthetics are commonly used for the induction and maintenance of general anesthesia and for sedation. The rapid onset and offset of these drugs is attributable to their physical translocation into and out of the brain. After a bolus IV injection, lipid-soluble drugs such as propofol, thiopental (not available in the United States), and etomidate rapidly distribute into the **vessel-rich group** of highly perfused tissues (eg, brain, heart, liver, and kidneys), causing an extremely rapid onset of effect. Plasma concentrations decrease as the drug is taken up by the less well-perfused tissues (eg, muscle and fat), and the drug rapidly leaves the brain. This **redistribution** from the brain is responsible for the termination of effects; the **clearance** of the active drug occurs mainly by hepatic **metabolism** and renal **elimination**. **Elimination half-life** is defined as the time required for the plasma concentration of a drug to decrease by 50% during the elimination phase of clearance. **Context-sensitive half-time (CSHT)** is defined as the time required for a 50% decrease in the central compartment drug concentration after a steady-state infusion of specified duration (duration is the "context").

A. Propofol (2,6-diisopropylphenol) is used for the induction or maintenance of general anesthesia and for procedural sedation. In the United States, it is marketed as a 1% isotonic oil-in-water emulsion, which contains 10% soybean oil, 2.25% glycerol, and 1.2% purified egg phosphatide. Bacterial growth is inhibited by ethylenediaminetetraacetic acid, diethylenetriamine pentaacetic acid, sulfite, or benzyl alcohol depending on the manufacturer. **Fospropofol** is an aqueous formulation of propofol available in other countries for procedural sedation. It is a prodrug of propofol, and its aqueous nature negates undesirable effects of the emulsion such as pain on injection and lipid disorders.

1. Mode of action. Facilitates inhibitory neurotransmission by enhancing the function of γ-aminobutyric acid type A ($GABA_A$) receptors in the central nervous system (CNS). The modulation of glycine receptors, N-methyl-D-aspartate (NMDA) receptors, cannabinoid receptors, and voltage-gated ion channels may also contribute to propofol's actions.

2. Pharmacokinetics

  a. Hepatic and extrahepatic metabolism to inactive metabolites that are renally excreted.

  b. CSHT remains below 15 minutes following 2-hour infusion, making propofol infusions useful for the maintenance of anesthesia, but CSHT may rise well above 30 minutes for infusions lasting over 8 hours.

3. Pharmacodynamics

a. CNS

1. Induction doses rapidly produce unconsciousness (30-45 seconds), followed by a rapid termination of effect due to redistribution. Emergence is rapid and often accompanied by mood elevation. Low doses produce sedation and amnesia.

2. Weak analgesic effects at hypnotic concentrations.

3. Decreases intracranial pressure (ICP) and also cerebral perfusion pressure (CPP) due to markedly decreased mean arterial pressure (MAP). Cerebral autoregulation, as well as vasoconstriction in response to hyperventilation, are unaffected.

4. Anticonvulsant properties raise the seizure threshold.

5. Propofol-induced anesthesia is associated with frontal alpha oscillations (8-12 Hz), delta oscillations (1-4 Hz), and slow oscillations (0.1-1 Hz) electroencephalogram (EEG). Higher doses cause burst suppression and isoelectric EEG.

6. Depresses somatosensory-evoked potentials (SSEPs) and motor-evoked potentials (MEPs), but little effect on brainstem auditory–evoked potentials (BAEPs).

7. Has antiemetic effects, even at subhypnotic doses. Postoperative nausea and vomiting (PONV) occurs less frequently after a propofol-based anesthetic compared with other techniques.

b. Cardiovascular system

1. Dose-dependent decreases in preload, afterload, and contractility lead to decreases in blood pressure (BP) and cardiac output. Hypotension may be marked in hypovolemic, elderly, or hemodynamically compromised patients.

2. Heart rate (HR) is minimally affected, and baroreceptor reflex is blunted.

c. Respiratory system

1. Dose-dependent decreases in respiratory rate (RR) and tidal volume (TV).

2. Ventilatory responses to hypoxia and hypercarbia are diminished.

4. Dosage and administration (Table 12.1)

a. Titrate with reduced incremental doses in hypovolemic, elderly, or hemodynamically compromised patients or if administered with other anesthetics.

b. Relatively larger induction and maintenance doses are required in infants and small children.

c. Propofol emulsion supports bacterial growth despite the addition of antimicrobials; prepare drug under sterile conditions, label with date and time, and discard unused propofol after **6 to 12 hours** to prevent inadvertent bacterial contamination.

d. Target-controlled infusion pumps have been developed, which, based on the patient's age and body weight, can titrate an initial bolus and variable infusion rate to achieve a desired plasma concentration (not available in the United States).

e. Systems have also been developed to measure propofol concentration by mass spectrophotometry in exhaled gas or by IV electrodes, but these modalities are not used in common practice.

5. Adverse effects

a. **Venous irritation.** May cause pain during IV administration, which can be reduced by administration in a large vein or by adding lidocaine to the solution (eg, 20 mg of lidocaine to 200 mg of propofol). The

TABLE 12.1	Dosages of Commonly Used IV Anesthetics and Induction Dose Onset and Duration				
Drug	**Dose**			**Onset (s)**	**Induction Dose Duration (min)**
	Induction (mg/kg)	**Maintenance (µg/kg/min)**	**Sedation (Titrate to Effect)**		
Propofol IV	1-3	100-150	25-75 µg/kg/min	<30	3-8
Midazolam IV	0.2-0.4	0.5-1.5	0.5-1.0 mg	30-60	15-30
Midazolam IM	—	—	0.07-0.1 mg/kg	—	—
Ketamine IV	1-2	15-90	0.1-0.8 mg/kg	45-60	10-20
Ketamine IM	5-10	—	2-4 mg/kg	—	—
Etomidate IV	0.2-0.4	10[a]	5-8 µg/kg/min[a]	<30	4-8
Dexmedetomidine IV	—	—	0.2–0.7 µg/kg/h[b]	—	—
Methohexital IV	1-1.5	—	0.5 mg/kg[c]	<30	4-7

IM, intramuscular; IV, intravenous.
[a]Off-label use, avoided due to risk of adrenal suppression.
[b]After loading dose of 0.5 to 1.0 µg/kg over 10 minutes.
[c]Off-label use, following initial loading dose of 0.75 to 1 mg/kg, redose every 2 to 5 minutes as needed.

most effective method to reduce pain is to give lidocaine (0.5 mg/kg, IV) 1 to 2 minutes before propofol injection with a tourniquet proximal to the IV site.

b. **Lipid disorders.** Propofol is a lipid emulsion and should be used cautiously in patients with disorders of lipid metabolism (eg, hyperlipidemia and pancreatitis).

c. **Myoclonus** and **hiccups** can occur after induction doses, although less frequently than with methohexital or etomidate.

d. **Propofol infusion syndrome** is a rare and often fatal disorder that occurs in critically ill patients (usually children) subjected to prolonged, high-dose propofol infusions. Typical features include rhabdomyolysis, metabolic acidosis, cardiac failure, and renal failure.

B. **Barbiturates** such as thiopental (not available in the United States) and methohexital rapidly produce unconsciousness (30-45 seconds) after IV administration, followed by rapid termination of effects due to redistribution. Barbiturate preparations for IV administration are highly alkaline (pH > 10) and are usually prepared as dilute solutions (1.0%-2.5%).

1. **Mode of action.** Similar to propofol, barbiturates facilitate inhibitory neurotransmission by enhancing $GABA_A$ receptor function, binding it at an allosteric site and increasing the amount of time Cl^- ions are open. At higher concentrations, they can cause direct stimulation of $GABA_A$ receptors. They also inhibit excitatory neurotransmission via glutamate and nicotinic acetylcholine receptors.

2. **Pharmacokinetics**

a. **Hepatic metabolism.** Methohexital has a much higher clearance than thiopental. Thiopental is metabolized to pentobarbital, an active metabolite with a longer half-life.

    b. Multiple doses or prolonged infusions may produce prolonged sedation or unconsciousness due to the reduced rate of redistribution, the return of the drug to the central compartment, and slow hepatic metabolism. The CSHT of thiopental is long, even after short infusions.

3. Pharmacodynamics

    a. CNS

        1. Dose-dependent CNS depression ranging from sedation to unconsciousness. Much higher doses are required to suppress responses to painful stimuli.

        2. Dose-dependent cerebral vasoconstriction and decrease in cerebral metabolic rate ($CMRO_2$) cause reductions in ICP and cerebral blood flow (CBF). Cerebral autoregulation remains unaffected.

        3. At high doses, thiopental will produce an isoelectric EEG. In contrast, methohexital can elicit seizure activity. This characteristic of methohexital, in addition to its favorable pharmacokinetic profile, makes it a suitable anesthetic agent for electroconvulsive therapy.

        4. Minimal effects on SSEPs or MEPs, but dose-dependent depression of BAEPs.

    b. Cardiovascular system

        1. Cause venodilation and depress myocardial contractility, leading to a dose-dependent decrease in BP and cardiac output, especially in patients who are preload dependent. Decrease in BP is less pronounced than with propofol.

        2. Baroreceptor reflexes remain largely intact; therefore, HR may increase in response to hypotension.

    c. Respiratory system

        1. Dose-dependent decreases in RR and TV. Ventilatory responses to hypoxia and hypercarbia are markedly depressed. Apnea may result 30 to 90 seconds after an induction dose.

        2. Laryngeal reflexes remain more intact relative to propofol; therefore, the incidence of cough and laryngospasm is higher.

4. Dosage and administration (Table 12.1)

    a. Doses should be reduced in hypovolemic, elderly, or hemodynamically compromised patients.

    b. May precipitate when mixed with drugs in lower pH solution (eg, succinylcholine) and cause the precipitation of other drugs (eg, vecuronium). Therefore, it is prudent to use a free-running IV and avoid simultaneous injection with other drugs.

5. Adverse effects

    a. Allergy. True allergies are unusual. Thiopental occasionally causes anaphylactoid reactions (ie, hives, flushing, and hypotension) due to histamine release.

    b. Porphyria

        1. Absolutely contraindicated in patients with acute intermittent porphyria, variegate porphyria, and hereditary coproporphyria.

        2. Barbiturates induce porphyrin synthetic enzymes such as δ-aminolevulinic acid synthetase; patients with porphyria may accumulate toxic heme precursors and suffer an acute attack.

    c. Venous irritation and tissue damage

        1. May cause pain at the site of administration due to venous irritation.

        2. Thiopental can cause severe pain and tissue necrosis if injected extravascularly or intra-arterially. If intra-arterial administration occurs, phentolamine (α-blocker), heparin, vasodilators, and regional sympathetic blockade may be helpful in treatment.

    d. Myoclonus and **hiccups** are often seen during induction with methohexital.

C. **Benzodiazepines** include midazolam, lorazepam, and diazepam. They are often used for sedation, amnesia, anxiolysis, or as adjuncts to general anesthesia. Midazolam is prepared in a water-soluble form at pH 3.5, while diazepam and lorazepam are dissolved in propylene glycol and polyethylene glycol, respectively.

1. **Mode of action.** Enhance inhibitory neurotransmission by increasing the affinity of $GABA_A$ receptors for GABA. In contrast to other agents (ie, barbiturates), benzodiazepines are unable to activate the $GABA_A$ receptor in the absence of GABA. Different clinical effects (eg, amnesia, sedation, and anxiolysis) appear to be mediated by different $GABA_A$ receptor subtypes.

2. **Pharmacokinetics**
   a. After IV administration, the onset of CNS effects occurs in 2 to 3 minutes for midazolam and diazepam (slightly longer for lorazepam). Effects are terminated by redistribution; therefore, durations of a single dose of diazepam and midazolam are similar. The effects of lorazepam are somewhat more prolonged.
   b. All three drugs are metabolized in the liver. Elimination half-lives for midazolam, lorazepam, and diazepam are approximately 2, 11, and 20 hours, respectively. The active metabolites of diazepam last longer than the parent drug and accumulate with repeated dosing. Hydroxymidazolam can accumulate and cause sedation in patients with renal failure.
   c. Diazepam clearance is reduced in the elderly, but this is less of a problem with midazolam and lorazepam. Obese patients may require higher initial doses of benzodiazepines, but clearance is not markedly different.

3. **Pharmacodynamics**
   a. **CNS**
      1. Amnestic, anticonvulsant, anxiolytic, muscle relaxant, and sedative-hypnotic effects in a dose-dependent manner. Amnesia may last for up to 1 hour following a single premedication dose of midazolam. Sedation may sometimes be prolonged.
      2. Unless combined with other agents, benzodiazepines are unable to inhibit the response to noxious stimulus sufficiently for surgical anesthesia to be achieved.
      3. Do not produce significant analgesia.
      4. Dose-dependent reduction of CBF and $CMRO_2$.
      5. Do not produce burst suppression or isoelectric EEG pattern, even at very high doses.
   b. **Cardiovascular system**
      1. Mild systemic vasodilation and decrease in cardiac output. HR is usually unchanged.
      2. Hemodynamic changes may be pronounced in hypovolemic or critically ill patients if rapidly administered in a large dose or with an opioid.
   c. **Respiratory system**
      1. Mild dose-dependent decreases in RR and TV. Some decrease in hypoxic ventilatory drive.
      2. Respiratory depression may be pronounced if administered with an opioid, in patients with pulmonary disease or in debilitated patients.

4. **Dosage and administration** (see **Table 12.1** for midazolam)
   a. Incremental IV doses of diazepam (2.5 mg) or lorazepam (0.25 mg) may be used for sedation.
   b. Appropriate oral doses are 5 to 10 mg of diazepam or 2 to 4 mg of lorazepam.

5. Adverse effects

a. Drug interactions. Administration of a benzodiazepine to a patient receiving the anticonvulsant **valproate** may precipitate a psychotic episode.

b. Pregnancy and labor

1. May be associated with a slightly increased risk of cleft lip and palate when administered during the first trimester.

2. Cross the placenta and may lead to CNS depression in the neonate.

c. Superficial thrombophlebitis and injection pain may be produced by the vehicles in diazepam and lorazepam.

6. Flumazenil (imidazobenzodiazepine) is a competitive antagonist at the benzodiazepine binding site of $GABA_A$ receptors in the CNS.

a. Reversal of benzodiazepine-induced sedative effects occurs within 2 minutes; peak effects occur at approximately 10 minutes. It does not completely antagonize the respiratory depressant effects of benzodiazepines.

b. Half-life is shorter than the benzodiazepine agonists, thus repeated administration may be necessary.

c. Metabolized to inactive metabolites in the liver.

d. Dose of 0.3 mg IV every 30 to 60 seconds (to a maximum dose of 5 mg).

e. Contraindicated in patients with tricyclic antidepressant (TCA) overdose (thought to be due to unmasking TCA-induced seizure activity) and in those receiving benzodiazepines for the control of seizures or elevated ICP. Use cautiously in patients who have had long-term treatment with benzodiazepines because acute withdrawal may be precipitated.

D. Etomidate is a benzylimidazole sedative-hypnotic agent most commonly used for IV induction of general anesthesia. It is supplied in a solution containing 35% of propylene glycol.

1. Mode of action. Facilitates inhibitory neurotransmission by enhancing $GABA_A$ receptor function.

2. Pharmacokinetics

a. After an induction dose, times to loss of consciousness and return of consciousness are similar to that for propofol. Effects of a single bolus dose are terminated by redistribution.

b. Very high clearance in the liver and by circulating esterases to inactive metabolites.

3. Pharmacodynamics

a. CNS

1. No analgesic properties.

2. CBF, $CMRO_2$, and ICP decrease, while CPP is usually maintained. Cerebral vasoconstriction in response to hyperventilation is preserved.

3. Induces burst suppression at high doses.

4. Less depression of evoked potentials compared to that with propofol or thiopental. BAEPs are unaffected, while SSEPs are enhanced.

a. Increases EEG activity in epileptogenic foci potentially precipitating with seizures.

b. Cardiovascular system

1. Minimal changes in HR, BP, and cardiac output. Often chosen to induce general anesthesia in hemodynamically compromised patients.

      2. Does not affect the sympathetic tone or the baroreceptor function. Will not effectively suppress hemodynamic responses to pain.

      3. Decreases myocardial oxygen consumption.

   c. Respiratory system

      1. Dose-dependent decreases in RR and TV; transient apnea may occur.

      2. The respiratory depressant effects of etomidate are less pronounced than those of propofol or barbiturates.

  4. Dosage and administration (Table 12.1)

  5. Adverse effects

   a. Myoclonus may occur after administration, particularly in response to stimulation. Can be avoided by premedication with benzodiazepines or opiates.

   b. Nausea and vomiting occur more frequently in the postoperative period than with other anesthetic agents.

   c. Venous irritation and superficial thrombophlebitis may be caused by the propylene glycol vehicle. Minimized by administration into a free-flowing IV carrier infusion. Pain at injection site has been described in 30% to 80% of patients.

   d. Adrenal suppression. Inhibits 11β-hydroxylase; a single induction dose suppresses adrenal steroid synthesis for up to 24 hours in elderly or debilitated patients. May not be clinically significant after a single dose, but repeated doses/infusions have been associated with increased mortality in the ICU.

   e. Hiccups and **nystagmus** are also relatively common side effects following induction with etomidate.

E. Ketamine is an arylcyclohexylamine (related to phencyclidine) sedative-hypnotic agent with potent analgesic properties. It is used for the induction of general anesthesia and for sedation and analgesia in the perioperative setting. It is a mixture of R+ and S− isomers. The S− isomer has higher potency and produces fewer side effects.

  1. Mode of action. Anesthetic effects are mainly attributed to noncompetitive antagonism of NMDA receptors in the CNS, although effects on opioid receptors, acetylcholine receptors, and voltage-gated sodium and calcium channels also have been reported.

  2. Pharmacokinetics

   a. Produces unconsciousness in 30 to 60 seconds after an IV induction dose. Effects are terminated by redistribution in 15 to 20 minutes. After intramuscular (IM) administration, the onset of CNS effects is delayed for approximately 5 minutes, with peak effect at approximately 15 minutes.

   b. Metabolized rapidly in the liver to multiple metabolites, some of which have modest activity (eg, norketamine). Elimination half-life is 2 to 3 hours.

   c. Repeated bolus doses or prolonged infusions result in accumulation.

  3. Pharmacodynamics

   a. CNS

      1. Produces a "dissociative" state accompanied by amnesia and profound analgesia. Analgesia occurs at much lower concentrations than hypnosis, so analgesic effects persist after the return of consciousness.

      2. Increases CBF, ICP, and $CMRO_2$; cerebral vasoconstriction in response to hyperventilation is preserved.

      3. Enhancement of SSEPs; depression of BAEPs and visual-evoked potentials.

    4. Dose-dependent EEG changes that differ from other anesthetics; high doses do not produce an isoelectric EEG. Gamma oscillations (25-40 Hz) are often observed.

b. Cardiovascular system

    1. Increases HR, cardiac output, and BP of systemic and pulmonary arteries by triggering the release of endogenous catecholamines.

    2. Often used for inducing general anesthesia in hemodynamically compromised patients, particularly those for whom HR, preload, and afterload should remain high. Should be used cautiously in patients with CAD or pulmonary hypertension.

    3. It has direct negative inotropic and vasodilation effects, usually outweighed by a potent sympathomimetic effect, but may act as a direct myocardial depressant in patients with maximal sympathetic nervous system stimulation or in patients with autonomic blockade.

c. Respiratory system

    1. Usually depresses RR and TV only mildly and has minimal effect on CO_2 response.

    2. Potent bronchodilator due to sympathomimetic effects.

    3. Laryngeal protective reflexes are relatively well maintained, although aspiration can still occur.

4. Dosage and administration (Table 12.1)

    a. Useful for IM induction in patients with no IV access (eg, children).

    b. A concentrated 10% solution is available for IM use only.

5. Adverse effects

    a. Oral secretions are markedly stimulated. The coadministration of an antisialagogue (eg, glycopyrrolate) may be helpful.

    b. Emotional disturbance. May cause agitation and unpleasant hallucinations during the early postoperative period. Incidence is higher with increased age, female gender, and dosages greater than 2 mg/kg but may be greatly reduced with the coadministration of a benzodiazepine or propofol. Children seem to be less troubled than adults by the hallucinations. Alternatives should be considered in patients with psychiatric disorders.

    c. Muscle tone. May lead to random myoclonic movements, especially in response to stimulation. Muscle tone is often increased.

    d. Increases ICP and is relatively contraindicated in patients with head trauma or intracranial hypertension.

    e. Ocular effects. May lead to mydriasis, vertical nystagmus, diplopia, blepharospasm, and increased intraocular pressure.

    f. Anesthetic depth may be difficult to assess. Common clinical signs of anesthetic depth (eg, HR, BP, and RR) as well as EEG-based monitors of anesthetic depth are less reliable when ketamine is used.

    g. PONV

F. Dexmedetomidine. Dexmedetomidine is a sedative agent with analgesic properties. It is used as an adjunct to general anesthesia and for sedation in the ICU and the OR. It is also used in regional anesthesia, in combination with local anesthetics to prolong the duration of the regional block, and for premedication of pediatric patients (nasal or oral). In some centers, it is also used routinely for awake craniotomies (off-label).

1. Mode of action. Highly selective α_2-adrenergic receptor agonist (α_2/α_1 1600:1). **Clonidine** is a less-selective and longer-acting α_2 agonist (α_2/α_1 200:1) with similar sedating and analgesic properties. Sedative effect mimics the mechanism of sleep. It decreases the inhibitory outflow from the locus coeruleus, causing an increase in the GABAergic outflow from the ventrolateral preoptic nucleus in the hypothalamus.

2. **Pharmacokinetics**
   a. Undergoes rapid redistribution after IV administration. Elimination half-life is approximately 2 hours.
   b. Metabolized extensively in the liver.
3. **Pharmacodynamics**
   a. **CNS**
      1. Elicits a sedated but arousable state similar to natural sleep.
      2. Potentiates CNS effects of propofol, volatile anesthetics, benzodiazepines, and opioids.
      3. Opioid sparing effect intraoperatively.
      4. Weak amnestic, lacking anticonvulsant properties.
         a. Low doses produce spindles on the EEG that are similar to those observed during non–rapid eye movement (REM) stage 2 sleep. Higher doses produce delta and slow oscillations similar to non-REM stage 3 sleep.
         b. Decreases the likelihood of emergence delirium in pediatric population.
   b. **Cardiovascular system**
      1. Decreases HR and BP, α_{2A} receptor–mediated decrease in catecholamine release.
      2. Transient hypertension may occur after an IV bolus, thought to be secondary to peripheral α_{2B} receptor activation.
      3. Baroreflex is well preserved.
   c. **Respiratory system**
      1. Minimal respiratory depression, although it may contribute to respiratory depressant effects of other anesthetics.
      2. Airway reflexes remain intact, making it useful for awake fiberoptic intubation.
   d. **Endocrine system.** May decrease adrenal response to adrenocorticotropic hormone after prolonged infusions, although clinical significance is unclear.
4. **Dosage and administration** (Table 12.1)
   a. Decreased dosage should be considered in patients with significant hepatic dysfunction. Because the activity of dexmedetomidine metabolites has not been studied, decreased dosage may be prudent for patients with severe renal dysfunction.
   b. Indicated only for infusions of less than 24 hours.
5. **Adverse effects.** Antimuscarinic effects (eg, dry mouth and blurred vision) may occur due to α_2 adrenal receptor–mediated inhibition of acetylcholine release.
G. **Opioids.** Morphine, meperidine, methadone, hydromorphone, fentanyl, sufentanil, alfentanil, and remifentanil are opioids commonly used in general anesthesia. Their primary effect is analgesia; they are used to supplement other agents during the induction or maintenance of general anesthesia. In high doses, opioids are occasionally used as the primary anesthetic (eg, cardiac surgery). Opioids differ in their potencies, pharmacokinetics, and side effects.
   1. **Mode of action.** Bind to specific receptors in the brain, spinal cord, and on peripheral neurons. The opioids listed above are all relatively selective for μ-opioid receptors, and most of the analgesic and side effects of opioid medications are mediated by μ-opioid receptors. Additional mechanism of action for specific opioids include NMDA antagonism, in the case of methadone, and inhibition of serotonin reuptake and $\alpha 2b$ agonism, in the case of meperidine.

2. **Pharmacokinetics**
   a. Pharmacokinetic data are presented in **Table 12.2**.
   b. After IV administration, the onset of action is within minutes for the fentanyl derivatives; hydromorphone and morphine may take 20 to 30 minutes for peak effect due to their lower lipid solubilities. The termination of effects for all opioids except remifentanil is by redistribution.
   c. Elimination is primarily by the liver and depends on hepatic blood flow. Remifentanil is metabolized by nonspecific esterases in tissues (primarily skeletal muscle). Morphine and meperidine have active metabolites, whereas hydromorphone and the fentanyl derivatives do not.
   d. Metabolites are primarily excreted in the urine. In patients with renal failure, the accumulation of morphine-6-glucuronide may cause prolonged narcosis and respiratory depression. Renal failure may also cause the accumulation of normeperidine, an active meperidine metabolite associated with seizure activity.
   e. CSHT of fentanyl derivatives: fentanyl > alfentanil > sufentanil > remifentanil
3. **Pharmacodynamics**
   a. **CNS**
      1. Produce sedation and analgesia in a dose-dependent manner; euphoria is common. Very large doses may produce amnesia and loss of consciousness, but opioids are not reliable hypnotics.

 Dose, Time to Peak Effect, and the Duration of Analgesia for Intravenous Opioid Agonists and Agonist-Antagonists[a]

Opioid	Dose (mg)[b]	Peak (minute)	Duration (hour)[c]
Morphine	10	30-60	3-4
Meperidine	80	5-7	2-3
Hydromorphone	1.5	15-30	2-3
Oxymorphone	1.0	15-30	3-4
Methadone	10	5-10	—
Fentanyl	0.1	3-5	0.5-1
Sufentanil	0.01	3-5	0.5-1
Alfentanil	0.75	1.5-2	0.2-0.3
Remifentanil	0.1	1.5-2	0.1-0.2
Pentazocine	60	15-20	2-3
Butorphanol	2	15-20	2-3
Nalbuphine	10	15-20	3-4
Buprenorphine	0.3	<30	5-6

[a]Data for fentanyl derivatives are derived from intraoperative studies, the remainder from postoperative pain studies.
[b]Approximately equianalgesic doses (see text).
[c]Average duration of first single dose.

2. Reduce the minimum alveolar concentration (MAC) of inhalational anesthetics and the requirements for IV sedative-hypnotic drugs.

3. Decrease CBF and $CMRO_2$.

4. Produce miosis by the stimulation of the Edinger-Westphal nucleus of the oculomotor nerve.

b. **Cardiovascular system**

1. All opioids except meperidine produce minimal changes in cardiac contractility. Baroreceptor reflexes are preserved.

2. Systemic vascular resistance (SVR) usually is moderately reduced because of reduced medullary sympathetic outflow. Bolus doses of meperidine or morphine may reduce SVR secondary to histamine release.

3. Produce bradycardia in a dose-dependent manner by the stimulation of the central vagal nuclei. Meperidine has a weak atropine-like effect and does not cause bradycardia.

4. The relative hemodynamic stability offered by opioids often leads to their use in sedation or anesthesia for hemodynamically compromised or critically ill patients.

c. **Respiratory system**

1. Produce dose-dependent respiratory depression. RR decreases initially; TV decreases with larger doses. The effect is accentuated in the presence of sedatives, other respiratory depressants, or preexisting pulmonary disease.

2. Decrease ventilatory response to hypercapnia and hypoxia. Effects are markedly increased if the patient falls asleep.

3. Opioids dose dependently decrease the cough reflex. Higher doses suppress tracheal and bronchial foreign body reflexes, so endotracheal intubation and mechanical ventilation are better tolerated.

d. **Gastrointestinal system**

1. Decrease gastric emptying and intestinal secretions. Colonic tone and sphincter tone increase and propulsive contractions decrease, resulting in constipation.

2. Increase biliary pressure and may produce biliary colic; the spasm of the sphincter of Oddi may prevent cannulation of the common bile duct. The incidence is lower with agonist-antagonist opioids.

4. **Dosage and administration.** Opioids are usually administered IV, either by bolus or by infusion. Appropriate dosages are presented in **Table 12.2**. Clinical dosing must be individualized and based on the patient's underlying condition and clinical response. Larger doses may be required in patients chronically receiving opioids. Opioids are also routinely utilized in neuraxial anesthesia techniques to optimize pain control.

5. **Adverse effects**

a. **Allergic reactions** are rare, although anaphylactoid reactions may occur with morphine and meperidine secondary to histamine release.

b. **Drug interactions.** The administration of meperidine or tramadol is contraindicated in patients taking monoamine oxidase inhibitor, as it may precipitate serotonin syndrome (clonus, hyperthermia, agitation).

c. **Nausea and vomiting** can occur because of the direct stimulation of the chemoreceptor trigger zone. Nausea is more likely if the patient is moving.

d. **Muscle rigidity** may occur, especially in the chest, abdomen, and upper airway, resulting in the inability to ventilate the patient. The incidence increases with drug potency, dose, rate of administration, and presence of nitrous oxide. Rigidity may be reversed by administering neuromuscular relaxants or opioid antagonists and is less likely after pretreatment with a benzodiazepine or propofol.

e. **Urinary retention** may occur because of increased tone in the vesical sphincter and inhibition of the detrusor (voiding) reflex. May also decrease awareness of the need to urinate.

6. **Naloxone** is a pure opioid antagonist used to **reverse** unanticipated or undesired opioid-induced effects such as respiratory or CNS depression.

   a. **Mode of action.** Competitive antagonist at opioid receptors in the brain and spinal cord.

   b. **Pharmacokinetics**

      1. Peak effects are seen within 1 to 2 minutes; a significant decrease in its clinical effects occurs after 30 minutes because of redistribution.

      2. Metabolized in the liver.

   c. **Pharmacodynamics**

      1. Reverses the pharmacologic effects of opioids such as CNS and respiratory depression.

      2. Crosses the placenta; administration to the parturient before delivery will decrease opioid-induced respiratory depression in the neonate.

   d. **Dosage and administration.** Perioperative respiratory depression in an adult can be treated with 0.04 mg IV every 2 to 3 minutes as needed. **Repeated administration may be necessary** due to short duration of action.

   e. **Adverse effects**

      1. May lead to the abrupt onset of **pain** as opioid analgesia is reversed. This may be accompanied by sudden hemodynamic changes (eg, hypertension and tachycardia).

      2. May precipitate **pulmonary edema** and **cardiac arrest** in rare cases.

II. PHARMACOLOGY OF INHALATION ANESTHETICS

Inhalation anesthetics are usually administered for the maintenance of general anesthesia, and also for "breathe-down" inhalation inductions. General properties of commonly used inhalation anesthetics are summarized in **Table 12.3**. Dosages of inhalation anesthetics are expressed as **MAC**, the **MAC** at 1 atm at which 50% of patients do not move in response to a surgical stimulus. MAC is additive (eg, 0.5 MAC nitrous oxide + 0.5 MAC isoflurane = 1 MAC total).

A. Mode of Action

   1. **Nitrous oxide.** Although exact mechanisms are unknown, anesthetic effects are mainly attributed to the antagonism of NMDA receptors in the CNS. It is the only inhaled anesthetic, which directly produces analgesia.

   2. **Volatile anesthetics.** Exact mechanisms are unknown. Various ion channels in the CNS involved in synaptic transmission (including $GABA_A$, glycine, and glutamate receptors) have been shown to be sensitive to inhalation anesthetics and may play a role.

B. Pharmacokinetics

   1. **Determinants of the speed of onset and offset.** The alveolar anesthetic concentration (F_A) may differ significantly from the inspired anesthetic concentration (F_I). The rate of rise of the ratio of these two concentrations

T A B L E

12.3 Properties of Inhalation Anesthetics

Anesthetic	Vapor Pressure (mm Hg, 20 °C)	Partition Coefficients		MAC (% With O$_2$ Only)
		Blood-Gas[a] (37 °C)	Brain-Blood (37 °C)	
Isoflurane	238	1.4	1.6	1.28
Desflurane	664	0.45	1.3	6.0
Sevoflurane	157	0.65	1.7	2.05
Nitrous oxide	43,879	0.47	1.1	105

MAC, minimum alveolar concentration.

[a]The blood-gas partition coefficient is inversely related to the rate of induction.

(F_A/F_I) determines the speed of induction of general anesthesia (**Figure 12.1**). Two opposing processes, anesthetic delivery to and uptake from alveoli, determine the F_A/F_I at a given time. Determinants of uptake include the following:

a. **Blood-gas partition coefficient.** A lower solubility in blood will lead to lower uptake of anesthetic into the bloodstream, thereby increasing the rate of rise of F_A/F_I. The solubility of halogenated volatile anesthetics in blood is increased somewhat with hypothermia and hyperlipidemia.

b. **Inspired anesthetic concentration.** This is influenced by the volume of the breathing circuit, fresh gas inflow rate, and the absorption of the volatile anesthetic by circuit components.

c. **Alveolar ventilation.** Increased minute ventilation, without the alteration of other processes that affect anesthetic delivery or uptake, increases F_A/F_I. This effect is more pronounced with the more blood-soluble agents.

d. **Concentration effect.** As F_I increases, the rate of rise of F_A/F_I also increases. For a gas with a high F_I like nitrous oxide, a large amount is taken up into blood, but this causes a large loss of the total gas volume. The remaining nitrous oxide is thus "concentrated," and the addition of more anesthetic with the next breath will increase the concentration further. The uptake of a large gas volume also creates a void that draws more fresh gas into the alveoli, thereby increasing F_A and augmenting the inspired TV. The concentration effect explains why the rate of rise of F_A/F_I is faster for nitrous oxide than for desflurane (**Figure 12.1**), even though the blood-gas partition coefficient for desflurane is smaller.

e. **The second gas effect.** This is a direct outcome of the concentration effect. When nitrous oxide and a potent inhalation anesthetic are administered together, the uptake of nitrous oxide concentrates the "second" gas (eg, isoflurane) and increases the input of additional second gas into the alveoli via the augmentation of inspired volume.

f. **Cardiac output.** An increase in the cardiac output (and therefore pulmonary blood flow) will increase anesthetic uptake and thus decrease the rate of rise in F_A/F_I. A decrease in the cardiac output will have the opposite effect. This effect of cardiac output is more pronounced with non-rebreathing circuits or highly soluble anesthetics and is most prominent early in the course of anesthetic administration.

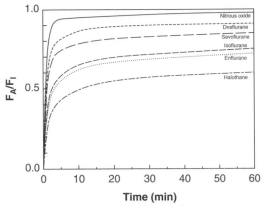

FIGURE 12.1 Ratio of alveolar to inspired gas concentration (F_A/F_I) as a function of time at constant cardiac output and minute ventilation.

g. **Gradient between alveolar and venous blood.** The uptake of anesthetic into the bloodstream will decrease as the anesthetic partial pressure gradient between the alveolar gas and the venous blood decreases. This gradient is particularly large early in the course of anesthetic administration.

2. **Distribution in tissues.** The rate of equilibration of anesthetic partial pressure between blood and a particular organ system depends on the following factors:

a. **Tissue blood flow.** Equilibration occurs more rapidly in tissues receiving increased perfusion. The **vessel-rich group** of highly perfused organ systems receives approximately 75% of the cardiac output. The remainder of the cardiac output perfuses predominantly into muscle and fat.

b. **Tissue solubility.** For a given arterial anesthetic partial pressure, anesthetic agents with high-tissue solubility are slower to equilibrate. Solubilities of anesthetic agents differ among tissues. Brain-blood partition coefficients of inhalation agents are shown in **Table 12.3**.

c. **Gradient between arterial blood and tissue.** Until equilibration is reached between the anesthetic partial pressure in the blood and a particular tissue, a gradient that leads to the uptake of anesthetic by the tissue exists. The rate of uptake will decrease as the gradient decreases.

3. **Elimination**

a. **Exhalation.** This is the predominant route of elimination. After discontinuation, an anesthetic's tissue and alveolar partial pressures decrease by reversing the processes that occurred when the anesthetic was introduced.

b. **Metabolism.** Significant biotransformation of nitrous oxide has not been demonstrated. Volatile anesthetics may undergo different degrees of hepatic metabolism.

c. **Anesthetic loss.** Inhalation anesthetics may be lost both percutaneously and through visceral membranes, although such losses are probably negligible.

C. **Pharmacodynamics**
  1. **Nitrous oxide**
     a. **CNS**
        1. Thought to act primarily by inhibiting NMDA receptors.
        2. Concentrations greater than 60% may produce amnesia, although not reliably.
        3. Because of its high MAC (105%), it is usually combined with other anesthetics to attain surgical anesthesia.
     b. **Cardiovascular system**
        1. Mild myocardial depressant and a mild sympathetic nervous system stimulant.
        2. HR and BP are usually unchanged.
        3. May increase pulmonary vascular resistance in adults.
     c. **Respiratory system.** Mild respiratory depressant, although less so than the volatile anesthetics.
  2. **Volatile anesthetics**
     a. **CNS**
        1. Produce unconsciousness and amnesia at relatively low inspired concentrations (25%-35% of MAC).
        2. At lower doses of halogenated ether anesthetics (isoflurane, sevoflurane, desflurane), alpha, delta, and slow oscillations are present. At higher doses, theta oscillations (4-8 Hz) appear, followed by burst suppression.
        3. Decreased amplitude and increased latency of SSEPs.
        4. Increase CBF and decrease $CMRO_2$; uncouple autoregulation of CBF.
     b. **Cardiovascular system**
        1. Produce dose-dependent myocardial depression and systemic vasodilation.
        2. HR tends to be unchanged, although desflurane can cause sympathetic stimulation, tachycardia, and hypertension at induction or when the inspired concentration is abruptly increased.
        3. Sensitize the myocardium to the arrhythmogenic effects of catecholamines, which is of particular concern during the infiltration of epinephrine-containing solutions or the administration of sympathomimetic agents.
     c. **Respiratory system**
        1. Produce dose-dependent respiratory depression with decrease in TV, increase in RR, and increase in arterial CO_2 pressure.
        2. Produce airway irritation and, during light levels of anesthesia, may precipitate coughing, laryngospasm, or bronchospasm, particularly in patients who smoke or have asthma. The lower pungency of sevoflurane makes it more suitable for use as an inhalation induction agent.
        3. Equipotent doses of volatile agents possess similar bronchodilator effects, with the exception of desflurane, which has mild bronchoconstricting activity.
        4. Inhibit hypoxic pulmonary vasoconstriction, which may contribute to pulmonary shunting.
     d. **Neuromuscular system**
        1. Dose-dependent decrease in skeletal muscle tone, often enhancing surgical conditions.
        2. May precipitate **malignant hyperthermia** in a susceptible patient.

e. **Hepatic system.** May cause a decrease in hepatic perfusion. Rarely, a patient may develop hepatitis secondary to exposure to a volatile agent, most notably with halothane ("halothane hepatitis").

f. **Renal system.** Decrease renal blood flow through either a decrease in MAP or an increase in renal vascular resistance.

D. **Adverse effects related to specific agents**

1. **Nitrous oxide**

a. **Expansion of closed gas spaces.** The predominant constituent in closed gas–containing spaces in the body is nitrogen. Because nitrous oxide is 35 times more soluble in blood than nitrogen, closed air spaces will expand as the amount of nitrous oxide diffusing into these spaces is greater than the amount of nitrogen diffusing out. Spaces containing air such as a pneumothorax, occluded middle ear, bowel lumen, or pneumocephalus will markedly enlarge if nitrous oxide is administered. Nitrous oxide will diffuse into the cuff of an endotracheal tube and may increase pressure within the cuff; this pressure should be assessed intermittently and, if necessary, reduced.

b. **Diffusion hypoxia.** After discontinuation of nitrous oxide, its rapid elimination from the blood into the lung may lead to a low partial pressure of oxygen in the alveoli, resulting in hypoxia and hypoxemia if supplemental oxygen is not administered.

c. **Inhibition of tetrahydrofolate synthesis.** N_2O inhibits methionine synthase, a vitamin B_{12}–dependent enzyme necessary for the synthesis of DNA. It should be used with caution in pregnant patients and those deficient in vitamin B_{12}.

2. **Desflurane** can be degraded to carbon monoxide in carbon dioxide absorbents (especially Baralyme). This is most likely to occur when the absorbent is new or dry.

3. **Sevoflurane** can be degraded in CO_2 absorbents (especially Baralyme) to fluoromethyl-2,2-difluoro-1-vinyl ether (**compound A**), which has been shown to produce renal toxicity in animal models. Compound A concentrations increase at low fresh gas rates. So far, there has been no evidence of consistent renal toxicity with sevoflurane usage in humans.

Suggested Readings

Brown EN, Purdon PL, Van Dort CJ. General anesthesia and altered states of arousal: a systems neuroscience analysis. *Annu Rev Neurosci.* 2011;34:601-628.

Dershwitz M, Rosow CE. Intravenous anesthetics. In: Longnecker DE, Mackey SC, Newman MF, Sandberg WS, Zapol WM, eds. *Anesthesiology.* 3rd ed. McGraw-Hill; 2017:636-649.

Eger EI. Uptake and distribution. In: Miller RD, ed. *Anesthesia.* 6th ed. Churchill Livingstone; 2005:131-153.

Forman SA, Benkwitz C. Inhalational anesthetics. In: Longnecker DE, Mackey SC, Newman MF, Sandberg WS, Zapol WM, eds. *Anesthesiology.* 3rd ed. McGraw-Hill; 2017:551-570.

McPhee LC, Badawi O, Fraser GL, et al. Single-dose etomidate is not associated with increased mortality in ICU patients with sepsis: analysis of a large electronic ICU database. *Crit Care Med.* 2013;41(3):774-783.

Patel HH, Pearn ML, Patel PM, Roth DM. General anesthetics and therapeutic gases. In: Brunton LL, Hilal-Dandan R, Knollmann BC, eds. *Goodman & Gilman's: The Pharmacological Basis of Therapeutics.* 13th ed. McGraw-Hill; 2018:387-404.

Rosow C, Dershwitz M. Opioid analgesics. In: Longnecker DE, Mackey SC, Newman MF, Sandberg WS, Zapol WM, eds. *Anesthesiology.* 3rd ed. McGraw-Hill; 2017:650-670.

13 Airway Evaluation and Management

Gregory H. Foos and Jean Kwo

I. APPLIED ANATOMY

A. The pharynx is divided into the nasopharynx, the oropharynx, and the laryngopharynx.

1. The **nasopharynx** consists of the nasal passages, including the septum, turbinates, and adenoids.

2. The **oropharynx** consists of the oral cavity, including the dentition and tongue.

3. The epiglottis separates the **laryngopharynx** into the larynx (leading to the trachea) and the **hypopharynx** (leading to the esophagus).

B. The larynx (see **Figure 13.1**)

1. The **larynx**, located at the level of the fourth to the sixth cervical vertebrae, originates at the laryngeal inlet and ends at the inferior border of the cricoid cartilage. It consists of nine cartilages: three unpaired (thyroid, cricoid, and epiglottis) and three paired (corniculates, cuneiforms, and arytenoids); ligaments; and muscles.

2. The **cricoid cartilage**, located just inferior to the **thyroid cartilage at the C5-6 vertebral level**, is the only complete cartilaginous ring in the respiratory tree. Because it is a complete ring, pressure is applied here (Sellick maneuver) to occlude the esophagus when performing a rapid sequence induction.

3. The **cricothyroid membrane** connects the thyroid and cricoid cartilages and measures 0.9×3.0 cm in adults. The membrane is superficial, thin, and devoid of major vessels in the midline, making it an important site for emergent surgical airway access (see Section VI.B.3).

4. **The laryngeal muscles** can be divided into two groups: muscles that open and close the glottis (lateral cricoarytenoid [adduction], posterior cricoarytenoid [abduction], and transverse arytenoid) and muscles that control the tension of the vocal ligaments (cricothyroid, vocalis, and thyroarytenoid).

5. **Innervation**

   a. **Sensory.** The **glossopharyngeal nerve** (cranial nerve IX) provides sensory innervation to the posterior one-third of the tongue, the oropharynx from its junction with the nasopharynx, including the pharyngeal surfaces of the soft palate, epiglottis, and the fauces, to the junction of the pharynx and esophagus. The **internal branch of the superior laryngeal nerve**, a branch of the vagus nerve (cranial nerve X), provides sensory innervation to the mucosa from the epiglottis to and including the vocal cords. The sensory fibers of the **inferior laryngeal nerve**, a branch of the recurrent laryngeal nerve (also a branch of the vagus nerve), provide sensory innervation to the mucosa of the subglottic larynx and trachea. A small branch of the **glossopharyngeal nerve, Hering nerve**, also serves to transmit information from baroreceptors in the carotid sinus and chemoreceptors in the carotid body to the brainstem.

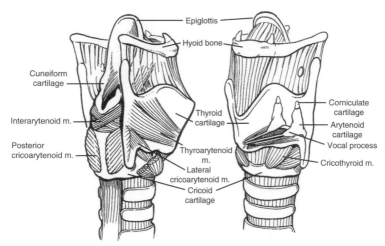

FIGURE 13.1 Laryngeal anatomy. (Reprinted from Garrett CG, Ossoff RH. Hoarseness. *Med Clin N Am.* 1999;83(1):115-123. Copyright © 1999 Elsevier. With permission.)

 b. Motor. The external branch of the **superior laryngeal nerve** provides motor innervation to the cricothyroid muscle. Activation of this muscle results in tensing of the vocal cords. The motor fibers of the **inferior laryngeal nerve** provide motor innervation to all other intrinsic muscles of the larynx. **Bilateral injury to the inferior laryngeal nerves** (eg, via injury to the recurrent laryngeal nerves) can produce unopposed activation of the cricothyroideus, leading to tensing of the vocal cords and airway closure.

C. The **glottis** is composed of the vocal folds (true and "false" cords) and the rima glottidis.

 1. The **rima glottidis** describes the aperture between the true vocal cords.

 2. The **glottis** is the narrowest point in the adult airway (more than 8 years of age), whereas the cricoid cartilage is the narrowest point in the infant airway (birth to 1 year of age). Of note, a recent MRI study showed the glottis is the narrowest portion of the sedated, unparalyzed pediatric (2 months-13 years).

D. The lower airway extends from the subglottic larynx to the bronchi.

 1. The subglottic larynx extends from the vocal folds to the inferior border of the cricoid cartilage (C6).

 2. The **trachea** is a fibromuscular tube that is 10 to 12 cm long with a diameter of approximately 20 mm in adults. It extends from the cricoid cartilage to the carina. The trachea is supported by 16 to 20 U-shaped cartilages, with the open end facing posteriorly. Noting the posterior absence of cartilaginous rings provides anterior-posterior orientation during fiberoptic exam of the tracheobronchial tree.

 3. The trachea bifurcates into the right and left main stem bronchi at the carina. The right main stem bronchus is approximately 2.5 cm long with a takeoff angle of approximately 25°. The left main stem bronchus is approximately 5 cm long with a takeoff angle of approximately 45°. Because the right main stem bronchus branches at a less acute angle, aspiration and accidental bronchial intubation are more likely to occur on the right side.

II. EVALUATION

A. History. A history of difficult airway management in the past may be the best predictor of a challenging airway. Prior anesthetic records should be reviewed for the ease of intubation and ventilation (the ability to mask ventilate and whether adjuncts to mask ventilation were required, the number of intubation attempts, the type of laryngoscope blade used, the size of the endotracheal tube [ETT], or if any specialty airway equipment, ie, video laryngoscopy or a bronchoscope were required). Particular importance should also be placed on diseases that may affect the airway. Specific symptoms related to airway compromise should be sought, including hoarseness, stridor, wheezing, dysphagia, dyspnea, and positional airway obstruction.

1. **Arthritis or cervical disk disease** may decrease neck mobility. Cervical spine instability and limitation of mandibular motion are common in rheumatoid arthritis. The temporomandibular and cricoarytenoid joints may also be involved. Aggressive neck manipulation in these patients may lead to atlantoaxial subluxation and spinal cord injury. The risk of atlantoaxial subluxation is highest in patients with severe hand deformities and skin nodules.

2. **Infections** of the floor of the mouth, salivary glands, tonsils, or pharynx may cause pain, edema, and trismus with limited mouth opening. **Epiglottitis** is a bacterial infection that causes an acute inflammation of the epiglottis and adjacent structures and can result in airway compromise. Because of routine vaccination against *Haemophilus*, epiglottitis has become more common in adults than children. In patients with airway compromise, intubation should be performed in the operating room with a specialist capable of performing rigid bronchoscopy or surgical airway, if needed, on standby.

3. **Tumors** may obstruct the airway or cause extrinsic compression and tracheal deviation.

4. **Increased body mass index** (BMI > 35) coupled with other anatomical findings (high Mallampati score, increased neck circumference, short thyromental distance) can be predictive for difficult mask ventilation and difficult tracheal intubation. The decreased functional residual capacity associated with an increased BMI can result in a precipitous oxygen desaturation with the apnea of induction.

5. A history of **snoring** or **obstructive sleep apnea** may be associated with difficult intubation.

6. **Trauma** may be associated with airway injuries, cervical spine injury, basilar skull fracture, or intracranial injury.

7. **Previous surgery, radiation, or burns** may produce scarring, contracture resulting in limited tissue mobility, and/or narrowed oral aperture.

8. The physiologic changes associated with **pregnancy** results in edema of the laryngeal and oral mucosa that can make obtaining a view of the glottis challenging, particularly at the end of the third trimester.

9. **Acromegaly** may cause mandibular hypertrophy and overgrowth and enlargement of the tongue and epiglottis. The glottic opening may be narrowed because of enlargement of the vocal cords.

10. **Scleroderma** may produce skin tightness and decrease mandibular motion and narrow the oral aperture.

11. **Trisomy 21 patients** may have atlantoaxial instability and macroglossia.

12. **Osteogenesis imperfecta and achondroplasia** may be associated with atlantoaxial instability and potentially difficult airway management because of mandibular hypoplasia (micrognathia).

13. **Other congenital anomalies** may complicate airway management, particularly pediatric and adult patients with craniofacial abnormalities such as Pierre Robin, Treacher Collins, Klippel-Feil, and Goldenhar syndromes. In contrast, children with isolated cleft palates are not specifically difficult to intubate if the condition is not associated with other airway or craniofacial abnormalities, but nasotracheal intubation should be avoided.

B. **Physical examination.** A normal airway exam does not completely exclude the likelihood of a difficult intubation.

1. **Specific findings** that may indicate a difficult airway include the following:

   a. Inability to open the mouth or small mouth opening: distance between upper and lower incisors <5 cm

   b. Poor cervical spine mobility

   c. Receding chin (retrognathia): length between angle of jaw to tip of chin <9 cm

   d. Large tongue (macroglossia)

   e. Prominent incisors

   f. Short thick neck

   g. Short thyromental distance

   h. Wilson score—combo of weight, cervical spine mobility, jaw mobility, retrognathia, prominent incisors.

2. **Injuries** to the face, neck, or chest must be evaluated to assess their contribution to airway compromise.

3. **Inhalational injury** to the airway due to direct thermal injury or chemical injury due to toxic gas inhalation can occur in patients with acute burns. The risk of inhalation injury increases with increased total body surface area burned. Upper airway swelling may not peak until 24 hours after the burn injury. Risk factors for impending airway obstruction include history of exposure to fire/smoke in an enclosed space, moderate to severe facial/oropharyngeal burns, circumferential neck burns, and evidence of airway injury on flexible nasoendoscopy.

4. **Head and neck examination**

   a. **Nose.** The patency of the nares or the presence of a deviated septum should be determined by occluding one nostril at a time and assessing ease of ventilation through the other nostril. This is especially important should nasotracheal intubation be required.

   b. **Mouth.** Identify macroglossia and conditions that reduce mouth opening (eg, facial scars or contractures, scleroderma, and temporomandibular joint disease). **Poor dentition** may increase the risk of tooth injury or avulsion during airway manipulation. Loose teeth should be identified preoperatively and protected or removed before initiation of airway management.

      1. The **upper lip bite test** (see **Figure 13.2**) assesses the range of motion of the mandible. Inability to bite upper lip with lower lip is associated with a 60% probability of difficult intubation.

   c. **Neck**

      1. A **thyromental distance** (the distance from the lower border of the mandible to the thyroid notch with the neck fully extended) of less than 6 cm (three to four finger breadths) is associated with difficulty visualizing the glottis. The mobility of laryngeal structures should be assessed. The trachea should be palpable in the midline above the sternal notch. Look for scars from previous neck surgery, an enlarged thyroid, other paratracheal masses, and indurated tissues suggestive of radiation therapy.

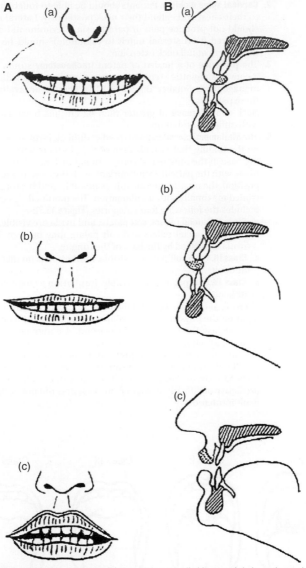

FIGURE 13.2 Frontal (A) and lateral (B) view of the upper lip bite test. Ask the patient to bite their upper lip with their lower incisors. a, Class 1—lower incisors able to bite entire upper lip, lip mucosa barely visible. b, Class 2—lower incisors bite upper lip partially, lip mucosa partially visible. c, Class 3—lower incisors cannot bite upper lip at all. (Reprinted with permission from Khan ZH, Kashfi A, Ebrahimkhani E. A comparison of the Upper Lip Bite Test (a simple new technique) with modified Mallampati classification in predicting difficulty in endotracheal intubation: a prospective blinded study. *Anesth Analg*. 2003;96(2):595-599. Copyright © 2003 International Anesthesia Research Society.)

2. **Cervical spine mobility.** Patients should be able to touch their chin to their chest and extend their neck posteriorly. Lateral rotation should not produce pain or paresthesia. Sternomental distance (measured from sternal notch to mandible) should be greater than 12 cm at full neck extension.

3. The presence of a healed or patent **tracheostomy** stoma may be a clue to subglottic stenosis or prior complications with airway management. Smaller diameter ETTs should be available for these patients.

4. **Neck circumference** of greater than 42 cm has been associated with difficult intubation.

5. The **Mallampati classification** to predict difficult intubation is based on the finding that visualization of the glottis is impaired when the base of the tongue is disproportionately large. Assessment is made with the patient sitting upright, with the head in the neutral position, the mouth open as wide as possible, and the tongue protruded maximally without phonation. The modified classification includes the following four categories (**Figure 13.3**):

   a. **Class I.** Faucial pillars, soft palate, and uvula are visible.

   b. **Class II.** Faucial pillars and soft palate may be seen, but the uvula is masked by the base of the tongue.

   c. **Class III.** Only soft palate is visible. Intubation is predicted to be difficult.

   d. **Class IV.** Soft palate is not visible. Intubation is predicted to be difficult.

6. There is no single best predictor of difficult airway management on the physical exam. **Multiple predictors** of difficult airway will increase the specificity of the exam. A combination of high Mallampati class, short thyromental or sternomental distance, and impaired mandibular protrusion increases the likelihood of difficult intubation. Composite scores (eg, Wilson score—see **Table 13.1**) are of limited utility because while a higher score is predictive of difficult intubation, lower scores did not exclude difficult intubation.

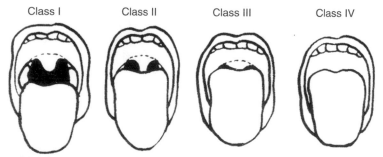

Class I   Class II   Class III   Class IV

FIGURE 13.3 Mallampati classification of the oropharyngeal structures as modified by Samsoon and Young, as defined in a patient sitting upright with mouth maximally opened and tongue protruded without phonation. (From Samsoon GLT, Young JRB. Difficult tracheal intubation: a retrospective study. *Anaesthesia.* 1987;42(5):487-490. Copyright © 1987 The Association of Anesthetists of Gt Britain and Ireland. Reprinted by permission of John Wiley & Sons, Inc.)

TABLE 13.1	Wilson Score		
	0	**1**	**2**
Weight	<90 kg	90-110 kg	>110 kg
Neck movement	>90°	90°	<90°
Jaw mobility	Interincisor gap ≥5 cm or able to protrude lower incisors beyond upper incisors	Interincisor gap <5 cm or able to protrude lower incisors to meet upper incisors	Interincisor gap <5 cm or unable to protrude lower incisors to meet upper incisors
Receding mandible	Normal	Moderate	Severe
Prominent incisors	Normal	Moderate	Severe

An example of a composite score to predict difficult intubation. Score is calculated by totaling numbers of parameters (total possible score 10). A score of ≥ 2 to 3 is strongly predictive of a difficult intubation. However, a low score rate does not reliably rule out a difficult intubation.
Reprinted from Wilson ME, Spiegelhalter D, Robertson JA, et al. Predicting difficult intubation. *Br J Anaesth.* 1988;61(2):211-216. Copyright © 1988 Elsevier. With permission.

C. **Special studies.** In most patients, a careful history and physical examination will be all that are needed to evaluate an airway. Useful adjuncts may include the following:

1. **Laryngoscopy** (direct, indirect, video, or flexible fiberoptic) will provide information about the hypopharynx, laryngeal inlet, and vocal cord function. It can be performed in a conscious patient with topical anesthesia or nerve blocks.

2. **Chest or cervical imaging** may reveal tracheal deviation or narrowing and bony deformities in the neck. Cervical spine films are particularly important in trauma cases and should be performed in case of an injury above the clavicle or serious multiple traumatic injuries. In patients with altered mental status or distracting injuries, a normal cervical radiograph cannot rule out a significant ligamentous injury. Cervical spine precautions should be applied during intubation. Computed tomography (CT) or MRI scans may provide additional information. Lateral cervical spine films may be useful in symptomatic patients with rheumatoid arthritis or Down syndrome to assess for atlantoaxial subluxation.

3. **Tracheal tomograms or CT** scan can delineate masses obstructing the airway.

4. **Pulmonary function tests** and flow volume loops can help determine the degree and site of airway obstruction (see Chapters 1 and 3).

5. **Baseline arterial blood gas tensions** can indicate the functional consequences of airway abnormalities and alert the clinician to patients with chronic hypoxemia or hypercarbia.

III. MASK AIRWAY
A. **Indications**
1. To preoxygenate (denitrogenate) a patient before endotracheal intubation.
2. To assist or control ventilation as part of initial resuscitation before an ETT is placed.
3. To provide inhalation anesthesia in patients not at risk for regurgitation of gastric contents.

B. Technique involves placing a face mask and maintaining a patent airway.

   1. **The mask** should fit snugly around the bridge of the nose, cheeks, and mouth. Clear plastic masks allow for observation of the lips (for color) and mouth (for secretions or vomitus).

   2. **Mask placement.** The mask is held in the left hand so that the little finger is at the angle of the mandible, the third and fourth fingers are along the mandible, and the index finger and thumb are placed on the mask in the shape of the letter "C." The right hand is available to control the reservoir bag. Two hands may be required to maintain a good mask fit, necessitating an assistant to control the bag. Alternatively, two hands may be applied with the ventilator functioning in pressure mode if an assistant is not available. Head straps may be used to assist mask fit. Peak inspiratory pressures should be kept below 20 cmH$_2$O in order to minimize gastric insufflation. There are certain airway environments that may require a reversal of the handedness of mask ventilation described above where the mask will be held in the right hand, and the left hand will control the reservoir bag. This should be an ambidextrous skill. Some face masks have a Luer lock, which allows air to be injected or removed to aid in fit.

   3. **Edentulous patients** may present a problem when attempting to achieve an adequate seal with the face mask because of decreased distance between the mandible and the maxilla. An oral airway will often correct this problem and the cheeks may be compressed against the mask to decrease leaks. Two hands may be required to do this. Alternatively, dentures may be left in place during mask ventilation and removed prior to intubation.

   4. **Airway obstruction** during spontaneous ventilation may be recognized by a paradoxical "rocking" motion of the chest and abdomen. During spontaneous ventilation, if the upper airway is obstructed as the diaphragm contracts, the abdomen distends as it normally does for each breath, but the thorax collapses instead of being insufflated. Stridor is a high-pitched noise associated with an extreme narrowing of the upper airway that is associated with diseases such as croup. It is also observed with **laryngospasm** after extubation. With airway obstruction, respiratory excursions in the reservoir bag will be decreased or absent, and peak airway pressures will be increased when positive-pressure ventilation is attempted.

   5. **Airway patency** may be restored by the following:
      a. Neck extension.
      b. Jaw thrust, by placing the fingers under the angles of the mandible and lifting forward.
      c. Turning the head to one side or the other.
      d. Insertion of an oral airway. An airway may not be tolerated if the gag reflex is intact. Complications from the use of oral airways include vomiting, laryngospasm, and dental trauma. A misfitting oral airway may worsen obstruction. If the oral airway is too short, it may compress the tongue and worsen obstruction; if it is too long, it may lie against the epiglottis. A proper fitting oral airway should extend from the midpoint of the incisors to the angle of the mandible when measured externally.
      e. A nasal airway helps maintain upper airway patency in a patient with minimal-to-moderate obstruction and is reasonably tolerated by awake or sedated patients. Nasal airways can cause epistaxis. Care should be taken when used with patients who are anticoagulated.

C. **Difficult mask ventilation.** Obesity (BMI > 30), edentition, beards, higher Mallampati classification (III or IV), limited jaw protrusion, cervical arthritis, larger neck circumference (>42 cm), or snoring/obstructive sleep apnea is associated with difficult mask ventilation. Appropriate oral and nasal airways and laryngeal mask airways (LMAs) should be immediately available when difficult mask ventilation is anticipated.

D. **Complications.** The mask can cause pressure injuries to soft tissues around the mouth, mandible, eyes, or nose. Mask ventilation does not protect the airway from aspiration of gastric contents. Loss of the airway may result from laryngospasm or vomiting. **Laryngospasm** is a tonic contraction of the laryngeal and pharyngeal muscles causing closure of the vocal cords and airway obstruction. It is relieved by jaw thrust and the application of constant positive airway pressure. If this fails, a small dose of succinylcholine (20 mg intravenously or intramuscularly in the adult) will relax the vocal cords and relieve the obstruction.

IV. LARYNGEAL MASK AIRWAY

A. LMAs are supraglottic airway management devices that can be used as an alternative to both mask ventilation and endotracheal intubation in appropriate patients. The LMA also plays an important role in the management of the difficult airway. When inserted appropriately, the LMA lies with its tip resting over the upper esophageal sphincter, cuff sides lying over the piriform fossae, and cuff upper border resting against the base of the tongue (see **Figure 13.4**). Such positioning allows for effective ventilation with minimal inflation of the stomach.

1. **Indications**

   a. As an alternative to mask ventilation or endotracheal intubation for airway management. The LMA is not a replacement for endotracheal intubation when endotracheal intubation is indicated.

   b. In the management of a known or unexpected difficult airway.

   c. In airway management during the resuscitation of an unconscious patient.

2. **Contraindications**

   a. Patients at risk of aspiration of gastric contents, such as patients with a full stomach or symptomatic gastroesophageal reflux disease.

   b. Patients with decreased respiratory system compliance. The low-pressure seal of the LMA cuff will leak at high inspiratory pressures resulting in gas entering the esophagus and gastric insufflation. Peak inspiratory pressures should be maintained at less than 20 cmH$_2$O to minimize cuff leaks and gastric insufflation.

   c. Patients in whom long-term mechanical ventilatory support is anticipated or required.

   d. Patients with intact upper airway reflexes because insertion can precipitate laryngospasm.

3. **Use**

   a. LMAs are available in a variety of pediatric and adult sizes (see **Table 13.2**). Using the proper size maximizes the probability of appropriate cuff fit. There are many techniques for inserting the LMA. A common maneuver for insertion of the LMA is shown in **Figure 13.5**. Alternatively, the cuff can be inserted partially inflated at a 90-degree angle to its final position. It is pinched as it passes between the tongue and hard palate and rotated into position while advancing until definite resistance is felt at the base of the hypopharynx.

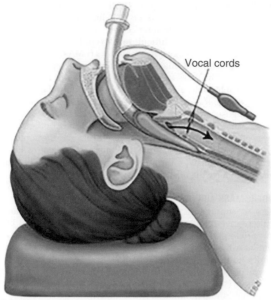

Vocal cords

FIGURE 13.4 Position of properly inserted laryngeal mask airway. (Reproduced with permission from Doyle DJ. Supraglottic devices (including laryngeal mask airways) for airway management for anesthesia in adults. In: Post TW, ed. *UpToDate*. UpToDate. Accessed May 12, 2020. Copyright © 2020 UpToDate, Inc. For more information visit www.uptodate.com.)

    b. The outer surface of the cuff may be lubricated to aid insertion. Lubrication of the LMA inner surface should be avoided because lubricant dripping into the larynx can precipitate laryngospasm.
    c. Follow usual preoxygenation and monitoring requirements.
    d. Ensure an adequate level of anesthesia and suppression of upper airway reflexes.

TABLE 13.2 Laryngeal Mask Airway Sizes[a]

Patient Age/Size	LMA Size	Cuff Volume	ETT Size (ID)
Neonates/infants up to 5 kg	1	Up to 4 mL	3.5 mm
Infants, 5-10 kg	1.5	Up to 7 mL	4.0 mm
Infants/children, 10-20 kg	2.0	Up to 10 mL	4.5 mm
Children, 20-30 kg	2.5	Up to 14 mL	5.0 mm
Children, 30 kg to small adults	3.0	Up to 20 mL	6.0 cuffed
Average adults	4.0	Up to 30 mL	6.0 cuffed
Large adults	5.0	Up to 40 mL	7.0 cuffed

ETT, endotracheal tube; ID, internal diameter; LMA, laryngeal mask airway.
[a]LMA sizes, cuff volume, and maximum ETT size differ with different manufacturers. Please consult manufacturer's instructions for use (IFU) for details.

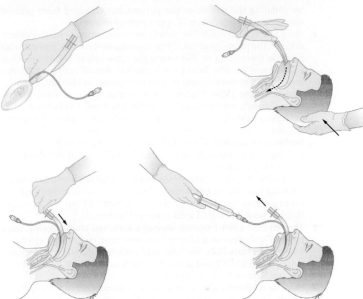

FIGURE 13.5 Technique for Insertion of LMA. Top left: Grasp the airway tube in the dominant hand and place the index finger between the tube and the deflated cuff of the mask. Top right: With the nondominant hand adjusting the head into the "sniffing" position, place the tip of the mask firmly against the palate and advance the LMA along the palate and into the posterior pharynx with the initial direction of force directed toward the operator's umbilicus. Lower left: The nondominant hand is then used to push the LMA further into the hypopharynx until resistance is encountered at the UES. Lower right: Once inserted, the cuff of the LMA is insufflated with just enough air to create a seal. (From Egan B. Supraglottic airway devices. In: Chu LF, Traynor AJ, Kurup V, eds. *Manual of Clinical Anesthesiology*. 2nd ed. Philadelphia, PA: Wolters Kluwer; 2021:190-199 and adapted from Walls RM, Murphy MF. *Manual of Emergency Airway Management*. 3rd ed. Philadelphia, PA: Lippincott Williams & Wilkins; 2008:125-127.)

  e. Position the patient's head appropriately. The "sniffing" position (slight flexion of the lower cervical spine with extension of C1-2) used to optimize endotracheal intubation also typically provides the best positioning for LMA insertion.
  f. Insert the LMA (see **Figure 13.5**). A soft bite block can be used to protect against a patient biting down on the LMA tube.
  g. Inflate cuff (see **Table 13.2**). Typically, one sees a smooth ovoid expansion of the tissues above the thyroid cartilage with adequate inflation of the appropriately positioned LMA.
  h. Ensure adequate ventilation with chest rise, end-tidal CO_2.
  i. Connect to anesthetic circuit. The LMA can be secured with tape if necessary.
  j. LMA removal. The LMA generally is well tolerated by a patient emerging from general anesthesia as long as the cuff is not overinflated (cuff pressure less than 60 cmH_2O). The LMA can be removed

by deflating the cuff once the patient has emerged from general anesthesia and has return of upper airway reflexes.

k. The LMA may be a suitable airway for some patients having procedures in the prone position. If this technique is chosen, patients can position themselves on the operating table before induction. After induction of anesthesia, the LMA can be inserted with the patient's head turned to the side and resting on a pillow or blankets.

4. **Second-generation LMAs.** Classic LMAs consist of a cuff, valve, airway tube, and circuit connection. "Second-generation" LMAs have additional functionality for unique situations and many include a widened proximal tube, which functions as a built-in bite-block.

a. **Intubating LMAs** are designed to facilitate intubation of the patient by passing an ETT through them, either blindly or with flexible bronchoscopic guidance.

b. The disposable, single-use air-Q LMA is similar in style to a standard LMA but has a larger reinforced tube and removable airway connector that allows the placement of any standard ETT (up to 8.5-mm ID) that has been lubricated with water gel lubricant.

c. The reusable LMA Fastrach includes a curved stainless-steel tube covered with silicone, a 15-mm end connector, cuff, and an epiglottic lifting bar (**Figure 13.6**). The tube is of sufficient diameter to accept a cuffed 8-mm ID ETT and is short enough to ensure that the ETT cuff will rest beyond the vocal cords.

d. Flexible-reinforced LMAs have small, wire-reinforced airway tubes, which allow significant manipulation of the airway tube without interference with mask seal. These are particularly useful in procedures involving the head and neck where a classic LMA could obstruct the surgical field.

e. The LMA ProSeal incorporates a high-pressure cuff and conduit for an orogastric tube for use in situations where risk of aspiration is elevated and has been employed successfully in laparoscopic surgery.

f. The LMA Gastro incorporates a large channel to allow passage of an endoscope.

5. Adverse effects. The most common adverse effect of using an LMA is a sore throat with an estimated incidence of 10%. The primary major adverse event is aspiration, which occurs at an incidence comparable to mask or endotracheal anesthesia. LMAs have been associated with lingual, recurrent laryngeal, and hypoglossal nerve injuries. LMA use for a duration greater than 3 hours should be avoided.

V. ENDOTRACHEAL INTUBATION
A. Orotracheal intubation
1. **Indications.** Endotracheal intubation is required to provide a patent airway when patients are at risk for aspiration, when airway maintenance by mask is difficult, and for prolonged controlled ventilation. Intubation also may be required for specific surgical procedures (eg, head/neck, intrathoracic, or intra-abdominal procedures).

2. **Technique.** Intubation is usually performed with a laryngoscope. The Macintosh and Miller blades are most commonly used.

a. The **Macintosh blade** is curved and the tip is inserted into the vallecula (the space between the base of the tongue and the pharyngeal surface of the epiglottis) (**Figure 13.7A**). It provides a good view of the oropharynx and hypopharynx, thus allowing more room for passage of the ETT with decreased trauma to the epiglottis. Blade sizes are designated as no. 1 through 4, with most adults requiring a Macintosh no. 3 blade.

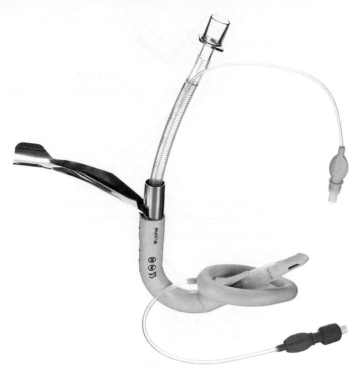

FIGURE 13.6 Features of the laryngeal mask airway fastrach. (Image courtesy of Teleflex Incorporated. Copyright © 2021 Teleflex Incorporated. All rights reserved.)

    b. The **Miller blade** is straight and it is passed so that the tip lies beneath the laryngeal surface of the epiglottis (**Figure 13.7B**). The epiglottis is then lifted to expose the vocal cords. The Miller blade provides excellent exposure of the glottic opening but provides a smaller passageway through the oropharynx and hypopharynx. Sizes are designated as no. 0 through 4, with most adults requiring a Miller no. 2 or 3 blade.

    c. Various modified laryngoscope blades provide better visualization of the cords through epiglottis lifting (eg, McCoy) or indirect visualization of the cords (eg, Siker and Truview EVO).

    d. The **sniffing position** with the occiput elevated by pads or folded blankets and the neck extended is the classic intubation position. On average, this improves the laryngoscopic view, although intubation and mouth opening may be facilitated in some patients by simple neck extension. Neck flexion may make it more difficult to open the mouth.

    e. The laryngoscope is held in the left hand near the junction between the handle and blade. After propping the mouth open with a scissoring motion of the right thumb and index finger, the laryngoscope is inserted into the right side of the patient's mouth while sweeping the tongue to the left. The lips should not be pinched by the blade

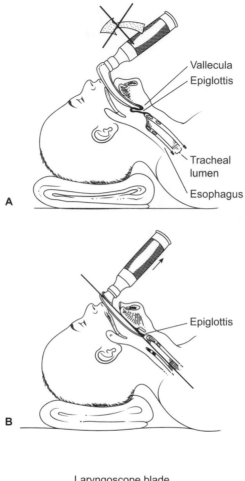

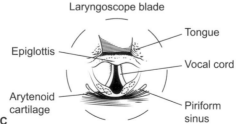

FIGURE 13.7 Anatomic relations for laryngoscopy and endotracheal intubation. A, Curved blade placement. B, Straight blade placement. C, Glottic exposure with curved blade placement.

and the teeth should be avoided. The blade is then advanced toward the midline until the epiglottis comes into view. The tongue and pharyngeal soft tissues are then lifted to expose the glottic opening. The laryngoscope should be used to lift (see **Figure 13.7B**) rather than act as a lever (see **Figure 13.7A**) to prevent damage to the maxillary incisors or gingiva.

f. An alternative to the classic sniffing position, the so-called **flexion-flexion** position, may be trialed if an appropriate glottic view cannot be obtained using conventional positioning. This technique involves first inserting the laryngoscope blade into the mouth as describe above. The head is then lifted, either using the anesthetist's right hand or the help of an assistant, and supported by the anesthetist's abdomen such that there is flexion both at the lower cervical level and at the atlantoaxial joint. The laryngoscope blade is then lifted such that the vector of force applied runs parallel to the body of the patient.

g. An appropriate ETT size depends on the patient's age, body habitus, and type of surgery. A 7.0-mm ETT is used for most women, and a 7.5-mm ETT is used for most men. The ETT is held in the right hand as one would hold a pencil and advanced through the oral cavity from the right corner of the mouth and then through the vocal cords. The anatomic view for visualization with a Macintosh laryngoscope is shown in **Figure 13.7C**. If visualization of the glottic opening is incomplete, it may be necessary to use the epiglottis as a landmark, passing the ETT immediately beneath it and into the trachea. External downward pressure on the cricoid and/or thyroid cartilage may aid in visualization. The proximal end of the ETT cuff is placed just below the vocal cords, and the markings on the tube are noted in relation to the patient's incisors or lips. The cuff is inflated just to the point of obtaining a seal in the presence of 20 to 30 cmH_2O positive airway pressure. Description of the visualization of the glottic opening should be recorded using the Cormack-Lehane scoring system (**Figure 13.8**).

h. **Proper placement of the ETT** must be verified by the detection of carbon dioxide in end-tidal or mixed expiratory gas as well as inspection and auscultation of the stomach and both lung fields during positive-pressure ventilation. If an ETT is inserted too deeply, it usually passes into the right mainstem bronchus. When breath sounds are heard on only one side of the thorax, an endobronchial intubation should be suspected, and the ETT should be withdrawn until breath sounds are heard bilaterally. (In trauma patients, unilateral breath sounds may be indicative of a pneumothorax.) Listening for breath sounds high in each axilla may decrease the chances of being misled by transmitted breath sounds from the opposite lung. A high index of suspicion of an esophageal intubation should be maintained until adequate oxygenation and ventilation are ensured.

i. The ETT should be fastened securely with tape, preferably to taut the skin overlying bony structures.

3. **Complications of orotracheal intubation** include injury of the lips or tongue, teeth, pharynx, or tracheal mucosa. Though rare, avulsion of arytenoid cartilages or damage to vocal cords or trachea can occur. High pressures in the cuff of the ETT can lead to ischemia of the tracheal mucosal. Ideally, the cuff pressure, measured with a manometer at the cuff inflation valve, should be between 20 and 30 cm of H_2O.

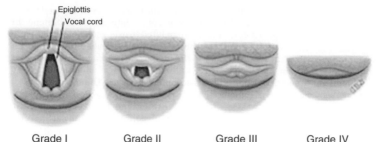

Grade I   Grade II   Grade III   Grade IV

FIGURE 13.8 Cormack-Lehane grade for view on direct laryngoscopy. Grade 1: Full view of glottis. Grade 2: Partial view of glottis. Grade 3: Only epiglottis seen. Grade 4: Unable to visualize the glottis and epiglottis. (Reproduced with permission from Orebaugh S, Snyder JV. Direct laryngoscopy and endotracheal intubation in adults. In: Post TW, ed. *UpToDate*. UpToDate. Accessed May 12, 2020. Copyright © 2020 UpToDate, Inc. For more information visit www. uptodate.com.)

B. Nasotracheal intubation

    1. Indications. Nasotracheal intubations are uncommon but may be required in patients undergoing an intraoral or oral maxillofacial facial procedure. Compared with oral ETTs, the maximal diameter that can be accommodated nasally is usually smaller and therefore, the resistance to breathing may be higher. The nasotracheal route is rarely used for long-term intubation because of increased airway resistance and the increased risk of sinusitis.

    2. Contraindications. Basilar skull fractures, especially of the ethmoid bone, nasal fractures, epistaxis, nasal polyps, coagulopathy, and planned systemic anticoagulation and/or thrombolysis (eg, patient with acute myocardial infarction), are relative contraindications to nasal intubation.

    3. Technique. Topical anesthesia and vasoconstriction of the nasal mucosa may be achieved by applying a mixture of 2% lidocaine and 0.25% phenylephrine using cotton-tipped pledgets. If both nares are patent, the right side is preferred because this will direct the bevel of most ETTs toward the flat nasal septum reducing risk of damage to the turbinates. The inferior turbinates can interfere with passage and limit the size of the ETT. Usually, a 6.0- to 6.5-mm ETT is used for women and a 7.0- to 7.5-mm ETT is used for men. After it passes through the nares into the pharynx, the tube is advanced through the glottic opening. Intubation may be performed blindly on spontaneously breathing patients. In anesthetized and apneic patients, the tube can be passed using direct laryngoscopy assisted by Magill forceps or with bronchoscopic assistance.

    4. Complications are similar to those described for orotracheal intubation (see Section V.A.3). Additionally, epistaxis, submucosal dissection, and dislodgement of enlarged tonsils and adenoids may occur. Compared with orotracheal intubation, the nasotracheal route has been associated with an increased incidence of sinusitis and bacteremia.

C. Bronchoscopic intubation. The flexible fiberoptic bronchoscope consists of glass fibers that are bound together to provide a flexible unit for the transmission of light and images. The fiberoptic bundle is fragile and excessive bending can damage the fibers. Flexible video bronchoscopes use a camera rather than conventional fiberoptic technology and are less prone to damage. Bronchoscopes have working channels that can be used to administer topical anesthetics and provide suction or oxygen. The visual field can become limited as the fiberoptic bronchoscope nears the glottic opening due to secretions, blood, or fogging of the lens. Immersing the tip of the bronchoscope in warm water helps to prevent fogging.

1. **Standard equipment** for oral or nasal flexible bronchoscopic intubation includes an oral bite block or Ovassapian airway, topical anesthetics and vasoconstrictors, suction, and a sterile bronchoscope with a light source.

2. **Indications**

    a. The flexible bronchoscope can be used in both awake and anesthetized patients to evaluate and intubate their airways. It can be used for both nasal and oral endotracheal intubations and should considered as a first option in an anticipated difficult airway rather than as a "last resort."

    b. Initial flexible bronchoscopic intubation should be considered in patients with known or suspected cervical spine pathology, head and neck tumors, or a history of difficult mask ventilation or intubation.

3. **Technique.** An ETT is placed over a lubricated bronchoscope, suction or oxygen tubing is attached to the working port, and the control lever is grasped with one hand while the scope is advanced or maneuvered with the other hand. The Ovassapian airway may be helpful oral bronchoscopic intubation. It is well tolerated in awake patients, has a channel to guide the ETT midline, and can be removed after the ETT is placed. It is important to keep the bronchoscope in the midline to avoid entering the piriform fossa. The tip of the scope is positioned anteriorly when in the hypopharynx and advanced toward the epiglottis. If mucous or secretions impair the view, the scope should be retracted or removed to clean the tip and then reinserted in the midline. Oxygen attached to the suction port can be used to blow secretions that may obstruct the view away. As the scope slides beneath the epiglottis, the vocal cords are seen. The scope is advanced with the tip in a neutral position until the tracheal rings are noted. The scope is then stabilized within the trachea, and the ETT is advanced over it and into the trachea. If there is resistance to passage, turning the ETT 90° counterclockwise to avoid the anterior commissure will often allow the ETT to pass through the vocal cords. "Flex-tip" ETTs have a tip that curves inward toward the lumen on the distal end that facilitates smoother passage through the vocal cords. The tracheal carina should be visualized prior to withdrawing the bronchoscope to ensure proper positioning of the tube.

D. **Alternative intubation equipment and techniques**

1. **Video laryngoscopy.** There are many specially designed laryngoscopes that incorporate a small video camera to further refine the concept of indirect visualization of the vocal cords on a video screen. These laryngoscopes include reusable systems that must be sterilized between each use and single-use systems, which involve a plastic sleeve that slips over a video wand that is discarded after use. Some systems consist of a laryngoscope and separate screen for viewing, while others consist of a blade with a small screen mounted at the base of the handle. These smaller portable systems may be more appropriate for use in remote locations outside of the operating room. When employed

properly, all of these systems result in vocal cord visualization in nearly 100% of patients. Despite optimal visualization of the vocal cords, ETT advancement can still occasionally be difficult.

- a. **Difficulty with ETT advancement** can occur because the laryngoscope occupies more space in the oropharynx than a conventional blade. One trick is to first advance the laryngoscope to obtain a glottic view and then partially withdraw the laryngoscope to allow the ETT to pass into the oropharynx. Then advance both the laryngoscope and ETT in parallel to visualize the ETT passing through the vocal cords.
- b. In cases where glottic visualization is achieved but there is significant difficulty in manuevering the ETT through the cords, a **gum elastic bougie** (described in the section that follows) may be easier to pass through the vocal cords. The ETT is then passed over the bougie and through the cords under direct visualization with the video laryngoscope.
- c. The different models of video laryngoscopes are all slightly different from each other. Proficiency with one model does not ensure proficiency with them all. Familiarization with the video laryngoscope by using it electively for intubations is recommended.
2. **The gum elastic bougie,** a 60-cm long, 15-French semi-rigid device with a slight J angle at its distal tip, exemplifies one of the various types of hollow and solid introducers that may facilitate passage of the ETT into the trachea when a partial view of the glottis is achieved with direct laryngoscopy. The bougie is advanced under the epiglottis under laryngoscopy and its angled end is directed anteriorly toward the glottic opening. If the bougie is inserted into the trachea, the tracheal rings can often be felt as a characteristic "clicking" sensation. The ETT is then advanced over the bougie and proper placement is confirmed as described above (see Section V.A.2.h). The bougie may also be used as an ETT exchanger.
3. **The light wand** consists of a malleable lighted stylet over which an oral ETT can be passed blindly into the trachea. To insert, the operating room lights are dimmed and the light wand and ETT are advanced following the curve of the tongue. A glow noted in the lateral neck indicates that the tip of the ETT lies in the piriform fossa. If the tip enters the esophagus, there is a marked diminution in the light's brightness. When the tip is correctly positioned in the trachea, a glow is noted in the anterior neck. At this point, the ETT is slid off the stylet and into the trachea.
4. **Retrograde tracheal intubation** can be performed when previously described techniques have been unsuccessful. It is performed in an awake or mildly sedated spontaneously breathing patient. For this technique, the cricothyroid membrane is identified, anesthetized with local anesthetic, and punctured in the midline with an 18-gauge intravenous (IV) catheter. An 80-cm, 0.025-inch guidewire is introduced and directed cephalad. A laryngoscope is used to visualize and retrieve the wire retrograde through the vocal cords. An ETT is then passed over the wire.

VI. THE DIFFICULT AIRWAY AND EMERGENCY AIRWAY TECHNIQUES
- A. **Difficult airway.** The 2013 revision of the American Society of Anesthesiologists (ASA) algorithm for managing difficult airways is shown in **Figure 13.9.** Familiarity with this algorithm is crucial for the anesthesiologist. Since its adoption in 1993, the number of death and brain death

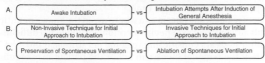

DIFFICULT AIRWAY ALGORITHM

1. Assess the likelihood and clinical impact of basic management problems:
   A. Difficult Ventilation
   B. Difficult Intubation
   C. Difficulty with Patient Cooperation or Consent
   D. Difficult Tracheostomy
2. Actively pursue opportunities to deliver supplemental oxygen throughout the process of difficult airway management
3. Consider the relative merits and feasibility of basic management choices:

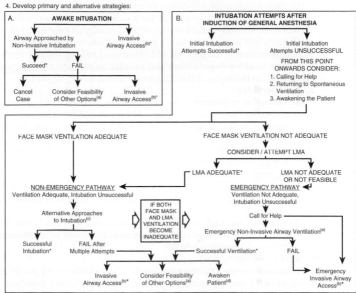

4. Develop primary and alternative strategies:

* Confirm ventilation, tracheal intubation, or LMA placement with exhaled CO_2

a. Other options include (but are not limited to): surgery utilizing face mask or LMA anesthesia, local anesthesia infiltration or regional nerve blockade. Pursuit of these options usually implies that mask ventilation will not be problematic. Therefore, these options may be of limited value if this step in the algorithm has been reached via the Emergency Pathway.

b. Invasive airway access includes surgical or percutaneous tracheostomy or cricothyrotomy.

c. Alternative non-invasive approaches to difficult intubation include (but are not limited to): use of different laryngoscope blades, LMA as an intubation conduit (with or without fiberoptic guidance), fiberoptic intubation, intubating stylet or tube changer, light wand, retrograde intubation, and blind oral or nasal intubation.

d. Consider re-preparation of the patient for awake intubation or canceling surgery.

e. Option for emergency non-invasive airway ventilation include (but are not limited to): rigid bronchoscope, esophageal-tracheal combitube ventilation, or transtracheal jet ventilation.

FIGURE 13.9 American Society of Anesthesiologists (ASA) difficult airway algorithm. (Reprinted with permission from American Society of Anesthesiologists Task Force on Management of the Difficult Airway. Practice guidelines for management of the difficult airway: an updated report by the American Society of Anesthesiologists Task Force on Management of the Difficult Airway. *Anesthesiology.* 2003;98(5):1269-1277. Copyright © 2003 American Society of Anesthesiologists, Inc.)

claims associated with airway-related events during induction of anesthesia has decreased significantly.

1. The difficult airway can be divided into the recognized difficult airway and the unrecognized difficult airway; the latter presents the greater challenge for the anesthesiologist.

2. The ASA defines **a difficult airway** as the situation in which an anesthesiologist experiences difficulty with mask ventilation, difficulty with tracheal intubation, or both. Another definition of a difficult airway is failure to intubate with conventional laryngoscopy after an optimal/best attempt. This optimal/best attempt is defined as an attempt with an experienced laryngoscopist, no significant resistive muscle tone, use of optimal sniffing position, use of external laryngeal manipulation, change of laryngoscope blade type a single time, and change of laryngoscope blade length a single time.

3. The use of **regional anesthesia** as a way to avoid the known or anticipated difficult airway deserves special mention. Although the difficult airway algorithm suggests considering regional anesthesia, it must be kept in mind that the regional block can fail or the patient may require rapid conversion to a general anesthetic for other reasons. Regional anesthesia generally should not be elected for a patient with a known difficult airway if the surgery cannot be terminated rapidly (in case of failed or inadequate block) or access to the patient's airway is compromised.

4. Supraglottic airway devices (eg, LMA) are used to keep the upper airway open to allow oxygenation and ventilation and are a prominent airway option throughout the 2013 ASA difficult airway algorithm:

   a. **Nonemergency**

      1. An airway in patients who can be mask ventilated after general anesthesia is induced but cannot be intubated. It is also an alternative if awake intubation has failed (but only when general anesthesia and mask ventilation are not considered problematic).

      2. A conduit for intubation in patients who can be mask ventilated but cannot be intubated with conventional laryngoscopy.

   b. **Emergency**

      1. An airway in patients who cannot be intubated and cannot be ventilated. The Combitube and transtracheal jet ventilation are other options.

      2. A conduit for intubation in patients who cannot be intubated and cannot be ventilated (when a supraglottic airway is insufficient and intubation is needed).

B. **Emergency airway techniques**

  1. **Percutaneous needle cricothyroidotomy** involves placing a 14-gauge IV catheter or 7.5-French introducer through the cricothyroid membrane into the trachea. Oxygen can be administered by connecting the breathing circuit to a 3-mm ID ETT adapter inserted directly into the IV catheter or to a 7.0-mm ID ETT adapter inserted into a 3-mL syringe barrel and connected to the IV catheter. Dedicated cricothyroidotomy catheters are preferred as the IV catheters have a very high rate of kinking and obstruction. Percutaneous needle cricothyroidotomy is a temporary maneuver until more stable airway access is achieved (tracheostomy or intubation). It is absolutely contraindicated in cases of complete upper airway obstruction because severe barotrauma may result.

   a. **Oxygenation**, but not ventilation, can be achieved by administering oxygen through the catheter at flow rates of 10 to 12 L/min.

   b. **Some ventilation** may be achieved by pressing the oxygen flush valve for 1 second and allowing for passive exhalation over 2 to 3 seconds.

   c. Once in place, the catheter must be carefully and firmly held in position to **avoid dislodgment**, which can be life threatening.

   d. **Complications** include barotrauma, pneumothorax, subcutaneous emphysema of the neck and anterior chest, loss of the airway, aspiration, and death.

2. **Rigid bronchoscopy** by a surgeon or interventional pulmonologist may be necessary to support an airway partially obstructed by a foreign body, traumatic disruption, stenosis, or mediastinal mass. General anesthesia is usually required. A range of bronchoscope sizes (including pediatric sizes) should be available (see Chapter 27).

3. **Cricothyroidotomy** is a rapid effective method for relieving severe upper airway obstruction. The cricothyroid membrane is an elastic tissue located between the inferior border of the thyroid cartilage and the superior border of the cricoid cartilage. With the neck extended, a small incision is made in this membrane in the midline. The handle of a scalpel or a Kelley forceps is used to separate the tissues, and a tube (eg, tracheostomy tube or ETT) is inserted. Alternatively, commercial kits are available, which allow cricothyroidotomy to be performed using Seldinger technique. An introducer needle is used to perforate the cricothyroid membrane and a guidewire is advanced through the needle. Next, a combined tissue dilator-airway catheter is advanced over the wire, the dilator is removed, and the airway catheter is left in the trachea.

4. **Tracheostomy** may be performed under local anesthesia before the induction of general anesthesia for a patient with a particularly difficult airway.
   a. **Technique.** After careful dissection of vessels, nerves, and the thyroid isthmus, a tracheal incision is made, usually between the third and fourth cartilaginous rings. Percutaneous dilational tracheostomy, using commercially available techniques and a modified Seldinger technique, may also be performed.
   b. **Complications** include hemorrhage, false passage, and pneumothorax.

VII. SPECIAL CONSIDERATIONS
A. Rapid sequence induction
1. **Indications.** Patients at risk for aspiration include those who have recently eaten (full stomach), pregnant patients, and those with bowel obstruction, acute abdomen, morbid obesity, or symptomatic reflux.
2. **Technique**
   a. **Equipment** necessary for a rapid sequence induction should include the following:
      1. Functioning tonsil-tip (Yankauer) suction
      2. Several different laryngoscope blades (Macintosh and Miller)
      3. Several ETTs with stylets, including one that is of size smaller than normal
      4. An assistant who can apply cricoid pressure effectively
   b. The patient is **preoxygenated** using high flow rates of 100% oxygen for 3 to 5 minutes (denitrogenation). Four to five vital capacity breaths of 100% oxygen achieve nearly similar results when time is of the essence. The patient can also be placed in a head up, reverse Trendelenburg position during preoxygenation, which may delay the onset of desaturation upon apnea.
   c. The neck is extended so the trachea is directly anterior to the esophagus. The administration of an induction agent (eg, propofol or ketamine) is immediately followed by succinylcholine (1-1.5 mg/kg IV). High-dose nondepolarizing neuromuscular blockers or remifentanil (3-5 µg/kg) can be used as an alternative for muscle relaxation when succinylcholine is contraindicated. An assistant places firm downward digital pressure on the cricoid cartilage, effectively compressing and occluding the esophagus (**Sellick maneuver**). This

maneuver theoretically reduces the risk of passive regurgitation of gastric contents into the pharynx and may bring the vocal cords into better view by displacing them posteriorly. It should not be used if the patient is actively vomiting, because high pressures could injure the esophagus. Of note, significant controversy exists regarding the use of cricoid pressure due to evidence showing that it may decrease lower esophageal sphincter tone and impair glottic view with unclear benefit in actually reducing aspiration. Regardless, cricoid pressure during rapid sequence induction remains the standard of care in anesthetic practice.

d. There should be no attempt to ventilate the patient by mask. Cricoid pressure is maintained until successful endotracheal intubation is verified.

e. Intubation should be performed within 30 seconds. If intubation attempts are unsuccessful, cricoid pressure should be maintained continuously during subsequent intubation maneuvers and while gentle mask ventilation is in progress.

B. Awake intubation

1. Indications. Awake oral or nasal intubation should be considered when there is:

a. A difficult intubation anticipated in a patient at risk for aspiration

b. Uncertainty about the ability to ventilate or intubate after induction of general anesthesia (eg, morbidly obese patients)

c. A need to assess neurologic function after intubation or positioning for surgery

2. Technique

a. To perform an awake intubation, a 4% lidocaine gargle, followed by a lidocaine spray or nebulizer, is used to decrease upper airway sensation.

1. Superior laryngeal nerve block may be used to anesthetize supraglottic structures. A 25-gauge needle is directed anterior to the greater cornu of the hyoid bone and inserted in the thyrohyoid membrane. After negative aspiration, 2 mL of 2% lidocaine is injected on each side.

2. Translaryngeal injection of local anesthetic can anesthetize the glottis and upper trachea. A 25-gauge needle is inserted through the cricothyroid membrane in the midline. After aspiration of air to confirm placement within the tracheal lumen, 2 mL of 2% lidocaine is injected, and the needle is withdrawn. The patient will cough when local anesthetic is injected aiding in anesthetic spread. This block may increase the risk for aspiration in a patient with a full stomach or may be difficult in a patient with a large neck where precise palpation of the cricothyroid membrane is difficult.

3. Glossopharyngeal nerve block may be useful in reducing the gag reflex during awake intubation. The tongue is swept to the opposite side, and a long 25-gauge needle is used to inject 2 mL of 2% lidocaine 0.5 cm deep just lateral to the base of the anterior tonsillar pillar.

b. Awake oral laryngoscopy often allows one to assess the airway. Sedatives such as midazolam, propofol, dexmedetomidine, and fentanyl may be used in addition to the nerve blocks described above.

    c. **Awake (blind) nasal intubation** may be performed after adequate topical anesthesia and regional airway blocks.

      1. Incremental doses of sedatives are useful adjuncts.

      2. A well-lubricated ETT is passed into the nasopharynx with gentle pressure.

      3. Deep resonant breath sounds may be noted as the tube is advanced toward the glottis. An exaggerated sniffing position may be useful. The ETT is usually passed into the trachea during inspiration.

      4. Successful intubation is noted when the patient is unable to phonate, breath sounds and humidification within the ETT are noted with ventilation, and carbon dioxide is noted on the capnograph.

   3. Complications are as described in Section V.A.3.

C. ETT changes. Occasionally, ETT cuff leaks or partial obstruction of the ETT necessitates changing an ETT in a patient with a difficult airway.

   1. The oropharynx is suctioned and the patient is ventilated with 100% oxygen.

   2. A **tracheal tube exchanger** is a specialized stylet that is placed through the ETT and into the trachea. The depth of insertion is carefully measured. While one person holds the tube changer and assures that it does not pass too distally, the second anesthetist slides the original ETT off the changer and passes a new one over the stylet into the trachea. The risks of using this technique are pneumothorax if the tube changer enters a distal airway and failure to pass the ETT through the cords.

   3. A **flexible bronchoscope** can also be used for reintubation. An ETT is placed over the bronchoscope, the tip of which is passed into the trachea alongside the existing tube. The cuff of the existing ETT is deflated, the bronchoscope is advanced, and tracheal rings are noted to confirm position. The existing ETT is removed (a tracheal tube changer may be left in its place), and the new one is advanced as described in Section V.C. The advantages of this technique are direct visualization of the trachea and oxygenation of the patient through the working port of the bronchoscope if there is difficulty passing the ETT through the vocal cords.

   4. An **Aintree intubation catheter** is similar to a tracheal tube exchanger, but it has a large channel that allows it to slide over a flexible bronchoscope. It has a second, smaller channel that allows the anesthetist to deliver oxygen to the patient during the tube change.

Suggested Readings

Adnet F, Baillard C, Borron SW, et al. Randomized study comparing the "sniffing position" with simple head extension for laryngoscopic view in elective surgery patients. *Anesthesiology.* 2001;95:836-841.

Apfelbaum JL, Hagberg CA, Caplan RA; American Society of Anesthesiologists Task Force on Management of the Difficult Airway. Practice guidelines for management of the difficult airway: an updated report by the American Society of Anesthesiologists Task Force on Management of the Difficult Airway. *Anesthesiology.* 2013;118:251-270.

Biro P. Difficult intubation in pregnancy. *Curr Opin Anesthesiol.* 2011;24:249-254.

Detsky ME, Jivraj N, Adhikari NK, et al. Will this patient be difficult to intubate? The rational clinical examination systematic review. *J Am Med Assoc.* 2019;321:493-503.

Hurford WE. Nasotracheal intubation. *Respir Care.* 1999;44:643-649.

Joffe AM, Aziz MF, Posner KL, Duggan LV, Mincer SL, Domino KB. Management of difficult tracheal intubation: a closed claims analysis. *Anesthesiology.* 2019;131(4):818-829.

Kheterpal S, Han R, Tremper KK, et al. Incidence and predictors of difficult and impossible mask ventilation. *Anesthesiology*. 2006;105:885-891.

Kheterpal S, Healy D, Aziz MF, et al. Incidence, predictors, and outcome of difficult mask ventilation combined with difficult laryngoscopy. *Anesthesiology*. 2013;119:1360-1369.

Lewis SR, Butler AR, Parker J, et al. Videolaryngoscopy versus direct laryngoscopy for adult patients requiring tracheal intubation: a Cochrane Systemic Review. *Br J Anaesth*. 2017;119:369-383.

Riad W, Vaez MN, Raveendran R, et al. Neck circumference as a predictor of difficult intubation and difficult mask ventilation in morbidly obese patients: a prospective observational study. *Eur J Anaesthesiol*. 2016;33:244-249.

Samsoon GLT, Young JRB. Difficult tracheal intubation: a retrospective study. *Anaesthesia*. 1987;42:490-497.

Sellick B. Cricoid pressure to control regurgitation of stomach contents during induction of anesthesia. *Lancet*. 1961;2:404-406.

14 | Neuromuscular Blockade

Aditi Balakrishna and Matthew W. Vanneman

The principal pharmacologic effect of **neuromuscular-blocking drugs (NMBDs)** is to interrupt transmission of synaptic signaling at **the neuromuscular junction (NMJ)** by interacting with **the nicotinic acetylcholine receptor (AChR)**.

I. NEUROMUSCULAR JUNCTION

A. The NMJ (**Figure 14.1**) is a chemical synapse located in the peripheral nervous system. The NMJ is composed of **the neuronal presynaptic terminal**, where **acetylcholine (ACh)** is stored in specialized organelles known as **synaptic vesicles**, and the postsynaptic muscle cell **(motor endplate)**.

B. In response to an action potential in the nerve, **voltage-dependent calcium channels** open and cause a rapid influx of calcium into the nerve terminal increasing its intracellular concentrations. This influx of calcium induces fusion of synaptic vesicles with the plasma membrane to release stored ACh. ACh then diffuses across the synaptic cleft where two molecules of ACh bind to a single nicotinic AChR.

C. Postjunctional nicotinic AChRs are glycoproteins composed of five subunits (two α and one each of β, δ, and ε) with the two α-subunits constituting the binding sites for ACh and NMBDs. When two molecules of ACh are bound, the AChR undergoes a conformational change (activation) that allows influx of sodium and calcium into the muscle cell to depolarize the membrane and causes contraction. Once depolarization occurs, repolarization begins with the efflux of potassium and the cessation of sodium and calcium entry. At this point, the AChR becomes inactivated. The amount of ACh released and the number of postsynaptic AChRs is much greater than that actually needed to induce contraction. This is termed the "safety factor" for neuromuscular transmission and plays a crucial role in certain pathologic conditions. After triggering depolarization, ACh diffuses into the synaptic cleft where it is rapidly hydrolyzed (within 15 milliseconds) by **acetylcholinesterase (AChE)** into choline and acetate. Choline is subsequently recycled to synthesize new ACh in the motor nerve terminal.

D. Prejunctional nicotinic AChRs are located on the presynaptic nerve terminal and are responsible for augmenting depolarization of the nerve terminal during high-frequency stimulation, thereby enhancing ACh release. Antagonism of these receptors by nondepolarizing NMBDs is the mechanism by which these agents produce fade on the train of four (TOF).

II. GENERAL PHARMACOLOGY

A. Cholinergic receptors are categorized as **nicotinic** and **muscarinic** by their responses to the alkaloids nicotine and muscarine, respectively. There are two main classes of nicotinic cholinergic receptors: muscular (found at the NMJ) and neuronal (found in autonomic ganglia, at end-organ sites of parasympathetic nerves, and in the central nervous system). Since the cholinergic receptors have different subunit composition, most drugs bind to them with different affinity and have different effects. Only ACh and drugs working by producing ACh (AChE inhibitors) are agonists at all of them.

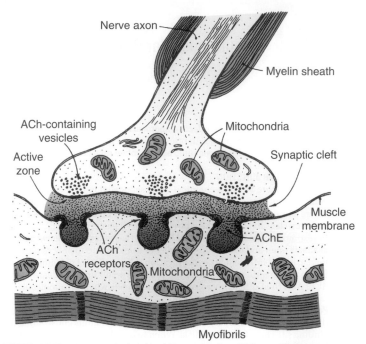

FIGURE 14.1 The neuromuscular junction. ACh, acetylcholine; AChE, acetylcholinesterase.

B. There are well-described signaling systems that regulate the **distribution and density of AChRs** at the NMJ. Pathologic conditions that affect AChR distribution are quite common. For example, denervation, prolonged inactivity, or prolonged mechanical ventilation decreases the density of AChRs at the NMJ, whereas extrajunctional AChRs (often referred to as immature or fetal postjunctional nicotinic AChRs) proliferate over the surface of the muscle membrane. This **"upregulation" of AChRs** increases sensitivity to agonists such as ACh and succinylcholine (SCh), but it decreases the sensitivity to competitive antagonists such as nondepolarizing NMBDs. In contrast, increased sensitivity to antagonists and decreased sensitivity to agonists develop under conditions associated with **downregulation of AChRs.** This can occur when the NMJ is exposed to excess ACh (eg, following chronic use of AChE inhibitors).

C. NMBDs can be classified by the duration of effect: **ultrashort-acting** (<10 minutes; SCh), **short-acting** (<20 minutes; mivacurium [not available in the United States]), **intermediate-acting** (45-60 minutes; atracurium, cisatracurium, rocuronium [0.6 mg/kg dose], and vecuronium), and **long-acting** (>1 hour; pancuronium, rocuronium >0.9 mg/kg dose). Nondepolarizing NMBDs can be further classified by chemical class: **aminosteroid derivatives** (eg, pancuronium, rocuronium, and vecuronium) and **benzylisoquinolines** (eg, atracurium, cisatracurium, and mivacurium). NMBDs differ substantially in their onset, duration of blockade, metabolism, side effects, and interactions with other drugs (**Tables 14.1** and **14.2**).

TABLE 14.1	Comparative Clinical Pharmacology of Neuromuscular-blocking Drugs[a]					
	ED_{95} (mg/kg)[b]	Intubating Dose (mg/kg)[c]	Time to Intubation (minutes)[d]	Time to 25% Recovery (minutes)[e]	Infusion Rate (µg/kg/min)[f]	Elimination
Depolarizing drug						
Succinylcholine	0.25	1-1.5	1	4-6	60-100	Plasma cholinesterase
Nondepolarizing drugs						
Atracurium	0.25	0.4-0.6	2-3	20-35	4-12	Ester hydrolysis, Hofmann elimination
Cisatracurium	0.05	0.15-0.2	2-3	40-60	1-3	Hofmann elimination
Mivacurium	0.08	0.15-0.25	2-3	15-25	3-15	Plasma cholinesterase
Pancuronium	0.06	0.06-0.1	3-4	60-100	—	Kidneys (70%-80%), biliary and hepatic (20%-30%)
Rocuronium	0.3	0.6-1.2	1.5-3	30-150	4-12	Primarily by liver
Vecuronium	0.05	0.08-0.12	2-3	25-40	0.8-2	Biliary and hepatic (70%-90%), kidneys (10%-30%)

[a]There is a large variability in the response to all relaxants, especially at the extremes of age and with profound illness. Therefore, all patients should be carefully monitored as described in the text. Doses shown here are intended for intravenous administration in adult patients.
[b]An ED_{95} dose of a relaxant provides adequate surgical relaxation with nitrous oxide–opioid anesthesia.
[c]These are customary intubating doses and not all equipotent. Neuromuscular blockade is potentiated by volatile anesthetics. For nondepolarizing agents, the intubating dose can be approximately double of the ED_{95}.
[d]These times reflect the use of customary intubating doses and may be substantially altered by the depth of anesthesia. For a rapid sequence induction with nondepolarizing agents, onset time can be shortened by administering a priming dose 3 to 5 minutes before the full dose. Alternatively, a dose of a nondepolarizing agent four times higher than the ED_{95} dose can be used.
[e]Maintenance bolus doses to be given when the train-of-four count reaches 2 to 3 are generally 20% to 25% of the initial bolus dose.
[f]Continuous infusion should be initiated only after early evidence of spontaneous recovery from the initial bolus dose.

III. NEUROMUSCULAR BLOCKADE

A. Depolarizing blockade

SCh, the only depolarizing NMBD, is composed of two ACh molecules linked together via an acetyl moiety. SCh binds to the α-subunits of the nicotinic AChR leading to depolarization of the postjunctional membrane. Because SCh is not degraded by AChE as rapidly as ACh, it persistently depolarizes the motor endplate, leading to inactivation of the voltage-gated sodium

TABLE 14.2	Cardiovascular Side Effects of Neuromuscular-Blocking Drugs			
Drugs	Histamine Release[a]	Ganglionic Effects	Vagolytic Activity	Sympathetic Stimulation
Atracurium	+	0	0	0
Cisatracurium	0	0	0	0
Mivacurium	+	0	0	0
Pancuronium	0	0	++	++
Rocuronium	0	0	+	0
Succinylcholine	±	+	0	0
Vecuronium	0	0	0	0

[a]Histamine release is dose and rate dependent and, therefore, less pronounced if drugs are injected slowly.

channels in the perijunctional zone that are necessary for propagation of the depolarization. Induction doses of SCh produce a rapid onset (about 1 minute) of a transient agonist effect (eg, muscle twitch) followed by skeletal muscle paralysis lasting 4 to 6 minutes. These characteristics make SCh a common choice for facilitating rapid tracheal intubation.

1. SCh's neuromuscular-blocking effect terminates when the drug diffuses away from the AChRs and is rapidly hydrolyzed by **plasma cholinesterase** (produced in the liver and also referred to as pseudocholinesterase) to succinylmonocholine and then, more slowly, to succinic acid and choline. This enzyme is not the same as AChE and is not found in the synaptic cleft. However, inhibitors of AChE affect both enzymes to different degrees.

2. **Side effects of SCh** are related to its agonist effects at both the nicotinic and muscarinic AChRs. These include the following:
   a. **Myalgias,** especially in the muscles of the abdomen, back, and neck. It is attributed to muscle fasciculations and observed more frequently in females and younger patients after minor surgical procedures.
   b. **Cardiac dysrhythmias.** SCh has no direct effect on the myocardium. However, ganglionic stimulation may increase heart rate and blood pressure in adults. Alternatively, SCh may stimulate muscarinic receptors at the sinus node, producing sinus bradycardia, a junctional rhythm, or even asystole, particularly in children and following repeated exposure within a short time interval (eg, 5 minutes) in adults. Pretreatment of children with intravenous (IV) atropine immediately before SCh reduces the occurrence of bradyarrhythmias.
   c. **Elevated serum potassium.** SCh-mediated depolarization may raise serum potassium by 0.5 to 1.0 mEq/L by exaggerating the usual transmembrane ionic flux. However, life-threatening **hyperkalemia and cardiovascular collapse may occur** in patients with major burns, massive tissue injuries, extensive denervation of skeletal muscle, or upper motor neuron diseases. This effect is attributed to a proliferation of extrajunctional AChRs or damaged muscle membranes and a massive release of potassium upon stimulation. In patients with burns, the period of greatest risk is from 2 weeks to 6 months after the burn has been sustained. However, it is recommended to avoid SCh after the first 24 hours and for 2 years from the time of the injury. Patients with mild elevations of potassium related to renal failure may usually safely receive SCh.

d. **Increased intraocular pressure,** by 5 to 10 mm Hg, which transiently occurs 2 to 4 minutes following SCh administration. The mechanism of this rise is not clear. The use of SCh in open eye injuries is still acceptable for rapid sequence inductions (Chapter 26).

e. **Increased intragastric pressure (IGP)** results from fasciculations of abdominal muscles. The risk for aspiration is related to the balance between this pressure and the lower esophageal sphincter (LES) pressure. There have been limited human studies that demonstrate an increase in LES tone that is greater than the increase in IGP. There has not been clinical evidence of an increased aspiration risk with use of SCh for RSI.

f. **Increase in intracranial pressure,** but the magnitude and clinical importance of this are unclear (Chapter 25). There have not been reports of cerebral herniation with use of SCh.

g. **A history of malignant hyperthermia (MH) is an absolute contraindication to the use of SCh.** Some degree of masseter muscle spasm may be a normal response to SCh, but severe jaw rigidity increases the risk that a fulminant MH episode may follow. Generalized muscle rigidity, tachycardia, tachypnea, and profound hyperpyrexia after SCh should alert the clinician to MH (Chapter 19).

h. **Pretreatment with a subparalyzing dose of a nondepolarizing NMBD** (eg, cisatracurium 1 mg IV or rocuronium 3 mg IV) 2 to 4 minutes before SCh may blunt visible fasciculations but is not uniformly effective in attenuating the abovementioned side effects. Moreover, awake patients pretreated with a nondepolarizing NMBD may experience diplopia, weakness, or dyspnea. When pretreating for a rapid sequence induction, the subsequent IV dose of SCh should be increased to 1.5 mg/kg.

3. **Phase I blockade.** Neuromuscular blockade (NMB) produced by SCh can be separated into two phases. Phase I blockade (**Figure 14.2**) is the usual response to SCh as previously described and is characterized by the following:

a. Transient muscle fasciculations followed by relaxation

b. Absence of fade to tetanic or TOF stimulation (Section IV.C)

c. Absence of post-tetanic potentiation (PTP; Section IV.C)

d. AChE inhibitors potentiate rather than reverse the block

4. **Phase II blockade** is most likely to occur after repeated or continuous administration of SCh when the total dose exceeds 3 to 5 mg/kg. Phase II blockade is thought to be secondary to repeated channel opening, causing distortion of the normal electrolyte balance and desensitizing the junctional membrane to further depolarization. It has some of the characteristics of a nondepolarizing blockade:

a. Fade after tetanic or TOF stimulation (Section IV.C)

b. Presence of PTP (Section IV.C)

c. Tachyphylaxis (increasing dose requirement to achieve same depth of NMB)

d. Prolonged recovery

e. Partial or complete reversal by AChE inhibitors

5. **Prolonged blockade** following SCh may be caused by low levels of plasma cholinesterase, a drug-induced inhibition of plasma cholinesterase activity, or a genetically atypical enzyme.

a. **Decreased plasma cholinesterase levels** are found in severe liver or kidney disease, starvation, carcinomas, hypothyroidism, burn patients, decompensated cardiac failure, the last trimester of pregnancy and several days postpartum, and after therapeutic radiation.

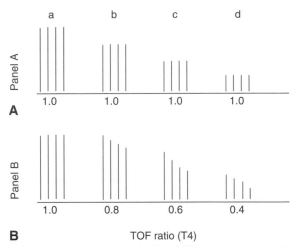

FIGURE 14.2 Schematic representation of train-of-four (TOF) responses to a depolarizing (A) and a nondepolarizing (B) muscle relaxant, showing the control response before the relaxant (a) and afterward (b, c, d). Note no fade with the depolarizing relaxant and progressive fade with the nondepolarizing relaxant.

b. **Inhibition of plasma cholinesterase** occurs with the use of organophosphorus compounds (eg, echothiophate eye drops and insecticides), AChE inhibitors (eg, neostigmine, pyridostigmine, and donepezil), chemotherapeutic agents (eg, cyclophosphamide and nitrogen mustard), oral contraceptives, glucocorticoids, esmolol, and monoamine oxidase inhibitors. Plasma cholinesterase levels are not usually altered by hemodialysis.

c. **Several genetic variants of plasma cholinesterase** exist: normal (N), atypical (A), fluoride resistant (F), and silent (S). **Homozygous atypical cholinesterase** (A–A, prevalence 0.04%) results in prolonged (2-3 hours) skeletal muscle paralysis and respiratory insufficiency following a conventional dose of SCh. Heterozygous atypical cholinesterase (N–A, prevalence 4%) results in only modest prolongation of effect.

d. The **dibucaine number** is a laboratory assay used to characterize plasma cholinesterase abnormality. Normally, the local anesthetic dibucaine inhibits plasma cholinesterase activity by about 80% (dibucaine number of 80), whereas A–A plasma cholinesterase is inhibited by about 20% (dibucaine number of 20). In N–A, dibucaine numbers range from 30 to 65. The comparable **fluoride number** ranges from 0 to 60. N–F individuals (prevalence 0.005%) have slight prolongation of SCh effect, a normal dibucaine number, and a reduced fluoride number. A heterozygous silent N–S individual (prevalence 0.005%) has slightly prolonged effect, but dibucaine and fluoride numbers are normal. Homozygotes F–F and S–S are extremely rare.

e. Patients exhibiting prolonged blocks after a single administration of SCh require sedation and continued intubation until there is a return of twitches. The NMB at this point is similar to that seen with nondepolarizing NMBD. Once fade with TOF is observed, reversal with neostigmine/glycopyrrolate is possible. Blood assays should be performed to determine total cholinesterase and, dibucaine number, and fluoride numbers.

B. **Nondepolarizing blockade** is produced by reversible competitive antagonism of ACh at the α-subunits of the AChRs.

1. It is **characterized** by the following (**Figures 14.2** and **14.3**):
   a. Absence of fasciculations
   b. Fade during tetanic and TOF stimulation (Section IV.C)
   c. Presence of PTP (Section IV.C)
   d. Antagonism of depolarizing blockade
   e. Potentiation by other nondepolarizing NMBDs and volatile anesthetic agents
   f. Reversal by AChE inhibitors

2. **The clinical pharmacology** of the commonly used nondepolarizing NMBDs is outlined in **Table 14.1**. Synergistic blockade may occur when aminosteroid NMBDs are administered together with benzylisoquinolines. When NMBDs with similar chemical class are combined, the effect is additive.

3. **Cisatracurium** is a benzylisoquinoline (see short description of fellow benzylisoquinolines atracurium and mivacurium in **Table 14.1**) of intermediate duration. High molar potency results in a relatively slow onset time (see rocuronium section). The drug is cleared primarily by Hofmann elimination, and its duration of action is largely independent of renal or hepatic function; it is, however, influenced by body temperature and pH given reliance on plasma enzymatic activity. Specifically, hypothermia may prolong duration of action, and hyperthermia may shorten duration of action.

4. **Vecuronium** is a lipophilic, aminosteroid NMBD that is readily absorbed by the liver and excreted into the bile. One of the metabolites, 3-desacetylvecuronium, has neuromuscular-blocking properties (about 50% to 70% of the potency of vecuronium) and is eliminated by the kidneys. Vecuronium has a prolonged clinical effect in elderly patients and those with liver disease and renal failure, as a result of reduced clearance and extended elimination half-life. Vecuronium has

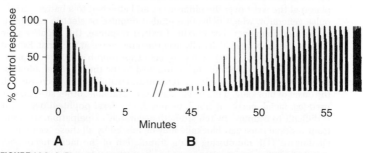

FIGURE 14.3 A, Electromyographic response to repeated train-of-four (TOF) stimulation after injection of a nondepolarizing agent. Each vertical bar is composed of four individual twitch responses. Fade of TOF response eventually leaves only one twitch (approximately 90% blockade). B, Reversal of the blockade by neostigmine and atropine given 45 minutes later shows a progressive recovery of the TOF response and reduction in fade with a TOF ratio of 0.9.

no significant effects on heart rate and blood pressure, but it inhibits histamine *N*-methyltransferase and might potentiate effects such as flushing and hypotension when histamine is released by drugs such as morphine and vancomycin.

5. **Rocuronium** is an analogue of vecuronium that has lower potency. The large intubating dose results in a fast onset time because a larger number of molecules reach the NMJ per circulation time. At a dose of 0.6 mg/kg, maximal blockade can be achieved between 1.8 and 2.7 minutes in adults, per product packaging. Increasing the dose to 1.2 mg/kg (four times the ED_{95}) shortens the time even more but significantly prolongs the duration of action, which can be highly variable among patients. This drug is often chosen when a rapid sequence induction is required but SCh is contraindicated. Clearance of rocuronium occurs as unchanged drug in bile and through renal excretion. Administration of the drug to patients with renal failure may result in a longer duration of action, especially after repeated doses or continuous infusion, though this effect is unpredictable and varied.

6. The **cardiovascular side effects** of nondepolarizing NMBDs are summarized in **Table 14.2**

IV. MONITORING OF NEUROMUSCULAR FUNCTION

A. There are several reasons to monitor neuromuscular function under anesthesia:
1. To facilitate timing of intubation
2. To provide an objective measurement of relaxation during surgery and degree of recovery before extubation
3. To titrate NMBD dosage according to patient response
4. To monitor for the development of phase II block for SCh
5. To permit early recognition of patients with abnormal plasma cholinesterase activity
6. To prevent sequelae of residual postoperative NMB

B. **Peripheral nerve stimulators** use various patterns of stimulation: single twitch, tetanus, TOF, and double-burst stimulation as well as the "posttetanic count." The **adductor pollicis response to ulnar nerve stimulation** at the wrist is most often used because it is easily accessible, and the results are not confused with direct muscle activation. Cutaneous electrodes are placed at the wrist over the ulnar nerve and attached to a battery-driven pulse generator, which delivers a graded impulse of electric current at a specified frequency. For maximal twitch response, the negative pole (active) should be placed distally over the ulnar nerve at the wrist. Evoked muscle tension can be estimated by feeling for thumb adduction or measured by using a force transducer attached to the thumb. After administration of a NMBD, the developed tension and twitch height decrease with the onset of blockade. If the ulnar nerve is unavailable, other sites may be used (eg, facial, posterior tibial, peroneal, or lateral popliteal nerves). It is difficult to estimate twitch strength accurately by palpation, so significant residual muscular blockade may be missed by all these techniques. Qualitative TOF monitoring using stimulation of the facial nerve with monitoring of eye muscle response has been shown to result in a fivefold greater risk of residual NMB compared with similar monitoring at the adductor pollicis.

C. The twitch response to various patterns of stimulation has been correlated with clinical end points, and these data are summarized in **Table 14.3**.

TABLE 14.3	Clinical Assessment of Neuromuscular Blockade
Twitch Response	**Clinical Correlate**
95% suppression of single twitch at 0.15-0.1 Hz	Adequate intubating conditions
90% suppression of single twitch; TOF count of one twitch	Surgical relaxation with nitrous oxide–opioid anesthesia
75% suppression of single twitch; TOF count of three twitches	Adequate relaxation with volatile agents
25% suppression of single twitch	Decreased vital capacity
TOF ratio >0.75; sustained tetanus at 50 Hz for 5 s	Head lift for 5 s; vital capacity of 15-20 mL/kg; inspiratory force of −25 cm H_2O; effective cough
TOF ratio >0.9	Sit up unassisted; normal pharyngeal function
TOF ratio of 1.0	Normal expiratory flow rate, vital capacity, and inspiratory force; diplopia resolves

TOF, train-of-four.

1. **Single twitch** is a supramaximal stimulus, typically lasting 0.2 milliseconds at a frequency of 0.1 Hz (one impulse every 10 seconds). The height of the muscle twitch (its amplitude for a given load and peak tension) is determined as a percent of control. A supramaximal stimulus ensures recruitment of all muscle fibers, while a short duration prevents repetitive nerve firing. The stimulus frequency is important because it affects twitch height and degree of fade. Single twitch is not a sensitive measure of onset or recovery from blockade because 75% of AChRs must be blocked before twitch height begins to decrease, and 75% of the receptors may still be blocked when it returns to control height.

2. **Tetanic stimulus** frequencies vary from 50 to 200 Hz. All NMBDs reduce twitch height, but with nondepolarizing and phase II blockades, a tetanic fade is also demonstrated. This occurs when NMBDs bind to presynaptic receptors and decrease mobilization of ACh during high-frequency stimulation. A tetanic stimulus at 50 Hz for 5 seconds is clinically useful because a sustained tension at this frequency corresponds to that achieved with maximum voluntary effort. However, tetanic stimuli are painful and can speed up recovery in the stimulated muscle, thus misleading the clinician with respect to the degree of recovery in respiratory and upper airway muscles.

3. **Post-tetanic single twitch** is measured by single-twitch stimulation 6 to 10 seconds after a tetanic stimulus. An increase in this twitch is called **PTP**, and it is due to increased mobilization and synthesis of ACh during and after tetanic stimulation. Both nondepolarizing and phase II blockade cause PTP, but depolarizing blockade does not.

4. **The TOF** is four supramaximal stimuli given at a frequency of 2 Hz (**Figure 14.2**). They could be repeated at intervals of at least 10 seconds. Responses at this frequency show fade during the onset and recovery of NMB. During nondepolarizing NMB, elimination of the fourth response

corresponds to 75% depression of a single twitch. Disappearance of the third, second, and first responses correspond to 80%, 90%, and 100% depression of a single twitch, respectively. The ratio of the height of the fourth to the first twitch (**TOF ratio**) correlates with several clinical parameters (**Table 14.3**). However, clinicians often overestimate TOF ratios and are unable to detect fade when the TOF ratio is greater than 0.4. Several commercially available TOF monitors quantify the TOF ratio using accelerometry, which measures the acceleration of muscle contraction in reaction to stimulus. Functional impairment of the muscles of the upper airway may exist up to TOF ratios as high as 0.9, with a significant risk of regurgitation and aspiration. NMBDs may also impair the carotid body hypoxic response, even at a TOF ratio of 0.7. Nevertheless, TOF is a very useful method for clinical monitoring because it does not require a control measurement, it is less painful than tetanic stimulation (may be performed in an awake patient to identify residual block), and it does not affect subsequent recovery. It provides a good measure of blockade required for surgical relaxation and is also useful in assessing recovery from blockade. It is not helpful in quantifying the degree of depolarizing blockade because no fade will be evident. However, TOF monitoring may be used to detect fade, indicating the onset of phase II blockade during continuous or repeated administration of SCh.

5. **Post-tetanic count** is used to quantify *deep* levels of nondepolarizing block. A 50-Hz tetanic stimulus is given for 5 seconds, followed 3 seconds later by repeated single stimuli at 1 Hz. The number of detectable responses predicts the time for spontaneous recovery. A response to post-tetanic twitch stimulation precedes the return of TOF responses.

6. **Double-burst stimulation** uses a burst of two or three tetanic stimuli at 50 Hz followed 750 milliseconds later by a second burst. A decrease in the second response indicates residual curarization. When using tactile evaluation, fade in response to double-burst stimulation is more easily detected than fade in response to TOF stimulation. When quantitative measurements are used, there is no advantage to using double-burst over TOF stimulation.

V. REVERSAL OF NMB

A. **Recovery from SCh-induced depolarizing blockade** usually occurs within 5 to 10 minutes following a 1 mg/kg IV dose. Patients with atypical or inhibited plasma cholinesterase could have a greatly prolonged duration of blockade. Reversal of phase II blockade occurs spontaneously within 10 to 15 minutes in approximately 50% of patients. It is advisable to allow patients with prolonged blockade to recover spontaneously for 20 to 25 minutes and then reversal with an anticholinesterase agent may be attempted if there is no further improvement in twitch strength. Earlier reversal could potentiate the block.

B. **Nondepolarizing blockade** spontaneously recovers when the drugs diffuse from the NMJ. Reversal can be accelerated by administering agents that inhibit AChE, thereby increasing the ACh available to compete for binding sites. Of note, a large multicenter, prospective observational study demonstrated an increased risk of postoperative pulmonary complications (PPCs) with use of any NMBD (compared to no NMBD), regardless of monitoring type or choice of reversal agent.

C. The most commonly used anticholinesterase drug is **neostigmine** (0.03-0.07 mg/kg; maximum dose up to a total of 5 mg). This drug acts by increasing ACh levels, producing nicotinic and muscarinic effects. Bradycardia, bronchoconstriction, salivation, tearing, and miosis can be minimized by administering an antimuscarinic drug; glycopyrrolate (0.02 mg/kg) is used with neostigmine. A meta-analysis of 15 studies suggests there is no evidence of increased postoperative nausea and vomiting (POVN) with use of neostigmine compared with no use of neostigmine. However, a subsequent small randomized controlled trial (RCT) demonstrated a higher risk of PONV with use of neostigmine compared with sugammadex, suggesting a possible effect. However, the potential harm associated with lack of reversal outweighs the risk of side effects.

D. **Encapsulating reversal agents** are novel muscle relaxant binding drugs that form tight water-soluble complexes with NMBDs, thereby reducing the amount of neuromuscular-blocking agent available to bind AChRs at the NMJ. **Sugammadex**, a modified γ-cyclodextrin, is the only such agent approved in the United States. Following IV administration, it binds steroidal NMBDs (rocuronium > vecuronium ≫ pancuronium) in a 1:1 molar ratio. In clinical trials, sugammadex has demonstrated the ability to rapidly reverse rocuronium- or vecuronium-induced NMB. For reversal of moderate NMB (1-2 twitches by TOF), 2 mg/kg is recommended; for reversal of deep blockade (1-2 post-tetanic counts), 4 mg/kg is recommended. If immediate reversal of rocuronium-induced RSI is required, a dose of 16 mg/kg is recommended.

E. In patients with severe renal failure (creatinine clearance <30 mL/min), the excretion of sugammadex or the sugammadex-rocuronium complexes is delayed, but no signs of recurrent NMB are observed. If readministration of rocuronium or vecuronium is required, a waiting time of 24 hours is recommended. Compared with neostigmine, sugammadex reverses blockade more quickly; it also was shown in a Cochrane review to be associated with 40% fewer adverse events than neostigmine, including decreased risks of bradycardia (relative risk [RR] 0.16), residual paralysis (RR 0.40), and PONV (RR 0.52). In addition, a recent blinded RCT of adults older than 70 years demonstrated a 40% reduction in residual neuromuscular block and a 10% reduction in 30-day hospital readmission rate when reversed with sugammadex versus neostigmine. There have, however, been numerous case reports of severe bradycardia as well as severe hypotension with sugammadex. There has also been evidence of bronchospasm and coronary arteriospasm in postmarketing analysis since the drug has been approved, though the incidence of these side effects is unclear. The FDA labeling for the drug describes a 0.3% anaphylaxis rate during a study with healthy volunteers, with reactions ranging from skin findings to shock. The drug may also interfere with hormonal contraceptive medications, so the FDA label states that patients should be advised to use alternative contraception for 7 days after use.

F. **Time to adequate reversal** is related to the degree of spontaneous recovery. Reversal may be more difficult with the use of long-acting NMBDs, large total doses, and high concentrations of inhalation anesthetics. Other factors that may prolong the blockade include hypothermia, antibiotics (particularly aminoglycosides, clindamycin, and tetracyclines), electrolyte disturbances (hypokalemia, hypocalcemia, and hypermagnesemia), and acid-base disturbances (alkalemia prolongs blockade, and acidemia impairs reversal). Reversal with an anticholinesterase agent should not be attempted unless at least one response to TOF stimulation is present. Attempts to reverse a deep or resistant block with excessive doses of neostigmine may increase the degree of residual weakness. If residual weakness is present after attempted reversal, the endotracheal tube should be left in place to provide adequate ventilation and airway protection. Sugammadex can be used to reverse even deep NMB, but larger doses are needed, as above. With sugammadex, drug-drug interactions are limited. Per FDA labeling, toremifene, an estrogen receptor modulator used in breast cancer treatment, has high binding affinity for sugammadex and can limit the availability of the molecule to bind NMB, thus potentiating blockade.

G. **Evidence of neuromuscular recovery**
1. The **TOF ratio corresponding to adequate neuromuscular recovery** is an objective standard for recovery, though the gold standard ratio has been a matter of debate. Historically, TOF ratios between 0.7 and 0.8 were deemed adequate; however, recent studies have demonstrated significant pharyngeal dysfunction associated with PPCs at these TOF ratios. A more stringent criterion, particularly for at-risk patients, would be a TOF ratio of >0.9. A previously described multicenter, prospective observational study did not demonstrate decreased PPCs when a TOF >0.9 cutoff was used. However, a post hoc analysis of the study suggested a significant risk reduction when using a cutoff of 0.95 compared to 0.9.
2. **Clinical signs of adequate neuromuscular recovery** include maintenance of a patient airway without assistance, adequate ventilation and oxygenation, sustained grip strength, the ability to sustain head lift or movement of an extremity without fade, the ability to clench down on an oral airway and prevent its withdrawal, and the absence of discoordinated muscle activity. While these signs have previously been cited as means of assessing recovery, they can correlate to variable objective degrees of reversal as defined by TOF ratio, thus conferring significant risk of residual blockade if used alone.

VI. EFFECTS OF NMB
A. **Surgical conditions** have been rated as superior by surgeons in blinded studies for laparoscopic and open surgery when deep NMB (post-tetanic count less than or equal to 1) was used compared with moderate block (1-2 twitches). Deep neuromuscular block has also been associated with more successful use of low-pressure pneumoperitoneum as well as reduced postoperative pain scores.
B. **EEG monitoring** has been cited as a means of reducing the probability of intraoperative awareness by assessing the depth of anesthesia. However, the commercially available EEG monitors can be influenced by use of NMBs. Facial muscle activity may be necessary for the devices' proprietary algorithms to produce reliable assessments of EEG activity, such that **readings may provide false security** by suggesting an inaccurately deeper level of anesthesia when paralytics are administered.

VII. DISORDERS THAT INFLUENCE THE RESPONSE TO NMBDS
Certain illnesses, both those confined to the NMJ and those affecting more general systems, dramatically affect the response to and safety of NMBDs. In general, transmission at the NMJ is abnormal in these disorders, and there are ultrastructural and biochemical changes in motor nerves, muscle, or both.
A. **Burns and immobilization**
1. **Thermal injury** affects fluid and electrolyte balance, cardiovascular and pulmonary function, drug metabolism, and musculoskeletal structure and function.

2. **Burn patients** and many **immobilized patients** have a greatly exaggerated response to depolarizing agents and a decreased responsiveness to nondepolarizing agents. Burn patients exhibit ultrastructural and biochemical alterations in both muscle cells and neuromuscular contacts. These effects can be seen for more than 1 year after the initial thermal insult. Administration of SCh can cause fatal hyperkalemia. Similar problems have been reported in patients with major crush injuries or large areas of devitalized tissue.

B. **Critical illness**
   1. **Myopathy of critical illness** is a collective group of disorders that can cause weakness in intensive care unit (ICU) patients. The prevalence is high (30%-70%). The underlying pathology is quite heterogeneous, ranging from pure neuropathies and myopathies to mixed neuromuscular transmission disorders. Sepsis and multiorgan system failure are commonly associated with myopathy of critical illness.
   2. **Weakness** is the common manifestation of all these myopathic disorders, and they contribute to ventilator dependence and increased morbidity and mortality. Myopathy may also produce altered deep tendon reflexes, increased creatine kinase levels, and electrophysiologic alterations in nerves, muscles, or both.
   3. **Corticosteroids, NMBDs, and certain antibiotics** can contribute to or precipitate weakness in ICU patients. One subtype of myopathy of critical illness, acute necrotizing myopathy, has been linked to the repeated administration of NMBDs, often in conjunction with high doses of corticosteroids.

C. **Myasthenia gravis (MG)**
   1. MG is an **autoimmune disease** with a prevalence of 14 to 20 per 100,000 population in the United States. It is most common in young adult women.
   2. **The loss of AChRs at motor endplates** in MG is induced by **antireceptor antibodies.** These antibodies are detectable in the serum of 90% of patients with MG, but antibody titers correlate poorly with clinical signs.
   3. MG often presents with the gradual onset of **pharyngeal or ocular weakness.** All muscle groups may be affected. The hallmark of MG is weakness that becomes worse with exercise.
   4. **Treatment** includes anticholinesterases (eg, pyridostigmine), corticosteroids, immunosuppressive drugs (eg, azathioprine and cyclophosphamide), plasmapheresis, and thymectomy. Remission of the disease is common after thymectomy.
   5. Special attention needs to be given to patients with MG receiving either regional anesthesia or general anesthesia.
      a. **Anticholinesterase therapy** should not be discontinued before surgery.
      b. **Neuraxial regional anesthesia** is associated with skeletal muscle relaxation and some degree of diaphragmatic weakness. This normal effect of regional anesthesia often unmasks underlying weakness. These patients, therefore, may suffer from profound respiratory weakness and need careful respiratory monitoring throughout anesthesia and recovery.
      c. These patients are often **resistant to depolarizing agents,** although clearance of SCh is inhibited by pyridostigmine. They are also **extremely sensitive to nondepolarizing agents.** Both longer-acting agents such as pancuronium and shorter-acting agents such as cisatracurium have been associated with prolonged blockade, refractoriness to reversal agents, and profound postoperative weakness.

    d. Monitoring of the degree of NMB is recommended, although complete recovery of the TOF does not ensure recovery of the muscles of the upper airway or adequate spontaneous ventilation.

    e. Surgery and anesthesia may exacerbate the underlying illness. Postoperative ventilatory support may be required even after minor surgical procedures.

D. Muscular dystrophies are a heterogeneous group of inherited muscle disorders characterized by a progressive loss of skeletal muscle function. **Duchene muscular dystrophy** is the most common and the most severe of the disorders. The responsible gene encodes a membrane-associated protein known as dystrophin that is critical for the stability of the muscular membrane. The disorder is X-linked recessive and clinically evident in males. The clinical course is characterized by painless degeneration and atrophy of skeletal muscle, which manifests as weakness by the age of 5 years. By the preteen years, the patient often is confined to a wheelchair, and death usually occurs by the mid-20s secondary to congestive heart failure.

    1. Cardiac (progressive systolic dysfunction and ventricular thinning) and smooth muscles (gastrointestinal hypomotility with delayed gastric emptying) are affected to various degrees. Although the diaphragm is spared, accessory muscle weakness produces a restrictive pattern on pulmonary function testing. Because coughing is impaired, pneumonia is a frequent complication.

    2. SCh can cause massive rhabdomyolysis, hyperkalemia, and death. Because the intensity and duration of drug effect are hard to predict, short-acting NMBDs may be preferable. **Volatile inhalational agents**, particularly halothane, can have exaggerated myocardial depressant effects. **MH** occurs with increased frequency. The delayed gastric emptying and ineffective cough place these patients at greater risk for regurgitation and aspiration. Postoperatively, these patients require aggressive pulmonary physiotherapy to ensure adequate secretion clearance. **Opioids**, which may further depress deep breathing and coughing, should be used cautiously.

E. The myotonic syndromes are a group of disorders characterized by a defect in skeletal muscle relaxation and persistent contraction of skeletal muscles after stimulation. The persistent contraction is a consequence of ineffective calcium removal from the cytoplasm to the sarcoplasmic reticulum. **Myotonic dystrophy** is the most common syndrome in this group of disorders.

    1. Patients with myotonic dystrophy have progressive involvement and deterioration of skeletal, cardiac, and smooth muscles throughout the body, with weakened respiratory effort, a restrictive pattern on pulmonary function testing, and diminished gastrointestinal motility. Other symptoms include cataracts, cardiac conduction abnormalities, baldness, and mental retardation.

    2. Regional anesthesia, neuromuscular-blocking agents, and increasing depth of general anesthesia do not relieve myotonic muscle rigidity. Pregnancy exacerbates this condition, and cesarean section is often indicated because of uterine muscle dysfunction. These patients are exquisitely sensitive to the respiratory depressant effects of opioids, benzodiazepines, and inhalational agents. Neuraxial opiates that have minimal effect on respiratory function in normal persons can have a substantial effect in these patients. Similar to patients with Duchene muscular dystrophy, these patients have frequent cardiac arrhythmias and are at increased risk for cardiac arrest during general anesthesia.

3. SCh should be avoided as it induces prolonged skeletal muscle contraction. **Nondepolarizing agents** can be used; however, the use of short-acting agents and careful titration of reversal agents are recommended.

Suggested Readings

Ali HH, Savarese JJ. Monitoring of neuromuscular function. *Anesthesiology*. 1976;45:216-249.

Berg H, Roed J, Viby-Mogensen J, et al. Residual neuromuscular block is a risk factor for postoperative pulmonary complications: a prospective, randomised, and blinded study of postoperative pulmonary complications after atracurium, vecuronium and pancuronium. *Acta Anaesthesiol Scand*. 1997;41:1095-1103.

Blobner M, Hunter JM, Meistelman C, et al. Use of a train-of-four ratio of 0.95 versus 0.9 for tracheal extubation: an exploratory analysis of POPULAR data. *Br J Anaesth*. 2020;124(1):63-72.

Briggs ED, Kirsch JR. Anesthetic implications of neuromuscular disease. *J Anesth*. 2003;17:177-185.

Bruintjes MH, van Helden EV, Braat AE, et al. Deep neuromuscular block to optimize surgical space conditions during laparoscopic surgery: a systematic review and meta-analysis. *Br J Anaesth*. 2017;118(6):834-842.

Cheng CR, Sessler D, Apfel CC. Does neostigmine administration produce a clinically important increase in postoperative nausea and vomiting? *Anesth Analg*. 2005;101(5):1349-1355.

Eriksson LI. Residual neuromuscular blockade. Incidence and relevance. *Anaesthesist*. 2000;49:S18-S19.

Eriksson LI. The effects of residual neuromuscular blockade and volatile anesthetics on the control of ventilation. *Anesth Analg*. 1999;89:243-251.

Kirmeier E, Eriksson LI, Lewald H, et al. Post-anaesthesia pulmonary complications after use of muscle relaxants (POPULAR): a multicentre, prospective observational study. *Lancet Respir Med*. 2019;7(2):129-140.

Kopman AF, Yee PS, Neuman GG. Relationship of the train-of-four fade ratio to clinical signs and symptoms of residual paralysis in awake volunteers. *Anesthesiology*. 1997;86:765-771.

Lien C. Development and potential clinical impact of ultra-short acting neuromuscular blocking agents. *Br J Anaesth*. 2011;107:i60-i71.

Martyn JA, Richtsfeld M. Succinylcholine-induced hyperkalemia in acquired pathologic states: etiologic factors and molecular mechanisms. *Anesthesiology*. 2006;104:158-169.

Murphy GS, Szokol JW, Marymont JH, et al. Residual paralysis at the time of tracheal extubation. *Anesth Analg*. 2005;100:1840-1845.

Murphy GS, Szokol JW. Monitoring neuromuscular blockade. *Int Anesthesiol Clin*. 2004;42:25-40.

Pandit L, Agrawal A. Neuromuscular disorders in critical illness. *Clin Neurol Neurosurg*. 2006;108:621-627.

Plaud B, Meretoja O, Hofmockel R, et al. Reversal of rocuronium-induced neuromuscular blockade with sugammadex in pediatric and adult surgical patients. *Anesthesiology*. 2009;110:284-294.

Shear TD, Martyn JA. Physiology and biology of neuromuscular transmission in health and disease. *J Crit Care*. 2009;24:5-10.

Thilen SR, Hansen BE, Ramaiah R, et al. Intraoperative neuromuscular monitoring site and residual paralysis. *Anesthesiology*. 2012;117(5):964-972.

15 Monitoring

Christopher M. Aiudi and Kyan C. Safavi

I. STANDARD MONITORING

The American Society of Anesthesiologists Standards for Basic Anesthetic Monitoring state that an anesthetist should be present during all anesthetics (general, regional, monitored anesthesia care [MAC]) and that oxygenation, ventilation, circulation, and temperature should be continually evaluated.

A. Standard monitoring for general anesthesia The minimal requirements for general anesthesia include an oxygen analyzer to confirm the administered FIO_2, pulse oximetry, electrocardiogram (ECG), blood pressure measurement, and the ability to assess temperature. Capnography (Chapters 11 and 13) is mandatory for general anesthesia and recommended for MAC and regional anesthesia.

B. Additional monitoring

The patient's comorbidities and operative procedure may require additional monitors to measure arterial and venous pressures, cardiac function (Chapters 3 and 29), neuromuscular blockade (Chapter 14), and central nervous system activity (Chapters 16 and 23).

II. CARDIOVASCULAR SYSTEM

Circulation may be assessed with clinical signs, ECG, noninvasive and invasive blood pressure monitoring, central venous pressure (CVP), pulmonary artery cannulation, and echocardiography.

A. Clinical signs and symptoms of perfusion abnormalities are often limited during general anesthetics but are important to assess in the preoperative period (Chapter 1) and may include clinical findings such as changes in mental status, neurologic deficits, dyspnea, chest pain, cool limbs, diminished pulses, and poor capillary refill.

B. ECG. The ECG is used to determine the heart rate and to detect and diagnose dysrhythmias, myocardial ischemia, pacemaker function, and electrolyte abnormalities. The presence of an ECG signal does not guarantee cardiac contraction and output.

1. **Mechanism of monitoring**

   a. **Electrode pads.** ECG electrodes measure a small electrical signal (about 1 mV). This makes the ECG prone to electrical interference from outside sources and requires proper electrode application to clean, dry skin.

   b. **Electrode locations.** To effectively detect dysrhythmias and ischemia, the pads must be placed in consistent locations on the body. Limb leads must be placed on or near their appropriate limbs and the precordial lead (V5) at the fifth intercostal space, anterior axillary line.

   c. **Modes and options**

      1. Monitors often have several choices for filtering of noise, commonly called "diagnostic" and "monitor" modes. The monitor mode filters out noise by using a narrowed bandpass (0.5-40 Hz), whereas the diagnostic mode filters less signal and noise by using

a wider bandpass (0.05-100 Hz). The diagnostic mode should be used when monitoring for ischemia.

2. Automatic trending of ST segment changes is useful monitoring for the development of ischemia over time.

2. **Rhythm detection.** The relationship between the P and QRS waves allows for dysrhythmia diagnosis; the P wave is best seen in lead II.

3. **Ischemia detection.** Monitoring leads II and V5 allows for detection of ischemia in 95% of patients since it monitors a large area of the myocardium. Lead II monitors the inferior portion of the heart, supplied by the right coronary artery. Lead V5 monitors the bulk of the left ventricle, supplied by the left anterior descending artery. Lead I may be monitored on patients in whom the left circumflex artery is at risk.

C. **Arterial blood pressure.** Arterial blood pressure is a function of vascular resistance and blood flow. Blood supply to an organ may be low despite adequate blood pressure because of high vascular resistance. Autoregulation in an individual organ may cause local changes in resistance to maintain a constant blood flow.

1. Measuring blood pressure

   a. **Mean arterial pressure** (MAP) may be measured directly or calculated (MAP = diastolic pressure + 1/3 pulse pressure [systolic − diastolic]).

2. **Automated noninvasive blood pressure** is the most common noninvasive method of measuring blood pressure in the operating room. **Manual blood pressure** directly measures the systolic and diastolic blood pressures by auscultation of Korotkoff sounds, palpation, or Doppler.

   a. **Limitations**

      1. An appropriate cuff size is required for correct determinations of blood pressure. A cuff that is too small may result in falsely high blood pressures, whereas a cuff that is too large may result in falsely low blood pressures. The cuff width should cover two-thirds of the upper arm or thigh.

      2. Dysrhythmias and motion artifact may result in erroneous values or may not give any values at all, resulting in a delay in accurate measurements when using an automated cuff.

      3. Venous congestion and ischemia may result from frequent blood pressure measurements during rapid or large blood pressure fluctuations.

      4. Very low or high blood pressures may not correlate with intra-arterial measurements; noninvasive blood pressure measurement often overestimates low blood pressure (ie, systolic blood pressure below 80 mm Hg).

3. **Palpation may be used to estimate systolic blood pressure** based on whether the pulse may be palpated at key points: radial artery (80 mm Hg), femoral artery (60 mm Hg), or carotid artery (50 mm Hg). This method is inaccurate and is only an estimation when the blood pressure is very low.

4. **Invasive blood pressure monitoring** uses an indwelling arterial catheter coupled through fluid-filled tubing to a pressure transducer. The transducer converts pressure into an electrical signal to be displayed.

   a. **Indications**

      1. Need for tight blood pressure control (eg, induced hypertension or hypotension).

      2. Hemodynamically unstable patient.

      3. Frequent arterial blood sampling.

      4. Inability to utilize noninvasive blood pressure measurements as during cardiopulmonary bypass when there is nonpulsatile flow.

b. **Materials** include appropriately sized arterial catheter and transducer apparatus. Generally, the catheter size is 22 to 24 gauge for infants, 20 to 22 gauge for children, and 18 to 20 gauge for adults.

1. The **transducer** is connected to a fluid-filled tubing and a pressurized bag of saline. The pressurized saline enables a continuous infusion at 3 mL/h to prevent clotting. The signal should have a flat frequency response below 20 Hz to monitor all physiologic heart rates.

2. The **tubing** should be rigid and as short as possible, with no kinks or air bubbles.

3. **Setup.** The transducer should be electronically zeroed while open to air and placed at the height of the coronary sinus for most patients (phlebostatic axis). Exceptions include placing the transducer at the level of the head during cerebral aneurysm surgery.

5. **Procedure: Arterial cannulation**

a. **Locations.** The radial artery is the most common site of insertion. Other locations include ulnar, brachial, axillary, femoral, and dorsalis pedis arteries. As distance from the heart increases, systolic blood pressure increases, diastolic pressure decreases, and MAP generally has little variation.

b. **Procedure: Radial artery cannulation**[a]

1. Hyperextend the wrist with an arm board, prep the skin, and use local anesthetic if placing in an awake patient (**Figure 15.1**).

2. Two approaches to insertion:

a. Catheter-over-needle technique: This technique is the same technique used for peripheral venous cannulation. For this procedure a standard intravenous catheter (ie, angiocatheter) is used. Advance the needle until blood flow is observed and then advance the catheter over the needle into the vessel. Remove the needle and attach the transducing tubing.

b. Transarterial: This approach requires the use of a guidewire. As above, the needle is advanced until blood flow is observed. It is then advanced further until it is through the back wall of the artery. The needle is then removed and the catheter is slowly withdrawn until arterial blood is spurting through the catheter in a pulsatile fashion. The guidewire is advanced, and the catheter is inserted into the artery. Alternatively, the short catheter may be removed and a longer one inserted over the wire.

3. Ultrasound guidance is helpful for arterial line placement in patients with poorly palpable arterial pulses.

4. Do not flush the line with more than 3 mL since retrograde flow into the cerebral circulation has been demonstrated.

c. **Considerations for placement**

1. Femoral and axillary artery cannulations are best performed with an 18- or 20-gauge catheter to enter the vessel followed by the insertion of a longer 6-inch catheter of corresponding gauge via the Seldinger technique.

2. The **modified Allen test** may assess the relative contribution of the radial and ulnar arteries to the blood supply to the hand, but the results are variable. Studies have demonstrated the validity of the modified Allen test as a screening test and would suggest that an

[a]Please refer clinical video at https://www.youtube.com/watch?v=7coTBnJt4iA.

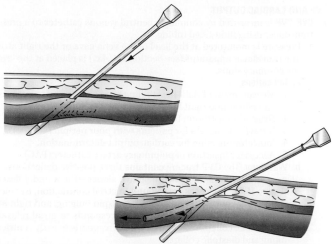

FIGURE 15.1 Radial artery cannulation using the transfixing technique. As shown in the upper drawing, the needle catheter is advanced through the artery. The lower drawing shows the needle withdrawn and the catheter removed until pulsatile flow is obtained. The catheter then is advanced into the artery with a guidewire using the Seldinger technique. (Reprinted with permission from Gerhardt MA, Walosik-Arenall KM. Monitoring the cardiac surgical patient. In: Hensley FA Jr, Gravlee GP, Martin DE, eds. *A Practical Approach to Cardiac Anesthesia*. 5th ed. Wolters Kluwer Health/Lippincott Williams & Wilkins; 2013.117-155.)

    abnormal test result should be followed up with ultrasonographic evaluation prior to arterial manipulation.

  3. Blood pressure and pulse should be assessed in both right and left sides; if disparity exists, the catheter should be placed on the side with the higher pressure since pressure artifacts tend to underestimate the correct blood pressure.

  4. Prior cannulation may result in thrombosis. Proximal pulsation should be assessed before placement. Distal pulsation may simply indicate collateral flow.

d. Complications

  1. An overdamped waveform will cause an artifactually low blood pressure measurement. This may result from arterial obstruction, catheter occlusion, excess tubing, stopcocks, air bubbles, or kinking of the pressure tubing.

  2. An underdamped waveform will result in an artifactually high systolic blood pressure measurement. This may result from use of nonrigid tubing or hyperresonance caused by reverberation of pressure waves.

  3. Rare complications include arterial thrombosis, ischemia, infection, and fistula or aneurysm formation. Pulse oximetry on the same hand as the arterial catheter may help to indicate impending vascular compromise. The catheter should be removed, and the opposite side used if new placement is indicated. The ipsilateral ulnar artery should not be cannulated in the event of radial artery complications.

III. CVP AND CARDIAC OUTPUT

A. CVP. CVP is measured by coupling a central venous catheter to a pressure transducer using fluid-filled tubing.

1. Pressure is monitored at the level of the vena cava or the right atrium. The transducer apparatus (see Section II.C.4.c.) is placed at the level of the coronary sinus.

   a. **Indications**

      1. Measurement of right heart filling pressures to assess intravascular volume and right heart function.
      2. Drug administration to the central circulation.
      3. Intravenous access for patients with poor peripheral access.
      4. Indicator injection for cardiac output determination.
      5. Access for insertion of pulmonary artery catheter (PAC).

   b. **Waveform.** The CVP tracing contains three positive deflections—the **a, c,** and **v** waves—and two negative slopes—the **x** and **y descents** (**Figure 15.2**). The waves correspond to atrial contraction, isovolemic ventricular contraction including tricuspid bulging, and right atrial filling, respectively. The x descent corresponds to atrial relaxation and systolic collapse. The y descent corresponds to early ventricular filling and diastolic collapse.

   c. **Analysis**

      1. **Range.** The CVP is read between the **a** and **c** waves at end expiration, thus minimizing the interaction of respiration. The **normal CVP is 2 to 6 mm Hg.**
      2. **Decreases in CVP.** When a CVP decrease is associated with an increase in blood pressure, without changes to the systemic vascular resistance, the CVP has fallen because of increased cardiac performance. If blood pressure is decreased, decreased CVP is due to decreased intravascular volume or venous return. Of note, however, the use of CVP for the evaluation of fluid responsiveness has been questioned. In general, CVP is a poor indicator of fluid responsiveness. Values of either low (<5 mm Hg) or high (>12 mm Hg) CVP may have some predictive value, but the predictive value is still poor.

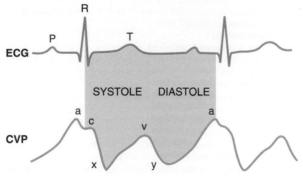

FIGURE 15.2 The normal central venous pressure (CVP) trace and electrocardiogram (ECG). (Reprinted from Mark JB. Central venous pressure monitoring: clinical insights beyond the numbers. *J Cardiothorac Vasc Anesth.* 1991;5(2):163-173. Copyright © 1991 Elsevier. With permission.)

3. **Increases in CVP.** When this increase is associated with increased blood pressure, without changes to the systemic vascular resistance, the cause of increased CVP is an increase in volume or venous return. With an associated decrease in blood pressure, the increased CVP is due to decreased cardiac performance.

d. **Pathology and CVP**

1. **Cannon a waves** are caused by the atrium contracting against a closed tricuspid valve, as during atrioventricular dissociation.

2. **Large v waves** are caused by regurgitant flow during ventricular contraction, as with tricuspid regurgitation.

e. **Positive-pressure ventilation** affects both cardiac output and venous return. According to the Starling rule, the transmural pressure, which is the difference between the atrial pressure and extracardiac pressure, correlates with the cardiac output. At low levels of PEEP, the CVP increases with increased PEEP. At high levels of PEEP (over about 15 cmH_2O), CVP increases as the cardiac output is depressed because of impaired right ventricular output.

2. **Procedure: CVP**

a. **Locations.** Common locations include the following veins: internal jugular (IJ), subclavian, external jugular, axillary, cephalic, and femoral.

b. **Materials** include a saline bag under pressure, fluid-filled tubing, and transducer. The transducer is placed at the level of the coronary sinus.

1. **Multiple lumen catheters** are directly inserted and are available with one to four lumens to provide access for multiple drugs, pressure monitoring, and blood sampling.

2. An **introducer** is a large-bore catheter with a septum valve. A special multiple-lumen catheter or a PAC is then placed through the introducer as described below.

3. **Ultrasound** can be used to identify anatomy, assist catheter insertion, and verify placement. After proper training and orientation, ultrasound assistance line placement has been shown to be superior to landmark technique by improving overall and first attempt success rates, reducing time for line placement and reducing the incidence of complications. Therefore, ultrasound-guided placement is considered the gold standard for most central access sites.

c. Catheter insertion into the right **IJ vein** is preferred because the vessel runs a straighter course to the right atrium (**Figure 15.3**).[b]

1. **Position and preparation.** There are three positions for placement of the CVP catheter into the IJ: anterior, medial, and posterior based on the location of insertion relative to the sternocleidomastoid muscle. The most common is the medial position. The patient is supine or in the Trendelenburg position with the head extended and turned toward the contralateral side of insertion. To reduce catheter-related infections, sterile drapes should cover the patient from head to toe, the proceduralist should wear sterile gown and gloves, and the neck should be prepped with chlorhexidine. Include a sterilely prepared linear array ultrasound probe in the field.

---

[b]Please refer to clinical video at https://www.youtube.com/watch?v=KSgw1V4bchM.

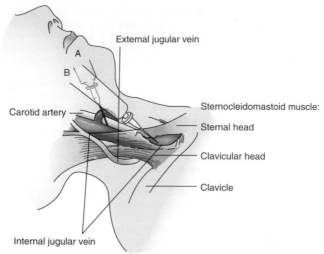

External jugular vein

A

B

Carotid artery

Sternocleidomastoid muscle:

Sternal head

Clavicular head

Clavicle

Internal jugular vein

FIGURE 15.3 Two methods for internal jugular cannulation. A, Anterior approach—insertion at the medial border of the sternocleidomastoid muscle medial head, 5 cm above the clavicle, directed toward the ipsilateral nipple. B, Central approach—insertion at the apex of the triangle formed by the lateral and medial head of the sternocleidomastoid muscle, directed toward the ipsilateral nipple. (Reprinted with permission from Gerhardt MA, Walosik-Arenall KM. Monitoring the cardiac surgical patient. In: Hensley FA Jr, Gravlee GP, Martin DE, eds. *A Practical Approach to Cardiac Anesthesia*. 5th ed. Wolters Kluwer Health/Lippincott Williams & Wilkins; 2013:117-155.)

2. Identify the vessel. Using the ultrasound, first identify the anatomy of the neck using a short-axis (cross-sectional) view of the vessels. Scan the neck with the ultrasound probe in a transverse orientation on the patient's neck. Scan the neck from cephalad to caudal to determine the location where the IJ vein is adequately lateral to the carotid artery (**Figure 15.4**). Confirm the venous versus arterial vessels by applying gentle downward pressure with the ultrasound probe. The IJ vein should collapse, whereas the carotid artery should remain pulsatile. Doppler ultrasound can also be used. Check for vein patency and ensure there are no preexisting anatomical variants or clot burden. There are several views that can be used with the ultrasound for this procedure.

3. Short axis. Using the cross-sectional view seen when scanning the neck, find the desired location on the IJ vein. This axis uses a needle out-of-plane technique. Insert the needle at a 60° angle to the vertical at the midline of the ultrasound probe. Advance the needle as directed below.

4. Long axis. Typically, a short-axis view is first obtained as previously described. Then rotate the probe 90° in a clockwise fashion to obtain the long-axis view. This method uses a needle in-plane technique. Insert the needle at 30° angle to the vertical at the proximal end of the ultrasound probe. Advance the needle as directed below.

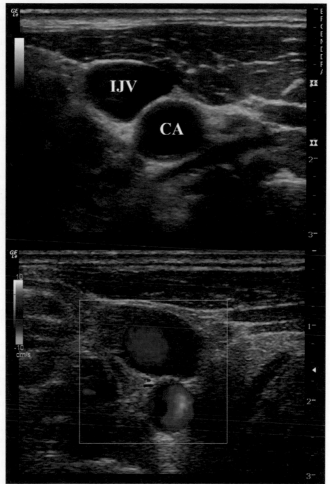

FIGURE 15.4 Ultrasound-guided internal jugular catheterization. The top picture demonstrates the two-dimensional examination showing the internal jugular vein (IJV) lateral to the carotid artery (CA). The bottom picture with the transducer-oriented caudad using color Doppler demonstrates the IJV with blue flow and CA with red flow. (Reprinted with permission from Barash PG, Cullen BF, Stoelting RK, et al. *Clinical Anesthesia*. 6th ed. Wolters Kluwer Health/ Lippincott Williams & Wilkins; 2009.)

5. Oblique axis. This axis is essentially a combination of the short- and long-axis views. First, obtain a short-axis view and then rotate the probe approximately 45° in a clockwise fashion. Both the IJ and carotid arteries should be visualized simultaneously. This axis uses a needle in-plane technique. Insert the needle in a 30° angle to the vertical at the proximal end of the ultrasound probe. Advance the needle as directed below.

6. Placement. Advance the needle at the desired angle (previously described) depending on the axis being used. Aspirate while advancing the needle until venous blood is aspirated. If using a short-axis view, only the tip of the needle will be seen. If using the long or oblique axis, the entirety of the needle shaft will be seen as it advances toward the vessel. Once the vein is located and blood is aspirated, the syringe is removed and a guidewire is passed through the needle or catheter.

7. Confirm intravenous position with ultrasound, echocardiography, fluoroscopy, or manometry. For manometry, a catheter should be placed in the vessel and connected to manometry tubing. The needle or catheter is then removed, and the insertion site is enlarged laterally by advancing the scalpel through the skin along the guidewire.

8. For triple- and quadruple-lumen catheters, a dilator is often not necessary when accessing the IJ vein. With countertraction, a rigid dilator is advanced over the wire with gentle twisting; the guidewire should still be easily mobile, indicating preserved intravascular position.

9. The dilator is removed while maintaining the guidewire, and a central catheter or introducer is inserted over the wire. Alternatively, an introducer and dilator are inserted simultaneously. The wire is removed, the ports are aspirated and flushed, and the catheter is secured to the skin.

10. A chest radiograph is required to confirm the position and exclude complications such as pneumothorax. The tip of the catheter should be at the junction of the superior vena cava (SVC) and right.

11. Landmark placement. Although the landmark technique is not the gold standard, it can still be used. Landmarks include the suprasternal notch, clavicle, lateral border of the sternocleidomastoid (SCM) muscle, and angle of the mandible. For insertion, locate the midpoint between the mastoid process and the sternal attachment of the SCM. Placement can vary based upon the needle insertion site in relation to the patient's neck anatomy (**Figure 15.3**). While aspirating, a finder needle is inserted at a 45° angle to the skin and advanced toward the ipsilateral nipple until venous blood is aspirated. Once the vein is located, the syringe is removed and a guidewire is passed through the needle or catheter.

d. The **SCV** (https://www.youtube.com/watch?v=RDtgzNWmYBw) may be easily accessed as the vessel passes under the clavicle at the midclavicular line. It is one of the most common central venous line locations. Although the artery is not compressible in case of puncture, coagulopathy is not a contraindication to placement. The SCV is often preferred for patient comfort, and the left SCV is often chosen because of the natural course of the brachial cephalic vein into the SVC.

1. **Landmarks** include the clavicle, suprasternal notch, and lateral border of the SCM as it inserts onto the clavicle. The insertion site is medial to the midclavicular line.

2. The thin-walled needle is placed at the insertion site and aimed at the suprasternal notch. It is used to identify the clavicle, and the tip is then "walked" posteriorly under the clavicle. The key to

avoid a pneumothorax is to always keep the needle parallel to the floor during insertion. Total insertion of the catheter should not be greater than 16 to 17 cm, as this may place the tip in the right atrium.

3. The **femoral vein** is one of the most easily accessible central veins and using it does not carry a risk of pneumothorax. Limitations include hip immobility and increased infection rate. As with most central access techniques, ultrasound guidance is preferred. However, this central vein access procedure is often done using landmark techniques in routine and emergency cases. **Landmarks** include the femoral artery, inguinal ligament, anterior superior iliac spine (ASIS), and pubic tubercle. The femoral vein is immediately medial to the femoral artery. A common mnemonic to remember the anatomic relationship of structure within the femoral triangle is "NAVeL" from lateral to medial indicating femoral nerve, artery, vein, and lymphatics. If the artery is not palpable, the vein is reliably located one-third of the distance from the pubic tubercle to the ASIS. In either case, the insertion point is just inferior to the inguinal ligament, 1 to 2 cm medial to the artery.

4. **Ultrasound technique.** Establish the relationship of vessels to each other and while using standard landmark findings to assist in choosing the ideal puncture site. As previously described, a short axis, long axis, or oblique axis can be used.

5. **Placement** uses the Seldinger technique.

e. The **external jugular vein** is cannulated similarly to an IJ vein placement described in Section II.D.2.b. It runs obliquely across the SCM, along a line running from the angle of the mandible to the midpoint of the clavicle. Occlusive pressure at the inferior portion of the vein near the clavicle may ease cannulation. Because the vessel bends to join the SCV, threading of a guidewire may be difficult and should not be forced. For this reason, IJ cannulation may be easier for central catheter placement.

f. **Basilic vein** may be used to access the central circulation with a long catheter. Passing the guidewire into the SCV may be difficult but may be facilitated by abducting the ipsilateral arm and turning the head toward the side of insertion.

3. **Complications**

a. **Dysrhythmias**, caused by the guidewire irritating the endocardium, typically resolve with withdrawal of the wire.

b. **Arterial puncture** can cause significant vessel damage and bleeding if the dilator or catheter is placed into the artery. Before dilation, intravenous position should be verified by ultrasound, echocardiography, manometry, or fluoroscopy. Blood gas measurement may be used as well. If an artery is punctured before dilation, the needle should be removed and pressure applied for at least 5 minutes (10 minutes in the case of coagulopathy) and a new site chosen. If the catheter is placed in the artery, it should remain in place and a vascular surgeon should be consulted.

c. The guidewire should not feel tethered with dilator placement, as this may signify venous damage or puncture of the posterior wall. Do not continue to advance a guidewire if it does not pass easily.

d. **Pneumothorax, hemothorax, hydrothorax, chylothorax, or pericardial tamponade** may become evident with vital sign changes. They are in part ruled out with chest radiography. The risk of pneumothorax is the highest with subclavian vein insertion.

e. Infection may develop at any time during the period that the catheter is in place. The longer the catheter remains in place, the greater the risk of developing an infection. The risk of infection is higher with femoral venous placement. Infections are best prevented through observance of strict sterile technique during catheter placement, antiseptic technique when accessing catheter ports, and expeditious removal of the catheter as as soon as is clinically appropriate.

f. **Air embolism** may occur at any time during catheter insertion or removal. To reduce air entrainment at the neck and subclavian sites, placing the patient in Trendelenburg position is helpful. To reduce the chance of air embolism upon catheter removal, the site is occluded with the patient performing a Valsalva maneuver.

4. **Pulmonary artery catheterization and pulmonary artery occlusion pressures.** The PAC gives information about ventricular function and vascular volume by measuring CVP, pulmonary artery pressure (PAP), pulmonary artery occlusion pressure (PAOP), mixed venous sampling, and cardiac output. Studies have demonstrated no hospital mortality benefit with the use of PACs in the intensive care unit setting and their placement can lead to catheter-related complications. Although PACs provide useful clinical data, they are not recommended for routine critical care.

a. **Mechanism.** The PAC is inserted through a central venous introducer catheter. It passes through the vena cava, right atrium, and right ventricle and into the pulmonary artery. Transducers are connected to separate ports to allow CVP and PAP measurements. Inflating the balloon at the tip of the catheter allows measurement of PAOP, or "wedge" pressure, reflecting the left atrial pressure and left ventricular preload. To minimize the effect of alveolar pressure on PAOP, the tip should rest in West zone III, where the pulmonary venous pressure is greater than the alveolar pressure. Fortunately, the tip usually ends up in this location.

b. **Indications**
   1. Unexplained hypotension.
   2. Access for cardiac pacing.
   3. Surgical procedures with significant physiologic changes (eg, open aortic aneurysm repair and lung or liver transplant).
   4. Acute myocardial infarction with shock.

c. **PAP and PAOP**
   1. **Waveform.** The PAP waveform is similar in shape to the systemic arterial waveform. Because of the location, the waveform is smaller and precedes the systemic waveform. With the balloon inflated, the PAC will measure the PAOP recording, which is similar to the CVP waveform, with **a** and **v** waves. This waveform approximates the left atrial pressures and is slightly delayed because of the interposed lung.
   2. **Range.** The **normal PAP is 15 to 30 mm Hg systolic and 5 to 12 mm Hg diastolic.** The **normal range for PAOP is 5 to 12 mm Hg.** At end expiration, this approximates the left atrial pressure and correlates with the left ventricular end diastolic volume.

d. **PAOP analysis** is used to assess the left-sided heart performance. A basic model of left-sided heart function is given by the relationship between the end-systolic pressure–volume curve and end-diastolic pressure–volume curve. Because the left ventricular end-diastolic pressure (LVEDP), which correlates with the left ventricular end-diastolic volume, is known, the following deductions are possible (**Figure 15.5**).

1. **Increase in PAOP** can be due to an increase in end-diastolic volume, decrease in compliance, or both.
2. **Decrease in PAOP** can be due to a decrease in end-diastolic volume, increase in compliance, or both.

e. **Pathology and PAOP**

1. **Large a waves** may be due to either left ventricular hypertrophy (LVH) or atrioventricular dissociation. LVH will decrease the compliance of the left ventricle and will elevate the LVEDP. Thus, the PAOP should be measured at the peak of the **a** wave. During atrioventricular dissociation, pressure should be measured before the **a** wave.
2. **Large v waves** are the result of mitral regurgitation.
3. **Right-sided heart dilatation** can cause shifting of the interventricular septum into the left ventricle, effectively decreasing the left ventricular end-diastolic compliance. Thus, LVEDP will be elevated.
4. **Pulmonary embolism** may cause an elevation of the PAP without a concomitant elevation of the PAOP.

f. **Materials/catheter types.** Most catheters are available with or without bonded heparin. Types of PACs include the following:

1. **Venous infusion** (VIP, VIP+) catheters provide extra ports for infusion and sampling.
2. **Paceports** allow placement of cardiac pacing wires.
3. **Continuous cardiac output** catheters perform frequent automated determinations of cardiac output by using frequent low-heat pulses to obtain a thermodilution curve; the values are usually an average over time.
4. **Oximetric** catheters monitor mixed venous O_2 saturation.
5. **Right ventricular ejection fraction** catheters use a rapid response thermistor to calculate the right ventricular ejection fraction in addition to cardiac output.

5. **Procedure: pulmonary artery catheter**

a. **Locations and preparation** are similar to those of the central venous catheter described in Section II.D.2. The PAC is invariably placed through an introducer catheter. The operator typically dons a fresh pair of sterile gloves between the introducer and PAC placement.

b. **Technique.** The PAC is prepared and examined as follows:

1. **Sheath placement** is done before balloon examination and placed at 70 cm. The sheath allows movement of the PAC to adjust to the optimum position while maintaining sterility.
2. **Balloon** examination includes inflating the balloon with 1.5 mL of air. The balloon should be symmetrical, inflate and deflate smoothly, and the tip of the PAC should not protrude past the balloon.
3. All ports are flushed to ensure patency and are attached to calibrated pressure transducers. Raising and lowering the PAC distal end should produce changes on the pressure tracing and serve as a quick test of the system before insertion.
4. **Placement** (**Figure 15.6**). The PAC is held so that it follows a natural curve through the heart during passage through the introducer. Once the 20-cm mark is reached, the balloon is inflated

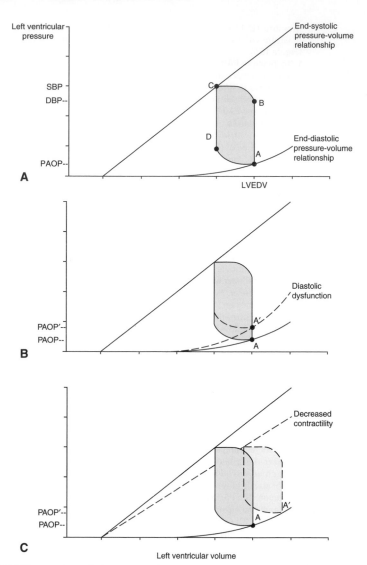

FIGURE 15.5 Left ventricular pressure-volume relationships. A, The cardiac cycle (A-B-C-D-A) is limited by the end-systolic pressure-volume relationship (describing the contractility) and the end-diastolic pressure-volume relationship. The PAOP approximates the LVEDP. An increase in PAOP may be ascribed to decreased diastolic compliance (B), an increase in left ventricular end-diastolic volume (LVEDV) (C), or a combination of both. An increase in LVEDV often results from decreased contractility in the setting of a properly performing right ventricle (C). DBP, diastolic blood pressure; SBP, systolic blood pressure.

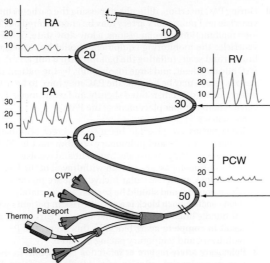

FIGURE 15.6 Pulmonary artery catheter (PAC) and pressure waveforms that will be encountered as it is inserted into the wedged position from the right internal jugular vein. Distances in centimeters on the catheter correspond to insertion distances read at the diaphragm of the introducer and are approximate. CVP, central venous pressure; PCW, pulmonary capillary wedge; RA, right atrium; RV, right ventricle; Thermo, thermistor connection for cardiac output determination. (Reprinted with permission from Gerhardt MA, Walosik-Arenall KM. Monitoring the cardiac surgical patient. In: Hensley FA Jr, Gravlee GP, Martin DE, eds. *A Practical Approach to Cardiac Anesthesia*. 5th ed. Wolters Kluwer Health/Lippincott Williams & Wilkins; 2013:117-155.)

with 1.5 mL of air and the CVP waveform is confirmed. As the catheter is advanced, the waveform will change to a right ventricular waveform and then to a pulmonary artery waveform (with a diastolic pressure step-up and down-sloping diastolic plateau). The PAC is advanced until a PAOP waveform is seen, and the balloon is then deflated. The waveform should return to a pulmonary artery tracing upon deflation. If it does not, then the PAC should be withdrawn about 5 cm with the balloon deflated, the balloon should be reinflated, and the PAC should be advanced until a PAOP tracing is encountered. The balloon should remain deflated normally.

5. **Securing** the sheath to the introducer proximally and at the 70-cm mark distally ensures the ability to manipulate the PAC aseptically. The introducer and PAC are secured to the patient, and an occlusive dressing is applied.

c. **Distances.** From the right IJ vein, each location appears "on the tens." The right atrium is reached at 20 cm, the right ventricle is reached at 30 cm, the pulmonary artery is reached at 40 cm, and the PAOP should be at 50 cm. For subclavian vein placement, subtract 5 cm from these distances; for femoral vein placement, add 20 cm to these distances.

   d. During PAC insertion, difficulty in passing the catheter into the right ventricle and pulmonary artery may be encountered because of balloon malfunction, valvular lesions, a low-flow state, or a dilated right ventricle. The monitoring equipment should be rechecked for calibration and scale. Inflating the balloon with a full 1.5 mL of air, slow PAC advancement, and large inspirations by the patient to augment venous return may be helpful. The PAC may have to be withdrawn to a depth of 20 to 30 cm, rotated slightly, and readvanced. Fluoroscopy can aid in the proper placement of the PAC.

   e. Complications

     1. Dysrhythmias are possible because of direct stimulation of the atrium, ventricle, and pulmonary outflow tract in 50% to 70% of placements. They are usually transient and resolve spontaneously with continued passage or with withdrawal of the PAC. Complete heart block and ventricular tachycardia are possible (up to 0.3% of placements) and should be treated appropriately.

     2. Right bundle branch block is a specific risk in patients with either a left bundle branch block or a first-degree heart block, as this may result in complete heart block. In this event, the PAC should be withdrawn and temporary pacing initiated.

     3. Pulmonary artery rupture or infarction is possible from overinflation or prolonged inflation of the balloon or from direct pressure by the PAC. Thus, the balloon should be slowly inflated, and volume to achieve PAOP should be monitored. Furthermore, the PAP should be monitored by default; if a persistent PAOP appears, the catheter should be pulled back immediately and repositioned.

     4. Pacemakers do not contraindicate PAC placement, although fluoroscopic guidance should be used if the pacemaker is less than 6 weeks old.

     5. Balloon rupture may occur with overinflation with more than the recommended 1.5 mL.

     6. Valve damage, thrombus formation, and infection can occur with PACs. Knotting of the catheter can happen when the catheter will not pass through the pulmonary valve and turns back on itself in the right ventricle.

6. Cardiac output is typically 4 to 8 L/min, whereas the cardiac index (CO/body surface area) is 2.4 to 4.0 L/min/m². CO is conventionally measured with a PAC using thermodilution. The risks of PAC placement have generated interest in alternative CO methods such as pulse contour analysis, whole body dilution techniques, esophageal Doppler, Fick methods, and impedance cardiography.

   a. Thermodilution with a PAC is the gold standard for CO measurement. A known volume of cold saline is injected into the CVP port. The resulting temperature change is monitored by the thermistor located at the PAC tip. The area under the temperature-time curve correlates with cardiac output.

     1. CO should be measured at end expiration. Changes in intrathoracic pressure affect the CO measurement. Negative intrathoracic pressure during the inspiration phase of spontaneous breathing increases venous return and left ventricular transmural pressure. Positive intrathoracic pressure during the inspiration phase of positive-pressure ventilation decreases venous return and left ventricular transmural pressure.

2. **Tricuspid regurgitation** often causes the CO and cardiac index to be underestimated by prolonging the time and increasing the area under the CO curve. Although underestimation is the most common error, values may be overestimated as well.

3. **Errors in CO measurement** may also be caused by injectate spillage, very slow injection, use of the wrong catheter constant, and intra-cardiac shunt.

b. **Pulse contour analysis** determines stroke volume and cardiac output by computer analysis of the arterial pulse pressure waveform. This method assumes that the aortic pulse pressure is proportional to stroke volume. The effects of vascular tone are included in the calculation as a conversion factor calculated from heart rate, MAP, and vessel compliance. The advantage is that central venous access is not needed. Available systems utilize patient demographics and physical characteristics for arterial impedance estimation (FloTrac System, Edwards Lifesciences, Irvine, CA) or injected indicators for calculation (see below). Limitations include:

1. **Nonlinearity of aortic compliance changes.** The compliance of the aorta changes nonlinearly with pressure. This may limit the accuracy of stroke volume estimates.

2. **Resonance and damping** may occur, as with use of any arterial catheter for invasive blood pressure monitoring.

3. **Does not accurately track changes in stroke volume.** Limited ability to clinically assess changes in SV after a volume challenge or the use of vasopressors.

4. Need for predefined optimal conditions for testing. The literature supports increased accuracy with a control mode mechanical ventilation (no spontaneous breaths) on a patient with a closed chest, a fixed respiratory rate, TV ≥ 8 mL/kg, and generally a PEEP ≥ 5.

c. **Whole body dilution techniques** were originally done using indocyanine green dye dilution. Currently available methods combine the use of an indicator dilution CO measurement for calibration and pulse contour analysis; examples include PiCCO and LiDCO.

1. **Transpulmonary thermodilution (PiCCO)** requires a central venous catheter and a specialized femoral arterial catheter with a thermistor. A cold saline bolus is injected through the central venous catheter. The femoral arterial thermistor records the temperature changes downstream. Analysis of the curve yields estimates of cardiac output and blood volume in the heart.

2. **Lithium dilution (LiDCO)** may be used with a radial or brachial artery catheter with a lithium sensor at the tip. A known concentration and volume of lithium chloride solution is injected through a central or peripheral vein. An arterial lithium concentration-time curve is generated. CO is calculated from the area under the curve.

3. **Limitations of dilution techniques.** Intracardiac shunt and aortic insufficiency may cause CO to be underestimated.

d. **Esophageal Doppler** measures descending thoracic aortic blood flow (ABF) with a Doppler beam and sensor positioned at a known angle in the esophagus. This measures ABF, but not CO, directly. Since ABF is roughly 70% of CO, CO may be estimated while avoiding the invasive risks of PAC placement. The probe requires minimal training to place and may be left in place for days. However, it cannot be performed easily on awake patients and does not provide direct information about cardiac filling pressures.

e. **Modified Fick techniques.** NICO (Philips Respironics, Pittsburgh, PA) uses sensors in the breathing circuit attached to an intubated patient to measure flow, airway pressure, and CO_2 concentration. During periods of rebreathing, CO_2 elimination is calculated from these measurements. The Fick principle is applied to calculate cardiac output, which is proportional to the change in CO_2 elimination divided by the change in end-tidal CO_2.

f. **Thoracic bioimpedance** uses skin electrodes placed along the neck and thorax to measure changes in voltage and impedance. Because blood is a stronger conductor than muscle, bone, and skin, changes in thoracic blood volume during the cardiac cycle result in impedance changes. Ohm's law is applied to use the change in impedance to determine CO. This method is completely noninvasive and the electrodes require minimal training to place. A large body habitus and fluid overload may result in inaccurate measurements.

g. **Thoracic bioreactance** (NICOM device, Cheetah Medical, Portland, OR) uses outer electrodes that apply an electric current of known frequency across the thorax and inner electrodes that record the signal after it interacts with the pulsatile blood flow within the thorax resulting in a time delay, or phase shift. The volume of pulsatile blood (stroke volume) that caused the specific time delay can be calculated and continually detected to create the NICOM signal. The continual, dynamic sensing results in less signal distortion than bioimpedance systems. Although further studies are needed, the CO as measured by bioreactance has been shown to be highly correlated with that measured by thermodilution.

7. **Echocardiography** (Chapter 2)

   a. **Mechanism.** Echocardiography is performed with ultrasonic waves to create a two-dimensional image of the heart and surrounding structures. This may be done from a transthoracic or transesophageal approach, depending on the targeted structures, patient compliance, and conditions during placement. It provides independent assessments of the same parameters that a PAC measures, but it also reveals cardiac valve function, ventricular contractility, diastolic function, and intracardiac structures.

   b. **Indications**
      1. **Hypotension** of unknown cause
      2. **Uninterpretable PAC values**
      3. **Suspected intracardiac masses or vegetations**
      4. **Valvular abnormalities**
      5. **Shunts**
      6. **Air embolism**
      7. **Pericardial disease**
      8. **Thoracic aneurysm/dissection**

   c. **Methods**
      1. **Transthoracic echocardiogram** can be performed with the patient awake and provides good visualization of right-sided heart structures and qualitative estimates of contractile performance, although visualization of the left side of the heart is limited and may not be allowed by the surgical location.
      2. **Transesophageal echocardiogram** requires that the patient be topically, locally, or generally anesthetized, but it may be performed intraoperatively and allows superior visualization of the left side of the heart.

IV. RESPIRATORY SYSTEM

The respiratory system is responsible for oxygen uptake and carbon dioxide removal and provides a conduit for delivery of anesthetic agents.

A. **Mandatory respiratory monitors** during general anesthesia include pulse oximetry, capnography, inspired oxygen analyzer, and a disconnect alarm. Direct visualization of the chest and a precordial or esophageal stethoscope may provide additional information. During regional anesthesia, respiration may be monitored with direct visualization, oximetry, and capnography.

B. **Oxygenation** is most easily measured by **pulse oximetry.** Other methods include qualitative assessment of skin color, transcutaneous oximetry, and arterial blood gas sampling.

1. **Method.** Oxygenated and deoxygenated hemoglobin absorb light differently at most wavelengths, including 660 and 960 nm, the wavelengths examined by most devices. The Beer-Lambert law allows the concentration of each species to be calculated from the absorption of light at those wavelengths. The ratio of absorption is processed to give the oxygen saturation of hemoglobin. The sensor has at least two light-emitting diodes (960 and 660 nm) and a light detector. This may be applied to fingers, toes, earlobes, tongue, or, with a special probe, the nose.

2. **Interpretation.** The normal range in a healthy adult is 96% to 99%, whereas values above 88% may be acceptable in patients with lung disease. A high pulse oximeter reading (SpO_2) generally indicates that oxygen is available in the lungs, taken up in the blood, and delivered to distal tissues. A low SpO_2 may be due to a problem along the above pathway or due to an error in monitoring.

3. **Limitations.**
   a. Oximetry may be a late indicator of inadequate gas exchange.
   b. **Carboxyhemoglobin** absorbs light similarly to oxygenated hemoglobin at 660 nm and will provide falsely elevated readings, although it does not contribute to oxygenation.
   c. **Methemoglobin** absorbs light at both 660 and 940 nm, resulting in a saturation of 85%, which does not correlate with the true saturation. Methemoglobinemia may often be treated with methylene blue.
   d. **Methylene blue, indocyanine green, indigo carmine,** and **isosulfan blue** injections transiently result in falsely low saturation readings.
   e. SpO_2 tends to be falsely overestimated at low saturations (below 80%).
   f. Low perfusion, motion, and nail polish (especially blue) may cause SpO_2 measurements to be uninterpretable or unreliable.

C. **Ventilation** is assessed by end-tidal carbon dioxide measurement (ie, capnography) and spirometry. Capnometry and capnography are often used as synonyms, as both analyze and record carbon dioxide, with the latter including a waveform. Capnography not only evaluates respiration but also confirms of endotracheal intubation and is diagnostic of pathologic conditions.

1. **Method.** The measurement of carbon dioxide is often based on infrared light absorption to determine concentration. Carbon dioxide may be measured either at the breathing circuit (mainstream capnograph) or via aspiration of gas samples by the capnograph (sidestream capnograph). Mainstream capnographs often cause traction on the endotracheal tube and can cause burns by radiant heat, whereas sidestream capnographs have a measurement delay based on sample volumes and

may result in significant leaks from sampling. Sidestream capnography may also be used on a nonintubated patient to give a qualitative assessment of respiration.

2. **Waveform.** The normal end-tidal carbon dioxide ($Petco_2$) waveform (**Figure 15.7**) contains the expiratory portion (phases I, II, III, and occasionally IV) and inspiratory portion (phase 0). Two angles, the α angle (between phases II and III) and the β angle (between phases III and 0), also aide in interpretation.

   a. **Phase 0** is the inspiratory segment.
   b. **Phase I** is the carbon dioxide–free gas that is not involved in gas exchange (dead space).
   c. **Phase II** is the rapid upswing and includes both alveolar gas and dead space gas.
   d. **Phase III** is a plateau that involves alveolar gas and has a small positive slope. $Petco_2$ is measured at the end of phase III.
   e. **Phase IV** is a terminal upswing seen in obese and pregnant patients with reduced thoracic compliance.
   f. The α **angle** is between phases II and III and is related to the ventilation: perfusion matching of the lung. The β **angle** is between phases III and 0 and usually is about 90°, and it may be used to assess rebreathing.

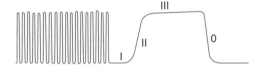

A

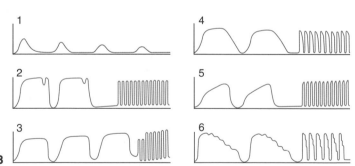

B

FIGURE 15.7 A, Normal capnograph. I, dead space expiration; II, mixed dead space and alveolar gas expiration; III, alveolar gas expiration and plateau; 0, inspiration. Phase IV is an upswing that occurs at the end of phase III. B, Capnographs that may be seen in practice. 1, rapidly extinguishing uncharacteristic waveform, compatible with esophageal intubation; 2, regular dips in end-expiratory plateau, seen in underventilated lungs or in patients recovering from neuromuscular blockade; 3, upward shift in baseline and plateau, seen with rebreathing of carbon dioxide, miscalibration, and so forth; 4, restrictive pulmonary disease; 5, obstructive pulmonary disease; 6, cardiogenic oscillations.

3. **Range and analysis**

   a. Normally, Petco$_2$ is 2 to 5 mm Hg lower than arterial CO$_2$ pressure, so the typical range for end-tidal carbon dioxide during general anesthesia is 30 to 40 mm Hg.

   b. Owing to swallowed gas, **esophageal intubation** may result in carbon dioxide return similar to that of endotracheal intubation, except that Petco$_2$ diminishes to zero with a few breaths.

   c. **An early sign of malignant hyperthermia** is a rapidly rising end-tidal carbon dioxide, especially if it is unresponsive to hyperventilation.

   d. Shock/low perfusion, embolism, auto-PEEP, airway obstruction, and system leaks will result in diminishing end-tidal carbon dioxide.

   e. Carbon dioxide absorption during laparoscopic procedures, reperfusion after releasing an arterial clamp or tourniquet, and absorbent exhaustion or channeling will result in rising end-tidal carbon dioxide.

   f. Widening of the β angle with an elevation of both phases 0/I and III is a sign of **inspiratory valve failure.**

   g. Elevation of both phase 0/I and phase III is a sign of **expiratory valve failure** or **absorbent malfunction.**

4. **Esophageal manometry.** Using an esophageal pressure probe to obtain a surrogate for pleural pressures. Esophageal manometry is used to calculate transpulmonary pressures and to optimize PEEP to reduce the risk of trauma and improve oxygenation for the lungs. Optimizing these pressures allows for the reduction of lung overdistention, prevention of lung atelectasis and atelectrauma, and increase of functional lung volumes. Changes in esophageal pressures reflect changes in pleural pressures. To accurately obtain the esophageal pressure, the esophageal probe should be placed approximately 40 cm or when cardiac oscillations are seen on the pressure tracing.

   When a patient is sedated, paralyzed, and mechanically ventilated, the airway pressures (peak and plateau) are generally used to guide ventilator parameters since these are assumed to closely approximate the pressure in the lung parenchyma. This assumption is reasonable in patients with normal chest wall elasticity and pleural pressure. As chest wall compliance decreases or pleural pressure increases, such as in conditions like ARDS, pleural effusion, ascites, or obesity, the portion of airway pressure that distends lungs decreases, resulting in atelectasis and overdistension in the nonatelectatic lung.

   a. Calculations to consider:

      1. Driving pressure = Plateau pressure − PEEP. This represents the pressure delivered to the respiratory system (includes the chest wall and lung parenchyma).

      2. Transpulmonary pressure = Plateau pressure − Pleural pressure. This represents the pressure to the lung parenchyma. Using esophageal manometry the optimal PEEP may be identified by estimating the transpulmonary pressure. Optimal PEEP can prevent atelectasis and improve oxygenation. In addition, it may prevent barotrauma in patients.

V. TEMPERATURE MONITORING

A. **Mechanism.** Temperature may be measured intermittently or continuously. The limitation of more external methods of temperature determination is that they may not reflect changes in the core body temperature, especially in the presence of vasoconstriction.

B. Indications

1. **Need to control temperature** during induced hypothermia and rewarming (eg, during cardiopulmonary bypass or vascular neurosurgery).
2. **Infants and small children** are prone to thermal lability owing to their high surface area-to-volume ratio.
3. **Adults subjected to large evaporative losses or low ambient temperatures** (as occurs with exposed body cavity, large volume transfusion of unwarmed fluids, or burns) are prone to hypothermia.
4. **Febrile patients** need to be monitored because of the risk of hyper- or hypothermia.
5. Patients with **autonomic dysfunction** are unable to autoregulate their body temperature.
6. **Malignant hyperthermia** is always a possible complication, and temperature monitoring should always be available.

C. Monitoring sites

1. **Skin temperature**, as measured on the forehead, is normally 3 °F to 4 °F below the core temperature, and this gradient may increase with further cooling.
2. **The axilla** is a common site for noninvasive temperature determination and is usually 1 °F below body temperature. The probe needs to be placed at the axillary artery with the arm adducted.
3. **Tympanic membrane temperature** correlates well with the core temperature. Intervening cerumen may enlarge the gradient with respect to core temperature.
4. **Rectal temperature** changes lag behind those of the core body temperature. This phenomenon is often noted during rewarming after hypothermia and indicates the slower peripheral, or "shell," rewarming. The risk of rectal perforation is a rare complication.
5. **Nasopharyngeal temperature**, measured at the posterior nasopharynx, reflects the brain temperature. This measurement is performed by measuring the distance from the external meatus of the ear to the external naris and inserting the temperature probe at that distance. This method may be associated with epistaxis in coagulopathic or pregnant patients or may result in skin necrosis if the probe is allowed to press on the naris during longer procedures. This method is discouraged in patients with head trauma or cerebrospinal fluid rhinorrhea.
6. **Esophageal temperature** monitoring reflects the core temperature well. The probe should be located at the lower third of the esophagus and rarely may be misplaced in the airway.
7. **Blood temperature** measurements may be obtained with the thermistor of a PAC.

Suggested Readings

Akoumianaki E, Maggiore SM, Valenza F, et al. The application of esophageal pressure measurement in patients with respiratory failure. *Am J Respir Crit Care Med.* 2014;189(5):520-531.

Jacobsohn E, Chorn R, O'Connor M. The role of the vasculature in regulating venous return and cardiac output: historical and graphical approach. *Can J Anaesth.* 1997;44:849-867.

Kodali BS. *Capnography: A Comprehensive Educational Website, May 2005.* Harvard Medical School. Accessed September 30, 2005. http://www.capnography.com

Lake CL. *Clinical Monitoring: Practical Applications for Anesthesia & Critical Care.* 1st ed. WB Saunders; 2001.

Marik PE. Noninvasive cardiac output monitors: a state-of the-art review. *J Cardiothorac Vasc Anesth.* 2012;27(1):121-134.

Mark JB. *Atlas of Cardiovascular Monitoring.* Churchill Livingstone; 1998.

Pagel PS, Grossman W, Haering JM, et al. Left ventricular diastolic function in the normal and diseased heart (1). *Anesthesiology*. 1993;79:836-854.

Pagel PS, Grossman W, Haering JM, et al. Left ventricular diastolic function in the normal and diseased heart (2). *Anesthesiology*. 1993;79:1104-1120.

Perret C, Tagan D, Feihl F, et al. *The Pulmonary Artery Catheter in Critical Care*. Blackwell Science; 1996.

Safavi KC, Driscoll W, Wiener-Kronish JP. Remote surveillance technologies: realizing the aim of right patient, right data, right time. *Anesth Analg*. 2019;129(3):726-734.

Sagawa K, Maughan L, Suga H, et al. *Cardiac Contraction and the Pressure-Volume Relationship*. Oxford University Press; 1988.

Monitoring Anesthetic Brain States

Johanna Lee and Oluwaseun Johnson-Akeju

I. GENERAL CONSIDERATIONS

General anesthesia is defined as a drug-induced reversible condition characterized by unconsciousness, amnesia, analgesia, immobility, and maintenance of physiological stability. Monitoring brain and behavioral states under general anesthesia is challenging, and the brain states of patients under general anesthesia are often tracked using physiologic signs and, at times, electroencephalography (EEG)-based markers of unconsciousness.

A. During the maintenance of general anesthesia, anesthesia providers often use changes in the physiologic measures of heart rate, blood pressure, and movement to track anesthetic states and guide the administration of anesthetic and analgesic medications.

B. The changes in heart rate and blood pressure that anesthetized patients show in response to a nociceptive stimulus can be explained in terms of the **nociceptive-medullary-autonomic (NMA) circuit**, which comprises the spinoreticular tract, the brainstem arousal circuits, and the sympathetic and parasympathetic efferent pathways.

   1. The **ascending nociceptive (pain) pathway** begins with A-delta and C-fibers whose free nerve endings bring nociceptive (painful) information from the periphery to the spinal cord.

   2. In the spinal cord, these fibers synapse in the dorsal horn on projection neurons that travel through the anterolateral fasciculus and synapse at multiple sites in the brainstem, including the nucleus of the tractus solitarius in the medulla.

   3. The **autonomic response to a painful stimulus** is initiated within the nucleus of the tractus solitarius, which mediates sympathetic output through the rostral ventral lateral medulla and the caudal ventral lateral medulla to the heart and peripheral blood vessels through projections to the thoracolumbar sympathetic ganglia. The parasympathetic output from the nucleus of the tractus solitarius is mediated through the nucleus ambiguus, which projects through the vagus nerve to the sinoatrial node of the heart.

C. A potentially nociceptive operative stimulus initiates an increase in sympathetic output and a decrease in parasympathetic output through the NMA circuit that rapidly results in an increase in heart rate and blood pressure. As such, these signs can be a rapid indicator of an inadequate level of analgesia.

D. Apart from physiologic signs, intraoperative EEG can be used to track altered levels of consciousness induced by general anesthesia and sedation.

II. ELECTROENCEPHALOGRAM-BASED INDICES OF LEVEL OF CONSCIOUSNESS

A. The EEG changes systematically in relation to the dose of anesthetic drug administered. As a consequence, the unprocessed EEG and various forms of processed EEG have been used to track the level of consciousness of patients receiving general anesthesia and sedation.

B. Basic biophysics of EEG

1. The EEG detects postsynaptic potentials, or local field potentials, in the cerebral cortex. As neurons synapse in a region of the cortex, they produce macroscopic extracellular currents that can be detected as potential differences by surface electrodes.

2. Subcortical structures, like the thalamus, produce smaller field potentials because the strength of the electrical field diminishes with distance from the surface recording electrodes.

3. However, cortical and subcortical structures are highly interconnected, and as a result, the EEG may reflect the dynamics of both cortical and subcortical structures.

4. EEG signals comprise oscillations of varying frequencies and amplitudes (**Figures 16.1** and **16.2**).

C. Several **EEG-based index systems** have been studied and used in clinical practice, including the bispectral index (BIS), patient state index (PSI), Narcotrend, and Entropy. These systems process the EEG and provide an index value or set of values in near real time to track the level of consciousness. In general, the indices are designed to decrease with decreasing levels of consciousness and increase as consciousness returns. The anesthesia provider can use these indices, along with physiologic signs such as changes in heart rate and blood pressure, to track the patient's state of unconsciousness and, to some degree, antinociception.

D. Bispectral index

1. The BIS uses a four-lead frontal EEG montage to record EEG signals for processing and analysis in near real time.

2. The BIS uses a proprietary algorithm that measures specific features of the spectrogram, bispectrum, and level of burst suppression to compute an index between 0 and 100 that indicates the patient's level of consciousness. A value of 100 corresponds to being completely awake, whereas 0 corresponds to a profound state of coma or unconsciousness that is reflected by an isoelectric or flat EEG.

3. **A patient is considered to be appropriately anesthetized when the BIS value is between 40 and 60.**

4. Along with the index value, the BIS monitor also displays the unprocessed EEG, the spectrogram, and the level of electromyographic (EMG) activity. The EMG indicator displays power in the frequency range of 70 to 110 Hz that is believed to be attributable to muscle activity.

5. The BAG-RECALL trial, which focused on patients at high risk for intraoperative awareness, found that patients with BIS-guided general anesthesia experienced a small but statistically significant increase in intraoperative awareness relative to patients receiving general anesthesia guided by an end-tidal anesthetic criterion.

E. Patient State Index

1. The PSI also uses a four-lead frontal EEG montage to record EEG signals for processing and analysis in near real time.

2. Like the BIS, a proprietary algorithm is used to compute an index between 0 and 100, where 0 reflects unconsciousness and 100 reflects complete alertness.

3. **A patient is considered to be unconscious and appropriately anesthetized when the PSI value is between 25 and 50.**

4. Like the BIS, the PSI monitor also shows the unprocessed EEG in real time with its spectrogram from the left and right sides of the head, the level of EMG activity, an artifact index, and a suppression ratio that measures the amount of time the EEG is in burst suppression.

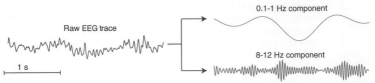

FIGURE 16.1 A typical electroencephalogram trace can be split into a slower oscillatory (0.1-1 Hz component **[top]**) with an overlying higher frequency (8-12 Hz component **[bottom]**).

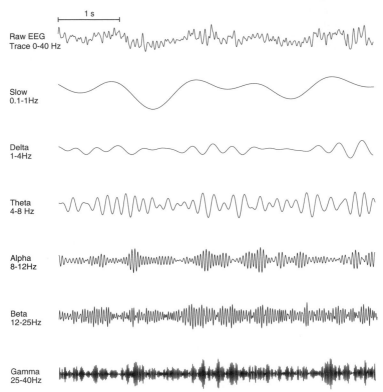

FIGURE 16.2 Anesthetic states and electroencephalogram signatures. Slow (0.1-1 Hz), delta (1-4 Hz), and alpha (8-12 Hz) oscillations are typically seen during unconsciousness at surgical planes. Beta (12-25 Hz) oscillations are frequently associated with an arousable state of sedation. Gamma (25-40 Hz) is associated with an awake pattern with eyes open.

5. Although the PSI correlates with BIS values in monitoring anesthetic states, the PSI monitor has been less frequently studied and has not received the same level of clinical use as the BIS monitor.

F. Narcotrend

1. Like the BIS and PSI, the Narcotrend uses a proprietary algorithm that converts the EEG into different states, reporting both a Narcotrend Stage (A-F) and Narcotrend Index (0-100).

   a. Narcotrend stage A corresponds to patients who are awake, whereas stage F corresponds to general anesthesia with increasing burst suppression. Target stages are D (general anesthesia) or E (general anesthesia with deep hypnosis).

   b. Like the BIS and PSI indices, a Narcotrend Index of 100 correlates with the awake state, whereas an index of 0 correlates with a suppressed EEG.

2. The monitor also displays the unprocessed EEG and its spectrogram.

3. Narcotrend has been less frequently used than either the BIS or PSI.

G. Entropy

1. Entropy is a measure of disorder within a system, and this concept has been more recently applied to EEG analysis to indicate the depth of anesthesia or level of unconsciousness. This measure relies on the observation that the EEG becomes highly structured and ordered under general anesthesia (ie, less disorder, and thus less entropy).

2. The Entropy monitor, which uses a publicly available algorithm, reports two values, the **response entropy (RE)** and **state entropy (SE)**.

   a. RE (range, 0-100) is computed from EEG power in frequencies from 0.8 to 47 Hz.

   b. SE (range, 0-91) is computed from EEG power in frequencies from 0.8 to 32 Hz.

   c. In general, EMG artifact due to facial muscle activity will have a higher frequency and will thus be reflected in the RE. As such, it has been proposed that the relative changes in RE and SE can be used to track brain states under anesthesia and distinguish recovery of consciousness from movement artifacts.

3. **Target RE or SE values for appropriate depth of anesthesia are from 40 to 60.**

H. Limitations of EEG-based indices

Although EEG-based indices have been available for nearly 20 years, there are several reasons why they are not part of standard practice in anesthesiology.

1. The use of EEG-based indices does not ensure that awareness under general anesthesia can be prevented.

2. Indices are considered less reliable in the elderly and pediatric populations.

3. Indices do not relate directly to the neurophysiology of how a specific anesthetic exerts its effects in the brain. Therefore, they cannot give an accurate picture of the brain's responses to the drugs. In particular, the above EEG-based indices tend to be unreliable with the use of ketamine, nitrous oxide, and dexmedetomidine. See Section V for more information.

4. Indices assume that the same index value reflects the same level of unconsciousness for all anesthetics.

III. END-TIDAL ANESTHETIC CONCENTRATION

A. The **median minimal alveolar concentration (MAC)** value (the MAC of inhaled anesthetic required for immobility, or more precisely lack of movement in response to a noxious stimuli, in 50% of patients) remains the gold standard for dosing inhaled anesthetics. However, MAC cannot be used to define or predict brain states in anesthetized patients. Animal experiments have demonstrated that there is no clear association between anesthetic-induced EEG patterns and immobility and that inhaled anesthetics produce immobility primarily by acting in the spinal cord, rather than in the brain.

B. Regardless, the end-tidal anesthetic concentration is widely used as a way to monitor the level of consciousness induced by inhaled anesthetics and guide anesthetic dosing.

   1. This use of MAC has been supported by the B-Unaware and BAG-RECALL trials that reported no difference or small increase, respectively, in the incidence of intraoperative awareness with an anesthetic protocol that maintained the BIS between 40 and 60 compared with a protocol that maintained the end-tidal anesthetic between 0.7 and 1.3 MAC.

C. Unlike the BIS, PSI, Narcotrend, and Entropy, which provide EEG-based measures of brain activity, the end-tidal anesthetic concentration is related very indirectly to brain activity through the concentration of anesthetic expired in the lungs.

D. Two concepts related to MAC are (1) MAC-awake, which is the MAC of inhaled anesthetic required for unconsciousness, which is approximately one-third of MAC; and (2) MAC-BAR (block of adrenergic response), which is the MAC of inhaled anesthetic required for the blunting of autonomic responses to nociception, and is approximately two times the MAC.

   1. The use of opioids can reduce MAC, MAC-awake, and, in particular, MAC-BAR, by decreasing nociception-induced arousal.

E. A key drawback with MAC is that it cannot be used with total intravenous anesthesia.

IV. THE SPECTRAL ANALYSIS OF THE EEG

A. The changes in brain states under sedation and general anesthesia are readily visible in the unprocessed EEG. However, it can be challenging to analyze the changes in frequencies and amplitudes in the unprocessed EEG in real time.

B. The **power spectrum** is a decomposition of a segment of EEG into its power (usually in dB) as a function of frequency. Because the spectrum captures only one instance in time it has limited utility during a dynamic anesthetic state (**Figure 16.3**).

C. Taking the spectrum plots at several adjacent time intervals and stacking them together forms a **spectrogram**. The spectrogram is a plot of power by frequency as a function of time.

D. The 3D spectrogram (also called the compressed spectral array) can be flattened into a 2D plot (also called the density spectral array), which is displayed on monitors in the operating room (**Figure 16.4**). These 2D spectrograms give a visual representation of the EEG structure in a manner that facilitates analysis and tracking of the brain states under anesthesia.

V. EFFECTS OF DIFFERENT ANESTHETICS ON THE BRAIN

A. Propofol

   1. Molecular mechanism

      a. Propofol is an agonist at postsynaptic gamma-aminobutyric acid type A ($GABA_A$) receptors, inducing an inward chloride current that hyperpolarizes postsynaptic neurons and enhances inhibition.

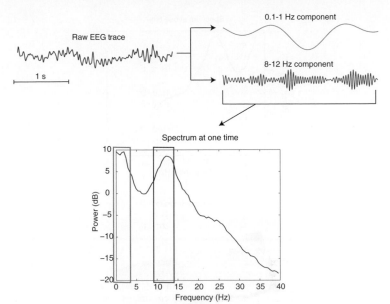

FIGURE 16.3 The plot of power (usually in decibels, dB) against the frequencies being analyzed is the power spectrum.

2. Neural circuit mechanism
   a. Propofol acts on GABA$_A$ receptors at multiple sites, including the cortex, thalamus, brainstem, and spinal cord.
   b. By enhancing GABAergic inhibition in the thalamus and brainstem, which are highly interconnected with the cortex, propofol decreases excitatory inputs and enhances the inhibition of cortical pyramidal neurons.
   c. The potentiation of GABAergic circuits is thought to produce the various features of anesthesia, including loss of consciousness, apnea, and atonia.
3. EEG signatures
   a. EEG signatures are markers of altered arousal states induced by each anesthetic.
   b. **Propofol-induced unconsciousness is characterized by slow-delta (0.1-4 Hz) and frontally coherent alpha (8-12 Hz) oscillations (Figure 16.5).**
   c. Slow-delta oscillations are thought to result from GABA-mediated inactivation of arousal circuits and appear to disrupt cortical integration by isolating local cortical networks and impairing intracortical communication. Specifically, slow-delta oscillations may be associated with neurons across the cortex being activated and inactivated at different times (up-down or on-off states). This fragments brain activity into asynchronous windows and impairs communication, which is also referred to as "cortical fragmentation" (**Figure 16.5**).
   d. Based on modeling studies, alpha oscillations are thought to reflect highly structured rhythms within thalamocortical circuits. During

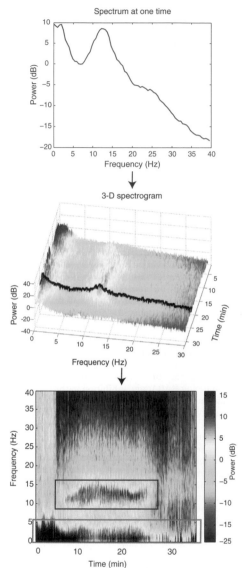

FIGURE 16.4 Construction of the spectrogram: The power spectrum plot at several points in time can be stacked together to form a 3D spectrogram **(middle)**. The spectrogram still retains the frequency and power axes but has the helpful addition of a time axis. The 3D spectrogram flattened into a 2D plot **(bottom)** is what is displayed intraoperatively on brain function monitors. Of note, as indicated on the power scale, red indicates high power and blue indicates low power.

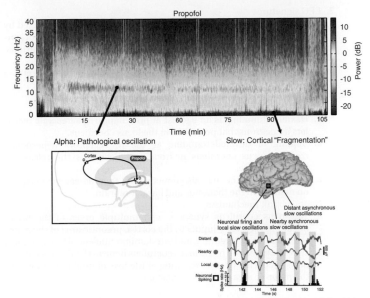

FIGURE 16.5 Spectrogram of propofol showing a pathologic alpha oscillation (8-12 Hz), which corresponds with prevention of communication between the thalamus and cortex, and slow wave (0.1-1 Hz) cortical fragmentation.

propofol-induced unconsciousness, these abnormally coherent or synchronous alpha oscillations are thought to interfere with communication between the thalamus and frontal cortex (**Figure 16.5**).

e. High concentrations of propofol (and several other anesthetics) can lead to **burst suppression**, which is characterized by alternating periods of brief bursts of high-amplitude activity and isoelectricity (suppression). Intraoperative burst suppression is generally avoided for routine cases owing to concerns about potential adverse effects but can be at times targeted for specific indications like status epilepticus, intracranial hypertension, or deep hypothermic circulatory arrest.

B. Ether-derived anesthetics (sevoflurane, isoflurane, desflurane)

1. Molecular mechanism

a. Ether-derived anesthetics bind at multiple targets within the central nervous system, including GABA$_A$ receptors, N-methyl-D-aspartate (NMDA) receptors, potassium channels, and others.

2. Neural circuit mechanism

a. Although the neural circuit mechanisms of ether-derived anesthetics have not been fully characterized, the EEG signature under general anesthesia with inhaled anesthetics is very similar to propofol-induced anesthesia, suggesting that the primary mechanism is GABA$_A$-mediated inhibition of similar thalamocortical and corticocortical dynamics.

3. EEG signatures
   a. Under sevoflurane general anesthesia, the EEG is characterized by prominent **alpha** and **slow-delta** oscillations, similar to propofol general anesthesia, with the addition of **theta** (4-8 Hz) oscillations, particularly at higher concentrations.
   b. The addition of theta oscillations creates a "fill in" effect between the slow and alpha oscillations (**Figure 16.6**).

C. Dexmedetomidine (Precedex)
1. Molecular mechanism
   a. Dexmedetomidine is an agonist at presynaptic α_2 **adrenergic receptors** on neurons that project from the locus coeruleus.
   b. Binding of dexmedetomidine at the α_2 receptors hyperpolarizes the locus coeruleus neurons and decreases the release of norepinephrine.
   c. Dexmedetomidine may also directly bind to α_2 **adrenergic receptors** on neurons in the thalamus and basal forebrain.
2. Neural circuit mechanism
   a. The locus coeruleus synapses with multiple areas of the brain, including excitatory inputs to the cortex, preoptic area of the hypothalamus, basal forebrain, and intralaminar nucleus of the thalamus.
   b. Hyperpolarization of the locus coeruleus neurons leads to decreased norepinephrine release, resulting in the loss of inhibitory inputs to the preoptic area of the hypothalamus.

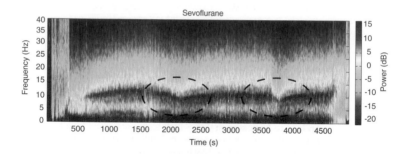

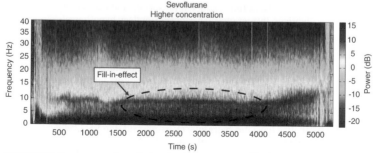

FIGURE 16.6 Spectrogram of sevoflurane showing an alpha (8-12 Hz) and slow wave (0.1-1 Hz) oscillation at low concentration and the "fill in" effect at high concentrations of anesthetic.

c. The loss of inhibitory inputs results in activation of the GABAergic inhibitory pathways from the preoptic area to arousal centers, leading to sedation.

d. This neural circuit mechanism is similar to the mechanism implicated in nonrapid eye movement (NREM) sleep.

3. EEG signatures

a. At **clinically recommended doses used for light sedation**, the EEG is characterized by **spindles** (intermittent bursts of 9- to 15-Hz oscillations) and **slow-delta oscillations** that resemble NREM stage II sleep (**Figure 16.7**).

b. The slow oscillations seen with dexmedetomidine likely result from decreased excitatory inputs to the cortex (owing to the disinhibition of inhibitory circuits, as described above).

c. The spindles observed with dexmedetomidine, like sleep spindles and propofol-induced alpha oscillations, are thought to be generated by thalamocortical mechanisms. Of note, spindles are brief intermittent bursts of EEG activity, in contrast to propofol alpha oscillations, which are continuous.

d. These slow oscillations and spindles are smaller in amplitude than the slow and alpha oscillations observed with propofol general anesthesia, likely reflective of a lower level of circuit inhibition and thus lighter levels of sedation.

D. Ketamine

1. Molecular mechanism

a. Ketamine is an **NMDA** receptor antagonist that binds to receptors within the brain and spinal cord. Ketamine also interacts with opioid, monoaminergic, cholinergic, nicotinic, and muscarinic receptors.

2. Neural circuit mechanism

a. At **low to moderate doses**, ketamine primarily **inhibits** excitatory glutamatergic inputs to inhibitory interneurons, thereby disinhibiting downstream excitatory neurons. This can lead to increased cerebral metabolism, as well as neuroexcitatory effects like hallucinations, dissociative states, and euphoria.

b. At **high doses**, ketamine will also block the NMDA receptors on the excitatory glutamatergic neurons and lead to loss of consciousness.

c. The antinociceptive effect of ketamine is likely due to its actions on NMDA receptors in the dorsal root ganglia and non-NMDA mechanisms (eg, monoaminergic) in supraspinal regions.

3. EEG signatures

a. In patients receiving ketamine, the EEG is characterized by **beta-gamma oscillations**, ranging approximately between 20 and 30 Hz (**Figure 16.8**).

b. For this reason, the numeric EEG-based index value associated with a ketamine anesthetic is often high, despite adequate anesthesia.

E. Nitrous oxide

1. Molecular mechanism

a. The mechanism of nitrous oxide is not completely understood, as it acts on many receptors. However, its anesthetic effects seem to be primarily due to antagonism of **NMDA** receptors.

2. EEG signatures

a. One common practice is to transition from an inhaled anesthetic (eg, sevoflurane, isoflurane) to high-concentration nitrous oxide (>50%) at the end of surgery to facilitate emergence from anesthesia.

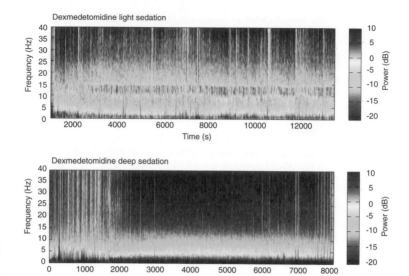

FIGURE 16.7 Spectrogram of dexmedetomidine showing both spindles (9-15 Hz) and slow wave (0.1-1 Hz) oscillations at low doses and a predominance of slow-wave oscillations at high doses.

b. During this transition to nitrous oxide, the EEG is characterized by transient, prominent slow-delta oscillations (lasting 3-12 minutes), followed by high-frequency beta-gamma (20-35 Hz) oscillations that are more commonly associated with nitrous oxide alone (**Figure 16.9**).

c. The beta-gamma oscillations observed under nitrous oxide are thought to be induced by a similar mechanism to ketamine, owing to the shared mechanism of NMDA antagonism.

d. The mechanism underlying the transient slow-delta oscillations is not fully understood.

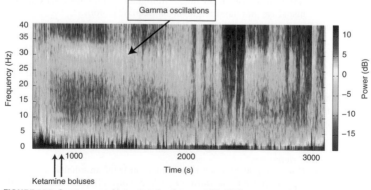

FIGURE 16.8 Spectrogram of ketamine showing a notable 30-Hz gamma oscillation.

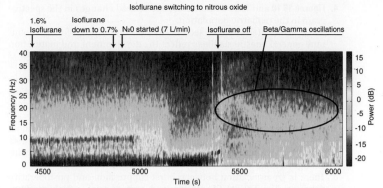

FIGURE 16.9 Spectrogram of nitrous oxide during a transition from isoflurane as the anesthetic to nitrous oxide, as may occur clinically toward the end of surgery to facilitate emergence. The spectrogram of nitrous oxide profound slow-delta oscillations that transition to gamma oscillations.

F. Sevoflurane plus ketamine

1. Patients will often receive a combination of medications under anesthesia, such as an inhaled anesthetic like sevoflurane for unconsciousness and ketamine for analgesia.

2. When ketamine is added to sevoflurane general anesthesia, the alpha and delta oscillations typically observed with sevoflurane are reduced in power, whereas beta oscillations are increased in power. These observed changes may be due to ketamine causing an excitatory effect on neurons with lower intrinsic spiking frequencies to higher-frequency spiking.

3. Of note, the use of ketamine as an adjunct in a patient already receiving an inhaled anesthetic or propofol may lead to burst suppression.

4. Although not all combinations of anesthetics and their adjuncts have been studied at this time, understanding their mechanisms and the neural circuits involved can help provide insight into predicted or observed EEG patterns, as well as possible limitations with certain combinations of medications.

VI. AGE-RELATED CHANGES IN ANESTHETIC-INDUCED EEG SIGNATURES

A. The EEG signatures of patients under general anesthesia vary with age, most notably in children and in the elderly.

B. Children

1. In infants from 0 to approximately 3 months of age, the EEG under propofol- or sevoflurane-induced general anesthesia consists of slow-delta oscillations but not alpha oscillations.

2. In children greater than approximately 3 months of age, the EEG consists of both slow-delta and alpha oscillations. The alpha oscillations become frontally coherent by approximately 1 year of age, reflecting patterns that are more similar to the adult EEG under general anesthesia.

3. The alpha band in children and young adults tends to be broader, encompassing 8 to 15 Hz, compared with a narrower band of 8 to 12 Hz in older adults. Power in the alpha band is also greater in children and young adults.

4. **Figures 16.10** and **16.11** demonstrate age-related changes in the spectrogram in the pediatric population.
5. These age-related changes seen in the EEG under propofol or sevoflurane general anesthesia likely reflect the development and maturation of underlying brain circuits, such as the thalamocortical circuit.

C. Elderly
1. The power and frontal coherence of the alpha oscillations decrease with age. This may reflect neurological changes that occur with aging, including but not limited to cortical thinning, decline in synaptic density, and decline in neurotransmitter synthesis (**Figure 16.12**).
2. The elderly appear to have a higher probability for burst suppression, characterized by alternating periods of isoelectricity and short bursts of high-amplitude activity, under general anesthesia compared with younger adults.
3. There is an association between burst suppression and postoperative delirium. The ENGAGES randomized clinical trial, which randomized patients to EEG-guided anesthetic administration or usual anesthetic care, did not show that the use of the EEG to guide anesthesia decreased the incidence of postoperative delirium. More recent studies suggest that a small portion of the total effect of previously described postoperative delirium risk factors (eg, cognitive status, physical function) is mediated by burst suppression.

D. There can be considerable interindividual differences in the EEG signature under general anesthesia. For example, some individuals may exhibit particular age-related changes, such as diminished alpha oscillations, at younger ages than others. These interindividual EEG differences may reflect underlying comorbidities.

VII. CLINICAL MONITORING OF ANESTHETIC STATES
A. The unprocessed EEG and spectrogram can be used to track brain states in patients under sedation or general anesthesia. EEG education resources have been developed by the following institutions and can be found at the following websites:
1. Massachusetts General Hospital in collaboration with the International Anesthesia Research Society (www.eegforanesthesia.iars.org)
2. International Consortium for EEG Training of Anesthesia Practitioners, Washington University (www.icetap.org)

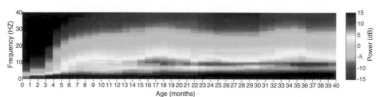

FIGURE 16.10 Age-varying spectral changes in the frontal spectrogram during infancy to childhood, showing the absence of alpha oscillation power from 0 to 3 months of age, with a gradual increase in alpha oscillation power thereafter, becoming more prominent and sustained at approximately 6 months of age. (Reprinted from Cornelissen L, Kim SE, Lee JM, et al. Electroencephalographic markers of brain development during sevoflurane anaesthesia in children up to 3 years old. *Br J Anaesth*. 2018;120(6):1274-1286. Copyright © 2018 Elsevier. With permission.)

Age-varying spectrogram under sevoflurane general anesthesia in children and young adults

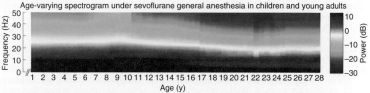

Age (y)

FIGURE 16.11 Age-varying spectral changes in the frontal spectrogram in children and young adults from 1 to 28 years of age, highlighting that, although the EEG structure is qualitatively preserved, the power of the oscillations changes as a function of age. (Reprinted from Akeju O, Pavone KJ, Thum JA, et al. Age-dependency of sevoflurane-induced electroencephalogram dynamics in children. *Br J Anaesth.* 2015;115(suppl 1):i66-i76. Copyright © 2015 Elsevier. With permission.)

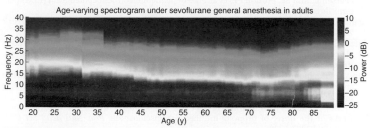

Age (y)

FIGURE 16.12 Age-varying spectral changes in the frontal spectrogram in adults ranging from 18 to 90 years of age, illustrating that alpha oscillation power decreases with age. (Reprinted from Purdon PL, Pavone KJ, Akeju O, et al. The Ageing Brain: age-dependent changes in the electroencephalogram during propofol and sevoflurane general anaesthesia. *Br J Anaesth.* 2015;115(suppl 1):i46-i57. Copyright © 2015 Elsevier. With permission.)

B. A personalized approach to monitoring brain states and guiding anesthetic management in patients may improve anesthetic care. Specifically, using these strategies to target specific brain states under general anesthesia may help avoid potential complications associated with overdosing or underdosing of anesthetic drugs.

VIII. CONCLUSION

A. Although the unprocessed EEG recordings of the anesthetics can be difficult to analyze, the spectrograms make clear that each anesthetic has a distinct EEG signature. These signatures can be related to the mechanisms by which the drugs act at specific receptors in specific neural circuits to alter arousal and can be used to monitor the brain states of patients under anesthesia care.

Suggested Readings

Akeju O, Westover MB, Pavone KJ, et al. Effects of sevoflurane and propofol on frontal electroencephalogram power and coherence. *Anesthesiology.* 2014;121:990-998.

Akeju O, Pavone KJ, Westover MB, et al. A comparison of propofol- and dexmedetomidine-induced electroencephalogram dynamics using spectral and coherence analysis. *Anesthesiology.* 2014;121:978-989.

Akeju O, Pavone KJ, Thum JA, et al. Age-dependency of sevoflurane-induced electroencephalogram dynamics in children. *Br J Anaes*. 2015;115(suppl 1):i66-i76.

Avidan MS, Jacobsohn E, Glick D, et al. Prevention of intraoperative awareness in a high-risk surgical population. *N Engl J Med*. 2011;365:591-600.

Avidan MS, Zhang L, Burnside BA, et al. Anesthesia awareness and the bispectral index. *N Engl J Med*. 2008;358:1097-1108.

Brown EN, Purdon PL, Akeju O, et al. Monitoring the state of the brain and central nervous system during general anesthesia and sedation. In: Gropper MA, Cohen NH, Eriksson LI, Fleisher LA, Leslie K, Wiener-Kronish JP, eds. *Miller's Anesthesia*. 9th ed. Eslsevier, Inc.; 2020:1279-1297.

Brown EN, Lydie R, Schiff ND. General anesthesia, sleep and coma. *N Engl J Med*. 2010;363:2638-2650.

Brown EN, Purdon PL, Van Dort CJ. General anesthesia and altered states of arousal: a systems neuroscience analysis. *Annu Rev Neurosci*. 2011;34:601-628.

Cornelissen L, Kim SE, Lee JM, et al. Electroencephalographic markers of brain development during sevoflurane anaesthesia in children up to 3 years old. *Br J Anaes*. 2018;120(6):1274-1286.

Cornelissen L, Kim SE, Purdon PL, et al. Age-dependent electroencephalogram (EEG) patterns during sevoflurane general anesthesia in infants. *Elife*. 2015;4:e06513.

Egan TE. Are opioids indispensable for general anaesthesia? *Br J Anaesth*. 2019;122(6):e127-e135.

Fritz BA, King CR, Ben Abdallah A, et al. Preoperative cognitive abnormality, intraoperative electroencephalogram suppression, and postoperative delirium: a mediation analysis. *Anesthesiology*. 2020;132(6):1458-1468.

Kim MC, Fricchione GL, Brown EN, et al. Role of electroencephalogram oscillations and the spectrogram in monitoring anaesthesia. *BJA Educ*. 2020;20(5):166-172. doi:10.1016/j.bjae.2020.01.004

Lewis LD, Weiner VS, Mukamel EA, et al. Rapid fragmentation of neuronal networks at the onset of propofol-induced unconsciousness. *Proc Natl Acad Sci USA*. 2012;109:E3377-E3386.

Pedemonte JC, Plummer GS, Chamadia S, et al. Electroencephalogram burst-suppression during cardiopulmonary bypass in elderly patients mediates postoperative delirium. *Anesthesiology*. 2020;133(2):280-292. doi:10.1097/ALN.0000000000003328

Purdon PL, Pierce ET, Mukamel EA, et al. Electroencephalogram signatures of loss and recovery of consciousness from propofol. *Proc Natl Acad Sci USA*. 2013;110:E1142-E1151.

Purdon PL, Sampson A, Pavone KJ, et al. Clinical electroencephalography for anesthesiologists. *Anesthesiology*. 2015;123(4):937-960.

Purdon PL, Pavone KJ, Akeju O, et al. The Ageing Brain: age-dependent changes in the electroencephalogram during propofol and sevoflurane general anaesthesia. *Br J Anaes*. 2015;115(suppl 1):i46-i57.

Wildes TS, Mickle AM, Abdallah B, et al. Effect of electroencephalography-guided anesthetic administration on postoperative delirium among older adults undergoing major surgery: the ENGAGES randomized clinical trial. *J Am Med Assoc*. 2019;321(5):473-483.

17 Intra-anesthetic Problems

Frances K. W. Chen, Ying Hui Low, and
Alexander Nagrebetsky

I. HYPOTENSION

Hypotension is a significant decrease of arterial blood pressure below the patient's usual range. It may be due to a decrease in cardiac function (contractility), systemic vascular resistance (SVR or afterload), venous return (preload), or the presence of dysrhythmias.

A. Contractility

Most anesthetic agents, including **inhalational agents**, **barbiturates**, **benzodiazepines**, and **etomidate** (see Chapter 12) cause dose-dependent direct myocardial depression. **Opiates** are not direct myocardial depressants in usual clinical doses, although clinically significant bradycardia and hypotension may be observed owing to decreased sympathetic outflow. Although **ketamine** can cause a dose-dependent increase in sympathetic nervous system discharge, its direct myocardial depressant effects may be unmasked in patients with depleted endogenous catecholamines, **myocardial depressants** such as β-adrenergic antagonists, calcium channel blockers, and lidocaine.

Acute cardiac dysfunction may occur with myocardial ischemia or myocardial infarction (MI), hypocalcemia, severe acidosis or alkalosis, hypothermia of less than 32 °C, cor pulmonale, vagal reflexes, and systemic toxicity from local anesthetics (particularly bupivacaine).

B. Decreased SVR

1. A decrease in SVR can be seen with many of the drugs administered during anesthesia.
   a. **Isoflurane** and, to a lesser extent, sevoflurane and desflurane produce a dose-dependent decrease in SVR.
   b. **Opiates** and **propofol** produce loss of vascular tone by reducing sympathetic nervous system outflow.
   c. **Benzodiazepines** may decrease SVR, particularly when administered at high doses in conjunction with opiates.
   d. **Direct vasodilators** (eg, nitroprusside, nitroglycerin, and hydralazine).
   e. α_1-**Adrenergic blockers** (eg, droperidol, chlorpromazine, phentolamine, and labetalol, prazosin, doxazosin).
   f. α_2-**Adrenergic agonists** (eg, clonidine and dexmedetomidine).
   g. **Histamine-releasing medications** (eg, d-tubocurarine, mivacurium, and morphine).
   h. **Calcium channel blockers.**
   i. **Angiotensin-converting enzyme inhibitors** and **angiotensin receptor blockers**.
   j. **Inodilators** (eg, milrinone).
2. **Sympathetic blockade** occurs during spinal and epidural anesthesia, particularly with blocks at higher dermatomes, leading to a reduction in SVR and/or preload.
3. **Sepsis** causes release of vasoactive substances that mediate peripheral vasodilation.

4. **Vasoactive metabolites** are released during bowel manipulation, aortic cross-clamp release, or tourniquet release.
5. **Allergic reactions** (see Section XVIII).
6. **Profound hypoxia.**
7. **Adrenal insufficiency** (including iatrogenic causes).

C. **Inadequate venous return (preload).**
1. **Hypovolemia** may be caused by blood loss, insensible evaporative losses, and preoperative deficits (eg, NPO (nothing by mouth) status, vomiting, diarrhea, nasogastric tube suction, enteric drains, and certain bowel preparations), or polyuria (eg, diuretic use, diabetes mellitus, diabetes insipidus, or postobstructive diuresis).
   a. *Positive pressure variation*: In patients undergoing positive-pressure ventilation, changes in cardiac output, and therefore the intra-arterial blood pressure trace, are correlated with volume responsiveness. Hypovolemia can be considered when the delta-down component (the difference between the systolic blood pressure during apnea and the lowest systolic blood pressure after a positive pressure breath) of the systolic pressure variation is greater than 10 mm Hg in a paralyzed and mechanically ventilated patient.
2. **Caval compression** may result from a gravid uterus, massive ascites, tumor, or surgical maneuvers or during laparoscopic insufflation of greater than 10 mm Hg leading to increased intra-abdominal pressure.
3. **Increased venous capacitance** may occur with the following:
   a. Sympathetic blockade (eg, ganglionic blockers or regional anesthesia).
   b. Direct vasodilators (eg, nitroglycerin).
   c. Histamine-releasing medications (eg, morphine, mivacurium).
   d. Medications that reduce sympathetic outflow (eg, propofol, inhalational agents, and opioids).
4. **Increased intrathoracic pressure** will impair venous return. Possible causes include mechanical compression (eg, positioning, surgeon leaning on patient), mechanical ventilation with large tidal volumes, positive end expiratory pressure (PEEP), auto-PEEP (air trapping or dynamic hyperinflation), and continuous positive airway pressure (CPAP).
5. **Acute primary increases in central venous pressure (CVP)** can cause a decrease in venous return as the increased CVP reduces the pressure gradient that drives blood from the periphery into the right side of the heart.
   a. **Tension pneumothorax** leads to compression of the heart and great vessels. The resulting elevation in CVP decreases preload and gives rise to hypotension.
   b. **Cardiac tamponade** is a collection of fluid or clot in the pericardial space causing compression of the heart, resulting in decreased filling due to elevated intrapericardial pressures.
   c. **Pulmonary embolism** obstructs right ventricular ejection and in turn raises right atrial pressure, which can drastically reduce venous return.
   d. **Intra-abdominal hypertension** causes increased intrathoracic pressure, which then compresses the heart and raises the CVP. Thus the CVP can be elevated while the heart is severely underfilled.

D. **Dysrhythmias (also see Section III)**
1. **Tachydysrhythmias** often result in hypotension secondary to a decreased diastolic filling time.
2. **Atrial fibrillation, atrial flutter, and junctional rhythms** cause hypotension from loss of the atrial contribution to diastolic filling. This is particularly pronounced in patients with valvular heart disease or diastolic

dysfunction, in whom atrial contraction may augment end-diastolic volume by more than 30%.

3. **Bradydysrhythmias** may cause hypotension if preload reserve is inadequate to maintain a compensatory increase in stroke volume.

E. **Treatment of hypotension** should be directed toward correcting the underlying cause. Depending on the etiology, appropriate maneuvers include:

1. **Decreasing anesthetic depth.**

2. **Volume expansion** (eg, administration of blood products, colloids, or crystalloids).

3. **Vasopressor support** to increase vascular resistance or decrease venous capacitance (eg, phenylephrine and vasopressin if acidemic) and increase stroke volume (eg, epinephrine).

4. **Correction of mechanical causes**, such as relief of pericardial tamponade, placement of a needle thoracostomy and chest tube for pneumothorax, reducing or eliminating PEEP or CPAP, decreasing mean airway pressure, relieving obstruction of the vena cava (eg, left uterine displacement for a pregnant patient), surgically relieving intra-abdominal hypertension, or surgically removing a massive pulmonary embolism (PE).

5. **Antidysrhythmic (see Section III)** may include β-blockers, calcium channel blockers, and amiodarone.

6. **Inotropic support** (eg, dobutamine, dopamine, norepinephrine, milrinone, and epinephrine).

7. **Anti-ischemic therapy** may include raising the systemic blood pressure with vasopressors and then treating the underlying ischemic myocardium (see Section XIV).

8. **In the case of refractory hypotension**, consider the use of additional noninvasive monitors (eg, transthoracic echocardiography (TTE)) and the placement of invasive monitors (eg, arterial line, central venous catheter, pulmonary artery catheter, transesophageal echocardiography (TEE)) to facilitate the identification of decreased cardiac output or SVR.

II. HYPERTENSION

A. **Etiologies:**

1. **Catecholamine excess** may be seen with inadequate anesthesia, especially with increased sympathetic stimulation during laryngoscopy, intubation, incision, emergence, patient anxiety, and pain or with hypoxia, hypercarbia, and prolonged tourniquet use.

2. **Preexisting disease** such as essential hypertension, secondary causes of hypertension such as pheochromocytoma, sleep apnea, or other endocrine, renal, or renovascular disorders.

3. **Increased intracranial pressure (ICP).** When ICP rises, blood pressure increases to maintain cerebral perfusion pressure.

4. **Systemic absorption of vasoconstrictors** (eg, injection of local anesthetic with epinephrine).

5. **Aortic cross-clamping,** which leads to a significant increase in SVR.

6. **Rebound hypertension** from discontinuation of clonidine or β-adrenergic blockers.

7. **Drug interactions.** The administration of ephedrine to patients receiving **tricyclic antidepressants** (eg, amitriptyline, nortriptyline, doxepin) and **monoamine oxidase inhibitors** (eg, isoniazid, rasagiline, selegiline) may cause an exaggerated hypertensive response.

8. **Bladder distension.** Sympathetic response with bladder distension leads to increased blood pressure.

9. **Administration of indigo carmine dye** (via an α-adrenergic effect).

B. The treatment of hypertension is directed toward correcting the underlying cause. It may include the following:

1. Optimizing oxygenation and ventilation.

2. Increasing the depth of anesthesia (eg, volatile and IV anesthetics and analgesics).

3. Sedating an anxious patient or emptying a full bladder.

4. Medications (for further discussion, see Chapter 18).

    a. *Combined α- and β-adrenergic blocking agents*: labetalol 5- to 10-mg increments IV.

    b. *β-Adrenergic blocking agents*: propranolol 0.5- to 1.0-mg increments IV; metoprolol 1.0 to 5.0 mg IV; or esmolol, 5- to 10-mg increments IV.

    c. **Vasodilators**: hydralazine 2.5- to 5-mg increments IV; nitroglycerin infusion, 30 to 50 μg/min IV and titrating to effect; nitroprusside infusion 30 to 50 μg/min IV and titrating to effect.

    d. **Calcium channel blockers**: verapamil 2.5 to 5 mg IV; diltiazem 5 to 10 mg IV.

III. DYSRHYTHMIAS

A. Sinus bradycardia is a sinus node–driven heart rate of less than 60 beats/min. Unless there is severe underlying heart disease, hemodynamic changes are minimal. With very slow rates, atrial and ventricular ectopic escape beats or rhythms may occur.

    1. Etiologies:

        a. Hypoxia.

        b. Intrinsic cardiac disease such as sick sinus syndrome or acute MI (particularly inferior wall MI).

        c. Medications such as **succinylcholine** (especially in young children via a direct cholinergic effect), **anticholinesterases**, **β-adrenergic blockers**, **calcium channel blockers**, **digoxin**, and synthetic **narcotics** (eg, fentanyl and remifentanil).

        d. Increased vagal tone occurs with traction on the peritoneum or spermatic cord; pressure on the globe via the oculocardiac reflex; pressure near the brainstem during craniotomies for posterior fossa lesions; direct pressure on the vagus nerve or carotid sinus during neck or intrathoracic surgery; acute distension of the peritoneal cavity during laparoscopy; centrally mediated vagal response from anxiety or pain (vasovagal reaction); and Valsalva maneuvers.

        e. Increased intracranial pressure (Cushing reflex).

        f. Reflex bradycardia. From baroreceptor reflex (eg, with phenylephrine administration), atrial stretch, or cardiopulmonary reflex.

    2. Treatment of sinus bradycardia

        a. Verify adequate oxygenation and ventilation.

        b. Bradycardia due to increased vagal tone requires discontinuation of the provocative stimulus. The vagal reflex may fatigue with repeat stimulus or be less pronounced with deeper anesthesia. Atropine 0.5 mg IV or low-dose epinephrine 10 to 50 μg IV may be needed if the patient is hypotensive. Glycopyrrolate 0.2 to 0.6 mg IV or ephedrine 5 to 10 mg IV may be given for hemodynamically stable bradycardia.

        c. In patients with intrinsic cardiac disease, treatment should proceed with atropine 0.5 mg IV, chronotropes (eg, ephedrine, dopamine), or cardiac pacing.

B. **Sinus tachycardia** is a sinus node–driven heart rate greater than 100 beats/min. The rate is regular and rarely exceeds 160 beats/min. Electrocardiogram (ECG) should demonstrate a P wave preceding each QRS complex with a fixed PR interval.
   1. Etiologies: Catecholamine excess, inadequate anesthesia or analgesia, hypercarbia, hypoxia, hypotension, hypovolemia, medications (eg, pancuronium, desflurane, atropine, and ephedrine), fever, MI, PE, tamponade, tension pneumothorax, malignant hyperthermia, pheochromocytoma, and thyrotoxicosis.
   2. Treatment should be directed toward correcting the underlying cause and may include the following:
      a. Correcting oxygenation and ventilation abnormalities.
      b. Increasing the depth of anesthesia and treating pain with analgesics.
      c. Correcting hypovolemia.
      d. Medications such as opioids and β-adrenergic blockers. Patients with active coronary artery disease and adequate blood pressure may benefit by treatment with β-adrenergic blockers to control the heart rate while the cause is being determined.

C. **Heart block**
   1. **First-degree atrioventricular (AV) block** is characterized by a PR interval of 0.2 seconds or longer. In first-degree block, every atrial pulse is transmitted to the ventricle.
   2. **Second-degree AV block** is divided into two types: Mobitz type 1 (Wenckebach) and Mobitz type 2.
      a. **Mobitz type 1** (Wenckebach) usually occurs when a conduction defect is in the AV node and is manifested by a progressive PR prolongation culminating in a nonconducted P wave. It is generally benign.
      b. **Mobitz type 2** is a conduction defect often distal to the AV node. It presents with a constant PR interval and frequent nonconducted P waves. It is more likely to progress to third-degree block.
   3. **Third-degree AV block** (complete heart block) may be caused by intrinsic AV nodal or His Purkinje disease and occurs when there is complete failure of any conduction from the atria to ventricles. It presents with AV dissociation (variable PR intervals) and either a junctional (narrow QRS) or ventricular (wide QRS) escape rhythm. For a quick reference, please see uptodate.com's ECG tutorial on atrioventricular block.
   4. **Treatment of heart block**
      a. **First-degree AV block** does not usually require specific treatment; however, temporary pacing should be available in the case of first-degree heart block in combination with a bifascicular block (so-called trifascicular block).
      b. **Second-degree AV block**
         1. **Mobitz type 1** requires treatment only if the patient becomes symptomatic or hemodynamically unstable. Temporary transcutaneous or transvenous pacing may be necessary, particularly during an inferior MI, although the block may resolve following revascularization
         2. **Mobitz type 2** may progress to complete heart block. Hemodynamically unstable patients should be urgently treated with atropine and often temporary cardiac pacing. Stable patients should be continuously monitored for progress to higher-grade conduction block warranting evaluation for pacemaker placement while being evaluated for stable causes.

    c. Third-degree AV block is treated with transcutaneous, transvenous, or epicardial pacing.

D. Supraventricular tachycardias (SVTs) originate at or above the bundle of His. The resulting QRS complexes are narrow (<120 ms) except during aberrant conduction.

    1. Atrial premature contractions (APCs or PACs) occur when ectopic foci in the atria fire before the next expected impulse from the sinus node. The P wave of an APC characteristically looks different from preceding P waves, and the PR interval may vary from normal. APCs may cause aberrant QRS complexes. If the AV node is still in a refractory period, an APC will not elicit a ventricular response. APCs are common, usually benign, and typically require no treatment.

    2. Junctional or AV nodal rhythms are characterized by absent or abnormal P waves and normal QRS complexes. Although they may indicate ischemic cardiac disease, junctional rhythms are commonly seen in healthy individuals receiving inhalational anesthesia. In the patient whose cardiac output depends heavily on the contribution from atrial contraction, stroke volume and blood pressure may decline precipitously. Treatment may include the following:

        a. Reduction of anesthetic depth.

        b. Increasing intravascular volume.

        c. Atropine in increments of 0.2 mg IV may convert a slow junctional rhythm to sinus rhythm, particularly if secondary to a vagal mechanism.

        d. Paradoxically, β-blockers may be used cautiously (eg, propranolol 0.5 mg IV and metoprolol 1-3 mg), especially with isorhythmic AV dissociation (independent atrial and ventricular rhythms that are similar in rate).

        e. If the dysrhythmia is associated with hypotension, increasing the blood pressure with vasopressors (eg, ephedrine or norepinephrine) may be required as a temporizing measure.

        f. If necessary, atrial pacing may be instituted to restore atrial contraction.

    3. Atrial fibrillation is an irregular rhythm with an atrial rate of 350 to 600 beats/min and a variable ventricular response. It may be seen with myocardial ischemia, mitral valvular disease, hyperthyroidism, PE, excessive sympathetic stimulation, and digitalis toxicity; after thoracic surgery; or when the heart has been manipulated. Treatment is based on the hemodynamic status.

        a. Rapid ventricular rate with stable hemodynamics can be treated initially with β-adrenergic blockade, such as propranolol 0.5-mg increments IV, metoprolol 2.5- to 5-mg increments, esmolol 5- to 10-mg increments, or a calcium channel blocker such as verapamil 2.5- to 5-mg increments or diltiazem 10 to 20 mg IV (see Chapters 18 and 39). Amiodarone 150 mg IV can be used to promote conversion back to sinus rhythm (anticoagulation prior to cardioversion is recommended in patients with atrial fibrillation for longer than 24 hours).

        b. Rapid ventricular rate with unstable hemodynamics requires synchronized cardioversion (50-100 J if biphasic or 200 J if monophasic) (see Chapters 18 and 39).

    4. Atrial flutter is usually a regular rhythm with an atrial rate of 250 to 350 beats/min and a characteristic sawtooth ECG configuration. It is often seen with underlying heart disease (ie, rheumatic heart disease and mitral stenosis). Conduction across the AV node is often 2:1 in patients not taking AV nodal blockers, but it may also be 1:1 or 4:1. A 2:1 block will result in a rapid ventricular rate (usually 150 beats/min). Treatment usually includes β-adrenergic, calcium channel blockade, or synchronized cardioversion (see Chapters 18 and 39).

5. **Paroxysmal SVT** is an abrupt-onset tachydysrhythmia (atrial and ventricular rates of 150-250 beats/min) with reentry usually through the AV node. This rhythm may be associated with **Wolff-Parkinson-White (WPW) syndrome,** thyrotoxicosis, or mitral valve prolapse. Patients without heart disease may develop this dysrhythmia owing to stress, caffeine, or excess catecholamines.

   a. Hemodynamically unstable patients with SVT should undergo synchronized cardioversion starting at 50 to 100 J. These patients are at high risk for ventricular fibrillation.

   b. For hemodynamically stable patients with SVT, treatment includes **adenosine** 6 to 18 mg IV, Valsalva maneuvers, carotid sinus massage, or propranolol 1 to 2 mg IV.

   c. For patients with WPW syndrome, AV nodal blockers (including adenosine, calcium channel, and β-blockers) are contraindicated for the treatment of atrial fibrillation or atrial flutter as they selectively slow conduction through the AV node, which can lead to increased conduction through the accessory pathway and cause ventricular fibrillation.

      1. Options for rhythm control in hemodynamically stable patients with WPW include procainamide 20 to 50 mg/min (until arrhythmia terminates, hypotension ensues, QRS is prolonged by >50%, or total of 17 mg/kg dose is reached) or ibutilide (for patients <60 kg, 0.01 mg/kg infused over 10 minutes; for patients >60 kg, 1 mg over 10 minutes). If the arrhythmia does not terminate within 10 minutes after the end of the infusion, a second bolus may be given).

E. **Ventricular dysrhythmias**

   1. **Ventricular premature contractions (VPCs or PVCs)** occur when ectopic foci in the ventricle fire before the next expected impulse arrives. They are characterized by widened QRS (>120 ms) complexes. When these are coupled alternately with normal beats, ventricular bigeminy exists. VPCs are occasionally seen in healthy individuals but carry a worse prognosis in patients with underlying heart disease. Under anesthesia, they frequently occur during states of catecholamine excess, hypoxia, or hypercarbia. They may also signify myocardial ischemia or infarction, heart failure, digitalis toxicity, hypokalemia, or hypomagnesemia. **VPCs may require therapy when a patient becomes hemodynamically unstable. Other concerning features include sustained durations, increase in frequency (>10% of all ventricular depolarizations), or occurrence on or near the preceding T wave (R-on-T phenomenon);** these situations may precede the development of ventricular tachycardia, ventricular fibrillation, and cardiac arrest.

      a. Treatment in an otherwise hemodynamically stable patient should begin with ensuring adequate depth of anesthesia, oxygenation, and ventilation and assessing for electrolyte abnormalities (especially potassium and magnesium). Patients with coronary artery disease who continue to have ventricular irritability should have any ischemia treated. If the ectopy continues, then **amiodarone** (150 mg IV over 10 minutes followed by an infusion at 1 mg/min for 6 hours then 0.5 mg/min thereafter) may be considered. Refractory ventricular ectopy may require further treatment (see Chapters 18 and 39).

2. **Ventricular tachycardia** is defined as three or more successive ventricular complexes. Nonsustained VT is three or more repetitive ventricular beats with a duration of <30 seconds. Sustained VT lasts for >30 seconds or is associated with hemodynamic impairment. Monomorphic VT is the repetition of the same basic QRS complex, whereas polymorphic VT refers to changing QRS morphology particularly if there is a change in axis. Polymorphic VT with a prolonged baseline QTc is called torsades de pointes.
   a. Hemodynamically unstable patients with a pulse should be treated as outlined in the advanced cardiac life support (ACLS) guidelines with cardiopulmonary resuscitation and cardioversion (120-200 J if biphasic, or 360 J if monophasic; if unresponsive, may increase energy in a stepwise fashion).
   b. For stable patients with sustained monomorphic VT, pharmacologic cardioversion can be attempted, but the patient should be monitored carefully as patients who are hemodynamically stable initially can rapidly become unstable. Underlying causes such as electrolyte disturbance, ischemia, and heart failure should also be treated.
   c. Polymorphic VT is usually a hemodynamically unstable rhythm requiring urgent defibrillation.
   d. In conscious, stable patients with torsades de points, intravenous magnesium sulfate is often an effective therapy.
3. **Ventricular fibrillation** is chaotic ventricular activity resulting in ineffective ventricular contractions. Prompt defibrillation is required with the same starting energy as above.
4. **Pre-excited atrial fibrillation.** In patients with a wide-complex tachycardia who are hemodynamically stable, consider pre-excited atrial fibrillation. Initial therapy with rhythm or rate control should be attempted (refer to WPW syndrome above).

IV. HYPOXEMIA
Hypoxemia occurs when oxygen delivery to the tissues is insufficient to meet metabolic demands.
A. Intraoperative etiologies
1. **Inadequate oxygen supply:**
   a. Loss of the main pipeline supply with an empty reserve oxygen tank.
   b. An oxygen flowmeter that is not turned to a sufficient flow.
   c. Breathing system disconnection.
   d. Large leaks in the anesthesia machine, ventilator, carbon dioxide absorber, breathing circuit, or around the endotracheal tube or laryngeal mask airway. This condition may be managed acutely by increasing oxygen flow or using a self-inflating (Ambu) bag to deliver oxygen to the patient.
   e. Obstructed endotracheal tube (eg, kinked or mucous plug).
   f. Malpositioned endotracheal tubes (eg, esophageal or mainstem bronchial intubation).
   g. Upper airway obstruction.
   h. Laryngospasm in the unintubated patient (see Section X).
2. **Hypoventilation** (see Section V).
3. **Ventilation-perfusion inequalities or shunting:**
   a. **Pulmonary shunt.** As seen with atelectasis, pneumonia, pulmonary edema, aspiration, pneumothorax, bronchospasm, mucous plugging, and other parenchymal pathologic states as well as with single lung ventilation. In some cases, these inequalities may be corrected by increasing mean airway pressure or applying PEEP.

    b. Cardiac shunt. Right-to-left cardiac shunt, as in ventricular septal defect (VSD), atrial septal defect (ASD), and tetralogy of Fallot.

  4. Reduction in oxygen carrying capacity. The oxygen carrying capacity is reduced with anemia, carbon monoxide poisoning, and hemoglobinopathies, despite a normal oxygen saturation as measured by pulse oximetry. Methemoglobin reduces the oxygen carrying capacity and at high levels will reduce oxygen saturation reading via pulse oximetry.

  5. A leftward shift of the hemoglobin-oxygen dissociation curve results from hypothermia, decreased 2,3-diphosphoglycerate concentration, alkalosis, hypocarbia, and carbon monoxide poisoning.

B. Treatment of hypoxemia

  1. If the patient is being mechanically ventilated, begin manual ventilation with 100% oxygen to assess pulmonary compliance. Evaluate breath sounds, check the surgical field for mechanical interference with ventilation, examine the endotracheal tube for obstruction or dislodgement, and confirm adequate movement of the chest wall or diaphragm. Elevated peak airway pressures may indicate bronchospasm, pneumothorax, an obstructed endotracheal tube, or endobronchial intubation.

  2. The breathing circuit, ventilator, and anesthesia machine should be checked for leaks. If a leak is present, ventilation should be started with high-flow 100% oxygen via an alternative source such as a self-inflating bag until the problem is rectified.

  3. Adequate oxygen delivery to the patient should be confirmed with an inline oxygen analyzer.

  4. Bronchoscopy may be valuable to help rule out obstructive causes.

  5. Ultrasound or bedside chest x-ray may help evaluate for a pneumothorax.

  6. Further treatment is outlined in Chapter 13.

V. HYPERCARBIA

Hypercarbia is due either to inadequate ventilation or to increased carbon dioxide production and can lead to respiratory acidosis, increased pulmonary artery pressure, and increased intracranial pressure.

A. Inadequate ventilation

  1. Central depression of the medullary respiratory center can be caused by medications (eg, opioids, barbiturates, benzodiazepines, and volatile anesthetics) or primary central nervous system pathology (eg, tumor, ischemia, and edema). Controlled ventilation and the administration of reversal agents (eg, naloxone and flumazenil) may be required.

  2. Neuromuscular depression may be seen with a high level of spinal anesthesia, phrenic nerve paralysis, and inadequate reversal of neuromuscular blockade.

  3. Inappropriate ventilator settings may result in low minute ventilation.

  4. Increased airway resistance may occur with bronchospasm, upper airway obstruction, mainstem intubation, obstructed endotracheal tube, severe chronic obstructive lung disease, congestive heart failure, and hemothorax or pneumothorax.

  5. Rebreathing of exhaled gases may occur owing to an exhausted carbon dioxide absorber, machine failure, inspiratory or expiratory valve failure, or inadequate fresh gas flow in nonrebreathing systems.

  6. One-lung ventilation in patients with preexisting pulmonary pathology can lead to significant hypercarbia.

B. Increased carbon dioxide production results from exogenous carbon dioxide (eg, absorption of carbon dioxide from insufflation during laparoscopy), reperfusion of ischemic tissue, and hypermetabolic states (eg, hyperthermia, sepsis, burns, and malignant hyperthermia).

C. Treatment of hypercarbia should be targeted to the cause. Depending on the etiology, treatment may include intubation, increasing minute ventilation, repositioning the endotracheal tube, suctioning, treatment of bronchospasm, diuresis, or placing a chest tube.

VI. ABNORMAL URINE OUTPUT

A. Oliguria is defined as urine output less than 0.5 mL/kg/h. Prerenal, renal, and postrenal causes are described in Chapter 5.

1. Treatment includes ruling out mechanical causes (eg, malpositioned, kinked, or obstructed Foley catheter) and renal dysfunction (can be accessed through renal ultrasound).

2. **Hypotension** should be corrected to ensure adequate renal perfusion pressure.

3. **Volume status should be assessed.** A fluid bolus may be given if hypovolemia is suspected. If oliguria persists, CVP measurement or systolic variation in arterial tracing in mechanically ventilated patients may help guide further fluid management. Patients with reduced ventricular function may require placement of a pulmonary artery catheter.

4. **If oliguria persists** despite an adequate volume status, urine output can be increased with the following drugs. Current evidence suggests that these medications do not affect renal function or outcome; however, they may aid in toxin elimination and reduce the formation of casts.

   a. Furosemide 2 to 20 mg IV.

   b. Dopamine infusion 1 to 3 μg/kg/min IV.

   c. Mannitol 12.5 to 25.0 g IV.

   d. Fenoldopam 0.1 to 0.4 μg/kg/min IV.

5. **Intraoperative diuretics** may be required to preserve urine output in patients on chronic diuretic therapy.

B. Anuria is a rare occurrence in the perioperative period. Mechanical causes, including Foley catheter malfunction or ureteral obstruction, damage, or transection, must be excluded, and hemodynamic instability must be treated.

C. High urine output may occur in response to iatrogenic causes (eg, vigorous fluid administration, mannitol, and Lasix), but other causes must be considered, including hyperglycemia and both neurogenic and nephrogenic diabetes insipidus (see Chapter 5). A high urine output is not a problem unless associated with hypovolemia or electrolyte abnormalities. Treatment should be directed at the underlying cause, maintaining volume status, and correcting electrolyte abnormalities.

VII. HYPOTHERMIA

Hypothermia is a common problem in the perioperative period.

A. Heat loss during general anesthesia and surgery may occur from any or all of the following mechanisms:

1. **Redistribution of heat from core areas** (eg, brain, heart) to peripheral tissues (eg, limbs, skin). Redistribution results in a reduction in the core temperature with maintenance of the mean body temperature.

2. **Radiation.** Radiant heat loss depends on cutaneous blood flow and exposed body surface area.

3. **Evaporation.** Energy is lost as liquid vaporizes from mucosal and serosal surfaces, skin, and lungs. Evaporative losses depend on the exposed surface area and the relative humidity of ambient gas.

4. **Conduction,** which is heat transfer from a warm to a cool object. This heat loss is proportional to the area exposed, difference in temperature, and thermal conductivity.

5. **Convection,** which is the loss of heat by conduction to a moving gas. High airflow rates in the operating rooms (10-15 room volume changes/hour) may result in significant heat loss.

B. **Pediatric patients** are particularly susceptible to intraoperative hypothermia (see Chapter 33).

C. **Geriatric patients** are also more prone to hypothermia.

D. **Anesthetic effects**

1. Volatile anesthetics impair the thermoregulatory center located in the posterior hypothalamus and predispose the patient to heat redistribution and heat loss due to their vasodilatory properties.

2. Opioids will reduce the vasoconstriction mechanism for heat conservation because of their sympatholytic properties.

3. Muscle relaxants reduce muscle tone and prevent shivering.

4. Regional anesthesia produces sympathetic blockade, muscle relaxation, and sensory blockade of thermal receptors, which inhibit compensatory responses.

E. **Severe hypothermia** is associated with a number of physiologic changes.

1. **Cardiovascular.** Increased SVR, ventricular dysrhythmias, and myocardial depression may occur with severe hypothermia.

2. **Metabolic.** Decreased metabolic rate and decreased tissue perfusion (from catecholamine response) may occur.

3. **Hematologic.** Increased blood viscosity, leftward shift of the hemoglobin dissociation curve, impaired coagulation, and platelet dysfunction occur.

4. **Neurologic.** Decreased cerebral blood flow, increased cerebrovascular resistance, decreased minimum alveolar concentration, delayed emergence from anesthesia, drowsiness, and confusion may occur.

5. **Drug disposition.** Decreased hepatic blood flow and metabolism coupled with decreased renal blood flow and clearance result in decreased anesthetic requirement.

6. **Shivering** can increase heat production, oxygen consumption, and sympathetic tone.

F. **Prevention and treatment of hypothermia**

1. **Maintain or increase ambient temperature.** Anesthetized patients frequently become hypothermic if the room temperature is below 21 °C.

2. **Cover exposed surfaces** to minimize conductive and convective losses. Forced warmed air blankets placed over the patient can provide both insulation and active warming. Active warming should not be attempted on ischemic tissues such as those found distal to the level of an aortic cross-clamp.

3. **Warming transfused fluids and blood** is essential in cases with large fluid requirements or rapid infusion rates (see Chapter 35). Doing so will reduce heat loss by about 0.25 °C/L of crystalloid.

4. **Use of closed or low-flow semiclosed circuit anesthesia** will decrease evaporative losses and modestly reduce heat loss.

5. **Heated humidifiers** can be added to the anesthetic circuit when high gas flows are used. These will warm and humidify the inspired gas, minimizing evaporative loss from the lungs. The temperature of the inspired gas

must be monitored and kept below 41 °C; otherwise, there is potential for airway burns. Alternatively, "artificial noses" (passive heat and moisture exchangers) can be placed between the endotracheal tube and the breathing circuit. These are hygroscopic membrane filters with large surface areas that trap the humidity of expired air.

6. **Warming blankets** placed beneath the patient can increase body temperature by conduction from warm water pumped through the blanket. This method is most effective in children weighing less than 10 kg. The temperature should be kept below 40 °C to avoid burns.

7. **Radiant warmers and heating lamps** warm the patients by infrared radiation and are useful only for infants. The warming lamps should be kept at least 70 cm from the patient to avoid burns.

8. **Warming irrigation solutions** prior to use.

VIII. HYPERTHERMIA

Hyperthermia is an increase in temperature of 2 °C/h or 0.5 °C/15 min. It is uncommon for a patient to become hyperthermic based solely on maneuvers to conserve body heat in the operating room. Therefore, any increase in temperature must be investigated. Hyperthermia and its accompanying hypermetabolic state produce an increase in oxygen consumption, cardiac work, glucose demand, and compensatory minute ventilation. Sweating and vasodilation may result in decreased intravascular volume and venous return.

A. **Etiologies**

1. **Malignant hyperthermia** must be considered during any perioperative temperature increase (see Section XVII).

2. **Inflammation, infection, and sepsis** with release of inflammatory mediators may cause hyperthermia.

3. **Hypermetabolic states** such as thyrotoxicosis may cause hyperthermia.

4. **Injury to the hypothalamic thermoregulatory center** from anoxia, edema, trauma, or tumor may affect temperature set points in the hypothalamus.

5. **Neuroleptic malignant syndrome** (NMS) triggered by neuroleptics such as phenothiazines (eg, haloperidol); it is a rare cause.

6. **Sympathomimetics**, such as monoamine oxidase inhibitors, amphetamines, cocaine, and tricyclic antidepressants, may produce a hypermetabolic state.

7. **Anticholinergics**, such as atropine, may suppress sweating.

B. **Treatment**

1. **If malignant hyperthermia is suspected**, dantrolene treatment must be initiated (see Section XVII).

2. **Severe hyperthermia** can be treated by cooling exposed body surfaces (eg, skin) with ice, cooling blankets, and reduced ambient temperature or by performing internal lavage (eg, stomach, bladder, bowel, and peritoneum) with cold saline.

   a. Volatile liquids, such as alcohol, applied to the skin will promote evaporative heat loss.

   b. Conductive heat loss can be increased with vasodilators such as nitroprusside and nitroglycerin.

   c. Centrally active agents such as aspirin and acetaminophen can be given by nasogastric tube or rectally.

   d. Shivering can be prevented by maintaining neuromuscular blockade.

   e. When hyperthermia is profound, **extracorporeal cooling** can be used. Cooling should be stopped when the body temperature reaches 38 °C to avoid hypothermia.

IX. DIAPHORESIS (SWEATING)

Diaphoresis (sweating) may occur in response to the sympathetic discharge caused by anxiety, pain, hypercarbia, or noxious stimuli in the presence of inadequate anesthesia. It may also be seen in conjunction with bradycardia, nausea, and hypotension as part of a generalized vagal reaction or as a thermoregulatory response to hyperthermia.

X. LARYNGOSPASM

A. **Laryngospasm** is most commonly caused by an irritative stimulus to the airway during a light plane of anesthesia. Common noxious airway stimuli that may elicit this reflex include secretions, vomitus, blood, inhalation of pungent volatile anesthetics, oropharyngeal or nasopharyngeal airway placement, laryngoscopy, painful peripheral stimuli, and peritoneal traction during light anesthesia. Laryngospasm can also result from sudden administration of high doses of synthetic narcotics (eg, fentanyl) during induction of anesthesia.

B. **Reflex closure of the vocal cords**, causing partial or total glottic obstruction, may be manifest in less severe cases by stridor and, when complete, by an obstructed pattern of breathing. In this situation, the abdominal wall rises with contraction of the diaphragm during inspiration, but because air entry is blocked the chest retracts or fails to expand. During attempted expiration, the abdomen falls as the diaphragm relaxes and the chest returns to its original position. With complete obstruction, the anesthetist will not be able to ventilate the patient.

C. The hypoxia, hypercarbia, and acidosis that result can cause hypertension and tachycardia. Hypotension, bradycardia, and ventricular dysrhythmias leading to cardiac arrest will ensue unless airway patency is restored within minutes. Children and pregnant women are particularly prone to these complications because of their small functional residual capacity and relatively high oxygen consumption.

D. **Treatment**

1. Deepening the anesthetic level and removing the stimulus (eg, by suction, withdrawal of an artificial airway, or stopping peripheral stimulation) while administering 100% oxygen may be adequate to relieve laryngospasm.

2. If laryngospasm is not relieved, **continuous positive pressure on the airway** with a jaw thrust may relieve the spasm; if not, a small dose of **succinylcholine** (eg, 10-20 mg IV in an adult) will relax the striated muscles of the larynx.

3. The lungs should be ventilated with 100% oxygen and the anesthetic level deepened before the noxious stimulation is resumed, or the patient may be allowed to awaken if laryngospasm has occurred during emergence.

4. Infrequently, laryngospasm may require reintubation.

5. Laryngospasm can result in negative-pressure pulmonary edema, which may need treatment after the laryngospasm resolves.

XI. BRONCHOSPASM

A. **Reflex bronchiolar constriction** may be centrally mediated or may be a local response to airway irritation. Bronchospasm is common in anaphylactoid or anaphylactic drug and blood transfusion reactions as well as in cigarette smokers and those with chronic bronchitis. Like laryngospasm, bronchospasm may be elicited by noxious stimuli such as secretions and endotracheal intubation.

B. **Wheezing** (usually more pronounced on expiration) characterizes bronchospasm and is associated with tachypnea and dyspnea in the awake patient. An anesthetized patient may be difficult to ventilate because of increased airway resistance. Decreased expiratory flow rates may produce air trapping and increase intrathoracic pressure, decreasing venous return, cardiac output, and blood pressure. End-tidal carbon dioxide curves often have an obstructive pattern (continual rise) during exhalation.

C. **Histamine-releasing drugs** (eg, morphine, mivacurium, vancomycin, and atracurium) may exacerbate bronchoconstriction.

D. **Treatment**

1. The **endotracheal tube position** should be checked and, if carinal stimulation is the cause, withdrawn slightly.

2. **Deepening the anesthetic level** will frequently reverse bronchospasm that is secondary to inadequate anesthesia. Deepening the level of anesthesia can usually be accomplished with an inhalational agent. An IV agent may be necessary when ventilation is significantly impaired. Propofol produces fewer symptoms of bronchoconstriction than barbiturates and is usually preferable. Ketamine has the advantage of causing bronchodilation by releasing endogenous catecholamines. The inspired oxygen concentration should be increased until adequate oxygenation is achieved.

3. **Medical treatment** includes administering inhaled or intravenous β_2-adrenergic agonists. Inhaled bronchodilators have limited systemic absorption, which may minimize cardiovascular side effects. Nebulized forms may contain large particles, which deposit to a large extent in tubing and upper airways. The dosage of metered dose inhalers should be titrated to effect when administered into a breathing circuit. Large doses (10-20 puffs) may be necessary. If the condition is severe, low-dose ketamine 0.1 to 0.15 mg/kg/h based on case reports or low-dose IV epinephrine 0.02 to 0.05 μg/kg/min based on case reports should be started.

4. **Adequate hydration and humidification** of inspired gases will minimize inspissation of secretions.

XII. ASPIRATION

General anesthesia causes depression of airway reflexes that predisposes patients to aspiration. Aspiration of gastric contents from vomiting or regurgitation may cause bronchospasm, hypoxemia, atelectasis, tachypnea, tachycardia, and hypotension. The severity of symptoms depends on the volume and pH of the gastric material aspirated. Conditions that predispose the patient to aspiration include gastric dysmotility, gastric outlet obstruction, gastroesophageal reflux, small-bowel obstruction, symptomatic hiatal hernia, pregnancy, and recent food ingestion.

A. **If vomiting or regurgitation occurs** in an anesthetized patient whose airway is not protected by an endotracheal tube, the patient should be placed in the Trendelenburg position to minimize passive flow of gastric contents into the trachea, the head should be turned to the side, the upper airway suctioned, and an endotracheal tube placed. Suctioning the endotracheal tube before instituting positive-pressure ventilation avoids forcing gastric contents into the distal airways. Evidence of significant aspiration includes wheezing, decreased lung compliance, and hypoxemia. A chest radiograph should be obtained; however, radiographic evidence of infiltrates may be delayed. Bronchodilators may be useful.

B. Bronchoscopy should be performed if a clinically significant aspiration is suspected. The airways should be suctioned clear, and foreign bodies such as teeth and food removed. Lavage with large volumes of saline is not helpful.

C. Aspiration of blood, unless of large volume, is usually benign.

D. Administration of antibiotics usually is not warranted unless the material aspirated contains a high bacterial load such as with bowel obstruction (see Chapter 8).

E. A sputum specimen should be obtained for Gram stain and culture.

F. Steroids are not useful for treating aspiration.

G. If significant aspiration has occurred, close postoperative observation should be undertaken. This includes pulse oximetry and repeat chest radiography. Ventilatory support and supplemental oxygen may be necessary (see Chapter 37).

XIII. PNEUMOTHORAX

Pneumothorax is the accumulation of gas within the pleural space.

A. Etiologies

   1. Spontaneous rupture of blebs and bullae.

   2. Blunt or penetrating chest trauma.

   3. Surgical entrance into the pleural space during thoracic, upper abdominal, or retroperitoneal surgery, tracheostomy, or surgery of the chest wall or neck.

   4. Iatrogenic complication of procedures such as subclavian or internal jugular vein catheter placement, thoracentesis, pericardiocentesis, or upper extremity nerve block.

   5. During positive-pressure ventilation using high pressures and volumes, causing barotrauma and alveolar rupture. Patients with chronic obstructive pulmonary disease are at particularly high risk.

   6. Malfunction of chest tubes.

B. Physiologic effects of a pneumothorax is largely a function of the gas volume and the rate of expansion. A small pneumothorax may have no significant cardiopulmonary effect, whereas a larger one may result in significant lung collapse and hypoxemia. A tension pneumothorax occurs when there is a one-way leak into the pleural space, causing a significant increase in intrapleural pressure. This can result in decreased venous return, mediastinal shift, and compression of the heart. A small tension pneumothorax can cause hypotension, whereas a large tension pneumothorax can cause a cardiac arrest.

C. The **diagnosis** of pneumothorax can be difficult.

   1. Signs of pneumothorax include decreased breath sounds on the affected side, a reduction in lung compliance, an increase in peak inspiratory pressure, and hypoxemia.

   2. Hypotension reflects the presence of a tension pneumothorax.

   3. A chest radiograph can usually reveal a pneumothorax as a hyperlucency between the chest wall, mediastinum, or diaphragm and lung parenchyma.

   4. Ultrasound imaging of the chest wall can provide a reliable and rapid diagnosis. Signs of a pneumothorax on ultrasound imaging will be the lack of parietal and visceral pleura sliding against each other respirations. Ultrasound can provide a reliable and rapid diagnosis.

D. Treatment. Nitrous oxide should be discontinued, and the patient should be ventilated with 100% oxygen. A tension pneumothorax requires immediate decompression. A large-bore catheter (14-16 gauge) can be inserted into the pleural space at the second intercostal space in the midclavicular line. A chest tube can then be placed at the fifth or sixth intercostal space in the midaxillary line.

XIV. MYOCARDIAL ISCHEMIA

A. Etiology. Myocardial ischemia is the result of an imbalance between myocardial oxygen supply and consumption and, if persistent, may lead to MI.

B. Clinical features

1. In the awake patient, myocardial ischemia may manifest as chest pain, dyspnea, nausea and vomiting, diaphoresis, or shoulder and jaw pain. **Asymptomatic ischemia is common** in the perioperative period, particularly in diabetic patients. In patients under general anesthesia, hemodynamic instability and ECG changes may occur with ischemia.

2. **ECG changes** such as **ST segment depression** greater than 1 mm or acute T-wave inversion may indicate subendocardial ischemia. **ST segment elevation** is usually seen with transmural myocardial ischemia. T-wave changes may also be seen with electrolyte abnormalities and thus are not particularly diagnostic of ischemia. Lead V_5 is the singlemost sensitive lead for detecting left ventricular ischemia (see Chapter 15).

3. **Other indicators of ischemia** include the following:
   a. Hypotension.
   b. Changes in central filling pressures or cardiac output.
   c. Regional wall motion abnormalities as detected with transesophageal echocardiography (TEE).
   d. Dysrhythmias, particularly ventricular ectopy.

C. Treatment

1. **Hypoxemia and anemia should be** optimally managed to maximize myocardial oxygen delivery.

2. **β-Adrenergic antagonists** (eg, metoprolol in 1- to 3-mg increments IV or propranolol in 0.5- to 1.0-mg increments IV or esmolol in 5- to 10-mg increments IV) decrease myocardial oxygen consumption by decreasing heart rate and contractility. The initiation of β-blockers should be delayed in patients with active heart failure.

3. **Nitroglycerin** (starting at 25-50 µg/min IV or 0.15 mg sublingually) reduces ventricular diastolic pressure and volume through venodilation and thus decreases the myocardial oxygen demand. In addition, nitroglycerin may improve oxygen delivery by enhancing collateral coronary flow. Nitrates should be avoided if there is suspected or known right ventricular ischemia, severe hypotension, marked bradycardia, phosphodiesterase inhibitor use in the last 24 hours, hypertrophic cardiomyopathy, and severe aortic stenosis.

4. **Myocardial ischemia occurring in the setting of hypotension** may require a vasopressor such as phenylephrine (40-80 µg/min IV) or norepinephrine (2-20 µg/min IV) to improve myocardial perfusion pressure. Anesthetic depth may need to be decreased and intravascular volume optimized.

5. When myocardial ischemia results in a significant reduction in cardiac output and hypotension (cardiogenic shock), positive **inotropes** such as dopamine 5 to 20 µg/kg/min IV, dobutamine 5 to 20 µg/kg/min IV, milrinone 0.375 to 0.75 µg/kg/min (after loading dose of 50 µg/kg), and norepinephrine 2 to 20 µg/min IV are indicated. Intra-aortic balloon counterpulsation may be lifesaving. A pulmonary artery catheter of

transesophageal echocardiogram may be helpful in assessing ventricular function and response to therapy.

6. **Aspirin** should be administered.

7. **Heparin treatment, thrombolytic therapy, angioplasty, and coronary revascularization** may be considered in selected patients under the guidance of a cardiologist.

XV. PULMONARY EMBOLISM

Pulmonary embolism (PE) is the obstruction of pulmonary arterial blood flow by thrombus, air, fat, or amniotic fluid. Large emboli may lead to a sudden decrease in end-tidal carbon dioxide tension owing to an **acute increase in dead space**. Other signs include an increase in end-tidal nitrogen tension, as well as an increased CVP, hypoxemia, hypotension, tachyarrhythmias or bradyarrhythmias, and ventricular ectopy.

A. **Thromboemboli** most commonly arise from the deep venous system of the pelvis and lower extremities. Predisposing factors for the development of thrombi are stasis, hypercoagulability, and vascular wall abnormalities. Associated conditions include pregnancy, trauma, carcinoma, prolonged bed rest, and vasculitis.

1. **Physical findings** are nonspecific and may include tachypnea and tachycardia, dyspnea, bronchospasm, and fever.

2. **Laboratory studies**

   a. The ECG reveals a nonspecific tachycardia unless embolization is severe, in which case right-axis deviation, right bundle branch block, and anterior T-wave changes may be seen. PE may cause atrial fibrillation.

   b. The chest radiograph may be unremarkable unless pulmonary infarction has occurred.

   c. Typically, hypotension and hypoxemia are present.

   d. In spontaneously breathing patients, hypocapnia and respiratory alkalosis may result from the increased respiratory rate.

   e. Definitive diagnosis requires a pulmonary angiogram or high-resolution computed tomography of the chest (spiral computed tomography).

3. **Intraoperative treatment** of a suspected PE is supportive. Oxygenation may be increased with increased FIO_2 and optimization of hemodynamic stability with inotropes and vasopressors as needed. Intraoperative anticoagulation therapy, eg, heparin treatment or thrombolytic therapy can be considered and weighed against the risk of hemorrhage. Catheter-directed thrombolysis or embolectomy, or surgical embolectomy with cardiopulmonary bypass, may also be considered particularly in hemodynamically unstable PE.

B. **Air embolism** occurs during entrainment of air into a vein or venous sinus. It occurs most commonly during intracranial surgery in the sitting position, where dural venous sinuses are stented open. Air embolism may also occur during central line placement or removal, liver transplantation, open cardiac procedures, and insufflation during laparoscopy.

1. **Additional signs indicating air embolism** include air seen by TEE or heard with a precordial Doppler. Possible vital sign changes include a sudden decrease in end-tidal CO_2, hypoxia, hypotension, or cardiovascular collapse.

2. **Treatment** begins with limiting the entrainment of additional air by flooding the surgical field with saline or repositioning the patient. Nitrous oxide should be discontinued to avoid enlarging air bubbles

within the circulation. FIO_2 should be increased to facilitate resorption of entrained air. Placing the patient in a head-down and left lateral decubitus position may help reduce an air collection from blocking right ventricular filling and limit air entering the pulmonary artery. If a central venous catheter is in place, it may be aspirated in an attempt to remove air. Fluid and especially vasopressors (such as norepinephrine) and inotropes are used to maintain blood pressure and support cardiac contractility. ACLS including chest compressions may be necessary.

3. **The use of PEEP** in the setting of air embolism is controversial. It will limit the entrainment of air by raising CVP but at the expense of reducing venous return and possibly cardiac output. **Hyperbaric oxygen** may be considered in cases where a large amount of gas has been entrained.

C. **Fat embolism** occurs after trauma or surgery involving the long bones, pelvis, or ribs.

1. **Clinical features** are related to mechanical obstruction of the pulmonary circulation and are similar to those found with pulmonary thromboembolism. The release of free fatty acids may lead to diminished mental status, worsening hypoxemia, fat globules in the urine, disseminated intravascular coagulation, thrombocytopenia, and petechial hemorrhages.

2. **Treatment is supportive**, with the administration of circulatory support plus supplemental oxygen and ventilation as necessary.

D. **Amniotic fluid emboli** (see Chapter 32).

XVI. CARDIAC TAMPONADE

Accumulation of fluid, clots, or loculations within the pericardial sac may prevent adequate ventricular filling and reduce cardiac output. When the accumulation is rapid, cardiovascular collapse may occur within minutes.

A. **Cardiac tamponade** may be associated with the following: chest trauma; cardiac or thoracic surgery; malignancy including lymphoma, leukemia, breast or lung cancer and radiation pericarditis; pericarditis (acute viral, pyogenic, uremic, or postradiation); myocardial perforation by a central venous or pulmonary artery catheter; and aortic dissection, acute MI, collagen vascular disease, and hypothyroidism with myxedema, or it may be idiopathic.

B. **Clinical features** include tachycardia, hypotension, jugular venous distention, muffled heart sounds, and a decrease in pulse pressure.

1. An ECG may reveal **electrical alternans** (ECG finding of alternating QRS amplitude or axis) and diffusely low voltage.

2. **Pulsus paradoxus** (>a 10-mm Hg inspiratory decrease in systolic blood pressure) may be appreciated.

3. There may be an **equalization of right- and left-sided heart pressures** as reflected in identical CVP, right ventricular end-diastolic pressure, pulmonary artery diastolic pressure, and pulmonary capillary wedge pressures.

4. Radiographic findings may include an enlarged cardiac silhouette.

5. An **echocardiogram** is usually diagnostic.

C. The **treatment** of a hemodynamically unstable patient with suspected cardiac tamponade is pericardiocentesis. Intravascular volume should be augmented, and vasopressors that maintain chronotropy and inotropy (ie, epinephrine) are administered to maintain blood pressure. A long needle is inserted between the xiphoid process and the left costal margin and directed toward the left shoulder. If the precordial lead of the ECG is attached to the needle, an injury current (ST segment elevation) will be observed when the needle contacts the epicardium. The needle should be withdrawn slightly and aspirated. Ultrasound-guided pericardiocentesis in the hands of a skilled operator can be accomplished by introducing a needle through the chest wall and aspirating the fluid accumulation where it is closest to the skin under continuous visualization.

1. **Complications of pericardiocentesis** include pneumothorax, coronary artery laceration, and myocardial perforation. A surgical pericardial window is a more permanent approach to alleviating tamponade.

XVII. MALIGNANT HYPERTHERMIA

A. Etiology. Malignant hyperthermia is a hypermetabolic syndrome occurring in genetically susceptible patients after exposure to an anesthetic triggering agent. **Triggering anesthetics** include all potent inhalational agents (eg, halothane, isoflurane, desflurane, and sevoflurane) and succinylcholine. The majority of cases are due to an inherited mutation in the ryanodine receptor, the calcium release channel in the sarcoplasmic reticulum. Abnormal function of this receptor causes reduction in the reuptake of Ca^{2+} by the sarcoplasmic reticulum necessary for the termination of muscle contraction. Consequently, muscle contraction is sustained, resulting in signs of hypermetabolism, including tachycardia, acidosis, hypercarbia, muscle rigidity, tachypnea, hypoxemia, and hyperthermia. Malignant hyperthermia usually occurs in the operating room, but onset may be delayed until the patient reaches the postanesthesia care unit or even the postoperative floor.

B. Clinical features
1. Unexplained tachycardia.
2. Hypercarbia in the mechanically ventilated patient or tachypnea in the spontaneously breathing patient who is unresponsive to increased minute ventilation.
3. Metabolic acidosis.
4. Muscle rigidity even in the presence of neuromuscular blockade. Masseter spasm after giving succinylcholine is associated with malignant hyperthermia. However, not all patients who develop masseter spasm will develop malignant hyperthermia.
5. Hypoxemia.
6. Ventricular dysrhythmias.
7. Hyperkalemia.
8. Fever is often a late sign.
9. Myoglobinuria.

C. Treatment
1. **Summon help** as soon as malignant hyperthermia is suspected. Discontinue all triggering anesthetics, and hyperventilate with 100% oxygen from a new source such as wall oxygen via an Ambu bag. Convert to a total intravenous anesthetic such as propofol. Surgery should be concluded as quickly as possible, and the anesthesia machine should be changed when feasible.
2. **Administer dantrolene or Ryanodex. Dantrolene** (Dantrium), 2.5 mg/kg IV is given initially and repeated to a total of 10 mg/kg or more if signs of malignant hyperthermia persist. Dantrolene is the only known specific treatment for malignant hyperthermia. Its efficacy is due to its ability to inhibit Ca^{2+} release from the sarcoplasmic reticulum. Each ampule contains 20 mg of dantrolene and 3 g of mannitol and should be reconstituted with 50 mL of warm sterile water. **Ryanodex** is a newer formulation of dantrolene sodium with increased solubility. Each vial

of Ryanodex contains 250 mg dantrolene sodium and 125 mg mannitol and should be reconstituted with 5 mL sterile water. Ryanodex dosing is the same as for the less-soluble dantrolene.

3. **Sodium bicarbonate administration** should be guided by pH and partial pressure of carbon dioxide (Pco_2) measurements.

4. **Hyperkalemia** may be corrected with insulin, glucose, and an inhaled β-agonist (eg, albuterol). However, hypokalemia may occur as the hypermetabolic state is brought under control. Calcium administration should be avoided.

5. **Dysrhythmias** generally subside with resolution of the hypermetabolic phase of malignant hyperthermia. Persistent dysrhythmias should be treated.

6. **Hyperthermia** is treated by a variety of methods (see Section VIII).

7. **Urine output** ideally should be maintained at 2 mL/kg/min to avoid renal tubular damage from myoglobin. A Foley catheter should be placed as soon as possible.

8. **Recrudescence, disseminated intravascular coagulation, and acute tubular necrosis** may occur after an acute episode of malignant hyperthermia. Therefore, dantrolene therapy (1 mg/kg IV or orally every 6 hours) and close observation should be continued for 48 to 72 hours after an episode of malignant hyperthermia.

9. Contact the malignant hyperthermia hotline if necessary at 1-800-MH-HYPER (1-800-644-9737) from within the United States. Information can also be obtained at www.mhaus.org.

D. **Anesthesia for malignant hyperthermia–susceptible patients**

1. A **family history** of anesthetic problems suggesting susceptibility, such as unexplained fevers or death during anesthesia, should be sought in every patient.

2. **Malignant hyperthermia (MH)** may be triggered in susceptible patients who have had previous uneventful exposures to triggering agents.

3. **Pretreatment with dantrolene** is not recommended for malignant hyperthermia–susceptible patients. A malignant hyperthermia cart or other dantrolene supply, however, should be immediately available.

4. **The anesthesia machine** should be prepared by changing the carbon dioxide absorbent and fresh gas tubing, disconnecting the vaporizers, using a disposable breathing circuit with charcoal filters if available, and flushing the machine with oxygen at a rate of 10 L/min for at least 20 minutes. The preparation of modern anesthesia machines is variable. Some are more difficult to prepare and may require prolonged flushing times with maximal fresh gas flows, whereas others only require carbon filters in inspiratory and expiratory limbs of the circuit.

5. **Local or regional anesthesia** should be considered, but general anesthesia with nontriggering agents is acceptable. **Safe drugs** for induction and maintenance of general anesthesia include barbiturates, propofol, benzodiazepines, opioids, and nitrous oxide. Nondepolarizing neuromuscular blockers may be used and safely reversed.

6. **Close monitoring** for early signs of malignant hyperthermia such as unexplained hypercarbia or tachycardia is crucial.

E. **Associated syndromes.** An increased risk of malignant hyperthermia has been reported in association with a number of disorders. In many of these cases, the association is not well established. However, patients with the following disorders should be treated as though they are susceptible to malignant hyperthermia:

1. **King-Denborough syndrome**, characterized by dwarfism, mental retardation, and musculoskeletal abnormalities.
2. **Central core disease**, a rare myopathy.
3. **Multiminicore disease**, another rare myopathy.
4. **Duchenne muscular dystrophy** and other **muscular dystrophies** are not associated with malignant hyperthermia but may be associated with hyperkalemia.

F. **Neuroleptic malignant syndrome (NMS)** is associated with the administration of neuroleptic drugs and shares many of the features of malignant hyperthermia.
  1. **Clinical features.** NMS typically develops over 24 to 72 hours and is clinically similar to malignant hyperthermia, presenting as a hypermetabolic episode consisting of hyperthermia, autonomic nervous system instability, pronounced muscle rigidity, and rhabdomyolysis. Creatine kinase and hepatic transaminases often are increased, and mortality approaches 30%.
  2. **Treatment** of NMS is with dantrolene, although benzodiazepines, dopamine antagonists such as bromocriptine, and nondepolarizing muscle relaxants will also decrease muscle rigidity.
  3. **Anesthetic implications.** The exact relationship between NMS and malignant hyperthermia is unclear. Some patients with a history of NMS may be at risk for malignant hyperthermia, and a conservative approach may be warranted (eg, avoidance of known triggering agents). Patients with NMS must be appropriately monitored for malignant hyperthermia during all anesthetics (eg, temperature and end-tidal carbon dioxide). They should not be pretreated with dantrolene.

XVIII. ANAPHYLACTIC AND ANAPHYLACTOID REACTIONS
A. **Anaphylaxis** is a life-threatening allergic reaction. It is initiated by antigen binding to preformed IgE antibodies on the surface of mast cells and basophils, which cause release of vasoactive substances (eg, histamine, leukotrienes, prostaglandins, kinins, and platelet-activating factor). Anaphylaxis is characterized by an acute elevation in tryptase levels.
B. **Anaphylactoid reactions** are clinically similar to anaphylactic reactions, but they are not mediated by IgE and do not require prior sensitization to an antigen.
C. **Clinical features** of anaphylactic or anaphylactoid reactions may include the following:
  1. Urticaria and flushing.
  2. Bronchospasm or airway edema, which can produce respiratory failure.
  3. Hypotension and shock due to peripheral vasodilation and increased capillary permeability.
  4. Pulmonary edema.
D. **Treatment**
  1. **Discontinue anesthetic agents** if circulatory collapse is present.
  2. **Administer 100% oxygen.** Assess the need to intubate and support ventilation. Airway edema can persist beyond the acute event.
  3. **Begin intravascular volume expansion.**
  4. **Treat hypotension by giving epinephrine** 50 to 100 µg IV. For overt cardiovascular collapse, epinephrine 0.5 to 1.0 mg IV is indicated, followed by an infusion if hypotension persists. Epinephrine is useful for treating hypotension and bronchospasm and for limiting mast cell degranulation. Other catecholamines such as norepinephrine may be added. Vasopressin should be added in refractory causes.

5. **Steroids** (eg, hydrocortisone 250 mg to 1.0 g IV, or methylprednisolone 1-2 g IV) may reduce the inflammatory response.
6. **Histamine antagonists** (eg, diphenhydramine 50 mg IV and ranitidine 50 mg IV in the adult) may be useful as second-line therapy.
7. **Consider** drawing a tryptase level after stabilization of the patient to aid in final diagnosis.

E. **Prophylaxis for drug hypersensitivity reactions**
1. **Histamine (H_1) antagonists.** Diphenhydramine 0.5 to 1.0 mg/kg or 50 mg IV in the adult the night before and morning of exposure.
2. **H_2 antagonists.** Ranitidine 50 mg IV or 150 mg orally in the adult the night before and the morning of exposure.
3. **Corticosteroids.** Prednisone 1 mg/kg or 50 mg for adults, four doses every 6 hours before exposure.

XIX. FIRE AND ELECTRICAL HAZARDS IN THE OPERATING ROOM

A. **Fire** in the operating room is a rare event that requires the presence of an ignition source, fuel, and an oxidizing agent.
1. **Lasers and electrocautery devices** are the most common ignition sources.
2. **Fuels** include alcohol, solvents, sheets, drapes, and plastic or rubber materials (including endotracheal tubes). Modern potent inhalation anesthetics are not fuels. During an electrical fire, it is important to unplug the electrical source.
3. **Oxygen** is by far the most common oxidizing agent, although nitrous oxide also supports combustion. Materials that are only marginally combustible in air can produce a massive flame in the presence of a high oxygen concentration. Supplemental oxygen can accumulate under surgical drapes and should be administered only when medically indicated.
4. **Fire extinguishers** should be readily available in all anesthetizing locations. Carbon dioxide and halon fire extinguishers offer the advantage of efficacy against a variety of fires without producing the particulate contamination associated with dry chemical extinguishers.

B. **Electrical safety**
1. **Macroshock** is an electrical injury caused when a large current passes through intact skin producing a thermal, neural, or muscular injury. It may disrupt normal physiologic function and cause cardiac or respiratory arrest. The level of injury varies with the source frequency and individuals, but, in general, the following guidelines can be applied for an alternating current of 60 cycles/s:
   a. **1 mA for 1 second**: threshold of perception
   b. **5 mA for 1 second**: accepted as maximum harmless current intensity. Level at which line isolation monitors alarm.
   c. **10 to 20 mA for 1 second**: current that results in sustained muscular contraction, referred to as the "Let go current."
   d. **100 mA for 1 second**: threshold for ventricular fibrillation.
2. **Microshock** occurs when small currents pass directly to the heart. This occurs intentionally when using cardiac pacemakers but can be harmful if it occurs inadvertently. Ventricular fibrillation can be produced by as little as **100 µA** of current applied to the myocardium. This current is well below the 2- to 5-mA threshold of the line isolation monitor alarm; thus, line isolation monitors do not protect a patient from microshock. To minimize the likelihood of microshock, all equipment should be properly grounded with a three-prong plug and connections to the patient should be electrically isolated. Battery operation does not ensure electrical isolation.

3. **Line isolation monitors** are designed to alert the anesthesiologist when faulty ground connections place patients and operating room personnel at risk of potential exposure to large currents (2-5 mA). The line isolation monitor alarms when one of the two "hot" power lines becomes grounded, creating a first fault. This event signals that someone in the operating room may receive a macroshock if they touch any electrical equipment supplied by this circuit, as they now serve as the ground for the system, creating the second fault. If the line isolation monitor alarms, unplug the last appliance that was plugged in. Further investigation into the appliance or circuit will be necessary. Although line isolation monitors continue to be used in operating rooms, most electrical equipment used today have built-in electrical isolation and many modern operating rooms contain ground fault interrupters on electrical outlets.

4. **Burns from electrosurgical units** may result from poor contact between the dispersive electrode (grounding pad) and the patient. Under such conditions, anything that is grounded may provide an alternative pathway for current, resulting in a burn at these sites. The risk of burns can be minimized by ensuring that the electrode gel is adequate, that the dispersive electrode is placed near the surgical site, and that the patient is insulated from possible alternative pathways for current flow.

XX. EQUIPMENT MALFUNCTIONS
For further information on monitoring, see Chapter 15. Below are discussed common technical challenges that arise with monitoring equipment and suggestions for troubleshooting.

A. Cardiovascular system

1. **ECG**
   a. Electrocautery, motion, or inadequate pad contact with skin may interfere with ECG reading.
   b. Magnetic resonance imaging (MRI)-safe ECG pads may encounter interference when the MRI is actively scanning.
   c. Placement of ECG pads will affect the morphology of the waveform. Check that ECF electrodes are appropriately placed to detect dysrhythmias and ischemia.

2. **Noninvasive blood pressure monitoring**
   a. Check that the blood pressure cuff size is appropriate for the patient. A cuff that is too small may result in a falsely high reading. A cuff that is too large may result in a falsely low reading.
   b. External compression (eg, surgeon leaning on patient's arm) may cause reading errors.

3. **Arterial line**
   a. **An overdampened waveform** will cause an artificially low blood pressure measurement with a narrowed pulse pressure. This may be due to arterial obstruction, catheter occlusion, excess tubing, stopcocks, air bubbles, or pressure tubing kinks.
   b. **An underdampened waveform** will cause an artificially high blood pressure measurement with a wide pulse pressure. This may be due to use of nonrigid tubing or hyperresonance caused by reverberation of pressure waves.

B. Respiratory system

1. Pulse oximeter
   a. Ensure proper placement of light-emitting diodes.
   b. Inadequate perfusion, motion, artificially colored or augmented fingernails, the presence of carboxyhemoglobin or methemoglobin,

and injections of methylene blue, indocyanine green, indigo carmine, and isosulfan blue may cause saturation readings to be uninterpretable or unreadable.

2. End-tidal CO_2

  a. Sampling can be obscured by moisture in sample line or water trap. Consider replacing clogged parts.

C. Neurological system

  1. EEG monitoring. Current methods of intraoperative electroencephalographic (EEG) recordings rely on surface electrodes placed on the frontal scalp.

  a. Ensure adequate contact between electrodes and the patient's skin.

  b. Adjust amplitude scale to maximize visualization of all frequencies.

  c. Use of electrocautery and patient movement may interfere with EEG monitoring.

Suggested Readings

Chacko T, Ledford D. Peri-anesthetic anaphylaxis. *Immunol Allergy Clin North Am*. 2007; 27(2):213-230.

Cottron N, Larcher C, Sommet A, et al. The sevoflurane washout profile of seven recent anesthesia workstations for malignant hyperthermia-susceptible adults and infants: a bench test study. *Anesth Analg*. 2014;119:67-75.

Ebo DG, Fisher MM, Hagendorens MM, et al. Anaphylaxis during anaesthesia: diagnostic approach. *Allergy*. 2007;62:471-487.

Flood P, Rathmell JP, Shafer S. *Stoelting's Pharmacology and Physiology in Anesthetic Practice*. 5th ed. Wolters Kluwer; 2014.

Fuchshuber P, Jones S, Josens D, et al. Ensuring safety in the operating room—the "fundamental use of surgical energy" (FUSE) program. *Int Anesthesiol Clin*. 2013;51:65-80.

Gaba DM, Fish KJ, Howard SN, et al. *Crisis Management in Anesthesiology*. 2nd ed. Churchill Livingstone; 2014.

Hines RL, Marschall KE. *Stoelting's Anesthesia and Co-existing Disease*. 6th ed. Saunders; 2012.

Kim TW, Nemergut ME. Preparation of modern anesthesia workstations for malignant hyperthermia-susceptible patients: a review of past and present practice. *Anesthesiology*. 2011;114:205-212.

Lobato EB, Gravenstein N, Kirby RR. *Complications in Anesthesiology*. Lippincott; 2007.

Marik PE. Aspiration pneumonitis and aspiration pneumonia. *N Engl J Med*. 2001;344: 665-671.

Marik PE, Cavallazzi R, Vasu T, et al. Dynamic changes in arterial waveform derived variables and fluid responsiveness in mechanically ventilated patients: a systematic review of the literature. *Crit Care Med*. 2009;36:2642-2647.

Simons ER, Ardusso LR, Bilo MB, et al. International consensus on (ICON) anaphylaxis. *World Allergy Organ J*. 2014;7:1-19.

Zacharias M, Mugawar M, Herbison GP, et al. Interventions for protecting renal function in the perioperative period. *Cochrane Database Syst Rev*. 2013;9:CD003590.

18 | Perioperative Hemodynamic Control

Devan Cote and William Benedetto

I. BLOOD PRESSURE

The aim of perioperative hemodynamic management strategies is to maintain adequate organ perfusion. Since organ perfusion itself is difficult to measure, systemic blood pressure is monitored as an indicator of blood flow and organ perfusion. The relationship between systemic blood pressure and systemic perfusion can be modeled by the mechanical analogue of Ohm's law: $MAP - CVP = CO \times SVR$, where MAP represents mean arterial pressure, CVP represents central venous pressure, CO represents cardiac output, and SVR represents systemic vascular resistance. By solving the equation for CO, it becomes apparent that changes in MAP do not always reflect changes in CO.

A. CO is influenced by heart rate, preload, afterload, myocardial compliance, and contractility. These variables are intimately interdependent and regulated by the autonomic nervous system and humoral factors.

II. AUTOREGULATION

Autoregulation describes the ability of an organ to maintain adequate blood flow despite varying **perfusion pressure**, the pressure gradient across an organ's vascular bed. Organs vary in autoregulatory reserve or the ability to increase or decrease vascular resistance in order to couple organ blood flow with metabolic demand. Vasodilating anesthetic agents interfere with organ autoregulation mechanisms. Accordingly, organ perfusion under anesthesia becomes more dependent on systemic blood pressure.

III. ADRENERGIC RECEPTOR PHYSIOLOGY (TABLE 18.1)

Adrenergic receptors bind **catecholamines** to mediate many physiologic functions. The endogenous catecholamines include epinephrine, norepinephrine, and dopamine. Many drugs used to control blood pressure perioperatively act on adrenergic receptors. α-adrenergic receptors are activated by norepinephrine, epinephrine, and isoproterenol in descending order of responsiveness. β-adrenergic receptors demonstrate the inverse, with the greatest activity in response to isoproterenol, followed by epinephrine, and finally norepinephrine. Receptors that interact with dopamine are termed **dopaminergic**. Adrenergic receptors can be further subdivided based on their anatomic location and downstream effects:

A. α_1-receptors are located postsynaptically in vascular smooth muscle, the uterus, skin, intestinal mucosa, iris, splanchnic bed, and myocardium. Activation causes arteriolar and venous constriction, mydriasis, and relaxation of the intestinal tract. Activation of cardiac α_1-receptors results in a mild increase in inotropy.

B. α_2-receptors exist in multiple subtypes and are found throughout the central nervous system (CNS) and autonomic nervous system, playing roles in wakefulness, attention, nociception, and autonomic modulation.

TABLE 18.1 Adrenergic Receptors and Their Effect Sites

Receptor	Site of Action	Effect	Agonists	Antagonists
α_1	Vascular smooth muscle	Inotropy	Phenylephrine[a]	Phenoxybenzamine
	Uterus	Vasoconstriction	Norepinephrine	Phentolamine
	Skin	Mydriasis	Epinephrine	Terazosin
	Intestinal mucosa	Uterine contraction	Methyldopa	Prazosin
	Iris	Sphincter constriction	Clonidine	Labetalol
	Splanchnic bed	Bronchoconstriction	Dexmedetomidine	Carvedilol
		Inhibition of insulin secretion		
α_2	Presynaptic:	Inhibit neurotransmitter release (NE, ACh, DA, 5-HT)	Dexmedetomidine	Phenoxybenzamine
	CNS	Hypnosis, sedation, analgesia	Clonidine	Phentolamine
	Adrenergic nerve terminals	↓ sympathetic tone (bradycardia, vasodilation)	Tizanidine	Labetalol
			Epinephrine	
	Postsynaptic:	Vasoconstriction	Norepinephrine	
	Vascular smooth muscle	↓ insulin release	Phenylephrine	
	Gastrointestinal tract	↓ salivation	Methyldopa	
	Pancreatic β cells	Hypnosis, sedation, analgesia		
	CNS	↓ sympathetic tone (bradycardia, vasodilation)		
β_1	Myocardium	Inotropy	Isoproterenol	Atenolol[c]
	SA node	Chronotropy	Epinephrine	Esmolol[c]
	Cardiac conduction system	Renin release	Dobutamine	Metoprolol[c]
	Kidneys	Lipolysis	Norepinephrine	Propranolol
	Adipose tissue		Dopamine	Labetalol
			Ephedrine[b]	
			Terbutaline	

Receptor	Site of Action	Effect	Agonists[a]	Antagonists
β_2	Vascular smooth muscle	Vasodilation	Isoproterenol	Labetalol
	Bronchial smooth muscle	Bronchodilation	Terbutaline	Propranolol
	Myocardium	Uterine relaxation	Epinephrine[b]	
	Uterus	Inotropy	Ephedrine[b]	
		Insulin release	Dopamine	
D_1	Renal smooth muscle	Vasodilation[d]	Fenoldopam	
	Mesenteric smooth muscle		Dopamine	
			Dopexamine	
D_2	CNS	Inhibit norepinephrine release[d]	Dopamine	
			Dopexamine	

[a]Agonists listed in descending order of effect.

[b]Primary mode of action for ephedrine is indirect stimulation of catecholamine release.

[c]Selective for β_1-receptors.

[d]Only hemodynamically significant drugs included in table.

5-HT, serotonin; ACh, acetylcholine; CNS, central nervous system; DA, dopamine; NE, norepinephrine; SA, sinoatrial.

1. **Presynaptic α_2-receptors** at peripheral adrenergic nerve terminals are involved in feedback inhibition to decrease sympathetic transmission. Their activation reduces norepinephrine release and has an overall vasodilating effect. Activation of presynaptic α_2-receptors within the CNS also inhibits the release of norepinephrine and other neurotransmitters and is associated with sedation, analgesia, and reduced sympathetic outflow, which contributes to vasodilation and bradycardia.

2. **Postsynaptic α_2-receptors** are located within the CNS and peripherally in vascular smooth muscle, the gastrointestinal (GI) tract, and pancreatic β cells. Activation of peripheral postsynaptic α_2-receptors causes vasoconstriction, decreased salivation, and decreased insulin release. Activation of central postsynaptic α_2-receptors is also associated with sedation, analgesia, and reduced sympathetic outflow.

C. **β_1-receptors** are located in the myocardium, sinoatrial (SA) node, ventricular conduction system, adipose tissue, and renal tissue. Activation increases inotropy, chronotropy, myocardial conduction velocity, renin release, and lipolysis.

D. **β_2-receptors** are located in the myocardium and smooth muscle of the vasculature, bronchi, uterus, and GI tract. Stimulation leads to vasodilation, bronchodilation, uterine relaxation, and a mild increase in inotropy. β_2-receptor activation also promotes gluconeogenesis, insulin release, and potassium uptake by cells.

E. **β_3-receptors** are involved in lipolysis and regulation of metabolic rate.

F. **Dopamine receptors** are divided into five subtypes (D_1, D_2, D_3, D_4, and D_5). These are further classified into a D_1-like family, consisting of D_1 and D_5 receptors, and a D_2-like family, consisting of D_2, D_3, and D_4 receptors.

1. **D_1-like family dopamine receptors** are mainly located postsynaptically in the peripheral nervous system and CNS. In the renal and mesenteric vascular smooth muscle cells, they directly mediate vasodilation.

2. **D_2-like family dopamine receptors** are mainly located presynaptically in the peripheral nervous system and CNS. Stimulation of some peripheral D_2-like receptors inhibits norepinephrine release, indirectly causing vasodilation.

G. **Receptor regulation.** There is an inverse relationship between exposure to circulating adrenergic agonists and adrenergic receptor availability through a process of **receptor upregulation and downregulation**. For example, chronic β-blocker therapy leads to the upregulation of β-adrenergic receptors. As a result, the sudden cessation of β-blocker therapy may be associated with hypersensitivity to endogenous catecholamines, resulting in rebound hypertension and tachycardia with increased risk for developing myocardial ischemia.

IV. ADRENERGIC AGONISTS (TABLE 18.2)

A. **α-agonists**

1. **Phenylephrine** is a direct-acting α_1-agonist at typical clinical doses of 40 to 200 μg/min. Phenylephrine causes both arterial and venous vasoconstriction. This dual action increases venous return and mean arterial blood pressure, frequently resulting in reflex bradycardia. Phenylephrine maintains CO in patients with normal myocardial function but may decrease cardiac performance in the presence of myocardial ischemia. Phenylephrine has a short duration of action, which makes it easily titratable.

2. **Midodrine** is an orally administered α_1-agonist approved for the treatment of symptomatic orthostatic hypotension at doses of 2.5 to 10 mg TID. It is a prodrug that mediates its clinical effect through its active metabolite, desglymidodrine. Midodrine is increasingly used off-label to prevent hemodialysis-related hypotension and to facilitate weaning of vasopressors in the ICU despite limited data on safety and efficacy. Mesenteric ischemia associated with midodrine administration has been reported.

3. **Clonidine** is a centrally acting antihypertensive with relative selectivity for α_2-adrenoreceptors. Its actions include reducing sympathetic tone, increasing parasympathetic tone, reducing anesthetic and analgesic requirements, causing sedation, and decreasing salivation. It may be administered intravenously, intramuscularly, orally, transcutaneously, epidurally, and intrathecally. Abrupt cessation of clonidine is associated with rebound hypertension, thus doses should be gradually tapered when discontinuing.

4. **Dexmedetomidine** is a selective α_2-adrenoreceptor agonist approved for intravenous (IV) sedation of mechanically ventilated patients in an intensive care setting. Its action on presynaptic receptors inhibits the release of norepinephrine, and its activation of postsynaptic α_2-receptors in the CNS inhibits sympathetic activity. These effects decrease blood pressure and heart rate. Dexmedetomidine offers potential advantages over other sedatives, including reduced respiratory depression, delirium, and hypotension.

B. **β-agonists (please refer to Table 18.2 for recommended dose ranges)**

1. **Isoproterenol** is a direct-acting, nonselective β-adrenergic agonist. It increases heart rate and contractility through its actions at β_1-receptors and reduces SVR through its actions on β_2-receptors. Its overall effect on CO is neutral. Other β_2-mediated effects of isoproterenol include bronchodilation and pulmonary vasodilation.

   a. **Indications**
      1. Hemodynamically significant, atropine-resistant bradycardia
      2. Atrioventricular (AV) nodal block, until temporary pacing can be instituted
      3. Maintenance of an elevated heart rate, such as in pediatric patients who have a fixed stroke volume and cardiac transplant recipients
      4. Status asthmaticus
      5. β-blocker overdose

   b. **Monitoring.** Continuous electrocardiographic monitoring is recommended with IV administration. Isoproterenol may be safely administered through a peripheral IV.

   c. **Adverse effects** include hypotension and tachydysrhythmias. Isoproterenol may contribute to an imbalance in myocardial oxygen supply and demand, leading to myocardial ischemia.

C. **Mixed agonists**

1. **Epinephrine** is a direct-acting α- and β-receptor agonist, produced by the adrenal medulla.

   a. **Indications**
      1. Cardiac arrest
      2. Anaphylaxis
      3. Bronchospasm
      4. Cardiogenic shock
      5. Symptomatic bradycardia or heart block

TABLE 18.2	Drug Dosages of Commonly Used Vasopressors and Inotropes								
		IV Infusion			**Receptor Selectivity**				
Drug Name (Trade Name)	**IV Bolus**	**Mix[a]**	**Kinetics[b]**	**Dose**	α_1	β_1	β_2	D_1	V_1
Arginine vasopressin (Pitressin)	NR	50 units/250 mL (0.2 units/mL)	O: <15 min D: 10-20 min	0.04 unit/min (range 0.01-0.1 unit/min)					+++
Dobutamine (Dobutrex)	NR	250 mg/250 mL (1000 μg/mL)	O: <10 min D: 5-10 min	2-20 μg/kg/min	+	+++	++		
Dopamine (Inotropin)	NR	200 mg/250 mL (800 μg/mL)	O: <5 min D: 5-10 min	1-5 μg/kg/min 5-10 μg/kg/min 10-20 μg/kg/min	+ +++	+ ++ ++	+ +	+++ ++ +	
Ephedrine	5-10 mg	NR	O: <5 min D: 15-20 min[c]	NR	++	++			
Epinephrine (Adrenaline)	20-100 μg (hypotension) 0.5-1 mg (cardiac arrest)	1 mg/250 mL (4 μg/mL)	O: <1 min D: 1-2 min	0.01-0.03 μg/kg/min 0.03-0.1 μg/kg/min >0.1 μg/kg/min	+ +++	++ +++ ++	+ + +		
Isoproterenol (Isuprel)	NR	1 mg/250 mL (4 μg/mL)	O: <1 min D: 10-15 min	2-10 μg/min		+++	+++		
Milrinone	NR	20 mg/100 mL (200 μg/mL)	O: 5-15 min D: 3-5 h	0.375-0.75 μg/kg/min[d]					
Norepinephrine (Levophed)	2-8 μg	4 mg/250 mL (16 μg/mL)	O: <1 min D: 1-2 min	1-30 μg/min	+++	++			
Phenylephrine (Neosynephrine)	40-100 μg	10 mg/250 mL (40 μg/mL)	O: <1 min D: 5-10 min	10-150 μg/min	+++				

[a]Massachusetts General Hospital infusion mix in 5% dextrose in water.
[b]O, onset; D, duration of action.
[c]Times given for single IV bolus dose.
[d]Optional 50 μg/kg IV load over 10 min; dosage adjustments required for renally impaired patients.
D, dopamine receptor; IV, intravenous; V, vasopressin receptor; NR, not recommended.

b. **Clinical use.** The clinical effect of epinephrine is determined by its activation of both α- and β-receptors, with β effects predominating at lower doses. At very low doses (eg, 0.01 µg/kg/min), epinephrine primarily causes bronchodilation. At usual clinical doses (0.03-0.1 µg/kg/min), epinephrine acts on α- and β-receptors to increase inotropy, chronotropy, and vasoconstriction. At even higher doses (>0.1 µg/kg/min), α effects predominate, and stroke volume may fall as SVR increases. Dose-limiting adverse effects include significant tachycardia, dysrhythmias, and myocardial ischemia. Volatile anesthetics, especially halothane, can sensitize the myocardium to circulating catecholamines leading to potentially life-threatening dysrhythmias. Epinephrine should be administered through central venous access whenever possible as extravasation may lead to tissue necrosis.

2. **Norepinephrine** is released by postganglionic sympathetic neurons and binds adrenergic receptors at target organs. Biosynthetically, it is the precursor of epinephrine. Norepinephrine is a potent α_1- and β_1-receptor agonist, with α effects predominating at lower doses. Compared to epinephrine, norepinephrine has minimal effects on β_2-receptors. Norepinephrine increases blood pressure by increasing SVR. However, organ perfusion may suffer despite increases in MAP due to increased vascular resistance across organs. CO remains relatively unchanged. As with most vasoactive agents, intra-arterial blood pressure monitoring and continuous cardiac rhythm monitoring are recommended. In most cases, norepinephrine should be administered centrally, although dilute concentrations (eg, 16 µg/mL) may be safely administered through reliable peripheral access temporarily. Adverse effects include arrhythmias and worsening microvascular perfusion (eg, digital ischemia), particularly at higher doses.

3. **Dopamine,** the biosynthetic precursor of norepinephrine, produces a dose-related combination of α-, β-, and dopamine receptor effects. It also causes the release of norepinephrine from nerve terminals in the heart. At lower doses (<5 µg/kg/min), dopamine primarily activates renal and splanchnic vessel D_1 receptors, resulting in increased renal blood flow, glomerular filtration, and sodium excretion. Although dopamine administration often increases urine output, it has not been shown to improve mortality outcomes or need for renal replacement therapy. At 5 to 10 µg/kg/min, β effects become more apparent, leading to increases in myocardial contractility, heart rate, and arterial blood pressure. At high doses (>10 µg/kg/min), α_1 effects predominate, leading to marked increases in arterial and venous blood pressure and decreases in renal blood flow. Dopamine is used in the management of cardiogenic shock, vasodilatory shock, heart failure, and refractory bradycardia. Adverse effects include tachycardia, ventricular arrhythmias, increased myocardial oxygen consumption, and profound vasoconstriction.

4. **Dobutamine** is a synthetic catecholamine available clinically as a racemic mixture of stereoisomers with the L(−)-isomer stimulating α_1-receptors and the D(+)-isomer stimulating β_1- and β_2-receptors. Through its effect on cardiac β_1-receptors, dobutamine increases myocardial contractility and chronotropy. In the peripheral vasculature, dobutamine generally has a vasodilatory effect owing to its more dominant β_2 action, despite its α_1 properties. Dobutamine is a useful agent for treating low CO states caused by acute myocardial infarction, cardiomyopathy, and myocardial depression after cardiac surgery. Dobutamine typically

reduces or has a neutral effect on pulmonary vascular resistance (PVR), which may be beneficial for patients with right ventricular failure. Systemic hypotension, increased myocardial oxygen consumption, and tachydysrhythmias are the most common side effects.

5. **Ephedrine** is a noncatecholamine, indirect adrenergic agonist that causes the release of norepinephrine and other endogenous catecholamines stored within nerve terminals. It is used primarily in the management of anesthetic-related hypotension and bradycardia. Administration is limited to intermittent boluses as tachyphylaxis develops quickly.

V. NONADRENERGIC AGENTS
A. Nonadrenergic vasopressors
1. **Arginine vasopressin (AVP)** is a synthetic analogue of antidiuretic hormone. AVP causes vasoconstriction by direct stimulation of vascular smooth muscle V_1 receptors. It is frequently used as a second pressor in septic shock requiring high-dose norepinephrine, although a mortality benefit has not been demonstrated. It may also be beneficial as a low-dose (0.04 unit/min) IV infusion in vasodilatory shock exacerbated by chronic angiotensin-converting enzyme (ACE) inhibitor therapy. AVP may be preferred in the setting of pulmonary hypertension as it preferentially constricts peripheral vasculature while sparing the pulmonary vasculature. AVP has a rapid onset with a duration of action of 10 to 20 minutes. Administration through a central venous catheter is recommended.

2. **Methylene blue** is used therapeutically as a redox agent in the treatment of methemoglobinemia (1 mg/kg IV over 5 minutes) and used diagnostically as an indicator dye in urologic surgery to assess the integrity of the urinary system. Methylene blue competitively inhibits guanylate cyclase, which decreases the production of cyclic guanosine monophosphate (cGMP), and renders the vascular endothelium less sensitive to cGMP-mediated vasodilators including **nitric oxide**. Methylene blue has been effective in the management of vasoplegia associated with cardiopulmonary bypass (eg, slow bolus of 2 mg/kg followed by an infusion of 0.5 mg/kg/h for 12 hours). As a reversible inhibitor of monoamine oxidase, methylene blue must be used with caution in patients on serotonergic medications including selective serotonin reuptake inhibitors, serotonin and norepinephrine reuptake inhibitors, and monoamine oxidase inhibitors, as fatal cases of serotonin syndrome have been reported. Other adverse effects include dysrhythmias, increased PVR, coronary vasoconstriction, and acute hemolytic anemia in patients with glucose-6-phosphate dehydrogenase deficiency. Administration of methylene blue may produce falsely low readings on pulse oximetry.

B. Nonadrenergic inotropes
1. **Cardiac glycosides** were the first inotropes to be used clinically. They are naturally occurring compounds found in plants (eg, foxgloves). Within this family of drugs, **digoxin** remains in clinical use today. The inotropic effect of digoxin derives from inhibition of the sodium-potassium ATPase, secondarily promoting an influx of calcium into cardiac myocytes via the sodium-calcium exchanger. It additionally has a direct suppressive effect on the AV node. Therapeutically, digoxin is reserved for rate control refractory to β-blockers and for refractory chronic heart failure symptoms despite maximal medical management. Its use is

limited by its narrow therapeutic window, many drug interactions, and lack of mortality benefit. Perioperatively, digoxin should be continued for patients on a stable regimen.

2. **Phosphodiesterase III inhibitors.** Inamrinone, milrinone, and enoximone are synthetic, noncatecholamine, nonglycosidic, bipyridine derivatives. They act by inhibiting type III phosphodiesterase (PDE3), thereby increasing cyclic adenosine monophosphate, leading to increased contractility and peripheral vasodilation. PDE3 inhibitors are synergistic with adrenergic agents.

   a. **Inamrinone** (name changed from amrinone to prevent confusion with amiodarone) was the first drug in the PDE3 inhibitor class. It is an inotrope and vasodilator that produces a dose-dependent improvement in cardiac index, left ventricular work index, and ejection fraction with a neutral effect on heart rate and MAP. Its clinical use was limited by thrombocytopenia and GI side effects and fell out of favor with the advent of its successor.

   b. **Milrinone** is a derivative of inamrinone with the same hemodynamic profile, yet 20 times more potent than its predecessor and with a more tolerable side effect profile. Typical dosing involves a loading dose of 50 µg/kg administered over 10 minutes followed by an infusion of 0.375 to 0.75 µg/kg/min. Adverse effects include hypotension, ventricular arrhythmias, cardiac ischemia, and torsades de pointes. Its prolonged elimination half-life of 2 to 4 hours requires that it be introduced with caution in unstable patients. Coadministration with a vasopressor is often necessary to counter vasodilation. Milrinone is frequently used for inotropic support after cardiac surgery.

   c. **Enoximone** is an orally available imidazolone derivative. At low doses (25-50 mg three times daily), it improves the exercise capacity of patients with chronic heart failure.

3. **Levosimendan** is a **calcium-sensitizing agent** that acts as a positive inotrope and a vasodilator. It sensitizes myofilaments to calcium through direct binding to cardiac troponin C, and it achieves vasodilation by facilitating the opening of ATP-dependent potassium channels. Despite achieving inotropy without increasing myocardial oxygen consumption, levosimendan has not demonstrated a mortality benefit over adrenergic agents in the treatment of acute decompensated low output heart failure. In cardiac surgical populations, levosimendan has not shown any mortality benefit. Despite its use in over 60 countries, levosimendan has not been approved for use in the United States or Canada. Adverse effects include hypotension, arrhythmias, myocardial ischemia, and hypokalemia.

VI. β-ADRENERGIC ANTAGONISTS (TABLE 18.3)

A. **β-blockers** are a mainstay of the perioperative management of sinus tachycardia, other tachyarrhythmias, hypertension, myocardial infarction, and heart failure. They can be distinguished by their adrenergic receptor selectivity and intrinsic sympathomimetic activity.

1. According to the 2014 American College of Cardiology and American Heart Association guidelines on the management of patients undergoing noncardiac surgery, patients should continue chronic β-blocker perioperatively as abrupt β-blocker cessation may be associated with increased adverse cardiac events. Preoperative initiation of β-blocker therapy may also be considered in patients with three or more revised

TABLE 18.3 β-Adrenergic Antagonists							
Drug Name (Trade Name)	**β_1-Selective**	**α_1-Blockade**	**Bioavailability**	**Half-Life**	**Elimination**	**Oral Dose**	**IV Dose**
Atenolol (Tenormin)	+	–	–	6-7 h	R (85%)	50-100 mg daily	5 mg q10min up to 10 mg total[a]
Esmolol (Brevibloc)	+	–	–	9 min	RBC esterase	–	1 mg/kg bolus; 50-200 µg/kg/min[b]
Metoprolol (Lopressor)	+	–	50%	3-4 h	H	25-100 mg q6h[c]	2.5-5 mg q5min up to 15 mg total
Carvedilol (Coreg)	–	+	30%	7-10 h	H	6.25-50 mg q12h	–
Labetalol (Trandate, Normodyne)	–	+	25%	3-8 h	H	100-800 mg q12h-q8h	5-20 mg initial bolus redosing 20-80 mg q10min up to 300 mg daily
Nadolol (Corgard)	–	–	30%	14-24 h	R (75%)	40-320 mg daily	–
Propranolol (Inderal)	–	–	30%-50%	3-6 h	H	10-40 mg q12h-q8h	0.25- to 1-mg increments
Timolol (Blocadren)	–	–	75%	2-4 h	H (80%)	5-20 mg q12h	NA

[a]Not available in the United States.
[b]Optional 0.25 to 0.5 mg/kg load prior to infusion.
[c]Dosing for metoprolol tartrate.
H, hepatic elimination; IV, intravenous; R, renal elimination; RBC, red blood cell.

cardiac risk index risk factors, which include prior stroke (or transient ischemic attack), diabetes mellitus requiring insulin, serum creatinine ≥2 mg/dL, congestive heart failure, coronary artery disease, and high-risk surgery (thoracic, abdominal, or suprainguinal vascular surgery). Both of these guidelines are supported by level B evidence.

2. β-blockers are contraindicated in patients with severe decompensated heart failure, symptomatic bradycardia in the absence of a pacemaker, and in patients with Wolff-Parkinson-White (WPW) syndrome in atrial fibrillation.

B. **Propranolol** is a nonselective β_1- and β_2-adrenergic receptor antagonist available in both IV and oral forms. Propranolol is highly lipophilic, almost entirely absorbed following oral administration, and undergoes up to 75% first-pass clearance by the liver. Hemodynamic effects of propranolol and other β-adrenergic antagonists are secondary to the reduction of CO and suppression of the renin-angiotensin system. Owing to their β_2-blocking action, nonselective β-blockers may induce bronchoconstriction in patients with asthma and chronic obstructive pulmonary disease, though studies have shown that this concern is largely theoretical.

C. **Metoprolol** is a selective β_1-adrenergic receptor antagonist available in both oral and IV forms. It is used to treat supraventricular tachycardia (SVT), such as for rate control of atrial fibrillation. It is also effective in the treatment of angina pectoris, in reducing mortality from myocardial infarction and heart failure, and in treating mild hypertension.

D. **Esmolol** is a selective β_1-adrenergic receptor antagonist that is metabolized rapidly by esterases within red blood cells. These esterases are distinct from plasma pseudocholinesterase and are not affected by anticholinesterases. Esmolol has a rapid onset and short duration of action, achieving its peak effect in 5 minutes with an elimination half-life of 9 minutes. These favorable kinetics make it a commonly used drug perioperatively. Prolonged infusions of esmolol in propylene glycol may lead to propylene glycol toxicity marked by encephalopathy and osmolal gap with or without an anion gap metabolic acidosis.

E. **Labetalol** is a combined α- and β-adrenergic receptor antagonist with a β- to α-adrenergic receptor blockade ratio of 3:1 when administered orally and 7:1 when administered intravenously. Its combined effect on both α- and β-receptors leads to decreased blood pressure without reflex tachycardia. Labetalol also decreases PVR and minimally affects CO. Labetalol is useful in the treatment of acute perioperative hypertension due to its rapid onset within 2 to 5 minutes. It is effective in the management of hypertension related to pregnancy, pheochromocytoma, and clonidine withdrawal.

VII. VASODILATORS (TABLE 18.4)

A. **Calcium channel antagonists,** or **calcium channel blockers (CCBs)**, bind L-type calcium channels that regulate calcium entry into vascular smooth muscle, myocardial cells, and cardiac pacemaker cells. They decrease the vascular resistance of peripheral organs, cause coronary artery vasodilation, and are myocardial depressants. CCBs are distinguished by their relative affinities for cardiac versus vascular L-type calcium channels.

1. **Dihydropyridine (DHP)** CCBs are more selective for vascular smooth muscle and are used to treat hypertension. Their physiologic effect is largely arterial vasodilation with minimal effects on venous capacitance.

a. **Clevidipine** is an ultrashort-acting antihypertensive administered by IV infusion ideal for perioperative use due to its rapid onset, titration, and elimination half-life of approximately 1 minute by serum esterases. After cessation, effects last 5 to 10 minutes, with a 90% return to baseline blood pressure by 7 minutes. Infusions are started at 1 to 2 mg/h and doubled every 90 seconds until blood pressure approaches target range. Usual doses are 4 to 8 mg/h. The maximum allowable dose is 21 mg/h.

b. **Nicardipine** is another short-acting antihypertensive administered in IV infusion perioperatively. Infusions are started at 5 mg/h, increased by 2.5 mg/h every 5 to 15 min until target blood pressure is reached, up to a maximum dose of 15 mg/h. Onset is within minutes. After cessation, effects may last up to 8 hours.

c. **Nifedipine** is limited to oral administration for the treatment of hypertension, including hypertension associated with pregnancy, at daily doses of 30 to 90 mg.

d. **Nimodipine** is an oral CCB approved for the prevention of vasospasm in subarachnoid hemorrhage at a dose of 60 mg q4h. Dose reductions are required in hepatic insufficiency.

e. **Amlodipine** is a common oral antihypertensive at daily doses of 5 to 10 mg.

2. **Non-DHP** CCBs are more selective for myocardial and pacemaker L-type calcium channels and are termed **cardioselective**. Verapamil and diltiazem are the two non-DHP CCBs in clinical use.

TABLE 18.4 Vasodilator Infusions

Drug Name (Trade Name)	IV Infusion			Mechanism of Action
	Mix[a]	Kinetics[b]	Dose	
Clevidipine (Cleviprex)	25 mg/50 mL lipid emulsion (0.5 mg/mL)[c]	O: 2-4 min D: 5-10 min	Initial: 1-2 mg/h[d] Usual: 4-8 mg/h	CCB; arterial > venous vasodilation
Nicardipine (Cardene)	40 mg/200 mL (0.2 mg/mL)[c]	O: 5-10 min D: 0.5-8 h	Initial: 5 mg/h[e] Usual: 5-15 mg/h	CCB; arterial > venous vasodilation
Nitroglycerin	50 mg/250 mL (400 µg/mL)	O: 1 min D: 5 min	Initial: 50 µg/min[f] IV bolus: 50-100 µg	NO; venodilation
Nitroprusside (Nipride)	50 mg/250 mL (200 µg/mL)	O: 1-2 min D: 5-10 min	Initial: 0.5 µg/kg/min[f] Usual: 0.5-4 µg/kg/min	NO; arterial > venous vasodilation
Fenoldopam (Corlopam)	10 mg/250 mL (40 µg/mL)	O: 5-10 min D: 1-4 h	Initial: 0.05 µg/kg/min[g] Usual: 0.05-1.5 µg/kg/min	D_1-agonism; arteriodilation

[a]Infusion mix in 5% dextrose in water unless otherwise specified.
[b]O, onset; D, duration of action.
[c]Manufacturer preparation.
[d]Double dose every 90 seconds until approaching blood pressure goal, up to maximum 21 mg/h.
[e]Increase dose by 2.5 mg/h every 5 to 15 min, up to maximum 15 mg/h.
[f]Increase dose every 5 min based on patient responsiveness, up to maximum dose of 400 µg/min.
[g]Increase dose by 0.05 to 0.1 µg/kg/min every 15 minutes, up to a maximum of 1.5 µg/kg/min.
CCB, calcium channel blocker; D_1, dopamine-1 receptor; NO, nitric oxide; NR, not recommended.

    a. Indications

       1. Antianginal therapy (by decreasing myocardial oxygen consumption and coronary vasospasm)

       2. Rate control (by depressing AV nodal conduction)

       3. Conversion of hemodynamically stable SVTs (by prolonging AV nodal repolarization, blocking reentry)

       4. Hypertension (by effecting vascular smooth muscle L-type calcium channels)

    b. Contraindications to CCBs are similar to those of β-blockers. CCBs are not appropriate antiarrhythmics for patients with WPW syndrome in atrial fibrillation/flutter, as they may allow for preferential conduction through the accessory pathway.

    c. Verapamil is initially dosed 2.5 to 5 mg IV over 2 minutes, with subsequent doses of 5 to 10 mg IV every 15 to 30 minutes.

    d. Diltiazem is initially dosed 10 to 20 mg IV over 2 minutes, which can be redosed up to 0.35 mg/kg after 15 minutes if needed. An infusion of 5 to 15 mg/h can be initiated in responders.

B. Sodium nitroprusside is a direct-acting vasodilator that acts on arterial and venous smooth muscle, reducing afterload through arteriolar dilation and reducing preload through venous dilation. Both SVR and PVR decrease.

    1. Mechanism of action. Nitroprusside decomposes to release **nitric oxide**, an endogenous vasodilator that activates guanylate cyclase, which increases cGMP, and leads to smooth muscle relaxation.

    2. Dosing. Infusions may be started at 0.5 µg/kg/min and titrated upward based on blood pressure response every 5 minutes up to a maximum per-minute dose of 400 µg/min (note: not weight-based).

    3. Kinetics. Nitroprusside is useful perioperatively because it has a fast onset within 2 minutes and its effects dissipate within 2 minutes of discontinuation.

    4. Adverse effects

       a. Reflex tachycardia. Nitroprusside's reduction of preload and afterload typically causes a reflex increase in heart rate and myocardial contractility and an increase in CO.

       b. Increased intracranial pressure (ICP). Nitroprusside dilates cerebral blood vessels and should be used with caution in patients with elevated ICP.

       c. Vascular steal phenomenon. Global vasodilation may give rise to unintentional imbalances in blood flow. Under normal conditions, ischemic regions are vasodilated by metabolic factors in order to maximize blood supply. Vascular steal phenomenon results when blood supply to a vasodilated ischemic region gets shunted to newly dilated nonischemic regions. This is of particular importance in the coronary vasculature where regional ischemia may be exacerbated by vasodilator-related steal, even when afterload reduction reduces overall myocardial oxygen consumption.

       d. Cyanide toxicity. Nitroprusside reacts nonenzymatically with sulfhydryl groups in hemoglobin to release five cyanide radicals. Cyanide toxicity results when cyanide radicals bind cytochrome oxidase, disrupting the electron transport chain, leading to cellular hypoxia and death even in the presence of oxygen. Cyanide radicals can be converted by tissue and liver rhodanese to thiocyanate, which is excreted in the urine. Thiocyanate accumulation in renal insufficiency can cause **thiocyanate toxicity**, which is characterized by abdominal pain, vomiting, and altered mental status.

1. **Clinical features.** Symptoms of cyanide toxicity include fatigue, nausea, muscle spasms, angina, and confusion. Cyanide toxicity typically occurs when more than 1 mg/kg sodium nitroprusside has been administered within 2.5 hours or when the blood concentration of cyanide reaches 100 µg/dL. Metabolic acidosis and elevated mixed venous oxygen tensions are early signs of cyanide toxicity.

2. **Treatment.** Sodium thiosulfate is a sulfur donor in the rhodanese reaction that converts cyanide to thiocyanate. After discontinuing nitroprusside and administering 100% oxygen, 150 mg/kg **sodium thiosulfate** should be administered over 15 minutes. Severe cyanide toxicity (base deficit >10 mEq, hemodynamic instability) may require the additional administration of **amyl nitrate** (0.3 mL by inhalation) or 3% **sodium nitrite** (5 mg/kg IV over 5 minutes). These two compounds create methemoglobin, which binds cyanide ion to form inactive cyanmethemoglobin.

C. **Nitroglycerin,** also known as trinitroglycerin, is a potent venodilator that also relaxes arterial, pulmonary, ureteral, uterine, GI, and bronchial smooth muscles. It mediates its effect via conversion to nitric oxide. Nitroglycerin decreases MAP primarily by increasing venous capacitance.

1. **Indications.** Nitroglycerin is useful for treating congestive heart failure and myocardial ischemia by increasing coronary flow and improving left ventricular performance. Nitroglycerin increases venous capacitance, decreases venous return, and consequently decreases ventricular end-diastolic volume. A decrease in end-diastolic volume is associated with a decrease in ventricular wall tension, which reduces myocardial oxygen consumption.

2. **Dosing.** Nitroglycerin can be administered as an IV bolus of 50 to 100 µg. The effects of a single bolus disappear within 5 minutes. An initial test dose of 50 µg or less is often useful to gauge patient responsiveness, which varies widely. Infusions may be started conservatively at 50 µg/min and titrated based on patient responsiveness every 5 minutes up to a maximum dose of 400 µg/min. Nitroglycerin is also available in oral, sublingual, and transdermal routes.

3. **Reflex tachycardia** frequently occurs and must be treated with β-blockers to avoid increasing myocardial oxygen consumption.

4. **Tachyphylaxis** often develops within 24 hours of continuous infusion.

5. **Complications.** Nitroglycerin is metabolized by the liver and has no known toxicity in the clinical dose range. High doses (>250 µg/min) and prolonged continuous use may produce methemoglobinemia. Nitroglycerin produces cerebral vasodilation and should be used with caution in patients at risk for elevated ICP.

D. **Hydralazine** is a direct-acting vasodilator that reduces arteriolar tone in the coronary, cerebral, renal, uterine, and splanchnic beds. It is commonly used to treat hypertensive emergencies or to augment the effect of other hypotensive agents.

1. **Reflex tachycardia.** The vasodilation induced by hydralazine triggers a reflex increase in heart rate and causes activation of the renin-angiotensin system. These effects can be attenuated by the concomitant use of a β-blocker.

2. **Dosing.** Hydralazine can be administered as an IV bolus of 5 to 20 mg.

3. **Kinetics and pitfalls.** Hydralazine's IV time to peak effect is 20 minutes, thus a reasonable initial bolus of 5 to 10 mg can be redosed in 20

minutes if blood pressure remains elevated. With its relatively longer elimination half-life of 3 to 7 hours, a single dose of hydralazine may act for up to 12 hours. Owing to its delayed onset, hydralazine can easily be dosed in excess of intention, resulting in hours of unwanted hypotension.

E. **Enalaprilat,** an active metabolite of enalapril, is currently the only ACE inhibitor available for IV use. It reduces systolic and diastolic blood pressure by inhibiting the conversion of angiotensin I to angiotensin II.

1. **Kinetics.** It has an onset of action of approximately 15 minutes, peak effect of 1 to 4 hours, and overall duration of action of about 4 hours. Elimination is primarily renal.

2. **Contraindications.** ACE inhibitors interfere with renal autoregulation and must be used with caution in patients with renal dysfunction.

F. **Fenoldopam** is a synthetic dopamine (D_1) receptor agonist that acts by selective dilation of arterial beds while maintaining renal perfusion.

1. **Uses.** A continuous IV infusion may be used perioperatively for the management of severe hypertension in patients with impaired renal function.

2. **Evidence.** Despite reducing the incidence of postoperative acute kidney injury (AKI), fenoldopam has not been shown to improve mortality or need for renal replacement therapy.

3. **Dosing.** "Renal dose" fenoldopam at 0.1 μg/kg/min has diuretic and natriuretic properties that increase renal blood flow without greatly effecting systemic blood pressure. For hypertension, it can be dosed up to 0.3 μg/kg/min.

4. **Kinetics.** Onset is within 5 to 15 minutes, and the dose should be adjusted every 15 to 20 minutes until optimal blood pressure control is achieved.

5. **Adverse effects** include dose-dependent tachycardia and occasional hypokalemia. Hypotension may occur with concomitant use of β-adrenergic receptor blockade.

G. **Adenosine** is a nucleoside that, in high doses, has inhibitory effects on cardiac impulse conduction through the AV node.

1. **Clinical uses**

a. Adenosine's ability to slow conduction through the AV node aids in diagnosing and treating SVT.

b. The transient asystole and hypotension from an adenosine bolus facilitate clipping of cerebral aneurysms by decompressing the aneurysm and improving visualization.

c. Adenosine dilates coronary arteries. Infusions of adenosine take advantage of coronary steal in pharmacologic stress testing to diagnose myocardial perfusion defects. Regadenoson (Lexiscan) is a more stable analogue of adenosine, which is commonly used for this purpose as a bolus dose of 0.4 mg.

2. **Dosing.** Because of rapid degradation by the vascular endothelium, adenosine boluses must be rapidly delivered and followed by flushes. The starting dose is 6 mg, which may be followed by up to two 12 mg boluses, if ineffective.

3. **Precautions.** Adenosine may induce acute myocardial ischemia, prolonged sinus pauses, and bradyarrhythmias, thus application of pads for transcutaneous pacing and defibrillation is recommended.

4. **Contraindications.** Adenosine should be avoided in patients with WPW syndrome in atrial fibrillation/flutter as it may allow for preferential conduction through the accessory pathway.

H. α-adrenergic antagonists
1. **Phentolamine** is a short-acting selective α-adrenergic receptor antagonist that causes predominantly arterial vasodilation.
   a. **Dosing.** It is used in 5 mg IV boluses to treat states of hypertension and catecholamine excess (eg, pheochromocytoma). It is additionally used for local infiltration to prevent tissue necrosis after extravasation of norepinephrine, phenylephrine, dopamine, or epinephrine (5-10 mg diluted in 10 mL of saline).
   b. **Kinetics.** Systemic doses have a rapid onset within 2 minutes and may last up to 30 minutes.
2. **Phenoxybenzamine** is an irreversible, long-acting α-adrenergic receptor antagonist approved for the preoperative management of patients with pheochromocytoma. While it effectively prevents intraoperative hypertension in patients with pheochromocytoma, postoperative hypotension is common given its long duration of action of up to a few days.
3. Selective α_1-adrenergic receptor antagonists including **tamsulosin, terazosin,** and **doxazosin** are used to induce prostatic smooth muscle relaxation in the management of benign prostatic hyperplasia. Orthostatic hypotension is an adverse effect common to this class of drugs.

I. Pulmonary vasodilators are used to treat pulmonary hypertension and right ventricular failure.
1. **Prostaglandin E$_1$ (alprostadil)** is a stable metabolite of arachidonic acid that causes peripheral and pulmonary vasodilation (Appendix I).
2. **Epoprostenol (Veletri, Flolan)** is a prostacyclin (PGI$_2$) analogue with vasodilating and antiplatelet effects (Appendix I).
3. **Inhaled nitric oxide** selectively delivers vasodilating nitric oxide to ventilated areas to improve V/Q matching, whereas systemic nitric oxide donors such as nitroprusside and nitroglycerin result in unselective pulmonary vasodilation.
4. **Sildenafil** is a selective phosphodiesterase-5 inhibitor that decreases cGMP degradation, increasing pulmonary levels of nitric oxide. It has been shown to improve exercise capacity and hemodynamics in patients with pulmonary hypertension.
5. **Bosentan** is an oral endothelin receptor antagonist that competitively blocks the binding of endothelin, a potent pulmonary vasoconstrictor. It is approved for pulmonary arterial hypertension.

VIII. CONTROLLED HYPOTENSION
Controlled hypotension (known alternatively as induced, permissive, and deliberate hypotension) is a technique used to improve surgical operating conditions by improving visualization in microsurgery (eg, middle ear, cerebral aneurysm clipping, and plastic surgery) or reduce the need for transfusion in orthopedic surgery or in patients with rare blood groups or religious objections to transfusion. While this technique was first described in the 1940s, there is a paucity of data to support or refute this hemodynamic technique as efficacious.
A. Patient selection. This technique is not appropriate for patients at risk for ischemia, including those with vascular insufficiency to vital organs, cardiac instability, uncontrolled hypertension, anemia, or hypovolemia. It should be utilized with caution as serious complications, while rare in healthy patients, include cerebral infarction, myocardial infarction, and AKI.
B. Hemodynamic goals. It is acceptable to target a MAP goal of around 30% below a patient's baseline, given that it is no lower than 50 mm Hg in an otherwise healthy patient or lower than 80 mmHg in an elderly patient.

C. Techniques. Hypotension can be achieved using neuraxial blockade, high concentrations of volatile anesthetics, potent short-acting opioids (eg, remifentanil), and peripheral vasodilators (eg, nitroprusside or nitroglycerin).

IX. DRUG DOSAGE CALCULATIONS

Drug concentrations must frequently be converted between various units of measurement prior to administration.

A. A drug concentration expressed as Z % contains

Z mg/dL = Z g/100 mL = $(10 \times Z)$ g/L = $(10 \times Z)$ mg/mL

Example: A 2.5% solution of sodium thiopental is equivalent to 25 g/L or 25 mg/mL.

B. A drug concentration that is expressed as a ratio is converted as follows:

1:1000 = 1 g/1000 mL = 1 mg/mL

1:10,000 = 1 g/10,000 mL = 0.1 mg/mL

1:100,000 = 1 g/100,000 mL = 0.01 mg/mL

C. Continuous drug infusions in 250 mL can be calculated based on a simple formula:

Z mg/250 mL = Z μg/min at an infusion rate of 15 mL/h

Standard drug mixes in use at Massachusetts General Hospital are shown in **Table 18.1**. The desired rate of infusion for any drug is easily calculated as a fraction or multiple of 15 mL/h.

Example: An 80-kg patient needs dopamine at 5 μg/kg/min. What is the infusion rate in mL/h using the standard MGH mix?

Desired rate in μg/min: 5 μg/kg/min × 80 kg = 400 μg/min

Find Z: There is 200 mg dopamine in the 250 mL solution. Thus, 200 μg/min = 15 mL/h

Desired rate in mL/h: 400/200 × 15 mL/h = 30 mL/h

Suggested Readings

Barak M, Yoav L, Abu el-Naaj I. Hypotensive anesthesia versus normotensive anesthesia during major maxillofacial surgery: a review of the literature. *Sci World J.* 2015; 2015:1-7.

Cardenas-garcia J, Schaub KF, Belchikov YG, Narasimhan M, Koenig SJ, Mayo PH. Safety of peripheral intravenous administration of vasoactive medication. *J Hosp Med.* 2015;10(9):581-585.

De Backer D, Biston P, Devriendt J, et al. Comparison of dopamine and norepinephrine in the treatment of shock. *N Engl J Med.* 2010;362(9):779-789.

Espinosa A, Ripollés-Melchor J, Casans-Francés R, et al. Perioperative use of clevidipine: a systematic review and meta-analysis. *PLoS One.* 2016;11(3):e0150625.

Fleisher LA, Fleischmann KE, Auerbach AD, et al. 2014 ACC/AHA guideline on perioperative cardiovascular evaluation and management of patients undergoing noncardiac surgery. Executive summary: a report of the American College of Cardiology/American Heart Association Task Force on Practice Guidelines. *Circulation.* 2014;130(24):2215-2245.

Jadadzadeh M, Hosseini SH, Mostafavi Pour Manshadi SM, et al. Effect of milrinone on short term outcome of patients with myocardial dysfunction undergoing off-pump coronary artery bypass graft: a randomized clinical trial. *Acta Med Iran.* 2013;51(10):681-686.

Lawson N, Meyer D. Autonomic nervous system: physiology and pharmacology. In: Barash PG, Cullen BF, Stoelting RK, eds. *Clinical Anesthesia.* 3rd ed. Lippincott-Raven Publishers; 1997:243-309.

Morozowich ST, Ramakrishna H. Pharmacologic agents for acute hemodynamic instability: recent advances in the management of perioperative shock – a systematic review. *Ann Card Anaesth.* 2015;18(4):543-554.

Onwochei DN, Ngan Kee WD, Fung L, Downey K, Ye XY, Carvalho JCA. Norepinephrine intermittent intravenous boluses to prevent hypotension during spinal anesthesia for cesarean delivery: a sequential allocation dose-finding study. *Anesth Analg.* 2017;125(1):212-218.

Rhodes A, Evans LE, Alhazzani W, et al. Surviving Sepsis Campaign. International Guidelines for Management of Sepsis and Septic Shock: 2016. *Intensive Care Med.* 2017;43(3):304-377.

Rizvi MS, Trivedi V, Nasim F, et al. Trends in use of midodrine in the ICU: a single-center retrospective case series. *Crit Care Med.* 2018;46(7):e628-e633.

Rodriquez MA, Kumar SK, De Caro M. Hypertensive crisis. *Cardiol Rev.* 2010;18(2):102-107.

Russell JA, Walley KR, Singer J, et al. Vasopressin versus norepinephrine infusion in patients with septic shock. *N Engl J Med.* 2008;358(9):877-887.

Santillo E, Migale M, Massini C, Incalzi RA. Levosimendan for perioperative cardioprotection: myth or reality? *Curr Cardiol Rev.* 2018;14(3):142-152.

Unverzagt S, Wachsmuth L, Hirsch K, et al. Inotropic agents and vasodilator strategies for acute myocardial infarction complicated by cardiogenic shock or low cardiac output syndrome. *Cochrane Database Syst Rev.* 2014;1:CD009669.

Wachter SB, Gilbert EM. Beta-adrenergic receptors, from their discovery and characterization through their manipulation to beneficial clinical application. *Cardiology.* 2012;122(2):104-112.

Local Anesthetics

Michael R. Fettiplace and Xiaodong Bao

I. GENERAL PRINCIPLES

A. **History:** Clinical local anesthetics refer almost exclusively to the ester and amide-linked **sodium channel blockers** synthesized from the benzoate ring of **cocaine** isolated from the coca plant of Peru. Other sodium channel blockers exist, but unless otherwise specified (in Chapter 19, Section IV.A) "local anesthetics" refers to the cocaine derivatives.

B. **Chemistry.** Local anesthetics are composed of a terminal amine attached to an aromatic ring via an ester or amide linkage, with both charged (protonated) and uncharged (unprotonated) forms at physiologic pH~7.4). Only uncharged moieties cross the lipid bilayer to block open-state sodium channels with stronger bases (eg, chloroprocaine pK_a 9.2) taking longer to take effect than weaker bases (eg, lidocaine pK_a 7.2). **Amide local anesthetics are preferred given their lower allogenicity and longer half-life.**

   1. **Esters.** Benzocaine, cocaine, chloroprocaine, procaine, and tetracaine. The ester linkage is cleaved by pseudocholinesterase. The half-life in the circulation is very short (about 1 minute). The degradation product of ester metabolism is p-aminobenzoic acid (PABA).

   2. **Amides.** Bupivacaine, etidocaine, lidocaine, mepivacaine, prilocaine, and ropivacaine. The amide linkage is cleaved through initial N-dealkylation followed by hydrolysis, which occurs primarily in the liver. The elimination half-life for most amide local anesthetics is 2 to 3 hours. In particular, **the elimination half-life of lidocaine is 90 to 120 minutes and it will remain in circulation for a prolonged period following cessation of intravenous infusions.**

C. **Mechanism of action**

   1. **Local anesthetics block nerve conduction** by impairing the propagation of the action potentials in axons. They do not alter the resting or threshold potentials but decrease the rate of increase of the action potential so that the threshold potential is not reached.

   2. **Local anesthetics inhibit specific receptors:** The therapeutic target of local anesthetics is the **voltage-gated Na^+ channel (NaV)**, inhibiting Na^+ ion influx. The charged form of the local anesthetic binds the intracellular pore of NaV. To access the intracellular portion, the uncharged molecule must traverse the lipid bilayer through passive nonionic diffusion. Local anesthetics also block other ionic channels (K^+, Ca^{2+}, etc.) and metabotropic channels; they also uncouple mitochondrial energy production and prevent excitation-contraction coupling in muscle.

   3. **Physiochemical properties** of the local anesthetics affect neural blockade.

      a. **Lipid solubility.** Defined by the **octanol/water coefficient (LogP)** with more lipophilic molecules exhibiting increased potency and prolonged duration of action since they take longer to unbind from channels.

      b. **Protein binding.** More protein binding prolongs the duration of the effect.

TABLE 19.1	Classification of Nerve Fibers			
Class	Myelin	Diameter (μm)	Local Anesthetic Sensitivity	Function
A-α	+++	12-20	++	Motor
A-β	+++	5-12	++	Touch/pressure
A-γ	++	1-4	+++	Proprioception/motor tone
A-δ	++	1-4	+++	Pain/temperature
B	+	1-3	++	Preganglionic autonomic
C	−	0.5-1	+	Pain/temperature

    c. pK$_a$. Agents with a lower pK$_a$ value will set up faster since a greater fraction of the drug will exist in the uncharged form, ready to diffuse across nerve membranes.

    d. pH of the drug solution. Higher pH will speed up the onset by increasing the proportion of molecules in the uncharged form.

    e. Drug concentration. Higher concentrations speed up onset owing to mass effect.

4. Differential blockade of nerve fibers

    a. Peripheral nerves are classified according to size and function (**Table 19.1**). Local anesthetics block conduction based on the number of NaV channels, with thin and myelinated fibers more susceptible to blockade than thick and unmyelinated fibers.

    b. Local anesthetics exert a **differential blockade**, reducing pain and temperature first, followed by fine touch and finally impairing motor function. However, the differential blockade is imperfect (eg, it is nearly **impossible to produce a full sensory block without loss of motor function**).

    c. Sequence of block progresses in the following order: Sympathetic ≥ pain and temperature ≥ proprioception ≥ fine touch and pressure ≥ motor.

5. Pathophysiologic factors affecting the neural block

    a. A decrease in the cardiac output reduces the plasma and tissue clearance of local anesthetics, increasing plasma concentration and the potential for toxicity.

    b. Severe hepatic disease may prolong the duration of action of amides.

    c. Renal disease has minimal effect.

    d. Reduced cholinesterase activity. Newborns and pregnant patients and patients with **atypical cholinesterase** may have decreased clearance of ester-type anesthetics, but this does not usually associate with toxicity.

    e. Fetal acidosis may cause an **ion-trapping** phenomenon (eg, accumulation of ionized local anesthetic in the fetal circulation) potentially resulting in fetal toxicity. This is more likely with amide forms not cleared rapidly by maternal liver enzymes.

    f. Sepsis, malignancy, and cardiac ischemia can increase plasma levels of α_1-**acid glycoprotein** and decrease the plasma concentration of free local anesthetics.

D. **Commercial preparations:** Most commercial preparations are solubilized with ethanol, chloroform, or acetone before dilution in sterile water. The pH is adjusted with hydrochloric acid or sodium hydroxide to a final value of 4 to 6 to maintain stability. Solutions with epinephrine are adjusted to pH 3 to 4 to keep the catecholamine in solution.

1. **Antimicrobial preservatives: Methylparaben** or other paraben derivatives are used as antiseptic agents for multidose vials. **Preservative-free solutions are used for neuraxial** anesthesia to minimize neurotoxic effects from preservatives.

2. **Epinephrine:** Following preservatives, the most common additive is epinephrine bitartrate to prolong the block and act as a marker for intravascular injection, which requires additional stabilizers (see Chapter 19, Section II.B).

3. **Antioxidants** (sodium metabisulfite, sodium ethylenediaminetetraacetic acid [EDTA]) are added to mixtures containing epinephrine **to slow the degradation by oxygen.**

4. **Liposomal bupivacaine:** Multivesicular bupivacaine sold under the trade name **Exparel** was designed for slow release of bupivacaine from liposomes to prolong its local anesthetic effects and reduce toxicity. It is approved by the US Food and Drug Administration (FDA) for TAP block and interscalene block. Data about its clinical benefit over standard bupivacaine are limited, and it holds potential for toxicity, especially when used improperly (eg, mixed with non-bupivacaine local anesthetics, which disrupts the liposomes).

II. CLINICAL USES OF LOCAL ANESTHETICS

The choice of local anesthetic must account for the duration of surgery, regional technique used, surgical requirements, potential for toxicity, and metabolic constraints (**Tables 19.2** and **19.3**).

A. **Combinations of local anesthetics**

1. **Mixtures of local anesthetics** (eg, mepivacaine bupivacaine) are asserted to accelerate onset, but data indicate that mixtures **do not speed onset but do reduce duration.**

2. Mixture of **non-bupivacaine** local anesthetics with **liposomal bupivacaine** will perturb liposomes and alter the release of bupivacaine. A mixture of **bupivacaine** with liposomal bupivacaine alters the pharmacokinetics of release.

3. **Eutectic mixture of local anesthetics (EMLA)** cream is a mixture of 2.5% lidocaine and 2.5% prilocaine for use as a topical skin anesthetic. It must be applied to unbroken, healthy skin for at least 30 minutes for an effect.

B. **Adjuncts** for local anesthesia

1. **Epinephrine:** the most common additive after preservatives

a. **Benefits** of epinephrine:

1. To assist in the **detection** of **intravascular injections.**

2. To **decrease systemic toxicity** by decreasing the rate of absorption of anesthetic into the circulation.

3. To **prolong the duration of anesthesia.** This varies with the anesthetic agent, concentration, and block performed. Prolongation is inferior to other adjuvants.

b. **Limitations** of epinephrine:

1. Epinephrine is neurotoxic in diabetic animal models. Systemic epinephrine is dangerous in patients with severe coronary artery disease, arrhythmias, uncontrolled hypertension, and hyperthyroidism; **it should be used with caution in susceptible populations.**

TABLE 19.2		Clinical Uses of Local Anesthetics				
Anesthetics	pK_a	Onset	Duration[a]	Relative Toxicity	Highest Recommended Dose (mg)[b]	Clinical Use/ Comments
Esters						
Procaine (Novocaine)	8.9	Slow	Short	Low	500 (600)	Infiltration, spinal Allergic potential
Chloro-procaine (Nesacaine)	9.1	Fast	Short	Low	800 (1000)	All,[d] rapid hydrolysis in plasma
Tetracaine (Pontocaine)	8.5	Slow	Long	High	10 (20)	Spinal, topical
Benzocaine	2.5	Moderate	Short	n/a[c]	n/a[c]	Topical only Methemo-globinemia
Amides						
Lidocaine (Xylocaine)	7.9	Fast	Medium	Medium	300 (500)	All[d]
Prilocaine (Citanest)	7.7	Fast	Medium	Medium	400 (600)	All,[d] methemo-globinemia
Mepivacaine (Carbocaine)	7.6	Fast	Medium	Medium	400 (550)	All[d]
Bupivacaine (Marcaine, Sensorcaine)	8.1	Moderate	Long	High	175 (225)	All,[d] differential block with low concentration
L-Bupi-vacaine (Chirocaine)	8.1	Moderate	Long	High	150 (n/a)	All[d] S-enantiomer of bupiva-caine—less cardiotoxic
Ropivacaine (Naropin)	8.1	Moderate	Long	High	225 (n/a)	All[d]
Etidocaine (Duranest)	7.7	Moderate	Long	High	300 (400)	All[d] Motor greater than sensory blockade

[a]Duration of dose depends on the site of administration and proximity to vasculature.
[b]Dose in epinephrine-containing solution in parenthesis. Maximum dose may require clinical judgment based on other comorbidities.
[c]The 20% spray has been removed from practice owing to high risk of methemoglobinemia.
[d]"All" indicates that the drug can be used for any type of local anesthesia (infiltration, local, regional, neuraxial).

TABLE 19.3	Local Anesthetic Agents			
Anesthetic Technique	Anesthetic	Concentration (%)	Duration (minutes)[a]	Usual Volume (mL; 70-kg Patient)[b]
Local infiltration	Procaine	1-2	20-30 (30-45)	
	Lidocaine	0.5-1	30-60 (120)	
	Mepivacaine	0.5-1	45-90 (120)	
	Bupivacaine	0.25-0.5	120-240 (180-240)	
	Ropivacaine	0.2-0.5	120-240 (180-240)	
Peripheral nerve blocks (drug with epinephrine 1:200,000)	Lidocaine	1-2	(120-240)	30-50
	Mepivacaine	1-1.5	(180-300)	30-50
	Bupivacaine	0.25-0.5	(360-720)	30-50
	Ropivacaine	0.2-0.5	(360-720)	30-50
Epidural (drug with epinephrine 1:200,000)	Chloroprocaine	2-3	(30-90)	15-30
	Lidocaine	1-2	(60-120)	15-30
	Mepivacaine	1-2	(60-180)	15-30
	Bupivacaine	0.25-0.5	(180-350)	15-30
	Levobupivacaine	0.25-0.75	(180-350)	15-30
	Ropivacaine	0.2-0.75	(180-350)	15-30
Spinal	Lidocaine + glucose (hyperbaric)	1.5, 5.0	30-60	1-2
	Bupivacaine (isobaric)	0.5	90-200	3-4
	Bupivacaine + glucose (hyperbaric)	0.75	90-200	2-3
	Tetracaine (hypobaric)	0.25	90-200	2-6
	Tetracaine (isobaric)	1.0	90-200	1-2
	Tetracaine + glucose (hyperbaric)	0.25-1.0	90-200	1-4

[a]Duration in epinephrine-containing solution in parenthesis.
[b]Doses should be reduced for patients with specific risk factors and when nonepinephrine–containing solutions are used.

2. Epinephrine should be **avoided** in peripheral nerve blocks in areas with **poor collateral blood flow** (eg, digits, penis, and nose) or in intravenous local-anesthetic techniques.

c. **Fresh epinephrine** can be added to make a 1:200,000 to 1:400,000 solution (2.5-5 µg/mL) prior to administration (while maintaining a high pH to speed onset of the block). Such a dilution is made by adding 0.5 to 0.1 mL (1 mg/mL) epinephrine to 20 mL of local anesthetic solution. These doses balance the detection of intravascular injection while minimizing the cardiovascular risk of higher doses of epinephrine.

   d. The **maximum dose of epinephrine** should not exceed **10 µg/kg in pediatric** patients and **5 µg/kg in adults** to avoid ventricular arrhythmias.

2. **Opioids** including fentanyl, morphine, and hydromorphone are particularly useful in spinal/epidural anesthesia to prolong pain relief given that they bind to opioid receptors in the spinal cord but are less useful in peripheral nerve blocks.

   a. **Buprenorphine** can generate a 1.5- to 3-fold increase in the duration of peripheral blocks (0.15-0.3 mg or 3 µg/kg) but is associated with an increased risk of postoperative nausea and vomiting (PONV).

   b. **Meperidine:** Given its opioid and local anesthetic properties, it is used as the sole anesthetic agent in spinal anesthesia but avoided in the United States given the risk for serotonin syndrome from its metabolite norpethidine.

3. **Sodium bicarbonate** raises the pH (from baseline of ~6 without epinephrine and ~4 with epinephrine) in order to increase the concentration of nonionized free base that can cross the membrane. This **speeds the onset** of neural blockade. Typically, 1 mEq of sodium bicarbonate is added to each 10 mL of lidocaine, chloroprocaine, or mepivacaine; only 0.1 mEq should be added to each 10 mL of bupivacaine to avoid precipitation.

4. **Alpha-2-agonists** are central acting adrenergic agonists that bind presynaptic receptors (in the locus ceruleus and other sites) to produce anesthesia and analgesia. Higher doses are associated with sedation and bradycardia.

   a. **Clonidine** prolongs the duration of neuraxial anesthesia (15-50 µg single dose) with less benefit to regional anesthesia duration (100-150 µg or 0.5-5 µg/kg).

   b. **Dexmetatomidine** prolongs both neuraxial (intrathecal 5-10 µg, epidural 1 µg/kg) and regional anesthesia (20-150 µg) duration.

5. **Dexamethasone**, an anti-inflammatory steroid extends the duration of regional blocks over intramuscular or intravenous injection of an equivalent dose of dexamethasone (neuraxial 4-8 mg, peripheral nerve block 1-8 mg).

6. **Magnesium,** the N-methyl-D-aspartate agonist, provides a prolonged block duration (100-500 mg) but with concerns of increased PONV at higher doses.

7. Other additives with little evidence and/or contraindications

   a. **Phenylephrine** has been used like epinephrine for local vasoconstriction but with limited clinical data and less utility as an intravascular marker.

   b. **Tramadol:** Multiple studies investigated tramadol with minimal benefit.

III. TOXICITY

A. Allergic reactions

True allergic reactions to local anesthetics are rare. Vasovagal episodes and responses to intravascular injection of local anesthetic/epinephrine are more common.

1. **Ester-type local anesthetics** may cause allergic reactions from the metabolite PABA. Patients allergic to PABA should avoid **methylparaben** owing to the structural similarity.

2. **Amide-type local anesthetics** are nearly devoid of allergic potential.
3. **Epinephrine containing solutions with sulfa-antioxidants** may cause allergic reactions in patients with sulfa allergies.
4. **Local hypersensitivity reactions** may produce local erythema, urticaria, edema, or dermatitis.
5. **Systemic hypersensitivity reactions** are rare and can present with generalized erythema, urticaria, edema, bronchoconstriction, hypotension, and cardiovascular collapse.
6. **Treatment** is supportive.

B. **Local toxicity**
1. **Tissue toxicity** is rare with short-term use.
2. **Post spinal pain syndrome** may occur after subarachnoid injection of local anesthetic with pain or dysesthesia in the buttocks or legs.
3. Large volumes of intrathecal or epidural chloroprocaine may cause intense back pain, potentially due to spasms of the paraspinal muscles from EDTA.

C. **Local anesthetic systemic toxicity (LAST)** results from intravascular accumulation of local anesthetic owing to inadvertent intravascular injection, absorption from a tissue depot, accumulation of metabolites, intentional intravenous infusion or a combination of these.
1. **Clinical characteristics**
   a. In the setting of **landmark-based anesthesia**, LAST is primarily due to **inadvertent intravascular injection**. Intravascular injection can be reduced by:
      1. Aspirating before injection
      2. Using an intravascular marker (eg, **epinephrine**)
      3. **Incremental injection** to establish the block (eg, 5 mL per injection)
      4. **Ultrasound guidance**
   b. **Ultrasound** has changed the clinical characteristics of LAST with increasing frequency of delayed toxicity from **depot absorption**.
   c. **Incidence** of systemic toxicity is ~1 to 2/1000 with 20% (2-4/10,000) representing severe cases with cardiac arrest and/or seizure.
   d. **Risk factors for toxicity** include total dose, vascularity of block site (penile > paravertebral > upper extremity block > lower extremity block), and prolonged infusions.
   e. **Patient risk factors** include diminutive stature (low body mass index), hypoalbuminemia, renal disease, liver failure, heart failure, mitochondrial disease, carnitine deficiency, and acidosis (which causes intracellular ion trapping of LA).
   f. **Perceived safety of local anesthesia** (particularly lidocaine) leads to overrepresentation of LAST in ASA I/II patients and **lidocaine as the causative agent**.
2. **Presentation of toxicity**: LAST presents with **neurological symptoms, cardiovascular symptoms**, or **both**. Early symptoms do not always precede late symptoms. The first observed symptom can be seizure or cardiac arrest.
   a. **Central nervous system** toxicity can include features of dizziness, lightheadedness, tinnitus, perioral numbness, metallic taste, and progress to muscle twitching, tremors, **seizures, and coma**. The first symptom can be seizures.
   b. **Cardiovascular toxicity** will present with electrocardiographic changes (bradycardia, prolonged PR interval, widened QRS), hypertension, and hypotension and can progress to complete heart block and/or cardiac arrest.

1. **Early cardiac toxicity** is due to sodium (and calcium) channel blockade with disruption of the conduction apparatus in the myocardium.
2. **Vascular toxicity** will cause a **bimodal effect** of early (and often unobserved) hypertension with subsequent hypotension (due to smooth muscle inhibition).
3. **Profound toxicity** is due to an **uncoupling of oxidative phosphorylation** in mitochondria.

c. Toxicity is **associated with lipophilicity (LogP)** with bupivacaine >>> ropivacaine > lidocaine > chloroprocaine.

d. **Pregnancy** increases sensitivity to cardiotoxicity.

e. **Acidosis and hypoxia** markedly worsen cardiotoxicity and neurotoxicity, making airway management a priority for treatment.

3. Treatment of LAST

a. **Secure** airway: **Ventilate with 100% O_2** and consider advanced airway technique to minimize respiratory and/or metabolic acidosis.

b. **Lipid emulsion therapy:** If LAST is suspected, **lipid emulsion is the definitive treatment**. Do not delay administration given that benefit far outweighs risks.

1. For a patient ≥ 70 kg, **bolus 100 mL 20% lipid emulsion** (eg, Intralipid) intravenously (or intraosseously) over 2 to 3 minutes followed by 0.25 mL/kg/min until 250 mL is infused.
2. For a patient < 70 kg, **bolus 1.5 mL/kg** (lean body mass) followed by 0.25 mL/kg for 10 minutes.
3. The provider can **repeat the bolus** for persistent cardiovascular collapse and **double the infusion rate** (0.5 mL/kg/min) for persistent hypotension.
4. Continue lipid emulsion infusion at least 15 minutes after patient is hemodynamically stable.
5. **An upper limit of 12.5 mL/kg is** recommended to comport with FDA guidelines.

c. **Treat seizures** with **benzodiazepines.** If only propofol is available, use small incremental dose such as 10 to 20 mg, especially in patients with cardiovascular instability.

d. If there is **cardiac arrest**, start chest compressions (basic life support/advanced cardiac life support).

1. **Epinephrine doses (<1 µg/kg) can be used.**
2. **Avoid vasopressin, calcium channel blockers, β-blockers, or local anesthetics.**

e. **Cardiopulmonary bypass (CPB):** If the patient fails to respond, the patient may require CPB. Given time required for CPB, notify CPB center ASAP if anticipated.

f. Monitor for **4 to 6 hours** for cardiovascular symptoms and **2 hours** for central nervous system symptoms given risk for recrudescence.

4. Emerging areas of concern for LAST: **local infiltration anesthesia** by surgeons, **intravenous lidocaine infusion** in unmonitored settings, prolonged **catheter infusions** especially in patients with risk factors and novel formulations (eg, **liposomal bupivacaine**) where mixing can lead to supratoxic dosing.

D. **Methohemoglobinemia results from** the oxidation of heme groups within deoxyhemoglobin (Fe^{2+}) to form methemoglobin (Fe^{3+}), which cannot transport oxygen.

1. **Causes: prilocaine** (in EMLA cream), which is metabolized to *o*-toluidine in the liver and oxidizes hemoglobin to methemoglobin; **benzocaine**, which is found in topical sprays.
2. **Treatment** is with **methylene blue** (1-2 mg/kg intravenously over 5 minutes), which converts methemoglobin back to reduced hemoglobin.

IV. NOVEL DEVELOPMENTS

Novel local anesthetics address the primary limitations of cocaine-derived anesthetics, specifically **limited duration** and **risk of systemic toxicity**.

A. Novel sodium channel blockers

1. **Neosaxitoxin** is a paralytic shellfish toxin that binds to the tetrodotoxin-binding site on the voltage-gated sodium channel. It **lacks cardiac toxicity** and produces a **longer block** in animal models, but there are currently no ongoing clinical trials on clinicaltrials.gov.
2. Other sodium channels blockers exist (tetrotodotoxin, alpha and beta-scorpion toxin, sea anemone toxin, brevetoxin, ciguatoxin, delta-conotoxin), with others in preclinical development, but no active candidates.

B. Extended-release formulations including liposomal bupivacaine

1. Multivesicular bupivacaine sold under the trade name **Exparel** as discussed in Chapter 19, Section I.D.4.
2. Sucrose acetate isobutyrate extended release **(SABER)-bupivacaine** is a formulation that improves pain relief compared with placebo but has not passed FDA review owing to safety concerns.
3. **HTX-011** is a biochromer-polymer of bupivacaine with meloxicam as an adjuvant. Phase III clinical trials support efficacy above bupivacaine alone.
4. Other extended-release formulations of bupivacaine exist in preclinical trials.

Suggested Readings

Aggarwal N. Local anesthetics systemic toxicity association with exparel (bupivacaine liposome)—a pharmacovigilance evaluation. *Expert Opin Drug Saf.* 2018;17:581-587.

Balocco AL, Van Zundert PGE, Gan SS, Gan TJ, Hadzic A. Extended release bupivacaine formulations for postoperative analgesia: an update. *Curr Opin Anaesthesiol.* 2018;31:636-642.

Berde CB, Strichartz GR. Local anesthetics. In: Miller RE, ed. *Anesthesia.* 8th ed. Elsevier; 2015:1028-1053.

Bhole MV, Manson AL, Seneviratne SL, Misbah SA. IgE-mediated allergy to local anaesthetics: separating fact from perception—a UK perspective. *Br J Anaesth.* 2012;108(6):903-911.

Clarkson C, Hondeghem L. Mechanism for bupivacaine depression of cardiac conduction: fast block of sodium channels during the action potential with slow recovery from block during diastole. *Anesthesiology.* 1985;62:396-405.

Fettiplace MR, Weinberg G. The mechanisms underlying lipid resuscitation therapy. *Reg Anesth Pain Med.* 2018;43:138-149.

Gadsden J, Hadzic A, Gandhi K, et al. The effect of mixing 1.5% mepivacaine and 0.5% bupivacaine on duration of analgesia and latency of block onset in ultrasound-guided interscalene block. *Anesth Analg.* 2011;112:471-476.

Gitman M, Barrington MJ. Local anesthetic systemic toxicity: a review of recent case reports and registries. *Reg Anesth Pain Med.* 2018;43:124-130.

Hamilton TW, Athanassoglou V, Mellon S, et al. Liposomal bupivacaine infiltration at the surgical site for the management of postoperative pain. *Cochrane Database Syst Rev.* 2017;2(2):1-63.

Hermanns H, Hollmann MW, Stevens MF, et al. Molecular mechanisms of action of systemic lidocaine in acute and chronic pain: a narrative review. *Br J Anaesth.* 2019;123:335-349.

Hiller N, Mirtschink P, Merkel C, et al. Myocardial accumulation of bupivacaine and ropivacaine is associated with reversible effects on mitochondria and reduced myocardial function. *Anesth Analg.* 2013;116:83-92.

Kirksey MA, Haskins SC, Cheng J, Liu SS. Local anesthetic peripheral nerve block adjuvants for prolongation of analgesia: a systematic qualitative review. *PLoS One.* 2015;10:e0137312.

Neal JM, Barrington MJ, Fettiplace MR, et al. The Third American Society of Regional Anesthesia and Pain Medicine Practice Advisory on local anesthetic systemic toxicity. *Reg Anesth Pain Med.* 2018;43:113-123.

Rodríguez-Navarro AJ, Berde CB, Wiedmaier G, et al. Comparison of neosaxitoxin versus bupivacaine via port infiltration for postoperative analgesia following laparoscopic cholecystectomy: a randomized, double-blind trial. *Reg Anesth Pain Med.* 2011;36:103-109.

Rosenberg PH, Veering BT, Urmey WF. Maximum recommended doses of local anesthetics: a multifactorial concept. *Reg Anesth Pain Med.* 2004;29(6):564-575.

Swain A, Nag DS, Sahu S, et al. Adjuvants to local anesthetics: current understanding and future trends. *World J Clin Cases.* 2017;5:307.

Vorobeichik L, Brull R, Abdallah FW. Evidence basis for using perineural dexmedetomidine to enhance the quality of brachial plexus nerve blocks: a systematic review and meta-analysis of randomized controlled trials. *Br J Anaesth.* 2017;118:167-181.

20 Spinal, Epidural, and Caudal Anesthesia

Erica L. Gee and Joseph L. McDowell

I. GENERAL CONSIDERATIONS

A. **Preoperative assessment** of the patient for regional anesthesia is similar to that for general anesthesia. The details of the procedure to be performed, including its anticipated length, patient position, and a complete review of any coexisting diseases, should be taken into account in determining the appropriateness of a regional technique.

B. **Review of systems:** A comprehensive review of cardiovascular and pulmonary systems should be performed. Preexisting neurologic abnormalities should be well documented. Any history of abnormal bleeding and a review of the patient's medications may indicate a need for additional coagulation studies.

C. **Physical examination:** Review of the patient's airway, cardiovascular, and pulmonary examinations should be performed The area where the block is to be administered should be examined for potential pathology, such as abnormal anatomy (kyphoscoliosis) or evidence of overlying infection.

D. **Informed consent** should be obtained including a detailed explanation of the planned procedure, with procedure-specific risks and benefits—these include bleeding, infection, nerve damage, paresthesias, and dural puncture headache. Patients should be reassured that additional sedation and anesthesia can be given during the operation and that general anesthesia is an option if the block fails or the operation becomes more prolonged or extensive than originally thought; therefore, general anesthesia must also be on the consent form. In some instances, it is planned from the onset to have a combination of regional and general anesthesia.

E. Monitoring: As with general anesthesia, patients should receive appropriate monitoring (see Chapter 15) and have an intravenous (IV) line in place. Oxygen, equipment for intubation and positive-pressure ventilation, and drugs to provide hemodynamic support must be available.

II. SEGMENTAL LEVEL REQUIRED FOR SURGERY

A. Knowledge of the sensory, motor, and autonomic distributions of spinal nerves will help the anesthetist determine the correct segmental level required for a particular operation and anticipate the potential physiologic effects of producing a block to that level. **Figure 20.1** illustrates the dermatomal distribution of the spinal nerves.

B. Afferent autonomic nerves innervate visceral sensation and viscerosomatic reflexes at spinal segmental levels much higher than would be predicted from skin dermatomes.

C. Minimal suggested levels for common surgical procedures are listed in **Table 20.1**.

III. CONTRAINDICATIONS TO NEURAXIAL ANESTHESIA

A. **Absolute**
1. Patient refusal
2. Localized infection at skin puncture site

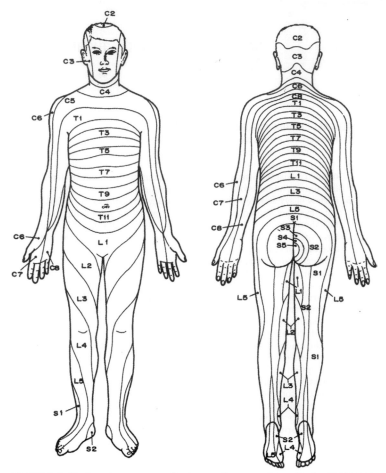

FIGURE 20.1 Skin dermatomes corresponding to respective sensory innervation by spinal nerves.

    3. Significant coagulopathy
    4. Increased intracranial pressure
  B. Relative
    1. Septicemia or bacteremia
    2. Hypovolemia
    3. Central nervous system disease

IV. SPINAL ANESTHESIA
  Spinal anesthesia involves administering local anesthetic into the subarachnoid space.
  A. Anatomy
    1. The **spinal canal** extends from the foramen magnum to the sacral hiatus. The boundaries of the bony canal are the vertebral body anteriorly,

Suggested Minimum Cutaneous Levels for Spinal Anesthesia

Operative Site	Level
Lower extremities	T12
Hip	T10
Vagina, uterus	T10
Bladder, prostate	T10
Lower extremities with tourniquet	T8
Testis, ovaries	T8
Lower intra-abdominal	T6
Other intra-abdominal	T4

the pedicles laterally, and the spinous processes and laminae posteriorly (**Figure 20.2**).

2. Three **interlaminar ligaments** bind the vertebral processes together:
   a. Superficially, the **supraspinous ligament** connects the apices of the spinous processes.
   b. The **interspinous ligament** connects the spinous processes on their horizontal surface.

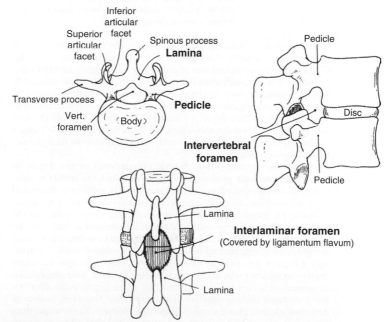

FIGURE 20.2 Vertebral anatomy.

    c. The **ligamentum flavum** connects the caudal edge of the lamina above to the cephalad edge of the lamina below. This ligament is composed of elastic fibers and is usually recognized by its increased resistance to the passage of a needle.

3. The **spinal cord** extends the length of the vertebral canal during fetal life, ends at about L3 at birth, and is moved progressively to a cephalad position as the vertebral column grows to reach near the adult L1 level by 2 years of age. The conus medullaris, lumbar, sacral, and coccygeal nerve roots branch out distally to form the cauda equina. Spinal needles are placed in this area of the canal (below L2) because the mobility of the nerves reduces the danger of trauma from the needle.

4. The spinal cord is invested in three **meninges**:
    a. The pia mater **directly invests the spinal cord**.
    b. The **arachnoid mater**, which lies between the pia and the dura mater.
    c. The **dura mater**, which is a tough fibrous sheath running longitudinally along the length of the spinal cord and is tethered caudally at S2.

5. The **subarachnoid space** lies between the pia mater and the arachnoid mater and extends from the attachment of the dura at S2 to the cerebral ventricles above. The space contains the spinal cord, nerves, cerebrospinal fluid (CSF), and blood vessels that supply the spinal cord.

6. **CSF** is a clear colorless fluid that fills the subarachnoid space. The total volume of CSF is 100 to 150 mL, and the volume that exists in the spinal subarachnoid space is ~25 to 35 mL. CSF is continuously formed at a rate of 450 mL/d by secretion or ultrafiltration of plasma from the choroid arterial plexuses located in the lateral, third, and fourth ventricles. CSF is reabsorbed into the bloodstream through the arachnoid villi and granulations that protrude through the dura to lie in contact with the endothelium of the cerebral venous sinuses.

B. Physiologic changes

1. **Neural blockade: Differential blockade** refers to the varying sensitivity of different types of nerve fibers to the effects of local anesthetics. Smaller C fibers conveying autonomic impulses are more easily blocked than the larger sensory and motor fibers. As a result, the level of autonomic blockade extends above the level of the sensory blockade by two to six segments. Similarly, fibers conveying sensation are more sensitive to local anesthetics than the larger motor fibers, and as a result, the sensory blockade will extend above the level of the motor blockade. Causes of this phenomenon are multifactorial and include nerve fiber diameter and myelination.

2. **Cardiovascular: Hypotension** is directly proportional to the degree of **sympathetic blockade** produced. Sympathetic blockade results in dilatation of arteries and venous capacitance vessels, leading to decreased systemic vascular resistance and decreased venous return. If the block is below T4, increased baroreceptor activity produces an increase in activity to the cardiac sympathetic fibers and vasoconstriction of the upper extremities. Blockade above T4 interrupts cardiac accelerator sympathetic fibers, leading to bradycardia, decreased cardiac output, and a further decrease in blood pressure. These changes are more marked in patients who are hypovolemic or elderly or have obstruction to venous return (eg, pregnancy). Risk factors for bradycardia after spinal anesthesia include baseline bradycardia, the American Society of Anesthesiologists physical status 1, use of β-blockers, age younger than 50 years, prolonged PR interval, and sensory level above T6.

3. **Respiratory:** Low spinal anesthesia has no effect on ventilation. With ascending height of the block into the thoracic area, there is progressive ascending intercostal muscle paralysis. This has little effect on ventilation in the supine surgical patient with intact diaphragmatic function mediated by the phrenic nerve (C3 to C5), but patients may report a sensation of dyspnea due to decreased sensation of chest wall expansion. Conversely, ventilation in patients with poor respiratory reserve, such as the morbidly obese, may be profoundly impaired. Paralysis of both intercostal and abdominal muscles decreases the efficiency of coughing, which may be important in patients with chronic obstructive pulmonary disease. Usually, a spinal level of T4 does not result in impaired ventilation, but respiratory compromise may occur in patients with limited respiratory reserve or higher spinal levels.

4. **Visceral effects**
   a. **Bladder:** Sacral blockade (S2 to S4) results in an atonic bladder that can retain large volumes of urine. Blockade of sympathetic afferent and efferent innervation of the sphincter and detrusor muscle produces urinary retention.
   b. **Intestine:** Sympathetic blockade (T5 to L1) produced by spinal anesthesia leads to contraction of the small and large intestines because of a predominance of parasympathetic tone.

5. **Neuroendocrine:** Peridural block to T5 inhibits part of the neural component of the stress response through its blockade of sympathetic afferents to the adrenal medulla and blockade of sympathetic and somatic pathways mediating pain. Other components of the stress response and central release of humoral factors are unaffected. Vagal afferent fibers from the upper abdominal viscera are not blocked and can stimulate release of hypothalamic and pituitary hormones, such as antidiuretic hormone and adrenocorticotropic hormone. Glucose tolerance and insulin release are normal.

6. **Thermoregulation:** Hypothermia may occur due to several mechanisms. The predominant cause is redistribution of the central heat to the periphery secondary to vasodilatation, which makes forced air warming particularly effective at raising the patient's temperature. Core temperature may drop even though surface temperature is preserved and patients can feel warm despite a decrease in temperature. Thermoregulation is impaired given the loss of vasoconstriction to preserve heat below the level of sympathectomy. Shivering is common.

7. **Central nervous system effects:** Spinal anesthesia may have direct effects to suppress consciousness, probably secondary to decreased afferent stimulation of the reticular activating system. During spinal or epidural anesthesia, doses of sedative agents may be decreased.

C. **Technique**
   1. **Spinal needle.** There are two main categories of spinal needles: those with a beveled tip that cut the dura ("cutting tip") and those with a conical tip ("pencil-point") with a lateral opening.
   2. **Sprotte** and **Whitacre** needles: Pencil-point needle; may reduce the incidence of postdural puncture headache (PDPH) (<1%) compared with traditional cutting-tip needles by splitting rather than cutting dural fibers during insertion. Twenty-four and 25-gauge needles are easily bent and are often inserted through a 19-gauge introducer needle.
   3. **Quincke needle:** Cutting tip. More prone to causing PDPH. The 22-gauge **Quincke** needle is more rigid and is easily directed when inserted. It can be useful in older patients in whom access may be more difficult and the incidence of PDPH is low.

4. **Patient position**. The lateral decubitus, prone, and sitting positions can be used for administration of spinal anesthesia.
   a. In the **lateral position**, the patient is placed with the affected side up if a hypobaric or isobaric technique is to be used and with the affected side down if a hyperbaric technique is to be used. The spine is horizontal and parallel to the edge of the table. The knees are drawn up toward the chest, and the chin is flexed downward onto the chest to obtain maximal flexion of the spine.
   b. The **sitting position** is useful for low spinal blocks required in certain gynecologic and urologic procedures and is commonly used in obese patients to assist in identification of the midline. It is often used in conjunction with hyperbaric anesthetics. The head and shoulders are flexed downward onto the trunk with the arms resting on a stand. An assistant should be available to stabilize the patient, and the patient should not be oversedated.
   c. The **prone position** is used in conjunction with hypobaric or isobaric anesthetics for procedures on the rectum, perineum, and anus. A prone jackknife position can be used for administration of spinal anesthesia and the subsequent surgery.

5. **Procedure**
   a. With all regional anesthetic procedures, the patient should be monitored with standard American Society of Anesthesiologists (ASA) monitors including electrocardiogram (ECG), blood pressure, and oxygen saturation.
   b. The L2–L3, L3–L4, or L4–L5 interspaces are commonly used for spinal anesthesia. The spinous process of L4 is aligned with the upper borders of the superior iliac crests.
   c. Disinfect a large area of skin with an appropriate antiseptic solution. Care must be taken to avoid contamination of the spinal kit with antiseptic solution as the solution is potentially neurotoxic.
   d. Check the stylet for correct fit within the needle; this can be done by pulling the stylet back and then replacing it.
   e. Raise a skin wheal with 1% lidocaine and a 25-gauge needle at the spinal puncture site.
   f. **Approaches**
      1. **Midline**. Place the spinal needle (or introducer) through the skin wheal and into the interspinous ligament. The needle should be in the same plane as the spinous processes and angulated slightly cephalad toward the interlaminar space (**Figure 20.3**).
      2. **Paramedian**. This approach is useful in patients who cannot adequately flex their backs because of pain or whose interspinous ligaments may be ossified. Place the spinal needle approximately 1 cm lateral and 1 cm caudad to the center of the selected interspace. Aim the needle medially and slightly cephalad, passing lateral to the supraspinous ligament. If the lamina is contacted, redirect the needle and walk the tip off the lamina in a medial and cephalad direction.
      3. **Needle placement**. Always keep the stylet in place when advancing the needle so that the needle's lumen does not become occluded with tissue. If paresthesias occur during placement, immediately withdraw the needle. Allow the paresthesia to pass and reposition the needle before proceeding again. Advance the needle until increased resistance is felt as it passes through the ligamentum flavum. As the needle is advanced beyond this ligament, a sudden loss of resistance will occur as the needle "pops" through the dura.

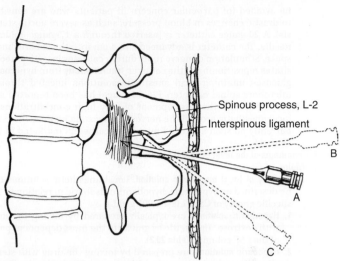

FIGURE 20.3 Spinal needle insertion, lateral view. For the classic midline approach, the needle is introduced in the middle of the interspace and advanced with a slight cephalad angulation. If correctly angled (A), it will enter the interspinous ligament, ligamentum flavum, and epidural space. If bone is contacted, it may be the inferior spinous process (B), and cephalad redirection will identify the correct path. If angling cephalad causes contact with bone again at a shallower depth (C), it is probably the superior spinous process. If bone is encountered at the same depth after several attempts at redirection (not shown), the needle is most likely on the lamina lateral to the interspace, and the position of the true midline should be reassessed. (Reprinted with permission from Mulroy MF. *Regional Anesthesia: An Illustrated Procedural Guide.* 2nd ed. Little, Brown and Company; 1996:79.)

4. Remove the stylet and confirm correct placement by noting free flow of CSF into the hub of the needle. Rotate the needle in 90-degree increments if necessary to confirm or reestablish good flow of CSF.

5. **Administration of anesthetic.** Connect the syringe containing the predetermined dose of local anesthetic to the needle. Gently aspirate CSF into the syringe, which produces birefringence within dextrose-containing solutions and confirms free flow. Inject the drug slowly. Repeat aspiration of CSF at the end of the injection confirms that the needle point is still within the subarachnoid space. Remove the needle and place the patient gently into the desired position.

g. **Closely monitor** (every 60-90 seconds) blood pressure, pulse, and respiratory function for 10 to 15 minutes. Determine the ascending anesthetic level by noting the response to a gentle pinprick, alcohol swab, or bag of ice. Stabilization of the local anesthetic level takes approximately 20 minutes.

h. **Continuous spinal anesthesia** allows small aliquots of drug to be injected repeatedly to produce the desired level of sensory blockade. With this technique, a high or rapid sympathetic block can be avoided (of particular concern in patients who are sensitive to drastic changes in blood pressure, such as severe aortic stenosis). A 20-gauge catheter is inserted through a 17-gauge epidural needle. The catheter is advanced 2 to 4 cm into the subarachnoid space. Stimulation of nerve roots during catheter insertion necessitates repositioning of the catheter. **Neurotoxicity** from hyperbaric glucose-containing local anesthetic solutions injected through microbore spinal catheters (26-32 gauge) has been reported and may be due to the development of very high concentrations of local anesthetic around the nerves of the cauda equina. There are currently no such approved microbore catheters marketed in the United States.

D. Determinants of the level of spinal blockade

1. Major

a. Baricity of local anesthetic solution. Local anesthetic solutions can be described as hyperbaric, hypobaric, or isobaric in relation to the specific gravity of CSF (1.004-1.007 g/mL).

1. Hyperbaric solutions are typically prepared by mixing the drug with dextrose. They settle by gravity to the most dependent parts of the CSF column (**Table 20.2**).

2. Hypobaric solutions are prepared by mixing the drug with sterile water. They slowly rise to the highest part of the CSF column.

3. Isobaric solutions may have the advantage of a predictable spread through the CSF that is less dependent on patient position. Increasing the dose of an isobaric anesthetic has more of an effect on the duration of anesthesia than on the dermatomal spread. Patient positioning can be altered to limit or increase the spread of these mixtures.

b. Drug dose. The anesthetic level varies directly with the dose of the agent used.

c. Drug volume. The greater the volume of the injected drug, the further the drug will spread within the CSF. This is especially applicable to hyperbaric solutions.

d. Patient position. This has a lesser effect on the spread of isobaric solutions.

2. Minor

a. Turbulence of CSF. Turbulence created within the CSF during or after the injection will increase the spread of the drug and the level obtained. Turbulence is created by rapid injection, barbotage

TABLE 20.2	Drugs and Dosages (in mg) for Spinal Anesthesia			
Drug	Level			Duration (minutes)
	T10	T8	T6	
Tetracaine[a]	10	12	14	90-120
Bupivacaine[a]	7.5	9.0	10.5	90-120
Mepivacaine	30	45	60	60-90

[a]Doses are based on a 66-inch patient. An additional 2 mg of tetracaine or 1.5 mg of bupivacaine should be added or subtracted for each 6 inches in height above or below 66 inches.

(the repeated aspiration and reinjection of small amounts of CSF mixed with drug), coughing, and excessive patient movement.

b. **CSF volume.** Lumbosacral CSF volume is inversely correlated with the extent of the spread of local anesthetic.

c. **Increased intra-abdominal pressure.** Pregnancy, obesity, ascites, and abdominal tumors increase pressure within the inferior vena cava. This pressure increases blood volume within the epidural venous plexus, concomitantly reducing the volume of CSF within the vertebral column, which permits greater spread of injected local anesthetic. In obese patients, this effect is potentiated further by increased fat within the epidural space.

d. **Spinal curvature.** Lumbar lordosis and thoracic kyphosis influence the spread of hyperbaric solutions. Drug injected above the L3 level will tend to spread cephalad but will be limited by the thoracic curvature at T4 (**Figure 20.4**).

E. **Determinants of the duration of the spinal blockade**
1. **Drugs and dose.** A characteristic duration is specific for each drug (see Chapter 19). The addition of opioids to the injected solution can modify the character of the block (see also Chapter 38). **Hydrophilic opioids** (eg, morphine) offer analgesia that is slow in onset and long in duration. Undesired side effects are more common, and delayed respiratory depression may occur. If hydrophilic opioids are given intrathecally, patients should be closely observed for at least 24 hours. **Lipophilic opioids** (eg, fentanyl) have a lower risk of delayed respiratory depression. Onset is fast, and duration is moderate.
2. **Vasoconstrictors.** The addition of epinephrine can prolong the duration of some spinal anesthetics by up to 50%. This effect has not been definitively demonstrated for bupivacaine, although there is evidence that epinephrine prolongs the analgesic effects of low-dose bupivacaine and fentanyl combinations used for labor analgesia. A typical concentration of epinephrine used in spinal anesthetics is 1:400,000 to 1:200,000 (2.5-5 µg/mL).

F. **Complications and side effects**
1. **Neurologic.** Nerve injury is infrequent but can be a serious problem. Several types of nerve injury may occur.
a. **Direct nerve injury related to needle or catheter placement.** Pain during insertion of the catheter or injection of the drug is a warning sign for potential nerve injury resulting from needle or catheter placement and requires repositioning of the needle or catheter. **Transient paresthesias reported by the patient** typically resolve immediately and are usually without any long-term sequelae.

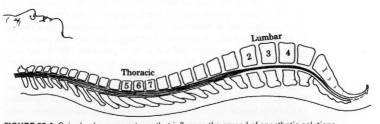

FIGURE 20.4 Spinal column curvatures that influence the spread of anesthetic solutions.

b. **Transient neurologic syndrome (TNS)** is a spontaneous severe radicular pain that occurs after resolution of the spinal anesthetic and may last for 2 to 7 days. Symptoms include buttock and thigh pain described as achy or burning in quality. TNS is usually responsive to conservative measures, such as nonsteroidal anti-inflammatory drugs and warm compresses. The incidence is highest with lidocaine administration but has also been observed with other local anesthetics, including tetracaine, bupivacaine, and mepivacaine. Obesity, ambulatory surgery, knee arthroscopic surgery, and lithotomy position are additional risk factors.

c. **Back pain** following spinal anesthesia may be related to the relaxation of the ligaments that occurs with anesthesia. There is a similar incidence of back pain following general anesthesia, again likely related to the effects of anesthetic agents and muscle relaxants on the structures of the back. Reassurance should be provided.

d. **Bloody tap.** Puncture of an epidural vein during needle insertion may result in either blood or a mixture of blood and CSF emerging from the spinal needle. If the fluid does not rapidly clear, the needle should be withdrawn and reinserted in a different space.

e. **Spinal hematoma** is a surgical emergency. Overall incidence is around 1/150,000. The signs and symptoms of severe back pain and persistent neurologic deficit usually present within 48 hours. Risk is higher among patients who are coagulopathic or anticoagulated. Bloody taps are not generally thought to cause a spinal hematoma in patients with normal coagulation. A bloody tap may be a risk factor for spinal hematoma in patients who undergo subsequent anticoagulation, but there are no data to support the mandatory cancellation of a case under these circumstances. Instead, we advocate direct communication with the surgeon and that a specific risk-benefit decision about proceeding be made on an individual basis. **Close postoperative monitoring** for signs consistent with hematoma is warranted. Diagnosis is usually made with magnetic resonance imaging (MRI), and treatment is via emergent hematoma evacuation. Because catheter removal as well as needle placement may cause spinal hematoma, anesthesiologists need to check a patient's coagulation status and the use of anticoagulants not only at the time of needle placement but also at the time of catheter removal. The approach to the use of anticoagulants, antiplatelet agents, and nonsteroidal anti-inflammatory drugs at Massachusetts General Hospital is listed in **Table 20.3**.

f. **PDPH** usually develops within 3 days; 70% of headaches resolve within 7 days and 90% within 6 months. The classic "spinal headache" is frontal and occipital in distribution, although the temporal area can be affected as well. The headache is exacerbated by upright posture and relieved by lying supine. Other manifestations can include visual disturbances or hearing impairment. Risk factors include younger age, female gender, larger needle size, pregnancy, multiple dural punctures, and a history of previous PDPH. The incidence may be reduced by using smaller needles and noncutting needles (eg, pencil-point needles). Initial treatments of symptoms include rehydration, maintenance of supine position, pain medication including opioids, and caffeine. Maintenance of supine position as a prevention is neither proven nor recommended. Caffeine exerts its effect by vasoconstriction of cerebral vessels. The recommended

TABLE 20.3 Anticoagulation and Epidural Anesthesia/Analgesia Guidelines				
Drug (Generic)	Common Trade Names	Time Interval for Catheter Placement or Neuraxial Procedure After Last Dose	Time Interval for Catheter Removal After Most Recent Dose	Time Interval to Restart Med After Neuraxial Procedure or Catheter Removal
Abciximab	ReoPro	48 h	48 h	24 h
Argatroban	Acova	At least 6 h; check for normal PTT or ACT	Check for normal PTT or ACT	2 h
Cilostazol[a]	Pletal	42 h	42 h	5 h
Clopidogrel[b]	Plavix	7 d	7 d if single 75 mg dose given	6 h
Eptifibatide	Integrilin	8 h	8 h	24 h
Fondaparinux[c]	Arixtra	7 d	4 d	6 h
Heparin subcutaneously (twice daily)	Heparin	4-6 h or assess AC status	4-6 h or assess AC status	Can be started immediately
Heparin IV	Heparin	IV: 4-6 h SC: 12 h and assess AC status	IV: 4-6 h SC: 12 h and assess AC status	1 h
Dalteparin (low-dose)[d]	Fragmin (≤5000 U daily)	12 h	12 h	4 h
Dalteparin (high-dose)[d]	Fragmin (5000 U twice daily or 120 U/kg twice daily or 175 U/kg daily)	24 h	24 h	4 h
Enoxaparin (low-dose)[d]	Lovenox (<60 mg daily)	12 h	BID dosing: indwelling catheter should be removed before initiation Daily dosing: 12 h after last dose	4 h after catheter removal and >12 h after needle/catheter placement
Enoxaparin (high-dose)[d]	Lovenox (>60 mg daily or 1 mg/kg twice daily)	24 h	Indwelling catheter should be removed before initiation	4 h after catheter removal and >24 h after needle/catheter placement

(*continued*)

TABLE 20.3	Anticoagulation and Epidural Anesthesia/Analgesia Guidelines (Continued)				
Drug (Generic)	**Common Trade Names**	**Time Interval for Catheter Placement or Neuraxial Procedure After Last Dose**	**Time Interval for Catheter Removal After Most Recent Dose**	**Time Interval to Restart Med After Neuraxial Procedure or Catheter Removal**
NSAID, ASA	Celebrex, Motrin, Naprosyn, Vioxx, etc.	No significant risk		
Thrombolytics: streptokinase, alteplase (tPA)	Streptase, Activase	10 d	10 d	10 d
Ticagrelor	Brilinta	5 d	5 d	6 h
Tirofiban	Aggrastat	8 h	8 h	24 h
Warfarin	Coumadin	3-5 d, INR ≤ 1.5	Check INR if treatment > 24 h, INR ≤ 1.5	Same day

ACT, activated clotting time; ASA, aspirin; NSAID, nonsteroidal anti-inflammatory drug; PTT, partial thromboplastin time.
[a]If cilostazol (Pletal) is the only anticoagulant given, then an epidural catheter placement is most likely safe. If cilostazol (Pletal) is combined with other anticoagulant medicines (eg, aspirin), neuraxial procedure or catheter placement should be delayed for at least 48 h.
[b]Clopidogrel (Plavix) has a 24- to 48-h window to remove an epidural catheter once the medication is given. If it has been more than 48 h since dosing of clopidogrel, you must wait for 7 d.
[c]Fondaparinux should not be given if regional anesthesia is anticipated or has been used. If, however, fondaparinux 2.5 mg is given, we suggest the above guidelines. For larger doses (5-10 mg), neuraxial procedure should not be done for 7 d.
[d]Low-molecular-weight heparin: single daily dosing may be started 6 to 8 h postoperatively. Twice-daily dosing should be started at least 24 h postoperatively. Epidural catheters should be removed before initiation of therapy.

dose of caffeine is 300 to 500 mg orally or IV. One cup of coffee contains 50 to 100 mg of caffeine. If initial therapy fails and severe symptoms persist more than 24 hours, an **epidural blood patch** can be done. Epidural needle insertion is done at the level of presumed dural puncture. Blood is drawn in a sterile fashion and injected into the epidural space. This procedure usually requires two providers. The typical blood volume is 20 to 30 mL or less if the patient complains of back discomfort during injection. The success rate ranges from 65% to 98%, and results are often immediate. A second blood patch can be tried with a success rate about the same as the first attempt. The use of a prophylactic epidural blood patch before the onset of headache symptoms is of controversial benefit, but is still performed by some anesthetists.

2. **Cardiovascular**
    a. **Hypotension.** The incidence of hypotension may be reduced by IV administration of 500 to 1000 mL of isotonic solution before performing the block. Patients with decreased cardiac function require

care in administering large volumes of IV fluid, because translocation of fluid from the peripheral to the central circulation during
cessation of the block and return of systemic vascular tone could
produce volume overload and pulmonary edema. Treatment of
hypotension includes increasing venous return and treating severe
bradycardia. Trendelenburg position, fluid administration, raising
lower extremities to autotransfuse blood, or the use of vasopressors
may be necessary.

b. Bradycardia. Bradycardia can be a sign of a vagal response or could
be indicative of a high spinal (less common). If present, bradycardia can be treated with atropine or glycopyrrolate. If bradycardia is
severe and accompanied by hypotension, ephedrine or epinephrine
may be used.

3. Respiratory

a. Dyspnea is a common complaint with high spinal levels. It is caused
by the proprioceptive blockade of afferent fibers from abdominal and chest wall muscles. Reassuring the patient may be all
that is required, although adequate ventilation must be ensured.
Supplemental O_2 can be provided for patient comfort.

b. Apnea can be caused by reduced medullary blood flow accompanying severe hypotension or from direct blockade of C3 to C5 ("total
spinal"), inhibiting phrenic nerve output. Immediate ventilatory
support is required in this scenario, so the provider should be prepared to mask ventilate and secure the airway if indicated.

4. Visceral

a. Urinary retention. The mechanism of urinary retention is described
in Section IV.B.4.a. Urinary retention may outlast the sensory and
motor blockade. A urinary catheter should be placed if anesthesia
or analgesia is maintained for a prolonged period.

b. Nausea and vomiting are usually caused by hypotension or unopposed
vagal stimulation. Treatment involves first restoring blood pressure,
followed by administering oxygen, and IV atropine if needed.

5. Infection after spinal anesthesia is exceedingly rare. Nevertheless, meningitis, arachnoiditis, and epidural abscess can occur. Possible etiologies include chemical contamination and viral or bacterial infection
due to lack of sterility. Consultation and prompt diagnosis and treatment are essential.

6. Pruritus commonly occurs with the use of neuraxial opioids and is more
frequent with intrathecal administration as opposed to epidural. The
exact mechanism is unclear. Pharmacologic treatments include nalbuphine (5-10 mg IV), naloxone (1-2 µg/kg/h), naltrexone (6-9 mg PO),
diphenhydramine (25-50 mg IV/PO), ondansetron (4-8 mg IV), and
propofol (10-20 mg IV bolus).

7. Shivering has a high incidence and may be treated with IV meperidine
(25 mg IV). Clonidine (65-300 µg IV) has been shown to have a similar
efficacy.

V. EPIDURAL ANESTHESIA

Epidural anesthesia is achieved by introducing local anesthetics into the
epidural space.

A. Anatomy. The epidural space is a potential space extending from the base
of the skull to the sacrococcygeal membrane. Posteriorly, it is bounded
by the ligamentum flavum, the anterior surfaces of the laminae, and the
articular processes. Anteriorly, it is bounded by the posterior longitudinal

ligament covering the vertebral bodies and intervertebral discs. Laterally, it is bounded by intervertebral foramina and the pedicles. It has direct communications with the paravertebral space. It contains fat and lymphatic tissue as well as epidural veins, which are most prominent in the lateral aspects of the space. The veins have no valves and directly communicate with the intracranial veins. The veins also communicate with the thoracic and abdominal veins through the intervertebral foramina and with the pelvic veins through the sacral venous plexus. The epidural space is widest in the midline and tapers off laterally. In the lumbar region, it is 5 to 6 mm wide in the midline; in the midthoracic region, the space is 3 to 5 mm wide.

B. **Physiology**
1. **Neural blockade.** Local anesthetic placed in the epidural space acts directly on the spinal nerve roots located in the lateral aspect of the space. These nerve roots are covered by the dural sheath. Local anesthetic gains access to the CSF by uptake through the dura. The onset of the block is slower than with spinal anesthesia, and the intensity of the sensory and motor block is less. Anesthesia develops in a segmental manner, and selective blockade can be achieved.
2. **Cardiovascular.** Physiologic changes from sympathetic blockade are similar to those described for spinal anesthesia (see Section IV.B.2), but usually, hemodynamic change is slower. Large doses of local anesthetic may be absorbed or inadvertently injected into the vasculature and could depress the myocardium. Epinephrine used to prolong the duration of the local anesthetics may also be absorbed or injected into the systemic circulation, producing tachycardia and hypertension.
3. **Respiratory.** Physiologic changes are similar to those described for spinal anesthesia. When we use postoperative epidural analgesia with dilute local anesthetics after major abdominal or thoracic surgery, the reduction in functional residual capacity and impairment of diaphragm function are minimized, which improves overall pulmonary outcome. With epidural anesthesia, the incidence of postoperative hypoxemia can be decreased by reducing the need for systemic opioids.
4. **Coagulation.** Epidural anesthesia has been reported to reduce venous thrombosis and subsequent pulmonary embolism. Proposed mechanisms include increased pelvic blood flow, decreased sympathetic response to surgery, and earlier mobility. Epidural anesthesia may reduce intraoperative blood loss during hip, pelvic, and lower abdominal surgeries.
5. **Gastrointestinal.** Epidural anesthesia can be administered for patients undergoing bowel resection with anastomosis. As with spinal anesthesia, the predominance of the parasympathetic system may cause contraction of the bowel. Patients often have earlier return of bowel function with the use of an epidural.
6. Other physiologic changes seen are similar to those described for spinal anesthesia (see Section IV.B).

C. **Technique**
1. **Epidural needles.** Most commonly, the 17-gauge **Tuohy** or **Weiss** needle is used for identification of the epidural space. These needles are styletted, have a blunt leading edge with a lateral opening, and have a thin wall to allow passage of a 20-gauge catheter.
2. **Patient position.** Patients can be positioned for epidural anesthesia in either the sitting or the lateral position. The same considerations apply as for spinal anesthesia (see Section IV.C.4).

3. **Monitoring.** The patient should be monitored with standard monitors including ECG, blood pressure, and oxygen saturation.

4. **Approaches.** Whether from a midline or paramedian approach, the needle should enter the epidural space in the midline, because the space is widest here and there is a decreased risk of puncturing epidural veins, spinal arteries, or spinal nerve roots, all of which lie predominantly in the lateral aspects of the epidural space. Palpation of landmarks, skin preparation, and draping are as described for spinal anesthesia (see Section IV.C.5) (**Figure 20.5**).

a. **Lumbar.** Use a long 25-gauge needle for superficial and deep infiltration of local anesthetic into the supraspinous and interspinous ligaments. This needle also assists in defining the direction in which the epidural needle should be inserted. Advance the epidural needle through the supraspinous and interspinous ligaments in a slightly cephalad direction, until it comes to lie within the "rubbery" ligamentum flavum.

1. **Loss-of-resistance techniques.** Remove the stylet and attach a glass or plastic loss-of-resistance syringe containing approximately 3 mL of air or saline to the needle hub. Apply constant pressure to the plunger of the syringe while slowly advancing the needle. When the bevel enters the epidural space, there is a marked "loss of resistance" to plunger displacement. Alternatively, an "intermittent" technique can be used, where the change in resistance is tested repeatedly in between small careful advances of

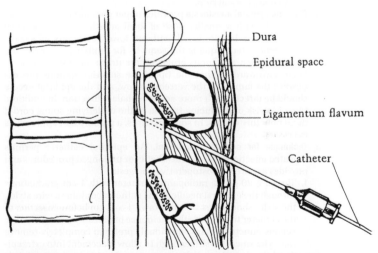

FIGURE 20.5 Insertion of an epidural catheter. The needle is secured by resting one hand on the back and grasping the hub firmly (not shown) while the other hand inserts the catheter into the hub and gently advances it beyond the tip of the needle. The bevel is usually directed cephalad, which produces the most reliable insertion; caudad orientation may allow the catheter to exit one of the intervertebral foramina. Ideally, the catheter is advanced 3 to 4 cm beyond the needle tip; further placement increases the potential for lateral misdirection or foraminal exit. (Reprinted with permission from Mulroy MF. *Regional Anesthesia: An Illustrated Procedural Guide.* 2nd ed. Little, Brown and Company; 1996:109.)

the epidural needle. When air is used for loss of resistance, the amount of air injected should be minimized. Patchy block, pneumocephalus, and air embolism have been reported with the loss of resistance with air technique.

2. The **hanging drop technique** relies on the principle that a drop of fluid placed on the hub of the epidural needle (once the ligamentum flavum has been entered) will retract into the needle as the tip of the needle is advanced into the epidural space. This negative pressure is provided by "tenting" of the dura by the needle tip but may be altered by transmitted changes in intra-abdominal and intrathoracic pressure (eg, pregnancy and obesity). Drop retraction occurs only about 80% of the time, so if a change in compliance is felt while advancing through the ligamentum flavum, it should be checked by loss of resistance to prevent unanticipated dural puncture.

3. In cases where landmarks are difficult to palpate, **ultrasound** can be used to identify the interspaces as well as midline. When placed perpendicular to the spinal cord (transverse approach), the spinous process can be identified as a hyperechoic signal close to the skin, continuing as a vertical acoustic shadow (can be triangular in shape), thus designating midline. The longitudinal paramedian approach involves placing the ultrasound probe parallel to the spinal cord just a few centimeters lateral and angled toward midline. This view allows visualization of the interspaces, as well as other structures including ligamentum flavum, vertebral body, and sacrum.

b. **Thoracic epidural anesthesia** provides upper abdominal and thoracic anesthesia with a smaller dose of local anesthetic. Postoperative analgesia can be produced without lower extremity blockade. Although the technique is the same as for lumbar placement, the thoracic vertebral spinous processes are much more sharply angulated downward so that the tip of the superior spinous process overlies the lamina of the vertebra below, and the epidural needle should be directed in a more acute cephalad direction. In addition, there is a risk of producing trauma to the underlying spinal cord if dural puncture occurs. In some patients, a paramedian approach is necessary.

c. **Technique for catheter placement.** An epidural catheter permits repeated injections of local anesthetic for prolonged procedures and provides a route for postoperative analgesia.

1. Thread a 20-gauge radiopaque catheter with 1-cm graduations through the epidural needle. If the catheter contains a wire stylet, the stylet should first be withdrawn 1 to 2 cm before insertion of the catheter to decrease the incidence of paresthesia and dural or venous puncture. Many individuals prefer to completely remove the stylet since it is stiff enough to allow placement into extraepidural tissue. If the catheter passes easily without the stylet, it is usually located in the epidural space. Polyvinyl chloride catheters are relatively stiff and resist kinking but can be associated with dural and venous puncture. Teflon catheters are very soft and flexible but may be more likely to kink and occlude. Newer catheters of nylon, polyamide, and polyvinyl offer compromises between flexibility and rigidity. Wire-reinforced soft catheters do not kink and are much less prone to slipping out. When multipore

catheters are used, the distance from the catheter tip to the most proximal lateral hole should be noted to ensure that all injected medication reaches the epidural space.

2. Make note of the depth at which loss of resistance occurred by counting the 1-cm markings on the Tuohy or Weiss needle that are exposed superficial to the patient's skin. A standard epidural needle measures 10 cm in length. By subtracting the number of 1-cm markings exposed superficial to the patient's skin from 10, an estimated distance between the skin and epidural space, or "depth" to the epidural space, can be obtained. Advance the catheter through the needle until the 15 cm marking on the catheter is within the shaft of the epidural needle to ensure that approximately 5 cm of catheter is exposed distal to the needle tip. The patient may experience an abrupt paresthesia, which is usually transient. If it is sustained, the catheter must be repositioned. If the catheter must be withdrawn, the catheter and needle should be removed together to avoid shearing the catheter tip.

3. Carefully withdraw the needle over the catheter making sure not to inadvertently withdraw the catheter as well. Make note of the marking on the catheter at the skin. Be sure to leave the catheter approximately 5 cm within the epidural space by securing the catheter at the skin 5 cm "deeper" than the "depth" to the epidural space (ie, if loss of resistance occurred at a "depth" of 6 cm, secure the catheter at the skin at a "depth" of 11 cm).

d. After aspirating for CSF using a 3 mL syringe, administer a **test dose** of local anesthetic agent through the needle if a single-dose technique is used or through the catheter for continuous techniques. A test dose usually consists of 3 mL of 1.5% lidocaine with 1:200,000 epinephrine. This should have little effect in the epidural space. If the solution has been injected into the CSF, a spinal block will occur rapidly. If the solution has been injected into an epidural vein, a 20% to 30% increase in heart rate may be seen. Other symptoms of an intravascular injection include perioral numbness, a metallic taste, tinnitus, and palpitations. The patient should be instructed to report any of these sensations if they arise. A corresponding increase in blood pressure can also be seen if the patient's heart rate is controlled with β-blockers.

e. **Injection of anesthetic.** Administer the anesthetic solution in 3 to 5 mL increments every 3 to 5 minutes until the desired total dose has been given. Aspirate the catheter or needle, checking for the appearance of blood or CSF, before each injection.

D. **Determinants of the level of the epidural blockade**

1. **Volume of local anesthetic.** A maximum dose of 1.6 mL of local anesthetic per segment has been suggested for the induction of epidural blockade. This maximum can be exceeded if dilute mixtures of medications are used, as for postoperative or labor analgesia.

2. **Age.** The volume of local anesthetic should be reduced by approximately 50% in the elderly and in neonates. Stenosis of intervertebral foramina in the elderly reduces the lateral paravertebral spread of the injected drug, allowing for a more cephalad spread.

3. **Pregnancy.** A 30% reduction in dose is expected in pregnant women. Hormonal effects during pregnancy render nerves more sensitive to the effects of local anesthetic, and inferior vena cava compression increases blood volume within the epidural venous plexus, reducing the potential volume of the epidural space.

4. **Speed of injection.** Rapid injection of drug into the epidural space may produce a less reliable block than a slow, steady injection at approximately 0.5 mL/s. Very rapid injection of large volumes of drug has the potentially hazardous effect of increasing pressure within the epidural space. Such a rise in pressure can produce headache, increased intracranial pressure, and possibly spinal cord ischemia by decreasing spinal cord blood flow.

5. **Position.** The position of the patient has a slight effect on the level of the epidural blockade. Patients sitting upright have greater caudad spread of blockade; patients in the lateral position have a higher level of block on the dependent side. This can be helpful if patients are reporting a "one-sided block," as the painful side can be positioned down during a bolus to overcome this.

6. **Spread of epidural blockade.** Onset of blockade occurs first and is most dense at the level of injection. Spread of the block usually occurs faster in a cephalad than in a caudad direction. This is likely because of the relative difference in size between the large lower lumbar and sacral nerve roots compared with the smaller thoracic nerve roots. L5–S1 are large nerve roots making them difficult to anesthetize and often leading to sparing of this area during epidural block.

E. **Determinants of the onset and duration of the epidural blockade**
   1. **Selection of drug** (see Chapter 19).
   2. **Addition of epinephrine.** Epinephrine, added at a concentration of 1:200,000, decreases the systemic uptake and plasma levels of local anesthetic, and prolongs its duration of action (see Chapter 19).
   3. **Addition of opioid.** The addition of fentanyl, 50 to 100 μg, to the local anesthetic solution speeds the onset, increases the level, prolongs the duration, and improves the quality of the block. Fentanyl is thought to produce this effect by having a selective action at the substantia gelatinosa of the dorsal horn of the spinal cord to modulate pain transmission. This action appears to be synergistic with the actions of the local anesthetics.
   4. **pH adjustment of solution.** The addition of sodium bicarbonate to the local anesthetic solution in a ratio of 1 mL of 8.4% sodium bicarbonate to each 10 mL of lidocaine (0.1 mL for each 10 mL of bupivacaine as excess bicarbonate will precipitate in bupivacaine) decreases the onset time for the blockade. It is thought that this effect is due to an increased amount of local anesthetic base, which increases the rate at which nonionized drug crosses axonal membranes.

F. **Complications**
   1. **Dural puncture** occurs in about 1% of epidural catheter placements. If dural puncture occurs during attempted epidural catheter insertion, the chance of PDPH is higher than with spinal anesthesia due to the larger size of the needle. Furthermore, it is important to minimize the amount of CSF leakage from the epidural needle by either covering the proximal hole of the needle with your finger or reinserting the stylet. Several management options are available after dural puncture. A conversion to spinal anesthesia can be made by injecting an appropriate amount of anesthetic into the CSF. Continuous spinal anesthesia can be performed by inserting an epidural catheter into the subarachnoid space through the epidural needle. If epidural anesthesia is required (eg, for postoperative analgesia), the catheter can be repositioned at a different interspace so that the tip of the epidural catheter lies well away from the site of dural puncture. The possibility of spinal anesthesia occurring with injection of the epidural catheter should be considered.

2. **Bloody tap.** If a bloody tap occurs during epidural needle placement, some practitioners advocate for epidural placement at a different interspace. Advantages include minimizing confounding effects of visualized blood on determination of correct catheter placement and potentially decreasing amounts of systemically absorbed local anesthetic that may be falsely interpreted as a positive test dose. In patients with normal coagulation, such bloody taps rarely lead to serious sequelae (eg, epidural hematoma). Bloody epidural taps may be risk factors for epidural hematoma in patients who undergo subsequent anticoagulation, but there are no data to support the mandatory cancellation of a case under these circumstances. Instead, we advocate direct communication with the surgeon and that a specific risk-benefit decision about proceeding be made on an individual basis. Close postoperative monitoring for signs consistent with hematoma is warranted.

3. **Catheter complications**

   a. **Inability to thread the epidural catheter** is relatively common. This problem can occur if the epidural needle is inserted into the lateral aspect of the epidural space rather than the midline or if the bevel of the needle is at too acute an angle to the epidural space for the catheter to emerge. It can also occur if the level of the needle is only partially through the ligamentum flavum when loss of resistance is found. In the latter case, slight (1 mm) advancement of the needle into the epidural space may facilitate catheter insertion.

   b. **The catheter can be inserted into an epidural vein.** Blood cannot always be aspirated back through the catheter. This may be noticed only when an initial test dose with epinephrine is administered, and tachycardia is noted. The catheter should be withdrawn until blood can no longer be aspirated, flushed with saline, and then retested. Withdrawal of the catheter more than 1 to 2 cm should prompt removal and reinsertion.

   c. **Catheters can break off or become knotted** within the epidural space. In the absence of infection, a retained catheter is no more reactive than a surgical suture. The patient should be informed of the problem and reassured. The complications of surgical exploration and removal of an asymptomatic catheter are greater than in conservative management.

   d. **Cannulation of the subdural space.** The subdural space is a potential space between the dura and the arachnoid membranes and may be entered with a needle or with a catheter. CSF is not aspirated but the effects of the local anesthetic are quite different from usual epidural anesthesia and are often quite variable. In the absence of myelography, it is a diagnosis of exclusion. It can result in dissociation of blocked modalities (eg, full sensory anesthesia without motor block or motor block with minimal sensory block). It should be suspected whenever an epidural dose produces a more extensive spread than expected. Subdural catheters should be removed and an epidural catheter should be placed.

4. **Unintentional subarachnoid injection.** The injection of a large volume of local anesthetic into the subarachnoid space can produce total spinal anesthesia. Treatment is similar to that described for spinal complications (see Section IV.F).

5. **Intravascular injection** of local anesthetic into an epidural vein causes central nervous system and cardiovascular toxicity and may result in convulsions and cardiopulmonary arrest. Resistant ventricular fibrillation with IV bupivacaine has been described. The treatment for

intravascular injection includes IV lipid emulsion for local anesthetic-related cardiotoxicity. A bolus of Intralipid 20%, 1.5 mL/kg, over 2 to 3 minutes followed by a continuous infusion (0.25 mL/kg/min) with repeat bolus doses once or twice for a total maximum dose of 12 mL/kg is the treatment of choice. Cardiopulmonary bypass is an option if ventricular fibrillation or cardiac arrest is resistant to pharmacologic therapy (see Chapters 19 and 39).

6. **Local anesthetic overdose.** Systemic local anesthetic toxicity may occur due to the relatively large amounts of drug required for anesthesia. Inadvertent intravascular injection is the most common cause of local anesthetic overdose. Vasoconstrictors such as epinephrine decreases the incidence of toxicity by decreasing the rate of absorption of local anesthetic.

7. **Direct spinal cord injury** is more likely if the epidural injection is above L2. The onset of a unilateral paresthesia during needle insertion suggests lateral entry into the epidural space. Further injection or insertion of a catheter at this point may produce trauma to a nerve root. Small feeder arteries to the anterior spinal artery also run in this area as they pass through the intervertebral foramen. Trauma to these arteries potentially may result in anterior spinal cord ischemia or an epidural hematoma. Placement of epidural catheters after the induction of general anesthesia negates the ability to appreciate symptoms of paresthesia and is done only when such potential risk is deemed necessary. Pediatric patients frequently have catheters placed after induction of general anesthesia, often at the caudal level.

8. **PDPH.** If the dura is punctured with a 17-gauge epidural needle, there is a greater than 75% chance of a young patient developing a PDPH. Management is the same as that described under spinal anesthesia (see Section IV.F.1.f.).

9. **Epidural abscess** is an extremely rare complication of epidural anesthesia. The source of infection usually is from hematogenous spread to the epidural space from an infection in another area. Infection can also arise from contamination during insertion, contamination of an indwelling catheter used for postoperative pain relief, or a cutaneous infection at the insertion site. The patient presents with fever, severe back pain, and localized back tenderness. Progression to nerve root pain and paralysis can occur. Initial laboratory investigations include evaluation for a leukocytosis and a lumbar puncture suggestive of a parameningeal infection. Definitive diagnosis is by MRI. Treatment includes antibiotics and sometimes urgent decompression laminectomy. Rapid diagnosis and treatment are associated with good neurologic recovery. Epidural catheter dressings should be inspected daily for signs of leakage and inflammation.

10. **Epidural hematoma** is an extremely rare complication of epidural anesthesia. An epidural hematoma is a surgical emergency. Trauma to epidural veins in the presence of a coagulopathy may result in a large epidural hematoma. The patient can present with severe back pain and persistent neurologic deficit after epidural anesthesia. Diagnosis is confirmed by MRI. A decompressive laminectomy within 8 hours from the onset of symptoms is required to preserve neurologic function.

11. **Horner syndrome** is seen in 1% to 4% of epidural anesthetics. The constellation of ptosis, miosis, anhidrosis, and enophthalmos occurs due to the sympathetic blockade of the upper thoracic spinal segments. Reassurance is provided to the patient as these symptoms resolve.

VI. COMBINED SPINAL-EPIDURAL ANESTHESIA

A. Spinal anesthesia offers the benefits of rapid onset. Placement of an epidural catheter at the same time offers the advantage of prolonged anesthesia and analgesia for longer procedures or postoperative pain management. This technique often is used in the labor and delivery setting (see Chapter 32).

B. **Technique.** Prepare the patient as for epidural placement (see Section V.C). After placing the epidural needle in the epidural space, advance a long spinal needle (Sprotte 24 gauge × 120 mm or Whitacre 25 gauge) through the epidural needle until the characteristic pop of dural penetration occurs. At this point, withdraw the stylet from the spinal needle and confirm free flow of CSF. Before withdrawing the stylet, it is recommended to grasp both the spinal needle and the epidural Tuohy needle at the same time to stabilize the position of the spinal needle. Inject medication into the subarachnoid space and withdraw the spinal needle. Thread an epidural catheter through the epidural needle in the standard fashion. If epidural anesthesia is used subsequently, a test dose is required (can be administered intraoperatively).

VII. CAUDAL ANESTHESIA

Caudal anesthesia is obtained by placing local anesthetic into the epidural space in the sacral region. This technique is often used for pediatric anesthesia. The details below are intended for the adult population.

A. **Anatomy.** The caudal space is an extension of the epidural space. The sacral hiatus is formed by the failure of the laminae of S5 to fuse. The hiatus is bounded laterally by the sacral cornua, which are the inferior articulating processes of S5. The **sacrococcygeal membrane** is a thin layer of fibrous tissue that covers the sacral hiatus. The caudal canal contains the sacral nerves, the sacral venous plexus, the filum terminale, and the dural sac, which usually ends at the lower border of S2. In neonates, the dural sac may extend to S4.

B. **Physiology.** The physiology of caudal anesthesia is similar to that described for epidural anesthesia (see Section V.B). It is indicated for surgical and obstetric procedures of the perineal and sacral areas.

C. **Technique**

1. Caudal epidural anesthesia is performed with the patient in the lateral, prone, or jackknife position.

2. Palpate the sacral cornua. If they are difficult to palpate directly, the location of the sacral hiatus in adults can be estimated by measuring 5 cm from the tip of the coccyx in the midline.

3. Skin preparation and draping are as described for spinal anesthesia (see Section IV.C.5).

4. Raise a skin wheal with 1% lidocaine between the sacral cornua.

5. Insert a 22-gauge spinal needle at an angle of 70° to 80° to the skin. Advance the needle through the sacrococcygeal membrane, which is identified by a characteristic pop. Avoid attempting to thread the needle up the caudal canal because this increases the likelihood of puncturing an epidural vein (**Figure 20.6**).

6. Withdraw the stylet and inspect the hub of the needle for passive CSF or blood flow. The needle can be aspirated as a further check. Reposition the needle if either blood or CSF appears.

7. Administer a test dose of 3 mL of local anesthetic solution with epinephrine (1:200,000), similar to that used for lumbar epidural anesthesia (see Section V.C.4.d), observing the patient for signs of subarachnoid

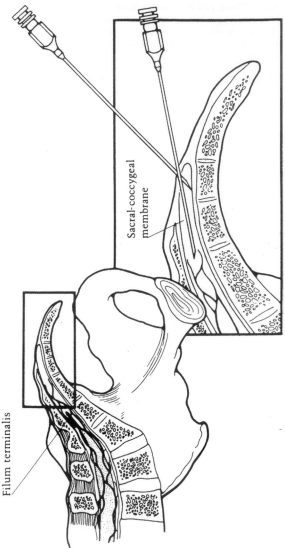

FIGURE 20.6 Sacral anatomy, lateral view. A needle directed through the sacral-coccygeal membrane at a 45-degree angle will usually "pop" through the ligament and contact the anterior bone of the sacral canal. The needle needs to be rotated so that the bevel does not scrape the periosteum of this layer, and the angle of advancement changed to allow passage directly 2 to 3 cm up the canal without contacting the bone again. This space is generously endowed with blood vessels, and the terminal point of the dural sac extends a variable distance in the sacral canal but usually lies at the S2 level. (Reprinted with permission from Mulroy MF. *Regional Anesthesia: An Illustrated Procedural Guide*. 2nd ed. Little, Brown and Company; 1996:124.)

or IV injection. Because the caudal canal has a rich epidural venous plexus, IV injections are seen frequently and can occur even though blood cannot be aspirated from the needle.

8. A caudal catheter can be placed in a manner analogous to that for lumbar epidural anesthesia with a 17-gauge Tuohy needle (see Section V.C.4.c). The catheter can be used for postoperative analgesia.

9. The level, onset, and duration for caudal anesthesia follow the same principles outlined for epidural anesthesia (see Sections V.D and V.E). The extent of caudal block is less predictable than other epidural techniques because of the variability in content and volume of the caudal canal and the amount of local anesthetic solution that leaks out of the sacral foramina. To obtain sacral anesthesia, a volume of 12 to 15 mL should be sufficient.

D. Complications. The complications of caudal anesthesia are similar to those of epidural anesthesia (see Section V.F).

VIII. ANTICOAGULATION AND NEURAXIAL BLOCKADE

Neuraxial blockade should be avoided in the presence of prophylactic or therapeutic anticoagulation because of the increased risk of epidural hematoma formation. Massachusetts General Hospital guidelines regarding neuraxial anesthesia in anticoagulated patients are listed in **Table 20.3**.

A. Oral anticoagulants. In patients receiving low-dose oral anticoagulants (warfarin), regional techniques may be performed if the thromboprophylaxis was initiated less than 24 hours previously. If epidural or spinal anesthesia is planned, hold warfarin 3 to 5 days before the operation, and the patient's international normalized ratio (INR) should be checked before the operation. An INR less than or equal to 1.5 is generally acceptable for many anesthesiologists, but there is no definite cutoff value above which epidural or spinal anesthesia is specifically discouraged.

B. Unfractionated heparin. Twice-daily subcutaneous heparin prophylaxis is not a contraindication for the use of neuraxial techniques. There is an unknown risk with prophylactic subcutaneous heparin dosed three times per day. In these cases, a coagulation profile should be obtained. Caution should be used in debilitated patients, in whom the action of the drug may be prolonged and in whom neurologic monitoring may be difficult. IV heparin should be stopped 2 to 4 hours before the initiation of neuraxial blockade, and a repeat coagulation profile should be obtained if there is any question about the state of anticoagulation. Administration of heparin should be delayed for at least 2 hours after placement. Removal of a catheter should be treated with the same anticoagulation guidelines as the placement of a catheter.

C. Low-molecular-weight heparin. Patients receiving low-molecular-weight heparin (LMWH) for thromboembolism prophylaxis have altered coagulation parameters. Spinal or epidural needle placement should not be done for at least 12 hours after the last dose. Patients receiving higher doses of LMWH (enoxaparin 1 mg/kg twice daily) will require longer delays (24 hours). In patients requiring continuing LMWH administration, spinal or epidural catheters should be removed before administration of LMWH. The subsequent administration of LMWH should be delayed for 4 hours after catheter removal.

D. Antiplatelet drugs. Patients receiving aspirin or nonsteroidal anti-inflammatory drugs do not appear to be at higher risk for epidural hematoma formation. These drugs could contribute to an increased bleeding risk, however, if they are used concurrently with other anticoagulants.

With regard to thienopyridine derivatives (ticlopidine and clopidogrel), the suggested time interval between discontinuation of medication and initiation of neuraxial block is 14 days for ticlopidine and 5 to 7 days for clopidogrel. Following platelet GPIIb/IIIa inhibitors, normal platelet function returns in 24 to 48 hours with abciximab and in 4 to 8 hours with eptifibatide and tirofiban.

E. **Fibrinolytic and thrombolytic agents.** Although the plasma half-life of thrombolytic drugs is only for hours, it takes several days before thrombolytic effects disappear. Surgery or puncture of noncompressible vessels within 10 days of thrombolytic therapy is contraindicated. There is no definitive guideline regarding the neuraxial anesthesia and thrombolytic therapy. Measurement of the fibrinogen level may be helpful in guiding the decision.

F. **Herbal medication (see Chapters 1 and 38).** Herbal medications including garlic, ginkgo, and ginseng are all known to affect coagulation. Currently, there are no specific guidelines for timing the neuraxial block in relation to herbal medication use. Because it is not known at which doses potential coagulopathies occur, management decisions are often based more on a clinical history of abnormal bleeding. Herbal medications are thought to be more problematic when taken concurrently with other conventional anticoagulant medications.

Suggested Readings

Aida S, Taga K, Yamakura T, Endoh H, Shimoji K. Headache after attempted epidural block: the role of intrathecal air. *Anesthesiology.* 1998;88:76-81.

Horlocker TT, Wedel DJ, Rowlingson JC, et al. Regional anesthesia in the patient receiving antithrombotic or thrombolytic therapy: American Society of Regional Anesthesia and Pain Medicine Evidence-Based Guidelines (Third Edition). *Reg Anesth Pain Med.* 2010;35(1):64-101.

Moen V, Dahlgren N, Irestedt L. Severe neurological complications after central neuraxial blockades in Sweden 1990-1999. *Anesthesiology.* 2004;101:950-959.

Moraca RJ, Sheldon DG, Thirlby RC. The role of epidural anesthesia and analgesia in surgical practice. *Ann Surg.* 2003;238:663-673.

Turnbull DK, Sheperd DB. Post-dural puncture headache: pathogenesis, prevention and treatment. *Br J Anaesth.* 2003;91(5):718-729.

21 Regional Anesthesia

Lucy T. Li, Shika Card, and A. Sassan Sabouri

ABBREVIATIONS

ASA American Society of Anesthesiologists
ASIS anterior superior iliac spine
BP brachial plexus
CPB cervical plexus block
EOM external oblique muscle
ESM erector spinae muscle
GA general anesthesia
IOM internal oblique muscle
IP in-plane
IV intravenous
LA local anesthetic
LAST local anesthetic systemic toxicity
LFC lateral femoral cutaneous
OOP out-of-plane
PCNT posterior cutaneous nerve of the thigh
PNS peripheral neurostimulation
QL quadratus lumborum muscle
RA regional anesthesia
SCM sternocleidomastoid muscle
SCN sciatic nerve
SCTL superior costotransverse ligament
TAM transversus abdominis muscle
TAP transversus abdominis plane
TP transverse process
TPVS thoracic paravertebral space
UGRA ultrasound-guided regional anesthesia

I. GENERAL CONSIDERATIONS

A. **Peripheral nerve blockade** can be an excellent addition or alternative to general anesthesia (GA) for many surgical procedures. Regional anesthesia (RA) may provide sensory and motor blockade without significantly disrupting systemic autonomic function. Single-shot blocks can provide postoperative analgesia that may last for hours.

B. **Continuous peripheral nerve catheters** prolong the analgesia of RA techniques beyond the maximum duration of a single injection block. This can be especially useful for patients with chronic pain or opioid tolerance. A nerve block catheter is inserted percutaneously adjacent to the peripheral nerves or fascia plane, often with ultrasound guidance. Local anesthetic (LA) is then infused through the catheter(s) providing analgesia for days or in certain circumstances even for weeks.

C. **The preoperative evaluation** includes patient history, particularly history of coagulopathy, and physical examination, with special attention to any preexisting neurological deficits. ASA guidelines for perioperative care are similar to those for patients receiving GA.

D. **Surgical considerations** must be incorporated into the regional anesthetic plan. These include intraoperative factors, such as projected surgical incision and extension, total surgical time, and tourniquet placement, and postoperative factors like anticipated level of pain and duration of recovery.

E. **Consent** for RA should include a thorough description of the risks, benefits, options, and common side effects. **Need for supplemental** LA, sedation, or potential for GA should always be discussed. **Laterality** of the procedure and thus block placement must be confirmed with the patient, case booking, available preprocedure imaging or notes, and markings made by the surgical team on the day of surgery.

F. **Preoperative anxiolysis** may be appropriate as long as the patient remains alert and cooperative. Conscious sedation is usually achieved by using short-acting agents such as midazolam and/or fentanyl.

G. **Standard ASA monitoring** of electrocardiogram, blood pressure measurement, and pulse oximetry with audible pitch tone must be used during placement of all blocks. Resuscitation medications and equipment should be readily available (see Section IV.G).

H. A **time-out** must be conducted prior to starting regional block placement to confirm patient identity, correct procedure site, and regional anesthetic to be performed.

I. **Aseptic technique** must be employed during performance of all blocks. This includes removal of jewelry; hand hygiene; use of caps, masks, and sterile gloves; use of individual packets of chlorhexidine solution (preferably alcohol based) for skin preparation and adequate drying time; sterile equipment; placement of sterile occlusive dressings over catheter insertion sites; and limiting disconnection and reconnection of LA delivery systems.

J. **Postoperative follow-up** should include assessment of block efficacy and duration, presence of residual sensory or motor blockade, paresthesia or other side effects, and patient satisfaction.

II. GENERAL CONTRAINDICATIONS

Absolute contraindications to RA include lack of patient consent, local skin infection at the site of needle insertion, or when nerve blockade would hinder the surgery or desired postoperative neurologic examination. Relative contraindications include coagulopathy, neuropathy, systemic infection, excessive patient anxiety, cognitive deficits or movement disorders, and anatomic distortion. Peripheral nervous system disorders such as diabetic neuropathy and inflammatory neuropathies may be aggravated by peripheral nerve blockade.

III. COMPLICATIONS COMMON TO ALL NERVE BLOCKS

A. **Complications of LAs** include intravascular injection, local anesthetic systemic toxicity (LAST) (see Chapter 19), and allergic reactions. Use of ultrasound, addition of epinephrine to LA solutions, and intermittent aspiration during injection may help identify intravascular injection.

B. **Nerve damage is rare**, with long-term neurologic injury occurring in 0.02% to 0.04% of peripheral nerve blocks. It may result from needle trauma, nerve compression, stretch, or ischemia, or be direct LA-induced neurotoxicity. Paresthesia with needle advancement or injection is not entirely predictive of nerve injury. However, if pain or paresthesia is encountered, one must consider this complication and redirect the needle. A combination of monitoring techniques, such as peripheral nerve stimulation, injection pressure monitoring, and ultrasound can be used for prevention.

C. **Hematomas** may result from vascular puncture but usually resolve without residual problems. When considering RA for an anticoagulated or coagulopathic patient, one should consider following neuraxial guidelines (see Chapter 20), particularly for deeper blocks (eg, infraclavicular, paravertebral) where vessel compression for bleeding control is challenging.

D. **Infection** risk is reduced with the use of aseptic technique (see Section I.I).

E. **Failure or incomplete block** can be identified with a careful neurologic examination prior to the beginning of the surgical procedure.

IV. EQUIPMENT

A. **Needles used for nerve blockade**

1. **Needle gauge** should be the smallest possible for patient comfort. A 22-gauge needle is used most commonly. **Short-beveled needles** (45°) have become standard for peripheral nerve blocks. **Insulated** needles used in nerve stimulator-guided techniques have a small conductive area at the needle tip allowing for more accurate nerve stimulation at lower amplitudes of current. Ideal **needle length** varies by block. Upper- and lower-extremity blocks are best performed with a 50- to 150-mm needle depending on nerve depth. **Echogenic needles** designed for use in ultrasound-guided techniques have modifications such as special coating, scoring of the needle's surface, and reflector placement to enhance reflection of ultrasound waves and improve needle visualization.

B. Connecting a large-volume (20-mL) **syringe** to the block needle with sterile extension tubing ensures stable needle position during aspiration and injection.

C. A variety of **continuous catheter kits** and infusion pumps for continuous nerve blockade are commercially available.

D. **Nerve stimulators (Figure 21.1)** designed for RA can deliver a current of 0.1 to 10.0 mA at a frequency of 0.5 to 4 Hz with a stimulus duration of 0.05 to 1.0 ms.

E. **Ultrasound machines** that are portable and utilize transducers of various shapes, sizes, and frequencies facilitate imaging of relevant anatomy and serve as an alternative/adjuvant to nerve stimulator approaches. Sterile transducer covers and gel allow for real-time imaging within a sterile field.

F. **Selection of LA** for a block depends upon the desired speed of onset and duration (see Chapter 19).

G. **Resuscitation drugs** should be immediately accessible for any provider performing RA. Medications include lipid emulsion with dosing guidelines and resuscitation medications including, but not limited to, epinephrine. **Emergency equipment** should include oxygen supply, airway management devices, suction, and defibrillators.

H. To provide for the safe and effective practice of RA, a designated and centralized **regional anesthesia bay** with equipment and nurses who are familiar and experienced with RA techniques is recommended (**Figure 21.2**).

V. NERVE LOCALIZATION TECHNIQUES

The classic approach uses anatomical landmarks, tactile feedback from fascial "clicks," elicited paresthesias, and transarterial approaches to guide needle advancement and LA injection. This technique has become less popular as many anesthetists have transitioned practice to either peripheral neurostimulation (PNS) or ultrasound-guided regional anesthesia (UGRA). **PNS techniques** allow the operator to estimate the distance of the needle tip from the target nerve based on the magnitude of current required to elicit the desired motor response. Although it does not require direct nerve contact,

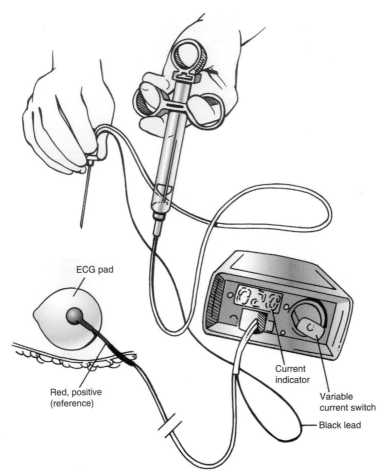

FIGURE 21.1 Nerve stimulator attached to the regional block needle. The negative (*black*) lead is attached to the exploring needle, whereas the positive (*red*) is connected to a reference electrocardiogram pad used as a "ground." (Reprinted with permission from Mulroy MF, Bernards CM, McDonald SB, et al. *A Practical Approach to Regional Anesthesia.* 4th ed. Wolters Kluwer Health/Lippincott Williams & Wilkins; 2009.)

nerve stimulation can cause patient discomfort especially in areas of injury, does not provide information about other structures like vasculature, and may be affected by variations in tissue impedance or peripheral neuropathy. **UGRA techniques** allow for real-time visualization of the desired anatomy, needle tip position and trajectory, and LA spread and have become widely used in recent years. Studies have shown that the use of ultrasound may reduce block performance time, number of needle passes, and volume of LA required for successful block and may also reduce the incidence of vascular puncture. Nevertheless, complications such as intravascular and intraneural injection have occurred even with the use of ultrasound, and visualization of

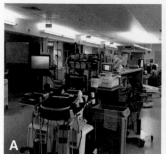
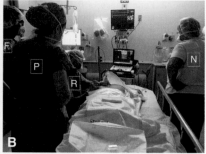

FIGURE 21.2 Regional anesthesia bay and team. A, A well-maintained and equipped regional anesthesia bay is essential to the safe practice of regional anesthesia techniques. B, A "block nurse" (N) who is familiar with regional anesthesia techniques is an important member of the team (physician [P], fellow [F], and resident [R]).

some structures like the lumbar plexus and smaller and deeper nerves may be limited.

A. PNS produces a motor response without significant pain.

1. Ground the positive lead of the stimulator to the patient and attach the negative terminal of the stimulator to the needle (**Figure 21.1**).

2. Set the nerve stimulator to an initial current of 0.5 to 1.0 mA and move the needle toward the nerve until a motor response in the desired muscle group occurs. Stimulation of the target nerve at a current of 0.5 mA suggests accurate needle placement for LA administration. Motor response at less than 0.5 mA is suggestive of intraneural placement, and the needle should be withdrawn slightly.

B. UGRA may supplement or replace the above techniques.

1. **Ultrasound** uses high-frequency sound waves (>20 kHz) to visualize structures and tissues in real time without ionizing radiation. Within the ultrasound transducer, electric current is applied to a piezoelectric crystal array, which vibrates at high frequency to generate sound waves. As these waves travel through the tissue being imaged, some are reflected back to the transducer. The intensity and delay in return of the reflected sound waves are used to construct a 2D gray-scale image. Denser structures such as bone reflect more sound waves and appear brighter or **hyperechoic**. Less dense substances such as air or fluid reflect less and appear darker or **hypoechoic**.

2. **"Knobology"**: Commercially available ultrasound machines allow the operator to adjust a number of parameters to optimize visualization. **Depth** should be set to the minimum that allows visualization of target structures. **Focus** of the ultrasound waves should be placed just beyond the depth of the target structures. **Gain** determines the overall brightness of the image and may be increased or decreased as needed. **Frequency** affects both image resolution and depth of penetration. Higher frequencies increase the resolution at the expense of penetration. Conversely, lower frequencies increase the depth of penetration at the expense of resolution. Most nerve blocks are performed at an intermediate depth and thus utilize intermediate frequencies. **Color Doppler** is mostly useful for identification of blood flow in vasculature.

3. **Performance** of the block depends on optimal visualization of target structures, proper needle positioning, and adequate spread of LA around the nerve(s).

   a. Initial positioning of the ultrasound transducer is determined by surface landmarks and refined by scanning to obtain the optimal view of the desired anatomy. The left-right orientation of the transducer in relation to the display should be confirmed prior to scanning. Basic scanning maneuvers include sliding the transducer in the horizontal plane, tilting its vertical axis to various angles in relation to the skin surface, rotating around its vertical axis, and applying more or less vertical pressure. Anatomic structures may be viewed in sagittal, transverse, or oblique planes.

   b. There are two options for needle visualization. In the "**out-of-plane**" (OOP) approach, the needle is inserted immediately above or below the midline of the transducer and advanced perpendicularly to the plane of the ultrasound beam. This provides a cross-sectional view of the needle tip as a hyperechoic dot. In the "**in-plane**" (IP) approach, the needle is inserted a few centimeters lateral to the transducer and advanced in the plane of the ultrasound beam, allowing continuous visualization of the length of the needle as a hyperechoic line.

   c. **Needle insertion angle** influences visibility of the needle tip. When the needle is nearly parallel to the ultrasound probe, the tip is easily identified. At steeper angles of entry, needle tip visibility can be more difficult. An echogenic needle can help improve visualization in those cases.

   d. The needle tip should be positioned near the target nerve. Injection of 0.5 to 1 mL of dextrose water or normal saline can help localize the needle tip (hydrolocalization). Spread of LA should be observed both for evidence of intraneural injection, which may result in nerve injury and should prompt adjustment of needle position, and for adequacy of spread. Circumferential spread of LA around the target nerve suggests injection in the proper fascial plane. For some blocks, multiple injection sites may be needed to achieve the desired distribution of LA.

VI. REGIONAL ANESTHESIA OF THE NECK

A. Cervical plexus block (CPB)

1. **Anatomy.** The cervical plexus lies in the paravertebral region of the upper four cervical vertebrae, formed from the anterior rami of the C1-C4 spinal nerve roots. The plexus is situated between the prevertebral muscle anteromedially and the muscles attached to the posterior tubercles of the cervical transverse processes (TP) posterolaterally. The plexus has cutaneous, muscular, and communicating branches. The **superficial cutaneous branches**, which include the lesser occipital, greater auricular, transverse cervical, and supraclavicular nerves, pierce the prevertebral fascia anteriorly, just deep to the sternocleidomastoid muscle (SCM) at the level of the C5 TP. They innervate the skin and fascia of the back of the head, lateral neck, top of the shoulder and chest, and the clavicle (**Figure 21.3**). The **deep muscular branches** are deep to the prevertebral fascia and supply the muscles and deep structures of the neck and form the phrenic nerve.

2. **Indications. Superficial CPB** (C2-C4) produces cutaneous anesthesia and is useful for superficial procedures on the neck and shoulder. It has been shown that superficial CPB is as effective as **paravertebral cervical**

root block, known previously as **deep CPB**, for carotid endarterectomy with fewer complications.

3. **Superficial CPB using UGRA** (see **Figure 21.5**): Position the patient supine with the neck slightly extended and the head turned toward the opposite side. Place the ultrasound probe transversely over the SCM at the level of the cricoid cartilage and scan posteriorly until the posterior edge of the SCM is visualized in the center of the screen. The SCP may be visualized as two to three small hypoechoic structures between the SCM and scalene muscles. Using an IP approach, insert a 23- to 25-gauge 50-mm needle lateral to the probe and advance until the needle tip is beneath the posterior border of the SCM and adjacent to the plexus. After negative aspiration, inject 10 mL of LA in a fan-like fashion along the posterior border of the SCM, 2 to 3 cm above and below the needle insertion site. LA should spread between the SCM and the underlying prevertebral fascia.

4. **Complications. Vagus nerve block** and **recurrent laryngeal nerve block** can occur if LA spreads too medially, causing hoarseness and vocal cord dysfunction.

VII. REGIONAL ANESTHESIA OF THE UPPER EXTREMITY

A. Anatomy (Figure 21.4)

1. The shoulder, axilla, and upper extremity are innervated by the **brachial plexus** (BP). Skin of the medial aspect of the upper arm is innervated by the **intercostobrachial nerve** formed by T2 and the **medial cutaneous nerve of the arm**. The **supraclavicular nerve**, which is formed by C3-C4, innervates the skin of the top of the shoulder (see Section VI.A.1).

2. The BP is formed from the ventral rami of the spinal nerves from C5 to C8 and T1, with frequent contributions from C4 and T2. It is traditionally divided into five parts: roots, trunks, divisions, cords, and branches.

3. Each **root** or ventral ramus exits posterior to the vertebral artery and travels laterally in the trough of its cervical TP, sandwiched between the fascial sheaths of the anterior and middle scalene muscles.

4. The **trunks** (superior, middle, and inferior) pass over the first rib through the space between the anterior and middle scalene muscles in association with the subclavian artery, which shares the same fascial sheath.

5. As the trunks pass over the first rib and under the clavicle, they split into the anterior (flexor) and posterior (extensor) **divisions**, which then reorganize to form the three **cords** (lateral, medial, and posterior, named for their usual positions relative to the axillary artery) of the plexus.

6. Branches of the lateral and medial cords form the **median nerve**. The lateral cord also gives off a branch that forms the **musculocutaneous nerve**. The medial cord also forms the **ulnar, medial antebrachial cutaneous**, and **medial brachial cutaneous nerves**. The posterior cord becomes the **axillary and radial nerves** (**Figure 21.4**). In the axilla, the median nerve classically lies lateral to the axillary artery, the radial nerve posterior and over the conjoint tendon (of the teres major and latissimus dorsi muscles), and the ulnar nerve medial, but variation in these relative positions may occur. The musculocutaneous and axillary nerves exit the sheath high up in the axilla. The musculocutaneous nerve travels through the coracobrachialis muscle before becoming subcutaneous below the elbow, and the axillary nerve travels through the quadrilateral space (bordered by the humeral shaft, long head of the triceps, and teres major and minor muscles) before dividing into its terminal branches.

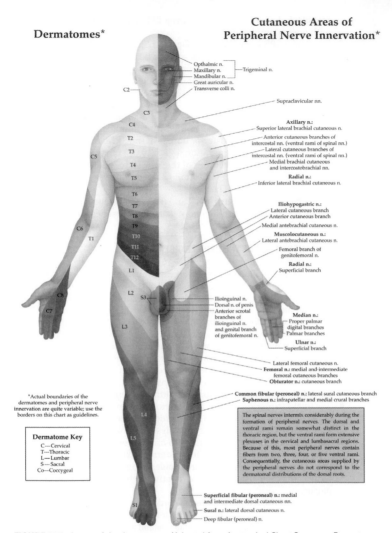

Dermatomes*

Cutaneous Areas of Peripheral Nerve Innervation*

Opthalmic n.
Maxillary n. ⎤ Trigeminal n.
Mandibular n. ⎦
Great auricular n.
Transverse colli n.

C2

C3

Supraclavicular nn.

C4

Axillary n.:
Superior lateral brachial cutaneous n.

T2

Anterior cutaneous branches of
intercostal nn. (ventral rami of spinal nn.)

T3

Lateral cutaneous branches of
intercostal nn. (ventral rami of spinal nn.)

C5

T4

Medial brachial cutaneous
and intercostobrachial nn.

T5

Radial n.:
Inferior lateral brachial cutaneous n.

T6

T7

Iliohypogastric n.:

T8

Lateral cutaneous branch
Anterior cutaneous branch

C6

T9

Medial antebrachial cutaneous n.

T10

Musculocutaneous n.:
Lateral antebrachial cutaneous n.

T1

T11

Femoral branch of
genitofemoral n.

T12

Radial n.:
Superficial branch

L1

L2

S3

Ilioinguinal n.
Dorsal n. of penis
Anterior scrotal
branches of
ilioinguinal n.
and genital branch
of genitofemoral n.

Median n.:
Proper palmar
digital branches
Palmar branches

L3

Ulnar n.:
Superficial branch

C8

C7

Lateral femoral cutaneous n.
Femoral n.: medial and intermediate
femoral cutaneous branches
Obturator n.: cutaneous branch

*Actual boundaries of the
dermatomes and peripheral nerve
innervation are quite variable; use the
borders on this chart as guidelines.

Common fibular (peroneal) n.: lateral sural cutaneous branch
Saphenous n.: infrapatellar and medial crural branches

The spinal nerves intermix considerably during the
formation of peripheral nerves. The dorsal and
ventral rami remain somewhat distinct in the
thoracic region, but the ventral rami form extensive
plexuses in the cervical and lumbasacral regions.
Because of this, most peripheral nerves contain
fibers from two, three, four, or five ventral rami.
Consequentially, the cutaneous areas supplied by
the peripheral nerves do not correspond to the
dermatomal distributions of the dorsal roots.

Dermatome Key
C—Cervical
T—Thoracic
L—Lumbar
S—Sacral
Co—Coccygeal

L4

L5

S1

Superficial fibular (peroneal) n.: medial
and intermediate dorsal cutaneous nn.
Sural n.: lateral dorsal cutaneous n.
Deep fibular (peroneal) n.

FIGURE 21.3 A map of the dermatomes. (Adapted from Anatomical Chart Company. *Dermatomes Anatomical Chart.* Wolters Kluwer; 2004 and Jaffe RA, Schmiesing CA, Golianu B, eds. *Anesthesiologist's Manual of Surgical Procedures.* 6th ed. Wolters Kluwer; 2020.)

Cutaneous Areas of Peripheral Nerve Innervation*

Dermatomes*

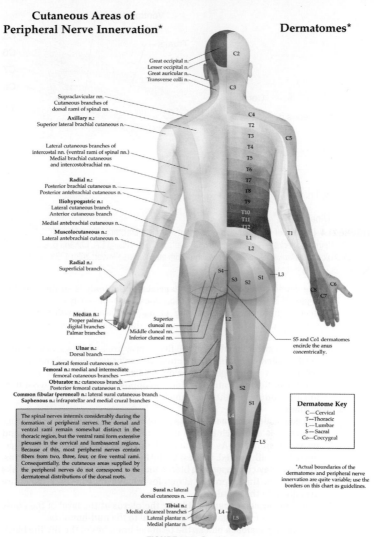

Great occipital n.
Lesser occipital n.
Great auricular n.
Transverse colli n.

C2

C3

Supraclavicular nn.
Cutaneous branches of
dorsal rami of spinal nn.

C4

Axillary n.:
Superior lateral brachial cutaneous n.

T2
T3
C5

Lateral cutaneous branches of
intercostal nn. (ventral rami of spinal nn.)
Medial brachial cutaneous
and intercostobrachial nn.

T4
T5
T6

Radial n.:
Posterior brachial cutaneous n.
Posterior antebrachial cutaneous n.

T7
T8
T9

Iliohypogastric n.:
Lateral cutaneous branch
Anterior cutaneous branch
Medial antebrachial cutaneous n.

T10
T11
T12

Musculocutaneous n.:
Lateral antebrachial cutaneous n.

L1
L2

T1

Radial n.:
Superficial branch

S4
S3 S2 S1 L3

C8 C6
C7

Median n.:
Proper palmar
digital branches
Palmar branches

Superior
cluneal nn.
Middle cluneal nn.
Inferior cluneal nn.

L2

Ulnar n.:
Dorsal branch

S5 and Co1 dermatomes
encircle the anus
concentrically.

Lateral femoral cutaneous n.
Femoral n.: medial and intermediate
femoral cutaneous branches
Obturator: cutaneous branch
Posterior femoral cutaneous n.
Common fibular (peroneal) n.: lateral sural cutaneous branch
Saphenous n.: infrapatellar and medial crural branches

L3

S2

S1

The spinal nerves intermix considerably during the
formation of peripheral nerves. The dorsal and
ventral rami remain somewhat distinct in the
thoracic region, but the ventral rami form extensive
plexuses in the cervical and lumbosacral regions.
Because of this, most peripheral nerves contain
fibers from two, three, four, or five ventral rami.
Consequentially, the cutaneous areas supplied by
the peripheral nerves do not correspond to the
dermatomal distributions of the dorsal roots.

L4

L5

Dermatome Key
C—Cervical
T—Thoracic
L—Lumbar
S—Sacral
Co—Coccygeal

*Actual boundaries of the
dermatomes and peripheral nerve
innervation are quite variable; use the
borders on this chart as guidelines.

Sural n.: lateral
dorsal cutaneous n.

Tibial n.:
Medial calcaneal branches
Lateral plantar n.
Medial plantar n.

L4 L5

FIGURE 21.3 Cont'd

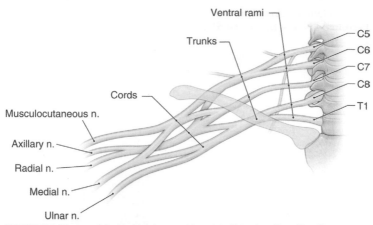

Ventral rami

Trunks

Cords

Musculocutaneous n.

Axillary n.

Radial n.

Medial n.

Ulnar n.

C5
C6
C7
C8
T1

FIGURE 21.4 Diagram of the brachial plexus and its terminal branches. (From Horn JL, Nasiri M. Regional blocks—A brief overview. In: Jaffe RA, Schmiesing CA, Golianu B, eds. *Anesthesiologist's Manual of Surgical Procedures.* 6th ed. Wolters Kluwer; 2020:1763-1799.)

7. The **dermatome distribution of the nerves** of the body is summarized in **Figure 21.3.** Cutaneous innervation does not necessarily correlate with deep structures, including the bones; therefore, knowledge of the osteotomes can be very useful in predicting the ultimate success of any regional technique.

8. The **major motor functions** of the five nerves are as follows: **axillary (circumflex nerve):** shoulder abduction; **musculocutaneous:** elbow flexion; **radial:** wrist and finger extension; **median:** forearm pronation, wrist and finger flexion, thumb flexion and opposition; and **ulnar:** wrist flexion and adduction, thumb adduction.

B. Indications

1. The **interscalene approach** blocks the BP at the level of the roots to upper trunks. This approach is most useful for surgeries of the shoulder and proximal humerus. As the inferior trunk (C8-T1) and therefore ulnar nerve is usually spared, it is less useful for forearm and hand operations.

2. The **supraclavicular approach** blocks the plexus at the level of the trunks to divisions. This approach allows for reliable anesthesia of the entire arm distal to the shoulder.

3. The **infraclavicular approach** blocks the plexus at the level of the cords and provides coverage for surgery distal to the mid-humerus.

4. The **axillary approach** blocks the terminal branches of the BP. The block is combined with blockade of the **musculocutaneous nerve** and is used for surgical procedures involving the forearm and hand.

5. The **intercostobrachial nerve** must be blocked in addition to the BP for procedures involving the medial arm or using a proximal humeral tourniquet.

6. **Suprascapular and axillary nerve blocks** provide shoulder analgesia similar to that of an interscalene block but avoid complications like phrenic nerve paralysis, which almost always occurs with interscalene block.

7. **Blockade of an individual peripheral nerve** may be useful when limited anesthesia is required or a BP block is incomplete and requires a rescue block.

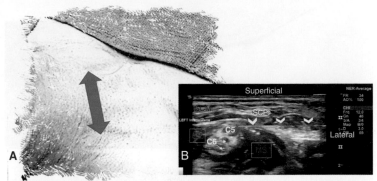

FIGURE 21.5 Superficial cervical plexus/interscalene block using ultrasound (US) guidance. A, The two-sided arrow shows the placement of the US probe. B, US image of brachial plexus (C5 and C6) at the level of interscalene. The yellow arrows delineate the path of the needle toward the plexus. AS, anterior scalene muscle; MS, middle scalene muscle; SCM, sternocleidomastoid; SCP, superficial cervical plexus.

C. Techniques and complications

1. **Interscalene block using UGRA** (Figure 21.5; ⊙ **Video 21.1**): Position the patient supine and semi-reclined or lateral decubitus with the arms at the side and head turned away from the side to be blocked. Place the probe over the SCM at the level of the cricoid cartilage (C6) and identify the internal carotid artery and internal jugular vein. Move the probe laterally and identify the anterior and middle scalene muscles. At this time, the roots and trunks, usually C5 and two branches of C6, will come into view as hypoechoic nodular structures often stacked in a "stoplight" configuration between the anterior and middle scalene. After centering the nerves on the screen, infiltrate with LA and insert a 22-gauge 50-mm needle just lateral to the probe site and advance with IP approach toward the target nerves in a lateral-to-medial direction. **Stimulation of the BP using PNS** will result in a muscle twitch in the deltoid, biceps, triceps, or pectoralis major muscles. After negative aspiration, deposit 15 to 20 mL LA solution between the two scalene muscles.
   a. **Complications. Phrenic nerve palsy** and hemidiaphragm paralysis almost always occurs. The **cervical sympathetic nerve block** can produce an ipsilateral Horner syndrome.
2. **Supraclavicular block using UGRA** (Figure 21.6; ⊙ **Video 21.2**): Position the patient similar to that for the interscalene block. A blanket roll or pillow behind the shoulder may facilitate visualization. Place the probe in the transverse plane with caudal tilt in the supraclavicular fossa. The BP will be visualized as a hypoechoic group of nerves ("cluster of grapes") located laterally and posterior to the subclavian artery. Deep to the artery, the hyperechoic first rib and part of the pleura are typically seen, with the portions of the pleura often obscured by the rib's acoustic shadow. Insert a 22-gauge 50-mm needle just lateral to the probe and advance IP in lateral-to-medial direction until it reaches the BP. **Stimulation of the BP using PNS** is manifested by a twitch of the fingers in flexion or extension. After negative aspiration, slowly administer 15 to 20 mL of LA solution. LA should spread

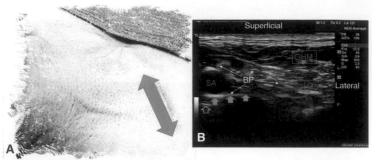

FIGURE 21.6 Supraclavicular block using ultrasound guidance. A, The two-sided arrow shows the placement of the US probe. B, The BP is at the posterolateral border of the SA and superior to the first rib (blue arrows). The pleura can be seen as a hyperechoic line deep to the first rib (white arrow). BP, brachial plexus; MS, middle scalene muscle; OHM, omohyoid muscle; SA, subclavian artery.

throughout the BP, between the middle scalene and subclavian artery, just above the first rib.

    a. Complications include pneumothorax (0.04% with UGRA), phrenic nerve block, and Horner syndrome.

3. **Infraclavicular block using UGRA** (Figure 21.7, ⊙ Video 21.3): Position the patient supine with arm supinated and abducted 90° at the shoulder, with the forearm supinated. Place the probe in the infraclavicular fossa (at the deltopectoral groove) and under the coracoid process. Identify the axillary artery and vein with hyperechoic lateral, posterior, and medial cords lying in a U-shape configuration around the artery. A needle-insertion site is identified approximately 1 cm superior to the probe, just inferior to the clavicle. A 22-gauge 100- to 150-mm needle is appropriate. Insert the needle and advance caudally at a steep angle to the skin in an IP approach until the tip is positioned posterior to the axillary artery (ie, in the 6-o'clock position). **PNS stimulation** of the posterior cord will produce extension at the wrist and/or finger (radial nerve) and stimulation of the medial cord produces flexor carpi ulnaris

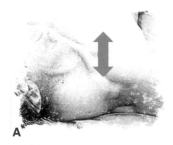
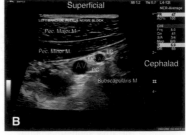

FIGURE 21.7 Infraclavicular block using ultrasound guidance. A, The two-sided arrow shows the placement of the US probe. B, The LC, MC, and PC are located around the AA. The PC can be obscured by the acoustic enhancement of the artery. The blue arrows designate the pleura. AA, axillary artery; AV, axillary vein; LC, lateral cord; MC, medial cord; PC, posterior cord.

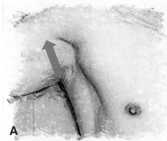 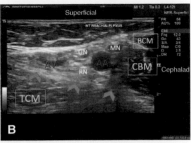

FIGURE 21.8 Axillary block using ultrasound guidance. A, The two-sided arrow shows the placement of the US probe. B, The axillary approach to the terminal branches of the brachial plexus is achieved by placement of the US probe over the axillary artery. The blue arrows trace the conjoined tendon of the latissimus dorsi and teres major muscle. AA, axillary artery; AV, axillary vein; BCM, biceps muscle; CBM, coracobrachialis muscle; MN, median nerve; RN, radial nerve; TCM, triceps muscle; UN, ulnar nerve.

movement with some flexion of the wrist and/or fingers (median and ulnar nerves); stimulation of the posterior cord generally results in a higher success rate. After negative aspiration, deposit 20 to 30 mL of LA solution with a goal of U-shaped spread around the axillary artery. This may require repositioning the needle to achieve the desired spread and coverage of the medial and lateral cords.

    a. Complications include pneumothorax in addition to those mentioned in Section III.

4. **Axillary block using UGRA (Figure 21.8; ⊙ Videos 21.4-21.7):** Position the patient supine with the arm abducted 90° at the shoulder, externally rotated and flexed at the elbow. Place the transducer over the axillary artery, perpendicular to the axis of the arm, and position the artery in the center of the screen. The hyperechoic median, ulnar, and radial nerves can be appreciated in the perivascular area. Special care should be taken to identify veins as pressure from the transducer may easily compress and obscure them from view. Insert a 22-gauge 25- to 50-mm needle superior to the transducer and advance toward the nerves with IP approach. **PNS stimulation** of each nerve will result in different motor stimulation (see Section VII.A.8). After negative aspiration, inject a total of 20 to 30 mL of LA near each terminal nerve. The goal is to cover each of the terminal nerves, which may be achieved by a single injection of 5 to 7 mL of LA around the median, radial, and ulnar nerves. Next, identify the **musculocutaneous nerve** as a hyperechoic oval or triangular structure between the coracobrachialis and biceps muscles or within one of the muscles. Without changing the needle entry site, redirect the needle adjacent to the nerve and inject 5 to 7 mL of LA solution. **PNS stimulation** of the musculocutaneous nerve leads to flexion of the elbow.

    a. Complications include LAST secondary to injection into the axillary artery or vein in addition to those mentioned in Section III.

5. **Intercostobrachial nerve block:** Insert a 25-gauge needle inferior to the axillary artery at the level of the axillary fossa. Subcutaneously infiltrate 5 mL of LA superiorly and inferiorly along the axillary crease. Complications are rare given the superficial nature of the block.

6. **Suprascapular and axillary nerve block:** A suprascapular nerve block with or without axillary nerve block is considered a phrenic nerve-sparing regional anesthesia technique for shoulder surgery.

   a. **Suprascapular nerve block using UGRA:** With the **posterior approach**, position the patient in the lateral position, with shoulder fully adducted. Place the ultrasound probe transversely over the supraspinous fossa, and trace it from the medial end of the spine of the scapula to the greater suprascapular notch laterally. Insert a 22-gauge needle and advance with an IP approach to the lateral aspect of the supraspinous fossa, beneath the supraspinatus muscle. After negative aspiration, inject 10 to 12 mL of LA. With the **anterior approach**, position the patient and the probe as for supraclavicular block. Identify the omohyoid muscle on the top of the brachial plexus. Follow the omohyoid muscle laterally and posteriorly. Locate the suprascapular nerve as it separates from the upper truck. Insert a 22-gauge needle and advance with an IP approach under the inferior belly of the omohyoid muscle. Inject 10 to 12 mL of LA adjacent to the nerve.

   b. **Axillary nerve block using UGRA:** Position the patient in the lateral position. Locate the humeral head and neck on the posterolateral aspect of the arm. Identify the humeral circumflex artery and visualize the axillary nerve located superior to the artery. Advance a 22-gauge needle IP through the deltoid muscle, and after negative aspiration, deposit 10 mL of LA solution around the axillary nerve. LA should fill the potential space between the deltoid and posterior surface of the humerus.

   c. **Complications** include concurrent radial nerve block due to spread of the LA proximally to the posterior cord in addition to those in Section III. As the suprascapular and/or the axillary nerve block do not anesthetize the other three terminal nerves of C5 and C6, supplemental analgesic is frequently necessary.

7. **Blockade of an individual terminal nerve of the BP**

   a. **Ulnar nerve block using UGRA: At the forearm,** the ulnar nerve is just lateral to the flexor carpi ulnaris and medial to the ulnar collateral artery, lying over the flexor digitorum profundus. Place the ultrasound probe transversally over the mid-forearm, and using an IP approach, inject 3 to 6 mL of LA around the nerve.

   b. **Median nerve block using UGRA: At the elbow,** the median nerve is just medial to the brachial artery and on the top of the brachialis muscle at the level of the epicondyles. Using the same approach as above for the ulnar nerve, inject 3 to 5 mL of LA around the median nerve, avoiding penetration of the brachial artery. **At the wrist**, the median nerve lies between the palmaris longus tendon and the flexor carpi radialis tendon. At this level, isolating the nerve from the tendons can be difficult with ultrasound. Sliding the probe alongside the forearm will help to visually separate tendons from the nerve, as tendons become muscles and their appearance will change while the nerve will stay the same. The approach is the same as above at the elbow.

   c. **Radial nerve block using UGRA: At the elbow,** the radial nerve lies lateral to the biceps tendon and medial to the brachioradialis muscle, at the level of the lateral epicondyle of the humerus. Place the ultrasound probe transversally about 3 to 4 cm above the lateral epicondyle to locate the radial nerve. Follow the radial nerve until it reaches the lateral margin of the humerus to confirm the nerve. Use an IP approach to reach the nerve and inject 3 to 5 mL of LA around it.

   d. **Lateral cutaneous nerve of the forearm block using UGRA:** This is the primary cutaneous branch of the musculocutaneous nerve. It may be blocked **in the axilla**, as described in Section VII.C.4, or **at the elbow**, where is it usually located on the lateral side of the forearm and can be seen between the biceps tendon and the brachioradialis muscle, usually accompanying the cephalic vein. Block technique is the same as above, but with 5 to 10 mL of LA.

D. Intravenous (IV) RA (Bier block): IV administration of LA distal to a tourniquet is a simple way to anesthetize an extremity for short procedures (60 minutes or less).

   1. Place a 20- to 22-gauge IV catheter as distally as possible in the extremity to be blocked. Apply a pneumatic double tourniquet proximally and exsanguinate the extremity by elevating it and wrapping it distally to proximally with an Esmarch bandage.

   2. Inflate the proximal cuff to 150 mm Hg greater than systolic pressure. Absence of pulses after inflation ensures arterial occlusion. Remove the Esmarch bandage and slowly inject the anesthetic into the previously placed IV catheter. Average drug doses are 50 mL of 0.5% lidocaine for an arm. Although Bier block has been described for the leg, it is generally not utilized as it is difficult to achieve complete vascular occlusion of the leg with a tourniquet and the volume of LA required increases the risk of systemic toxicity.

   3. Anesthesia occurs within 5 minutes of LA injection. Tourniquet pain generally becomes unbearable after 1 hour and is the limiting factor for the success of this technique. When the patient complains of pain, the distal tourniquet that overlies the anesthetized skin should be inflated and the proximal tourniquet released.

   4. The major **complication** associated with IV RA is LA toxicity. It may occur during injection if the tourniquet fails or after tourniquet deflation, particularly with a short inflation time.

VIII. REGIONAL ANESTHESIA OF THE LOWER EXTREMITY

A. Anatomy. There are two major plexuses that innervate the lower extremity: the lumbar plexus and the sacral plexus.

   1. The **lumbar plexus (Figure 21.9A)** is formed within the psoas muscle from the anterior rami of the L1-4 spinal nerves, with contribution from the 12th thoracic nerve (subcostal nerve). The most cephalad nerves of the plexus are the **iliohypogastric, ilioinguinal,** and **genitofemoral.** These nerves pierce the abdominal musculature anteriorly before supplying the skin of the hip, groin, and genital regions. The three caudal nerves of the lumber plexus are the **lateral femoral cutaneous (LFC), femoral,** and **obturator.**

   a. The **LFC nerve** passes under the lateral end of the inguinal ligament, supplying sensory innervation to the lateral thigh and buttock.

   b. The **femoral nerve** passes under the inguinal ligament just lateral to the femoral artery and vein, under the fascia iliaca, on the surface of the iliacus muscle. It supplies the muscles and skin of the anterior thigh as well as the knee and hip joints. From there, it courses with the femoral artery and vein through the **adductor canal,** an anatomic tunnel bounded by the fascial planes of the sartorius, the vastus medialis, and the adductor longus and magnus muscles. The

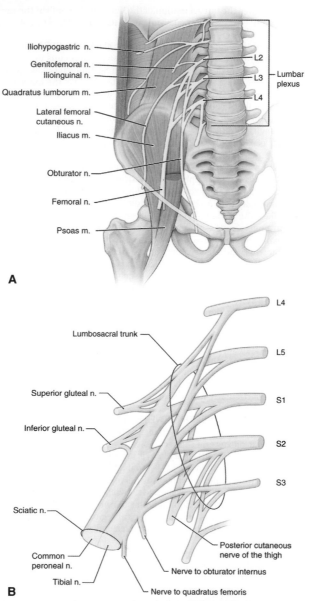

FIGURE 21.9 Diagram of the lumbar (A) and sacral plexus (B). (From Horn JL, Nasiri M. Regional blocks—A brief overview. In: Jaffe RA, Schmiesing CA, Golianu B, eds. *Anesthesiologist's Manual of Surgical Procedures*. 6th ed. 2020:1763-1799.)

nerve and vessels exit the canal at the adductor hiatus just above the medial femoral condyle. The **saphenous nerve** is the cutaneous termination of the nerve, supplying the skin of the medial leg and foot. It is the only nerve of the lumbar plexus that innervates below the knee (**Figure 21.3**).

   c. The **obturator nerve** exits from the pelvis through the obturator canal of the ischium, innervating the adductor muscles of the thigh, the hip and knee joints, and a portion of the skin of the medial thigh.

2. The **sacral plexus** (**Figure 21.9B**) is formed from the anterior rami of the L4-5 nerves and the S1-3 nerves (lumbosacral trunk). The two major nerves of the sacral plexus are the **sciatic nerve (SCN)** and the **posterior cutaneous nerve of the thigh (PCNT)**. Other branches of the sacral plexus are the pudendal, superior, and inferior gluteal nerves.

   a. The **PCNT** travels with the SCN in its proximal extent and supplies the skin of the posterior thigh, extending sometimes to the posterior calf.

   b. The **SCN** passes out of the pelvis through the greater sciatic foramen, becomes superficial at the lower border of the gluteus maximus, descends along the medial aspect of the femur supplying branches to the hamstrings, and becomes superficial again at the popliteal fossa, where it lies between the semimembranosus and semitendinosus muscles medially and biceps femoris muscle laterally. There, it divides into the tibial nerve and the common peroneal nerve.

      1. The **tibial nerve** travels down the posterior calf and passes under the medial malleolus before dividing into its terminal branches. It supplies the skin of the medial and plantar foot and causes plantar flexion (**Figure 21.3**).

      2. The **common peroneal nerve** winds around the head of the fibula before dividing into the superficial and deep peroneal nerves.

         a. The **superficial peroneal nerve** is a sensory nerve that passes down the lateral calf, dividing into its terminal branches just medial to the lateral malleolus, supplying the dorsal aspect of the foot (**Figure 21.3**).

         b. The **deep peroneal nerve** enters the foot just lateral to the anterior tibial artery, lying at the superior border of the malleolus, in between the anterior tibialis tendon and the extensor hallucis longus tendon. Although primarily a motor nerve causing dorsiflexion of the foot, it also sends a sensory branch to the web space between the first and second toes (**Figure 21.3**).

         c. The **sural nerve** is a sensory nerve formed from branches of the common peroneal and tibial nerves. It passes under the lateral malleolus, supplying the lateral foot (**Figure 21.3**).

B. **Indications.** Anesthetizing the entire lower extremity requires blocking components of both the lumbar and sacral plexuses.

   1. Innervation of the **hip joint** includes many nerves from both lumbar and sacral plexuses including genitofemoral, LFC, femoral, obturator, sciatic, superior cluneal, and superior gluteal nerves and the nerve to the quadratus femoris muscle. This complex innervation makes it difficult to find one single RA technique for hip surgery operation. However, the **lumbar plexus block**, **femoral nerve block** (including **fascia iliaca block**), **SCN block**, and **periarticular injection techniques** have been used for post–hip surgery pain control.

   2. An **LFC nerve block** provides excellent analgesia for skin graft donor sites on the anterior thigh. An isolated **femoral nerve block** is useful for

providing postoperative analgesia for femoral shaft fractures as well as quadricepsplasty or repair of a patellar fracture.

3. **Knee joint** innervation is also complex. Branches of the LFC, tibial, common peroneal, and obturator nerves as well as the nerves to the vastus lateralis and intermedius and femoral branches like the saphenous and medial femoral cutaneous nerves contribute to knee joint innervation. This complex innervation makes it difficult to find one single RA technique for open knee surgery. Blocks of the lumbar plexus, femoral nerve, SCN, and **adductor canal** and **periarticular injection between the popliteal artery and posterior capsule of the knee (IPACK)** have been used for postoperative analgesia for open knee surgeries.

4. **Operations distal to the knee** can be performed under **sciatic and saphenous nerve blocks.**

C. **Complications** specific to lower extremity blocks are common to all nerve blocks (see Section III).

D. **Techniques**

1. **Lumbar plexus (psoas) block using UGRA (Figure 21.10):** Place the patient in the lateral position, hips flexed, with the surgical side up. Place a curved array transducer in the transverse plane along the posterior axillary line above the iliac crest at the level of L2-4. Scan from medial to lateral and identify the TP, erector spinae muscle (ESM) superficial to the TP, psoas muscle (deep to the TP), and peritoneum, noting the depth of all structures. Identify the posterior one-third of the psoas muscle, where the lumbar plexus is located. The plexus itself may not be visualized inside the psoas muscle. Insert a 22-gauge 150-mm needle medial to the transducer and advance IP from medial to lateral until the needle tip lies in the posterior one-third of the psoas muscle. PNS is helpful for localization and will cause quadriceps contraction. After negative aspiration, inject 25 to 30 mL of LA. **Complications** specific to this block include epidural blockade with potential sympathectomy, vascular injury, perforated viscus, and renal injury.

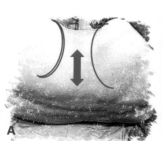 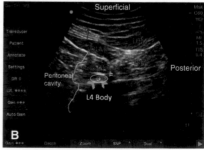

FIGURE 21.10 Lumbar plexus (psoas)/quadratus lumborum block using ultrasound guidance. A, The two-sided arrow shows the placement of the US probe, between the iliac crest (one blue line) and costal margin (two blue lines). B, The red bracket delineates the three abdominal muscle layers (1: external oblique, 2: internal oblique, 3: transversus abdominis). The TP of the lumbar vertebra separates the psoas muscle from the ESM. The LP is embedded within the psoas muscle. ESM, erector spinae muscle; LDM, latissimus dorsi muscle; LP, lumbar plexus; QLM, quadratus lumborum muscle; TP, transverse process.

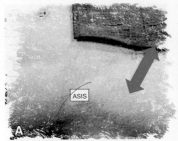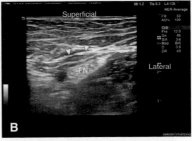

FIGURE 21.11 Femoral nerve/fascia iliaca block using ultrasound guidance. A, The two-sided arrow shows the placement of the US probe, parallel and caudad to the inguinal ligament. The blue lines show the iliac crest. B, The FN is located deep to the fascia lata (yellow arrows) and fascia iliaca (blue arrow) and lateral to the FA. ASIS, anterior superior iliac spine; FA, femoral artery; FN, femoral nerve.

2. **LFC nerve**
   a. **LFC nerve block using landmark:** Insert a 22-gauge 25-mm needle 1 to 2 cm caudal and medial to the anterior superior iliac spine (ASIS). Direct the needle in a slightly lateral and cephalad direction, striking the iliac bone medially just below the ASIS, and inject 5 to 10 mL of LA.
   b. **LFC nerve block using UGRA:** Place the probe inferior to the ASIS, parallel to the inguinal ligament. The LFC nerve is localized on the "fat pad" between the tensor fasciae lata and sartorius muscles. Insert a 22-gauge 25-mm needle with IP approach and inject 5 to 10 mL of LA around the nerve. Note that the nerve may pass through the sartorius muscle in up to 22% of the population.
3. **Femoral nerve block using UGRA (Figure 21.11):** With the patient supine, place the probe over the femoral artery at the level of the femoral crease and move approximately 1 cm laterally so that the artery is at the medial edge of the image. Two separate fascial layers can be visualized overlying the iliopsoas muscle: the superficial fascia lata and the deeper fascia iliaca. The nerve can be visualized just deep to the fascia iliaca and lateral to the artery. Insert a 22-gauge needle at least 50-mm in length and advance medially at a 60° angle to the skin using an IP approach. As the needle is advanced, two distinct "pops" are felt and seen as the two fascial layers are traversed. At this point, the needle tip should lie between the fascia iliaca and the iliopsoas muscle, on the lateral side of the nerve. If the needle is in the proper plane, with **PNS** a quadriceps twitch (patella dance) is elicited and LA spread is seen mostly in the horizontal direction, easily reaching the femoral nerve.
4. **Fascia iliaca block using UGRA (Figure 21.11):** This technique can block the LFC and femoral nerves. The approach is essentially the same as the femoral nerve block. Approximately 35 to 40 mL of diluted LA is injected at the lateral edge under the fascia iliaca and will spread medially toward the femoral nerve.
5. **Adductor canal block using UGRA (Figure 21.12; ⊙ Video 21.8):** This block anesthetizes the terminal branches of the femoral nerve (saphenous nerve and nerve to the vastus medialis) and the branches of the obturator nerve at the level of the mid-thigh as they course through the adductor canal. Blocking the femoral nerve terminal branches here as

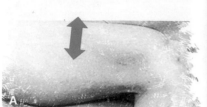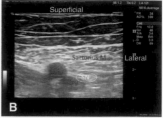

FIGURE 21.12 Adductor canal block using ultrasound guidance. A, The two-sided arrow shows the placement of the US probe. B, The FA and FV are located beneath the sartorius muscle, with the SN usually located lateral to the artery. FA, femoral artery; FV, femoral vein; SN, saphenous nerve.

opposed to at the inguinal crease has been shown to result in equivalent analgesia with potentially less motor blockade of the quadriceps. Place the patient in the supine position, with the operative leg externally rotated and slightly flexed at the knee. Scan with the ultrasound probe to identify the femoral artery deep to the sartorius at the medial aspect of the mid-thigh. The nerve bundles can be visualized as echo-dense structures lateral to the femoral artery. Insert a 22-gauge 80- to 100-mm needle lateral to the probe and advance toward the target structures. After negative aspiration, deposit a total of 15 to 20 mL of LA on each side of the femoral artery.

6. **Saphenous nerve block using UGRA:** The adductor canal approach is used for saphenous nerve block at the level of the mid-thigh. For saphenous nerve block below the knee, position the patient supine with the leg straight. Place the probe at the level of the tibial tuberosity. Visualize the saphenous vein and fascia lata and inject LA around the saphenous nerve close to the saphenous vein. Using a tourniquet above the knee may help to engorge the saphenous vein.

7. **Obturator nerve block using UGRA:** Position the patient supine. Place the transducer on the medial thigh just below the inguinal crease. Identify the anterior branch of the obturator nerve in the fascial plane between the adductor longus and brevis muscles. Identify the posterior branch in the fascial plane between the adductor brevis and magnus muscles. Advance a 22-gauge 80-mm needle with the IP or OOP approach until the tip lies in the appropriate fascial plane. **PNS** of the obturator nerve will elicit an adductor twitch. Inject 5 to 10 mL of LA around each branch (total of 10-20 mL).

8. **SCN block**
   a. **Gluteal/subgluteal approach using UGRA:** Place the patient in the Sims position, a lateral decubitus position with the leg to be blocked uppermost and flexed at the hip and knee. Place a curved transducer between the greater trochanter and ischial tuberosity. Visualize the hyperechoic SCN in the transverse plane at the level of the ischial spine, deep to the gluteus maximus muscle and superficial to the quadratus femoris muscle. Insert a 22-gauge 80- to 100-mm needle lateral to the transducer and advance in plane until the needle tip is in proximity to the nerve. **PNS** elicits a motor response in the SCN distribution (contraction of hamstring or gastrocnemius, foot dorsiflexion or plantar flexion) or paresthesia in the leg or foot. After negative aspiration,

inject 15 to 25 mL of LA with the goal of circumferential spread around the nerve. In the **subgluteal approach** (Figure 21.13; 🔘 **Video 21.9**), the needle is inserted a few centimeters more distally where the gluteus maximus is thinner and the SCN is more superficial.

b. **Popliteal approach using UGRA (Figure 21.14; 🔘 Video 21.10):** This may be performed posteriorly with the patient in the prone, lateral, or supine position with the leg elevated. The linear or curved probe is placed at the level of the popliteal crease, and the popliteal artery should be seen in cross-section. The artery is then followed cephalad 5 to 7 cm. The popliteal vein classically lies superficial and lateral to the artery, and the SCN lies even more superficial and lateral to the vein. The semimembranosus muscle is seen medially and the biceps femoris is seen lateral to the nerve. The nerve should be traced to identify the site of bifurcation into the tibial and common peroneal nerves. With the SCN centered in the image and taking an IP approach, a needle insertion site is chosen approximately 1 cm lateral to the probe. Insert a 22-gauge 80-mm needle and advance the needle tip adjacent to the nerve at the point of bifurcation and between common peroneal and tibial nerves. A distinct pop is felt with entry into the perineural sheath. **PNS** causes foot dorsiflexion or plantar flexion and/or paresthesia in the leg or foot. After negative aspiration, inject 20 to 30 mL of LA to achieve circumferential spread around the nerve.

9. **Ankle block**
   a. The five nerves supplying the foot can be blocked at the ankle. These include two deep nerves (tibial and deep peroneal) and three superficial nerves (superficial peroneal, sural, saphenous) (**Figure 21.15**). The ankle block can be performed with the landmark technique or UGRA with a small linear high-frequency probe.
      1. At the superior border of the malleoli, the **deep peroneal nerve** is situated between the anterior tibialis tendon and the extensor hallucis longus tendon, which are easily palpable with dorsiflexion of the foot and extension of the great toe. Place the transducer transversely at the level of the extensor retinaculum on the anterior ankle and identify the nerve lateral to the anterior tibial artery. Insert a 25-mm needle just lateral to the anterior tibial artery while depositing 5 to 10 mL of LA close to the nerve.

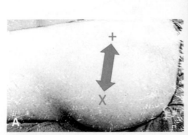
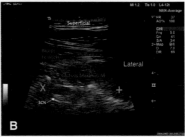

FIGURE 21.13 Sciatic nerve block with subgluteal approach using ultrasound guidance. A, The two-sided arrow shows the placement of the US probe between the ischial tuberosity (X) and the greater trochanter (+). B, The nerve is located deep to the gluteus maximus muscle. SCN, sciatic nerve.

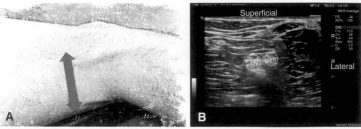

FIGURE 21.14 Sciatic nerve block with popliteal fossa approach using ultrasound guidance. A, The two-sided arrow shows the placement of the US probe at the popliteal fossa. B, The SM/STM is seen medially, and the BFM is seen lateral to the sciatic nerve, which is composed of the TN and CPN. BFM, biceps femoris muscle; CPN, common peroneal nerve; SM, semimembranosus muscle; STM, semitendinosus muscle; TN, tibial nerve.

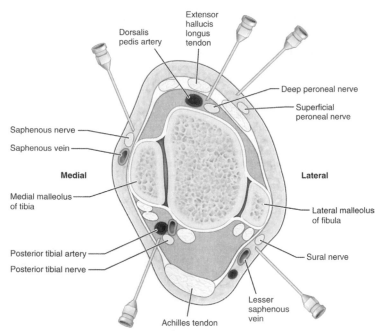

FIGURE 21.15 Cross-section of anatomic structures at the level of the ankle. The deep peroneal nerve is located lateral to the extensor hallucis longus tendon and dorsalis pedis artery. The posterior tibial nerve is posterior to the distal medial malleolus and posterior tibial artery. (From Horn JL, Nasiri M. Regional blocks—A brief overview. In: Jaffe RA, Schmiesing CA, Golianu B, eds. *Anesthesiologist's Manual of Surgical Procedures.* 6th ed. 2020:1763-1799.)

2. Block the **superficial peroneal nerve** by placing the transducer transversely 5 to 10 cm proximal and anterior to the lateral malleolus. Identify the nerve in the subcutaneous tissue superficial to the fascia. Alternatively, inject 10 mL of LA subcutaneously across the anterior surface of the tibia, from malleolus to malleolus. The latter approach will block the **superficial peroneal nerve** laterally and the **saphenous nerve** medially.

3. To block the **posterior tibial nerve**, place the transducer transversely at the level of the medial malleolus and visualize the nerve posterior to the posterior tibial artery. Insert a needle OOP posterior to the medial malleolus, directed toward the posterior tibial nerve, and inject 5 to 10 mL of LA in a fan-shaped plane.

4. Block the **sural nerve** by placing the probe lateral and proximal to the lateral malleolus. Find the small saphenous vein, identify the nerve superficial to the deep fascia and adjacent to the saphenous vein, and inject 5 mL of LA.

IX. REGIONAL ANESTHESIA OF THE TRUNK
A. Anatomy

1. The **thoracic spinal nerves** exit from the intervertebral foramina and divide into dorsal and ventral rami. The **ventral rami** become the **intercostal nerves**, which travel within the intercostal spaces below the inferior border of the superior rib and innervate the thoracic and abdominal walls. All intercostal nerves except for T1 give off a lateral cutaneous branch, which innervates the lateral chest. The anterior cutaneous branches of intercostal nerves T2-5 provide sensory innervation to the **medial breast**, and the lateral cutaneous branches innervate the **lateral breast**, while the supraclavicular nerve innervates the **superior pole of the breast**. Other nerves that contribute to breast innervation are lateral and medial pectoral, long thoracic, intercostobrachial (which innervates the axilla and axillary tail of the breast), and thoracodorsal nerves (**Figure 21.3**).

2. The **thoracic paravertebral space (TPVS)** is a wedge-shaped space that exists on both sides of the thoracic vertebra and is limited anterolaterally by the pleura, medially by vertebra, and posteriorly by the superior costotransverse ligament (SCTL). It contains the ventral and dorsal rami, sympathetic chain, and intercostal vessels.

3. The intercostal nerves arising from T6-11 ultimately terminate in the **anterolateral abdominal wall** and are known as the **thoracoabdominal nerves**. The ventral ramus of T12 is known as the subcostal nerve and travels entirely in the abdominal wall. The anterior abdominal wall receives sensory innervation from the ventral rami of the T6-L1 spinal nerves. The terminal branches of these nerves travel through the lateral abdominal wall within the **transversus abdominis plane** (TAP), the fascial plane between the internal oblique muscle (IOM) and the transversus abdominis muscle (TAM), and generate a plexus. The upper T6-9 segmental nerves exit the intercostal space and enter the TAP lateral to the linea alba. The anterior cutaneous branches of the thoracoabdominal nerves enter the rectus muscle and sheath lateral to the linea semilunaris and form a plexus with each other. The presence of both TAP and rectus sheath plexuses explains why the precise dermatomal map may not be accurate. The L1 nerve divides into iliohypogastric and ilioinguinal nerves (see Section VIII.A.1).

B. RA of the thorax using UGRA

1. **Indications.** Thoracic wall blocks are useful for analgesia for the chest and upper abdomen, including patients with rib fractures or those undergoing thoracotomy, breast surgery, gastrostomy, cholecystectomy, and herniorrhaphy.

2. **Complications** specific to thoracic wall blocks include pneumothorax and intrathecal or epidural injection for paravertebral blocks.

3. **Techniques**

   a. **Thoracic paravertebral block**: The TPVS can be accessed to provide unilateral somatic and sympathetic sensory loss. The block may be performed with a **sagittal paramedian approach**. With the patient prone, place the probe parasagittally, lateral to the spinous processes, and scan medially until the TP and TPVS are visualized, as well as the pleura and the SCTL. Insert a 22-gauge 80-mm needle and advance OOP until the SCTL is pierced. A depression of the pleura with LA injection should be visualized if the SCTL has been traversed. Alternatively, a **transverse approach (Figure 21.16; ⊚ Video 21.11**) may be used to allow continuous visualization of the needle. Place the probe transversely, lateral to the spinous processes. The rib is visualized as a shallow hyperechoic structure with acoustic shadowing below it. Move the probe slightly cranially or caudally off the rib into the intercostal space and visualize the hyperechoic pleura and the shadow of the TP. The TPVS appears as a hypoechoic triangle bounded by the pleura below, the hyperechoic innermost intercostal membrane above, and the TP medially. Insert a 22-gauge 80- to 100-mm needle lateral to the probe and advance IP medially toward the TPVS. Continuous visualization of the needle tip is essential to avoid pleural puncture. Hydrolocalization may be used to help find the needle tip. After negative aspiration, 3 to 5 mL of LA may be injected at multiple single levels or a larger volume (up to 20 mL) may be injected at a single midpoint level. A catheter may be placed to provide continuous analgesia. Depression of the pleura is observed with injection of LA, and spread can be traced cranially and caudally.

   b. **Thoracic interfascial plane blocks** are newer UGRA techniques that rely on the spread of LA on the target fascial plane and were developed initially as safer alternatives to epidural, thoracic paravertebral, and intercostal blocks.

      1. **Pectoral nerve block (Pecs):** The pectoral nerves innervate the pectoral major and minor muscles, providing analgesia for postoperative pectoral muscle spasm and myofascial pain. The **Pecs I block (⊚ Video 21.12**) involves LA injection between the pectoralis major and minor muscles to block the lateral and medial pectoral nerves. Position the patient supine with the arm next to the chest or abducted to 90°. Place the probe parasagittally, similar to the infraclavicular approach to the BP (**Figure 21.7**). Rotate the transducer slightly from medial to lateral to help locate the pectoral branch of the thoracoacromial artery and allow for an IP approach. Hydrodissection is used to confirm the correct fascial plane. After negative aspiration, inject 10 mL of LA. The **Pecs II block (⊚ Video 21.13**) involves two separate LA injections along two fascial planes and is essentially a combination of the Pecs I and injection between the serratus anterior muscle and

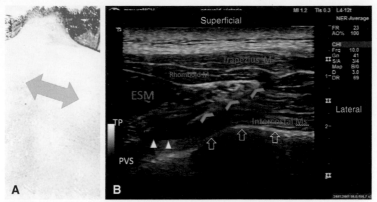

FIGURE 21.16 Thoracic paravertebral block with transverse approach using ultrasound guidance. A, The two-sided arrow shows the placement of the US probe. B, The PVS is located ventral to the superior costotransverse ligament (yellow arrows) and posterior to the TP. The blue arrows show the needle approaching the PVS, and the white arrows designate the pleura. ESM, erector spinae muscle; PVS, paravertebral space; TP, transverse process.

pectoralis minor muscle. Both injections can be performed with a single needle pass. Positioning is the same as for Pecs I. The first injection is made in the same manner as Pecs I. The transducer is then moved laterally to identify the pectoralis minor and serratus anterior, and the second injection is made between these two muscles at the anterior axillary line at the level of the fourth rib. This will block the lateral cutaneous branches of T2-4 and the intercostobrachial nerves.

2. **Serratus anterior plane block:** This block is performed in the axillary region, in a more lateral and posterior position than the Pecs blocks, and between the second and seventh ribs. The block targets the lateral cutaneous branches of the intercostal nerves and the thoracic and thoracodorsal nerves. Coverage may extend from T2 to T7, and this block is used for breast analgesia and thoracotomy. Place the probe between the fourth and fifth ribs to locate the latissimus dorsi. Identify the thoracodorsal artery, which runs in the fascial plane between the serratus anterior and latissimus dorsi. LA may be injected superficial or deep to the serratus anterior.

3. **Erector spinae block (Figure 21.17; ⊚ Video 21.14):** This block has been used for rib fractures and truncal analgesia. LA is injected in the fascial plane deep to the ESM and superficial to the tips of the TP. The block relies on the spread of LA to the paravertebral and epidural spaces. Place the probe parasagittally over the tip of the TP. Insert a 22-gauge 80-mm needle using an IP approach until the needle tip is in contact with the TP. A single injection of 20 mL provides coverage to 6 to 10 levels in the intercostal area.

4. **Retrolaminar block:** This block has been used for TP fractures and truncal analgesia, and although similar to the erector spinae

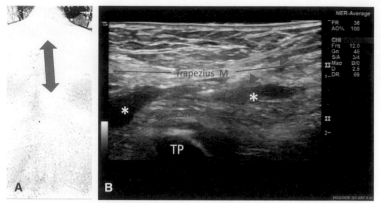

FIGURE 21.17 Erector spinae block using ultrasound guidance. A, The two-sided arrow shows the placement of the US probe. B, The ESM is located dorsal to the TP. The blue arrows show the needle and hydrodissection (*) above the ESM. ESM, erector spinae muscle; TP, transverse process.

block, it targets the vertebral laminae rather than TP. Place the probe closer to the midline to visualize the lamina. A single injection of 20 mL provides coverage to 2 to 4 sensory levels in the paravertebral and epidural spaces.

c. **Intercostal nerve block:** This block involves LA injection in the proximal intercostal space between the internal intercostal membrane and endothoracic fascial/parietal pleura. It can be performed with the patient in prone, sitting, or lateral decubitus positions. Place the probe in a paramedian, sagittal orientation and identify the tip of the TP, then laterally to visualize the rib. Insert a 22-gauge 25- to 50-mm needle using an IP approach until the tip of the needle is below the internal intercostal membrane and above the pleura. After negative aspiration, a 3- to 5-mL injection of LA will spread laterally and in a single intercostal level. Multiple injections may be needed to provide extensive analgesia.

C. RA of the abdomen using UGRA

1. **Indications.** Abdominal wall blocks provide analgesia for periumbilical abdominal incisions, including laparoscopy, laparotomy for colorectal surgery, appendectomy, retropubic prostatectomy, abdominal hysterectomy, Cesarean section, and hernia repair. Bilateral blocks are required for midline incisions.

2. **Complications** specific to these blocks include perforated viscus, intravascular injection into epigastric arteries, and LAST given the large amount of LA injection required.

3. **Techniques**

a. **TAP block:** The TAP block provides analgesia of the anterior abdominal wall including the skin, muscles, and parietal peritoneum. Theoretically, T7-L1 block can be achieved; however, the extent of this block is variable clinically. There are two approaches to the TAP block.

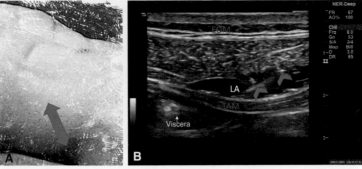

FIGURE 21.18 Transverse abdominis block with lateral approach using ultrasound guidance. A, The two-sided arrow shows the placement of the US probe. B, LA is deposited by the block needle (blue arrows) between the IOM and TAM. EOM, external oblique muscle; IOM, internal oblique muscle; LA, local anesthetic; TAM, transversus abdominis muscle.

1. **Lateral (Figure 21.18; ⊙ Video 21.15):** This approach targets the lateral abdominal wall between the mid- and anterior axillary lines. Position the patient supine with the abdomen exposed from costal margin to iliac crest. Place the probe along the midaxillary line between the subcostal margin and the iliac crest. Identify the three muscular layers of the abdominal wall: the external oblique (EOM), IOM, and TAM. The parietal peritoneum can be visualized deep to the TAM with loops of bowel sliding beneath it. Insert a 22-gauge 80- to 100-mm blunt-tipped needle 2 cm medial to the probe at a 30° angle to the skin. Advance the needle IP until the needle tip is in the fascial plane between the IOM and TAM. After negative aspiration, inject 20 to 30 mL of LA per side or thread a catheter for continuous analgesia. The spread can be traced superiorly and inferiorly.

2. **Subcostal:** The subcostal approach targets the anterior abdominal wall from the xiphoid process to the ASIS and is typically used for upper abdominal sensory block (T6-10). Positioning is the same as above. Place the probe along the subcostal margin. Identify the rectus abdominis muscle and posterior rectus sheath. Deep to the rectus sheath is the TAM. Insert the needle until the tip is between the posterior rectus sheath and the TAM, and inject LA and follow it laterally toward the ASIS.

b. **Rectus sheath block (Figure 21.19):** The rectus sheath block is useful for analgesia after umbilical hernia repair and other midline abdominal incisions. The rectus abdominis muscle is located beneath the superficial fascia of the abdomen. Position the patient supine with the abdomen exposed. Place the probe transversely just lateral to the umbilicus. Insert a 22-gauge 80- to 100-mm needle medial to the probe and advance IP in a medial-to-lateral direction through the anterior rectus sheath and rectus abdominis muscle until the tip rests against the posterior rectus sheath. After negative aspiration, inject 10 to 20 mL of LA per side. Take care to avoid the inferior epigastric vein and artery.

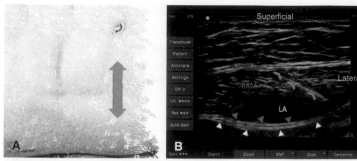

FIGURE 21.19 Rectus sheath block using ultrasound guidance. A, The two-sided arrow shows the placement of the US probe. B, LA is injected by the block needle (blue arrows) between the RAM and the rectus sheath (red arrows). The yellow arrows show the endoabdominal fascia. EA, epigastric artery; LA, local anesthetic; RAM, rectus abdominis muscle.

   c. **Iliohypogastric/ilioinguinal block:** This block provides excellent analgesia for groin operations (eg, hernia repair). Place the transducer medial to the ASIS along a line connecting the ASIS and umbilicus. Identify the nerves as hyperechoic structures in the fascial plane between the IOM and TAM. The superficial iliac circumflex vein and artery may present in the same plane and can be used to identify the plane. Insert a 22-gauge 25-mm needle medial to the probe and advance IP in a medial-to-lateral direction until the needle tip is within the previously described fascial plane. After negative aspiration, inject 10 mL of LA.

   d. **Quadratus lumborum (QL) block:** This block involves LA injection adjacent to the QL and covers T7-L1. There are several different variations of the block that are named based on the location of the needle tip and deposition of LA relative to the muscle. The patient may be positioned supine, lateral, sitting, or prone for any type.

      1. **QL type 1 (lateral):** Using a linear transducer, place the probe in the midaxillary line and move it laterally until the aponeurosis of the TAM is visualized. Using an IP approach, insert a 22-gauge 80- to 150-mm needle lateral to the probe with an anterior-posterior needle trajectory. Advance the needle tip until it crosses the transversus abdominis aponeurosis but is superficial to the transversalis fascia. LA is injected at the lateral border of the QL.

      2. **QL type 2 (posterior):** The approach is similar to type 1 with the same probe positioning and needle insertion. The difference is that LA is injected on the posterior surface of the QL, at the fascial layer separating the QL and ESM.

      3. **Transmuscular QL (anterior)** (**Figure 21.10;** ⊙ **Video 21.16**): Using a curved array transducer, place the probe just cranial to the iliac crest. Visualize the "shamrock sign," which contains the TP of L4 as the stem, QL laterally, ESM posteriorly, and psoas major anteriorly. Insert the needle using an IP approach in a posterior-to-anterior fashion. Inject the LA in the fascial plane between the QL and psoas major muscle and visualize the spread of LA to the paravertebral space.

ACKNOWLEDGMENTS

The editors and publisher would like to thank Dr. Lane Crawford and Dr. Lisa Warren for their contributions on this topic in the prior edition, which has served as the foundation for this current chapter. We would also like to thank Dr. Trudy Van Houten for her anatomic instructions.

Suggested Readings

Abell DJ, Barrington MJ. Pneumothorax after ultrasound-guided supraclavicular block. *Reg Anesth Pain Med*. 2014;39(2):164-167.

Adhikary SD, Bernard S, Lopez H, et al. Erector spinae plane block versus retrolaminar block: a magnetic resonance imaging and anatomical study. *Reg Anesth Pain Med*. 2018;43(7):756-762.

ASA House of Delegates. *Standards for Basic Anesthetic Monitoring*; 2015:1-4.

ASA Task Force. Practice advisory for the prevention, diagnosis, and management of infectious complications associated with neuraxial techniques. *Anesthesiology*. 2010;112:530-545.

Bigeleisen PE, Moayeri N, Groen GJ. Extraneural versus intraneural stimulation thresholds during ultrasound-guided supraclavicular block. *Anesthesiology*. 2009;110:1235-1243.

Chin KJ. Thoracic wall blocks: from paravertebral to retrolaminar to serratus to erector spinae and back again. A review of evidence. *Best Pract Res Clin Anaesthesiol*. 2019;33(1):67-77.

Chin KJ, McDonnell JG, Carvalho B, Sharkey A, Pawa A, Gadsden J. Essentials of our current understanding: abdominal wall blocks. *Reg Anesth Pain Med*. 2017;42(2):133-183.

Elsharkawy H, El-Boghdadly K, Barrington M. Quadratus lumborum block: anatomical concepts, mechanisms, and techniques. *Anesthesiology*. 2019;130(2):322-335.

Elsharkawy H, Pawa A, Mariano E. Interfascial plane blocks: back to basics. *Reg Anesth Pain Med*. 2018;43(4):341-346.

Greengrass RA, Narouze S, Bendtsen TF, et al. Cervical plexus and greater occipital nerve blocks: controversies and technique update. *Reg Anesth Pain Med*. 2019;44:623-626.

Hadzic A. *Textbook of Regional Anesthesia and Acute Pain Management*. 2nd ed. McGraw-Hill Education; 2017.

Horlocker TT, Vandermeulen E, Kopp SL, et al. Regional anesthesia in the patient receiving antithrombotic or thrombolytic therapy: American Society of Regional Anesthesia and Pain Medicine evidence-based guidelines (fourth edition). *Reg Anesth Pain Med*. 2018;43:263-309.

Hussain N, Golder G, Ragina N, et al. Suprascapular and interscalene nerve block for shoulder surgery. *Anesthesiology*. 2017;127(6):998-1013.

Ilfeld BM. Continuous peripheral nerve blocks: a review of the published evidence. *Anesth Analg*. 2011;113:904-925.

Kandarian B, Indelli PF, Sinha S, et al. Implementation of the IPACK (Infiltration between the Popliteal Artery and Capsule of the Knee) block into a multimodal analgesic pathway for total knee replacement. *Korean J Anesthesiol*. 2019;72(3):238-244.

Ladak A, Tubbs RS, Spinner RJ. Mapping sensory nerve communications between peripheral nerve territories. *Clin Anat*. 2014;27(5):681-690.

Neal JM, Bernards CM, Hadzic A, et al. ASRA practice advisory on neurologic complications in regional anesthesia and pain medicine. *Reg Anesth Pain Med*. 2008;33:404-415.

Neal JM, Gerancher JC, Hebl JR, et al. Upper extremity regional anesthesia. *Reg Anesth Pain Med*. 2009;34:134-170.

Pandit JJ, Bree S, Dillon P, et al. A comparison of superficial versus combined (superficial and deep) cervical plexus block for carotid endarterectomy: a prospective, randomized study. *Anesth Analg*. 2009;91:781-786.

Sabouri AS, Crawford L, Bick SK, Nozari A, Anderson TA. Is a retrolaminar approach to the thoracic paravertebral space possible?: a human cadaveric study. *Reg Anesth Pain Med*. 2018;43(8):864-867.

Singelyn FJ, Lhotel L, Fabre B. Pain relief after arthroscopic shoulder surgery: a comparison of intraarticular analgesia, suprascapular nerve block, and interscalene brachial plexus block. *Anesth Analg*. 2004;99:589-592.

Sites BD, Taenzer AH, Herrick MD, et al. Incidence of local anesthetic systemic toxicity and postoperative neurologic symptoms associated with 12,668 ultrasound-guided nerve blocks: an analysis from a prospective clinical registry. *Reg Anesth Pain Med.* 2012;37(5):478-482.

Tran DQ, Bravo D, Leurcharusmee P, Neal J. Transversus abdominis plane block: a narrative review. *Anesthesiology.* 2019;131(5):1166-1190.

Tran DQ, Salinas F, Benzon HT, et al. Lower extremity regional anesthesia: essentials of our current understanding. *Reg Anesth Pain Med.* 2019;44:143-180.

Woodworth GE, Ivie RMJ, Nelson S, et al. Perioperative breast analgesia: a qualitative review of anatomy and regional techniques. *Reg Anesth Pain Med.* 2017;42(5):609-631.

Anesthesia for Orthopedic Surgery

Susan A. Vassallo, Philipp Gerner, and Shauna Williams

I. GENERAL CONSIDERATION

There are multiple features of orthopedic surgery that mandate special consideration. Orthopedic anesthesia requires mastery of a wide range of anesthetic techniques: general anesthesia, neuraxial anesthesia, and regional anesthesia. It is critical to know the indications, limitations, and potential complications for each type of anesthesia and surgery. The anesthetist also must be comfortable caring for patients throughout many age ranges, who may range from young and completely healthy to nearing the end of life with multiple medical comorbidities. These patients may require simple elective surgery, major reconstructive surgery, or palliative surgery.

II. ANESTHESIA FOR TOTAL HIP AND KNEE ARTHROPLASTY

Total hip and total knee arthroplasties are two of the most common surgical procedures performed in the United States. An aging population has increased the prevalence of degenerative and traumatic disease in both healthy and frail patients. Modern medicine now offers the hope of maintaining a reasonable quality of life even for those patients who previously may have been deemed nonoperative candidates.

A. Neuraxial anesthesia is a staple of anesthetic practice in orthopedic surgery, especially for total hip arthroplasty (THA) and total knee arthroplasty (TKA). Neuraxial anesthesia is described in Chapter 20, and its use for specific orthopedic operations is described here. Bupivacaine 0.5% is the most common drug used for hip and knee arthroplasties at the Massachusetts General Hospital (MGH); the dose is adjusted for the patient's height, weight, complexity of case, and estimated surgical time. We strive to provide neuraxial anesthesia sufficient for the entire operation. This usually can be achieved with doses of 2.5 to 3.0 mL for THA and 1.6 to 2.0 mL for TKA. Early recovery of motor function allows for physical therapy the evening post surgery.

B. Pneumatic tourniquets often are used in TKA and produce optimal surgical conditions by creating a bloodless field. This device is inflated to 100 mm Hg above the patient's systolic pressure.

1. Significant pain despite profound neuraxial anesthesia can occur. This **"tourniquet pain"** may manifest as a sympathetic nervous system response, necessitating pharmacologic treatment and, rarely, conversion to general anesthesia. Usually, this response is seen when the tourniquet time is greater than 60 minutes. Multiple expert opinions have suggested deflating the tourniquet for 10 minutes and then reinflating the tourniquet in this situation. Severe postoperative neuropraxias may occur if the inflation time exceeds 120 minutes.

2. Deflation of the pneumatic tourniquet anytime during the procedure can cause multiple physiologic changes; the anesthetist should be prepared to manage these events. Release will lower CVP and MAP as the extremity is perfused. The washout of metabolic products from the

extremity will increase $Paco_2$, $Etco_2$, and potassium and lactate levels and decrease pH and body temperature. These changes can cause an increase in minute ventilation in the spontaneously breathing patient. Rarely, cardiac arrhythmias, ST segment changes, and T wave changes can occur.

C. **Tranexamic acid (TXA)** is an antifibrinolytic drug often used to reduce perioperative blood loss and minimize transfusion requirements in orthopedic surgery. Its use has been studied widely in joint arthroplasty, spine surgery, and trauma surgery. At MGH we routinely use TXA over aminocaproic acid, although the mechanism of action and outcomes are similar.
   1. Mechanism of action: TXA is a synthetic analogue of lysine. It binds the lysine receptor sites on plasminogen and thereby inhibits conversion to plasmin.
   2. Dosing: in adults undergoing joint arthroplasty, TXA is given as two infusions of 1 g intravenously over 10 minutes; one is given 20 minutes before incision, and a subsequent infusion 15 minutes before closure.
   3. Contraindications: (1) a history of arterial or venous thromboembolic disease; (2) recent cardiac stent placement within 3 months; (3) a history of severe ischemic heart disease (New York Heart Association class III or IV) or myocardial infarction; (4) allergy to TXA; (5) recent cerebrovascular accident (within 3 months); (6) renal impairment (serum creatinine concentration above 1.5 mg/dL); (7) pregnancy; (8) vision loss or retinal disease.

D. **Multimodal analgesia mixture** is often injected by the surgical team prior to closure of the incision. This consists of ropivacaine 0.5% (300 mg), ketorolac (30 mg), epinephrine (1 mg), and clonidine (80 μg) diluted in 150 mL of normal saline.

E. **Cement implantation syndrome** is a feared complication of joint arthroplasty. "Cement" is polymethyl methacrylate and is a synthetic resin. It is prepared on the surgical field by mixing a liquid with a powder, which results in the polymerization of methyl methacrylate. This exothermic reaction creates a paste, which is placed in the femoral canal and on the femoral and tibial prosthesis components during THA and TKA, respectively. Placement can cause intramedullary hypertension, which can then cause embolization of cement, bone marrow, or fat. The primary pathophysiology is an increase in pulmonary vascular resistance. Hence, patients with pre-existing right-sided heart dysfunction or pulmonary hypertension are especially vulnerable.
   1. **Clinical presentation** includes hypotension, hypoxia, and arrhythmias.
   2. To avoid these complications, our practice is to increase the Fio_2 and volume status prior to cement placement. Clear communication between the surgical and anesthesia teams is paramount; if the patient is unstable, then cement placement should be delayed. A discussion about the suitability of cement should occur before surgery in patients with complex condition who require hemiarthroplasty or THA for repair of a hip fracture. The team should consider an uncemented prosthesis in patients with known pulmonary hypertension or right-sided heart failure; in patients with a dire prognosis; and when palliative surgery is necessary to allow transfer to home or hospice care.

F. **Bilateral TKA/THA**, defined as same-day bilateral hip or knee arthroplasty, is less frequently performed. Several studies have reviewed outcomes of bilateral arthroplasty surgery. The benefits of decreased rehabilitation time and patient convenience must be weighed against the potentially

increased risk of perioperative complications of bilateral procedures when compared with their staged, unilateral counterparts.
1. A consensus statement by leading experts recommended the use of the following exclusion criteria for patients considering bilateral arthroplasty: (1) age over 75 years; (2) ASA class III or higher; (3) presence of a number of comorbidities, especially morbid obesity and a history of cardiopulmonary disease.

III. ANESTHESIA FOR SHOULDER SURGERY
Shoulder surgery can be performed with general anesthesia, regional anesthesia, or both. These operations include total shoulder arthroplasty, anterior acromioplasty, rotator cuff repair, and repair of humeral or clavicular fractures. Surgery may be performed via an arthroscopic or open approach. Elderly, frail and high-risk patients especially may benefit from regional anesthesia, when administered solely or as adjunct to general anesthesia.

A. Positioning is a critical consideration in shoulder surgery. The sitting or "beach chair" position has gained immense popularity and replaced the traditional lateral position (**Figure 22.1**). The sitting position has implications for airway management and hemodynamic stability. The patient's head is supported on a mobile head rest and then the operating table is turned 45° within the room. It is essential to protect the patient's head and eyes throughout surgery. Periodic inspection of the patient is essential to prevent injury.

B. Blood pressure measurement in the upright position: Recall that actual blood pressure will change by 1 mm Hg for every 1.36 cm difference in vertical height. For example, if the blood pressure measurement for a cuff placed at the level of the heart is 120/80 mm Hg, and the circle of Willis is now at a 25 cm elevation above the heart, the cerebral perfusion pressure will be 102/62 mm Hg. Aiming for a higher blood pressure to offset this change in vertical height is a strategy we employ. The surgeon may request permissive hypotension for improved hemostasis, but this request must be considered carefully in patients with cerebrovascular disease. Invasive

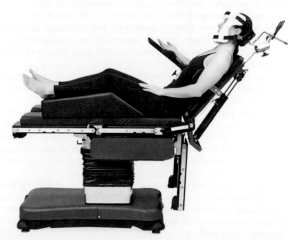

FIGURE 22.1 Beach chair positioning, shown on the T-MAX table by Smith & Nephew. (Courtesy of Smith & Nephew, Inc.)

measurement of arterial pressure may be necessary to manage hemodynamics in a patient with complex condition or sepsis.

C. **The Bezold-Jarisch reflex** can complicate up to 20% of sitting cases in patients who receive preoperative regional anesthesia prior to shoulder surgery, caused by a combination of bradycardia and hypotension. The sudden onset of these hemodynamic alterations begins about 60 minutes after block placement and is likely the result of a hyperdynamic heart and may be associated with epinephrine used in the block or due to anxiety in a conscious patient. This heart vigorously contracts against a volume-depleted ventricle owing to decreased preload in the sitting position. These conditions combine to activate mechanoreceptors in the ventricular wall, and reflexive bradycardia occurs. Studies show conflicting results as to whether pre-emptive beta blockade is effective in mitigating this reflex.

D. **Airway management** usually necessitates use of an endotracheal tube in these patients, as the upright position and operative field can make it difficult to reposition a malfunctioning laryngeal mask airway.

E. **Interscalene nerve block** is often ideal when considering regional anesthesia, as most of the deep shoulder is innervated by the C5-C6 nerve roots. A catheter also can be inserted for prolonged postoperative analgesia. Occasionally, an intercostobrachial nerve block can help augment anesthesia in the posterior shoulder.

F. **Intense muscle relaxation** often is needed in total shoulder arthroplasty and repair of dislocated humeral fractures; this provides optimal conditions for proper realignment and fixation. Regional anesthesia has the benefit of offering excellent muscle relaxation without the necessity for dense neuromuscular blockade.

IV. ANESTHESIA FOR FOOT AND ANKLE SURGERY

Surgery of the distal lower extremities offers unique opportunities for regional anesthesia. Many procedures can be accomplished with peripheral nerve block (PNB) and sedation alone, whereas others may require general anesthesia; in the absence of contraindications, PNB should be considered for all patients, keeping in mind contraindications, discussed below. This approach can provide excellent intraoperative anesthesia and postoperative analgesia. In addition, neuraxial anesthesia may be used in procedures of the lower extremities.

A. The **decision between general anesthesia and monitored anesthesia care,** with a nerve block as the primary anesthetic or as an adjunct to general anesthesia, is based on procedure, operative plan, length of surgery, and patient factors.

1. The intraoperative use of **a thigh tourniquet** often will necessitate general anesthesia, because the pain from the applied pressure is not covered by many lower extremity nerve blocks.

2. **Positioning** plays a role in anesthetic choice. Most foot and ankle surgeries can be performed in the supine or lateral position. Achilles' tendon surgery and calcaneal fractures often are performed in the prone position. Regional anesthesia may be appropriate if airway management is safe and comfortable for the patient. However, general anesthesia with controlled airway management may be necessary.

3. The surgeon may need to evaluate the neurovascular integrity of a distal extremity after a procedure; this concern may influence the choice of regional anesthesia or general anesthesia. The aging of our patient population, who often have advanced cardiovascular and pulmonary disease, may shift our anesthetic practices toward regional anesthesia. **It is essential to remember that the perceived benefits of regional**

anesthesia, such as less postoperative delirium, decreased hospital stay, and faster rehabilitation may not be apparent if excessive sedation is used.

4. **Other nerve blocks** to consider:

a. **Sciatic nerve block (popliteal block)** is one of the most common blocks used in foot and ankle surgery. Anesthetizing the sciatic nerve in the popliteal fossa proximal to its bifurcation into the tibial and common peroneal nerves provides complete sensory loss below the knee, with the exception of the *medial* aspects of the leg and foot.

b. The **saphenous nerve** innervates the medial leg and foot and can be anesthetized in the adductor canal, at the tibial tuberosity or the ankle. The nerve is commonly targeted next to the femoral artery, beneath the sartorious muscle.

c. **Ankle block** can be utilized for foot surgeries when sensory loss above the ankle is not needed. Five nerves innervate the foot and can be blocked with a circumferential ring at the level of the malleolus. These include the saphenous, sural, tibial, and superficial and deep peroneal nerves.

5. **Contraindications** to regional techniques include the following: (1) infection at the site of injection; (2) allergy to local anesthetic; (3) risk for compartment syndrome; (4) acute neurologic deficit.

V. ANESTHESIA FOR ELBOW, ARM, AND HAND SURGERY

Regional anesthesia, alone or as an adjunct to general anesthesia, should be considered for upper extremity surgery. The same discussion surrounding patient position, tourniquet use, length of surgery, and need for muscle relaxation influences the type of anesthesia (see above, Section IV).

A. **Elbow and upper arm surgery** often can be performed with an interscalene or lower brachial plexus nerve block (see Section III). The former does have a higher incidence of incomplete blockade of the inferior trunk of the brachial plexus and can result in inadequate blockade within the ulnar nerve distribution.

1. **Axillary block,** often with separate musculocutaneous nerve block, will provide reliable anesthesia of the upper extremity from the mid arm down to the hand. The area above the deltoid is not anesthetized because the axillary nerve leaves the posterior cord more proximally in the axilla.

2. Of note, **intercostobrachial** and **medial cutaneous nerve blocks** may be used to augment an axillary block if medial incision of the upper arm will be performed. This is performed by injecting local anesthetic into the subcutaneous tissue overlying the axillary (brachial) artery at the level of the major pectoral muscle.

3. Absolute **contraindications** are similar to all regional techniques; axillary lymphadenopathy is a relative contraindication to regional anesthesia.

4. For a complete description of techniques, drugs, and doses please see Chapter 21. The New York Society of Regional Anesthesia (NYSORA) website, listed in suggested readings, has detailed descriptions of many regional anesthesia techniques.

B. **Forearm and hand surgery** often can be performed with regional anesthesia and sedation. Tourniquet use and its placement will influence the specific block.

1. **Lower brachial plexus blocks (supraclavicular, infraclavicular, and axillary)** can be used for operations of the hand and elbow; they can also be useful for most forearm operations.

2. Use of a tourniquet will usually also require an **additional block of the intercostobrachial nerve and medial brachial cutaneous nerves (T1-T3 nerve**

roots) as they innervate the medial aspect of the upper arm and are not blocked by a brachial plexus block (see above).

3. **PNBs** at the wrist often are used for minor procedures that do not require a forearm or upper arm tourniquet. The median, ulnar, and radial nerves are easily accessible.

4. **Intravenous regional anesthesia or Bier block** can be used for minor surgical procedures of the wrist and hand, including carpal tunnel release. A smaller volume of local anesthetic drug can be used if a forearm, rather than an upper arm, tourniquet is used.

VI. ANESTHESIA FOR ORTHOPEDIC ONCOLOGY

Significant preoperative, intraoperative, and postoperative concerns must be considered in this patient population. Bone, cartilage, and soft tissue malignancy can occur in every age group. Over the past 3 decades, aggressive surgical treatment and creative reconstructive techniques have revolutionized care, and limb salvage is a reality for many patients. Orthopedic malignancies include primary tumors—osteogenic sarcoma, chondrosarcoma, and Ewing sarcoma—and metastatic tumors, which are usually breast, prostate, and melanoma cancers.

A. **Preoperative concerns**

1. **Chemotherapy** is a critical concern; patients may have had extensive treatment prior to surgery. Myelosuppression, anemia, thrombocytopenia, and leukopenia, as well as end organ chemotherapy side effects may be present. Preoperative erythropoietin, red blood cell, and platelet transfusion may be necessary.

B. The **specific chemotherapy regimen** must be reviewed; doxorubicin is an anthracycline drug and frequently is administered preoperatively to patients with bone tumors. Its cardiac side effects are dose related and include arrhythmias, electrocardiographic changes such as ST-segment and T wave abnormalities, congestive heart failure, and cardiomyopathy. Cumulative doses greater than 550 mg/m^2 are associated with a greater risk of cardiomyopathy. Echocardiography is performed prior to the start of doxorubicin therapy; serial cardiac examinations are part of the regimen.

1. **Radiation** is an equally important consideration, as previous radiation of a tumor can result in scarred tissue, which poses the risk of large intraoperative hemorrhage.

2. **Highly vascularized tumors** pose an additional risk of large blood loss. Preoperative embolization of the tumor should be considered. Multidisciplinary management of complex tumors is now our standard approach; for example, the team will include an orthopedic oncologic surgeon and usually a spine surgeon. A general surgeon may isolate the bowel, a urologic surgeon may place ureteral stents, a vascular surgeon may identify arterial and venous vessels, a thoracic surgeon may assist in resection of chest tumors, and a plastic or reconstructive surgeon may create a "free flap" for coverage of an extensive wound.

C. **Intraoperative considerations** include precise identification of the tumor, the anticipated length of surgery, the potential for staged surgery, patient positioning, and the possible need for electrophysiological monitoring such as somatosensory evoked potentials and motor evoked potentials. For cross-reference, please see Chapter 24.

1. **Anesthetic technique** will depend on tumor location and burden. Often, isolated tumors of distal extremities lend themselves to excision with a regional anesthetic technique unless an immediate postoperative

neurovascular examination is planned. The postoperative plan for thromboprophylaxis must be discussed prior to choosing a technique that may interfere, such as neuraxial or other regional anesthetic techniques.

2. **Massive blood loss should be anticipated** from highly vascularized tumors; major peripheral and central venous access, ability for rapid blood product transfusion, blood component availability, arterial access, and additional anesthesia staff are essential. These patients may have significant airway edema and vasopressor requirements, so postoperative transfer to an intensive care unit is ideal.

3. **Postoperative pain control** may be difficult and usually involves a multi-modal approach to analgesia. Oncology patients often have significant pain prior to surgery and may be taking high doses of opioid, tricyclic antidepressants, and anticonvulsant (eg, gabapentin) medications. The anesthetist should understand the patient's tolerance and preoperative requirements, as this regimen likely will need to be escalated in the postoperative period.

VII. ANESTHESIA FOR ORTHOPEDIC TRAUMA

Orthopedic trauma is often one component of a multitrauma, and all standard procedures should be followed for triage and patient preoperative evaluation. If possible, investigation of underlying comorbidities, current medications, allergies, and previous surgeries should be attempted. Along with standards of trauma care, including appropriate intravenous access, control of the airway, and management of comorbid disease and implanted devices, some unique considerations are described.

A. **Emergent** and **urgent** orthopedic procedures are those that should be started immediately or within 4 to 6 hours, respectively. Emergent cases include those that threaten loss of limb or life and include vascular injuries, traumatic amputations, pelvic fractures accompanied by major blood loss, long bone fractures, and compartment syndrome; urgent cases are those at risk for complications without prompt fixation or repair. These include open fractures with the potential for soft tissue or bone infection and joint injuries that may lead to avascular necrosis.

B. **Monitoring.** The potential for hemodynamic instability, blood loss, and frequent laboratory tests will dictate the need for arterial and central venous access. Transesophageal or transthoracic echocardiography and, occasionally, a pulmonary artery catheter, can be considered for detailed information on cardiac function and volume status. Radiographic and ultrasound examination of the heart, chest, and lungs can be quite useful if pneumothorax, hemothorax, and lung or cardiac contusions are suspected.

C. **Hip fracture** is one of the most common orthopedic trauma injuries. In the United States, each year 300,000 people suffer a hip fracture. Worldwide, 1.6 million hip fractures occur annually. To give some meaning to these numbers, the lifetime risk of hip fracture is 14% to 18% for women and 3% to 6% for men. This injury can have devastating consequences in the elderly. The mortality following hip fracture can be considered at two time points—acute inpatient mortality and mortality at 1 year. Death is rare after orthopedic surgery. In the United States, the rate of acute mortality after in-patient surgery is approximately 1% for all patients, 3.1% for patients with a hip fracture, and 0.5% for patients without a hip fracture. Significant preoperative risk factors for death include chronic renal failure, congestive heart failure, chronic obstructive pulmonary disease, and age greater than 70 years. The mortality of patients with hip fracture is 20%

to 25% 1 year later. This is the most significant number to remember when speaking to medical colleagues, patients, and their families.

1. The care of the patient with a hip fracture can range from reasonably simple to profoundly complex. Although the surgery may be straightforward, the patient's comorbidities often present challenges to the anesthesia team. In addition, the type of repair planned by the orthopedic team will have implications for anesthetic management; these can include fixation of a femoral neck fracture with cannulated screws; fixation of a hip fracture with a dynamic hip screw (DHS); a cephalomedullary nail such as the trochanteric femoral nail (TFN) or Gamma Nail; hip hemiarthroplasty or THA. A DHS or TFN repair requires traction, and the patient must be positioned on an appropriate fracture table (**Figure 22.2**). Hemiarthroplasty or THA is performed while the patient is in the lateral position. More manipulation and intraoperative fluoroscopy can extend surgical time, which influences the choice of regional anesthesia or general anesthesia.

2. Although there may be several issues to consider when devising a plan for repair of a hip fracture, the two long-standing questions have been:

   a. Does the type of anesthesia—general anesthesia or regional anesthesia—influence acute and long-term morbidity, mortality, and other outcomes?

      1. Early retrospective reviews, like Neuman et al (2012), suggested that regional anesthesia was associated with lower odds of inpatient mortality and pulmonary complications among patients with hip fracture when compared with general anesthesia. This benefit was more apparent in patients with intertrochanteric fractures but not in patients with femoral neck fractures. A second study published by the same authors looked at a similar population cohort of 56,729 patients where 28% of patients received regional anesthesia and 72% of patients received general anesthesia. This analysis did not demonstrate lower 30-day mortality with regional anesthesia when compared with general anesthesia but did show a modest overall decrease in length of stay with regional

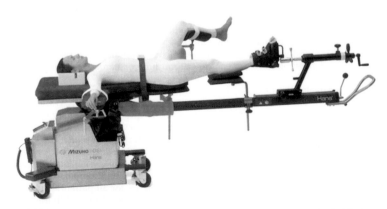

FIGURE 22.2 An example of fracture table positioning on the Hana orthopedic table by Misuho OSI. (Courtesy of Mizuho OSI, Union City, CA.)

anesthesia (6.2 days) when compared with general anesthesia (6.6 days). The findings in this very large study, Neuman et al 2014, led the authors to conclude that there is no observed benefit in mortality for regional anesthesia after hip fracture.

2. Studies have thus far supported similar outcomes for general or spinal anesthesia. See *Suggested Readings* for detailed reviews of this topic.

b. Does the timing of surgery affect similar outcomes?

1. A second point of discussion is the timing of hip fracture surgery. Although it seems intuitive that earlier surgery may lead to superior postoperative results, how does one define "earlier surgery?" Several factors may preclude earlier surgery such as a patient's medical condition (eg, acute myocardial infarction), delays in transfer from a referral hospital, operating room availability, and patient and family wishes.

2. At the MGH, we strive to repair frailty fractures within 48 to 72 hours of injury. We will delay surgery if the patient has the following conditions: acute myocardial infarction with increasing troponin levels, acute congestive heart failure, acute pneumonia with worsening saturation levels, acute metabolic derangements, and acute mental status changes necessitating evaluation and imaging.

D. There are **several complications** relevant to orthopedic trauma:

1. **Fat embolism syndrome (FES)** is estimated to occur in 3% to 10% of orthopedic trauma patients. With high levels of mortality (10%-20%), care should be taken for prevention, early diagnosis, and treatment.

a. **Pathophysiology of FES** usually is considered to be either mechanical or biochemical in origin. In the *mechanical* theory, large fat droplets are released into the venous system during injury and circulate through pulmonary capillaries and through arteriovenous shunts into the cerebral circulation. This microvascular lodging then produces inflammation and local ischemia. In the *biochemical* theory, these physiologic reactions are caused by inflammation due to injury, which causes bone marrow to release fatty acids into the circulation. Fatty acids and resultant inflammation combine to damage the capillary beds of the lungs and other organs.

b. **Clinical presentation** usually occurs 12 hours to 3 days after long bone or pelvic trauma. The characteristic triad of respiratory distress, neurologic dysfunction, and skin petechiae may be present in varying degrees.

c. **Diagnosis** is clinical in nature but aided by the use of either of two separate classification schemes, Gurd's Diagnostic Criteria, or the Schonfeld FES Index.

1. Gurd's Diagnostic Criteria

a. Major criteria

i. Respiratory insufficiency ($PaO_2 < 60$, FiO_2 0.4)

ii. Central nervous system depression disproportionate to hypoxemia

iii. Petechial rash

iv. Pulmonary edema

b. Minor criteria

i. Tachycardia > 110 bpm

ii. Fever > 38.5 °C

iii. Jaundice

iv. Retinal changes

v. Renal changes

       vi. Microglobulinemia (required)

      vii. Thrombocytopenia

      viii. Elevated erythrocyte sedimentation rate

      ix. Anemia

    At least two positive major criteria and one minor criteria or four positive minor criteria are suggestive of FES.

  2. Schonfeld Fat Embolism Syndrome Index

    a. Five points: Petechial rash

    b. Four points: Diffuse alveolar infiltrates

    c. Three points: Hypoxemia (PaO_2 < 70 mm Hg with an FiO_2 100%)

    d. One point: Confusion, fever, tachycardia, tachypnea

    e. Five or more points are needed for the diagnosis of FES.

  d. Prevention consists of early operative fixation of long bone fractures; this intervention has been shown to reduce the incidence of FES by >75%, especially with internal fixation. If internal fixation is delayed, then external fixation for pelvic and long bone fractures should be considered.

  e. Treatment focuses on supportive measures, which will depend upon the severity of lung and other end-organ dysfunction. Steroids, heparin, and vena cava filters all have been proposed, but prospective, randomized, controlled studies are currently nonconclusive.

2. Acute compartment syndrome (ACS) is a true orthopedic emergency. Regional anesthesia may potentially delay diagnosis, and therefore, anesthetists must be aware of its presentation and management selecting an anesthetic technique. ACS develops most commonly in the forearm and lower leg, although it can occur in the upper arm and upper leg.

  a. Early clinical signs are variable, although pain out of proportion to injury is an important symptom. The other classic "P's" of pulselessness, pallor, and paresthesia have been found to be nonspecific in predicting compartment syndrome.

  b. Diagnosis should be made by objective measurements of compartment pressures. An absolute value above 20 mm Hg in a normotensive patient is indicative of ACS.

  c. Definitive treatment of ACS is emergent fasciotomy, which is indicated if compartment pressures reach 30 mm Hg or within 30 mm Hg of diastolic blood pressure. Prompt treatment confers a good chance of complete recovery. Incisions are left open for a minimum of 3 to 5 days.

3. Crush injury and muscle compression can cause rhabdomyolysis. These injuries can lead to acute renal failure, which has a significant mortality rate.

  a. Serum creatinine kinase levels correlate with the degree of muscle damage and are useful for diagnosis and monitoring.

  b. Therapy includes measures to avoid myoglobin precipitation in the renal tubules. Aggressive treatment of hypovolemia and diuresis are often employed.

4. The treatment of intraoperative hypotension and shock and the process of massive transfusion is discussed in Chapter 35.

VIII. ANESTHESIA FOR SPINE SURGERY

This topic is covered separately in Chapter 24: "Anesthesia for Spine Surgery."

Suggested Readings

Anderson MR, Jeng CL, Wittig JC, et al. Anesthesia for patients undergoing orthopedic oncologic surgeries. *J Clin Anesth.* 2010;22(7):565-572.

Donaldson AJ, Thomson HE, Harper NJ, Kenny NW. Bone cement implantation syndrome. *Br J Anaesth.* 2009;102(1):12-22.

Fingerman M, Benonis JG, Martin G. A practical guide to commonly performed ultrasound-guided peripheral-nerve blocks (Review). *Curr Opin Anaesthesiol.* 2009;22(5):600-607.

Guay J, Parker MJ, Gajendragadkar PR, Kopp S. Anaesthesia for hip fracture surgery in adults (Review). *Cochrane Database Syst Rev.* 2016;2:CD000521.

Kahn RL, Hargett MJ. β-Adrenergic blockers and vasovagal episodes during shoulder surgery in the sitting position under interscalene block. *Surv Anesthesiol.* 1999;43(6):356.

Kwiatt E, Mark J, Seamon. Fat embolism syndrome. *Int J Crit Illn Inj Sci.* 2013;3(1):64-68.

Liguori GA, Kan RL, Gordon J, et al. The use of metoprolol and glycopyrrolate to prevent hypotensive/bradycardic events during shoulder arthroscopy in the sitting position under interscalene block. *Anesth Analg.* 1998;87(6):1320-1325.

Memtsoudis SG, Hargett M, Russell LA, et al. Consensus statement from the consensus conference on bilateral total knee arthroplasty group. *Clin Orthop Relat Res.* 2013;471(8):2649-2657.

Neuman MD, Rosenbaum PR, Ludwig JM, Zubizarreta JR. Anesthesia technique, mortality, and length of stay after hip fracture surgery. *J Am Med Assoc.* 2014;311(24):2508-2517.

Neuman MD, Silber JH, Elkassabary NM, Ludwig JM, Flesicher LA. Comparative effectiveness of regional anesthesia versus general anesthesia for hip fracture surgery in adults. *Anesthesiology.* 2012;117(1):72-92.

Papadonikolakis A, Wiesler ER, Olympio MA, Poehling GG. Avoiding catastrophic complications of stroke and death related to shoulder surgery in the sitting position, *Arthrosc J Arthrosc Relat Surg.* 2008;24(4):481-482.

Perlas A, Chan VW, Beattie S. Anesthesia technique and mortality after total hip or knee arthroplasty. *Anesthesiology.* 2016;125(4):724-731.

Rains DD, Rooke GA, Wahl CJ. Pathomechanisms and complications related to patient positioning and anesthesia during shoulder arthroscopy. *Arthroscopy.* 2011;27(4):532-541.

Rashid HH, Shah AA, Shakoor A, et al. Hip fracture surgery: does type of anesthesia matter? *Biomed Res Int.* 2013;2013:252356.

Ryan DJ, Yoshihara H, Yoneoka D, Egol KA, Zuckerman JD. Delay in hip fracture surgery: an analysis of patient-specific and hospital-specific risk factors. *J Orthop Trauma.* 2015;29(8):343-348.

Shaikh N. Emergency management of fat embolism syndrome. *J Emerg Trauma Shock.* 2009;2(1):29-33.

Triplet JJ, Lonetta CM, Everding NG, Moor MA, Levy JC. Association between temporal mean arterial pressure and brachial noninvasive blood pressure during shoulder surgery in the beach chair position during general anesthesia. *J Shoulder Elbow Surg.* 2015;24:127-132.

Warltier DC, Campagna JA, Carter C. Clinical relevance of the Bezold–Jarisch reflex. *Anesthesiology.* 2003;98(5):1250-1260.

Anesthesia for Neurosurgery

Eleanor M. Mullen and Daniel Ankeny

I. PHYSIOLOGY

   A. Cerebral blood flow (CBF) is equal to cerebral perfusion pressure (CPP) divided by the cerebral vascular resistance. **CPP is defined as the difference between the mean arterial pressure (MAP) and intracranial pressure (ICP) or central venous pressure, whichever is higher.** CBF averages 50 mL/100 g of brain tissue per minute in the normal brain and is affected by blood pressure, metabolic demands, $Paco_2$, Pao_2, blood viscosity, vasoactive agents, and neurogenic regulation. The brain receives approximately 15% of the cardiac output.

   1. **CBF** is maintained at a constant level by constriction and dilation of arterioles (autoregulation) (**Figure 23.1**) when the MAP is between 50 and 150 mm Hg. This concept is known as **cerebral autoregulation.** When MAP is outside these limits, CBF varies directly with the MAP. Chronic hypertension shifts the autoregulatory curve to the right, rendering hypertensive patients susceptible to cerebral ischemia at blood pressures considered normal in healthy individuals. Chronic antihypertensive therapy likely normalizes the autoregulatory range. Cerebral ischemia, trauma, hypoxia, hypercarbia, edema, mass effect, and volatile anesthetics attenuate or abolish autoregulation and may make blood flow to the affected area dependent on MAP.

   2. **$Paco_2$** has profound effects on CBF by its effect on the pH of the brain extracellular fluid (ECF). CBF increases linearly with increasing $Paco_2$ in the range from 20 to 80 mm Hg, with an absolute change of 1 to 2 mL/100 g/min for each mm Hg change in $Paco_2$. The effect of $Paco_2$ on CBF decreases over 6 to 24 hours because of slow adaptive changes in the brain ECF bicarbonate concentration. Sustained hyperventilation causes cerebrospinal fluid (CSF) bicarbonate production to decrease, allowing CSF pH to gradually normalize. Rapid normalization of $Paco_2$ after a period of hyperventilation results in a significant CSF acidosis with vasodilation and increased ICP.

   3. **Pao_2.** Hypoxia is a potent cerebral vasodilator. CBF increases markedly below a Pao_2 of 60 mm Hg. Pao_2 above 60 mm Hg has little influence on CBF. However, hyperoxia may be deleterious under conditions of neuropathology, via promotion of oxidative injury.

   4. **Neurogenic regulation.** The cerebral vasculature receives extensive cholinergic, adrenergic, serotonergic, and VIPergic innervation, though the exact role these systems play in regulation of CBF is not clear. Evidence suggests, however, that increased sympathetic tone in hemorrhagic shock shifts the lower end of the autoregulatory curve to the right and results in lower CBF at a given MAP.

   5. **Viscosity.** Normal hematocrit (33%-45%) in a healthy brain has little influence on CBF. During focal cerebral ischemia, however, reduction in viscosity by hemodilution (hematocrit 30%-34%) may increase CBF to ischemic territories.

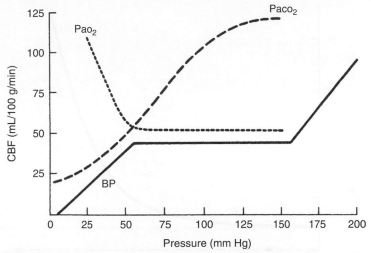

FIGURE 23.1 Autoregulation maintains a constant level of cerebral blood flow (CBF) over a wide range of carotid artery mean blood pressures. Independent of this effect, CBF is elevated by hypercarbia ($Paco_2$) and hypoxemia (Pao_2); hypocarbia diminishes CBF.

B. **Cerebral metabolic rate** ($CMRO_2$) and CBF are tightly coupled because the brain requires a constant supply of energy to meet its high metabolic demands. Regional or global increases in $CMRO_2$ elicit a corresponding increase in CBF, probably mediated by signaling molecules such as nitric oxide. Other factors that modulate $CMRO_2$ (and CBF through this mechanism) include the following:
   1. **Anesthetics.** Variable effect (Sections II.A and B).
   2. **Temperature.** Hypothermia decreases $CMRO_2$ by 7% per 1 °C below 37 °C, while hyperthermia increases $CMRO_2$.
   3. **Seizures.** Increases $CMRO_2$.
   4. **Pain or arousal.** Increases $CMRO_2$.
C. **ICP** reflects the relationship between the volume of the intracranial contents (brain, blood, and CSF) and the volume of the cranial vault. **Normal ICP varies between 5 and 15 mm Hg.** A sustained elevation of ICP greater than 15 to 20 mm Hg in the setting of intracranial pathology is considered abnormal.
   1. **The cranial vault is rigid**, and its capacity to accommodate increases in intracranial volume is limited. A developing intracranial mass (eg, tumor, edema, hematoma, or hydrocephalus) initially displaces blood and CSF, and ICP remains relatively normal (**Figure 23.2**). As intracranial volume increases further, intracranial compliance decreases, and ICP rises rapidly (**Figure 23.2**). Thus, patients with decreased compliance may develop marked increases in ICP even with small increases in intracranial volume (eg, cerebral vasodilation due to anesthesia, hypertension, or carbon dioxide retention) (**Figure 23.2**).
   2. **Clinical features of elevated ICP.** ICP elevation usually decreases CPP and may cause ischemia in regions of the brain where autoregulation is defective and CBF depends on CPP. Early signs and symptoms

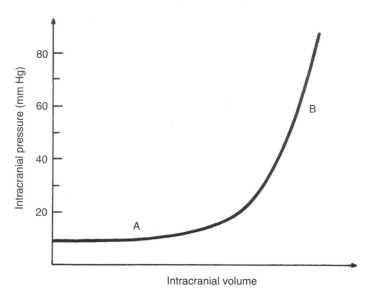

FIGURE 23.2 The intracranial compliance curve. In the normal intracranial pressure (ICP) range (A), increases in intracranial volume produce minimal changes in ICP. Further, small increases in ICP after the "elbow" of the curve can produce abrupt increases in ICP (B).

of increased ICP include headache, nausea, vomiting, blurred vision, papilledema, and decreased levels of consciousness. As ICP increases, brain herniation may occur causing mechanical injury and/or ischemia to the brainstem and cranial nerves. This may result in hypertension with bradycardia or tachydysrhythmia, irregular respiration, oculomotor (third cranial nerve) palsy leading to ipsilateral pupillary dilation with absent light reflex, abducens (sixth cranial nerve) palsy, contralateral hemiparesis or hemiplegia, and ultimately, coma and respiratory arrest.

3. **Treatment of elevated ICP** involves strategies aimed at decreasing the volume of the intracranial components, as outlined below:

a. **Hyperventilation to a Paco$_2$ of 25 to 30 mm Hg produces cerebral vasoconstriction and may be used as a temporizing measure in the management of acutely increased ICP.** Hyperventilation is potentially deleterious, however, and can cause ischemia in injured brain and penumbra where CBF is low. Therefore, hyperventilation should be withdrawn when effective definite therapy is established. Moreover, the effect of hyperventilation on ICP decreases as CSF pH normalizes. Conversely, **hypoxia and hypercarbia cause cerebral vasodilation** and should be avoided.

b. **Decrease jugular venous pressure.** Elevating the head at least 30° from supine promotes venous drainage and decreases intracranial venous blood volume, thereby lowering ICP. Avoid excessive flexion or rotation of the neck and prevent increases in the intrathoracic pressure (eg, coughing, straining, and elevated intrathoracic pressure), since each of these may decrease jugular outflow. Similarly, positive end-expiratory pressure should be minimized to the lowest level that maintains adequate lung recruitment.

c. **Control CMRO₂.** Barbiturates are potent vasoconstrictors that decrease cerebral blood volume while decreasing $CMRO_2$. Prevent increases in $CMOR_2$ due to arousal/seizures with adequate sedation and seizure prophylaxis where indicated.

d. **Maintaining high serum osmolality** (305-320 mOsm/kg) may reduce cerebral edema and decrease brain volume via promotion of favorable fluid gradients (hydrostatic and oncotic pressures). Fluid management is designed to achieve this goal (Section V.D). In addition, **mannitol** (0.5-1.0 g/kg intravenous [IV]) and **furosemide** produce a hyperosmolar state and are effective in the acute reduction of ICP. **Hypertonic saline** is an alternative to mannitol for managing raised ICP.

e. **CSF volume can be reduced by** draining the CSF through ventriculostomy catheter or needle aspiration intraoperatively, or even preoperatively when ICP is dangerously elevated.

f. Surgical removal of tumor, hematoma, or decompressive craniectomy reduces intracranial volume and ICP.

g. Steroids may reduce cerebral edema associated with tumors, though this is a gradual process and likely does not contribute to acute ICP management.

II. PHARMACOLOGY

Agents used in anesthesia may affect $CMRO_2$ and CBF.

A. **Inhalation anesthetics** produce a dose-related reduction in $CMRO_2$ while causing an increase in CBF.

1. **Nitrous oxide** can increase $CMRO_2$, CBF, and ICP. These effects are greatly attenuated or abolished when N_2O is administered in conjunction with IV anesthetic agents. Nitrous oxide should be avoided when air-filled intracranial airspaces (eg, pneumocephalus) exist because it diffuses more rapidly into these spaces than nitrogen diffuses out and may thereby produce an acute increase in ICP.

2. Volatile agents cause increases in CBF due to their direct vasodilatory actions. Autoregulation can be attenuated or abolished by increasing the concentrations of these drugs, but cerebrovascular responsiveness to carbon dioxide is preserved (**Table 23.1**). The vasodilatory effect of inhalational agents is clinically insignificant in patients with normal

TABLE 23.1	Cerebral Physiologic Effects of Inhalational Anesthetics			
	Nitrous Oxide	**Desflurane**	**Sevoflurane**	**Isoflurane**
CBF	↑	↑↑	↑	↑↑
CPP	↓	↓↓	↓	↓↓
ICP	↔/↑	↔/↑	↔/↑	↔/↑
Metabolic demands	↑	↓	↓	↓
CO₂ reactivity	↔	↔	↔	↔
Seizure threshold	↓	↓	↓	↓

CBF, cerebral blood flow; CPP, cerebral perfusion pressure; ICP, intracranial pressure.

intracranial compliance. These agents should be used with caution in patients with compromised intracranial compliance (eg, large intracranial mass lesion and acute intracranial hematoma).

3. Volatile anesthetics produce dose-dependent reductions in metabolism ($CMRO_2$), probably by depressing neuronal electrical activity. Isoflurane is the most potent in this respect and is the only volatile agent that induces an isoelectric electroencephalogram (EEG) at clinically relevant concentrations (2 × minimum alveolar concentration).

B. **IV anesthetics** generally cause coupled reduction in CBF and $CMRO_2$ in a dose-dependent manner. This is due to the depression of cerebral metabolism. **Barbiturates, etomidate,** and **propofol** markedly decrease CBF and $CMRO_2$ and can produce isoelectric EEGs. Etomidate has been associated with seizures and is best avoided in seizure-prone patients. **Lidocaine** in therapeutic doses decreases both CBF and $CMRO_2$. **Ketamine,** by contrast, increases CBF and $CMRO_2$ and is used infrequently in neuroanesthesia. **Opioids** and **benzodiazepines** produce minimal changes in CBF and $CMRO_2$. Autoregulation and carbon dioxide responsiveness appear to be preserved with IV agents.

C. **Muscle relaxants** have no direct effect on CBF and $CMRO_2$ but may alter cerebral hemodynamics indirectly through their effects on blood pressure. **Succinylcholine** produces a transient, modest increase in ICP, likely caused by arousal phenomena, which can be attenuated by prior administration of a barbiturate or a defasciculating dose of a nondepolarizing muscle relaxant.

D. **Vasoactive drugs**

1. **Adrenergic agonists.** α-Adrenergic agonists and low-dose β-adrenergic agonists have little influence on CBF if MAP is within the limits of autoregulation. Larger doses of β-adrenergic agonists can produce an increase in $CMRO_2$ and CBF that can be exaggerated in the setting of a defect in the blood-brain barrier. Dopamine causes an increase in CBF with little change in $CMRO_2$.

2. **Vasodilators.** Sodium nitroprusside, nitroglycerin, hydralazine, nimodipine, and nicardipine can increase CBF and ICP by direct cerebral vasodilation if MAP is maintained. β-Adrenergic–blocking agents probably have minimal effects. Despite these profiles, all these agents have been used safely during neuroanesthesia, particularly if CPP is maintained.

E. **Cerebral protection**

1. **Focal versus global cerebral ischemia**

a. **Focal ischemia** is characterized by an area of densely ischemic tissue that is surrounded by nonischemic brain, which may provide collateral flow to the penumbral margins. This residual blood flow may allow neurons to survive for varied periods of time (eg, thrombolysis within 3 hours after stroke onset may prevent a full infarct due to reperfusion).

b. **Complete global ischemia** is characterized by absent CBF (eg, cardiac arrest). Tolerance for surviving global ischemia is on the order of minutes. Therapeutic hypothermia (see section on hypothermia, below) after cardiac arrest may improve survival and decrease neural dysfunction.

2. **Agents**

a. **IV anesthetic agents:** High-dose **barbiturates** may slightly improve neurologic recovery from focal ischemia, possibly by decreasing metabolic rate or more likely by a direct pharmacologic effect.

Propofol may also reduce focal ischemic cerebral injury, although it is not as extensively studied as barbiturates. Etomidate aggravates ischemic brain injury. Early clinical reports suggest that prophylactic low-dose **lidocaine** may have neuroprotective effects in nondiabetic patients.

b. **Volatile anesthetic agents** may provide some cerebral protection, but data are conflicting, and it is unclear whether this neuroprotection is sustained.

c. The 1,4-dihydropyridine calcium channel blocker **nimodipine** has beneficial effects on cerebral vasospasm after subarachnoid hemorrhage (SAH). These effects are well established and are likely mediated through neuronal rather than vascular effects. Clinical trials failed to detect a beneficial effect for patients with acute stroke.

d. **Steroids** have not been found to be beneficial after stroke or severe head injury. Their effects on recovery after traumatic spinal cord injury are also controversial.

e. **Magnesium** confers significant neuroprotection in animal studies. However, a large clinical trial did not show protection in acute stroke victims.

f. **Hypothermia** reduces metabolism for both neuronal and cellular functions and therefore may be beneficial in the setting of decreased cerebral perfusion. Induced mild hypothermia (maintaining core temperature between 34 °C and 36 °C for 12-24 hours) has been shown to be effective in reducing morbidity in patients who sustain cardiac arrest. By contrast, two clinical studies did not demonstrate improved outcome when induced mild hypothermia was used in patients after significant head injury or intraoperatively for aneurysm surgery.

g. **Hyperthermia** profoundly worsens outcome from focal cerebral ischemia and should be avoided.

h. Moderate **hyperglycemia** (>170 mg/dL) exacerbates neurologic injury after an ischemic insult. There are human data suggesting that normalizing blood glucose causes higher incidence of good outcome in patients with stroke.

i. **Other physiologic variables:** In addition to the abovementioned variables of temperature and glucose, meticulous management of perfusion pressure, PCO_2, PO_2, pH normalization, and seizure prophylaxis contributes significantly to improved neurologic outcome in the setting of cerebral ischemia. Maintenance of a high-normal CPP can augment collateral CBF. By contrast, hypotension reduces CBF and exacerbates the injury. Normocapnia should be maintained. Seizures, which can increase CBF and ICP and decrease CPP, should be prevented and rapidly treated.

3. There is preliminary evidence that female sex hormones may confer some neuroprotection after traumatic brain injury or spinal cord injury.

III. ELECTROPHYSIOLOGIC MONITORING

A. **Electroencephalography** (EEG) measures the electrical activity of neurons in the cerebral cortex and is thus used as a threshold marker for detecting ischemia due to inadequate CBF. EEG is used frequently during procedures that jeopardize cerebral perfusion, such as carotid endarterectomy, or to ensure electrical silence before circulatory arrest.

1. Normal CBF in gray and white matter averages 50 mL/100 g/min. With most anesthetic techniques, the EEG becomes abnormal when CBF decreases to 20 mL/100 g/min. Isoflurane is distinct as the EEG

becomes abnormal when CBF is much lower at 8 to 10 mL/100 g/min. Cellular survival is endangered when CBF decreases to 12 mL/100 g/min (lower with isoflurane). Thus, EEG changes can warn of ischemia before CBF becomes insufficient to maintain tissue viability. Prompt detection of EEG changes may be treated with increases in perfusion pressure or shunting to restore CBF, thereby preventing infarction.

2. The EEG may exhibit changes intraoperatively with no demonstrable neurologic deficit during postoperative examination. Cerebral ischemia can produce electrical dysfunction without causing neuronal cell damage because the blood flow threshold for electrical failure is higher than that needed to maintain cellular integrity.

3. Factors other than anesthetics that may affect the EEG include hypothermia (which may limit the usefulness of EEG during cardiopulmonary bypass), hypotension, hypoglycemia, hypoxia, tumors, vascular abnormalities, and epilepsy. An abnormal EEG in patients with preexisting neurologic deficits, an evolving stroke, or recent reversible ischemic neurologic deficits can also make it difficult to interpret new changes.

4. **Anesthetic effects on the EEG** are generally global, which often helps distinguish them from the focal changes of ischemia. A predominance of slow activity is seen as the anesthetic depth increases. "Deep" anesthesia may cause marked EEG slowing, making detection of superimposed ischemic changes during critical periods difficult to interpret. Maintaining a constant level of anesthesia during critical periods (eg, carotid clamping) facilitates EEG interpretation.

B. **Evoked potential monitoring**

1. **Sensory-evoked potentials** are electrical potentials generated within the neuraxis in response to stimulation of a peripheral or cranial nerve. As they travel from the periphery to the brain, these potentials can be recorded by electrodes placed over the scalp and along the transmission pathway. Evoked potentials (EPs) have lower voltage than background EEG activity, but summation of hundreds using neurophysiologic recording devices allow the neurophysiologist to visualize them by averaging and subtracting out the random background EEG. A normal response implies that the conduction pathway is intact. **Damage to the pathway generally decreases the amplitude and/or prolongs latency** (ie, the time from peripheral stimulus to arrival of potentials at the recording site) of the electrical waveform peaks. EPs are classified according to the nerve tract being evaluated.

a. **Somatosensory-evoked potentials (SSEPs)** are obtained by stimulating a peripheral nerve (eg, median nerve at the wrist or posterior tibial nerve at the ankle or in the popliteal fossa) and recording the elicited signals over the spinal cord (spinal SSEPs) or cerebral cortex (cortical SSEPs). SSEPs are used most commonly to monitor spinal cord function during spinal cord or vertebral column surgery (eg, major spine surgery with instrumentation) and may be used during peripheral nerve, brachial plexus, or thoracic aortic surgery (to detect spinal ischemia during aortic cross-clamping). Because SSEPs are conducted primarily by the spinal cord dorsal column, there are concerns about the reliability of SSEP monitoring for detecting threatened motor function (ie, anterior spinal cord ischemia). For this reason, the "wake-up test" is used in some centers (Section VII.B.2), and the neurophysiologist can also perform motor-evoked potential (MEP) monitoring.

b. **Brainstem-auditory evoked potentials (BAEPs)** are recorded by delivering an auditory stimulus to one ear through an ear-insert headphone. BAEPs reflect the transmission of electrical impulses along the auditory pathway and are monitored during posterior fossa surgery in an attempt to avoid brainstem or auditory (eighth cranial) nerve damage.

2. **MEPs.** Monitoring the integrity of the motor tracts within the spinal cord may be more reliable than SSEP monitoring during spinal surgery, as indicated above. The ventral motor columns of the spinal cord may be more susceptible to ischemia than the posterior proprioceptive fibers. Motor impulses can be generated by transcranial electrical stimulation. The evoked responses are measured as a potential over the spinal cord below the surgical field and in the muscle of interest. Anesthetics substantially modify transcranial-induced potentials but less so if the stimulus is measured in the spinal cord below the surgical field.

3. **Electromyography** (EMG) records muscle responses to the stimulation of motor nerves. EMG is used frequently when there is risk of facial nerve injury during cerebellopontine angle surgery (eg, posterior fossa surgery for meningioma). Because the EMG records motor responses to stimulation, neuromuscular-blocking agents are avoided during the periods of electrical stimulation and monitoring.

4. **Confounding factors.** Interpretation of EP changes is confounded by factors similar to those that affect the EEG (eg, anesthetics, temperature, hypotension, hypoxia, anemia, and preexisting neurologic lesions). Volatile anesthetics can depress SSEPs by reducing the amplitude or prolonging the latency of the SSEPs and can abolish the far more sensitive MEPs. BAEPs are more resistant to the depressive effects of anesthetics than cortical SSEPs. IV anesthetics have smaller effect than volatile anesthetics; barbiturates, propofol, and fentanyl/or remifentanil are compatible with effective monitoring of cortical SSEPs, BAEPs, and MEPs.

5. **False positives.** Changes in EPs occur frequently and often are not associated with postoperative neurologic complications. Further work is required to establish the nature, magnitude, and duration of EP changes associated with irreversible damage.

IV. **PREOPERATIVE CONSIDERATIONS FOR NEUROSURGICAL PROCEDURES**

A. **Intracranial compliance** may be decreased by intracranial mass lesions (eg, tumor, hematoma, or abscess). Surrounding normal brain tissue may be compressed, leading to blood-brain barrier compromise, cerebral edema, loss of cerebral autoregulation, and local ischemia and inflammation. Signs and symptoms of increased ICP are discussed in Section I.C.2.

B. **A computed tomography (CT) or magnetic resonance imaging scan** should be reviewed. Midline shift, basal cistern obliteration, loss of cortical sulci, and ventricular effacement suggest the presence of increased ICP. The degree of brain edema surrounding the mass and the site of the lesion in relation to major intracranial vessels and structures should be noted. Lesions near the dural venous sinuses may require exposure of the sinuses to the atmosphere and may be associated with elevated risk of venous air embolism (Section VI.D.3).

C. **The pathology of the mass** is important in anticipating possible perioperative problems. Vascular lesions (eg, meningiomas and some metastatic brain tumors) may bleed profusely, prompting alterations of the anesthetic planning. Infiltrating malignant tumors may render the patient particularly prone to postoperative cerebral edema.

D. **Preoperative fluid and electrolyte imbalances and glucose intolerance may be present due to poor oral intake, use of diuretics and steroids, and centrally mediated endocrine abnormalities.**

E. **Anticonvulsants** may be required to control seizures. **Corticosteroids** may be necessary to treat edema. These drugs should be continued perioperatively.

F. **Premedication** with anxiolytics such as benzodiazepines and opioids should be prescribed cautiously because patients with intracranial disease may be extremely sensitive to the effects of central nervous system (CNS) depressants. Frequently, no premedication is given. If sedation is needed, diazepam (0.1-0.2 mg/kg orally) can be used. Additional sedation can be given once the patient arrives in the operating room. If the patient has impaired intracranial compliance and/or a high ICP, opioids should be avoided because of their respiratory-depressant effects and the increases in CBF that occur with hypercarbia.

G. In addition to standard anesthetic monitoring (Chapter 10), arterial catheters are used in most patients undergoing craniotomy. Capnography is particularly useful when reducing ICP by hyperventilation. A urinary catheter is placed to aid fluid management and diuretic therapy. Invasive monitoring (eg, pulmonary artery catheter or transesophageal echocardiography) may be indicated for patients with severe cardiac, renal, or pulmonary disease in the context of marked diuretic-induced fluid shifts. Because access to the neck is limited during neurosurgery, placing central lines by brachial or subclavian approaches should be considered. A second IV catheter for drug administration is often useful.

V. INTRAOPERATIVE MANAGEMENT

Anesthetic goals for intracranial procedures include hypnosis, amnesia, immobility, control of ICP and CPP, and a "relaxed brain" (ie, optimal surgical conditions). Whenever possible, promptly following the procedure, the anesthetist should endeavor to provide an awake and interactive, extubated patient who can be evaluated neurologically by the neurosurgical team.

A. **Induction of anesthesia** must be accomplished without increasing ICP or compromising CBF. Hypertension, hypotension, hypoxia, hypercarbia, and coughing should be avoided.

1. While thiopental ([not available in the United States] 3-7 mg/kg), propofol (1.0-2.5 mg/kg), midazolam (0.2-0.4 mg/kg), and etomidate (0.3-0.4 mg/kg) are all reasonable IV induction agents, the hemodynamic effects caused by these agents should be carefully considered.

2. **An adequate mask airway** is essential to prevent hypoventilation and increased $Paco_2$. After induction, hyperventilation by mask can be started with either a nitrous oxide–oxygen mixture or 100% oxygen.

3. An intubating dose of muscle relaxant is given. Nondepolarizing agents are commonly chosen. Adequate relaxation should be obtained before laryngoscopy and intubation to avoid coughing and straining.

4. **Opioids** cause minimal changes in cerebral hemodynamics and are useful in blunting responses to intubation and craniotomy. Because intubation, placement of head pins, and craniotomy (skin incision and manipulation of the periosteum) are the most physiologically stimulating periods during intracranial procedures, generous doses of narcotics are given before these manipulations. Fentanyl (5-10 µg/kg) and remifentanil are most commonly used because both have rapid onset

and high potency. Lidocaine (1.5 mg/kg IV) or esmolol (~0.5 mg/kg IV) can also be used to attenuate the cardiovascular and ICP responses to intubation.

5. **Low concentrations of a potent volatile agent** are occasionally added to prevent hypertension during the initial surgical stimulation.

6. After intubation, the eyes are covered with watertight patches to prevent irritation from surgical preparation solutions, and the head is carefully checked after final positioning to ensure good venous return. Because **access to the airway is limited during neurosurgical procedures**, breath sounds and ventilation should be checked after final positioning to ensure proper placement of the endotracheal tube, the tube should be adequately secured, and all connections in the breathing circuit should be securely tightened.

B. **Maintenance**

1. **Adequate brain relaxation** is necessary before opening the dura. This is achieved by ensuring adequate oxygenation, venous return, muscle relaxation, anesthetic depth, a $PaCO_2$ of 33 to 35 mm Hg (hyperventilation if dictated by surgical field), and often the administration of furosemide (10-20 mg IV), mannitol (0.5-1.5 g/kg IV), and dexamethasone before the craniotomy is completed. The surgeon can then assess the need for further brain relaxation by checking the tension of the dura. If necessary, additional IV thiopental can be administered or CSF can be drained through a previously placed lumbar subarachnoid catheter.

2. **Anesthetic requirements** are substantially lower after craniotomy and dural opening because the brain parenchyma is devoid of sensation. If supplemental narcotics are needed, small doses of morphine or fentanyl can be given. A continuous infusion of propofol (50-150 μg/kg/min) and/or remifentanil (0.1-0.5 μg/kg/min) produces a stable level of anesthesia and allows for a rapid emergence. Large doses of **long-acting narcotics and sedatives are usually avoided during the last 1 to 2 hours of the procedure** to facilitate neurologic examination at the end of surgery and avoid potential drowsiness and hypoventilation.

3. **Muscle relaxants** are frequently continued throughout the procedure to prevent movement. Patients receiving anticonvulsants (eg, phenytoin) may require more frequent administration of muscle relaxants.

C. **Emergence** should occur promptly without straining or coughing. IV lidocaine may be administered to suppress the cough reflex but may delay emergence. Toward the end of the procedure, $PaCO_2$ is normalized gradually if hyperventilation was employed. Hypertension should be controlled to minimize bleeding; rapidly acting IV agents such as labetalol, esmolol, sodium nitroprusside, and nitroglycerin are often used. Muscle relaxation is usually maintained until the head dressing is completed and then reversal agents are administered. Before leaving the operating room, the patient should be awake and responsive so that a brief neurologic examination can be performed. The differential diagnosis of persisting unconsciousness after discontinuation of all anesthetics should include residual anesthesia, narcosis, hypothermia, hypoxia, hypercapnia, partial neuromuscular blockade, metabolic causes, and surgically induced increases in ICP (bleeding, edema, and hydrocephalus). Physostigmine (0.01-0.03 mg/kg IV) or naloxone (0.04-0.4 mg IV) may help antagonize pharmacologically induced CNS depression. The presence of new localized or generalized neurologic deficits should be immediately addressed and may be evaluated by CT and/or surgical reexploration.

D. **Perioperative fluid management** is designed to decrease brain water content, thereby reducing ICP and providing adequate brain relaxation, while maintaining hemodynamic stability and CPP.
1. **The blood-brain** barrier is selectively permeable. Gradients for osmotically active substances ultimately determine the distribution of fluids between the brain and intravascular spaces.
   a. **Water freely passes through the blood-brain barrier.** Intravascular infusion of free water may increase brain water content and may elevate ICP. Isoosmotic glucose solutions (eg, 5% dextrose in water) have the same effect because the glucose is metabolized, and free water remains. As such, these are usually avoided during neurosurgery.
   b. **The blood-brain barrier is impermeable to most ions** including Na^+. Unlike the peripheral vasculature, total osmolality, rather than colloid oncotic pressure, determines the osmotic pressure gradient across the blood-brain barrier. Consequently, maintenance of high-normal serum osmolality can decrease brain water content, while administration of a large amount of hypoosmolar crystalloid solution may increase brain fluid content.
   c. **Large, polar substances cross the blood-brain barrier poorly.** Albumin has little effect on brain ECF because the colloid oncotic pressure contributes to only a small portion of total plasma osmolality (approximately 1 mOsm/L).
   d. If the blood-brain barrier is disrupted (eg, by ischemia, head trauma, or tumor), permeability to mannitol, albumin, and saline increases so that these molecules have equal access to brain ECF. Under such circumstances, isoosmolar colloid and crystalloid solutions seem to have similar effects on edema formation and ICP.
2. **Severe fluid restriction** can produce marked hypovolemia, leading to hypotension, reduced CBF, and ischemia of the brain and other organs, while only modestly decreasing brain water content. **Excessive hypervolemia** may cause hypertension and cerebral edema.
3. **Specific treatment recommendations are outlined below.** The overarching goal is to maintain normal intravascular volume and to produce a hyperosmolar state.
   a. **Fluid losses.** The fluid deficit incurred by an overnight fast is usually not replaced. Physiologic maintenance fluids are given. Third spacing of fluids during intracranial surgery is minimal and usually does not warrant replacement. Two-thirds to total intraoperative urine output is replaced with crystalloid. If signs of hypovolemia develop, additional fluid is administered.
   b. **Assessment of blood loss** may be difficult during intracranial procedures because significant amounts can be hidden under the drapes. Also, irrigating solutions are used generously by the neurosurgeon. As such, the anesthetist should keep track of total irrigation fluids used during the procedure.
   c. **The serum osmolality** is increased to 305 to 320 mOsm/kg. If large fluid requirements are anticipated, isoosmolar crystalloid solutions such as 0.9% normal saline (309 mOsm/kg) may be preferable to hypoosmolar solutions such as lactated Ringer (272 mOsm/kg). However, large volumes of 0.9% normal saline may cause a metabolic acidosis that can be deleterious to end-organ function. Therefore, it is prudent to follow the arterial blood gases and change to lactated Ringer if indicated. Mannitol (0.5-2.0 g/kg IV) and/or furosemide (5-20 mg IV) are also often administered. The marked diuresis produced by

these agents demands close monitoring of intravascular volume and electrolytes.

d. **Hypokalemia** may develop from the use of steroids or potassium-wasting diuretics and is exacerbated by hyperventilation. Nevertheless, intraoperative administration of potassium is rarely necessary.

e. **Hyponatremia** may be produced by diuretics or syndrome of inappropriate antidiuretic hormone secretion (SIADH).

f. **Hyperglycemia** may worsen neurologic outcome after ischemia (Section II.E.2.d). Glucose-containing solutions are avoided in patients at risk for CNS ischemia.

E. **Immediate postoperative care.** Patients are observed closely in an intensive care setting after most intracranial neurosurgical procedures.

1. **The head of the bed** should be elevated 30° to promote venous drainage.

2. **Neurologic function**, including the level of consciousness, orientation, pupillary size, and motor strength, should be assessed frequently. Deterioration of any of these may indicate development of cerebral edema, hematoma, hydrocephalus, or herniation.

3. **Adequate ventilation and oxygenation** are essential in patients with reduced consciousness.

4. **Continuous monitoring of ICP** may be indicated if intracranial hypertension exists at the time of dural closure or is anticipated in the postoperative period.

5. **Serum electrolytes and osmolarity** should be checked and corrected as appropriate.

6. **SIADH** can be diagnosed by hyponatremia and low serum osmolality with high urine osmolality and is treated by restricting free water intake.

7. **Cerebral salt-wasting syndrome** can occur in the setting of brain tumors or injury to the brain. It is characterized by hyponatremia and polyuria. Polydipsia, extreme salt cravings, and dehydration may also be seen. It is a diagnosis of exclusion and can be difficult to distinguish from SIADH, with the main difference being volume status (hypovolemia in cerebral salt wasting syndrome and normal to hypervolemia in SIADH).

8. **Diabetes insipidus** may occur after any intracranial procedure but is most common after pituitary surgery. **Polyuria** is associated with hypernatremia, serum hyperosmolality, and low urine osmolality. Conscious patients can compensate by increasing their fluid intake; otherwise, adequate IV replacement is mandatory. **Aqueous vasopressin** (5-10 USP units subcutaneously or 3 units/h by IV infusion) may be given. Larger doses may cause hypertension. Alternatively, **desmopressin** (1-2 mg IV or subcutaneously every 6-12 hours) can be used and is associated with a lower incidence of hypertension than vasopressin.

9. **Seizures** may indicate the presence of an expanding intracranial hematoma or cerebral edema. If a seizure occurs, airway patency, oxygenation, and ventilation must be ensured. The patient should be protected from injury and the IV secured. For acute therapy, thiopental (50-100 mg IV), midazolam (2-4 mg IV), or lorazepam (2 mg) may be used. Fosphenytoin (15-20 mg/kg IV, 100-150 mg/min) can be administered to prevent recurrence.

10. **Tension pneumocephalus** may occur and should be suspected after failure to awaken from anesthesia. Skull radiographs or head CT scans confirm the diagnosis; treatment consists of opening the dura to release the air.

VI. SPECIFIC NEUROSURGICAL PROCEDURES

A. Patients with **intracranial aneurysms** present for surgery electively or emergently following **SAH.**

1. Preoperative evaluation of patients with SAH should include all components of a routine anesthetic preoperative evaluation (Chapter 1), with attention to known associated physiologic perturbations. These include the **neurologic grade** (**Table 23.2**), presence of **vasospasm** (and the hemodynamic parameters that have been effective in relieving clinical symptoms), degree of hydrocephalus, ICP elevation, and concurrent drug therapy such as calcium channel blockade with nimodipine, which may moderately lower systemic blood pressures intraoperatively. **Electrocardiographic changes** are common after SAH and include arrhythmias and fluctuating ST-segment, QT-interval, and T-wave changes. These are probably caused by subendocardial injury following the autonomic discharge that occurs in association with the initial SAH. Provided these are not associated with cardiac dysfunction, no modification of patient management is necessary, although recent data suggest that a heart rate of either less than 60 or greater than 80 or the presence of nonspecific ST/T wave abnormalities are independently associated with increased mortality in patients with SAH receiving aneurysm clipping. Cardiac biomarkers may be increased as well.

2. Current practice is to intervene early during the first 72 hours after SAH for patients with neurologic grades I to III, which decreases the risk of rebleeding and facilitates the hypertensive management of vasospasm.

3. **Specific anesthetic considerations** include the following:

   a. **Avoidance of hypertension**, which may increase the risk of aneurysm rupture before aneurysm clipping. Prophylactic use of agents such as IV nicardipine, fentanyl, β-adrenergic blockers, lidocaine, or additional doses of barbiturates or propofol will often attenuate the blood pressure response to noxious stimulus such as laryngoscopy and intubation.

   b. **Avoidance of hypotension** to maintain adequate CPP in the recently insulted brain with resultant altered autoregulation and often marginal perfusion in the penumbra.

   c. **Providing adequate brain relaxation** to optimize surgical exposure. Rapid reductions in ICP may affect transmural pressure and increase the risk of aneurysm rupture. This should be done cautiously before opening the dura.

TABLE 23.2	Classification of Patients With Intracranial Aneurysms According to Surgical Risk (Hunt and Hess Classification)
Grade	**Characteristics**
I	Asymptomatic or minimal headache and slight nuchal rigidity
II	Moderate to severe headache, nuchal rigidity, no neurologic deficit other than cranial nerve palsy
III	Drowsiness, confusion, mild focal deficit
IV	Stupor, moderate to severe hemiparesis, possibly early decerebrate rigidity, vegetative disturbances
V	Deep coma, decerebrate rigidity, moribund

  d. **Induced hypertension** may be requested during temporary clipping to improve collateral blood flow to regions that were perfused by the clipped arteries. Often, IV phenylephrine is used for this purpose. It is critical that hypertension be induced only **after** the temporary clip has been placed, otherwise the risk of aneurysm rupture is markedly increased.

  e. **Intraoperative aneurysm rupture** can produce rapid and **massive blood loss** requiring large-bore IV access for volume resuscitation. Accurate estimation of blood loss is essential to guide volume repletion. Induced hypotension, adenosine-mediated cardiac standstill, or, occasionally, manual pressure on the ipsilateral carotid artery may be helpful during the desperate situation of a large and uncontrolled premature rupture.

  f. **Mild hypothermia** (34 °C) has been traditionally used as a protective strategy for the brain during periods of cerebral ischemia. **Data from the Intraoperative Hypothermia for Aneurysm Surgery Trial, however, suggest that hypothermia does not improve either neurologic or neuropsychologic outcome in patients with good-grade surgical SAH.** Given the cardiac and infectious morbidity associated with hypothermia, it is now controversial whether hypothermia is the desired physiologic goal for aneurysm surgery.

  g. Once the permanent clips have been placed on the aneurysm, prevention of postoperative vasospasm becomes important. Blood pressure is increased moderately, and fluids are administered to achieve a mildly positive fluid balance.

  h. When appropriate, the anesthetic should be designed for a prompt emergence from anesthesia to enable an immediate neurologic examination to ensure that clip placement does not compromise the parent vessel.

B. **An arteriovenous malformation** (AVM) is a direct communication between cerebral arteries and veins without an intervening capillary bed. Because an AVM is a high-flow, low-resistance system, surrounding brain regions may be hypoperfused by the diversion of blood through the AVM ("steal" phenomenon). The most common presentations of an AVM are SAH, seizures, headaches, and, rarely, progressive neurologic deficits due to steal phenomenon.

  1. Patients with AVMs may require anesthetic care for embolization procedures or surgical resection.

    a. **Embolizations** are usually done to decrease blood flow to the AVM prior to surgical resection. Embolization may decrease the risk of intraoperative bleeding and postoperative reperfusion hyperemia.

    b. Embolizations can be done under general anesthesia or monitored anesthesia care, which has the advantage of permitting continuous neurologic evaluation.

    c. The anesthetist should be prepared for adverse reactions to the contrast dye (eg, anaphylaxis and osmotic load that may cause congestive heart failure), vessel perforation (sudden and rapid blood loss requiring immediate craniotomy), and neurologic changes.

  2. **Anesthetic management for surgical resection** of an AVM is similar to that for cerebral aneurysms.

    a. The primary focus is on tight blood pressure control because hypotension can lead to ischemia of hypoperfused regions. Hypertension can exacerbate perfusion pressure breakthrough, a poorly understood phenomenon that is thought to be caused by abrupt diversion of the AVM's blood flow to adjacent, previously marginally perfused brain, which produces sudden cerebral engorgement and hemorrhage. Should perfusion pressure breakthrough and brain swelling occur, they are commonly treated with barbiturates, hypothermia, and modest lowering of blood pressure.

b. Potential for large blood loss occurs in cases in which the AVM is large and has arterial feeders from more than one part of the cerebral arterial vasculature or when the preoperative embolization has been unsuccessful.

c. **Postoperative angiography** to confirm complete AVM resection is usually done immediately after surgery. Should any residual AVM be detected, further resection is indicated.

C. Posterior fossa surgery

1. **Posterior fossa tumors** may cause cranial nerve palsies, cerebellar dysfunction, and hydrocephalus due to obstruction of the fourth ventricle. Tumors or surgery around the glossopharyngeal and vagus nerves may impair the gag reflex and increase the risk of postoperative aspiration. Tumor resection that results in edema in the floor of the fourth ventricle may damage respiratory centers and necessitate postoperative mechanical ventilation.

2. **Cardiovascular instability** resulting from surgical manipulation is common. Sudden severe bradycardia and hypertension occur if the trigeminal nerve is stimulated. Bradycardia, asystole, or hypotension may follow stimulation of the glossopharyngeal or vagus nerve. In such cases, the surgeon should be notified immediately because the instability usually resolves with cessation of the stimulus. Pharmacologic treatment (eg, atropine, glycopyrrolate, or ephedrine) is rarely necessary.

3. **A sitting position** is occasionally used for posterior fossa surgery. The advantages include better surgical exposure, improved venous and CSF drainage, diminished bleeding due to lower venous pressures, and improved access to the airway, chest, and extremities for the anesthetist. The sitting position is also associated with a higher incidence of venous air embolism and cardiovascular instability. Modified supine, prone, and three-quarter prone positioning may be substituted for the sitting position because of these concerns.

a. **Venous air embolism** is a risk whenever the operative site is above the level of the heart and there is an open vein. Under these circumstances, an open venous sinus can entrain air and produce hypoxia, hypercarbia, bronchoconstriction, hypotension, and ultimately, cardiovascular collapse. Systemic arterial air embolism is a risk whenever right-to-left shunts occur and can cause myocardial and cerebral ischemia. Monitoring devices for the detection of air embolism and central venous catheters for aspiration of air are often placed when there is risk for venous air embolism.

b. **Methods used to monitor for venous air embolism** include Doppler ultrasound (which reveals a characteristic "mill wheel" murmur when air is entrained), capnography (which may reveal a sudden decrease in end-tidal CO_2), end-tidal nitrogen monitoring, and transesophageal echocardiography (TEE). Of these, TEE is the most sensitive of the invasive monitors and Doppler ultrasound the most sensitive of noninvasive monitors.

c. **If air is detected**, the focus is to prevent further air aspiration and treatment of the adverse consequences. First, the surgeons are notified so they can eliminate the source of air (close the dural opening, place bone wax, or flood the surgical field), nitrous oxide is discontinued, and air is aspirated from the central venous pressure catheter. If possible, patient positioning should be modified to place the surgical site below the level of the heart to reverse the pressure gradient facilitating air entry. If the patient remains stable, the prevention of further air entry may be all that is needed. If hypotension develops, Trendelenburg positioning, fluid administration, and inotropic support may be required.

4. At the end of surgery, the adequacy of the airway and respiration should be verified before extubation. Surgical manipulation may damage the cranial nerves or respiratory centers in the brainstem with resulting pharyngeal or respiratory dysfunction. Postoperative infarction, edema, or hematoma formation in the posterior fossa can cause rapid clinical deterioration. Close observation and prompt support including intubation, mechanical ventilation, and circulatory management may be required.

D. Awake craniotomy

1. Recommended for removal of tumors involving or adjacent to speech centers and/or motor cortex and for epileptogenic focus resection. Intraoperative cortical mapping allows maximal resection with minimal postoperative neurologic dysfunction.

2. The goals are to provide adequate analgesia and sedation as well as to ensure hemodynamic stability, a patent airway, and patient cooperation with neurologic testing during cortical stimulation. Adequate local anesthesia is required. Conscious sedation with propofol, dexmedetomidine, remifentanil, or other agents may be used. Alternatively, an "asleep-awake-asleep" technique may be used as long as the patient is fully cooperative during testing. A laryngeal mask airway (LMA) may be necessary for airway patency during the "asleep" portions of the case.

3. Be prepared to treat a **cortical stimulation–induced seizure**. If one occurs, ask the neurosurgeons to irrigate the cortex with iced saline. Next, the seizure may be aborted with either midazolam, propofol, or a small amount of barbiturate (thiopental 50 mg IV). These small doses may stop the seizure and not overly sedate the patient so that testing may continue. It is important that the IV catheter is not placed across a joint, which may be flexed and ineffective during a grand mal seizure. Before the procedure, the patient's anticonvulsant level should be checked to ensure that it is therapeutic.

4. **Allow adequate access to the patient's airway.** This should include sufficient room to provide mask ventilation and LMA insertion should the circumstances require these interventions.

E. Transsphenoidal resection of the pituitary gland is performed through either a nasal or a labial incision.

1. Although nonfunctioning **pituitary adenomas** are the most common tumor type, some patients have endocrine deficiencies due to hypothalamopituitary compression. Various hyperpituitarism syndromes may accompany functioning adenomas, including Cushing syndrome, acromegaly (with associated airway difficulties), and amenorrhea-galactorrhea.

2. ICP is not a concern as these tumors are usually small and unlikely to compromise intracranial compliance.

3. **Uncontrollable bleeding** is rare but can be massive and catastrophic due to lack of exposure. Frontal craniotomy ultimately may be required to achieve hemostasis.

4. **Monitoring.** The operating microscope obstructs access to the patient's head, so the endotracheal tube must be firmly secured. Continuous monitoring of ventilation is essential. Arterial monitors are usually not indicated unless indicated by other medical comorbidities.

5. **Throat packs** will prevent blood from accumulating in the stomach and may reduce postoperative vomiting. The throat pack must be removed before extubation.

6. At the conclusion of surgery, nasal breathing will be obstructed by packs. Patients should be prepared for this preoperatively.

7. **Diabetes insipidus** may occur after transsphenoidal hypophysectomy (usually 4-12 hours postoperatively). Treatment with IV fluids or vasopressin may be necessary (Section V.E.7). Some patients may develop postoperative adrenal insufficiency and require corticosteroids postoperatively.

F. **Stereotactic surgery** is usually performed through a burr hole, using a three-dimensional reference grid attached to the head with pins placed in the outer table of the skull. This approach allows localization of a discrete area of brain for biopsy or ablation. In most cases, the procedure can be performed under local anesthesia with IV sedation. Because the stereotactic apparatus precludes full access to the airway, sedation must be given with caution. If general anesthesia is needed after the frame is placed, the technique for securing the airway is selected based on the urgency of airway management and whether the stereotactic frame interferes with the mask or LMA. Because the frame may also prevent optimal head positioning for mask ventilation and direct laryngoscopy, LMAs and equipment for awake intubation, preferably with a fiberoptic laryngoscope, should be available. The stereotactic frame can be removed in an emergency; newer models can be quickly removed to provide more rapid access to the airway.

G. **Deep brain stimulators** are inserted in patients with movement disorders (mostly Parkinson disease) who have failed medical therapy. Microelectrodes are inserted through burr holes to a precise location in the subthalamic nuclei, globus pallidum, or thalamus. A stereotactic headframe with image-guided navigation is required to identify and locate the electrode target.

1. Patients often do not receive their morning dose of either dopaminergic or anticholinergic medications to improve electrode recordings that guide electrode placement to a specific cell layer.

2. Patients are awake and often not sedated during the electrode placement, since most sedatives can alter the electrode recordings. Once the electrodes are secure, appropriate sedation is may be implemented.

H. **Epilepsy surgery** is performed in patients with epilepsy of focal origin who are refractory to medical therapy or intolerant of the side effects of anticonvulsants.

1. **Excision of a seizure focus.** Electrophysiologic mapping of the epileptic focus and other cortical areas (eg, language, memory, or sensorimotor) is often performed to maximize the resection of the epileptogenic lesion while minimizing the neurologic deficits. Awake craniotomy with IV sedation and local anesthesia of the scalp permits performance of the mapping procedure, which requires patient cooperation. General anesthesia offers the advantages of patient comfort, immobility, a secure airway, and ability to control $PaCO_2$ and other variables. The anesthetic technique is chosen for its ability to augment (eg, enflurane, methohexital, etomidate, alfentanil, or ketamine) or attenuate (eg, benzodiazepines, barbiturates, or isoflurane) the seizure focus and

its compatibility with intraoperative monitoring (Section III). Because there is often an initial increase in seizure activity postoperatively, anticonvulsants should be resumed promptly.

2. **Vagal nerve stimulators** (VNS) may be placed for medically refractory epilepsy. The electrodes are typically placed through an incision in the left neck and then tunneled to a generator located above the left pectoralis fascia. VNS are typically placed under general anesthesia with endotracheal intubation. Patients frequently are taking multiple antiepileptic drugs, which may cause resistance to neuromuscular-blocking drugs. Additionally, medications that may trigger seizure activity (eg, ketamine) should be avoided. Postoperatively, monitoring for peritracheal hematoma and vocal cord paralysis should be performed.

I. Head trauma. Anesthetic management of the patient with head trauma is complicated by the challenging combination of a "tight" head, full stomach, and potentially unstable cervical spine. While following the "ABCs" of resuscitation, the anesthesiologist should ascertain the mechanism and extent of injury. **Cervical spinal cord injury** must be suspected, and the neck stabilized until cervical vertebral fracture is excluded.

1. Patients who are responsive and ventilating adequately should receive supplemental oxygen and be observed closely for evidence of neurologic deterioration.

2. Comatose patients require immediate endotracheal intubation for airway protection and to avoid hypercarbia and hypoxia, which can exacerbate increases in ICP and contribute to secondary brain injury.

3. **Endotracheal intubation** should be accomplished rapidly, with blood pressure stability and without coughing or straining.
   a. **A rapid sequence induction** is usually performed. If a cervical spine fracture has not been excluded, the neck should be immobilized with manual in-line stabilization (MILS). The anterior part of the cervical collar may be removed to apply gentle cricoid pressure (excessive pressure may displace a fracture) and obtain sufficient mouth opening. A short-acting induction agent such as propofol, thiopental, or etomidate is used to induce anesthesia, which is immediately followed by an intubating dose of muscle relaxant. Succinylcholine can be used safely unless contraindicated for other reasons (Section II.C and Chapter 13). Nondepolarizing relaxants also may be used. When MILS is used, the laryngoscopist should anticipate an increased likelihood of poor glottic visualization due to limited extension of the occiput, C1, and C2.
   b. **Awake intubation** (eg, blind nasal or fiberoptic) may be advocated because of full-stomach considerations, the potential for worsening neck injuries during manipulation of the airway, and anticipation of a difficult airway due to associated facial injuries. Awake approaches are often impractical or unwise in head-injured patients because of lack of cooperation, airway bleeding, and increases in ICP that can be induced by hypertension, coughing, and straining.
   c. **Nasal intubation and nasogastric tube placement** are relatively contraindicated in the presence of a basilar skull fracture (eg, CSF rhinorrhea, otorrhea, or Le Fort III facial fracture).

4. **Hypertension** in head-injured patients may be the body's compensatory effort to maintain CPP in the face of increased ICP. CPP should be maintained at 60 mm Hg. **Hypotension can be detrimental** in patients with elevated ICP and, when combined with tachycardia, should lead one to suspect bleeding from other injuries. Interventions to stop bleeding

and restore intravascular volume should precede or proceed in concert with surgical treatment of the head injury.

5. **Hypoxia should be aggressively treated** as its presence dramatically worsens neurologic outcome in head-injured patients.

6. **Hyperglycemia should be treated** to improve neurologic outcome.

7. **ICP monitoring** can be performed if severe or progressive intracranial hypertension is suspected.

8. **Seizures** may accompany direct cerebral injury or signal the expansion of an intracranial hematoma.

9. **Brain contusion** is the most common type of head injury. Surgery is usually reserved for acute epidural hematomas and acute subdural hematomas. Subdural hematomas are much more common than epidural hematomas and carry a worse prognosis. Intracranial hypertension is frequently seen even after evacuation of hematomas because of severe brain swelling.

10. **Penetrating brain injuries** require early débridement of injured tissue and removal of bone fragments and hematoma. Skull fractures may require débridement, cranioplasty, and repair of dural lacerations.

11. **Anesthetic management** follows the general rules of maintaining CPP and reducing ICP and cerebral edema. Postoperative intubation and ventilatory support are frequently required for ICP control and airway protection in patients with prolonged loss of consciousness or an inadequate gag reflex. Preoperative alteration in the level of consciousness is helpful in predicting the need for postoperative intubation.

12. **Disseminated intravascular coagulation** is a frequent complication of an acute head injury, particularly those associated with a subdural hematoma. Frequent monitoring of the patient's coagulation status is recommended throughout the procedure and early postoperative period.

13. **Corticosteroids are not indicated for head trauma** and may increase morbidity and mortality.

J. **CSF shunts** are inserted in patients with hydrocephalus. A ventriculoperitoneal (VP) shunt is the most common treatment for hydrocephalus. A ventricular catheter is placed through a frontal burr hole and is attached to a subcutaneous reservoir and valve. These are then attached to the draining catheter that is tunneled subcutaneously to the upper abdomen where a minilaparotomy is performed to insert the catheter under direct supervision.

1. The anesthetic management of these patients is determined primarily by the acuity of their disease. Acute hydrocephalus is a neurosurgical emergency where rapidly rising ICP could cause ischemic neurologic damage. Management should focus on measures that will reduce the patient's ICP, maintain a CPP of at least 60 mm Hg, and enable rapid neurosurgical decompression. Anesthetic management of elective VP shunt insertion or revision employs a standard, well-managed, and safe anesthetic where factors that cause extreme ICP elevation are avoided.

2. Some patients with a trapped ventricle can be treated with a ventriculostomy that is inserted through a frontal burr hole. A perforation is made in the ventricular septum under direct vision. These patients are anesthetized with general anesthesia as the ICP sometimes increases with the infused irrigating solution. This could potentially cause patient discomfort or altered consciousness.

VII. SURGERY ON THE SPINE AND SPINAL CORD

Surgery on the spine and spinal cord is undertaken for a variety of conditions, including intervertebral disk disease, spondylosis, stenosis, neoplasm, scoliosis, and trauma. The physiology of the spinal cord and brain is similar, even though absolute rates of blood flow and metabolism are lower in the spinal cord. Maintaining spinal cord perfusion pressure (which equals MAP minus extrinsic pressure on the cord) and reducing cord compression are clinical management objectives.

A. The prone position is frequently used. Most patients can be anesthetized on a stretcher and "logrolled" onto the operating room table after endotracheal intubation. Awake intubation should be considered for patients with tenuous neurologic conditions that may be worsened by laryngoscopy/ intubation or positioning (eg, patients with unstable cervical or thoracic spine injuries). Under these circumstances, an abbreviated neurologic examination should be performed after intubation and transfer to ensure that injury has not occurred. The anesthetist should ensure that all pressure points are padded; neck and extremities are in neutral positions; eyes, ears, nose, breasts, and genitalia are free from pressure; and all monitors and lines are secured in place and functioning. Special attention should be paid to the endotracheal tube, since it can move or kink in the process of positioning. **Ischemic optic neuropathy is a potential complication** of prone cases associated with length of procedure (usually >5 hours), blood loss (usually >2 L), hypotension, medical comorbidities, and fluid resuscitation. Increased facial swelling may alter venous hemodynamics in the globe, leading to optic nerve ischemia and postoperative visual deficits. There are no standard preventive guidelines, but maintenance of systemic blood pressure near baseline values, frequent eye checks to assess for direct pressure on the globe, and maintenance of adequate perfusion are likely beneficial.

B. Surgery to correct scoliosis can be accompanied by significant blood loss. Various techniques can be used to reduce homologous blood transfusion, including preoperative autologous donation, intraoperative hemodilution, use of intraoperative blood-scavenging techniques, and meticulous patient positioning to prevent increased abdominal and intrathoracic pressures that can increase venous bleeding. Because of concern of neurologic sequelae, induced hypotension may not be advantageous in this procedure. Scoliosis surgery is accompanied by a 1% to 4% incidence of serious postoperative neurologic complications. Spinal instrumentation and distraction can cause spinal cord ischemia and result in paraplegia. Intraoperative monitoring of spinal cord function is used routinely.

1. **SSEP and MEP monitoring** provide continuous evaluation of spinal cord function (Section III.B).

2. **The selective wake-up test.** Intraoperatively, if there is uncertainty about the neurophysiologic monitoring, the presence of neuromuscular function is assured when patients are awakened briefly and asked to move their legs. If there is no leg movement, the spine distraction is released until movement is observed. Patients should be prepared for this event preoperatively. Wake-up tests can be performed in older children and adults.

3. **Total IV anesthesia** with propofol and remifentanil is often selected because it is less likely to interfere with neurophysiologic monitoring than volatile anesthetics; however, it does not provide for a reliably fast intraoperative wake-up test. Alternatively, children, who often have robust nerve conduction, may be anesthetized with desflurane, with or without nitrous oxide and short-acting narcotics to achieve

a much faster intraoperative wake-up. Communication of anesthetic interventions with the clinical neurophysiologist or technician is important.

C. **After acute spinal cord injury**, surgery may be required to decompress and stabilize the spinal cord. The primary goal in the initial management of acute spinal cord injury is to prevent secondary damage to the injured cord. This is accomplished by stabilizing the spine and correcting circulatory and ventilatory abnormalities that can exacerbate the primary injury. The presence of cervical cord injury should lead one to suspect associated head, face, or tracheal trauma; thoracic and lumbar spine injuries often are associated with chest or intra-abdominal trauma.

1. **Spinal shock** is characterized by systemic vasodilation and hypotension from impaired activation of the sympathetic nervous system. If the lesion involves the sympathetic cardiac accelerator nerves (T1-T4), bradycardia, bradyarrhythmias, atrioventricular block, and cardiac arrest can occur due to unopposed vagal activity. Spinal shock occurs because of functional transection of sympathetic innervation below the level of the injury and may persist for days to weeks. Bradycardia can be treated by atropine. Hypotension can be treated by fluid, vasopressors, or both. A pulmonary artery catheter may be helpful when other injuries are present and volume status is uncertain. Patients with high spinal cord injury may be unusually sensitive to the cardiovascular depressant effects of anesthetics because of an inability to increase sympathetic tone.

2. **Lesions above C3-C4 necessitate intubation and mechanical** ventilatory **support** because of loss of innervation to the diaphragm (C3-C5). Lesions below C5-C6 may still cause as much as 70% reduction in vital capacity and FEV_1 with impaired ventilation and oxygenation.

3. **Atony of the gastrointestinal tract and urinary bladder** necessitates a nasogastric tube and indwelling urinary catheter, respectively. These patients are also **prone to heat loss** because of inability to vasoconstrict.

4. **Methylprednisolone** (30 mg/kg IV loading dose, followed by an infusion of 5.4 mg/kg/h for 23 hours) may improve the functional recovery of patients with acute spinal cord injuries if treatment is begun within the first 3 hours after injury. There is considerable controversy surrounding this therapy for spinal cord injury, and some centers do not follow this protocol.

5. **Chronic spinal cord injuries** are discussed in Chapter 27.

6. **Airway management** of patients with cervical spine injury is discussed in Section VI.I.

D. Neuroradiologic procedures are performed in suites often remote from the main operating room. For a detailed discussion of anesthetic issues pertaining to the patient having a magnetic resonance imaging or interventional radiologic procedures, see Sections IV and V in Chapter 33.

Suggested Readings

Cottrell JE, Young WL, eds. *Cottrell and Young's Neuroanesthesia*. 5th ed. Mosby; 2010.

Drummond JC, Patel PM. Neurosurgical anesthesia. In: Miller RD, ed. *Miller's Anesthesia*. 7th ed. Churchill Livingstone; 2010:2045-2088.

Koht A, Sloan TB, Toleikis JR, eds. *Monitoring the Nervous System for Anesthesiologists and Other Health Care Professionals*. Springer; 2012.

Mashour GA, Farag E. *Case Studies in Neuroanesthesia and Neurocritical Care*. Cambridge; 2011.

Newfield P, Cottrell JE. *Handbook of Neuroanesthesia*. 5th ed. Lippincott; 2012.

Patel PM, Drummond JC. Cerebral physiology and the effects of anesthetic drugs. In: Miller RD, ed. *Miller's Anesthesia*. Churchill Livingstone; 2010:305-339.

Seubert CN, Mahla ME. Neurologic monitoring. In: Miller RD, ed. *Miller's Anesthesia*. Churchill Livingstone; 2010:1477-1514.

24 Anesthesia for Spine Surgery

John Marota and Raissa Quezado da Nobrega

Pathological conditions of the spine treated with surgical intervention include intervertebral disk disease, spinal stenosis, scoliosis, spondylosis, spondylolisthesis, kyphosis and lordosis, tumors and trauma. The number of these procedures has increased exponentially in the United States as a consequence of the low back pain epidemic, aging population, and development of less invasive surgical techniques. It is imperative that anesthetists be familiar with the challenges associated with these procedures including prone position, fluid shifts, prolonged surgeries and manipulations adjacent to nerves and major blood vessels. General anesthesia is the most common technique for surgery of the spine, although regional anesthesia is a potential option for lumbar microdiskectomy or laminectomy.

A. Spinal cord injury

1. Acute spinal cord injury may present with neurogenic shock, more commonly with lesions above T6. Presentation is hemodynamic instability due to sympathectomy and resultant vasodilation; hypotension and increased heat loss are common. Weeks to months after the acute phase of spinal shock, autonomic dysreflexia may develop, characterized by hypertension and bradycardia in response to stimulation; these may result in myocardial ischemia, retinal/cerebral hemorrhage, and seizures.

2. Cervical spine injury is commonly associated with head trauma. Notable lesions are C5 injury presenting with weakness of the deltoid, biceps, brachialis, brachioradialis and partial diaphragmatic paralysis; C4 lesions can result in paralysis of respiratory muscles including the diaphragm and necessitate positive pressure ventilation.

3. Prolonged immobility secondary to paraplegia/quadriplegia leads to increased extrajunctional receptors at the neuromuscular junction. Succinylcholine is, therefore, contraindicated from 48 hours after spinal cord injury due to risk of hyperkalemia.

B. Airway

1. In addition to the standard concerns for securing the airway, additional caution is required for patients with cervical spine injuries to prevent or not worsen damage to the spinal cord. Hard cervical collars permit 72% to 73% of normal extension and flexion of the cervical spine.

2. Video laryngoscopy has emerged as a useful technique for intubation of patients with cervical spine injury because it requires less cervical spinal motion during laryngoscopy.

3. For patients with severely unstable cervical spine injury, awake fiberoptic intubation followed by awake positioning should be considered; pointed neurological examination is performed immediately before and after intubation to confirm that no change has occurred with manipulation. The sequence of events should be explained to the patient in advance. Intubation is achieved with minimal or no sedation and adequate topicalization of the upper and lower airway with local

anesthetic, after which a brief neurological examination is repeated. The patient can be positioned on the operating (OR) table awake and then general anesthesia induced after confirming postposition neurological examination.

4. **Manual inline stabilization** can be performed to limit cervical motion; a second provider holds the shoulders and head to limit motion of the neck during intubation and positioning. The position is standing aside the patient with forearms resting on the chest. Although this technique has gained wide acceptance and is a component of Advanced Trauma Life Support, effectiveness has been questioned due to potential increase in craniocervical motion and worsening view during laryngoscopy.

5. In emergency situations where there is no evidence of facial/basal skull fractures, blind nasotracheal intubation is an acceptable option.

C. Prone position

1. For patients undergoing posterior procedures, induction of general anesthesia and intubation is performed supine, typically on a stretcher or hospital bed, and then the patient rolled prone onto OR table. Before turning prone, eyes are protected with tape or clear plastic adhesive; bite blocks, orogastric tube, and temperature probe are placed. Nasogastric or nasal temperature probes are discouraged because of potential for bleeding when prone.

2. There are several options to support the head in the prone position. It can be placed on a commercially available foam head and/or face rest in which there are cut out spaces for the eyes and nose to remain free from compression; endotracheal tubes may be positioned either straight down through a hole in the rest or accessed to the side. Alternatively, the head can be supported by sharp pins screwed into the outer table of skull; Gardner-Wells tongs use two pins; Mayfield skull clamp system uses three pins. Gardner-Wells tongs system provides continuous traction; the Mayfield skull clamp system holds the head rigidly in place attached to the OR table. Alternatively, the halo of a halo vest can be used either with traction or fixed to the OR table.

3. The physiologic changes associated with prone positioning may include depressed cardiac index from reduced filling pressures, inferior vena cava obstruction with decreased venous return to the heart, peripheral pooling of blood volume, increase in airway ventilation pressure with increase in intrathoracic pressure, increased functional residual capacity, and redistribution of pulmonary blood flow and lung ventilation to dependent areas.

4. Care should be taken so that the eyes, abdomen, genitalia, and breasts are free from compression; the stomach and bladder can be decompressed with an orogastric tube and urinary catheter. Improper positioning of arms can result in vascular compromise or brachial plexus injury, specifically increased pressure within the cubital tunnel with elbow flexion greater than 130°. Complications such as shoulder dislocation, facial and laryngeal edema, eye injuries, and peripheral nerve palsy have been reported. The greatest risk for injury to the spinal cord occurs during turning from supine to prone; care should be taken to maintain good alignment of the spine across the area of instability.

D. Monitoring

1. **Intraoperative monitoring** of spinal cord functional integrity involves electrophysiologic monitoring of the sensory and/or motor pathway transmission, changes in functional activity could result from direct compression or ischemia produced by compromise or distortion of

blood vessels. Different methods to monitor spinal cord function include somatosensory-evoked potentials (SSEPs), motor-evoked potentials (MEPs), epidural electrodes, direct stimulation of spinal roots, F-responses, H-reflexes, testing specific reflexes, electromyography, transcranial electrical stimulation with screw electrodes, neuromuscular junction monitoring, and electrical impedance testing. Combining multiple methods increases sensitivity when risk of ischemia is high. Use of intraoperative monitoring has been shown to reduce postoperative neurologic morbidity and may identify in real-time compromise with surgical manipulation (ie, retractor or pedicle screw placement) to permit correction of a reversible deficit.

2. **SSEPs and MEPs** are the two most commonly utilized modalities for monitoring integrity of the spinal cord and peripheral nervous system; amplitude and latency of the electrophysiological complex wave generated by depolarization of either nerve or muscle, respectively, are detected from multiple electrodes placed on the patient. Peripheral nerves at sites distal to the surgical site are stimulated repetitively to obtain SSEPs; interruption of blood supply of the posterior spinal arteries or nerve compression causes loss of these signals. Transcranial electrical stimulation of the motor cortex or direct stimulation of the spinal cord or nerve roots generates MEPs detected as action potentials within specific muscles; spinal cord motor pathways are supplied by the single anterior spinal artery.

3. Intraoperative **"wake-up test"** can be used to assess motor function. Patients are coached about testing before induction of general anesthesia. At the appropriate time, typically immediately after distraction of the spinal cord, the anesthetic is reduced sufficiently to permit patient response to command to move the hands and feet; the anesthetic is deepened after confirming adequate neurological function. The procedure requires adequate analgesia and reversal of muscle relaxation before the "wake-up." The test carries the potential complications of coughing, displacement or loss of the endotracheal tube, venous air embolism (VAE), and awareness.

4. All general anesthetics decrease the effectiveness of neuromonitoring in a dose-dependent manner by increasing latency and/or decreasing amplitude of the electrophysiological signal detected from depolarization; these same changes are suggestive also of ischemia. Hypothermia and burst suppression on EEG suppress SSEPs; hypothermia and neuromuscular blockers suppress MEPs. Low concentrations of isoflurane, desflurane, and N_2O permit intraoperative monitoring but with reduced signal. Intravenous anesthesia with propofol, remifentanil, ketamine, midazolam, and etomidate, or some combination of these drugs, also permit adequate signal for neuromonitoring with less suppression of signal; etomidate increases SSEP amplitude.

I. BLOOD LOSS

Epidural vessel bleeding and decortication of bone during instrumentation and fusion of the vertebral column account for the majority of blood loss during spinal surgery. Factors predicting blood loss requiring transfusion include type of surgery (fusion, laminectomy, pedicle subtraction osteotomy, osteotomy), low preoperative hemoglobin, tumor surgery, number of spine levels involved and underlying cardiopulmonary disease. Factors likely to decrease blood loss include use of the Jackson table, hypotensive techniques, and use of tranexamic acid or epsilon-aminocaproic acid. In nontumor surgery, use of a "cell saver" to capture blood cells for reinfusion decreases requirement for transfusion. Monitoring for development of intraoperative coagulopathy includes testing prothrombin time/international normalized ratio, partial thromboplastin time, platelet count, and thrombin level.

II. SPINAL CORD PERFUSION

Spinal cord perfusion may be compromised by the initial trauma, surgical manipulation, hematoma formation, and reductions in blood pressure and cardiac output. Similar to cerebral perfusion pressure, spinal cord perfusion pressure (SCPP) is determined by mean arterial pressure (MAP) and intraspinal pressure (ISP) (or central venous pressure [CVP] if CVP > ISP): SCPP = MAP − ISP. Blood vessel injury (decreased local blood flow), systemic hypotension (decreased MAP), and obstruction to blood flow (either segmental or elevated ISP) will decrease SCPP. Methods to maximize SCPP include elevating MAP to maximize perfusion, monitoring cerebrospinal fluid (CSF) pressure within the thecal sac, and CSF drainage to maximize perfusion pressure.

A. Complications

1. Spinal surgery carries significant risks with complication rates that are accordingly higher than many other procedures; major complications occur in 11% of cases and minor complications in 24%. The lowest complication rates were among adolescents undergoing idiopathic scoliosis surgery and highest among patients with neuromuscular scoliosis. Surgeries that combine anterior/posterior approach carry greater complication rate than staged procedures. Age older than 60 years increases the rate of complications.

2. **VAE** can be fatal during spinal surgery. Risk is elevated because of the large surface area of exposed and decorticated bone and the surgical site elevated relative to the heart. Routine monitoring is accomplished with capnography and/or precordial Doppler. Transesophageal echocardiography is the most sensitive monitor for detection. If VAE is suspected, treatment includes irrigating the wound with saline, discontinuing N_2O, vasopressors to treat hypotension, turning from prone to supine (difficult with an open surgical exposure), institution of advanced life support, and potentially initiating cardiopulmonary bypass in cases refractory to resuscitation attempts.

3. **Bone cement embolism** is a rare complication of vertebroplasty or kyphoplasty to treat vertebral compression fractures; cement emboli migrate to the pulmonary vasculature from leakage of bone cement into the low-pressure venous drainage system of vertebrae. Most emboli are incidental findings, <1% present with symptoms, typically dyspnea. Diagnosis is made with imaging demonstrating cement in a vascular distribution with chest x-ray or CT; treatment is typically conservative monitoring but may require systemic anticoagulation and surgical embolectomy based on the severity of symptoms.

4. **Postoperative visual loss** occurs in approximately 0.2% of cases and has been postulated to involve optic nerve ischemia by venous engorgement, decreased arterial perfusion pressure from hypotension, hemodilution or increased intraocular pressure in the prone position. Risk factors include vascular disease, preoperative anemia, prolonged procedure time, substantial blood loss, obesity, and tobacco use. The American Society of Anesthesiologists recommends continuous blood

pressure monitoring, use of colloids or crystalloids for substantial blood loss, periodic hemoglobin/hematocrit monitoring and case-by-case consideration for use of deliberate hypotension, central venous pressure monitoring and staging surgical procedures in high-risk patients.

5. **Peripheral nerve injury:** Ulnar nerve injury is the most common peripheral nerve injury during spine surgery. Elbow flexion greater than 130° results in increased pressure within the cubital tunnel, which may compress the ulnar nerve.

6. **Spinal cord injury** can result in postoperative paraplegia and may occur despite monitoring SSEPs and MEPs. Cervical traction has been demonstrated as an effective method to decrease motion at the occipitocervical junction to prevent cervical spine injury. Immobilization for positioning/turning the patient and fiber-optic intubation for orotracheal intubation reduce cervical motion.

7. **Vascular injury** can occur in major vasculature structures adjacent to and within the spine. The major vessels at risk are summarized in **Table 24.1**.

III. DISPOSITION

Immediate postsurgical care is dependent upon procedure and patient comorbidities. For all patients, frequent neurologic checks are preferred to assess for development of edema, compressive hematomas, or vascular compromise. Factors determining disposition to an ICU include extensive surgery, significant blood loss, significant facial and airway edema, and requirement for postoperative ventilation and endotracheal intubation to maintain airway patency.

TABLE 24.1	Major Blood Vessels at Risk of Injury During Common Surgical Spine Procedures
Surgical Procedure	**Vessel(s)**
Anterior screw fixation of the odontoid fracture	Vertebral artery Internal carotid artery
Anterior cervical spine surgery	Vertebral artery
Posterior C1-C2 arthrodesis	Vertebral artery
Posterior cervical spine surgery	Vertebral artery
Anterolateral approach for thoracolumbar spine fracture	Aorta Inferior vena cava
Posterior thoracic spine surgery	Thoracic aorta
Scoliosis surgery	Superior mesenteric artery
Anterior lumbar interbody fusion	Inferior vena cava Iliac veins and arteries (L > R)
Lumbar disk surgery	Inferior vena cava Iliac veins
Posterior lumbar spine surgery	Epidural venous bleeding

IV. POSTOPERATIVE PAIN MANAGEMENT

A. Postoperative pain management may be a significant issue for patients with chronic pain, specifically back pain, who present with history of long-term high dose opioid therapy prior to surgical intervention.

B. Intraoperative methadone has been reported to reduce pain scores and analgesic requirements with acceptable side effects after complex spine surgery. Continuous infusions of short-acting opioids during surgery, such as fentanyl or remifentanil, have been demonstrated to provide adequate intraoperative analgesia and may facilitate an intraoperative "wake-up test." Postoperative pain is typically managed initially with intravenous opioids, either by patient-controlled analgesia or continuous infusion, if necessary. Injection of long-acting local anesthetic at the site of surgical incision at closure and intravenous acetaminophen may be helpful for immediate postprocedure pain control.

C. Adjuncts with demonstrated efficacy to reduce postprocedure analgesic requirements include preoperative acetaminophen, celecoxib, and either gabapentin or pregabalin as well intraoperative administration of dexamethasone and ketamine infusion. Ketamine 0.15 mg/kg bolus before surgical stimulus followed by infusion of 0.015 to 0.02 mg/kg/min has been shown to reduce opioid requirements.

Suggested Readings

American College of Surgeons. *Advanced Trauma Life Support: Student Course Manual.* American College of Surgeons; 2012.

Manoach S, Paladino L. Manual in-line stabilization for acute airway management of suspected cervical spine injury: historical review and current questions. *Ann Emerg Med.* 2007;50(3):236-245.

Edgcombe H, Carter K, Yarrow S. Anaesthesia in the prone position. *Br J Anaesth.* 2008;100(2):165-183.

Lennarson PJ, Smith D, Todd MM, et al. Segmental cervical spine motion during orotracheal intubation of the intact and injured spine with and without external stabilization. *J Neurosurg.* 2000;92:201-206.

Raw DA, Beattie JK, Hunter JM. Anaesthesia for spinal surgery in adults. *Br J Anaesth.* 2003;91(6):886-904.

Lo YL, Dan YF, Tan YE, et al. Intraoperative motor-evoked potential monitoring in scoliosis surgery: comparison of desflurane/nitrous oxide with propofol total intravenous anesthetic regimens. *J Neurosurg Anesthesiol.* 2006;18(3):211-214.

Banoub M, Tetzlaff JE, Schubert A. Pharmacologic and Physiologic influences affecting sensory evoked potentials. *Anesthesiology.* 2003;99(3):716-737.

Scheufler KM, Zentner J. Total intravenous anesthesia for intraoperative monitoring of the motor pathways: an integral view combining clinical and experimental data. *J Neurosurg.* 2002;96:571-579.

Nuttall GA, Horlocker TT, Santrach PJ, et al. Predictors of blood transfusions in spinal instrumentation and fusion surgery. *Spine.* 2000;25(5):596-601.

Werndle M, Saadoun S, Phang I, et al. Monitoring of spinal cord perfusion pressure in acute spinal cord injury: initial findings of the injured spinal cord pressure evaluation study. *Crit Care Med.* 2014;42(3):646-655.

Kong CY, Hosseini AM, Belanger LM, et al. A prospective evaluation of hemodynamic management in acute spinal cord injury patients. *Spinal Cord.* 2013;51:466-471.

McDonnell MF, Glassman SD, Dimar JR, et al. Perioperative complications of anterior procedures on the spine. *J Bone Joint Surg.* 1996;78(6):839-847.

American Society of Anesthesiology. Practice advisory for perioperative visual loss associated with spine surgery: an updated report by the American Society of Anesthesiologists Task Force on Perioperative Visual Loss. *Anesthesiology.* 2012;116(2):274-285.

Lennarson PJ, Smith DW, Sawin PD, et al. Cervical spinal motion during intubation: efficacy of stabilization maneuvers in the setting of complete segmental instability. *J Neurosurg.* 2001;94(2 suppl):265:270.

Inamasu J, Guiot BH. Vascular injury and complication in neurosurgical spine surgery. *Acta Neurochir (Wien)*. 2006;148(4):375-387.

Klatt JWB, Mickelson J, Hung M, et al. A randomized prospective evaluation of 3 techniques of postoperative pain management after posterior spinal instrumentation and fusion. *Spine*. 2013;38(19):1626-1631.

Reynolds RA, Legakis JE, Tweedie J, et al. Postoperative pain management after spinal fusion surgery: an analysis of the efficacy of continuous infusion of local anesthetics. *Global Spine J*. 2013;3(1):7-14.

Urban MK, Ya Deau JT, Wukovits B, et al. Ketamine as an adjunct to postoperative pain management in opioid tolerant patients after spinal fusions: a prospective randomized trial. *HSS J*. 2007;4:62-65.

Schmid RL, Sandler AN, Katz J. Use and efficacy of low-dose ketamine in the management of acute postoperative pain: a review of current techniques and outcomes. *Pain*. 1999;82(2):111-125.

Farag E. Airway management for cervical spine surgery. *Best Pract Res Clin Anaesthesiol*. 2016;30(1):13-25.

Li G, Sun TW, Luo G, Zhang C. Efficacy of antifibrinolytic agents on surgical bleeding and transfusion requirements in spine surgery: a meta-analysis. *Eur Spine J*. 2017;26(1):140-154.

Murphy GS, Avram MJ, Greenberg SB, et al. Postoperative pain and analgesic requirements in the first year after intraoperative methadone for complex spine and cardiac surgery. *Anesthesiology*. 2020;132(2):330-342.

Murphy GS, Szokol JW, Avram MJ, et al. Clinicaleffectiveness and safety of intraoperative methadone in patients undergoing posterior spinal fusion surgery: a randomized, double-blinded, controlled trial. *Anesthesiology*. 2017;126(5):822-833.

Alboog A, Bae S, Chui J. Anesthetic management of complex spine surgery in adult patients: a review based on outcome evidence. *Curr Opin Anaesthesiol*. 2019;32(5):600-608.

Anesthesia for Transplant Surgery

Elisa C. Walsh and Hovig V. Chitilian

I. HISTORY AND ETHICAL CONSIDERATIONS

A. The first successful human organ transplant (kidney) was performed in 1954. Since that time, the **heart, lungs, liver, pancreas, intestine, stomach, testis, penis, hand, thymus,** and **uterus** have all been successfully transplanted.

B. From the mid-1950s to the early 1970s, individual hospitals and organ procurement organizations managed all aspects of organ donation and transplantation. In 1984, the **United Network for Organ Sharing (UNOS)** was created to coordinate the allocation of organs and collect data about donors, transplant candidates, and transplant recipients in the United States.

C. Although demand continues to exceed supply, modifications of the organ allocation system, expansion of criteria for acceptable donor organs, and advances in organ preservation techniques have increased the availability of organs and improved allograft survival.

   1. The LifePort Kidney Transporter is a perfusion preservation machine for donor kidneys that works by pumping the vasculature continuously with a cold perfusate, reducing the odds of delay in kidney function and improving first-year posttransplant success compared with static storage.

   2. US Food and Drug Administration–approved transport systems have been developed for donor lungs (eg, TransMedics' OCS Lung, a "lung-in-a-box" device). This machine maintains normothermia, breathing, and perfusion throughout transport, allowing expanded retrieval ranges and successful use of organs that had been rejected by transplant centers using cold storage.

   3. Similar devices are now under investigation for donor hearts and livers.

D. The success of solid organ transplantation critically depends on the careful selection of transplant recipients. The suitability of candidates is typically determined by a multidisciplinary committee and based on national criteria.

   1. Patients require a thorough **history and physical examination** as well as **psychosocial evaluation** to identify any behavioral, social, or financial issues that may preclude adherence to immunosuppressive therapy and medical follow-up after transplantation.

   2. In addition to **standard laboratory tests**, **serologic tests** for varicella, measles, mumps, rubella, HIV, hepatitis, tuberculosis, syphilis, cytomegalovirus, Ebstein-Barr virus; **drug screening**; **ABO-Rh blood typing**; **age-appropriate screening**; and **electrocardiography** are required.

   3. As of 2020, all recipients must be tested for novel coronavirus (SARS-CoV-2) via nucleic acid test from either the upper or lower respiratory tract as close to the time of transplantation as possible.

   4. The need for additional cardiac and pulmonary testing is dependent on patient comorbidities as well as the type of transplant to be performed.

5. **Absolute contraindications** include active infection, active malignancy, substance abuse, uncontrolled psychiatric disease, life expectancy less than 1 year, and ongoing nonadherence to treatment.

6. **Ethical issues** in transplantation are numerous and include the definition of death and brain death, financial incentives and organ trafficking, and coerced donation. A full discussion is beyond the scope of this chapter.

II. ANESTHESIA FOR KIDNEY TRANSPLANTATION

A. In 2019, 23,401 kidney transplants were performed in the United States from 16,534 deceased donors and 6867 living donors. The 5-year survival is estimated to be 83.3% and 92.1% for recipients of cadaveric and living grafts, respectively.

B. Indications and recipient selection

1. A kidney transplant may be indicated for patients with **end-stage renal disease (ESRD)** from any cause.

2. Patients are generally referred to a transplantation center when the **estimated glomerular filtration rate is under 30 mL/min/1.73 m^2** in order to ensure timely completion of evaluation and any interventions required to address candidacy for transplantation.

3. The scheduling of a deceased donor kidney transplantation should take into consideration the limited viability of the donated kidney (**Table 25.1**). Transplantation from a living donor is generally elective, although in some instances transplants are conducted as part of a donor chain and thus timing is more critical.

C. Preanesthetic considerations

1. Preoperative evaluation for the patient with ESRD is discussed in **Chapter 5.**

2. Patients presenting for kidney transplantation will have undergone a thorough preoperative evaluation prior to listing. In the patient presenting for surgery, we recommend a tailored evaluation of the following:

   a. **Volume status** can be assessed through a number of modalities including physical examination, comparison with estimated dry weight, and chest radiographs.

   b. **Electrolyte imbalances** including hyponatremia, hyperkalemia, hypocalcemia, hyperphosphatemia, and metabolic acidosis can be diagnosed with a comprehensive metabolic panel and arterial blood gas.

TABLE 25.1	UNOS Guidelines for Maximum Cold Ischemic Times for Commonly Transplanted Organs
Organ	**Cold Ischemic Time (Hours)**
Kidney	24-36
Pancreas	12-18
Liver	8-12
Heart/Lung	4-6

   c. Anemia can be assessed with a complete blood count. **Coagulopathy** arising from uremic platelet dysfunction is difficult to measure but should be anticipated.

   d. Relevant medications (diuretics, antihypertensives, nephrotoxins) and **dialysis schedule** should be confirmed.

   e. Comorbid cardiovascular disease may be assessed through history, physical examination, and electrocardiogram with additional testing as indicated.

D. Monitoring

1. **Standard monitors** (see **Chapter 15**) including continuous electrocardiography (ECG) display of leads II and V5 with ST segment analysis and temperature monitoring are required.

2. For patients with a significant cardiac history, **intra-arterial blood pressure monitoring** may be necessary.

3. Intraoperative fluid management remains a challenge. Urine output will not be a reliable measurement of volume status. Traditionally, **central venous pressure** or **pulmonary arterial pressure monitoring** has been used. The use of **transesophageal echocardiography, arterial pulse waveform analysis,** and **thoracic electrical bioimpedance** has also been described.

E. Preoperative management

1. **Peripheral venous access** should be established with two intravenous catheters in separate venous systems. One catheter will be reserved for the administration of rabbit antithymocyte globulin.

2. For patients undergoing regular dialysis, it is important to confirm their most recent session as well as the method of dialysis (eg, hemodialysis, peritoneal dialysis), and to assess their volume status. If a patient is deemed to be hypovolemic, **volume expansion** may be necessary prior to anesthetic induction with 250 to 500 mL of non-potassium-containing isotonic fluid. A patient who is floridly hypervolemic may require **immediate dialysis.**

3. It is essential to confirm that the patient has received **oral immunosuppressant** (usually mycophenate mofetinil) prior to arrival to the operating room.

4. If there are no contraindications, patients should be consented for a **transversus abdominis plane block** for postoperative pain management. Neuraxial techniques are typically avoided owing to concern for uremic platelet dysfunction.

F. Intraoperative management

1. **Rapid sequence induction** is indicated for patients receiving peritoneal dialysis or patients with a diagnosis of autonomic neuropathy. It may also be considered for patients with comorbidities such as obesity and diabetes that may predispose to delayed gastric emptying.

2. For immunosuppression, **methylprednisolone** 125 to 250 mg is administered as a bolus after intubation followed by **rabbit antithymocyte globulin** 1.5 mg/kg over 6 hours via dedicated intravenous catheter with a filter. Lower-risk patients may receive basiliximab instead of thymoglobulin.

   a. Rabbit antithymocyte globulin can produce a cytokine release syndrome due to activation of T cells manifesting in fevers, hypotension, and rigors. **Diphenhydramine** 50 mg is often given to reduce the risk of this reaction.

3. **Maintenance anesthesia** can be established with either **volatile agents** or **propofol.** Owing to the theoretical risk of renal toxicity from compound A, it is advised to use fresh gas flows greater than 2 L/min when

administering sevoflurane. **Processed electroencephalography** can be used to appropriately titrate the anesthetic.

4. **Analgesia** can be maintained with intermittent doses of nonrenally cleared opioids such as **fentanyl** and **hydromorphone**. Morphine and meperidine are contraindicated owing to the accumulation of active renally cleared metabolites (morphine-6-glucuronide and normeperidine, respectively) (see Chapter 5).

5. **Neuromuscular blockade** is best accomplished with **cisatracurium** owing to its organ-independent elimination.

6. The surgery typically takes **3 to 5 hours.** The procedure begins with a vertical curvilinear incision extending from the pubis symphysis to above the anterior superior iliac spine. During incision and dissection, there is increased surgical stimulation and potentially exaggerated hemodynamic response. Analgesics, anesthetics, and relaxants should be titrated accordingly.

7. After exposure and mobilization, the external iliac vein is clamped and anastomosed to the donor renal vein. The external iliac artery is then clamped and anastomosed to the donor renal artery.

   a. In order to increase renal blood flow and promote allograft function, the mean arterial pressure (MAP) should be maintained in the range of **70 to 90 mm Hg or within 15% to 20% of the patient's baseline.**

8. **Intraoperative volume expansion** with isotonic crystalloid or albumin 5% and **titration of anesthetic agents** is favored over the administration of vasopressors owing to concern for graft malperfusion with alpha agonists.

   a. **Mannitol** (12.5 g) is often administered after the vascular anastomoses and prior to reperfusion to decrease the incidence of acute tubular necrosis in the allograft. **Furosemide** (60-100 mg) is also often administered at this time to promote diuresis after reperfusion.

   b. Rarely, removal of the vascular clamps is associated with significant blood loss requiring resuscitation and transfusion.

9. The donor ureter is then implanted into the recipient bladder, which is filled with antibiotic saline irrigation solution. The surgeon will request that the Foley be clamped prior to retrograde infusion of a methylene blue solution into the bladder to check for leaks.

10. During closure, it is **essential that neuromuscular blockade is maintained** until closure of the fascial layer owing to the risk of damage to the vascular anastomoses with coughing or other unexpected movement.

11. The majority of patients are **extubated** in the operating room.

G. **Postoperative management**

1. **Urine output is strictly monitored.** Suspected hypovolemia is managed with volume resuscitation. Ureteral obstruction, vascular thrombosis, and hemorrhage are managed with early surgical re-exploration.

2. **Delayed graft function**, defined as a need for dialysis within 7 days of transplant, is a common complication with a rising incidence due to the increasing use of marginal donor organs. In addition to urine output monitoring, patients should have a basic metabolic panel postoperatively to check for electrolyte imbalances that may require immediate dialysis.

3. Analgesia is generally achieved with **patient-controlled analgesia** with intravenous fentanyl or hydromorphone. Morphine and meperidine are avoided owing to the accumulation of renally excreted toxic metabolites. Nonsteroidal anti-inflammatory drugs are avoided owing to nephrotoxicity. **Transversus abdominis plane blocks** may reduce postoperative opioid requirements.

III. ANESTHESIA FOR PANCREAS TRANSPLANTATION
A. Indications and recipient selection
1. The goal of pancreas transplantation is to **restore euglycemia and halt the progression of diabetic complications** in patients who are unable to produce insulin owing to dysfunction of the beta cells of the pancreas.
2. Pancreas transplantation is most commonly performed as a **simultaneous kidney-pancreas transplant** or **pancreas after kidney transplant** for patients with ESRD and type 1 diabetes mellitus. Select patients with insulin-dependent type 2 diabetes mellitus may also be candidates for pancreas transplantation.
3. **Pancreas transplant alone** is generally reserved for patients with severe complications of type 1 diabetes mellitus including a history of frequent severe metabolic complications (eg, diabetic ketoacidosis) and failure of exogenous insulin therapy to prevent these complications.
4. **Islet cell transplantation** is an experimental therapy wherein islet cells from a deceased donor pancreas are harvested and then injected percutaneously into the portal vein.
5. In 2019, 143 pancreas transplants and 872 kidney-pancreas transplants were performed in the United States. The 5-year survival rates are estimated at greater than 88%.

B. Preanesthetic considerations
1. Preoperative evaluation for the patient with pancreatic disease is discussed in **Chapter 7**.
2. For patients presenting for pancreatic transplant, we recommend a tailored evaluation including the following:
   a. **Macro- and microvascular complications of diabetes** should be confirmed by history and physical examination. Special attention should be paid to cardiac, neurologic, and renal comorbidities. Patients with **comorbid end-stage renal disease** presenting for dual kidney-pancreas transplant should be evaluated as described in the prior section.
3. **Acute metabolic abnormalitie**s such as diabetic ketoacidosis or hypoglycemia can be identified with a basic metabolic panel and frequent blood glucose measurements.
4. **Recent insulin administration and baseline insulin requirements** should be assessed and documented.

C. Monitoring
1. **Standard monitors** (see Chapter 15) including continuous ECG display of leads II and V5 with ST segment analysis and temperature monitoring are recommended.
2. For patients with a significant cardiac history, **intra-arterial blood pressure monitoring** may be necessary.
3. Owing to the necessity of frequent intraoperative glucose monitoring, a **glucometer** or an intra-arterial catheter must be available.

D. Preoperative management
1. **Peripheral venous access** should be established with two intravenous catheters in separate venous systems. One catheter should be reserved for administration of immunosuppression induction agent, most often rabbit antithymocyte globulin.
2. It is essential to confirm that the patient has received oral immunosuppressant prior to arrival in the operating room.
3. Patients may benefit from the preoperative placement of a **thoracic epidural** at the T5-T8 level if there are no contraindications. In patients with significant comorbid renal disease, neuraxial anesthesia may be

deferred owing to concern for uremic platelet dysfunction. A postoperative **transversus abdominis plane block** is a reasonable alternative.

E. **Intraoperative management**
   1. **Rapid sequence induction** is recommended owing to risk of gastroparesis from long-standing diabetes and administration of oral immunosuppressants preoperatively.
   2. Immediately after intubation, **methylprednisolone** 125 to 250 mg is administered as a bolus followed by **rabbit antithymocyte globulin** 1.5 mg/kg over 6 hours via dedicated intravenous catheter with a filter.
   3. **Maintenance anesthesia** can be maintained with either volatile agents or propofol infusion.
   4. **Analgesia** is usually accomplished with intermittent opioid dosing or epidural anesthesia/analgesia.
   5. **Neuromuscular blockade** is best accomplished with cisatracurium or rocuronium.
   6. **Insulin and dextrose (D5W or D10W) infusions** should be titrated to maintain blood glucose levels of **110 to 180 mg/dL** to prevent hyperglycemia-induced islet cell dysfunction intraoperatively.
   7. Case length is typically **3 hours** for a pancreas transplant and **up to 6 hours** for a combined kidney-pancreas transplant. A midline surgical incision is used for both procedures. After dissection and mobilization, three anastomoses for the donor pancreas must be performed: (1) **arterial**, typically from the recipient iliac artery; (2) **venous**, typically to the recipient iliac vein; and (3) **exocrine**, most commonly to the intestine or bladder.
      a. Following allograft perfusion, pancreatic beta cells begin secreting insulin within 5 minutes. **Blood glucose levels** should be assessed **every 15 minutes** for the first hour after reperfusion, then **every 30 minutes** thereafter.
      b. To promote graft perfusion after reperfusion, **intraoperative volume expansion** with isotonic crystalloid or albumin 5% and **titration of anesthetic agents** is favored over the administration of vasopressors owing to concern for graft malperfusion with alpha agonists.
      c. Rarely, there is significant blood loss associated with the vascular anastomoses requiring resuscitation and transfusion.
   8. During closure, it is essential that **neuromuscular blockade is maintained** until the fascial layer owing to the risk of damage to the vascular anastomoses with coughing or other unexpected movement.
   9. The majority of patients **are extubated** in the operating room.

F. **Postoperative management**
   1. **Blood glucose and electrolytes are strictly monitored.** Exogenous insulin is administered as necessary for delayed graft function, defined as hyperglycemia exceeding 200 mg/dL.
   2. Technical failures such as pancreatic thrombosis, leaks, and bleeding may require early reoperation.
   3. In the absence of a working thoracic epidural, pain control is generally achieved with **patient-controlled analgesia** with intravenous hydromorphone or morphine, or regional anesthesia.

IV. **ANESTHESIA FOR LIVER TRANSPLANTATION**
   A. **Introduction**
      1. In 2019, 8896 liver transplants were performed in the United States from 8372 deceased donors and 524 living donors.
      2. The 5-year survival is estimated at 75% and 83.9% for recipients of cadaveric and living grafts, respectively.

B. **Indications** for liver transplantation include but are not limited to:
1. Acute fulminant hepatic failure (highest priority).
2. Cirrhosis with evidence of portal hypertension and markers of serious decompensation including variceal hemorrhage, ascites, hepatic encephalopathy, and hepatorenal syndrome. Etiologies include chronic hepatitis B or C, alcoholic liver disease, biliary cirrhosis, cryptogenic cirrhosis, autoimmune hepatitis, hemochromatosis, nonalcoholic steatohepatitis.
3. Hepatocellular carcinoma (HCC), stage I or II.
4. Budd-Chiari syndrome (hepatic vein thrombosis).
5. Sclerosing cholangitis.
6. Biliary atresia and inborn errors of metabolism.

C. **Recipient selection**
1. Priority on the liver transplant waitlist is based on a patient's **Model for End-Stage Liver Disease (MELD)** score, an objective and accurate predictor of short-term survival in patients with cirrhosis. The MELD score is derived from the patient's **serum bilirubin, serum creatinine, and international normalized ratio.** For patients who are on hemodialysis, the score is calculated using a serum creatinine value of 4 mg/dL. For patients with a MELD score greater than 11, the serum sodium concentration is also factored in to yield the **MELD-Na score**, which reflects the vasodilatory state in cirrhosis and predicts mortality independent of the MELD score.
2. Exception points
   a. Certain conditions are associated with a higher mortality than reflected in the MELD score. Patients with **stage I or II HCC, hepatopulmonary syndrome, portopulmonary hypertension**, and **hereditary hemorrhagic telangiectasia** receive **exception points** in addition to their calculated MELD score that lead to higher prioritization on the waitlist.
   b. Patients with other complicating medical conditions related to their liver disease but not qualifying for standard MELD exception points may **petition** for additional points.

D. **Preanesthetic considerations**
1. Preoperative evaluation for the patient with liver disease is discussed in **Chapter 6.**
2. Preoperative testing is typically initiated at a MELD score of **10 to 15 points**. The goals of this assessment are to determine the extent of **hepatic dysfunction**; to screen for cardiac, pulmonary, and renal **comorbidities** unique to cirrhotic patients; and to evaluate for **fitness to survive** after transplantation. The decision to list a patient is based on the review of the test results by a **multidisciplinary committee** that includes liver transplant anesthesiologists.
3. For cardiac clearance, each patient is screened for **structural heart disease, coronary artery disease**, and **portopulmonary hypertension**.
   a. Our institutional approach for patients under age 50 years is to acquire a **transthoracic echocardiogram**, with special attention paid to the estimated right ventricular systolic pressure (RVSP), right ventricular function, and right ventricular size. Contrast-enhanced echocardiography may be employed to identify intrapulmonary shunting. **Right heart catheterization** is necessary for any patient with elevated RVSP to ascertain the mean pulmonary arterial pressure (mPAP) and pulmonary vascular resistance (PVR). The RVSP cutoff varies by institution but is usually either **40 or 50 mm Hg.**

   b. **Portopulmonary hypertension** is defined by an mPAP greater than 25 mm Hg, pulmonary capillary wedge pressure (PCWP) less than 15 mm Hg, and a PVR greater than 240 dynes/s/cm^5.

   c. Patients with an **mPAP greater than 35 mm Hg or a PVR greater than 250 dynes/s/cm**^{5} have a 36% mortality rate within 18 days of transplantation.

   d. Patients over age 50 years or with significant cardiac risk factors undergo **dobutamine stress echocardiography** to assess cardiac function in response to an elevated heart rate. For patients on a beta-blocker who are unable to mount a heart rate response, we obtain a **nuclear stress test** with a coronary vasodilator. **Cirrhotic cardiomyopathy** is a syndrome defined by increased cardiac output and contractility at rest with a blunted contractile response and/or diastolic dysfunction with stress.

  4. For pulmonary clearance, we acquire **pulse oximetry, pulmonary function testing**, and **arterial blood gas testing** for age-adjusted alveolar-arterial gradient.

   a. **Hepatopulmonary syndrome** is defined by a triad of portal hypertension with or without cirrhosis, arterial hypoxemia (Pao_2 less than 60-80 mm Hg with room air at rest in a sitting position), and the presence of intrapulmonary shunts. The degree of hypoxemia is directly related to the perioperative mortality.

  5. **Chest** and **abdominal imaging** is generally required to rule out the presence of occult malignancy and to assess the presence of any anatomic barriers to transplantation. **Multiphase contrast-induced computed tomography or contrast-enhanced magnetic resonance imaging** is preferred to assess hepatic vasculature and stage hepatocellular carcinoma, if present.

  6. **Upper endoscopy** is performed to assess for the presence of significant esophageal varices.

E. Monitoring

  1. **Standard monitors** (see **Chapter 15**) including continuous ECG display of leads II and V5 with ST segment analysis and temperature monitoring are required.

  2. **Intra-arterial blood pressure monitoring** is essential both for hemodynamic management and frequent laboratory draws.

  3. **Pulmonary arterial catheter monitoring** is frequently used to assess pulmonary arterial pressure and cardiac output intraoperatively.

  4. **Transesophageal echocardiography** is increasingly used to assess intraoperative cardiac output and chamber function, particularly in the presence of cirrhotic cardiomyopathy or other preexisting cardiac disease. It is necessary to first exclude significant esophageal variceal disease.

F. Preoperative management

  1. A **large-bore peripheral venous access** should be established. Insertion of a short 7.5-French catheter may be considered for rapid infusion. The left arm is preferred as the right arm is often tucked. The largest catheter should be attached to a rapid transfusion system capable of delivering 1.0 to 1.5 L/min at 38°C.

  2. A **radial artery catheter** is placed in the left arm. We suggest the ultrasound-guided single-puncture technique to avoid through-and-through technique in the setting of coagulopathy.

  3. **Blood products** should be ordered prior to induction in anticipation of significant bleeding during the initial stages of surgery. Blood loss during a liver transplant is highly variable, ranging from 500 mL to several patient blood volumes. A number of variables have been associated with increased transfusion during liver transplantation, including (but not limited to) the **severity of liver disease**, **history of prior abdominal procedures**, and **cold ischemic time** of the donor organ. Knowledge of the patient blood antibody status and ability to cross-match large volumes of blood are critical. We suggest starting with the following:

   a. **5 to 10 units of packed red blood cells** in the room and **10 units crossed**.
   b. **5 to 10 units of fresh frozen plasma** in the room and **10 units crossed**.
   c. **Five aliquots of 5% albumin** (250 mL each).

   4. It is essential to confirm that the patient has received oral immunosuppressant (usually mycophenate mofetinil) prior to arrival in the operating room.

G. **Intraoperative management**
   1. **Induction: Rapid-sequence induction** is advised owing to the emergent nature of surgery, preoperative administration of oral immunosuppressants, and the presence of ascites.
   2. **Maintenance anesthetic** is most often established with a balanced technique including a volatile agent and opioid administration. In the setting of even mild encephalopathy, a lower concentration of anesthetic is often sufficient and can be titrated using processed electroencephalography.
   3. **Central venous access** should be established for drug administration as well as monitoring of central venous pressure. Depending on the adequacy of peripheral volume access and expected blood loss, a single- or double-lumen 9-French cannula may be inserted. If a need for **venovenous bypass (VVBP)** is anticipated, a 15-French VVBP inflow cannula can be inserted ideally in the right internal jugular vein.
   4. The ideal agent for **neuromuscular blockade** is cisatracurium owing to its organ-independent elimination, but rocuronium may also be used with twitch-guided dosing. Liver failure produces a large volume of distribution that may lead to delayed onset and recovery from neuromuscular blockade.
   5. **Preanhepatic stage**
      a. The case length is typically **6 to 8 hours.**
      b. The preanhepatic stage begins with the **bisubcostal (Chevron) incision** and ends with **cross-clamping of the portal vein.** The diseased liver is dissected and mobilized.
      c. If **VVBP** is being used, the surgical team will place outflow cannulas in the femoral and portal veins. Bypass is initiated prior to the anhepatic phase.
      d. During the preanhepatic stage, the most common problem encountered is **hypotension.**
      e. **Drainage of large-volume abdominal ascites** can be managed with anticipatory administration of colloid-containing fluid to minimize changes in preload.
      f. **Bleeding** is related to the degree of preexisting coagulopathy, presence and severity of portal hypertension, and duration and complexity of surgical procedure (eg, severe adhesions).
      g. **Compression of the inferior vena cava** with the manipulation of the liver during dissection can lead to hypotension owing to a reduction in venous return.
      h. Along with hemodynamic monitoring, the patient's hemoglobin and metabolic status should be assessed regularly.
      i. **Methylprednisolone 125 to 250 mg** is given for immunosuppression when the recipient liver is removed.

6. **Anhepatic stage**
   a. The anhepatic stage begins with **portal vein cross-clamp** and ends with **graft reperfusion.** The recipient liver and a portion of the inferior vena cava is removed, and the donor liver is inserted with caval and portal anastomoses.
   b. Approaches (**Figure 25.1**).
      1. In the **bicaval or "classic" technique,** the suprahepatic and infrahepatic cava are clamped prior to removal of the liver. To preserve venous return, **VVBP** allows diversion of blood flow from the recipient's inferior vena cava and portal vein to the axillary vein

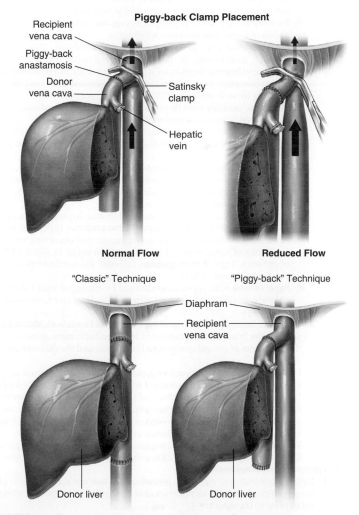

Piggy-back Clamp Placement

Recipient vena cava

Piggy-back anastamosis

Donor vena cava

Satinsky clamp

Hepatic vein

Normal Flow

"Classic" Technique

Reduced Flow

"Piggy-back" Technique

Diaphram

Recipient vena cava

Donor liver

Donor liver

FIGURE 25.1 "Classic" versus piggyback technique for donor liver implantation.

and attenuates the decrease in preload. However, the use of VVBP may increase the risk of postoperative acute renal failure, air embolism, thromboembolism, and inadvertent decannulation.

2. Once VVBP has been initiated, if the patient becomes hypotensive with caval cross-clamping, the VVBP flows should be increased to maintain adequate venous return. If the flows cannot be increased ("line chatter"), additional volume should be administered to the patient.

3. In the **"piggyback" technique,** a side-biting clamp is placed across the base of the hepatic vein, preserving caval flow and venous return. The suprahepatic cava of the donor liver is then anastomosed to the base of the hepatic vein. This technique preserves the recipient's inferior vena cava and avoids VVBP.

4. **Fibrinolysis** may occur during this stage owing to the unopposed action of tissue plasminogen activator.

5. Hypocalcemia may occur as citrate, administered with blood product transfusion, is not metabolized with the complete absence of hepatic function. Citrate binds to calcium reducing its serum concentration. Serum ionized calcium less than 1 mg/dL is typically treated with 100 to 200 mg of calcium chloride.

6. Metabolic acidosis may develop in patients with preexisting acidosis, renal failure, or a prolonged anhepatic phase.

7. **Reperfusion** is defined as the release of portal venous clamp following completion of caval anastomosis and portal venous anastomosis.

8. Prior to completion of the anastomosis and graft reperfusion, the donor liver is flushed into the field to wash out the preservative solution. It may be flushed with a colloid/crystalloid solution or with blood through the portal vein.

9. Reperfusion is associated with hypotension, hyperkalemia, acidemia, and arrhythmias. **Postreperfusion syndrome** is defined as a >30% decrease in MAP lasting over 1 minute and occurring within 5 minutes of reperfusion. It is estimated to occur in 15% to 30% of patients. Typical management includes the administration of vasopressors and volume.

10. **Hyperkalemia** with reperfusion should be managed with calcium chloride, insulin (and glucose), hyperventilation, and furosemide.

7. **Neohepatic stage**

a. This stage begins following **graft reperfusion** and ends with **abdominal closure.** The primary considerations for anesthetic management are the treatment of coagulopathy and fibrinolysis and the maintenance of low CVP.

b. **Fibrinolysis,** caused by rising tissue plasminogen activator from graft endothelial cells, is often managed with the administration of fresh frozen plasma, cryoprecipitate, and platelets as guided by **frequent laboratory testing, thromboelastography, or thromboelastometry.** In cases of profound coagulopathy, infusion of antifibrinolytic agents such as aminocaproic acid and tranexamic acid may be necessary.

c. **Volume resuscitation** is carried out in a judicious manner to target a **CVP <10 mm Hg** to prevent hepatic congestion and graft dysfunction.

H. **Postoperative management**

1. Patients are transported to the **intensive care unit** upon completion of surgery. If clinically stable, patients may be extubated in the operating room prior to transport.

2. Immediate complications of liver transplantation include **postoperative bleeding, biliary leaks, graft dysfunction,** and **vascular thromboses (hepatic artery or portal vein)** that may require emergent reoperation.

3. **Infection** is a later complication due to immunosuppression.

V. ANESTHESIA FOR ORGAN PROCUREMENT

A. Types of donors[a]

1. **Donation after brain death (DBD)** donors are patients who have had a terminal neurologic insult and have been declared brain dead in accordance with the American Academy of Neurology guidelines and any institutional policies.

2. **Donation after cardiac death** donors are patients who have had a terminal neurologic insult but do not meet criteria for brain death. Death is declared based on cardiopulmonary criteria after life support is withdrawn. A period of 5 minutes is allowed to elapse prior to procurement to ensure no autoresuscitation.

3. **Living donors** are patients who willingly donate an organ, most often a kidney. Living liver donation can occur with left lateral segment or lobe donation to a pediatric recipient or a right lobe in adult-to-adult transplants.

   a. Living organ donation boasts improved survival rates, reduced waiting times, and opportunity to electively schedule surgery. However, it presents a significant **ethical challenge** as it is the only surgery from which a patient derives no benefit for the risk they take.

   b. Living liver donations should involve a liver transplant anesthesiologist who is familiar with the anesthetic considerations for dissection and mobilization of the hepatic segment, which can present significant risk to the donor.

B. Preanesthetic considerations for DBD procurement

1. For the purposes of our discussion, we will focus on the **DBD donor** presenting for organ procurement as these cases directly involve the anesthesiology team and present unique challenges.

2. **Brain death** precipitates a number of **profound physiologic changes** affecting nearly every organ system, as summarized in **Table 25.2.**

C. Preoperative management for DBD procurement

1. **Peripheral venous access** should be established with at least two large-bore intravenous catheters in each arm.

2. **Intra-arterial pressure monitoring** is favored owing to hemodynamic instability and the potential need for laboratory draws during the dissection.

3. **Central venous catheter access** should be established for dynamic measurement of central venous pressure and vasopressor administration.

4. **Pulmonary arterial catheter** monitoring may be indicated.

D. Intraoperative management for DBD procurement

1. **Neuromuscular blockade** is necessary to inhibit spinal motor reflexes.

---

[a]As of 2020, all donors should undergo nucleic acid testing for SARS-CoV-2 from the upper or lower respiratory tract within 3 days of procurement. Living donors are encouraged to self-quarantine for 14 days prior to organ donation surgery. Organ donations from patients with known SARS-CoV-2 is not recommended at this time, although the rate of transmission from donor to recipient is unknown.

Organ System	Pathology
	Pathological Changes in Donation After Brain Death Donors by Organ System
Pulmonary	• Increased pulmonary capillary permeability • Pulmonary edema
Cardiovascular	• Profound vasoplegia • Myocardial injury • Hypovolemia • Autonomic storming
Hematologic	• Coagulopathy progressing to disseminated intravascular coagulation
Endocrine	• Pituitary infarction leading to diabetes insipidus, adrenal insufficiency, and hypothyroidism • Insulin resistance leading to hyperglycemia

Adapted by permission from Springer: Anderson TA, Bekker P, Vagefi PA. Anesthetic considerations in organ procurement surgery: a narrative review. *Can J Anaesth.* 2015; 62(5):529-539. Copyright © 2015 Springer Nature.

2. **Analgesia** via intravenous opioids and a low to moderate dose of volatile anesthetic is often employed to minimize hemodynamic response to incision.

3. A **lung-protective ventilator strategy** with tidal volumes of 6 to 8 mL/kg of predicted body weight, positive end-pulmonary pressure of 8 to 10 mm Hg, and inspiratory pressures below 35 cmH$_2$O is recommended.

4. **Hemodynamic goals** of systolic blood pressure greater than 100 mm Hg, central venous pressure of 4 to 8 mm Hg, mean arterial pressure greater than 70 mm Hg, and heart rate of 60 to 120 bpm are accomplished with the use of **continuous vasopressor infusions and boluses** as needed. **Vasopressin** is the vasopressor of choice as it both raises systemic vascular resistance and treats comorbid diabetes insipidus.

5. In the presence of significant diabetes insipidus, **intravascular volume replacement** is necessary with administration of colloids such as albumin 5% or packed red blood cells (for a hemoglobin goal of greater than 7 g/dL) preferred over balanced crystalloids. Synthetic colloids are avoided entirely. **Desmopressin (ddAVP)** (1-4 µg every 6 hours intravenously) may also be employed.

6. **Heparin** is delivered immediately prior to **thoracic and abdominal aortic cross-clamping.** After this, the organs are cooled and removed in the following order: heart, lung, liver, pancreas, and kidneys.

7. After aortic cross-clamping, the anesthesiologist closes the intraoperative record and turns off the ventilator as well as all ongoing infusions.

Suggested Readings

Anderson TA, Bekker P, Vagefi PA. Anesthetic considerations in organ procurement surgery: a narrative review. *Can J Anesth.* 2015;62:529-539.

Aniskevich S, Perry D. Anesthesia for pancreas transplantation. *Pancreatic Dis Ther.* 2013;3:1-3.

Carton EG, Plevak DJ, Kranner PW, et al. Perioperative care of the liver transplant patient. Part I and II. *Anesth Analg.* 1994;78(120-133):382-399.

Deshpande R, Chadha RM. Tutorial 377. Anaesthesia for orthotopic liver transplantation. In: Doane MA, Poon C, ed. *Anesthesia Tutorial of the Week*. 2018. Accessed March 29, 2020. https://www.wfsahq.org/components/com_virtual_library/media/c7978058d48874571f25ee46e1c8864c-377-Anaesthesia-for-Liver-Transplantation.pdf

Gruessner RWG, Gruessner AC. The current state of pancreas transplantation. *Nat Rev Endocrinol*. 2013;9:555-562.

Krowka M, Wiesner RH, Heimbach JK. Pulmonary contraindications, indications, and MELD exceptions for liver transplantation: a contemporary view and look forward. *J Hepatol*. 2013;59(2):367-374.

Moers C, Pirenne J, Paul A, Ploeg RJ; Machine Preservation Trial Study Group. Machine perfusion or cold storage in deceased-donor kidney transplantation. *N Engl J Med*. 2009;360:7-19.

Organ Procurement and Transplantation Network (OPTN). *U.S. Department of Health and Human Services*. Last updated March 29, 2020. Accessed March 29, 2020. https://optn.transplant.hrsa.gov/data/

Schmid S, Jungwirth B. Anesthesia for renal transplant surgery: an update. *Eur J Anaesthesiol*. 2012;29:552-558.

Steadman RH. Anesthesia for liver transplant surgery. *Anesthesiol Clin North Am*. 2004;22:687-711.

Steadman RH, Wray CL. Anesthesia for abdominal organ transplantation. In: Miller RD, ed. *Miller's Anesthesia*. 8th ed. Elsevier; 2015:2262-2289.

TransMedics OCS: Science That Mirrors life. TransMedics; 2020. Accessed April 5, 2020. https://www.transmedics.com/ocs-hcp/

United Network for Organ Sharing (UNOS). 2020. Accessed April 1, 2020. https://unos.org/

Xia V, Steadman RH. Anesthesia for organ procurement. In: Miller RD, ed. *Miller's Anesthesia*, 8th ed. Elsevier; 2015:2262-2289.

David Hao and Triffin J. Psyhojos

I. PREANESTHETIC CONSIDERATIONS

Patients undergoing abdominal surgery necessitate a complete history and physical examination as outlined in Chapter 1. Additional concerns germane to abdominal surgery should be considered including:

A. Preoperative volume status. Surgery in the abdomen has the potential to cause severe derangements in volume status and fluid homeostasis. The main sources of perioperative fluid deficits include preoperative fasting, interstitial sequestration of intravascular volume (via inflammation or edema), and surgical bleeding.

1. Assessment of volume status

   a. Postural changes in vital signs (increased heart rate and decreased blood pressure) and clinical signs including dry mucous membranes, decreased skin turgor or mottling, and delayed capillary refill may suggest hypovolemia or dehydration.

   b. Laboratory analysis of base excess or deficit, hematocrit, serum osmolality, BUN (blood urea nitrogen) to creatinine ratio, serum and urine electrolyte concentrations, and urine output may be helpful in estimating volume deficits.

   c. Dynamic hemodynamic monitoring may also be considered to guide assessment of intravascular volume status. Pulse pressure variation (PPV) and systolic pressure variation (SPV) obtained from an arterial catheter waveform may aid in estimating volume-responsiveness. Generally, a delta-down component of 5 mm Hg for SPV or 13% to 15% for PPV is indicative of volume-responsiveness. Traditional assessments of volume status including central venous pressure (CVP) and pulmonary artery occlusion pressures have been questioned in the context of guiding intraoperative fluid management.

2. Etiologies of hypovolemia

   a. Reduced oral intake, malabsorption, or gastrointestinal tract dysmotility may predispose a patient to hypovolemia or dehydration in the perioperative period.

   b. Emesis, gastric drainage, or diarrhea may produce significant fluid and electrolyte derangements. Monitoring the quantity, quality, duration, and frequency of output is recommended.

   c. Bleeding from the gastrointestinal tract may be occult and include sources like ulcers, neoplasms, esophageal varices, diverticula, angiodysplasia, and hemorrhoids.

   d. Sequestration of fluid may occur either into the bowel lumen from ileus or into the interstitium from peritonitis.

   e. Fever increases insensible fluid loss.

B. Metabolic derangements occur frequently in patients requiring emergency abdominal surgery. Hypokalemic metabolic alkalosis is common in patients with large gastric losses (emesis or nasogastric [NG] tube drainage). Severe hypovolemia or septicemia may cause profound metabolic acidosis.

C. **Length of surgery** is influenced by the history of previous abdominal surgery, intra-abdominal infection, radiation therapy, steroid use, surgical technique, and surgeon experience.

D. **All patients for emergency abdominal procedures should be considered as high risk for aspiration and induced as a "full stomach."** A rapid sequence induction (RSI) is indicated with the goal of minimizing aspiration risk. Cricoid pressure is an area of active controversy with respect to its role and efficacy in minimizing aspiration. Premedication with histamine (H_2) antagonists and oral nonparticulate antacids may decrease gastric acidity.

II. ANESTHETIC TECHNIQUES

A. **General anesthesia (GA)** is the most commonly employed technique.

1. Advantages particularly relevant to abdominal surgery include airway protection and control of ventilation parameters.

2. Disadvantages include loss of airway reflexes, which increases the risk of aspiration during routine or emergency surgery, and potential adverse hemodynamic consequences.

B. **Regional anesthetic techniques** for abdominal surgery include neuraxial anesthetics (ie, spinal, epidural, and caudal anesthesia) and peripheral nerve blocks performed on the trunk. The innervation of the abdominal wall is via the anterior divisions of the thoracolumbar nerves (T6-L1). Blocks that target various divisions of the nerves include rectus sheath, transversus abdominis plane (TAP), subcostal TAP, ilioinguinal, and iliohypogastric nerve blocks.

1. **Lower abdominal procedures** (eg, inguinal hernia repair) may be performed solely with regional anesthesia techniques.

   a. Epidural anesthesia usually is performed with a continuous catheter technique. A "single-dose" technique may be applicable for surgery of less than 3 hours but rarely used in practice.

   b. Spinal anesthesia usually is performed with a single-dose technique, though spinal catheters may be placed. The duration of block is determined by the choice of local anesthetic and adjuvants (see Chapter 17).

   c. Peripheral nerve blocks (discussed in the section that follows) may provide adequate anesthesia for abdominal surgery but are more commonly used as adjuvant techniques for postoperative analgesia.

   d. Vaginal and intrauterine procedures may be performed under neuraxial anesthesia alone. A T10 level is usually sufficient for these, while a T4 level is usually necessary for a vaginal hysterectomy to cover the expected peritoneal traction associated with the procedure.

2. **Upper abdominal procedures** (above the umbilicus at T10) are unlikely to be well tolerated under regional anesthesia alone. Spinal or epidural anesthesia for upper abdominal procedures may necessitate a sensory level of T2 to T4. Paralysis of intercostal muscles from a high thoracic level impairs deep breathing. Although minute ventilation is maintained, patients often complain of a sensation of dyspnea. Intraperitoneal air or upper abdominal exploration commonly generates a dull pain referred to the C_5 dermatomal distribution (usually over the shoulders) that may not prevented by regional anesthesia and thus, require supplementation with intravenous (IV) analgesics.

3. **Advantages**

   a. If awake for the procedure, patients maintain the ability to communicate symptoms (eg, chest pain).

   b. Airway reflexes are maintained.

    c. Profound muscle relaxation and bowel contraction optimizes surgical exposure.

    d. Sympathectomy increases blood flow to the bowel.

    e. Continuous catheter techniques provide a ready means for postoperative analgesia.

    f. Regional techniques are opioid sparing.

    g. There is some evidence to support earlier return of bowel function in patients with prolonged postoperative ileus when epidural catheters are used for postoperative analgesia.

4. Disadvantages

    a. Local anesthetic toxicity from inadvertent IV injection or rapid absorption.

    b. Patient cooperation is necessary for the institution of block and positioning during surgery.

    c. Failure necessitates intraoperative conversion to GA.

    d. Regional nerve blockade may be contraindicated in patients with abnormal bleeding profile or localized infection at the site of injection.

    e. Sympathectomy with neuraxial techniques may lead to vaso/venodilation and bradycardia that can precipitate profound hypotension, especially in patients who are hypovolemic. Unopposed parasympathetic activity causes the bowel to contract and may make construction of bowel anastomoses more difficult; this can be reversed with glycopyrrolate, 0.2 to 0.4 mg IV, or 1 mg glucagon.

    f. Blockade of upper thoracic nerves may compromise pulmonary function.

    g. Awake patients often require frequent communication and reassurance; this may distract the anesthesiologist during complicated cases.

C. A combined technique makes use of a regional technique along with a general anesthetic. This technique is commonly used for extensive upper abdominal surgeries and may include an epidural or a nerve block + GA. Peripheral nerve blocks of the abdominal wall may be done awake, but more commonly immediately after induction or just prior to emergence (postprocedure) from GA. The nerve blocks can provide significant intraoperative and postoperative analgesia, creating an opioid-sparing technique. The blocks may be viable options when neuraxial techniques are contraindicated due to concerns for sepsis, severe spinal stenosis, severe peripheral nerve disease, or patient refusal. The most common peripheral nerve blocks performed on the abdominal wall include the following:

    1. TAP blocks can be used for most lower abdominal procedures, often as an alternative for epidural anesthesia. A regional needle is placed in the anterior axillary line, between the costal margin and the iliac crest. The local anesthetic spreads between the transversus abdominis and internal oblique muscle planes. Catheters are often used for TAP blocks to provide postoperative analgesia, providing a significant opioid-sparing effect.

    2. Rectus sheath blocks are appropriate for midline procedures, particularly periumbilical procedures. Local anesthetic is deposited via a regional needle between the rectus muscle and posterior rectus sheath.

    3. Subcostal TAP blocks are similar to the TAP block described above, but the needle is placed more superiorly and laterally, below the costal margin. The upper nerve fibers, in particular T8 to T10, are more likely anesthetized with this modification of the TAP block.

III. MANAGEMENT OF ANESTHESIA

A. Standard monitors are used as described in Chapter 10.

B. Induction of anesthesia

1. Restoration of volume deficits prior to induction should be considered (discussed in the section that follows).

2. RSI or awake intubation is indicated for all patients considered to have full stomachs. Additional indications include conditions in which gastric emptying is delayed, intra-abdominal pressure is increased, or lower esophageal tone is compromised. Examples include trauma, bowel obstruction or ileus, hiatal hernia, gastroesophageal reflux disease, pregnancy beyond the first trimester, significant obesity, ascites, and diabetes with gastroparesis and autonomic dysfunction.

C. Maintenance of anesthesia

1. Fluid replacement is guided by clinical judgment and may be aided by invasive monitoring. Traditionally, extended operative cases with significant bowel exposure and preoperative hypovolemia have necessitated fluid replacement of up to 10 to 15 mL/kg/h. Emerging evidence, though, suggests that a more restrictive approach to fluid resuscitation may be associated with faster recovery and fewer complications.

2. A "protocol-based" strategy for fluid administration is claimed to reduce impairment of bowel motility, cardiopulmonary complications, and bowel edema. It may also improve anastomosis healing and reduce hospital length of stay (LOS). Currently, no clear consensus exists on definitions or protocols for fluid-restrictive strategies. Literature has been published measuring multiple parameters including volume of fluid, perioperative weight, and hemodynamic responsiveness. A deliberate and planned strategy for intraoperative fluid administration on a case-by-case basis would seem to be the most prudent approach.

    a. Bleeding may be estimated both by direct observation of the surgical field and suction traps and by weighing sponges. Blood loss may be concealed (eg, beneath drapes or within the patient) and labs should be checked as clinically indicated.

    b. Insensible losses may range from 0.5 to 1 mL/kg/h for larger abdominal cases.

    c. In spite of an overnight NPO period, blood volume is possibly near normal in many patients, and perceived fluid deficits may not necessitate IV fluid repletion. Clinical judgment will guide the need for resuscitation prior to starting the case.

    d. Abrupt drainage of ascitic fluid with surgical entry into the peritoneum has the potential to cause acute hypotension from a sudden decrease of intra-abdominal pressure and pooling of blood in mesenteric vessels, reducing venous return to the right heart. Postoperative re-accumulation of ascitic fluid may produce significant intravascular fluid losses.

    e. NG and other enteric drainage should be quantified and replaced appropriately.

3. Fluid losses should be replaced with crystalloids, colloids, or blood products.

    a. Initially, fluid should be replaced by administration of an isotonic salt solution. When an isotonic crystalloid solution is used to replace blood loss, goal-directed therapy and fluid responsiveness is likely more optimal than traditional 3:1 replacement. Evidence suggests that aggressive normal saline resuscitation may cause nonanion gap metabolic acidosis.

    b. Colloids are fluids with particles large enough to exert oncotic pressure with the theory of remaining in the intravascular space longer than crystalloids. Multiple studies comparing fluid resuscitation with crystalloids to colloids have reported no benefit with colloids. Colloid solutions are more expensive than crystalloids, and routine use may not be justified. Albumin may be superior to crystalloid in certain patients including significant burns, hepatorenal disease, or acute lung injury. Hydroxyethyl starch solutions (eg, Hextend or Hespan) are non–blood-derived colloids that may also be used as methods of volume expansion but are increasingly less favorable due to deleterious effects on renal function, coagulation, and potentially all-cause mortality.

4. Muscle relaxation is required for all but the most superficial abdominal procedures. Sufficient relaxation is critical for abdominal closure as bowel distention, edema, and organ transplantation may increase the volume of abdominal contents.

    a. Titrating relaxants to obtain a single twitch by train-of-four monitoring is generally sufficient for surgical closure and allows for reversal of muscle relaxants for extubation.

    b. Potent inhalational agents are synergistic with muscle relaxants in blocking neuromuscular conduction.

    c. Flexing the operating table may decrease tension on transverse abdominal and subcostal incisions and facilitate surgical closure without the need for profound muscular relaxation as may be requested by the surgeons.

5. Use of nitrous oxide (N_2O) may cause bowel distention as N_2O diffuses into the bowel lumen. The amount of distention depends on the concentration of N_2O delivered, blood flow to the bowel, and duration of N_2O administration. Under normal conditions, the initial volume of bowel gas is small; doubling or tripling of this volume does not pose a significant problem. Studies have shown that N_2O may be used in lower fractions and shorter (<3 hours) open and laparoscopic surgeries, without causing clinically significant bowel distention. Use of N_2O is relatively contraindicated in bowel obstruction because the initial volume of bowel gas may be large.

6. NG tubes are frequently placed in the perioperative period.

    a. Preoperative placement is indicated for decompression of the stomach, especially in trauma victims and patients with bowel obstructions. Although suction via a large-bore NG tube may reduce the volume of gastric contents, it does not completely evacuate the stomach and may facilitate aspiration by stenting open the lower esophageal sphincter. NG tubes may also compromise mask fit. Before induction, suction should be applied to NG tubes. During induction, tubes should be allowed to drain. Cricoid pressure may help to prevent passive reflux when an NG tube is present.

    b. Intraoperative placement is required to drain gastric fluid and air during abdominal surgery. NG and orogastric tubes should never be inserted with excessive force. Lubrication and head flexion facilitate insertion. Tubes can be directed into the esophagus by using a finger within the oropharynx or using Magill forceps under direct visualization with a laryngoscope.

    c. Complications of NG tube insertion include bleeding, submucosal dissection of the retropharynx, and placement in the trachea. Intracranial placement has been described in patients with basilar skull fracture. The NG tube should be secured carefully to avoid excessive pressure on the nasal septum or nares, as this may cause ischemic necrosis.

d. As discussed in the previous section, the need for a gastric tube should be discussed with the surgeon as placement for elective procedures is not recommended in many cases.

D. Enhanced recovery after surgery (ERAS)

ERAS is a concept of multimodal evidence-based care designed to enhance postoperative recovery and optimize patients for discharge. Core tenets center on a continuum of preoperative, intraoperative, and postoperative pathway strategies.

Current literature suggests that ERAS protocols may be associated with reduced hospital LOS, faster recovery, reduced overall morbidity and nonsurgical complications, and similar rates of readmission compared to traditional care. As most ERAS pathways are instituted as a "bundle" there is a paucity of evidence as to which elements of a specific bundle are more or less meaningful than others.

E. Notable highlights of ERAS protocols for elective colorectal surgery are discussed in the section that follows. Specific components continue to be increasingly mapped to ERAS protocols for other surgeries.

1. Minimization of preoperative fasting. Clear liquids and carbohydrate drinks are encouraged up to 2 hours before surgery. Modifications may be based on disease state (eg, bowel obstruction).

2. Avoidance of routine preoperative sedative premedications due to the potential impairment of postoperative psychomotor function and ability to mobilize and begin PO intake.

3. Avoidance of routine mechanical bowel preparation due to adverse physiologic effects related to dehydration and association with prolonged ileus and spillage of bowel contents.

4. Avoidance of routine postoperative NG tubes to minimize patient discomfort and delay in time to oral intake. NG tubes placed intraoperatively should be removed prior to emergence.

5. Intraoperative maintenance of normothermia.

6. Intraoperative fluid management strategy continues to be an area of active research and debate. Goal-directed fluid management guided by administration of fluid to a physiologic objective is a cornerstone of ERAS protocols but the specific goals continues to be ill-defined. Noninvasive methods of measuring cardiac output, stroke volume, and stroke volume variation may be employed with no evidence currently suggesting any method as being superior or better than rational management by clinical judgment.

7. Minimization of postoperative fluids to maintain normovolemia and minimize fluid overload.

8. Use of multimodal analgesia and regional techniques to minimize opioids and, thus, facilitate early postoperative ambulation and rehabilitation.

IV. ANESTHETIC CONSIDERATIONS FOR SPECIFIC ABDOMINAL PROCEDURES

A. Laparoscopic surgery. Laparoscopic approaches are utilized for an increasing number of surgical procedures including appendectomy, cholecystectomy, hernia repair, fundoplication, nephrectomy, weight loss surgery, liver resection, and colon resection. Benefits of laparoscopic surgery include smaller incisions, reduced postoperative pain, decreased postoperative ileus, early ambulation, shorter hospital LOS, and earlier return to function.

1. Operative technique involves intraperitoneal insufflation of CO_2 through a needle inserted into the abdomen via a small incision.

Insufflation typically increases intra-abdominal pressure to 12 to 15 mm Hg. Trendelenburg or reverse Trendelenburg positioning is often necessary to facilitate operative exposure.

2. Anesthetic considerations

 a. Hemodynamic changes associated with laparoscopy are generally mediated by the intra-abdominal pressure related to pneumoperitoneum, volume of CO_2 absorbed, intravascular volume status, patient positioning, and anesthetic agents. Mean arterial pressure and systemic vascular resistance generally increases with the creation of pneumoperitoneum due to catecholamine release and activation of the renin-angiotensin system. Patients with coexisting cardiac disease may be susceptible to the physiologic effects of pneumoperitoneum and manifest with decreased cardiac output and hypotension. Absorption of CO_2 across the peritoneal surface typically causes hypercarbia and acidosis, thus increasing sympathetic nervous system stimulation and decreasing cardiac contractility.

 b. Reduction in functional residual capacity (FRC) associated with GA is compounded by the creation of pneumoperitoneum, and FRC may be further compromised by the Trendelenburg position and patient body habitus. Frequent recruitment and titration of positive end-expiratory pressure (PEEP) may be necessary to mitigate against alveolar collapse.

 c. Attention to cardiovascular function with positioning in steep Trendelenburg or reverse Trendelenburg is essential due to change in venous return.

 d. Embryonic channels between the peritoneal and pleural or pericardial cavities may open with increased intraperitoneal pressure, resulting in pneumomediastinum, pneumopericardium, and pneumothorax. Diffusion of gas cephalad from the mediastinum may lead to subcutaneous emphysema of the face and neck.

 e. Vascular or other internal organ injuries due to incorrect introduction of the needle or trocar may produce sudden blood loss and necessitate conversion to an open procedure and vascular repair to control bleeding.

 f. Clinically significant venous gas embolism is rare but may occur on induction of pneumoperitoneum if the needle or trocar is placed into a vessel or abdominal organ, or if gas is trapped in the portal circulation. The high capacity of blood to absorb CO_2 and rapid elimination in the lungs increases the margin of safety in cases of accidental IV injection of CO_2. Insufflation of gas under high pressure can lead to a "gas lock" in the vena cava and right atrium; this will decrease venous return and cardiac output and produce circulatory collapse. Embolization of gas into the pulmonary circulation leads to increased dead space, ventilation-perfusion mismatch, and hypoxemia. Systemic gas embolization (with occasionally devastating effects on cerebral and coronary circulation) may occur with massive gas entrainment or via a patent foramen ovale. Treatment is supportive and includes immediate cessation of gas insufflation, increasing FiO_2 to minimize hypoxemia, positioning the patient in steep head-down left-lateral decubitus to displace gas from the right ventricular outflow tract (see Chapter 19), and inotropic right ventricular support.

3. Anesthetic management. Although laparoscopic procedures have been performed under neuraxial techniques, GA is usually required for laparoscopy. Creation of pneumoperitoneum and steep Trendelenburg

positioning may compromise ventilatory function and are generally not tolerated in an awake patient. Rescue IV and radial artery access may be limited by draping and position of the patient.

B. Robotic surgery is increasingly utilized as a telemanipulator technique in surgical specialties with the goal of affording the surgeon a higher degree of precision and control with purported benefits of decreased hospital LOS and improved postoperative recovery.

1. Advantages of the robotic systems include affording surgeons' true three-dimensional depth perception and magnification of the operative field. In addition, the system filters natural hand tremors and scales movements for precision work. Compared to laparoscopic surgery, the surgeon is afforded a cumulative six degrees of freedom of movement.

2. Anesthetic considerations and management

   a. Positioning for robotic surgery often entails steep Trendelenburg positioning and intraperitoneal insufflation, which has the potential for serious physiologic derangements. Patients with coexisting cardiovascular, respiratory, intraocular, or central nervous system pathology may be considered for alternative approaches.

   b. Any lines, monitors, or patient-protective devices must be placed and secured beforehand as access to the patient is limited after robot positioning and engagement. Depending on the robotic model and equipment, the position of the operating table may need to be maintained stationary throughout the procedure.

   c. Deep neuromuscular blockade must be maintained until the robot is undocked at the end of the procedure. A continuous infusion of a nondepolarizing neuromuscular blocking agent may be indicated. The robotic arms have minimal flexibility, and any movement has the potential for serious morbidity to organs and vasculature. Sugammadex may be indicated to reverse deep neuromuscular blockade in a timely fashion.

   d. Vigilant assessment of patient positioning and paddling is imperative as the patient is often in a steep position for several hours.

   e. Shoulder supports and other patient-protective devices for securing the patient on the operating table during steep positioning may create suboptimal conditions for airway access on induction.

   f. Steep Trendelenburg positioning and carbon dioxide pneumoperitoneum may have synergistic cardiovascular and respiratory effects.

   g. Abdominal contents are translocated cephalad with a corresponding reduction of FRC and lung compliance. Patients may be prone to ventilation-perfusion mismatch, increased peak airway pressures, and atelectasis.

   h. CVP, pulmonary artery pressure, and pulmonary capillary wedge pressure are increased and correspond to the degree of head-down tilt. Arterial vasculature compression increases systemic and pulmonary vascular resistance.

   i. Swelling of the face and upper airway may be seen with the steep and prolonged positioning. A restrictive fluid management strategy may be beneficial. A small period of reverse Trendelenburg at the end of the case may allow venous drainage of airway structures and may be particularly helpful in patients with difficult airways on induction.

C. Esophageal surgery for gastroesophageal reflux disease can be performed via either an abdominal approach (see below) or a thoracic approach.

1. The Nissen fundoplication is the most common surgical treatment for reflux disease. It involves wrapping the fundus of the stomach around the lower part of the esophagus. This creates a collar in which

intragastric pressure serves to constrict the wrapped esophagus rather than push the gastric contents into the esophagus. Hiatal hernias, if present, are repaired at the time of surgery. This procedure is often performed using laparoscopic techniques to decrease the duration of postsurgical hospitalization.

    a. Anesthetic considerations. This procedure is performed most commonly with GA or combined GA-epidural (for open procedures). Patients who come to surgery often have been treated medically with proton pump inhibitors, H_2-receptor antagonists, or prokinetic agents. These should be continued until the day of surgery. An RSI is generally indicated because of the high risk of gastroesophageal reflux and the potential for aspiration.

    b. An esophageal bougie may be placed to calibrate fundoplication; this ensures an adequate esophageal lumen to minimize postoperative dysphagia. The stomach or esophagus may be perforated by passage of the bougie or NG tube. With the laparoscopic method, the bougie is directed into the stomach by observation alone. Correct angulation of the esophagus or stomach during this maneuver is extremely important in preventing injury. The dilator or NG tube should be passed slowly and should be directly visualized. Particular attention should be paid to patients with esophageal strictures.

D. Gastric surgery for gastric cancer, lymphoma, and uncontrolled bleeding is usually performed with combined GA-epidural. The high likelihood of aspiration in these patients necessitates rapid-sequence intubation.

    1. Gastrectomy or hemigastrectomy with gastroduodenostomy (Billroth I) or gastrojejunostomy (Billroth II) is usually performed for gastric adenocarcinoma, lymphoma, or intractable bleeding from gastric or duodenal ulcers. Rarely, it is necessary in Zollinger-Ellison syndrome.

    2. Gastrostomy tube placement can be performed through a small upper abdominal incision or percutaneously with an endoscope. Local anesthesia with sedation is often adequate in the debilitated elderly patient, although some require GA.

E. Intestinal and peritoneal surgery. Indications for small bowel resection include infection, penetrating trauma, Crohn disease, obstructing adhesions, Meckel diverticulum, carcinoma, and infarction (from volvulus, intussusception, or thromboemboli). Patients are often hypovolemic and are considered to have a full stomach.

    1. Appendectomy is performed through a small lower abdominal incision or via laparoscopy. IV hydration before induction is indicated because fever, poor oral intake, and vomiting may produce hypovolemia. GA with rapid-sequence intubation is generally indicated. TAP blocks may be opioid sparing and can be considered as an adjuvant for this procedure.

    2. Colectomy or hemicolectomy is used to treat colon cancer, diverticular disease, Crohn disease, ulcerative colitis, trauma, ischemic colitis, and abscess. Emergency colectomy on unprepared bowel carries a high risk of peritonitis from fecal contamination. Some emergencies involving the colon are treated with an initial diverting colostomy, followed later by bowel preparation and elective colectomy. Patients must be evaluated for hypovolemia, anemia, and sepsis. All emergency colectomies and colostomies should be treated as if at risk for aspiration. Combination general/regional anesthetics are common, although epidural analgesia use is decreasing with laparoscopic techniques and the intraoperative use of adjuvants.

3. Perirectal abscess drainage, hemorrhoidectomy, and pilonidal cystectomy are relatively noninvasive and brief procedures. Pilonidal cysts are excised with patients positioned prone; abscess drainage and hemorrhoidectomy can be performed in either a prone or a lithotomy position. If GA is used, deep planes of anesthesia or use of muscle relaxants may be necessary to achieve adequate sphincter relaxation. Hyperbaric spinal anesthesia can be used for procedures in the lithotomy position, whereas a hypobaric technique is useful for the flexed prone (jackknife) or knee-chest position. A caudal block may be performed for either position.

4. Inguinal, femoral, or ventral herniorrhaphies can be performed under local anesthesia, regional anesthesia (spinal, epidural, caudal, or nerve block), or GA. Maximum stimulation and profound vagal responses may occur during spermatic cord or peritoneal retraction. Communication with surgeons is important, as they may need to reduce traction if necessary. Techniques to minimize coughing on emergence that can strain the repair are indicated, and deep extubation can be considered in patients where is not contraindicated (ie, difficult mask airway, difficult intubation, high risk of aspiration, etc).

F. Hepatic surgery

1. Partial hepatectomy is performed for hepatoma, unilobar metastasis of a carcinoma, arteriovenous malformation, or echinococcal cysts. Extensive hemorrhage should be anticipated and standard monitors are supplemented with placement of arterial and large-bore IV access and/or central venous catheters. Blood loss during hepatic parenchymal division can be reduced by temporary occlusion of portal venous and arterial inflow at the level of the hepatic pedicle (Pringle maneuver). Low CVP techniques have been shown to reduce blood loss during the case and improve survival. The CVP is generally kept in the range of 2 to 5 mm Hg. CVP essentially represents the back pressure which causes bleeding during the resection, since there are no valves between the right atrium and the liver. Fluids should be restricted with a goal of maintaining a nonzero urine output and an acceptable blood pressure (variable depending on patient). If fluid restriction is not adequate, nitrates and opioids can be used as well. Resuscitation of the patient after the resection is completed and hemostasis has been achieved is indicated. This can be guided by signs of hypovolemia such as the respiratory variation of arterial systolic pressure, arterial PPV, cardiac output, CVP, and stroke volume variation. The normal liver has considerable reserve, and extensive resection is required before clinical impairment of drug metabolism is evident. The effects of liver disease on anesthetic management are discussed in Chapter 5. Epidural or paravertebral catheters can be placed in patients with normal coagulation status.

2. Transjugular intrahepatic portosystemic shunts (TIPS) procedure has replaced portacaval or splenorenal shunt procedure for patients with portal hypertension because of superior outcome. The procedure entails access of internal jugular vein (most on right side). A shunt between portal vein and hepatic vein will be created after verifying position with both contrast and pressure measurement. TIPS procedure can be performed under monitored anesthesia care, but is usually performed under GA. Although the anesthetic for a TIPS is simple, a high-level vigilance is required because of potential bleeding.

G. Biliary tract procedures

  1. Cholecystectomy is a common procedure performed via either open laparotomy or laparoscopic techniques. GA is favored for either technique. During laparoscopic cholecystectomy, the patient is placed in a steep reverse Trendelenburg position, and the gallbladder is dissected from the liver bed by using either cautery or laser. Muscle relaxants are required for adequate abdominal wall relaxation. The amount of hemorrhage is difficult to assess because of the limited field of view and high magnification of the laparoscope; heavy bleeding from the cystic or hepatic arteries may occur.

  2. Biliary drainage procedures include transduodenal sphincteroplasty for extensive choledocholithiasis; cholecystojejunostomy for distal common bile duct obstruction from pancreatic cancer; and choledochojejunostomy for chronic pancreatitis, stone disease, and benign strictures of the distal bile duct. Endoscopic and transhepatic techniques are increasingly common, but open surgical drainage is occasionally required. Blood loss is usually minimal but fluid loss may be significant.

H. Pancreatic surgery

  1. Although the initial treatment of acute pancreatitis is supportive, surgical intervention may be necessary for complications of pancreatitis. Surgical management is indicated for infected pancreatic necrosis and hemorrhagic pancreatitis unresponsive to resuscitation with blood products and correction of coagulopathy. Pancreatic pseudocysts may require drainage either surgically or via endoscopy. The cyst may be anastomosed to a Roux-en-Y limb of jejunum, the posterior wall of the stomach, or duodenum. Surgical intervention can produce significant bleeding and third-space fluid losses. In severe acute pancreatitis, activation of inflammatory mediators can produce sepsis and multiple organ dysfunction that require fluid resuscitation, mechanical ventilation, and vasopressor support.

  2. Pancreaticojejunostomy with gastrojejunostomy and choledochojejunostomy (Whipple procedure) is typically performed for resection of adenocarcinoma of the pancreas, malignant cystadenoma, or refractory pancreatitis confined to the head of the pancreas. These procedures have a high potential for hemorrhage and fluid loss. Epidural catheters and other regional techniques such as paravertebral blocks are generally helpful for postoperative pain control in the absence of contraindications. Intraoperative neurolytic celiac plexus blocks can be used in unresectable cases where significant postoperative pain is expected.

 I. Splenectomy may be performed emergently after blunt or penetrating trauma or electively for the treatment of idiopathic thrombocytopenic purpura or Hodgkin lymphoma. GA and muscle relaxation are required. Large-bore IV access is necessary because major blood loss requiring transfusion can be encountered. A combined epidural and general anesthetic technique is appropriate with the caveat that a sympathectomy may significantly potentiate hypotension from hemorrhage. Occasionally, a transthoracic approach to gain control of the hilar vessels of a very large spleen may be necessary. Splenectomy patients should receive polyvalent pneumococcal vaccine in the postoperative period.

 J. Intraoperative radiation therapy for pancreatic, colonic, or other carcinomas may be performed during laparotomy for primary resection or tumor debulking. Specially designed operating rooms have been constructed to facilitate intraoperative radiotherapy. The patients must be hemodynamically stable and have a stable ventilatory status as they are monitored by remote television outside the radiation area. Aortic or inferior vena cava (IVC) compression may occur when the sterile cone of the radiation therapy device is positioned in the abdominal wound. Ventilation with 100% oxygen can maximize the sensitivity of the tumor to radiation therapy. Treatments usually last just a few minutes and can be interrupted in the event of problems with hemodynamics or ventilation. Wound closure is performed after the radiation therapy is complete, and any necessary anastomoses are made.

K. Surgery for the obese patient. As the prevalence of obesity in the US population continues to rise, the perioperative management of the obese patient is increasingly relevant. Obesity is defined by the body mass index (BMI) and is calculated as follows: BMI = body weight (kg)/height (m²). Patients are typically defined as obese if BMI exceeds 30 kg/m².

1. Preanesthetic considerations

   a. Obese patients have increased circulating blood volume and cardiac output to meet increased oxygen consumption. Depressed left ventricular function related to left ventricular hypertrophy may be seen even in young asymptomatic patients and is often correlated to the duration of obesity.

   b. Obese individuals have an increased risk for cardiovascular disease and may require additional cardiac evaluation or consultation to optimize management in the perioperative period.

   c. Respiratory system compliance is decreased in obesity due to reduced chest wall compliance. FRC and expiratory reserve capacity are also likely to be reduced. In the supine position, FRC may be less than the closing volume, leading to ventilation-perfusion mismatch and hypoxemia. The higher metabolic demand of the obese person coupled with increased oxygen consumption and CO_2 production necessitates an increase in minute ventilation to maintain normocapnia.

   d. Increased submucosal fat in the pharynx increases collapse of the hypopharynx with normal sleep, thus predisposing to obstructive sleep apnea. Long-standing hypoxemia may result in pulmonary hypertension and right heart failure. Obstructive sleep apnea increases the risk of perioperative complications and screening may be accomplished with validated tools including the STOP-Bang questionnaire.

   e. Increased gastric emptying time and elevated intra-abdominal pressure and volume predisposes to a higher incidence of symptomatic gastroesophageal reflux.

   f. Type 2 diabetes with hyperglycemia, hyperinsulinemia, and insulin resistance is common in obesity. Because perfusion of adipose tissue is variable, IV insulin infusions may be necessary to control hyperglycemia. Guidelines for the management of glucose and insulin are covered in Chapter 6.

   g. Airway management is a challenge in obesity including difficulty with intubation and mask ventilation. Careful assessment of neck and jaw mobility, inspection of the oropharynx, and examination of dental status are required. If intubation is expected to be difficult, an airway management strategy should be discussed and awake intubation considered.

   h. Positioning of the upper body with the external auditory meatus in line with the sternal notch has been shown to provide a better view for direct laryngoscopy. This is often accomplished by making a "ramp" of blankets under the thorax, which facilitates alignment of the thorax with the trachea. In addition, a reverse Trendelenburg position should be used in morbidly obese patients to increase FRC and utilize gravity to displace soft tissue away from the neck and airway.

2. **Surgical techniques.** Bariatric surgery is currently the most effective treatment of morbid obesity. Patients with a BMI ≥ 40 kg/m^2 or with a BMI ≥ 35 kg/m^2 with obesity-related comorbidities may be candidates for surgery. Currently, two basic types of bariatric surgery are performed.

   a. Vertical banded gastroplasty (gastric sleeve) produces a small gastric pouch that restricts the volume of food that can be ingested. Long-term weight loss may be limited by maladaptive eating patterns (liquids with high caloric content) or by staple line disruption. Gastroplasty procedures, particularly the laparoscopic sleeve gastrectomy, are becoming increasingly popular due to lower complications than formal bypass procedures.

   b. Roux-en-Y gastric bypass surgery consists of formation of a small gastric pouch and anastomosis of the pouch to the proximal jejunum. Weight loss occurs due to both a restrictive anatomy as well as decreased absorption of calories because of the bypassed small intestine. Patients who undergo this surgery may experience a "dumping" syndrome in which ingestion of high-energy-density food leads to nausea, abdominal cramping, and diarrhea. The Roux-en-Y gastric bypass is often performed laparoscopically.

3. **Anesthetic management**

   a. Standard operating tables are often unable to accommodate the size and weight of the obese patient; tables specifically designed for obese patients should be used. Extra padding and skin protection are necessary even for short procedures.

   b. Standard noninvasive monitoring, with a urinary catheter, is acceptable in obese patients without significant comorbidities. An appropriately sized blood pressure cuff is critical; a regular-sized cuff placed on the forearm may be more effective than an oversized cuff on the upper arm. IV access may be challenging.

   c. Regional and neuraxial anesthetic techniques may be challenging due to less defined anatomic landmarks. For neuraxial techniques, the midline of the spine may be more readily apparent in the sitting position than in lateral decubitus, thus facilitating catheter placement. Long epidural needles (5 inches) may be necessary. The volume of local anesthetic volume injected may need to be decreased in obese patients. The volume of the epidural space is thought to be decreased due to adipose infiltration and increased blood volume in the epidural venous system.

   d. The combination of increased metabolic demand and decreased FRC leads to rapid and sometimes refractory desaturation with apnea. Preoxygenation for a minimum of 3 to 5 minutes and targeting an end-tidal concentration of O$_2$ greater than 90% is recommended. Mask ventilation may be challenging and adequate gas exchange is often limited. Use of an oral or nasopharyngeal airway or two-person bag-mask technique is frequently required.

   e. Morbidly obese patients have greater reductions in lung volumes than nonobese patients on induction of GA. Physiologically, this manifests as increasing atelectasis, airway closure, and hypoxemia. Titration of PEEP may be necessary to counteract this.

f. Drug dosing is a challenge and subject of controversy in the obese patient. Obese patients have increased total body weight (TBW) and lean body weight (LBW). However, the ratio of LBW to TBW decreases with increases in TBW. Physiologically, obese patients have increased cardiac output, total body volume, glomerular filtration rate (GFR), and regional alterations in blood flow that alter pharmacokinetics and pharmacodynamics. Generally, lipid-soluble drugs have an increased volume of distribution, but exceptions exist.

1. In obese patients, LBW is highly correlated with cardiac output, which determines early distribution kinetics, and drug clearance. Most anesthetic drugs should be dosed by LBW.

2. LBW is determined by individual's height and weight and is best determined in obese patients by a modified LBW equation: $LBW_{men} = [9 \times 103 \times \text{body weight}/7 \times 103 + (216 \times BMI)$; $LBW_{women} = [9 \times 103 \times \text{body weight}/9 \times 103 + (244 \times BMI)$.

3. Induction doses of propofol should be based on LBW, and maintenance dosing should be based on TBW.

4. Doses of opioids, including remifentanil, should be based on LBW.

5. With increased amount of pseudocholinesterase and extracellular fluid, succinylcholine administration should be based on TBW.

6. Nondepolarizing muscle relaxants should be dosed on ideal body weight.

g. The patient should be extubated in the operating room when awake, with adequate cough reflexes, and after confirmation of adequate reversal of muscle relaxation. Because the supine position decreases FRC, obese patients should be placed in a sitting position as soon as possible. Patients requiring continuous positive airway pressure for sleep apnea can resume this treatment as soon as necessary; gastric distention does not appear to be a problem.

h. Postoperative intensive care or step-down unit should be considered for patients with severe coronary artery disease, poorly controlled diabetes, and severe sleep apnea. Studies have shown that patients who are male, older (>50 years), heavier (BMI > 60 kg/m²), and who have complications requiring reoperation are more likely to need intensive care.

L. Recovery of organs for transplantation after brain death

1. A significant gap exists between the supply of suitable donated organs and the demand for these organs to treat end-stage disease. To increase the donor pool, strict exclusion criteria (age and coexisting illnesses) are no longer used. In addition, some centers use aggressive care regimens for potential donors to prevent common perturbations in homeostasis that accompany brain death. An alternative is the non–heart-beating donor, who does not meet brain death criteria but has such a poor prognosis that the family might consider withdrawing life support. A transplant coordinator from an organ procurement organization must screen all potential donors.

2. Organs may be deemed unsuitable based on donor age, organ injury, disease, or gross abnormalities.

3. Hormonal therapy using methylprednisolone, arginine vasopressin, and triiodothyronine can increase the number of successfully implanted organs and reduce graft dysfunction when administered to brain-dead donors who demonstrate resistance to conventional resuscitation as manifested by low cardiac output, inadequate organ perfusion, or worsening lactic acidosis.

4. Anesthetic management for harvesting organs should focus on optimizing organ perfusion and oxygenation. Volatile anesthetics may help to blunt spinal reflex, reduce the adrenergic storm, and provide some ischemic preconditioning to the vital organs, although studies have not been done to confirm clinical significance. Opioids will also help with reduction in response to stimulation.

   a. Dissection of organs usually occurs in the following order: heart (30 minutes), lungs (1-1.5 hours), liver (1-1.5 hours), pancreas (1-1.5 hours), and kidneys (30 minutes-1 hour).

   b. Once all organs are mobilized, heparin (20,000-30,000 units IV in adult donors) is administered and the aorta is cross-clamped. The distal aorta and IVC are cannulated, and the harvested organs are perfused in situ, topically cooled, and exsanguinated via the IVC.

   c. Ventilatory support is discontinued after the aorta is cross-clamped, and the anesthesiologist's role is completed with the discontinuation of all monitoring and supportive care, except during heart and lung procurement.

   d. Non–heart-beating organ donation, also referred to as donation after cardiac death (DCD), is reserved for patients who are not declared brain dead but whose family has chosen to remove them from life support because their condition is considered "hopeless." Life-sustaining treatment (mechanical ventilation and vasopressors) is discontinued after the patient is prepared for surgery to remove the organs. Five minutes after asystole occurs, a physician who is not part of the transplant team declares death. The body is rapidly cooled with preservative solution via an aortic cannula, and the abdomen entered and organs removed expeditiously. This technique has the disadvantage of significant warm ischemia time before organ procurement begins. In addition, there are ethical debates about the appropriateness of interventions (heparin treatment) aimed at improving grafts before the donor's death. Usually, anesthesiologists are not involved in DCD. However, if the lungs are donated, an anesthesiologist may be asked to intubate the deceased and briefly ventilate.

5. Specific management problems

   a. Hypoxemia may be caused by atelectasis, pulmonary edema, aspiration, or pneumonia. The FiO_2 and minute ventilation should be adjusted to maintain a $Pao_2 \leq 100$ mm Hg and $Paco_2 = 35$ to 45 mm Hg with pH 7.35 to 7.45. Arterial blood gases should be determined every 30 to 60 minutes. High levels of PEEP should be avoided to preserve cardiac output and avoid barotrauma. High FiO_2 should be avoided in potential lung donors to minimize possible oxygen toxicity.

   b. Poikilothermia is common, and early aggressive measures should be taken to minimize heat loss.

   c. Hypertension often transiently accompanies brain death and can be dramatic. Reflex hypertensive responses to surgical stimulation may occur. Short-acting agents such as nitroprusside or esmolol should be used anticipating hypertension that is often more challenging to control during organ procurement.

   d. Hypotension is common and is due to a combination of hypovolemia and neurogenic derangement of vasomotor control. Central venous or pulmonary artery catheterization may be necessary to optimize filling pressures. Hypovolemia can be treated with crystalloid, colloid solutions, and blood products as necessary. Hematocrit should be maintained greater than 30%. After restoration of intra-vascular volume, a vasopressor such as dopamine, epinephrine, or norepinephrine may be necessary.

e. Dysrhythmias occur frequently, especially in the setting of elec-trolyte imbalance, hypothermia, increased intracranial pressure, hypoxemia and acidosis, and derangement of brainstem cardiovas-cular control centers. Standard therapy is indicated. Bradycardia is often resistant to atropine and may require pacing therapy.

f. Polyuria may be secondary to volume overload, osmotic diure-sis, or the diabetes insipidus resulting from derangement of the hypothalamic-pituitary axis. An IV infusion of vasopressin or desmopressin may be titrated to treat severe diabetes insipidus (see Chapter 6) and should be done in consultation with the sur-gical team. If used, it is prudent to discontinue these infusions 1 hour before aortic cross-clamping to minimize the risk of uneven distribution or ischemic injury with the infusion of preservative solution.

g. Oliguria should be treated by ensuring adequate intravascular vol-ume. Dopamine is preferred for the initial treatment of hypotension. A brisk diuresis is preferred when the kidneys are to be harvested. If volume repletion and vasopressors are not effective in restor-ing adequate urine output, mannitol and/or furosemide may be administered.

Suggested Readings

Ahmad S, Nagle A, McCarthy RJ, Fitzgerald PC, Sullivan JT, Prystowsky J. Postoperative hypoxemia in morbidly obese patients with and without obstructive sleep apnea undergoing laparoscopic bariatric surgery. *Anesth Analg.* 2008;107(1):138-143.

Akca O, Lenhardt R, Fleischmann E, et al. Nitrous oxide increases the incidence of bowel distention in patients undergoing elective colon resection. *Acta Aanesthesiol Scand.* 2004;48:894-898.

Ballantyne JC, Carr DB, deFerranti S, et al. The comparative effects of postoperative analge-sic therapies on pulmonary outcome: cumulative meta-analyses of randomized, con-trolled trials. *Anesth Analg.* 1998;86:598-612.

Boldt J, Haisch G, Suttner S, Kumle B, Schellhaass A. Effects of a new modified, balanced hydroxyethyl starch preparation (Hextend) on measures of coagulation. *Br J Anaesth.* 2002;89:722-728.

Brodsky JB, Lemmens HJ, Brock-Utne JG, Vierra M, Saidman LJ. Morbid obesity and tra-cheal intubation. *Anesth Analg.* 2002;94(3):732-736.

Brodsky JB, Lemmens HJ, Collins JS, Morton JM, Curet MJ, Brock-Utne JG. Nitrous oxide and laparoscopic bariatric surgery. *Obes Surg.* 2005;15:494-496.

Chappell D, Jacob M, Hofmann-Kiefer K, Conzen P, Rehm M. A rational approach to periop-erative fluid management. *Anesthesiology.* 2008;109(4):723-740.

Choi PT, Yip G, Quinonez LG, Cook DJ. Crystalloids vs. colloids in fluid resuscitation: a systematic review. *Crit Care Med.* 1999;27:200-210.

Corcoran T, Rhodes J, Clarke S, Myles PS, Ho KM. Perioperative fluid management strat-egies in major surgery: a stratified meta-analysis. *Anesth Analg.* 2012;114(3):640-651.

Doherty M, Buggy DJ. Intraoperative fluids: how much is too much? *Br J Anaesth.* 2012;109(1):69-79.

Ebert TJ, Shankar H, Haake RM. Perioperative considerations for patients with morbid obe-sity. *Anesthesiol Clin.* 2006;24(3):621-636.

Gridelli B, Remuzzi G. Strategies for making more organs available for transplantation. *N Engl J Med.* 2000;343:404-410.

Gustafsson UO, Scott MJ, Schwenk W, et al. Enhanced recovery after surgery society. Guidelines for perioperative care in elective colonic surgery: enhanced Recovery After Surgery (ERAS®) Society recommendations. *World J Surg.* 2013;37(2):259-284.

Hartog CS, Bauer M, Reinhart K. The efficacy and safety of colloid resuscitation in the critically ill. *Anesth Analg.* 2011;112:156-164.

Hebbard PD, Barrington MJ, Vasey C. Ultrasound-guided continuous oblique subcostal transversus abdominis plane blockade: description of anatomy and clinical technique. *Reg Anesth Pain Med.* 2010;35(5):436-441.

Huntington JT, Royall NA, Schmidt CR. Minimizing blood loss during hepatectomy: a literature review. *J Surg Oncol.* 2014;109:81-88.

Ingrande J, Lemmens HJ. Dose adjustment of the anaesthetics in the morbidly obese. *Br J Anaesth.* 2010;105(suppl 1):i16-i23.

Lobo SM, Ronchi LS, Oliveira NE, et al. Restrictive strategy of intraoperative fluid maintenance during optimization of oxygen delivery decreases major complications after high-risk surgery. *Crit Care.* 2011;15(5):R226.

Lowham AS, Filipi CJ, Hinder RA, et al. Mechanisms and avoidance of esophageal perforation by anesthesia personnel during laparoscopic foregut surgery. *Surg Endosc.* 1996;10:979-982.

McKeown DW, Bonser RS, Kellum JA. Management of the heart beating brain-dead organ donor. *Br J Anaesth.* 2012;108(suppl 1):i96-i107.

Molenaar IQ, Warnaar N, Groen H, Tenvergert EM, Slooff MJ, Porte RJ. Efficacy and safety of antifibrinolytic drugs in liver transplantation: a systematic review and meta-analysis. *Am J Transplant.* 2007;7:185-194.

Myles PS, Leslie K, Chan MT, et al; ANZCA Trials Group for the ENIGMA-II Investigators. The safety of addition of nitrous oxide to general anesthesia in at-risk patients having major non-cardiac surgery (ENIGMA II): a randomised, single blind trial. *Lancet.* 2014;384(9952):1446-1454.

Neligan PJ, Porter S, Max B, et al. Obstructive sleep apnea is not a risk factor for difficult intubation in morbidly obese patients. *Anesth Analg.* 2009;109(4):1182-1186.

Ogunnaike BO, Jones SB, Jones DB, Provost D, Whitten CW. Anesthetic considerations for bariatric surgery. *Anesth Analg.* 2002;95(6):1793-1805.

Patel T. Surgery in the patient with liver disease. *Mayo Clin Proc.* 1999;74:593-599.

Pelosi P, Ravagnan I, Giurati G, et al. Positive end-expiratory pressure improves respiratory function in obese but not in normal subjects during anesthesia and paralysis. *Anesthesiology.* 1999;91:1221-1231.

Qadan M, Akca O, Mahid SS, Hornung CA, Polk HC Jr. Perioperative supplemental oxygen therapy and surgical site infection: a meta-analysis of randomized controlled trials. *Arch Surg.* 2009;144:359-366.

Robertson KM, Cook DR. Perioperative management of the multiorgan donor. *Anesth Analg.* 1990;70:546-556.

Shenkman Z, Shir Y, Brodsky JB. Perioperative management of the obese patient. *Br J Anaesth.* 1993;70:349-359.

Sinha AC. Some anesthetic aspects of morbid obesity. *Curr Opin Anaesthesiol.* 2009;22(3):442-446.

Spanjersberg WR, Reurings J, Keus F, van Laarhoven CJ. Fast track surgery versus conventional recovery strategies for colorectal surgery. *Cochrane Database Syst Rev.* 2011;(2):CD007635.

Strunden MS, Heckel K, Goetz AE, Reuter DA. Perioperative fluid and volume management: physiological basis, tools and strategies. *Ann Intensive Care.* 2011;1(1):2.

Tympa A, Theodoraki K, Tsaroucha A, Arkadopoulos N, Vassiliou I, Smyrniotis V. Anesthetic considerations in hepatectomies under hepatic vascular control. *HPB Surg.* 2012;2012:720-754.

White PF. The changing role of non-opioid analgesic techniques in the management of postoperative pain. *Anesth Analg.* 2005;101(5 suppl):S5-S22.

Zhuang CL, Ye XZ, Zhang XD, Chen BC, Yu Z. Enhanced recovery after surgery programs versus traditional care for colorectal surgery: a meta-analysis of randomized controlled trials. *Dis Colon Rectum.* 2013;56(5):667-678.

27 Anesthesia for Thoracic Surgery

Peter O. Ochieng and Ryan J. Horvath

I. PREOPERATIVE EVALUATION

A. **Patients scheduled for thoracic surgery** should undergo the usual preoperative assessment as detailed in Chapter 1.

   1. Any patient undergoing elective thoracic surgery should be carefully screened for underlying bronchitis or pneumonia and treated appropriately before surgery.

   a. **Diagnostic procedures** such as bronchoscopy and lung biopsy may be indicated for persistent infection.

   2. In patients with **tracheal stenosis or mediastinal masses**, the history should focus on symptoms or signs of positional dyspnea, static versus dynamic airway collapse, and evidence of hypoxemia. The history may also suggest the probable location of the lesion.

B. An **arterial blood gas (ABG)** may help clarify the severity of underlying pulmonary disease but is not routinely necessary.

C. **Pulmonary function tests (PFTs)** are useful for assessing the pulmonary risk of lung resection. Forced expiratory volume in 1 second (FEV1) and diffusion capacity of the lung for carbon monoxide (DLCO) serve as initial predictors of postoperative outcomes. If either of these values is less than 80% of predicted, it should prompt additional studies beginning with postoperative predicted (PPO) FEV1 and DLCO. If both PPO FEV1 and PPO DLCO are ≥60%, then the patient is considered low risk for surgery. If either is <60% but both are ≥30%, then the patient undergoes stair-climbing test (SCT) or shuttle walk test (SWT). If SCT is ≥22 m or SWT ≥25 shuttles, the patient is considered low risk. If either PPO FEV1 and DLCO are <30% or performance on SCT and SWT is not satisfactory, cardiopulmonary exercise test to calculate maximum oxygen consumption (Vo_2 max) is needed. Vo_2 max >20 mL/kg/min or >75% indicates low-risk, while Vo_2 max of <10 mL/kg/min or <35% is high-risk group and surgery is not recommended. Vo_2 max 10 to 20 mL/kg/min or 35% to 75% indicates moderate-risk and Vo_2 max <10 mL/kg/min or <35% indicates high-risk group and surgery is not recommended. Quantitative ventilation/perfusion (V/Q) scan can also be used to calculate PPO FEV1 in patients scheduled to undergo pneumonectomy.

D. **Cardiac function** should be assessed if there is a question about the relative contribution of cardiac and pulmonary diseases to the patient's functional impairment. Echocardiography can be used to assess right ventricular function. Echocardiographic estimation of right ventricular systolic pressure can be used as a screening tool for pulmonary hypertension, although right heart catheterization is required for definitive diagnosis. This is especially important for procedures requiring clamping of a pulmonary artery (eg, pneumonectomy).

E. **Chest radiography, computed tomography (CT)**, and **magnetic resonance imaging (MRI)** are useful to determine the presence and extent of tracheobronchial, pulmonary and mediastinal pathology. Imaging studies can also reveal the nature and degree of involvement of other thoracic structures in the disease process. **Three-dimensional CT reconstruction** can be used to assess caliber of stenotic airway to guide anesthetic airway plan. These studies can also be helpful in planning for lung isolation if required.

II. PREOPERATIVE PREPARATION
A. Preoperative sedation should be given carefully to patients with tracheal or pulmonary disease.
1. **Heavy sedation** may impair postoperative deep breathing, coughing, and airway protection. Patients with poor pulmonary function will be more prone to hypoxemia when their respiratory drive is suppressed. When sedating these patients, it is prudent to monitor oxygenation and administer supplemental oxygen.
2. **In the presence of airway obstruction**, sedation must be carefully balanced. It is crucial to maintain spontaneous ventilation. Oversedation may profoundly suppress ventilation, but an anxious patient may make exaggerated respiratory efforts. In this case, the increased turbulence may worsen airway obstruction, leading to increased anxiety. Benzodiazepines, reassuring words, careful monitoring, and an expeditious start to the procedure are the best approach. In patients with airway stenosis, **Heliox**, a mixture of 79% helium and 21% oxygen, will lower the density of the respiratory gas and reduce airway resistance, however, at the cost of lower FIO_2. **Additionally, glycopyrrolate** (0.2 mg intravenously) may be given to decrease oral secretions.

III. MONITORING
A. Standard monitoring should be used as described in Chapter 15.
B. Intra-arterial blood pressure monitoring should be used if, based on the patient's condition or the nature of the surgical procedure, rapid hemodynamic alterations are anticipated, or frequent ABG evaluation is needed.
1. Compression of the heart and great vessels may occur during thoracic surgical exposure. Continuous blood pressure monitoring allows for the immediate diagnosis of hemodynamic instability.
2. Manipulations during surgical procedures on peripheral lung tissue, such as thoracoscopic wedge resection, are less likely to compress the heart or great vessels. Intermittent blood pressure monitoring may be sufficient in these cases.
3. Arterial line is helpful for hemodynamic monitoring of patients undergoing thoracic surgery.
4. In the lateral position, it is possible for blood flow to the dependent arm to be impaired by compression of the axilla. Pulsatile flow to the dependent arm should be monitored with an arterial catheter or a pulse oximeter.
5. During mediastinal surgery (eg, mediastinoscopy), it is possible for the innominate artery to be compressed, restricting flow to the right carotid and brachial arteries. Perfusion to the right arm should be monitored by pulse oximeter. Immediate feedback to the surgeon will allow decompression of the innominate artery. Blood pressure monitoring of the left arm should be available to allow monitoring of systemic arterial pressure in the event that the surgeon is unable to relieve compression of the innominate artery.
C. The use of additional invasive monitors is dictated by the patient's comorbidities. If a pulmonary artery catheter is placed:
1. It is customarily inserted from the nondependent side of the neck. If the catheter interferes with the surgical resection, it can be retracted into the main pulmonary artery and readvanced when the artery on the operative side is clamped.

2. Pressure measurements referenced to the atmosphere may be affected by lateral positioning and opening the chest. Trends in central venous pressure, pulmonary artery pressure, and pulmonary artery occlusion pressure should be monitored for these changes. Cardiac output and stroke volume measurements should remain accurate.

IV. ENDOSCOPIC PROCEDURES

Endoscopic procedures include direct or indirect visualization of the pharynx, larynx, esophagus, trachea, and bronchi. Endoscopy may be undertaken to obtain biopsy samples, delineate airway anatomy, remove obstructing foreign bodies, assess hemoptysis, place stents and guidewires, position radiation catheters, apply photodynamic therapy, and perform cryotherapy and laser surgery.

A. **Flexible bronchoscopy** permits visualization from the larynx to the segmental bronchi.

1. A "working lumen" is used for suctioning, administering drugs, and passing wire instruments.

2. Ventilation must occur around the flexible bronchoscope. Bronchoscopes range in external diameter from approximately 5 mm (standard adult size) to 2 mm (neonatal bronchoscopes that lack a working lumen). Larger "therapeutic" bronchoscopes and ultrasound-equipped scopes have diameters ranging to 7 mm.

3. **Topical anesthesia** is a common anesthetic approach.

   a. The patient should meet the American Society of Anesthesiologists preoperative fasting guidelines.

   b. Lidocaine (various formulations from 1% to 4%) is applied to the oropharynx or nasopharynx, larynx, and vocal cords. The trachea can be sprayed with anesthetic through the bronchoscope or by transtracheal injection. If good topicalization of the airway is achieved, no further anesthesia is required.

   c. Care should be taken with the total dose of local anesthetic due to high systemic absorption from the orotracheal mucosa.

   d. Premedication with atropine or glycopyrrolate will limit salivary dilution of the anesthetic and may improve the onset and efficacy of the anesthetic.

   e. Nerve blocks may be used to supplement airway anesthesia (see Chapter 13).

   f. The patient should have nothing by mouth until tracheal and laryngeal reflexes return, 2 to 3 hours following administration, to prevent postprocedure aspiration.

4. **General anesthesia** may be indicated in anxious or uncooperative patients; in more extensive bronchoscopic procedures; or if bronchoscopy is part of a larger surgical procedure.

   a. Bronchoscopy is very stimulating but does not cause significant postoperative pain, so a potent short-acting anesthetic is preferable.

   b. Muscle relaxation or topical anesthesia to the trachea is generally needed to prevent coughing during the procedure.

   c. The endotracheal tube (ETT) used should be sufficiently large (7 mm inner diameter for a standard scope, 8.5 or 9 mm if ultrasound will be used) to permit ventilation in the annular space around the scope.

   d. If there are no contraindications to its use, a laryngeal mask airway (LMA) offers the advantages of a large lumen and the ability to visualize the vocal cords and proximal trachea.

B. **Endobronchial ultrasound** involves the use of ultrasound during bronchoscopy to visualize structures within the lungs, airway, and mediastinum. It is used to biopsy lesions (such as enlarged mediastinal lymph nodes) that are close to the airway.

1. Although topical anesthesia with mild sedation can be used, the procedure is typically done under general anesthesia using a large ETT or LMA.

2. Whichever anesthetic technique is used, it is imperative to prevent coughing and movement as this can increase risk to injury of major vessels within the thorax during the procedure.

C. **Rigid bronchoscopy** permits visualization of the airway from the larynx to the mainstem bronchi.

1. A rigid bronchoscope has better optics and a larger working channel than a flexible bronchoscope. It can be used to establish an airway, visualize the trachea, and treat tracheal pathologies such as obstruction, stenosis, and hemorrhage.

2. Ventilation is accomplished through the lumen of the scope, allowing better control of a marginal airway.

3. Rigid scopes are not cuffed, so a variable leak will occur depending on the size of the scope, lumen of the airway, and depth of insertion.

4. General anesthesia is required for rigid bronchoscopy. It is important to prevent coughing or movement to avoid tracheal disruption. Either deep inhalation anesthesia or muscle relaxation is required to prevent movement and coughing.

5. Conventional ventilation can be used, with the anesthesia circuit attached to a side arm of the rigid bronchoscope. The proximal end of the rigid bronchoscope is closed by a clear lens or by a gasket through which telescopes may be passed.

   a. The potentially large leak requires an anesthesia machine capable of delivering high oxygen flows.

   b. An intravenous anesthetic technique is preferred. It can be difficult to maintain adequate anesthesia with an inhalational technique due to leak and interruption of ventilation. There will also be considerable operating room contamination with volatile anesthetics.

   c. Close coordination between the surgeon and anesthetist is needed because ventilation may need to be interrupted for surgery, and surgery in turn may be interrupted by the need to ventilate.

6. In cases of severely compromised airways (eg, severe airway stenosis or airway disruption), maintenance of spontaneous ventilation is indicated. The patient may be given an inhalational induction with sevoflurane, and the rigid bronchoscope may be introduced under a deep plane of anesthesia. After securing the airway, intravenous agents could be substituted.

7. Ventilating gas usually leaks out around the bronchoscope so that measurements of end-tidal carbon dioxide may be inaccurate. Adequacy of ventilation should be assessed by observation of chest excursion, pulse oximetry, and, if necessary, blood gas analysis.

8. Rigid bronchoscopes are available that are designed for jet ventilation through a special small side lumen.

   a. The central lumen remains open. Severe barotrauma and pneumothorax may occur if gas is not allowed to escape. Observation of chest movement during the expiratory phase is critical. Conversely, ventilation may be ineffective with noncompliant lungs.

   b. An intravenous anesthetic technique (see Chapter 11) must be used. Muscle relaxation is required for the jet to inflate the lungs adequately.

    c. The inspired oxygen concentration is uncertain because the amount of room air entrained cannot be controlled.

    d. During laser surgery, the fractional inspired oxygen concentration should be reduced to below 0.3, either by jetting air or by using a gas blender for the jet intake.

    e. The advantage of the jet technique is that ventilation is not interrupted by suctioning or surgical manipulations because the proximal end of the bronchoscope is always open. This makes the bronchoscope suitable for use during laser surgery of the larynx, vocal cords, or proximal trachea.

    f. Automated jet ventilators carry the added safety feature of automatic hold when the expiratory airway pressure rises above a set threshold. This prevents breath stacking and subsequent barotrauma.

  9. Complications of bronchoscopy include dental and laryngeal damage from intubation, injuries to the eyes or lips, airway rupture, pneumothorax, and hemorrhage. Airway obstruction may be caused by hemorrhage, a foreign body, or a dislodged mass.

D. Flexible esophagoscopy may be performed under local anesthesia as described for flexible bronchoscopy (see Section IV.A) or after the induction of general anesthesia and endotracheal intubation. Use of a smaller caliber ETT will allow the surgeon more room to work in the pharynx and proximal esophagus.

E. Rigid esophagoscopy is commonly performed under general anesthesia with muscle relaxation. As with flexible esophagoscopy, a smaller ETT is used.

F. Laser surgery is performed on upper and lower airway lesions, including laryngeal tumors, subglottic webs, and laryngeal papillomatosis. A laser's wavelength determines its penetration and biologic effect. The surgery may be performed via rigid bronchoscopy, laryngoscopy with jet ventilation, or traditional endotracheal intubation. The patient is often in laryngeal suspension, and this requires muscle relaxation. Postoperative pain is minimal.

  1. During laryngeal suspension, it is important to monitor vital signs as this maneuver can trigger vagal response and lead to severe bradycardia. Glycopyrrolate can be given and the surgeon can also be asked to remove the laryngoscope out of suspension until the bradycardia resolves.

V. MEDIASTINAL OPERATIONS

A. Mediastinoscopy is conducted to evaluate the extrapulmonary spread of pulmonary tumors and to investigate mediastinal masses. Mediastinoscopy is performed through an incision just superior to the manubrium. A rigid endoscope is then introduced beneath the sternum, and the anterior surfaces of the trachea and the hilum are examined. The patient is supine with the neck extended.

  1. Any general anesthetic technique may be used, provided the patient remains immobile. Although the procedure is not very painful, intermittent stimulation of the trachea, carina, and mainstem bronchi occurs.

  2. Complications include pneumothorax, rupture of the great vessels, and damage to the airways. Large-bore IV access is required, and the patient should have blood cross-matched in the case of hemorrhage. IV access should be placed in the right upper extremity as the left innominate vein may be compressed during mediastinoscopy. If there is concern for trauma to the superior vena cava (SVC) intraoperatively, lower extremity IV access should be established. There is a risk of stroke from innominate artery occlusion by compression between the mediastinoscope and the posterior surface of the sternum. As stated previously, perfusion to the right arm should be monitored by pulse oximetry or blood pressure measurement. Blood pressure monitoring in the left arm is essential to monitor systemic blood pressure in the event of innominate arterial compression. Should innominate arterial compression occur and the surgeon be incapable of relieving the pressure (ie, while managing hemorrhage through the mediastinoscope), the mean systemic pressure must be increased to encourage collateral flow to the right cerebral hemisphere. The trachea may be intermittently compressed by the mediastinoscope, and the position of the patient and surgeon increases the chance of accidental disconnection of the breathing circuit.

B. **Chamberlain procedure** uses an anterior parasternal incision to obtain lung or anterior mediastinal tissue for diagnostic purposes or to drain abscesses. The incision is typically in the left second intercostal interspace. The patient is supine.

1. Following the induction of general anesthesia, the procedure is performed with the patient in the supine position. If no ribs are resected, the procedure is usually not very painful. Infiltration of the incision with local anesthetic or administration of small doses of opioids and/or IV nonsteroidal anti-inflammatories is usually sufficient for analgesia.

2. One-lung ventilation is not required for lung biopsy, but manual ventilation in cooperation with the surgeon(s) can facilitate the procedure.

3. If the pleural space is evacuated as it is closed, a chest tube generally is not required postoperatively, although the patient should be monitored carefully for any signs of pneumothorax.

C. **Mediastinal surgery**

1. Median sternotomy is performed for resection of mediastinal tumors and for bilateral pulmonary resections. In descending order of frequency, mediastinal masses include neurogenic tumors, cysts, teratodermoids, lymphomas, thymomas, parathyroid tumors, and retrosternal thyroids.

2. Thymectomy is performed by median sternotomy and may be performed to treat myasthenia gravis. Anesthetic considerations for the patient with myasthenia gravis are detailed in Chapter 14.

3. General anesthesia may be induced and maintained with any technique.

   a. Neuromuscular blockers are not required to maintain surgical exposure but may be a useful adjunct to general anesthesia. Both nondepolarizing and depolarizing muscle relaxants are best avoided in the myasthenic patient (although using rocuronium and reversal with sugammadex is currently under debate).

   b. During the actual sternotomy, the patient's lungs should be deflated and motionless. Even so, complications of sternotomy include laceration of the right ventricle, atrium, or great vessels (particularly the innominate artery) and unrecognized pneumothorax in either side of the chest.

   c. Postoperative pain from a median sternotomy is significantly less than from a thoracotomy and may be managed with either an epidural or parenteral opioids.

D. **Anesthesia for mediastinal mass resection**

1. General consideration:

   a. Anterior mediastinal masses can be associated with hemodynamic collapse due to great vessel cardiac compression. Additionally mass can obstruct venous drainage from upper chest leading to SVC syndrome as well as airway obstruction leading to airway compromise.

   b. A thorough preoperative assessment and discussion with the surgeon about operative plan, possible perioperative complications, and management approach to cardiovascular or airway compression is essential.

c. Sedation and paralysis during induction of anesthesia can lead to airway collapse due to bronchial smooth muscle relaxation.

d. CT scan and patient's signs and symptoms are the most important determinants of patient's risk for general anesthesia.

2. Preoperative:

a. Preoperative PFTs are not routinely obtained, as they offer minimal clinical benefit. Additionally, studies have shown that flow-volume loops are not useful clinically because of poor correlation with airway obstruction.

b. A focused history on patient's symptoms is important and can be graded based on patient's ability to lie flat. Symptomatic, mild: can lie supine with some pressure/cough sensation, moderate: can lie supine for short periods, and severe: cannot tolerate supine. Additionally, the patients' most comfortable position should be assessed as it can be used as "rescue position" in the event of airway obstruction.

c. CT scan assesses relationship of the mass to heart (compression or pericardial effusion), tracheobronchial compression, and major blood vessels. CT scan showing >50% tracheobronchial obstruction indicates high risk.

d. Arterial line and at least one large bore peripheral IV should be placed depending on additional cannulation strategy. If there is concern for occlusion of upper body vasculature, they should be placed on the lower extremity.

e. If epidural analgesia is planned for postoperative pain control (eg, thoracotomy, clamshell), it should be placed preoperative as well; however, caution should be used in dosing prior to induction and mass removal.

f. Depending on patient's comorbidities and nature of the mass, central venous catheter may also be placed prior to induction. Again placement is dependent on mass effect of major vasculature.

g. If the is a high probability of complete airway obstruction or cardiovascular collapse during induction process, femoral cannulas for **cardiopulmonary bypass (CPB)** or **extracorporeal membrane oxygenation (ECMO)** are inserted and can be initiated prior to induction. This is done under local anesthesia, but minimal sedation with midazolam 1 to 4 mg and ketamine 0.5 to 1 mg/kg may be given during the cannulation process.

3. Induction/intubation:

a. Induction technique and airway management depends upon patient's severity of symptoms and airway pathology. The surgeon should be present during this time and appropriate rescue airway equipment including **rigid bronchoscopy** should be immediately available as well in case airway collapse occurs.

b. Patient should be placed in backup position for comfort until airway is secured.

c. Maintaining spontaneous ventilation until airway is secured or during the procedure if possible is the safest approach.

d. Awake fiberoptic intubation is done in patients who have moderate-severe symptoms or if the mass is proximal on CT scan. This can be done with local or regional techniques (see Chapter 13).

e. Inhalation induction using sevoflurane prior to intubation with fiberoptic bronchoscopy (FOB) can be done in patients with mild symptoms.

f. In patients with no symptoms or no evidence of airway or cardiovascular compression, routine IV induction can be done carefully.

g. Reinforced ETT is preferred if there is tracheal compression by the mass. However, it is important to have an array of ETTs including microlaryngoscopy tubes, double-lumen tubes (DLTs), and bronchial blockers if one-lung ventilation might be required (see section that follows). It is important that the ETT should also be placed distal to obstruction.

h. If airway obstruction or hemodynamic collapse occurs after induction and ventilation is not possible, steps to take include position change or rigid bronchoscopy. The surgeon should also be prepared for emergency sternotomy to lift the mass and alleviate compression.

4. Intraoperative/postoperative:

a. Transesophageal echocardiogram can be used to assess global function, especially if the mass is compressing the major vessels or the heart if mass does not affect the esophagus.

b. Blood products should be immediately available for transfusion.

c. The patient might require mechanical ventilation and should be transferred to ICU for monitoring.

VI. PULMONARY RESECTION

A. Anesthetic technique. General anesthesia, in combination with epidural or regional anesthesia, is the preferred technique. If an epidural is used, it should be placed at the thoracic level (**see Chapter 20**).

1. General anesthesia can be maintained with volatile anesthetic or total intravenous anesthesia (TIVA).

2. Muscle relaxants are useful adjuncts to general anesthesia. Although surgical exposure does not require muscle relaxation, movement and coughing carry some risk.

3. One-lung ventilation is typically necessary to isolate and collapse the operative lung to provide optimal surgical exposure. This can be achieved with DLT or bronchial blocker as described in the section that follows.

4. Epidural analgesia is an effective method for postoperative pain relief after thoracotomy. The epidural may be used intraoperatively to augment the general anesthetic.

B. Positioning. Operations for lung resection are most commonly performed in the lateral decubitus position with the bed sharply flexed and the hemithorax on the operative side parallel to the floor.

1. The arms are usually extended in front of the patient and must be carefully padded to avoid compression of the radial and ulnar nerves or obstruction of arterial and venous cannulas. This can usually be avoided by placing cannulas in the dependent arm. The dependent brachial plexus must be checked for excessive tension. Various devices exist for supporting the upper arm securely above the lower, leaving the anesthetist with good access to the lower arm. Neither arm should be abducted more than 90°.

2. The neck should remain in a neutral position, which requires constant support of the head during the movement of the bed into the flexed position. The dependent eye and ear should be carefully checked to ensure that they are not under any direct pressure.

3. The lower extremities should be padded appropriately to avoid compression injuries. In male patients, the scrotum should be free of compressive forces.

4. During the positioning process, the vital signs should be closely observed because pooling of blood in dependent extremities may cause hypotension.

5. Changes in position can move the endobronchial tube or blocker and change V/Q relationships.

6. Lung compliance, lung isolation, and oxygenation should be reassessed after any change in position.

C. Emergence and extubation. The goal of the anesthetic technique selected is to have an awake, comfortable, and extubated patient at the end of the procedure.

1. Before closing the chest, the operative lung is inflated with 20 to 30 cm H_2O pressure for 15 to 30 seconds to reinflate the atelectatic areas and check for significant air leaks.

2. Chest tubes are inserted to drain the pleural cavity and promote lung expansion. Chest tubes usually are placed under water seal and up to 20 cm H_2O suction, except after a pneumonectomy. After pneumonectomy, a chest tube, if used, should be placed under water seal only. Applying suction could shift the mediastinum to the draining side and reduce venous return, causing tension physiology.

3. At the conclusion of the procedure with both lungs ventilated, nitrous oxide, in concentrations up to 70%, can provide a smooth emergence. It is essential that the chest tubes are functioning. Ensuring complete reversal on paralysis is also key in these patients.

4. Prompt extubation avoids the potential disruptive effects of endotracheal intubation and positive-pressure ventilation on fresh suture lines. If postoperative mechanical ventilation is required, the DLT should be exchanged for a conventional ETT with a high-volume low-pressure cuff. Inspiratory pressures should be kept as low as possible.

D. Surgical techniques

1. **Lateral or posterolateral thoracotomy** is an approach for the resection of large pulmonary neoplasms or abscesses. Thoracotomy is often preceded by staging procedures such as bronchoscopy, mediastinoscopy, or thoracoscopy. If the staging procedures are performed at the same sitting, the anesthetic should be planned to accommodate the possibility of a shortened procedure if metastatic disease is discovered.

2. **Video-assisted thoracoscopic surgery (VATS)** is a common approach for wedge resection, segmentectomy, and lobectomy. Thoracoscopic surgery may result in less postoperative pain and a shorter recovery time. Lung isolation is required for adequate visualization of the surgical field.

3. **Robot-assisted thoracoscopic surgery (RATS)** is a growing technique that is theoretically superior to VATS in that the accuracy of the robotic arm facilitates lymph node resection with the conservation of nerves and improved cure rates.

a. As with VATS, positioning is in lateral decubitus and complete collapse of the operative lung must be maintained. Low-pressure CO_2 is often used to augment this collapse.

b. Good pressure point padding must be ensured due to extremes of positioning with robotic surgery.

c. It has been previously stated that once the robot is docked, the surgical bed must not be moved at all. However, newer robotic system allows the robot and the surgical bed to be moved as one unit, decreasing the risk for patient injury when the bed position is changed.

d. It is important to ensure that adequate muscle relation during RATS as patient coughing or movement during surgery can be dangerous.

E. **Endobronchial tubes.** Placement of a DLT is indicated for lung protection (for significant hemoptysis or unilateral infection), bronchoalveolar lavage, or surgical exposure.

1. **Choice of tube**

   a. DLTs range in size from 26 to 41 French. In general, a 39- or 41-French tube is chosen for adult males and a 35- or 37-French is chosen for adult females. Selection is also based on the patient's height. In general, for men, 70 inches is used for a cutoff height between the 39- or 41-French tubes. For women, 65 inches is a cutoff between 35 or 37 French.

   b. **Right- and left-sided DLTs** are available and are designed to conform to either the right or the left mainstem bronchus. Each tube has separate channels: one for ventilation of the bronchus and the other for the trachea and nonintubated bronchus. Right-sided tubes have a separate opening (Murphy eye) in the bronchial lumen to permit ventilation of the right upper lobe.

   c. **The choice of a left- or right-sided tube** depends on the type and side of operation. If a mainstem bronchus is absent, stenotic, disrupted, or obstructed, the DLT must be placed on the opposite side, preferably under direct fiberoptic guidance. In most cases, the choice of a left- versus right-sided tube is not so absolute. Most surgical procedures can be performed with a left-sided DLT. It is our practice, however, to selectively intubate the dependent (nonoperative) bronchus. This ensures that the endobronchial tube will not interfere with resection of the mainstem bronchus if this is necessary. Also, if the nondependent lung is intubated, ventilation of the dependent lung through the tracheal lumen may be compromised by mediastinal pressure pushing the tube against the tracheal wall and creating a "ball-valve" obstruction.

2. **Insertion**

   a. The endobronchial tube, including both cuffs and all necessary connectors, should be carefully checked before placement. The tube may be lubricated, and a stylet should be placed in the bronchial lumen.

   b. After laryngoscopy, the endobronchial tube should be inserted initially with the distal curve facing anteriorly. Once in the trachea, the stylet should be removed and the tube rotated so that the bronchial lumen is toward the appropriate side. The tube is then advanced to an average depth of 29 cm at the incisors or gums (27 cm in females) or less if resistance is met.

   c. Alternatively, a fiberoptic bronchoscope can be passed down the bronchial lumen as soon as the tube is in the trachea and then used to guide the tube into the correct mainstem bronchus.

   d. Once the tube has been inserted and connected to the anesthesia circuit, the tracheal cuff is inflated, and manual ventilation is initiated. Endotracheal placement is confirmed by the presence of end-tidal CO_2 and the auscultation of bilateral breath sounds. The tracheal side of the adapter is then clamped, and the distal tracheal lumen is opened to atmospheric pressure via the access port. The bronchial cuff is inflated to a point just sufficient to eliminate air leak from the tracheal lumen, and the chest is auscultated. Breath sounds should now be limited to the side that has been endobronchially intubated. Moving the clamp to the bronchial side of the adapter and closing the tracheal access port should cause only the nonintubated side to be ventilated.

e. Fiberoptic bronchoscope should be used to confirm tube position. When passed down the tracheal lumen, the bronchoscope should reveal the carina with the proximal edge of the bronchial cuff just visible in the mainstem bronchus. Passing the bronchoscope down the bronchial lumen should reveal either the left mainstem bronchus or the bronchus intermedius, depending on whether a left- or right-sided tube has been placed. The orifice of the right upper lobe should be visible through the side lumen of a right-sided tube. A bronchoscope should be kept available throughout the case.

f. Lung isolation can be monitored continuously if the anesthesia machine is able to measure inspiratory and expiratory volumes independently and display the leak.

3. DLT tube malposition commonly has a few patterns.

a. The tube is placed too far into the bronchus so that the distal lumen ventilates a single lobe.

b. The tube is too shallow such that the bronchial balloon obstructs the entire tracheal lumen.

c. A left-sided tube is misplaced into the right mainstem bronchus, with the right upper lobe mistakenly thought to be the entire right bronchus. This malposition can be corrected under bronchoscopic guidance via the bronchial lumen, withdrawing the tube to the trachea and directing toward the left mainstem bronchus.

4. Prior to extubation or any significant manipulation of the endobronchial tube, the bronchial cuff should be deflated.

5. The procedure for passing an endobronchial tube through an existing tracheostomy stoma is identical. Bronchoscopy will help to determine how far the tube should be advanced once it is in the trachea.

F. **Univent tubes** are large-caliber ETTs encompassing a small integrated channel for a built-in bronchial blocker. Indications for a Univent tube include the need for post-op intubation, the desire to avoid changing from a DLT to a single-lumen tube, and situations in which placement of a DLT is difficult or contraindicated. A potential complication is inadvertent advancement and insufflation of the bronchial blocker into the trachea, causing complete obstruction to ventilation.

1. **Insertion.** The Univent tube is inserted into the trachea in the usual fashion and is rotated toward the operative lung. After inflation of the tracheal cuff, the bronchial blocker is advanced into the operative mainstem bronchus under fiberoptic guidance. After appropriate positioning, the cuff of the bronchial blocker is inflated. Because the Univent tube is made of Silastic rather than polyvinyl chloride, thorough lubrication of the bronchoscope is required.

2. **Collapse of the operative lung** occurs through both exhalation via the small distal opening in the blocker and progressive absorption of oxygen from the lung, which will produce alveolar collapse. This is a slow process but may be hastened by deflating the blocker and disconnecting the anesthesia circuit while observing the lung. Once collapse has occurred, the blocker can be reinflated and the circuit reconnected.

G. **Bronchial blockers** may be used routinely, but especially in situations in which it is not possible to place an endobronchial tube, including in pediatric patients, in those with difficult airway anatomy, or where satisfactory lung isolation cannot be achieved by other means.

1. **Vascular occlusion catheters, such as the Fogarty, are an older source for bronchial blocker.** An appropriately sized Fogarty catheter (8- to 14-French venous occlusion catheter with a 10-mL balloon) is selected

and placed into the trachea before endotracheal intubation. After intubation, the balloon tip is positioned with a fiberoptic bronchoscope in the appropriate mainstem bronchus and inflated. Lung collapse occurs slowly, via absorption of gases. There is no ability to suction or perform maneuvers such as continuous positive airway pressure (CPAP) to the nonventilated lung.

2. The **Arndt blocker** is a bronchial blocker especially designed for lung isolation. Placement is facilitated by a distal loop that can be snared with a bronchoscope. The airway connector is well designed, with separate access ports for the blocker, bronchoscope, and ventilation circuit. Like the Univent tube, the blocker has a small central lumen that can be used for lung collapse or CPAP.

3. The Y-shaped **EZ-blocker** is designed to simplify positioning. Like the Arndt blocker, it includes an airway connector that allows simultaneous ventilation, bronchoscopic visualization, and blocker placement. This blocker terminates at a Y shape that mimics the carinal division into the mainstem bronchi, terminating with a cuff on each extension. The blocker is placed such that the Y sits at the carina with the extensions in each mainstem bronchus. Each cuff can be inflated by its corresponding balloon. Like the other blockers, each extension has a small central lumen.

H. Complications of lung isolation techniques include collapse of obstructed segments of the lung, airway trauma including bronchial rupture, bleeding, and aspiration during prolonged efforts at intubation. Hypoxia and hypoventilation may occur both during placement efforts and as a result of malpositioning.

I. One-lung ventilation. General anesthesia, the lateral position, an open chest, surgical manipulations, and one-lung ventilation all alter ventilation and perfusion.

1. **Oxygenation**

   a. The amount of pulmonary blood flow passing through the unventilated lung (pulmonary shunt) is the most important factor determining arterial oxygenation during one-lung ventilation.

   b. Diseased lungs often have reduced perfusion secondary to vascular occlusion or vasoconstriction. This may limit shunting of blood through the nonventilated operative lung during one-lung ventilation.

   c. Perfusion of the unventilated lung is also reduced by hypoxic pulmonary vasoconstriction (HPV). HPV is the pulmonary vascular mechanism that diverts blood flow away from poorly ventilated areas of the lung, minimizing V/Q mismatch.

   d. **Positive end-expiratory pressure (PEEP)** has variable effect on the PVR, and PEEP has not been definitively shown to improve oxygenation during one-lung ventilation, but it is used as part of lung-protective strategies.

   e. The lateral position (as opposed to supine) reduces pulmonary shunting, because gravity decreases blood flowing to the nondependent lung.

   f. Oxygenation should be continuously monitored by pulse oximetry.

2. **Ventilation**

   a. **Arterial carbon dioxide tension** during one-lung ventilation is generally maintained at the same level as on two lungs. This should not be at the expense of hyperinflating or overdistending the ventilated lung.

    b. Controlled ventilation is mandatory during open-chest operations.

    c. Plateau (or end-inspiratory) airway pressure should generally be maintained below 25 cm H_2O to avoid overdistention of the lung. The occurrence of high airway pressure should be investigated immediately, including with a fiberoptic bronchoscope and is usually due to malpositioning of the endobronchial tube or the presence of secretions.

    d. Tidal volume should be maintained in the 4 to 6 mL/kg range for protective one-lung ventilation.

    e. A moderate increase in partial pressure of carbon dioxide in arterial blood is usually well tolerated. Respiratory rate can be increased to maintain minute ventilation if necessary (as long as intrinsic PEEP and air trapping are minimal).

    f. When switching from two-lung to one-lung ventilation, manual ventilation allows instantaneous adaptation to the expected changes in compliance and facilitates assessment of lung isolation. Once tidal volume and compliance have been assessed by hand and lung collapse has been confirmed visually, mechanical ventilation can be reinstituted.

J. Management of one-lung ventilation

  1. Anesthetic management. During one-lung ventilation, the use of nitrous oxide is limited or discontinued if there is any evidence of a significant decrease in partial pressure of oxygen in arterial blood (eg, a decrease in oxygen saturation).

  2. Difficulties with oxygenation during one-lung ventilation may be treated with a variety of maneuvers directed at decreasing blood flow to the nonventilated lung (decreasing shunt fraction), minimizing atelectasis in the ventilated lung, or providing additional oxygen to the operative lung.

    a. Tube position should be reassessed by fiberoptic bronchoscopy and repositioned if necessary. Additionally, the bronchial lumen should be suctioned to clear secretions and ensure patency.

    b. CPAP can be applied to the nonventilated lung with a separate circuit. Under direct visualization, the collapsed lung is inflated and then allowed to deflate to a volume that will not interfere with surgical exposure (usually 2-5 cm H_2O CPAP).

    c. PEEP may be increased to the ventilated lung to treat atelectasis, but this may lower arterial oxygen saturation if a greater proportion of blood flow is forced into the unventilated lung as a result.

    d. Recruitment maneuvers to overcome atelectasis have been shown to be effective.

    e. Apneic oxygenation may be provided to the nonventilated lung by partially inflating it with 100% oxygen and then capping the exhalation port. In this way, a motionless partially collapsed lung is maintained. **Reinstallation** of oxygen will be necessary every 10 to 20 minutes.

    f. In the event of persistent hypoxemia that is uncorrectable by combinations of the aforementioned therapies or a sudden precipitous desaturation, the surgeon must be notified and the operative lung reinflated with 100% oxygen. Two-lung ventilation should be maintained until the situation has stabilized, after which the operative lung can be allowed to collapse again. Periodic reinflations or manual two-lung ventilation may be required to maintain an adequate arterial oxygen saturation throughout some procedures.

Consideration should also be given to nonpulmonary etiology of the shunt (ie, PFO with right to left shunt) in the setting of elevated right-sided pressures on OLV.

g. **TIVA** may be preferred to the administration of a volatile anesthetic, because it is easier to maintain a constant depth of anesthesia while performing maneuvers to improve oxygenation and ventilation. TIVA has not been shown to decrease hypoxia, and unlike inhalation agents, it does not attenuate the inflammatory response.

h. **If hypoxemia persists**, the surgeon can minimize shunt by compressing or clamping the pulmonary artery of the surgical lung or any of its available lobes.

i. **CPB** or **ECMO** can be instituted to provide oxygenation (see Chapter 29) in extreme situations.

3. When switching from one-lung back to two-lung ventilation, a few manual breaths with a prolonged inspiratory hold will help to reexpand collapsed alveoli.

K. **Postoperative analgesia.** Posterolateral thoracotomy is a painful incision, involving multiple muscle layers, rib resection, and continuous motion as the patient breathes. Therapy for postoperative pain should begin before the patient emerges from general anesthesia.

1. **Epidural analgesia** has been long considered the preferred approach for postthoracotomy pain management (see Chapter 39). Ipsilateral shoulder pain that thoracotomy patients commonly note is referred pain from phrenic nerve irritation and is not covered by epidural analgesia but is well treated with adjuncts, such as nonsteroidal analgesics and acetaminophen.

2. **Paravertebral nerve blocks**
   a. Recent studies have suggested that paravertebral nerve blocks are an effective alternative to epidural analgesia in thoracotomy patients.
   b. Preoperative blocks are usually performed to provide sensory block from approximately T4 to T9. These blocks can be placed intraoperatively in the surgical field or percutaneously using anatomic landmarks, or ultrasound for guidance. The block may be conducted with the patient in either the sitting or prone position. Ultrasound-guided paramedian sagittal or transverse intercostal techniques may be used. For both ultrasound percutaneous techniques, the end point of the block is visualization of depression of the pleura by the local anesthetic into the paravertebral space. If landmark technique is used, the endpoint of the block is loss of resistance. A single-shot block provides analgesia for 12 to 24 hours depending on choice of local anesthetic. Additionally, an infusion catheter may be placed in the paravertebral space for continuous postoperative analgesia.
   c. Intercostal nerve blocks can be placed under direct thoracoscopic guidance, or percutaneously by following landmarks. The neurovascular bundle travels in a groove inferior to each rib. These nerve blocks provide analgesia for 6 to 8 hours. Care to avoid intravascular injection is important.

3. Parenteral opioids, if required, should be administered judiciously.

4. **Nonsteroidal anti-inflammatory agents**, such as **ketorolac**, have proved effective as a supplemental analgesic but should be used with caution in the elderly, in patients with renal insufficiency, and in those with a history of gastric bleeding. **Acetaminophen** is also effective for the treatment of referred shoulder pain as described above.

VII. TRACHEAL RESECTION AND RECONSTRUCTION

A. **General considerations.** Surgery of the trachea and mainstem bronchi involves significant anesthetic risks, including interruption of airway continuity and the potential for total obstruction of an already stenotic airway.

1. The surgical approach depends on the location and extent of the lesion. Lesions of the cervical trachea are approached through a transverse neck incision. Lower lesions necessitate an upper sternotomy. Lesions of the distal trachea and carina may require a median sternotomy or a right thoracotomy.

2. Extubation at the conclusion of the surgical procedure is the goal of the anesthetic to avoid trauma to the fresh tracheal anastomosis from an ETT.

3. **The anesthetic technique** must include a plan for preserving airway patency throughout induction and intubation and emergency plans and equipment for dealing with any sudden loss of airway control, ranging from rigid bronchoscopy to CPB based on the clinical assessment and experience of the team.

4. **If the airway is critically stenotic,** it is important to have a skilled rigid bronchoscopist/thoracic surgeon and necessary equipment immediately available during induction. Spontaneous ventilation should be maintained throughout the induction because it may not be possible to ventilate the lungs by mask ventilation if apnea occurs. A volatile agent is the preferred anesthetic, and no muscle relaxants are used. Sevoflurane, with its lack of airway irritability, is suitable for inhalational induction. A deep plane of anesthesia must be established before instrumentation, and this may require 15 to 20 minutes in a patient with small tidal volumes and a large functional residual capacity. Hemodynamic support with phenylephrine may be required for an elderly or debilitated patient to tolerate the necessary high concentration of volatile agent.

5. **Patients with preexisting mature tracheostomies** may be induced with intravenous agents followed by cannulation of the tracheostomy with a cuffed, flexible, armored ETT. The surgical field around the tube is prepared, and the tube is removed and replaced with a sterile one by the surgeon.

B. **Intraoperative management** is complicated by periodic interruption of airway continuity by the surgical procedure.

1. **Rigid bronchoscopy** is commonly performed before the surgical incision to delineate tracheal anatomy and caliber.

   a. If the surgeon determines that an ETT can be placed through the stenotic segment, this should be done as soon as the bronchoscope is withdrawn. Controlled ventilation can then be used safely.

   b. If the stenotic segment is too narrow or friable to allow intubation, spontaneous ventilation and anesthesia must continue through the bronchoscope until surgical access to the distal trachea is achieved. Alternatives include having the surgeon "core out" the tracheal lesion with the rigid bronchoscope, placing a tracheostomy distal to the stenotic segment, intubating the trachea above the lesion or placing an LMA and allowing spontaneous ventilation to continue, or using a jet ventilation system to ventilate the patient from above the lesion.

   c. Flexible bronchoscopy via an LMA is an alternative to rigid bronchoscopy immediately prior to tracheal resection.

2. When the airway is in jeopardy or ventilation is intermittent, 100% oxygen should be administered.

3. **For lower tracheal or carinal resections**, a long ETT with a flexible armored wall can be used. This allows the surgeon to position the tip in the trachea or either mainstem bronchus and to operate around it without interrupting ventilation.

4. **When the trachea is surgically divided**, the ETT must be retracted proximal to the division and a sterile armored tube placed into the distal trachea by the surgeon. A suture may be placed in the distal end of the orotracheal tube before pulling it back into the pharynx to facilitate replacing it in the trachea at the end of the procedure.

   a. The tube is frequently removed and reinserted by the surgeons as they work around it. Close coordination during this portion of the procedure will help avoid leakage of gas from the circuit.

   b. Once the stenotic segment has been removed and the posterior tracheal reanastomosis completed, the transtracheal tube is removed, and the ETT is readvanced from above. The distal trachea should be suctioned to remove accumulated blood and secretions. The patient's neck is then flexed forward, reducing tension on the trachea, and the anterior portion of the anastomosis is completed.

5. **Jet ventilation** through a catheter held by one of the surgeons may be required during carinal resection if the distal airways are too small to accommodate an ETT.

   a. It is difficult to administer volatile agents by a jet ventilator so intravenous agents are needed during this portion of the surgery.

   b. Jet ventilation rate and pressure should be carefully titrated by direct observation of the surgical field. Obstruction of exhalation will lead to "stacking" of breaths, increased airway pressure, and barotrauma.

6. **At the conclusion of the procedure**, a single large suture is placed from the chin to the anterior chest to preserve neck flexion and thereby minimize tension on the tracheal suture line. Several blankets under the head will help maintain flexion. Close attention to neck position during emergence, extubation, and transfer is essential.

C. **Emergence and extubation**

1. **Spontaneous ventilation** should be resumed as soon as possible after the procedure to minimize trauma to the tracheal suture line. Most patients may be safely extubated, but in those for whom difficult anatomy or copious secretions make this undesirable, a small tracheostomy may be placed below the tracheal repair.

   a. The patient should be awake enough to maintain spontaneous ventilation and avoid aspiration but should be extubated before excessive head movement can damage the surgical repair.

   b. Fiberoptic examination of the surgical repair via LMA may be planned for the conclusion of the case, or done if there is suspicion of obstruction after extubation.

   c. If tracheal collapse, airway edema, or secretions cause persistent respiratory distress after extubation, the patient should be reintubated fiberoptically with a small uncuffed ETT, preferably with the head maintained in forward flexion.

2. Frequent bronchoscopies at the bedside under local anesthesia may be required to remove secretions from the lungs in the postoperative period.

3. Only relatively small amounts of intravenous opioids are usually needed to treat the mild pain from the neck incision. Analgesia usually is administered after the patient is wide awake and responsive and while monitoring for undesirable respiratory depression.

D. Tracheal disruption may be caused by airway instrumentation or thoracic trauma and may be signaled by hypoxia, dyspnea, subcutaneous emphysema, pneumomediastinum, or pneumothorax.

1. **The point of injury** is commonly at the cricoid, midtrachea, carina, or either mainstem bronchus. Several mechanisms of injury have been proposed, including high airway pressures, lateral stretch of the thoracic cavity, and deceleration injury.

2. **Positive-pressure ventilation** will exacerbate the air leak and rapidly worsen symptoms from pneumothorax or pneumomediastinum. If possible, the patient should be allowed to breathe spontaneously, following the protocol for the patient with critical tracheal stenosis.

3. **Tracheal damage** in the already anesthetized patient may be treated initially by advancement of a small ETT past the point of injury. In the case of a difficult airway in which the tube causes the injury, an immediate surgical tracheostomy must be performed and access to the distal trachea secured.

4. Once a tube has been placed across or distal to the site of tracheal disruption, controlled positive-pressure ventilation can begin. Further management is as for the patient undergoing elective airway surgery.

VIII. INTRAPULMONARY HEMORRHAGE

Massive hemoptysis may be caused by thoracic trauma, pulmonary artery rupture secondary to catheterization, or erosion into a vessel by a tracheostomy, abscess, or airway tumor.

A. The trachea must be immediately intubated and the lungs ventilated with 100% oxygen.

B. An attempt should be made to suction the airway clear, ideally by rigid bronchoscopy.

C. If a unilateral source is identified, lung isolation may be undertaken to protect the uninvolved lung and facilitate corrective surgery.

1. **Lung isolation** may be achieved by placing an endobronchial blocker or a double-lumen endobronchial tube. Choice of technique depends on experience, equipment at hand, and the extent of active bleeding. Active bleeding may obscure airway visualization during flexible bronchoscopy. Obstruction of the ETT is an ever-present danger, and frequent suctioning may be necessary.

2. In an emergency, the existing ETT can be advanced into the mainstem bronchus of the uninvolved lung and the cuff inflated.

3. **Fiberoptic bronchoscopy** is essential for suctioning blood and confirming isolation.

   a. Frequently, the source of bleeding is from the bronchial circulation. **Embolization** in the radiology suite is often attempted if the patient is stable.

   b. Definitive treatment may require a thoracotomy and surgical repair.

IX. BRONCHOPLEURAL FISTULA

Bronchopleural fistula is a connection between a bronchial stump and the surrounding pleura. Symptoms include dyspnea, subcutaneous emphysema, persistent air leak, and purulent discharge from the chest tube.

A. General considerations

1. Small fistulas may close spontaneously; a persistent leak indicates involvement of a larger bronchus.

2. Treatment of subsequent sepsis involves antibiotics and chest tube drainage.

3. Surgical approach varies, ranging from application of fibrin glue via bronchoscopy to thoracoplasty with a pedicled muscle flap.

B. Anesthetic management

1. Positive-pressure ventilation may be inadequate if most ventilation escapes through the fistula. A functional chest tube must be in place before induction and positive-pressure ventilation.

2. Patients often undergo inhalation induction with spontaneous ventilation and lung isolation via endobronchial intubation to minimize the amount of time spent ventilating the fistula.

3. **High-frequency jet ventilation (HFJV)** has been used as an alternative to lung isolation to successfully decrease gas leak through the fistula by providing lower peak and mean airway pressures than with traditional positive-pressure ventilation. HFJV is not as effective in patients with noncompliant lungs such as those with acute respiratory distress syndrome. If mechanical ventilation via a standard ETT is to be used, flow redistribution may not be used to signal the end of a breath: the fistula will allow for gas flow at a constant velocity, causing the mechanical breath to continue indefinitely.

X. ESOPHAGEAL SURGERY

Esophageal surgery includes procedures for resecting esophageal neoplasms, for treating reflux, and for repairing traumatic or congenital lesions.

A. General considerations

1. Patients may be chronically malnourished both from systemic illness (carcinoma) and anatomic interference with swallowing. Enteral or parenteral nutrition may have been initiated preoperatively.

2. Both esophageal carcinoma and traumatic disruption of the distal esophagus are associated with ethanol abuse; patients may have impaired liver function, elevated portal pressures, anemia, cardiomyopathy, and bleeding disorders.

3. Patients who have difficulty swallowing may be significantly hypovolemic. Cardiovascular instability may be further exacerbated by preoperative chemotherapy with cardiotoxins.

4. Most patients presenting for esophageal procedures will be at risk for aspiration. Rapid sequence induction or awake intubation should be planned.

5. Monitors should include a radial artery and urinary catheters. Central venous access may be desirable.

6. Temperature conservation measures should be aggressively pursued. The use of a warmed air blanket over the lower body is routine.

B. Operative approach and anesthesia

1. **An upper esophageal diverticulum** (Zenker diverticulum) is approached through a lateral cervical incision, similar to that for carotid surgery. This incision may also be used for upper esophageal myotomies for swallowing disorders.

   a. **Positioning.** The patient is positioned supine with the neck extended and the head turned to the contralateral side.

   b. **General anesthesia** may be induced and maintained with any technique after rapid sequence intubation. Postoperative pain and fluid shifts are usually minimal with a cervical incision, and patients may be safely extubated at the conclusion of the procedure. The surgeons may or may not elect to leave a nasogastric tube in place.

2. **Carcinoma**

   a. General considerations

   1. Mid case repositioning and lung isolation using double-lumen ETT is required for most of the surgical approaches that involve entering the thorax.

2. Large-volume blood loss is uncommon. However, large-bore intravenous access and a preoperative type and screen should be acquired.

3. Postoperative endotracheal extubation is performed when patients can protect their own airway from aspiration and they are fully awake. Immediate postoperative extubation can be considered in healthier patients after uncomplicated procedures.

4. Virtually, any anesthetic technique may be used. Epidural analgesia is commonly used in the postoperative period both for analgesia from large incisions and to avoid any risk of aspiration from somnolence secondary to parenteral narcotics.

5. Epidural analgesia has been shown to improve esophageal blood flow, as long as hypotension and hypovolemia are treated.

6. If postoperative intubation is deemed necessary, it is usual to change from a double-lumen to a conventional ETT at the conclusion of the resection. Dependent tissue edema may significantly narrow the airway, rendering reintubation difficult.

b. **Lesions of the upper esophagus** are approached by a "three-hole" approach, which includes a transverse cervical incision, a laparotomy, and a right thoracotomy. Sometimes the lesion is high enough to be removed with a **transhiatal approach**, including only the anterior cervical incision and the laparotomy, avoiding the thoracotomy. The laparotomy (and sometimes the right thoracotomy) is required to mobilize the stomach and lower esophagus. A cervical incision allows for anastomosis of the proximal esophagus and distal stomach.

c. **Lesions of the middle esophagus** are commonly approached with a laparotomy followed by a right-sided thoracotomy. This procedure is known as an **Ivor Lewis esophagectomy**. Mobilization of the stomach or jejunum is accomplished through a midline abdominal incision. The right thoracotomy allows for a proximal anastomosis above the level of the aortic arch. There are also minimally invasive versions of this procedure that use laparoscopic and thoracoscopic equipment for the abdominal and thoracic portions of the procedure, respectively.

d. **Lower esophageal lesions** are approached through an extended left thoracoabdominal incision. After resection, the surgeon will perform a primary anastomosis of the esophagus and stomach. Occasionally, the stomach does not provide an adequate distal anastomosis, and the surgeon instead brings up a Roux-en-Y loop of jejunum.

3. **Trauma to the entire esophagus**, as with lye ingestion, may necessitate a total esophagectomy with subsequent interposition of a segment of colon or jejunum to serve as a conduit between the pharynx and stomach.

a. Surgical exposure may require two or three incisions, as described previously.

b. These patients may have a prolonged postoperative course with significant fluid shifts and nutritional depletion and are at risk for aspiration pneumonia. The trachea may remain intubated at the conclusion of the surgery, if a complex procedure has been done.

4. **Fundoplication** (eg, Belsey Mark IV, Hill, or Nissen) is performed to relieve gastroesophageal reflux; the specific procedure depends on the surgeon's preference and the patient's anatomy.

    a. The surgical approach is transabdominal for the Hill and Nissen procedures, and transthoracic for the Belsey. Collapse of the left lung is required for the latter procedure.

    b. Fluid shifts are usually less than after other esophageal surgeries, and the patients may be safely extubated at the conclusion of the procedure. Postoperative analgesic requirements are determined by the specific incision made; most patients benefit from epidural medications.

Suggested Readings

Roy PM. Preoperative pulmonary evaluation for lung resection. *J Anaesthesiol Clin Pharmacol.* 2018;34(3):296-300.

Detterbeck FC, Lewis SZ, Diekemper R, Addrizzo-Harris D, Alberts WM. Executive summary: diagnosis and management of lung cancer, 3rd ed. American College of Chest Physicians evidence-based clinical practice guidelines. *Chest.* 2013;143(5 suppl):7S-37S.

Brunelli A, Kim AW, Berger KI, Addrizzo-Harris DJ. Physiologic evaluation of the patient with lung cancer being considered for resectional surgery: diagnosis and management of lung cancer, 3rd ed. American College of Chest Physicians evidence-based clinical practice guidelines. *Chest.* 2013;143(5 suppl):e166S-e190S. Published correction appears in *Chest.* 2014;145(2):437.

Yoo ID, Im JJ, Chung YA, Choi EK, Oh JK, Lee SH. Prediction of postoperative lung function in lung cancer patients using perfusion scintigraphy. *Acta Radiol.* 2019;60(4):488-495.

Subramanyam P, Sundaram PS. Which is better – a standalone ventilation or perfusion scan or combined imaging to predict postoperative FEV_1 in one seconds in patients posted for lung surgeries with borderline pulmonary reserve. *Indian J Nucl Med.* 2018;33(2):105-111.

Duthie DJ. Anesthetic agents for thoracic surgery: what's best?. *Curr Opin Anaesthesiol.* 2013;25:53-57.

Ahuja S, Cohen B, Hinkelbein J, Diemunsch P, Ruetzler K. Practical anesthetic considerations in patients undergoing tracheobronchial surgeries: a clinical review of current literature. *J Thorac Dis.* 2016;8(11):3431-3441.

Lederman D, Easwar J, Feldman J, Shapiro V. Anesthetic considerations for lung resection: preoperative assessment, intraoperative challenges and postoperative analgesia. *Ann Transl Med.* 2019;7(15):356.

Castillo M, Slinger P. Myths of anterior mediastinal masses. *South Afr J Anaesth Analg.* 2013;19(1):38-40.

Ku CM. Anesthesia for patients with mediastinal masses. In: Slinger P, eds. *Principles and Practice of Anesthesia for Thoracic Surgery.* Springer; 2011.

Erdös G, Tzanova I. Perioperative anaesthetic management of mediastinal mass in adults, *Eur J Anaesthesiol.* 2009;26(8):627-632.

Hobai IA, Chhangani SV, Alfille PH. Anesthesia for tracheal resection and reconstruction. *Anesthesiol Clin.* 2012;30:709-730.

Lennox PH, Umedaly HS, Grant RP, et al. A pulsatile pressure waveform is a sensitive marker for confirming the location of the thoracic epidural space. *J Cardiothorac Vasc Anesth.* 2006;20(5):659-663.

Pawlowski J. Anesthetic considerations for interventional pulmonary procedures. *Curr Opin Anaesthesiol.* 2013;25:6-12.

Vidal Melo MF, Musch G, Kaczka DW. Pulmonary pathophysiology and lung mechanics in anesthesiology: a cased-based overview. *Anesthesiol Clin.* 2012;30:759-784.

Pauli H, Eladawy M, Park J. Anesthesia for robotic thoracic surgery. *Ann Cardiothorac Surg.* 2019;8(2):263-268.

Ahmad S, Taneja A, Kurman J, Dagar G, Kumar G. National trends in lung volume reduction surgery in the United States: 2000 to 2010. *Chest.* 2014;146(6):e228-e229.

28

Anesthesia for Vascular Surgery

Christopher J. Mariani and James Taylor Lloyd

I. PREOPERATIVE ASSESSMENT AND MANAGEMENT

Patients undergoing vascular surgery frequently have multiple comorbid conditions that should be optimized prior to surgery.

A. Cardiovascular system. Major adverse cardiac events (MACE) such as stroke, myocardial infarction (MI), cardiac arrest, and death are the leading cause of morbidity and mortality in patients undergoing vascular surgery. MI accounts for about one-half of early postoperative deaths. Accurate risk stratification based on preoperative patient characteristics remains a significant challenge in vascular surgery. Commonly used risk calculators such as the Revised Cardiac Risk Index (RCRI) and Gupta Myocardial Infarction or Cardiac Arrest have reduced performances in vascular surgery. Alternate scoring systems such as the Geriatric-Sensitive Perioperative Risk Calculator, Vascular Surgery Group of New England Cardiac Risk Index, and Vascular Quality Initiative Cardiac Risk Index tools have been proposed to address these shortcomings, but have their own limitations. Below are some specific considerations with regard to vascular surgical patients.

1. **Cardiac stress testing.** For nonemergent cases, in patients estimated to be at elevated risk (>1% risk of perioperative MACE) with poor functional capacity (<4 METS), noninvasive cardiac stress testing should be carried out if the results will impact patient care. Dobutamine stress echocardiogrpahy or myocardial perfusion imaging will be necessary for patients with physical limitations such as claudication or disability from prior stroke. The need for coronary artery catheterization is determined based on the results of the stress test, in consultation with a cardiologist.

2. **Echocardiography** may be indicated if the patient has a new murmur, dyspnea of unknown etiology, valvular heart disease, or heart failure with new or worsening symptomatology.

3. **Blood pressures** should be measured in both arms to determine whether there is a difference. Due to the systemic nature of atherosclerosis, patients may have subclavian or axillary arterial stenoses. Blood pressure should be monitored in the extremity with the higher reading.

4. **Coronary revascularization** should be carried out only if medically indicated. According to the Coronary Artery Revascularization Prophylaxis trial, coronary revascularization in advance of major vascular surgery has not been shown to improve outcome when compared with medical management. This trial excluded patients with left main coronary artery disease, ejection fraction less than 20%, and severe aortic stenosis.

5. **β-Blocker therapy** should be maintained in patients already on chronic therapy. Initiation of β-blocker therapy is reasonable in patients with three or more RCRI risk factors or in patients with reversible ischemia on preoperative testing. However, improper timing and dose titration

may increase risk of stroke and mortality. β-Blocker therapy should be started at least 2 days prior to surgery; 7 days is preferred. Therapy should be started at a low dose and titrated slowly to achieve target heart rate of 60 to 80 bpm and should be held for hypotension.

6. **Antiplatelet therapy.** Aspirin therapy should be continued in patients with coronary stents, cerebrovascular disease, or high-risk coronary artery disease. Continuation should be considered in all vascular surgical procedures in discussion with the surgical team. Aspirin therapy is associated with an increased risk of bleeding. POISE-2, a randomized, controlled trial of 10,000 patients undergoing noncardiac surgery, did not show a benefit of aspirin initiation or continuation with respect to MACE or death. However, it excluded patients who had recently received coronary stents and those undergoing carotid endarterectomy (CEA). Furthermore, only a small proportion of the study population underwent vascular surgery. Continuation of **clopidogrel** therapy depends on patient factors (eg, presence and type of coronary stents and when they were placed) as well as surgical factors.

7. **Statins** should be continued perioperatively. The initiation of statin therapy is reasonable in patients undergoing vascular surgery. The statin should ideally be started 1 week to 30 days prior to the surgical procedure. There is evidence that statins decrease coronary inflammation regardless of low-density lipoprotein level. Withdrawal prior to surgery has been associated with increased cardiac events.

8. **Warfarin,** depending upon the indication and in consultation with the surgical team and prescribing provider, should be discontinued at least 3 to 5 days before surgery, and heparin therapy initiated.

9. If **regional anesthesia** is planned, anticoagulant and antiplatelet agents should be held according to the most recent American Society of Regional Anesthesia (ASRA) guidelines and in consultation with the surgeon and cardiologist.

B. **Respiratory system.** Many vascular patients have histories of significant tobacco use and may have compromised pulmonary function (see Chapter 4). Routine pulmonary function testing is not indicated. Aortic cross-clamping and associated ischemia-reperfusion can produce a systemic inflammatory response that may contribute to postoperative lung injury.

C. **Renal system.** Preexisting renal dysfunction is common. It is related to atherosclerosis, hypertension, diabetes, and advanced age and may exist even in the absence of an abnormal serum creatinine value. Due to a decreased number of functioning glomeruli, these patients have a reduced capacity to autoregulate renal perfusion in the setting of hypotension and are often intolerant to perioperative insults such as ischemia-reperfusion, atheroembolism, and nephrotoxins like contrast dye. Patients with chronically elevated serum creatinine levels (>2 mg/dL) have substantially greater morbidity and mortality following vascular surgery. Open aortic and renal arterial surgeries carry the highest risk for postoperative renal dysfunction. Patients undergoing endovascular procedures are at risk for **contrast-induced acute kidney injury (CI-AKI).** CI-AKI is diagnosed by an increase in serum creatinine beginning 24 to 48 hours following contrast exposure in a patient with no other reason for AKI. In otherwise healthy patients, the risk of CI-AKI is low and its clinical relevance is debated. The risk of CI-AKI is increased in patients with chronic kidney disease, diabetes, anemia, heart failure, and hemodynamic instability. Procedures using high-osmolar contrast or high volumes of contrast are higher risk. In patients at risk, crystalloid administration and the use of low volumes of iso-osmolar or low-osmolar contrast agents are recommended. Treatment with sodium bicarbonate and N-acetylcysteine has also been used to prevent CI-AKI. However, results of the PRESERVE trial demonstrated neither a benefit of sodium bicarbonate over saline nor a benefit of NAC over placebo in preventing AKI.

D. Central nervous system. Patients should be examined for carotid bruits and questioned for a history of transient ischemic attacks (TIAs) and cerebrovascular accidents. Symptomatic carotid disease may warrant revascularization prior to other elective procedures.

E. Endocrine system. In addition to accelerated atherosclerosis, patients with long-standing diabetes may have extensive microvascular disease resulting in autonomic dysfunction, silent myocardial ischemia, and nephropathy. In consultation with the patient's endocrinologist, **metformin** should be discontinued prior to procedures that involve IV contrast dye or renal or hepatic ischemia due to the potential for the development of severe lactic acidosis. It should also be held in patients with preexisting renal dysfunction or heart failure.

F. Hematologic system. The vascular surgical patient is at particularly high risk to develop **heparin-induced thrombocytopenia (HIT)** due to the need for repeated and occasionally prolonged exposure to heparin (see Chapter 24). This syndrome is characterized by thrombocytopenia and/or thrombosis in the setting of heparin exposure and is due to the formation of antibodies to the heparin-platelet factor 4 (PF4) complex. The 4T score helps determine the pretest probability of a HIT diagnosis and should guide clinical management (eg, suspension of heparin administration if the probability is intermediate or high). Generally, if the pretest probability of HIT is intermediate or high, heparin administration should be suspended and laboratory testing pursued. Anti-PF4 antibody levels are a sensitive but not specific test for HIT and are generally checked first. A negative anti-PF4 antibody test makes HIT unlikely. If anti-PF4 levels are elevated, a serotonin release assay (SRA) is recommended. If the SRA is negative, heparin can be used intraoperatively irrespective of the result of the anti-PF4 antibody test. If both the anti-PF4 antibody test and the SRA are positive, surgery should be delayed or an alternative anticoagulant should be used. The **acute management** of the patient with HIT includes discontinuation of all heparins, suspension of warfarin, avoidance of platelet transfusions, and the initiation of alternative, nonheparin, anticoagulant therapy.

II. PERIPHERAL ARTERIAL SURGERY

A. General considerations. Peripheral arterial procedures include the bypass or stenting of stenotic arteries; embolectomy of occluded arteries; and the repair of peripheral arterial aneurysms. Endovascular approaches are employed whenever possible and are typically performed in the operating room, angiography suites, or hybrid operating rooms. Special considerations for the provision of anesthesia outside of the operating room are discussed in Chapter 34.

B. Percutaneous balloon angioplasty and stenting. Limb patency and amputation-free survival rates are similar to open bypass surgery. Patients must have a target lesion amenable to the endovascular approach: typically a focal short-segment occlusion with patent vessels distal to the treated lesion (ie, "good runoff"). Advantages of percutaneous therapy include faster patient recovery, shorter hospital stay, smaller wounds with lower complication rates, and potential cost savings. Procedures on the upper and lower extremities are typically performed in the operating room angiography suites and are frequently done under local anesthesia with sedation.

1. **Surgical approach** may be percutaneous or through a cutdown to the artery. Brachial artery access may be required necessitating IV placement and blood pressure monitoring on the contralateral arm.

2. **Large amounts of intravenous contrast dye** may be administered and may require prophylaxis for CI-AKI (see Section I.C).

3. **Anesthetic technique** frequently involves monitored anesthesia care with standard monitors. Local anesthesia typically provides sufficient analgesia. Provisions should be made to allow for conversion to general anesthesia in the case of an unplanned conversion to open repair.

4. **IV unfractionated heparin** is often used as an adjunct and is given prior to arterial cannulation. A **vasodilator** may be administered intra-arterially by the surgeon to treat catheter or wire-induced vasospasm. Treatment of systemic effects may be required.

5. **Distal embolization** is a potential serious complication with aggressive endovascular instrumentation.

C. **Lower-extremity bypass grafting.** In the presence of multisegment disease or poor distal runoff, open **surgical bypass** of the lower extremity is preferred over the endovascular approach. An autologous saphenous vein graft is the most commonly used conduit. If this is not available, or is of unacceptable quality, an upper extremity vein from the patient or cryopreserved cadaveric vein may be used. Preparation of the vein and subsequent anastomoses to the arterial circulation may be time consuming but rarely place significant hemodynamic stress on the patient. The use of synthetic grafts in selected patients may reduce the length of these procedures; however, long-term patency rates with prosthetic grafts are generally reduced relative to autologous vein grafts. **Blood loss is usually minimal,** but may be significant with revision of a previous bypass. **Routine monitoring** is usually sufficient. Patient comorbidities or surgical complexity may warrant placement of invasive monitors. **No significant differences in morbidity or mortality have been demonstrated between regional anesthesia and general anesthesia** for lower limb revascularization.

1. **General anesthesia.** Any technique is appropriate provided hemodynamic stability is maintained.

2. **Regional anesthesia.** Potential advantages may include sympathetic blockade, improved pain control, lack of airway instrumentation, improved ability to detect symptoms of myocardial ischemia in an awake patient, and reduced incidence of pneumonia. However, long procedures under regional anesthesia can pose a challenge for patients who may become uncomfortable and restless.

   a. A continuous **lumbar epidural catheter** is commonly used. It provides excellent analgesia and muscle relaxation as well as the ability to administer postoperative analgesia. Spinal anesthesia may be used if the length of the procedure is appropriate. For **femoral-popliteal** and distal lower extremity bypass limited to a single limb, combined lumbar plexus and sciatic nerve block may be used as an alternative to neuraxial anesthesia. For **iliofemoral bypass**, a spinal or epidural will require a higher level (ie, T8-T10) because of proximal extension of the incision and peritoneal retraction for exposure of the iliac artery. **Femoral-femoral bypass grafting** is used to treat symptomatic unilateral iliac occlusive disease.

   b. An α-adrenergic agent (eg, phenylephrine) should be available to treat the hypotension associated with sympathetic blockade.

D. **Peripheral embolectomy and femoral pseudoaneurysm.** Femoral pseudoaneurysms are most often iatrogenic, occurring in the setting of femoral artery catheterization (eg, for coronary angiography or intra-aortic balloon pump placement). As such, these patients often have unstable cardiovascular disease (eg, recent MI with stent placement). Some are anticoagulated or have recently received thrombolytic agents, thus precluding regional anesthesia. Field blocks with local anesthesia may be most appropriate in the setting of cardiovascular instability. Embolectomy of an obstructed artery may be associated with significant blood loss and hypotension.

E. **Peripheral aneurysms.** Peripheral arterial aneurysms, such as popliteal artery aneurysms, rarely rupture but are associated with a high rate of thrombosis and embolism. Either general or neuraxial anesthesia may be used to manage their repair.

F. **Axillofemoral bypass grafting.** An axillofemoral bypass graft restores arterial blood flow to the lower extremities in patients with occluded aortoiliac vessels who are not candidates for aortic reconstruction for various reasons including high anesthetic risk, significant intra-abdominal adhesions due to prior abdominal surgeries, active abdominal infection, or an infected aortic prosthesis. A prosthetic graft is tunneled under the pectoralis muscle and positioned in the subcutaneous layer of the thorax and abdomen and anastomosed distally to the femoral artery. General anesthesia is most appropriate.

G. **Vascular surgery of the upper extremity.** Vascular surgery of the upper extremity usually includes distal embolectomy and repair of traumatic injuries. The surgery is localized, but there may be a need to harvest a vein graft at a site distant from the vascular repair. Possible anesthetic techniques include field block and regional or general anesthesia.

III. CAROTID REVASCULARIZATION

A. **General considerations.** Carotid revascularization is performed in patients with stenotic lesions of the internal carotid artery. These lesions often present as carotid bruits and may produce TIAs or strokes. The indication for surgical revascularization takes into account patient life expectancy, surgical complication rates, the presence of symptoms, and the degree of stenosis. CEA is indicated for patients with nondisabling stroke or TIA who have greater than 70% stenosis by noninvasive imaging, as long as their life expectancy is greater than or equal to 5 years and the surgeon's perioperative stroke and death risk is less than 6%. 2014 American Heart Association/American Stroke Association guidelines also suggest CEA be considered in patients with symptomatic stenosis of 50% to 69% depending on age, sex, and comorbidities. The data are less clear for patients with asymptomatic disease. CEA may be indicated in asymptomatic males with greater than 70% stenosis and a life expectancy in excess of 5 years if the surgeon's perioperative stroke and death risk is less than 3%. It is not clear that CEA is more effective than medical therapy in women with asymptomatic carotid artery stenosis. If the patient does not meet criteria for surgical revascularization, risk factor modification with medical therapy and lifestyle changes is instituted. This consists of statin and antiplatelet therapy, smoking cessation, blood pressure control, and management of diabetes. CEA is the preferred modality for operative therapy of carotid artery stenosis. The role of carotid artery stenting (CAS) is still being defined. Evidence suggests that CAS and CEA have similar long-term results, but CAS is associated with a higher rate of periprocedural morbidity and mortality. In symptomatic patients, CAS is recommended for patients with difficult surgical access (ie, prior neck dissections) or radiation-induced carotid stenosis as long as the surgeon's postoperative stroke and death risk is less than 6%. CAS is not recommended for patients with asymptomatic carotid artery stenosis. Along with the standard history and physical, the preoperative anesthetic assessment should focus on the documentation of **existing neurologic deficits** as well as the **range of motion of the patient's neck**.

B. **Carotid artery stenting**
1. **Indications.** CAS may be preferred over CEA in patients with neck anatomy that is unfavorable for open surgery, such as with prior neck surgery or radiation, or in patients with higher operative risk due to severe cardiac or pulmonary disease. Due to the potential for CI-AKI, CAS is generally avoided in patients with renal dysfunction.
2. **Monitoring.** An arterial catheter is indicated for continuous hemodynamic monitoring and facilitates frequent blood draws for monitoring of activated clotting time (ACT). Close observation of the patient's **mental status** is necessary to detect new-onset stroke resulting from plaque embolization.
3. **Anesthetic management** usually consists of monitored anesthesia care combined with local anesthesia at the vascular access site. Care should be taken to maintain the patient's level of alertness to facilitate intraoperative neurologic monitoring. The femoral artery is typically accessed percutaneously. The awake patient may feel pain during balloon angioplasty and arterial dilation that resolves immediately with balloon deflation.
4. **IV contrast dye** and fluoroscopy are used intermittently throughout the procedure.
5. **Heparin** is administered prior to arteriotomy.
6. Vagally mediated **bradycardia** can occur following stent deployment. Pretreatment with glycopyrrolate is helpful.
7. **Complications** include stroke, vascular access site injuries, device malfunction, restenosis, and CI-AKI. Microembolic injuries are more frequent after CAS compared with CEA; embolic protection devices can reduce neurologic injuries if the operator is experienced with the apparatus.

C. **Carotid endarterectomy**
1. **Monitoring.**
   a. **Intra-arterial blood pressure monitoring is necessary.**
   b. **CNS monitoring** is necessary, especially during carotid cross-clamp application, to evaluate the adequacy of cerebral perfusion and to identify patients who may require **shunting**. The awake patient is the gold standard for intraoperative CNS monitoring. If the procedure is being conducted under general anesthesia, the CNS can be monitored using **electroencephalography** (EEG), transcranial Doppler ultrasound, or arterial stump pressure measurement. CEA can also be conducted with routine shunting without continuous CNS monitoring. There are no data to support the use of routine versus selective shunting. No particular method of CNS monitoring in selective shunting has been shown to produce better outcomes.
2. **Anesthetic technique.** The superiority of general versus regional anesthesia has been debated. Retrospective observational studies have suggested a benefit to regional techniques, including in a meta-analysis. However, pooled analysis of available randomized trials did not find a difference between the techniques. If a clinical difference exists, it is

likely small and anesthetic technique is usually based on the preferences of the surgeon and the patient.

a. Regional anesthesia

1. Regional anesthesia may be performed with a combined **super-ficial** and **deep cervical plexus block** or with a superficial plexus block that is supplemented in the field by the surgeon (see Chapter 18). Both have potential complications.

2. CEA under regional anesthesia **requires an alert, cooperative patient** who is able to tolerate lying still, with the head rotated to the side, under the drapes.

3. **Access to the airway** may be necessary at any time, and the patient should be positioned and draped with this in mind. An appropriately sized laryngeal mask airway should be readily available.

4. **Continuous neurologic** assessment is possible in the awake patient.

b. General anesthesia

1. **Prior to induction, neuromonitoring baselines** are established.

2. **Blood pressure** should be maintained at the patient's **high-normal** range that may require a vasopressor.

3. **A hemodynamically stable induction** is desired to preserve cerebral perfusion.

4. Minute ventilation should be adjusted to avoid hypocapnic cere-bral vasoconstriction. Hypercarbia has no clinical benefit.

5. When employing intraoperative EEG monitoring, communica-tion with the neuromonitoring team is essential. Goals include a stable anesthetic plane to facilitate EEG interpretation and the avoidance of burst suppression. **Neuromuscular blockade** mini-mizes muscle artifact that can interfere with EEG interpretation and with inadvertent patient movement during delicate portions of the procedure.

6. The goals during emergence are twofold: to minimize straining, which poses a risk to the arteriotomy closure, and to facilitate a **prompt neurologic examination** in case of new neurologic or cra-nial nerve deficit. This is best summarized as a crisp, smooth emergence.

3. Carotid cross-clamping

a. Systemic heparin is administered before cross-clamping.

b. Prior to cross-clamp, **blood pressure** is typically increased by the use of a vasopressor, with the intention of maintaining ipsilateral cere-bral perfusion through the Circle of Willis from the contralateral carotid.

c. Surgical manipulation of the carotid sinus may cause intense vagal stimulation, leading to hypotension and bradycardia. Release of traction or infiltration with local anesthetic will typically abolish the response. Administration of anticholinergics is seldom required. Prophylactic infiltration of local anesthetic infiltration should be considered for patients with significant preoperative cardiac con-duction delay, critical aortic stenosis, and significant coronary disease.

d. Routine shunting, selective shunting, or no shunting. Shunting involves the placement of a temporary arterial graft to span the arteriotomy and preserve ipsilateral, antegrade cerebral perfusion during carotid artery cross-clamping. The approach to shunting is based on surgi-cal preference. A number of case series have shown similar stroke risk with the three approaches. Selective shunting describes the practice of shunt placement upon EEG evidence of cerebral ischemia following carotid cross-clamping.

  e. **Unclamping** may produce reflex vasodilation and bradycardia. Vasopressors may be required as the baroreceptors adapt, which may continue into the postoperative period.

D. **Postoperative considerations**

  1. Immediate postoperative complications include **neurologic deficits, blood pressure lability, and airway obstruction.**

  2. **Neurologic deficits** are typically due to emboli related to the surgical procedure. They should be managed aggressively with increased blood pressure and consultation with the surgeon and a stroke specialist.

  3. **Labile blood pressures** may be observed secondary to alterations in the carotid baroreceptor response brought about by the endarterectomy. Hypertension requiring administration of vasodilator (labetalol or hydralazine boluses or escalating to nitroglycerin or nicardipine as an IV infusion) may be a result of surgical denervation of the carotid sinus. Hypotension requiring a vasopressor (phenylephrine) may be a result of baroreceptor hypersensitivity and typically does not reflect hypovolemia.

  4. **Postextubation airway compromise** can be secondary to dehiscence at the arteriotomy suture line leading expanding hematoma. The immediate release of the superficial sutures with evacuation of the hematoma is necessary to prevent airway compromise.

  5. Other etiologies for postextubation airway compromise include **injury to the recurrent laryngeal, superior laryngeal, or hypoglossal nerves.** Unilateral recurrent laryngeal nerve injury manifests with a hoarse voice. Bilateral recurrent laryngeal nerve injury is rare but must be considered in patients who have undergone previous contralateral CEA or neck surgery.

  6. **Cerebral hyperperfusion syndrome** typically occurs several days postoperatively and may manifest as ipsilateral headache, seizure, focal neurologic signs, or intracranial hemorrhage. It is related to an abrupt increase in blood flow with loss of autoregulation in the surgically reperfused brain. Based on the pathophysiology of the syndrome, **it is reasonable to target postoperative blood pressures in the normal to slightly subnormal range** (often systolic blood pressure [SBP] < 140 mm Hg).

IV. **ABDOMINAL AORTIC REPAIR**

  Abdominal aortic repair may be required for atherosclerotic occlusive disease or aneurysmal dilation of the aorta. Aorto-occlusive disease usually presents as claudication. An abdominal aortic aneurysm (AAA) may be found incidentally. Alternatively, it may present with back pain or, if ruptured, severe shock. Ninety-five percent of all AAAs occur below the level of the renal arteries. Indications for repair are largest diameter greater than 5.5 cm; rate of expansion exceeding 1 cm/y; or symptoms secondary to the AAA. In females, repair of asymptomatic AAA may be indicated at a lower diameter threshold due to a higher rate of rupture, although females may also be at a higher perioperative risk. The annual risk of rupture of an expanding 5-cm aneurysm is about 4%. The operative mortality for elective AAA repair is less than 2%, while the overall mortality of aneurysm rupture is 70% to 80%.

  A. **Endovascular abdominal aortic repair (EVAR)**

    1. **Overview.** The majority of infrarenal AAA are treated by EVAR. The procedure involves the endovascular placement of an expandable stent graft spanning the aneurysm under fluoroscopic guidance. The stent

graft excludes the aneurysm from the circulation preventing its expansion and rupture. The application of an aortic **cross clamp is not required** consequently. **EVAR leads to greater intraoperative hemodynamic stability.** There is a lower incidence of postoperative pulmonary, cardiovascular, and renal morbidity and significantly reduced 30-day operative mortality for EVAR compared to open surgery. The early survival benefit is lost over time. At about 2 years postprocedure, mortality rates are the same as those for patients who have undergone open aneurysm resection. Patients with endovascular repair also require regular follow-up imaging and may require additional EVAR-related interventions.

2. **Patient suitability** for EVAR depends on the size and morphology of the AAA. Most infrarenal AAAs with favorable neck anatomy are repaired endovascularly. EVAR has lower short-term, perioperative mortality, but higher incidence of leak and other long-term complications, and requires a lifetime of imaging surveillance. Younger patients with better risk profile may more suited for open repair.

3. **Monitoring and access.** Intra-arterial blood pressure monitoring is required in addition to standard monitors. Large bore peripheral access (16 gauge or 14 gauge) is desirable. Central venous access is rarely required.

4. **Surgical considerations.** Systemic **heparinization** is required. If the aneurysm involves the renal or mesenteric arteries, a more complex endovascular stent graft with branches or fenestrations can be used. For infrarenal aneurysms, **surgical access is usually via bilateral common femoral arteries**. Exposure of the arteries followed by arteriotomies is typically performed with surgical repair afterward. Percutaneous access with subsequent closure using a specialized device is possible for select patients in the absence of femoral artery disease or stenosis. There is significant **radiation exposure** with **fluoroscopy** and a **contrast** dye load. **Ensuring the patient does not move** during digital subtraction angiography will reduce the patient's exposure by minimizing the need for repeated studies. Following stent graft deployment, an intra-aortic balloon is inflated to expand the stent graft and anchor it in place. Balloon inflation leads to temporary aortic occlusion. The occlusion is short lived, typically lasting 3 to 4 heartbeats. Hypertension may be observed during the period of balloon occlusion; however, it usually does not last long enough to warrant therapy. **Controlled hypotension** may be requested by the surgeon during stent graft deployment to prevent proximal hypertension and stent graft displacement.

5. **Anesthetic technique.** EVAR may be performed under **local, regional**, or **general anesthesia.** Factors such as anticoagulant use, patient comfort, surgeon preference, and anticipated length of surgery will influence the choice of anesthetic. There is some evidence to suggest lower morbidity and mortality, shorter hospital stays, and fewer ICU admissions with local or regional anesthesia as compared to general anesthesia. Bilateral ilioinguinal or iliohypogastric nerve blocks are alternatives along with local infiltration. Of note, in contrast to neuraxial anesthesia, local anesthesia will not alleviate the ischemia pain associated with femoral artery occlusion, and supplementation with systemic analgesics may be required.

6. **Conversion to open repair is rare (<1%).** It may be necessary in the setting of difficult arterial access (eg, with severely atherosclerotic arteries); vessel dissection at the arterial access site; tortuous iliac arteries that prevent passage of the deployment system; stent malposition or

migration; and aneurysm rupture. Resuscitation equipment such as a red blood cell salvage device and a rapid infusion device should be available in centers performing EVAR.

7. **Bleeding** may occur around the femoral sheaths and is often difficult to quantify or track. Massive hemorrhage is rare.

8. **Complications of EVAR** include failure to exclude the AAA from the arterial system (endoleak), embolism, arterial injury, graft kinking, groin access injury, limb ischemia and infection. AKI can result from contrast administration and embolization of debris dislodged by catheters and wires (see Section I.C).

   a. **Endoleak (Figure 28.1)** is the persistence of blood flow into the aneurysm sac leading to expansion. It occurs in 20% to 25% of EVARs. Types I and III endoleaks are considered at high risk for aneurysm sac pressurization and rupture and should be treated as soon as diagnosed. Type II endoleaks may spontaneously resolve and are followed closely with serial imaging. If they persist, they may require a subsequent procedure to embolize the responsible vessel. Treatment is not recommended for type IV endoleaks.

B. Open abdominal aortic surgery

   Patient selection. Open surgical repair is indicated for patients whose aortic anatomy does not meet the specified minimum requirements for standard, commercially available endografts; for patients in whom delaying repair to wait for a custom-made endograft may result in significant risk of rupture; and for patients unlikely to comply with long-term imaging surveillance protocols following EVAR.

1. **Surgical approach.** Compared with a **transabdominal** approach, the **retroperitoneal (RP)** approach may result in a lower incidence of postoperative ileus, pulmonary complications, cardiovascular complications, and fluid shifts. The RP approach is technically advantageous in morbidly obese patients and in those who have had previous abdominal procedures.

2. **Monitoring.** A large peripheral IV, arterial line, central venous catheter, and Foley catheter are indicated. Procedures that require a supraceliac cross-clamp entail greater hemodynamic perturbations and blood loss. Enhanced intraoperative monitoring of cardiac function with TEE or PA catheter may be beneficial. Vasopressors and vasodilators must be available.

3. **Anesthetic technique.** Most patients receive combined general and epidural anesthesia using a low-thoracic to midthoracic epidural catheter. Although general anesthesia alone is acceptable, a combined technique reduces anesthetic requirements, facilitates earlier extubation, and provides effective postoperative analgesia. Retrospective data suggests a mortality benefit with epidural use in elective AAA repair.

4. The hemodynamic goal of **induction** is to **avoid hypertension.** It is helpful to establish a sensory level with the epidural catheter prior to the induction of general anesthesia.

5. **Heat conservation.** Heat loss during aortic procedures may be considerable. Strategies for heat conservation are discussed in Chapter 19. Forced air warmers should **never** be used **below the level of the aortic cross-clamp**. Severe burns may develop during cross-clamping due to the absence of heat redistribution by normal blood flow.

6. **Bowel manipulation** is necessary to gain access to the aorta during the transabdominal approach and may be accompanied by skin flushing, decreased systemic vascular resistance, and profound hypotension.

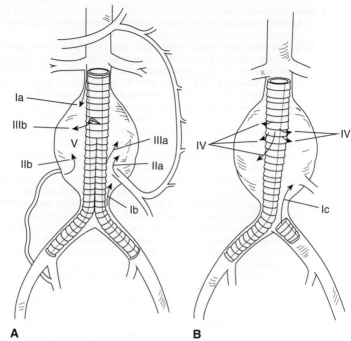

FIGURE 28.1 A and B, Schematic demonstrating the different types of endoleak after endovascular aneurysm repair. Type I endoleaks occur because of inadequate graft seal resulting in perigraft flow and include (Ia) perigraft flow occurring proximally, (Ib) perigraft flow occurring distally, and (Ic) perigraft flow around an iliac artery occlusion device. Type II endoleaks occur when branch arteries backbleed because of collateral flow. These endoleaks include (IIa) backbleeding inferior mesenteric artery and (IIb) backbleeding lumbar artery. Type III endoleaks occur when flow persists between the segments of a modular graft and include (IIIa) leaks between iliac limbs or an iliac limb and main body component and (IIIb) leaks between main body components. Type IV endoleaks (IV) occur when flow is present through endograft material (graft porosity). Type V endoleak, or, "endotension" (V), occurs when persistent or recurrent pressurization of the aortic aneurysm exists in the absence of demonstrable endoleak. (Drawings prepared by H. Fischer, MFA.)

These changes may be caused by the release of prostaglandins and vaso-active peptides from the bowel and last for 20 to 30 minutes. Treatment consists of vasopressor administration and volume expansion.

7. **Fluid management.** There is the potential for significant intravascular volume depletion due to hemorrhage; insensible losses into the bowel and peritoneal cavity; and evaporative losses associated with the lapa-rotomy. Volume resuscitation is guided by the patient's hemodynamics. Aortic cross-clamp application will give rise to renal insufficiency, even with an infrarenal cross-clamp.

8. **Blood product administration** should be guided by the patient's labora-tory values.

 9. **Aortic cross-clamping**
   a. **Systemic heparin** is administered several minutes prior to the application of the aortic cross-clamp.
   b. **Hypertension** will occur with aortic cross-clamping. The degree of hypertension is a function of the cross-clamp location. A more proximal cross-clamp is associated with a greater increase in blood pressure. Consideration can be given to inducing mild hypotension prior to the application of the cross-clamp. The **increased afterload** is well tolerated by patients with normal cardiac function, but those with compromised left ventricular function may develop myocardial ischemia and hypotension. Hypotension with the application of the aortic cross-clamp may indicate left ventricular failure secondary to increased afterload or retrograde dissection into the coronary arteries. Cardiac function must be evaluated and supported.
   c. Avoidance of excessive hypertension is important during aortic cross-clamp to minimize the **risk of retrograde aortic dissection.**
   d. Following proximal clamping, **vascular control distal to the aneurysm** is established. If the vasculature distal to the aneurysm has been surgically exposed, distal control may be achieved via the application of a cross-clamp on the aorta or common iliac arteries distal to the aneurysm. If the distal vasculature is not exposed, endovascular control is achieved. Once the aneurysm sac is opened, a balloon-tipped catheter is advanced distal to the aneurysm. Balloon inflation occludes the vessel and prevents backbleeding, establishing distal control. Significant retrograde hemorrhage may occur during this maneuver.
   e. There is no compelling evidence to support the use of renal protective adjuncts such as **mannitol and fenoldopam.** The application of an aortic cross-clamp at any level may lead to decreased renal cortical blood flow and urine output. With suprarenal clamping, renal perfusion is at even greater risk due to longer cross-clamp times and potential for cholesterol embolization. The maintenance of adequate hydration and urine output is paramount.

10. **Aortic unclamping**
   a. Unclamping will produce immediate **hypotension** due to a fall in systemic vascular resistance.
   b. The degree of hypotension is a function of clamp duration and the proximal extent of the clamp.
   c. Prior to release of the aortic cross-clamp, steps should be taken to optimize the patient's intravascular **volume status** and **increase vascular tone.** Inspired oxygen concentration should be increased to 100%. **Minute ventilation** may also be increased to induce a mild respiratory alkalosis.
   d. Following unclamping, reperfusion of the ischemic organs and tissues leads to acidemia and systemic vasodilation. The magnitude of these disturbances is a function of the duration of the aortic cross-clamp and the metabolic activity of the organs that were ischemic. **Cross-clamping above the celiac or superior mesenteric artery can produce profound visceral ischemia and acidosis. Sodium bicarbonate** may be administered at unclamping to mitigate the effects of acidosis. In the setting of profound hypotension that is unresponsive to fluids or vasopressors, the aortic cross-clamp may be reapplied to maintain adequate perfusion pressure while additional volume and vasopressors are administered.

11. **Emergence.** Most patients with working epidurals and infrarenal or juxtarenal cross-clamps can be extubated at the end of the procedure. Patients with hemodynamic instability, persistent hemorrhage, persistent acidosis, or severe hypothermia (<33 °C) are left intubated. Hypertension, tachycardia, pain, and shivering should be anticipated and treated.

C. **Emergent repair of a ruptured AAA.** Patients may be **hemodynamically stable or unstable** depending on the degree to which the rupture is contained. Rupture can occur into the peritoneal cavity or the RP space. Some measure of tamponade will temporarily reduce the volume of blood loss.

1. The priority for anesthetic management is the establishment of adequate **IV access** for large volume resuscitation.

2. **Blood products** should be ordered immediately. If type-specific blood and FFP are unavailable, universal donor-type blood (type O negative for women of childbearing age and type O positive for all others) and FFP (type AB) should be obtained, and a **blood bank sample** should be sent immediately to the lab for cross-matching. **Colloid solutions** should be ordered. A red blood cell salvage system as well as a rapid transfuser should be immediately available.

3. **Standard monitors** should initially be applied if the patient is unstable, so as not to delay definitive surgical control. The immediate priority is to control bleeding surgically by cross-clamping the aorta through a laparotomy or thoracotomy. Alternatively, the aorta may be occluded endovascularly using a balloon-tipped catheter. Invasive monitors (arterial line, central line, PA catheter) may be placed as time and hemodynamics permit. **Clear communication with the surgical team** regarding the surgical and anesthetic plans is essential. If the patient's hemodynamics permit, placement of a central venous catheter is often performed while the patient is awake.

4. **Hypotensive resuscitation** that involves restricting intravascular volume administration to maintain SBP in the 70 to 100 mm Hg range has been recommended. Evidence for this management strategy is borrowed from the trauma literature, and this strategy has not been studied in ruptured aortic syndromes. The physiologic rationale behind this strategy is to limit hypothermic and dilutional coagulopathy while avoiding clot disruption caused by increases in SBP.

5. Based on the clinical circumstances, the surgical plan, and the available equipment, it may be preferable to insert an occlusive balloon-tipped catheter into the aorta above the level of the aneurysm prior to the induction of general anesthesia. Such a catheter may be inserted percutaneously using local anesthesia. It can then be used to occlude the aorta in the event of circulatory collapse following anesthetic induction.

6. **Surgical technique: endovascular versus open**
   a. **Open repair**
      1. **Induction.** In moribund patients, endotracheal intubation should be performed immediately. Hypotensive patients should be preoxygenated and induced expeditiously. Hemodynamics may allow for only small doses of scopolamine, etomidate, ketamine, and a benzodiazepine. **Severe hypotension on induction may occur** as a result of vasodilation, loss of sympathetic drive, and loss of peritoneal tamponade with abdominal wall relaxation. The patient should be prepped and draped prior to induction and the surgeon ready to make incision if needed.

2. Care must be taken to **avoid hypertension** during induction.
3. Once the aorta has been clamped and hemodynamic stability achieved, incremental doses of opioids and supplemental anesthetics may be given as tolerated.
4. Blood component therapy should be guided by the laboratory values. In the event of massive hemorrhage, packed red blood cells and FFP should be administered in a ratio of at least 2:1.
5. **Hypothermia** contributes to acidosis, coagulopathy, and myocardial dysfunction and should be treated.
6. **Renal protective strategies** such as aggressive hydration and the maintenance of appropriate perfusion pressure should be instituted. The administration of mannitol and fenoldopam may be considered, although there is no compelling evidence to support their use. Mortality in patients developing renal failure following a ruptured AAA is high.

b. **Endovascular repair** can be considered as an alternative to open repair provided anatomy is suitable, the center is appropriately equipped, and the team is appropriately experienced. The procedure may be performed under local anesthesia. Retrospective studies have shown a survival benefit in patients treated with EVAR, but evidence from prospective randomized trials is lacking.

7. **Complications and prognosis.** Under the best of circumstances, there is a 40% to 50% mortality rate. The incidence of MI, acute renal failure, respiratory failure, and coagulopathy is high.

V. THORACOABDOMINAL AORTIC ANEURYSM REPAIR

A. **Etiology of thoracic aortic disease**. Causes of thoracic aortic disease include atherosclerosis, degenerative disorders of connective tissue (eg, Marfan and Ehlers-Danlos syndromes and cystic necrosis), infection (eg, syphilis), congenital defects (eg, coarctation and congenital aneurysms of the sinus of Valsalva), trauma (eg, penetrating and deceleration injuries), and inflammatory processes (eg, Takayasu aortitis). The most common problem affecting the thoracic aorta is **atherosclerotic aneurysm** of the descending portion, accounting for about 20% of all aortic aneurysms. When such aneurysms dissect proximally, they may involve the aortic valve or coronary ostia. Distal dissection may involve the abdominal aorta with renal or mesenteric involvement. The next most frequent problem is **traumatic disruption** of the thoracic aorta. Adventitial false aneurysms may form distal to the left subclavian artery at the insertion of the ligamentum arteriosum, because of penetrating or deceleration injuries. These false aneurysms may dissect proximally and involve the arch and its major branches.

B. **Crawford classification** of thoracoabdominal aneurysms (**Figure 28.2**).
1. **Type I.** Aneurysm of the descending thoracic aorta distal to the subclavian artery, ending at or above the origin of the visceral vessels.
2. **Type II.** Aneurysm from the origin of the subclavian artery to the distal abdominal aorta. This is the highest risk type in terms of paralysis, renal failure, and mortality.
3. **Type III.** Aneurysm from the mid-descending thoracic aorta to the distal abdominal aorta.
4. **Type IV.** Aneurysm from the diaphragm down to the distal aorta.

C. **Associated findings**
1. **Airway deviation or compression**, particularly of the left mainstem bronchus, producing atelectasis.

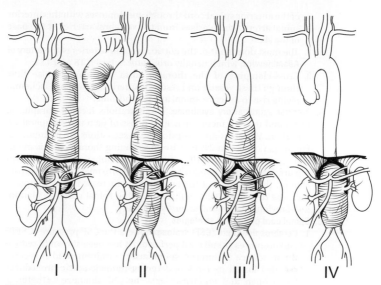

FIGURE 28.2 Crawford classification of thoracic and thoracoabdominal aortic aneurysms. (From Crawford ES, Crawford JL, Safi HJ, et al. Thoracoabdominal aortic aneurysms preoperative and intraoperative factors determining immediate and long-term results of operations in 605 patients. *J Vasc Surg.* 1986;3:389-404.)

2. **Tracheal displacement or disruption**, producing difficulties with endotracheal intubation and ventilation. Long-standing aneurysms may give rise to recurrent laryngeal nerve damage, resulting in vocal cord paralysis and hoarseness.
3. **Hemoptysis**, due to the erosion of the aneurysm into an adjacent bronchus.
4. **Esophageal compression** with dysphagia and an increased risk of aspiration.
5. **Distortion and compression of the central venous and arterial anatomy**, producing markedly asymmetric pulses and difficult internal jugular vein cannulation.
6. **Hemothorax and mediastinal shift** from rupture or leakage, producing respiratory and circulatory compromise.
7. **Reduced distal perfusion** secondary to aortic branch vessel occlusion, producing renal, mesenteric, spinal cord, or extremity ischemia.

D. **Open thoracic aortic aneurysm repair**
   1. **Surgical technique.** During repair of the aneurysm, the affected aortic segment is isolated, and an interposition graft is inserted. During aortic cross-clamping, distal aortic perfusion may be provided by atrial-femoral bypass. The **inclusion technique** involves using the portion of native aorta containing the celiac, superior mesenteric, and renal ostia as a component of the bypass graft.
   2. **Spinal cord protection**
      a. **Anatomy**
         1. **Aortic radicular arteries**, arising segmentally from the lumbar and lower thoracic regions of the aorta, contribute to the blood supply

of the anterior spinal cord through anastomoses with the anterior spinal artery, which arises from the vertebral arteries at the base of the skull.

2. The most dominant of the aortic radicular arteries is the **artery of Adamkiewicz**, which usually originates between T8 and T12.

3. Cross-clamping of the thoracic aorta may compromise flow through these vessels and result in anterior spinal cord ischemia giving rise to anterior spinal artery syndrome.

b. **Anterior spinal artery syndrome.** Manifestations include paraplegia, rectal and urinary incontinence, and loss of pain and temperature sensation. Vibratory and proprioceptive sensations are maintained. Paraplegia occurs in 2% to 4% of descending thoracic aortic aneurysm repairs and 3% to 10% of thoracoabdominal aortic aneurysm repairs. **Risk factors** include the location of proximal and distal cross-clamps; the duration of the cross-clamp; increased body temperature; the degree of collateralization of the spinal cord circulation; and previous abdominal aneurysm surgery.

c. **Spinal cord protection strategies**

1. **Cerebrospinal fluid (CSF) drainage** lowers the CSF pressure (CSFP) and promotes spinal cord perfusion. It has been shown to reduce the incidence of anterior spinal artery syndrome and is recommended for all patients undergoing thoracic aortic procedures (both open and endovascular). The CSF drainage catheter is inserted at the L4-5 level and advanced 8 to 12 cm into the subarachnoid space. CSFP is monitored throughout the procedure and CSF drained to a goal pressure of less than 10 mm Hg. Complications include spinal headache, intracranial hypotension, subdural hemorrhage, epidural or spinal hematoma, meningitis, and persistent CSF leak.

2. **Maintaining a mean arterial pressure (MAP) greater than 80 mm Hg** is recommended. Spinal cord perfusion pressure (SCPP) is the difference between MAP and CSFP (or CVP if it is greater). The target SCPP is greater than 70 mm Hg. This goal can be achieved by maintaining a MAP greater than 80 mm Hg, CSFP less than 10 mm Hg, and CVP less than 10 mm Hg.

3. **Moderate systemic hypothermia** is reasonable for spinal cord protection.

4. **Distal aortic perfusion** using atrial-femoral bypass may be used to minimize ischemic time to the spinal cord and visceral organs.

5. **Motor-evoked potential (MEP) monitoring** and/or somatosensory-evoked potentials (SSEPs) monitoring can be used to detect spinal cord ischemia. In response to the degradation of MEPs or SSEPs, MAP can be raised to encourage collateral perfusion to the spinal cord. Furthermore, the surgeon may reimplant intercostal arteries into the graft.

3. **Renal protection.** Lasix, mannitol, and dopamine have not been demonstrated to reduce the incidence of renal insufficiency. Distal aortic perfusion when the distal clamp is proximal to the renal arteries reduces renal ischemic time. Perfusion of a cold crystalloid (sometimes including mannitol or methylprednisolone and cooled to 4 °C, "renal cold") directly into the renal arteries can reduce the incidence of renal injury.

4. **Monitoring** includes a right upper extremity intra-arterial cannula as application of the aortic cross-clamp proximal to the left subclavian artery is occasionally necessary. A femoral intra-arterial catheter

connected to a pressure transducer is used to monitor distal aortic perfusion pressures during atrial-femoral bypass. CSF pressure transducer is necessary. TEE or PA catheter may be used to monitor cardiac function. Care must be exercised with insertion of the TEE probe as the aneurysm may compress the esophagus.

5. **Anesthetic technique**

   a. **Vasopressors** (phenylephrine and norepinephrine) and **vasodilators** (nitroglycerin and nitroprusside) should be available prior to induction.

   b. **General anesthesia** is induced as detailed in Section IV.B.5 to 6. When MEPs are used for spinal cord monitoring, paralytics and volatile anesthetics must be avoided. Total intravenous anesthesia (TIVA) is required.

   c. **Lung isolation** is achieved to facilitate surgical access and protect the left lung from trauma during left thoracotomy. Lung isolation can be accomplished using a double-lumen tube (DLT) or an endobronchial blocker (see Chapter 27). A right-sided DLT is preferred in case where the aneurysm distorts the left bronchial anatomy. The advantage of using a bronchial blocker is that it avoids the need to change from a DLT to a single-lumen endotracheal tube at the conclusion of the procedure.

   d. **Positioning.** The patient is turned to the right lateral decubitus position with the pelvis at a small degree of tilt to facilitate femoral access. Bite blocks are placed between the molars bilaterally with the tongue free to prevent injury during MEP monitoring.

6. **Maintenance**

   a. **TIVA** with propofol and opioid (and avoidance of neuromuscular blockade) is used for these cases because volatile anesthetics can interfere with spinal cord monitoring.

   b. **Fluid management** is based on the patient's hemodynamics. Fluid administration is limited to FFP, red blood cells, platelets, and colloids in an attempt to limit the development of a coagulopathy and edema brought about by excessive crystalloid administration. A red blood cell salvage system and a rapid infuser should be used.

7. **Aortic cross-clamping**

   a. Prior to cross-clamping, a target CSFP of 6 to 10 mm Hg is maintained.

   b. **Marked hypertension** is universal with a proximal aortic cross-clamp application and is treated with clevidipine or nitroprusside.

   c. **Renal ischemia is minimized** by the infusion of cold crystalloid directly into the renal arteries.

8. **Use of shunts**

   a. Perfusion of the mesentery can be maintained either using a shunt from a limb of the atrial-femoral bypass circuit or through a side-arm shunt (Gott shunt) on the graft.

   b. Distal aortic perfusion through atrial-femoral bypass maintains blood flow to organs distal to the distal aortic clamp. The adequacy of perfusion is monitored using a femoral arterial line. **Table 28.1** summarizes the management consideration for atrial-femoral bypass.

9. **Aortic unclamping** produces hypotension by the mechanism discussed in Section IV.B.13. Volume administration before and during unclamping, slow release of the cross-clamp, and use of vasopressors are continued until myocardial function and vascular tone have returned to baseline.

	Management of Flow Through the Atrial-to-Left-Femoral-Artery Bypass Shunt	
Radial Artery Pressure	**Femoral Artery Pressure**	**Intervention**
↑	↓	Increase pump flow
↓	↑	Decrease pump flow
↓	↓	Administer volume or vasopressor
↑	↑	Administer vasodilator

10. **Systemic acidosis** is universal after the release of the aortic cross-clamp. The degree of acidosis depends on the ischemic time to the organs. An infusion of bicarbonate during the cross-clamping period may minimize the acidemia and preserve the function of the myocardium and vasopressor agents.

11. At the conclusion of the procedure, the patient is kept intubated and sedated. If a double-lumen endotracheal tube was employed for lung isolation, consider exchange to a single-lumen ETT. An appropriately sized airway exchange catheter can mitigate the risk of airway loss: proceed with as there may be significant airway and oropharyngeal edema. An elevated MAP should be maintained to maximize collateral perfusion to the spinal cord.

E. **Endovascular thoracic/thoracoabdominal aortic aneurysm repair (TEVAR)**

1. **Benefits and patient selection.** Endovascular thoracic aortic aneurysm repair leads to significantly lower morbidity than open repair. Patients with significant comorbidities who would be poor candidates for open surgical repair may particularly benefit from endovascular repair. Patients must have suitable aortic anatomy to accommodate a stent graft as well as suitable vascular access sites free from significant atherosclerotic disease to allow large-bore sheath insertion.

2. **Spinal cord and bowel preservation.** To minimize risk of spinal cord ischemia and paraplegia, **CSF monitoring and drainage** are recommended for all thoracic aortic procedures (see Section V.D.2.c.). For thoracoabdominal aortic aneurysm repairs, preservation of mesenteric perfusion may be achieved through the construction of extra-anatomic bypass grafts prior to endograft implantation. Creation of these extra-anatomic grafts via open surgical techniques, performed in combination with endovascular aortic stent grafting, is referred to as **hybrid repair.**

3. **Monitoring** includes an arterial line and central venous or PA catheter, based on patient indications. **TEE** is reasonable for cardiac monitoring as well as for procedural guidance.

4. **Surgical considerations** for TEVAR are similar to those for EVAR (Section IV.A.4).

5. **Anesthetic technique.** TEVAR is almost exclusively performed under general anesthesia. Neuraxial anesthesia may interfere with postoperative motor examination and neurologic monitoring.

6. Following the deployment of the stent graft, an elevated MAP should be maintained to encourage collateral perfusion to the spinal cord.

7. **Complications of TEVAR** include **paraplegia** as well as those discussed in Section IV.A.6 to 7 for EVAR: injury to the vascular access site and

thromboemboli to the lower extremities, kidneys, or mesentery. Endoleaks occur in 10% to 20% of patients. Six to seven percent of patients require reintervention. Hypotension in the postoperative period increases the risk of delayed-onset paraplegia and should be avoided.

VI. AMPUTATIONS

A. General considerations. Amputations can be performed under general or regional anesthesia. There is no mortality difference between regional and general anesthesia. Regardless, insertion of an epidural catheter or perineural block is typically recommended for postoperative pain control. Postoperative stump pain is effectively treated with either continuous perineural infusion of bupivacaine or epidural infusion of bupivacaine combined with an opioid.

B. Phantom limb pain (PLP) has been reported to occur in 60% to 70% of patients undergoing amputation. It is controversial whether the use of perioperative neuraxial anesthesia decreases the risk of development of chronic PLP. The literature suggests that good perioperative pain control, starting in the preoperative period and extending postoperatively, may be associated with a reduced incidence of PLP. Further studies are needed.

Suggested Readings

Bardia A, Sood A, Mahmood F, et al. Combined epidural-general anesthesia vs general anesthesia alone for elective abdominal aortic aneurysm repair. *JAMA Surg.* 2016;151(12):1116-1123.

Brott TG, Halperin JL, Abbara S, et al. 2011 ASA/ACCF/AHA/AANN/AANS/ACRA/ASNR/CNS/SAIP/SCAI/SIR/SNIA/SVM/SVS guideline on the management of patients with extracranial carotid and vertebral artery disease: executive summary. *J Am Coll Cardiol.* 2011;57(8):1002-1044.

Chaikof EL, Brewster DC, Dalman RL, et al. Society for Vascular Surgery practice guidelines for the care of patients with an abdominal aortic aneurysm: executive summary. *J Vasc Surg.* 2009;50(4):880-896.

Chery J, Semaan E, Darji S, et al. Impact of regional versus general anesthesia on the clinical outcomes of patients undergoing major lower extremity amputation. *Ann Vasc Surg.* 2014;28(5):1149-1156.

De Bruin JL, Baas AF, Buth J, et al. Long-term outcome of open or endovascular repair abdominal aortic aneurysm. *N Engl J Med.* 2010;362:1881-1889.

Duncan D, Wijeysundera D. Preoperative cardiac evaluation and management of the patient undergoing major vascular surgery. *Int Anesthesiol Clin.* 2016;54(2):1-32.

Erickson KM, Cole DJ. Carotid artery disease: stenting vs. endarterectomy. *Br J Anaesth.* 2010;105:i34-i49.

Fedorow CA, Moon MC, Mutch AC, et al. Lumbar cerebrospinal fluid drainage for thoracoabdominal aortic surgery: rationale and practical considerations for management. *Anesth Analg.* 2010;111:46-58.

Fleisher LA, Beckman JA, Brown KA, et al. 2009 ACCF/AHA focused update on perioperative beta blockade incorporated into the ACC/AHA 2007 guidelines on perioperative cardiovascular evaluation and care for noncardiac surgery. *J Am Coll Cardiol.* 2009;54(22):e13-e118.

Fleisher LA, Fleischmann KE, Auerbach AD, et al. 2014 ACC/AHA guideline on perioperative cardiovascular evaluation and management of patients undergoing noncardiac surgery: executive summary. A report of the American College of Cardiology/American Heart Association Task Force on Practice Guidelines. *J Am Coll Cardiol.* 2014;130(24):2215-2245.

GALA Trial Collaborative Group; Lewis SC, Warlow CP, Bodenham AR, et al. General anaesthesia versus local anaesthesia for carotid surgery (GALA): a multicentre, randomised controlled trial. *Lancet.* 2008;372:2132-2142.

Gelman S. The pathophysiology of aortic cross-clamping and unclamping. *Anesthesiology.* 1995;82:1026-1060.

Guarracino F. Cerebral monitoring during cardiovascular surgery. *Curr Opin Anaesthesiol.* 2008;21(1):50-54.

Gutsche JT, Szeto W, Cheung AT. Endovascular stenting of thoracic aortic aneurysm. *Anesthesiol Clin.* 2008;26(3):481-499.

Hajibandeh S, Anoniou SA, Torella F, Antoniou GA. Meta-analysis and trial sequential analysis of local vs. general anaesthesia for carotid endarterectomy. *Anaesthesia.* 2018;73(10):1280-1289.

Hiratzka LF, Bakris GL, Beckman JA, et al. 2010 ACCF/AHA/AATS/ACR/ASA/SCA/SCAI/SIR/STS/SVM guidelines for the diagnosis and management of patients with thoracic aortic disease. *Circulation.* 2010;121(13):e266-e369.

IMPROVE Trial Investigators. Endovascular or open repair strategy for ruptured abdominal aortic aneurysm: 30 day outcomes from IMPROVE randomised trial. *Br Med J.* 2014;348:f7661.

Kent KC. Abdominal aortic aneurysms. *N Engl J Med.* 2014;371:2101-2108.

Lamuraglia GM, Houbballah R, Laposata M. The identification and management of heparin-induced thrombocytopenia in the vascular patient. *J Vasc Surg.* 2012;55:562-570.

Mehran R, Dangas GD, Weisbord SD. Contrast-associated acute kidney injury. *N Engl J Med.* 2019;380:2146-2155.

McFalls EO, Ward HB, Moritz TE, et al. Coronary artery revascularization before elective major vascular surgery. *N Engl J Med.* 2004;351:2795-2804.

Moll FL, Powell JT, Fraedrich G, et al. Management of abdominal aortic aneurysms clinical practice guidelines of the European Society for Vascular Surgery. *Eur J Vasc Endovasc Surg.* 2011;41(suppl 1):S1-S58.

Moreno DH, Cacione DG, Baptista-Silva JC. Controlled hypotension versus normotensive resuscitation strategy for people with ruptured abdominal aortic aneurysm. *Cochrane Database Syst Rev.* 2018;6(6):CD011664.

Nicolaou G, Ismail M, Cheng D. Thoracic endovascular aortic repair: update on indications and guidelines. *Anesthesiol Clin.* 2013;31(2):451-478.

Reddy U, Smith M. Anesthetic management of endovascular procedures for cerebrovascular atherosclerosis. *Curr Opin Anaesthesiol.* 2012;25(4):486-492.

Smaka TJ, Cobas M, Velazquez OC, et al. Perioperative management of endovascular abdominal aortic aneurysm repair: update 2010. *J Cardiothorac Vasc Anesth.* 2011;25(1):166-176.

United Kingdom EVAR Trial Investigators. Endovascular versus open repair of abdominal aortic aneurysm. *N Engl J Med.* 2010;362:1863-1871.

United Kingdom EVAR Trial Investigators. Endovascular repair of aortic aneurysm in patients physically ineligible for open repair. *N Engl J Med.* 2010;362:1872-1880.

Vaughn SB, LeMaire SA, Collard CD. Case scenario: anesthetic considerations for thoracoabdominal aortic aneurysm repair. *Anesthesiology.* 2011;115:1093-1102.

Vaniyapong T, Chongruksut W, Rerkasem K. Local versus general anaesthesia for carotid endarterectomy. *Cochrane Database Syst Rev.* 2013;12:CD000126.

Wesner L, Marone LK, Dennehy KC. Anesthesia for lower extremity bypass. *Int Anesthesiol Clin.* 2005;43(1):93-110.

Weisbord SD, Gallagher M, Jneid H, Garcia S. Outcomes after angiography with sodium bicarbonate and acetylcysteine. *N Engl J Med.* 2018;378:603-614.

29 Anesthesia for Cardiac Surgery

Maximilian Frank Lang and Jason Zhensheng Qu

I. CARDIOPULMONARY BYPASS

Cardiopulmonary bypass (CBP) is used to temporarily perform the functions of the heart (circulation of blood) and lungs (gas exchange) during surgical procedures on the heart and great vessels. It involves a pump and oxygenator connected through an extracorporeal circuit that provides oxygenated blood flow to the systemic circulation, bypassing the heart and lungs.

A. Components of circuit

1. Venous blood is drained from the venous cannula (inserted into the right atrium) to a **venous reservoir.** Maintaining an adequate fluid level in the venous reservoir is critical to prevent air entrainment.

2. A **pump** (roller or centrifugal) propels the venous blood forward. Unlike roller pumps, centrifugal pumps are afterload sensitive and will decrease flow if resistance increases (eg, with outflow obstruction). Centrifugal pumps are less traumatic to blood and do not pump air.

3. Venous blood enters a **heat exchanger** and an **oxygenator** that adds oxygen and removes carbon dioxide by adjusting the FiO_2 and sweep rate. A volatile anesthetic (eg, isoflurane) is added to the oxygenator gas mixture. The arterialized blood enters the systemic circulation via an aortic cannula, which is usually inserted in the ascending aorta. The femoral artery is sometimes used for aortic cannulation for emergency or redo sternotomy situations.

4. Cardioplegic solution containing high potassium is infused into the coronary circulation to induce and maintain cardiac arrest. Cardioplegia can be infused via the aortic root or coronary ostia (antegrade) or through the coronary sinus (retrograde).

5. **Left ventricular (LV) vent** removes blood that accumulates in the LV to decrease wall tension by suctioning on the same catheter placed for antegrade cardioplegia or one inserted into the LV via the right pulmonary vein across the mitral valve (MV).

B. CPB pathophysiology.
Contact of blood with the CPB circuit can lead to an intense systemic inflammatory response via the complement, kallikrein and coagulation cascades. A prolonged CPB time is associated with multisystem compromise including neurologic dysfunction, acute respiratory distress syndrome, coagulopathy, hepatic insufficiency, and acute kidney injury. A number of approaches have been tested to decrease inflammation in CPB including leukocyte depletion, hemofiltration, administration of monoclonal antibodies against inflammatory mediators, and the coating of circuitry with heparin. None have shown definitive clinical benefit in humans.

C. CPB effects on pharmacokinetics.
CPB results in increased volume of distribution and decreased protein binding. Acid-base shifts can affect the ionized and unionized concentrations of drugs. Decreased perfusion pressures during CPB can lead to reduced hepatic and renal clearance. Hypothermia further decreases hepatic enzyme function.

II. PREOPERATIVE ASSESSMENT FOR CARDIAC SURGERY

A. Issues **pertinent to the cardiac procedure** and the physiologic impact of CPB and circulatory arrest include the following:

   1. **Prior surgery** in the chest, which technically complicates surgery.
   2. **Evidence of aortic and cerebrovascular disease**—symptomatic or documented carotid arterial disease may warrant endarterectomy. Aortic disease can affect cannulation strategies for bypass and may sometimes require concomitant repair with the cardiac operation.
   3. **History of bleeding, anticoagulation regimens, and prothrombotic** tendencies may reveal a condition responsive to perioperative therapy.
   4. A history of **heparin-induced thrombocytopenia** (HIT) alerts to the potential for the development of life-threatening thrombotic complications when exposed to heparin. HIT is discussed later in the chapter.
   5. **Renal insufficiency** may indicate the need for intraoperative renal protective measures.
   6. Patients with **pulmonary disease** can develop severe **post-CPB pulmonary dysfunction** and may benefit from preoperative antibiotics, bronchodilators, steroids, or chest physical therapy.
   7. **Liver dysfunction** (eg, cardiac cirrhosis) may indicate derangements in coagulation and platelet function and the need for transfusion of coagulation factors, platelets, and fibrinogen.

B. **Cardiac evaluation** determines the major anatomic and physiologic characteristics of the cardiovascular system, to predict of intraoperative ischemia and functional reserve of the heart.

   1. **Radionuclide imaging** may demonstrate the regions and extent of myocardium at risk for ischemia. Radionuclide ventriculography characterizes cardiac chamber volume, ejection fraction, and right-to-left stroke volume ratios.
   2. **Viability studies** in patients with severe LV dysfunction can help distinguish areas of myocardial necrosis from hibernation; the latter may recover after revascularization. Current modalities include nuclear imaging (SPECT or PET), dobutamine stress echocardiography, and magnetic resonance imaging (MRI).
   3. **Echocardiography** provides an assessment of ventricular function and valve function. Regional wall motion abnormalities (WMAs) may reflect ischemia or prior myocardial infarction.
   4. **CT scan and f-MRI** are noninvasive modalities to assess for coronary vascular disease. They can be useful in patients who are not candidates for cardiac catheterization.
   5. **Cardiac catheterization** remains the gold standard diagnostic test for most forms of cardiac disease.

      a. **Anatomic data.** Coronary angiography reveals the location and extent of coronary stenoses, distal runoff, collateral flow, and coronary dominance. **Significant stenosis** implies a greater than 70% reduction in luminal diameter. The **dominant coronary artery** supplies the atrioventricular node and the posterior descending coronary artery.

      b. **Functional data.** Ventriculography may demonstrate WMA, mitral regurgitation (MR), and intracardiac shunts. Left ventricular ejection fraction is normally greater than 0.6. Impaired ventricular performance is a useful predictor of increased surgical risk.

      c. **Hemodynamic data** are compiled from both right and left heart catheterization. Intracardiac and pulmonary vascular pressures reflect volume status, valvular function, and the presence of pulmonary

TABLE 29.1	Normal Intracardiac Pressure and Oxygen Saturation	
	Pressure (mm Hg)	**O₂ Saturation (%)**
Superior vena cava	—	71
Inferior vena cava	—	77
Right atrium (mean)	1-8	75
RV (systolic/diastolic)	15-30/0-8	75
PA (systolic/diastolic)	15-30/4-12	75
PA occlusion pressure (mean)	2-12	—
Left atrium (mean)	2-12	98
LV (systolic/diastolic/end diastolic)	100-140/0-8/2-12	98
Aorta (systolic/diastolic)	100-140/60-90	98

LV, left ventricle; PA, pulmonary artery; RV, right ventricle.

vascular disease (normal values are presented in **Table 29.1**). An elevated LV end-diastolic pressure (LVEDP) may be due to ventricular failure and dilation, volume overload (mitral or aortic insufficiency [AI]), poor compliance from ischemia or hypertrophy, or a constrictive process. The LVEDP may rise substantially in patients with coronary artery disease (CAD) after dye injection for ventriculography or coronary angiography, despite otherwise normal hemodynamic values.

    d. Left-to-right intracardiac shunts are demonstrated by an arterial oxygen saturation (SaO_2) "step up" in the right heart.

    e. Cardiac output is determined by thermodilution and can be used to derive the hemodynamic indices (**Table 29.2**).

C. Other studies

    1. Routine labs for patients undergoing a cardiac operation usually include a CBC, prothrombin time, activated partial thromboplastin time (aPTT), platelet count, electrolytes, blood urea nitrogen, creatinine, glucose, liver function tests, and thyroid-stimulating hormone level. A heparin-platelet factor 4 antibody detection assay should be considered for patients with a low or rapidly falling platelet count associated with heparin, as these patients are at risk for developing HIT.

    2. Chest radiograph and a 12-lead ECG with a rhythm strip.

    3. Pulmonary function tests may be appropriate in patients with underlying lung disease.

    4. Vascular studies such as carotid duplex and vein mapping.

D. Cardiac medications

    1. *β*-**Adrenergic antagonists, calcium channel blockers, antiarrhythmics,** and **nitrates,** including intravenous nitroglycerin, are routinely continued on schedule until the patient's arrival in the operating room (OR).

    2. Digoxin is commonly held for 24 hours preoperatively due to potential toxicity (especially in the presence of hypokalemia) and a long elimination half-life. When rate control is critical, however, as in mitral stenosis (MS), digoxin should be continued.

	Ventricular Function Indices		
Formula		**Units**	**Normal Value**
$SV = \dfrac{CO}{HR} \times 1{,}000$		mL/beat	60-90
$SI = \dfrac{SV}{BSA}$		mL/beat/m^2	40-60
$LVSWI = \dfrac{1.36\left(MAP - PCWP\right)}{100} \times SI$		g-m/m^2/beat	45-60
$RVSWI = \dfrac{1.36\left(PAP - CVP\right)}{100} \times SI$		g-m/m^2/beat	5-10
$SVR = \dfrac{\left(MAP - CVP\right)}{CO} \times 80$		dyne-s/cm^5	900-1500
$PVR = \dfrac{\left(PAP - PCWP\right)}{CO} \times 80$		dyne-s/cm^5	50-150

TABLE 29.2

BSA, body surface area; CO, cardiac output; CVP, mean central venous pressure; HR, heart rate; LVSWI, left ventricular stroke work index; MAP, mean arterial pressure; PAP, mean pulmonary artery pressure; PCWP, pulmonary capillary wedge pressure; PVR, pulmonary vascular resistance; RVSWI, right ventricular stroke work index; SI, stroke index; SV, stroke volume; SVR, systemic vascular resistance.

3. **Angiotensin-converting enzyme (ACE) inhibitors**, angiotensin receptor blockers, and **diuretics** are usually held before surgery. Patients with significant LV dysfunction are prone to vasodilatory shock when they receive an ACE inhibitor preoperatively.

4. **Aspirin** has a positive effect on graft patency and should be continued in most patients who have significant CAD. Bleeding related solely to aspirin therapy can be overcome with platelet transfusion provided the drug has been cleared from the circulation. Patients receiving multiple antiplatelet agents may or may not be rapidly reversible (**Table 29.3**). Clopidogrel or prasugrel is stopped 5 to 7 days prior to surgery. If a bare-metal stent was placed within the past month or a drug-eluting stent within the last year, clopidogrel is often continued up until the time of surgery. Short-acting IIb/IIIa inhibitors should be stopped 4 hours preoperatively.

5. **Warfarin** is held 3 to 5 days preoperatively to allow normalization of the international normalization ratio. Intravenous vitamin K (5-10 mg) or fresh-frozen plasma (FFP) may be used emergently to correct coagulopathy. However, FFP will only transiently correct a warfarin-induced coagulopathy due to the relatively longer half-life of warfarin compared with the vitamin K–dependent cofactors (factors II, VII, IX, and X), thus putting the patient at risk for rebound coagulopathy. Oral anticoagulants such as dabigatran, rivaroxaban, and apixaban should be stopped 5 days before cardiac surgery. Unlike warfarin, their actions cannot be

Drug	Inhibits	Half-Life	Duration	Reversible	Methods to Restore Function
Aspirin	Cyclooxygenase	15-20 min	7 d	No	Platelet transfusion
Abciximab (Reopro)	Glycoprotein IIb/IIIa receptor	30 min	48 h	Partially	Platelet transfusion
Eptifibatide (Integrilin)	Glycoprotein IIb/IIIa receptor	2.5 h	4-8 h	Yes	Delay surgery 8 h after stopping drug
Tirofiban (Aggrastat)	Glycoprotein IIb/IIIa receptor	1.5-3 h	4-8 h	Yes	Discontinue drug 8 h before surgery
Clopidogrel (Plavix)	Adenosine diphosphate receptor	8 h	7 d	No	Platelet transfusion
Prasugrel (Effient)	Adenosine diphosphate receptor	2-15 h	7 d	No	Platelet transfusion
Cangrelor	Adenosine diphosphate receptor	2-5 min	1 h	Yes	Platelet transfusion or wait 6 h before surgery
Ticagrelor (Brilinta)	Adenosine diphosphate receptor	6-9 h	5 d	No	Platelet transfusion
Ticlopidine (Ticlid)	Adenosine diphosphate receptor	12 h-5 d with repeated dosing	7 d	No	Platelet transfusion
Dipyridamole[a] (Persantine)	Adenosine uptake; phosphodiesterase	9-13 h	4-10 h	Yes	Platelet transfusion
Cilostazol (Pletal)	Phosphodiesterase III	11-13 h	48 h	Yes	Platelet transfusion
Vorapaxar	Protease-activated receptor-1	7-13 d	4 mo	Yes	Platelet transfusion
Herbal therapies[b]	Platelet aggregation	Variable	Variable	Variable	Limited data available

TABLE 29.3 Antiplatelet Agents

[a]Dipyridamole is available in a formulation with aspirin (Aggrenox).
[b]Includes garlic, ginkgo, ginseng, ginger, feverfew, fish oil, and dong quai.

reversed by the administration of vitamin K or FFP. Emergent reversal requires the administration of four-component prothrombin complex concentrates. In the case of dabigatran, hemodialysis may be used. Rivaroxaban and apixaban are too highly protein bound to be removed by dialysis.

6. **Heparin** infusions initiated for unstable angina or left main CAD are continued preoperatively. The anticoagulant effects of unfractionated heparin are reversible with IV protamine administration. In contrast, the anticoagulant effects of low molecular weight heparin (LMWH) preparations are not fully reversible with protamine. LMWH has been associated with increased perioperative hemorrhage in cardiac surgical patients.

III. ANESTHETIC MANAGEMENT
A. Monitoring
1. **Standard monitors**
   a. Continuous **ECG** display of both leads II and V_5 with ST segment trend analysis.
   b. **Temperature monitoring** includes that of the oral or nasopharynx (core temperature), the blood temperature (measured from pulmonary artery [PA] catheter), and bladder or rectal temperature, which represents the average body temperature.
2. **Central venous and PA pressures**
   a. **Patients with normal ventricular function** can be effectively managed with either central venous pressure (CVP) monitoring with or without transesophageal echocardiography (TEE) or a PA catheter.
   b. **PA catheter** provides helpful data in managing hemodynamics of patients with valvular and redo surgeries. **Mixed venous oxygen saturation** ($SmvO_2$) monitoring is available continuously with PA catheters specially equipped with a fiberoptic-linked oximeter. A decrease in $SmvO_2$ is the result of decreased cardiac output, decreased hemoglobin, increased oxygen consumption, or decreased SaO_2.
3. **Intraoperative TEE** can help surgical and anesthetic decision-making. The Society of Cardiovascular Anesthesiologists/American Society of Echocardiography TEE guidelines recommend the use of intraoperative TEE in all open heart (eg, valvular procedure) and thoracic aortic surgical procedures and to be considered in coronary artery bypass grafting (CABG) surgery. TEE provides guidance during catheter-based intracardiac procedures (eg, transcatheter aortic valve replacement [TAVR] and MitraClips).
   a. The routine examination consists of **20 standard views**. The probe is advanced into the esophagus (upper and midesophageal views) and then into the stomach for transgastric views.
   b. **Application** of intraoperative TEE includes confirmation of the placement of guidewire or cannula, assessment of global and regional ventricular function, chamber sizes, and valvular anatomy and function. TEE is very sensitive for detecting ischemia. It is also used to assess ventricular function, the presence of intracardiac air, and the presence of paravalvular leaks.
   c. **Absolute contraindications** to TEE:
      1. Esophageal stricture
      2. Tracheoesophageal fistula
      3. History of recent esophageal surgery and esophageal trauma.

      4. TEE must be used cautiously in patients with esophageal vari-ces and altered anatomy (eg, from gastric bypass surgery) and in those who have had radiation therapy to the neck and mediasti-num. The incidence of severe complications such as esophageal perforation is on the order of 0.1%.

     d. 3-Dimensional TEE can provide detailed images of valve and other structures.

  4. Neurologic monitors such as transcranial Doppler, multichannel electro-encephalography (EEG), and near-infrared spectroscopy may improve neurologic outcome by alerting the clinician of cerebral ischemia. Processed EEG (BIS or Sedline) monitor is a useful guide to predict the depth of anesthesia.

B. Preinduction

  1. Peripheral venous access is established with one large-bore (14- or 16-gauge) intravenous (IV) catheter. If excessive bleeding is expected (eg, a redo operation or a patient with a preexisting coagulopathy), a second volume line will facilitate blood product administration.

  2. Sedation and analgesia: Benzodiazepines should only be given to extremely anxious patient. Patients with severe aortic stenosis (AS), MS, pulmonary hypertension, or left main CAD may not tolerate even small degrees of hypotension and respiratory depression; minimal or no premedication is administered until the patient arrives in the OR.

  3. Arterial cannulation is performed with a 20-gauge catheter into right radial artery.

     a. Left radial or femoral artery cannulation is used for systemic blood pressure monitoring when right axillary artery cannulation is planned for antegrade cerebral protection during deep hypothermic circula-tory arrest (DHCA).

     b. Cannulation distal to a previous brachial artery cutdown site should be avoided.

     c. If blood pressure measurements are asymmetric, the arterial cathe-ter should be placed on the side with the higher value.

     d. Be certain to note whether the surgeon will use the radial artery for CABG surgery.

     e. Femoral artery cannulation is a safe and reliable alternative to radial artery cannulation. Preoperative femoral artery cannulation can also be accessed for emergency CPB and intra-aortic balloon pump (IABP) insertion in patients with redo, severe CAD and poor LV func-tion. Brachial and axillary artery cannulations are third and fourth choices.

     f. Intra-aortic balloon central lumen pressure can be transduced as a monitor of central arterial pressure.

  4. Central venous access may be established before or after induction.

  5. A defibrillator and an external pacemaker generator must be available. Permanent pacemaker or implantable cardioverter defibrillator (ICD) should be interrogated and a magnet should be available.

  6. Typed and cross-matched packed red blood cells (2-4 units) must be pres-ent and checked.

  7. Baseline hemodynamics values, including cardiac output, are recorded.

  8. Available medications should include heparin, calcium chloride, lido-caine, amiodarone, inotropes, vasopressors, vasodilators, and nitro-glycerin. Protamine should never be drawn up until the patient is safely separated from CPB.

IV. INDUCTION

A. **During induction,** a surgeon should be available, and the CPB pump should be ready in the event of severe hemodynamic instability during induction. A systematic and gradual induction involves minimizing the degree of cardiovascular depression while maintaining an adequate anesthetic depth.

1. **Induction agents:**

   a. **IV opioids** produce various degrees of vasodilation and bradycardia without significant myocardial depression. Fentanyl (50-100 µg/kg) or sufentanil (10-20 µg/kg) can be used as both the induction and primary maintenance agents. Alternatively, a smaller induction bolus (fentanyl 25-50 µg/kg) may be supplemented with a continuous opioid infusion. Alternatively, even lower doses (fentanyl 10-25 µg/kg, or sufentanil 1-5 µg/kg) may be used in conjunction with other central nervous system depressants as part of a balanced technique.

   b. **Sedative hypnotics and amnestics,** including propofol, etomidate, and dexmedetomidine, may be useful as coinduction agents in particular situations. Of these drugs, etomidate causes the least myocardial depression.

   c. **Volatile inhalation anesthetics** are useful supplementary and maintenance agents.

   d. **Muscle relaxants** with minimal cardiovascular effects are commonly chosen (eg, vecuronium, cisatracurium, and rocuronium). Pretreatment with a "priming dose" and early relaxant administration help to counteract chest wall rigidity often encountered during opioid-based inductions.

2. **Specific considerations for valvular heart disease** (see also Chapter 2).

   a. **Aortic stenosis (AS).** Physiologic goals include the maintenance of adequate intravascular volume, sinus rhythm, contractility, and systemic vascular resistance (SVR) and the avoidance of tachycardia. Patients with AS typically have a hypertrophied and noncompliant ventricle and require higher filling pressures (LVEDP of 20-30 mm Hg). Anesthetic agents that reduce vascular tone or myocardial contractility should be avoided. An infusion of phenylephrine can be started 1 to 2 minutes before induction to decrease the risk of developing significant hypotension associated with induction. Dysrhythmias must be treated aggressively.

   b. **Aortic regurgitation (AR).** Physiologic goals include maintenance of adequate intravascular volume and adequate contractility. Bradycardia and increases in SVR must be avoided. Patients with AR are often highly dependent on endogenous sympathetic tone. Patients with coexisting CAD may decompensate with significant bradycardia due to very low diastolic perfusion pressure. A means for rapid pacing should be available.

   c. **Mitral stenosis (MS).** Hemodynamic goals mandate the maintenance of a slow rhythm, preferably sinus, and adequate intravascular volume, contractility, and SVR. Patients with severe MS and elevated pulmonary vascular resistance (PVR) are challenging to induce. Elevated PVR, often secondary to hypoventilation or positive end-expiratory pressure (PEEP), must be avoided. Atrial fibrillation with rapid ventricular response must be treated aggressively, such as with immediate cardioversion.

   d. **Mitral regurgitation (MR).** Physiologic goals include the maintenance of adequate intravascular volume, myocardial contractility, a normal or elevated heart rate, and a reduction of systemic vascular tone. Increased SVR should be avoided. Anesthesia-induced decreases in SVR are usually well tolerated.

e. **Mixed valvular lesions**, the most hemodynamically significant lesion, dominate the management goals. The addition of CAD to mixed valvular lesions makes planning even more complex (eg, AS with AR and CAD). In all situations, determine the three most likely problems that could occur during induction and plan the management for each.

3. **Specific considerations for emergent inductions**

   a. **Pulmonary embolus.** Induction of general anesthesia and the institution of positive-pressure ventilation can precipitate cardiovascular collapse. It is prudent to prepare and drape the unstable patient prior to induction. In patients with compromised RV function, cannulation of the femoral vessels under local anesthesia should be performed prior to induction to allow for the emergent institution of CPB if needed.

   b. **Pericardial tamponade.** Similar concerns are present for patients with pericardial tamponade. Adequate volume administration is essential. Starting an inotropic agent and a vasopressor before induction may be helpful. A rapid sternotomy may be required if hemodynamic collapse occurs with anesthesia induction. If possible, the pericardial effusion should be drained under local anesthesia prior to induction.

   c. **Aortic dissection.** Hypertension can precipitate aortic rupture. Packed red blood cells must be available in the OR before induction. Proximal extension of the dissection into the coronary arteries can occur, leading to myocardial ischemia or tamponade.

   d. **Ventricular septal defect (VSD) and papillary muscle rupture after myocardial infarction.** Patients may present with extreme hypotension. Rapid initiation of CPB is essential. Preinduction initiation of intra-aortic balloon counterpulsation therapy is indicated in many of these patients.

B. **The pre-bypass period** is characterized by variable levels of stimulation during the preparation for CPB initiation. Stimulating periods include incision, sternotomy, and sternal retraction and pericardiotomy.

1. **Baseline** Pao_2, $Paco_2$, pH, hematocrit (Hct), and activated clotting time (ACT) should be obtained.

2. Consider **acute normovolemic hemodilution in** patients with a starting Hct of 35% or greater. 1 to 2 units of whole blood may be removed with maintenance of normovolemia using cystalloid and/or colloid replacement fluid. The blood is later transfused into the patient following conclusion of CPB and heparin reversal.

3. **The lungs are deflated** during sternotomy. Physical alterations of the chest wall can produce ECG changes (especially T-wave changes), which should be noted to avoid confusion with ischemia.

4. **Left internal mammary artery dissection** may cause ispilateral hemothorax and negatively affect pulmonary mechanics in patients with reduced pulmonary reserve.

5. **Anticoagulation for cannulation and bypass**

   a. **Prior to the induction of anesthesia**, bolus dose of heparin should be drawn up and kept readily available in case the emergent initiation of CPB is necessary. The dose may be calculated by body weight (300-500 units/kg) or heparin dose responsive formula. The heparin should be administered through a centrally placed catheter.

b. **Hypotension** often follows the heparin bolus and should be anticipated.

c. The **ACT** is used to monitor the degree of anticoagulation and measured approximately 5 minutes after administering full-dose heparin. Baseline values are 80 to 150 seconds. Heparin treatment sufficient to prevent microthrombus formation during CPB correlates with an ACT of more than 400 seconds (at higher than 35 °C). Antithrombin concentrate (500-1000 units) or 2 to 4 units of FFP administration may be necessary to achieve ACT target in patients with antithrombin III deficiency.

d. **Patients with a diagnosis of HIT type 2 (also known as HIT with thrombotic syndrome [HITTS])** require alternative anticoagulation management during CPB. The classification of HIT is determined by immune involvement. HIT type 1 is a nonimmunologic reaction of heparin with platelets that causes a mild thrombocytopenia. HIT type 2 is an immune-mediated phenomenon that activates platelets, resulting in platelet aggregation. Biochemical mediators from activated platelets can induce the generation of thrombin, leading to diffuse arterial and venous clotting. The diagnosis requires serologic and clinical evidence. Patients with a positive functional assay (serotonin release assay or platelet aggregation study), greater than 50% reduction in platelets (irrespective of starting platelet count), drop in platelet count less than 150k, or history of a thrombotic event associated with heparin use are more likely to have an adverse outcome when reexpose to heparin. Patients with a positive ELISA test in the absence of a positive functional assay or clinical symptoms have a lower likelihood of having an adverse reaction to heparin.

e. For patients with HIT type 2 or HITTS, **alternatives to standard heparin treatment** exist (**Table 29.4**); each has significant limitations that should be discussed with the surgeon and a hematologist before use.
   1. All forms of heparin are removed preoperatively. Saline is used to flush pressure transducers, and citrated saline is used to wash salvaged blood during the centrifugation process.
   2. A heparin-free PA catheter is used.
   3. Alternative anticoagulant regimens may be used. These include bivalirudin, or unfractionated heparin in combination with an antiplatelet agent (see **Table 29.4**).
   4. If unfractionated heparin is used, then a bypass dose of porcine heparin is administered before aortic cannulation (to minimize the likelihood of a repeat dose of heparin).
   5. Aspirin is administered early in the postoperative period, and initiation of systemic anticoagulation with a direct thrombin inhibitor and warfarin may be indicated to prevent both early and late postoperative thromboembolic complications.

6. **Antifibrinolytic drugs** such as ε-aminocaproic acid (Amicar) are usually given as a bolus 10 g followed by an infusion 2 g/h during all on-pump procedures, with the intention of inhibiting excessive fibrinolysis (ie, plasmin activity and D-dimer formation) and possibly preserving platelet function. Tranexamic acid can be used to substitute Amicar with different dose.

7. **Aortic cannulation** is conducted in the ascending aorta. **Epiaortic scanning** is used to sonographically direct the cannulation site in patients with atherosclerotic disease. Maintaining a slightly low systolic blood pressure (90-100 mm Hg) during aortic cannulation decreases the risk of dissection.

TABLE 29.4	Alternative CPB Anticoagulation in Patients With HIT				
Drug	**Mechanism**	**Half-Life**	**Lab Monitor**	**Reversible?**
Bivalirudin (Angiomax)	Direct thrombin inhibitor	25 min (normal renal function)	ACT	No
Argatroban	Direct thrombin inhibitor	40-50 min (prolonged in hepatic insufficiency)	ACT	No
Tirofiban (Aggrastat) + unfractionated heparin[a]	Glycoprotein IIb/IIIa receptor inhibitor prevents platelet aggregation in HIT	1.5-3 h	ACT (platelets and D-dimer if heparin-induced thrombosis is suspected)	No

ACT, activated clotting time; CPB, cardiopulmonary bypass; HIT, heparin-induced thrombocytopenia.
[a]Additional training is required to safely use this anticoagulation technique for patients requiring CPB.

8. **Venous return cannulas** are inserted via the right atrium. A single cavoatrial catheter is placed in the right atrial appendage, with the tip in the inferior vena cava (IVC) and fenestrations in the midatrium. For open-heart procedures (ie, mitral and tricuspid valve surgeries), bicaval cannulation, consisting of separate superior vena cava (SVC) and IVC cannulas, is conducted.

9. **Retrograde autologous priming (RAP)** can be used to reduce the hemodilution from the crystalloid priming solutions of the bypass circuit. During RAP, the patient's blood pushes the crystalloid prime out of the circuit, often necessitating use of α-agonist agents to maintain vascular tone and prevent hypotension.

C. **Cardiopulmonary bypass**

1. **Initiation of CPB.** After an ACT greater than or equal to 400 seconds is obtained, the clamp on the venous line is released and CPB is initiated. The pump flow progressively increases to 2.0 to 2.4 L/min/m^2 with target mean arterial pressure (MAP) of 60 to 80 mm Hg. Ventilation is discontinued. Anesthesia is maintained using IV agents or inhalational agents administered through a vaporizer in the fresh gas line of CPB circuit. It is advisable to withdraw the PA catheter 2 to 5 cm to prevent the catheter tip from migrating into a wedge position during CPB. If two venous return lines are used and tourniquets are applied to achieve complete CPB, the CVP measured above the tourniquet is the SVC pressure. High CVP may indicate obstruction of SVC cannula. A vent cannula may be inserted via right pulmonary vein to drain the LV.

2. **Maintenance of CPB**

a. **Myocardial protection** during the cross-clamp period is achieved primarily by reducing myocardial oxygen consumption through hypothermia, hyperkalemic arrest, or both.

1. **Intermittent cold cardioplegia** is a commonly used technique. Cold (4 °C-6 °C) hyperkalemic solution with or without blood is delivered to the coronary circulation approximately every 20 minutes

as needed. Systemic cooling of the patient and topical cooling of the heart augment myocardial protection.

2. The **warm cardioplegia technique** delivers a warm (32 °C-37 °C) hyperkalemic solution mixed with blood at approximately a 1:5 ratio. The solution is delivered continuously during the cross-clamp period with a few interruptions to allow visualization of the anastomotic sites. Mild systemic cooling to 32 °C-34 °C is frequently performed. Blood glucose levels should be monitored and controlled between 80 and 180 mg/L with IV insulin bolus and infusion as needed.

b. **Hypothermia** (20 °C-34 °C) is commonly used during CPB. Oxygen consumption and blood flow requirements are reduced while blood viscosity is increased, thus counteracting prime-induced hypoviscosity. Adverse effects of hypothermia include impaired autoregulatory, enzymatic, and cellular membrane function; decreased oxygen delivery (leftward shift of the hemoglobin oxygen dissociation curve); and potentiation of coagulopathy. Metabolic requirements decrease about 7% for every degree Celsius reduction in body temperature below 37 °C.

c. **Hemodynamic monitoring**

1. **Hypotension** during the initiation of CPB is usually due to hemodilution, hypoviscosity, and cardioplegia administration. Other causes include inadequate pump flow, vasodilation, aortic dissection, and aortic cannula mispositioning. A phenylephrine infusion may be required to treat transient hypotension. During the course of CPB, a pressure gradient (as high as 40 mm Hg) may develop between the radial artery and the aorta. The lower radial artery pressure could lead to unnecessary administration of vasopressors if the discrepancy is not recognized. In the presence of carotid stenosis, MAP should be maintained at a higher level than usual (eg, 70-80 mm Hg), and hypocarbia should be avoided.

2. **Hypertension** (MAP > 90 mm Hg) may be due to excessive flow rates or increased vascular resistance, which may be treated with vasodilators or anesthetics.

3. **Elevated PA pressures** indicate left heart distention, which may be due to inadequate venting, AI, or inadequate isolation of venous return. Severe distention may result in myocardial injury.

d. **Acid-base management.** In the setting of hypothermia, gas solubility increases and the dissociation constant for water decreases, resulting in a lower $[H^+]$ and $[OH^-]$ and a higher pH. While total CO_2 content remains constant, the partial pressure of CO_2 decreases.

1. **pH-stat** corrects the patient's blood gas for temperature and strives to maintain a neutral pH of 7.4 and CO_2 near 40 mm Hg by adding CO_2 to the CPB circuit. This strategy results in cerebral vasodilatation and more uniform cerebral cooling, however at an increased risk of cerebral microembolism.

2. **Alpha-stat** involves the use of uncorrected gas tensions during hypothermia. No CO_2 is added to the oxygenator. The basis of the approach is that the total CO_2 content of blood and the intracellular electroneutrality (as primarily governed by the imidazole rings of histidine residues) are unchanged during hypothermia. Cerebral blood flow is autoregulated and coupled to cerebral oxygen demand.

3. Most studies fail to reveal any significant difference in patient outcomes between the two methods. Generally, alpha-stat is used in adults and pH-stat in children when circulatory arrest is used.

e. **Metabolic acidosis and oliguria** may suggest inadequate systemic perfusion. Additional volume (blood or crystalloid depending on Hct) may be required to achieve increased flow. Brisk urine output should be established within the first 10 minutes of CPB.

1. **Oliguria** (<1 mL/kg/h) may be treated with a trial of increased perfusion pressure and/or flow, mannitol (0.25-0.5 g/kg). Patients on chronic furosemide therapy may require their usual dose during CPB to sustain diuresis.

2. **Hemolysis** during CPB is usually due to mechanical trauma to red blood cells from the bypass machine and the pump suction. Released pigments may cause acute renal failure postoperatively. For hemoglobinuria, diuresis is maintained using IV fluids with mannitol or furosemide. In severe cases, the urine is alkalinized by administering sodium bicarbonate at 0.5 to 1.0 mEq/kg.

f. **Additional heparin** bolus and/or infusion may be needed for prolonged CPB. The duration of heparin anticoagulation may be shorter in patients on chronic heparin therapy or during cases in which systemic hypothermia is not used. The ACT does not correlate well with plasma heparin levels when the patient is on CPB, but many centers routinely monitor the ACT during hypothermic (25 °C-34 °C) CPB.

g. **Blood glucose** should be controlled between 80 and 180 mg/dL during bypass. Hyperglycemia may be associated with an increased risk of neurologic injury. Diabetic patients following a warm cardioplegia technique will typically require an insulin infusion.

h. **Table 29.5** lists some of the **problems** that can be encountered during CPB.

D. **Discontinuing CPB** implies transferring cardiopulmonary function from the bypass system back to the patient. In preparation for this transition, the anesthesiologist must examine and optimize the patient's metabolic, anesthetic, and cardiorespiratory conditions.

TABLE 29.5	Potential Problems During CPB
Problem	**Possible Cause**
Inadequate systemic pressures	Vasoplegia, inadequate flow, hemodilution
Poor gas exchange	Oxygenator failure, hypoxic gas mixture, inadequate coagulation, poor perfusion
High arterial line pressure	Mechanical obstruction, malpositioned aortic cannula, aortic dissection, inadequate anticoagulation, or cold agglutination
Distension of heart	Poor venous drainage, inadequate venting, increased regurgitation, or shunting
High coronary sinus pressure (during retrograde cardioplegia)	Small coronary sinus, malpositioning of catheter

CPB, cardiopulmonary bypass.

1. **Preparation for discontinuing CPB begins during rewarming.** The arterial blood is warmed but not exceed 37 °C before discontinuation from CPB.
   a. **Laboratory data** to be acquired during rewarming include PaO_2, $PaCO_2$, pH, potassium, calcium, glucose, Hgb, and ACT. Clinical decisions concerning pH are usually made according to the values measured at 37 °C (alpha-stat management).
   b. **Adequate anticoagulation** during rewarming and separation from CPB is ensured with additional heparin if necessary.
   c. **Metabolic acidosis** should be treated with sodium bicarbonate, and the perfusionist may elect to increase the sweep rate to remove CO_2. **Hyperkalemia** frequently corrects spontaneously by redistribution and diuresis. If not, the administration of IV insulin/glucose with sodium bicarbonate will lower serum potassium.
   d. Usually, a **Hct** of over 21% should be achieved before separation, either by transfusion or by hemoconcentration, as indicated by the CPB reservoir volume.
   e. **FFP** and **platelets** should also be readily available to correct coagulopathy.
2. **Separation from CPB**
   a. **De-airing maneuvers** under TEE guidance are used to prevent air embolism to the cerebral or coronary circulations. Air in the left ventricle can be liberated and suctioned out via aortic root vent by manipulation of the heart and ventricular filling.
   b. **Aortic cross-clamp removal** reestablishes coronary perfusion.
   c. **Defibrillation** may be spontaneous; ventricular fibrillation is treated with internal paddles delivering 5 to 10 J of energy with a biphasic waveform defibrillator. Failure may indicate inadequate warming, graft problems, a metabolic disturbance, or inadequate myocardial protection. Additional lidocaine, magnesium (1 g IV slowly), or amiodarone (150-mg IV bolus followed by infusion at 1 mg/min for 6 hours, then 0.5 mg/min) may be required.
   d. **Rhythm is assessed.** With bradycardia, atrial pacing is established through epicardial wires. Ventricular pacing is added if there are atrioventricular conduction abnormalities. Hypothermia as well as hypocalcemia, hyperkalemia, and hypermagnesemia caused by cardioplegia solutions may contribute to a high incidence of reversible heart block immediately after CPB. Other atrial dysrhythmias may be treated with overdrive pacing, cardioversion, and antiarrhythmics (eg, esmolol, propranolol, amiodarone, verapamil, or rarely digoxin).
   e. **The ECG should be inspected** for evidence of ischemia possibly related to intracoronary air or inadequate revascularization.
   f. During separation from CPB, volume administration may be guided by monitoring LV filling using TEE, mean PA or wedge pressure. RV filling is indicated by the CVP or direct RV visualization. Patients without LVH will most likely need an LA pressure of 10 mm Hg or a mean PA pressure of 20 mm Hg. A patient with severe LVH and inadequate revascularization may need an LA pressure of 20 mm Hg or a mean PA pressure of 30 mm Hg.
   g. **If a gradient** between central (aortic) and peripheral (radial) arterial pressures is present, a femoral arterial line can be placed.
   h. **Compliance and resistance of the lungs** are tested with a few trial breaths. Ventilation should be reestablished when LV ejection begins even if the patient is still on CPB. To facilitate reexpansion of the lungs, the pleural cavities are drained if they have been opened

previously or fluid is detected by TEE. If the lungs are difficult to ventilate, tracheobronchial suctioning and the administration of bronchodilators may be indicated.

  i. **Visual inspection of the heart** confirms atrioventricular synchrony. Contractility is assessed both by gross appearance and by systolic performance, as estimated by peak systolic and pulse pressure (taking into account pump flow and LA and PA pressures). If poor myocardial performance is demonstrated or anticipated (eg, impaired preoperative function or intraoperative ischemia), initiation of inotropic support before separation from CPB may be indicated. Pump flow rate is checked and compared with the patient's preoperative cardiac output. Significantly higher flows indicate the need to increase vascular tone.

  j. **Ionized Ca²⁺** may be corrected slowly after heart is reperfused. Rapid Ca²⁺ administration, especially in the presence of myocardial ischemia, is associated with Ca²⁺-induced myocardial injury. Calcium will increase both contractility and SVR.

E. **At the time of separation from CPB**, venous lines to the pump are slowly clamped, allowing the heart to gradually fill and eject with each contraction. Prolonged partial venous line occlusion allows for "partial bypass," during which time cardiopulmonary function is shared and hemodynamics are assessed. After complete venous line occlusion, once adequate filling pressures are achieved, perfusion through the aortic cannula is stopped, and the heart alone provides systemic perfusion.

  1. **Pressure maintenance.** Transfusion from the CPB reservoir maintains an optimal filling condition assessed by MAP, PA, CVP, and TEE. Care is taken not to overdistend the heart. Should overdistention occur, the surgeon may "empty" the heart by transiently unclamping a venous line. Alternatively, the patient may be temporarily placed in reverse Trendelenburg position to decrease venous return to the overdistended heart.

  2. **At termination of bypass, it is important to assess** the ECG, systemic blood pressure, filling of the ventricles, and the cardiac output. These values are compared with target values for the patient. If the patient is unstable, correct any pacing problems, have the surgeon assess the patency of the grafts, and use TEE to assess the valve replacement or repair. Assuming there is no surgical cause for hemodynamic instability, the unstable patient will usually fall into one of the categories listed in **Table 29.6. If a return to CPB is necessary**, adequate anticoagulation must be ensured. A **full dose** of heparin is indicated if protamine has been administered.

F. **Post-bypass period**

  1. **Hemodynamic stability** is the primary goal. CPB gives rise to myocardial functional impairment and a systemic inflammatory response. Maintain adequate volume status, perfusion pressure, and appropriate rate and rhythm. Continuously monitor and reassess the surgical field.

  2. **Hemostasis.** Once cardiovascular stability has been achieved and surgical bleeding is controlled, **protamine** administration begins. Initially, 25 to 50 mg is given over 2 to 3 minutes, and the hemodynamic response is observed. Protamine often causes systemic vasodilation (type I reaction) that can be avoided by slow administration over 10 to 15 minutes with or without α-agonist support. Rarely, an anaphylactic or anaphylactoid reaction (type II reaction) resulting in hypotension, bronchospasm, and pulmonary edema is encountered. Type II reactions are

TABLE 29.6	Hemodynamic Changes and Management After CPB				
Clinical Scenarios	SBP	CO	PAP	CVP	Management Options
Hypovolemia	↓	↓	↓	↓	Volume administration
LV failure	↓	↓	↑	↑	Inotropes, IABP, CPB, and LVAD
RV failure	↓	↓	↓	↑	Inotropes, increase MAP, decrease PVR, CPB, and RVAD
Biventricular failure	↓	↓	↑	↑	Treatment for LV and RV failure
Low SVR	↓	↑	Normal	Normal	Vasopressors; decrease anesthetic
High SVR	↑	↓	Normal	Normal	Vasodilators; deepen anesthetic
pHTN	↓	↓	↑	↑	Inotropes with pulmonary dilating properties (eg, milrinone), nitrous oxide; reinstitute CPB

CO, cardiac output; CPB, cardiopulmonary bypass; CVP, central venous pressure; IABP, intra-aortic balloon pump; LV, left ventricle; LVAD, left ventricular assist device; MAP, mean arterial pressure; PAP, pulmonary artery pressure; pHTN, pulmonary hypertension; PVR, pulmonary vascular resistance; RV, right ventricle; RVAD, right ventricular assist device; SVR, systemic vascular resistance.

more likely observed in diabetic patients taking subcutaneous injections of protamine-containing insulin preparations (ie, NPH) and men who have had a vasectomy. Finally, catastrophic pulmonary hypertension (type III reaction) can occur, manifested by elevated PA pressures, right ventricular dilatation, systemic hypotension, and myocardial depression. Upon severe reaction, protamine is immediately discontinued, appropriate resuscitative measures are used, and, if necessary, the patient is retreated with heparin (with a full loading dose), and CPB is reinitiated. If forward flow is compromised, ask the surgeon to inject the heparin into the right atrium.

   a. The protamine dose is calculated based on the patient's whole blood heparin level. Automated heparin-protamine titration assays calculate the protamine dose for complete heparin neutralization; this method is associated with reduced protamine requirement. Alternatively, 1 to 1.3 mg of protamine is administered for each 100 units of heparin administered throughout the procedure.
   b. ACT monitoring is useful for titrating protamine after initial dose. Thromboelastography may be used to provide information about coagulation factor activity, platelet function, and degree of fibrinolysis during and after CPB.
   c. Normothermia reduces post-CPB coagulopathy
3. Pulmonary dysfunction may follow CPB. Aggressive treatment of bronchospasm before sternal closure is imperative.

4. **Pulmonary hypertension** may arise during the post-CPB period. See **Table 29.6** for approaches to management.
5. **Sternal closure** may precipitate acute cardiovascular decompensation. **Cardiac tamponade** may develop from compression of the heart and great vessels in the mediastinum. Severe hemodynamic compromise may necessitate transport to ICU with open sternum.
   a. Volatile anesthetics and other negative inotropes are reduced in anticipation of sternal closure. Intravascular volume should be optimized.
   b. Immediately after sternal closure, the filling pressures and cardiac output are compared with preclosure values, and appropriate adjustments in volume or drug infusions are made.
   c. Mediastinal and pleural tubes are placed on suction to prevent tamponade and quantify blood loss.
   d. Epicardial pacing is rechecked to assure reliable capture and optimal pacing setting.
G. **Transfer to the ICU**
   1. Patients should always be hemodynamically stable before transport. Transport with full monitors and defibrillator.
   2. Upon arrival to the ICU, mediastinal and pleural drainage tubes are attached to suction. Detailed sign out should be given before transfer care to the ICU team.

V. POSTOPERATIVE CARE
A. **Warming.** Most cardiac surgical patients will be hypothermic upon arrival to the ICU, and their initial course is notable for warming and vasodilation. Adequate sedation will prevent unwanted waking and shivering during this period.
B. **Complications**
   1. **Dysrhythmias and myocardial ischemia** are common in the immediate postoperative period. Diagnosis and management are discussed in Chapter 36.
   2. **Unexplained profound hypotension**, unresponsive to volume and pharmacologic resuscitation, is an indication for immediate reopening of the chest in the ICU. The OR should be notified, and blood products requisitioned.
   3. **Cardiac tamponade** may occur insidiously. Most often, an accumulation of blood in the mediastinum and inadequate chest tube drainage secondary to clot are responsible. Placing mediastinal tubes on suction as soon as the sternum is closed will help to prevent the development of tamponade. Reopening the sternum may be lifesaving. The diagnosis is considered with hypotension or low-output state. TEE is very helpful to make quick diagnosis.

VI. PEDIATRIC CARDIAC ANESTHESIA
A. **Transition from fetal to adult circulation.** The transition from fetal to adult circulation is a transformation from a parallel to a series circulation. In utero, there is right-to-left shunting of blood across the ductus arteriosus. After birth, as the lungs are expanded and alveolar oxygen tension rises, the PVR decreases. Simultaneously, the SVR increases in association with the loss of the low-resistance placental circulation. The net effect of the PVR falling below the SVR is a reversal of ductus flow. The ductus arteriosus will contract and functionally close in the first 10 to 15 hours of life. This is caused by a loss of placental-produced prostaglandins and an

increase in neonatal blood oxygen tension. Accompanying the decrease in PVR is an increase in pulmonary blood flow, an improvement in RV compliance, and a decrease in right-sided pressures relative to the left. This drop in right atrial pressure results in the closure of the foramen ovale. With the closure of the ductus arteriosus and the foramen ovale, the circulation assumes an adult configuration. These changes in the neonatal period are tentative; however, and reversion to a fetal circulation can occur during periods of abnormal physiologic stress. Persistence of elements of fetal circulation is common in many cases of congenital heart disease (CHD) and can occasionally be lifesaving.

B. **Differences between neonatal and adult cardiac physiology**
   1. In infants, there is **parasympathetic nervous system dominance** that reflects the relative immaturity of the sympathetic nervous system. Infant hearts are more responsive to circulating catecholamines than to sympathetic nervous stimulation.
   2. Neonatal hearts have more inelastic membrane mass than elastic contractile mass. Consequently, infant hearts have less myocardial reserve, a greater sensitivity to myocardial depressants, and a greater sensitivity to volume overload. The relatively noncompliant ventricles make stroke volume less responsive to increases in preload or demand. As such, **increases in cardiac output largely depend on increases in heart rate**.
   3. The RV and LV are equal in muscle mass at birth. A left-to-right muscle mass ratio of 2:1 is not achieved until the age of 4 to 5 months.

C. **Congenital Heart Disease (CHD)**. The clinical presentation depends on both the anatomy and the physiologic changes secondary to intracardiac shunts and obstructive lesions. In general, there are three categories of lesions: shunt, mixing lesion, and flow obstruction.
   1. **Shunt**. A shunt is an abnormal communication between the systemic and pulmonary circulations. Examples are atrial septal defect (ASD), VSD, and patent ductus arteriosus (PDA). The direction of blood flow is dependent on the pressures on either side of the shunt and the size of the shunt orifice.
      a. **Left-to-right shunt**—occurs when the PVR is lower than the SVR, resulting in increased pulmonary blood flow. This can cause pulmonary circulation congestion, volume overload, and increased work for the LV. Prolonged exposure to increased pulmonary blood flow results in progressive elevations in PVR, eventually leading to pulmonary vascular obstructive disease.
      b. **Right-to-left shunt**—occurs when PVR or RV outflow tract resistance exceeds SVR, thereby reducing pulmonary blood flow and manifesting as hypoxemia and cyanosis. Pure right-to-left shunting due to high PVR is seen in Eisenmenger syndrome and persistent pulmonary hypertension of the newborn with atrial and ductal shunting.
      c. **Simple versus complex shunts:** Simple shunts are not associated with anatomic obstruction to ventricular outflow. Pulmonary and systemic blood flow is determined by both the size of the shunt and the relative PVR/SVR ratio. Most left-to-right shunts are simple shunts. In contrast, most right-to-left shunts are **complex shunts**. These shunts are accompanied by an anatomic obstruction to blood flow. Shunt flow depends less on the PVR/SVR ratio and more on the resistance of the obstructive lesion. For example, tetralogy of Fallot is a complex right-to-left shunt since shunting occurs through the VSD because of pulmonary outflow obstruction while PVR remains low.

d. **Shunt flow calculation.** Measuring the Q_p/Q_s (ratio of pulmonary to systemic blood flow) quantifies the direction and degree of shunting.

$$Q_p/Q_s = (SaO_2 - SmvO_2)/(SpvO_2 - SpaO_2)$$

$Q_p/Q_s > 1$ indicates left-to-right shunt

$(1-1.5$ small shunt; $1.5-2.0$ moderate shunt; > 2.0 large shunt$)$.

$Q_p/Q_s < 1$ indicates right-to left shunt

where Q_p is pulmonary blood flow, $SmvO_2$ is mixed venous oxygen saturation, Q_s is systemic blood flow, $SpvO_2$ is pulmonary venous oxygen saturation, SaO_2 is systemic arterial oxygen saturation, and $SpaO_2$ is PA oxygen saturation. When calculating the ratio, oxygen saturation can be conveniently used instead of oxygen content. To simplify the calculation, if systemic blood is fully saturated, one can approximate that there is no significant right-to-left shunting and that pulmonary venous oxygen saturation is equal to systemic oxygen saturation ($SpvO_2 = SaO_2$).

2. **Mixing lesions.** In these lesions, there is large mixing between the pulmonary and systemic circulation as if they act as a common chamber. The Q_p/Q_s is independent of the shunt size and entirely dependent on relative vascular resistance or outflow obstruction. In cases of LV outflow obstruction, the pulmonary blood flow may be excessive enough to impair systemic perfusion. Examples of mixing lesions include truncus arteriosus, single ventricle, and total anomalous pulmonary venous return.

3. **Obstructive lesions.** These include AS, pulmonic stenosis, coarctation of the aorta, and asymmetrical septal hypertrophy. These lesions have ductal-dependent circulations. For example, in left-sided obstructive defects, systemic perfusion is dependent on blood flow from the RV via the PDA. In right-sided obstructive lesions, pulmonary blood flow is supplied from the aorta via the PDA.

D. **Anesthetic management**
   1. **Preoperative evaluation**
      a. The **history** should provide an assessment of the extent of cardiopulmonary impairment. Documentation should be made of the presence of cyanosis or CHF, exercise tolerance, cyanotic spells, activity level, feeding and growth patterns, associated syndromes, and anatomic abnormalities.
      b. **Physical examination** should make note of skin color, activity level, respiratory pattern and frequency, heart and lung sounds, and appropriateness of development for given age. Peripheral pulses should be palpated and blood pressure measurements obtained in both arms as well as the lower extremities to rule out coarctation.
      c. The **chest radiograph** should be examined for evidence of cardiomegaly, CHF, abnormalities in heart position, and the presence of any thoracic cage abnormalities.
      d. The **ECG** may be normal; however, abnormalities can be important clues to underlying cardiac lesions.
      e. **Cardiac catheterization** can define the cardiopulmonary anatomy and quantify pulmonary and systemic shunt flows, vascular resistance, and intracardiac chamber pressures.
   2. **Premedication.** Infants younger than 6 months of age, cyanotic or dyspneic children, and patients who are critically ill should generally

receive no premedication. Older or more vigorous children may be given oral midazolam (0.5-1.0 mg/kg) with or without oral ketamine (5-7 mg/kg). An alternative intramuscular regimen is ketamine (3-5 mg/kg) in combination with midazolam (0.5-1.0 mg) and glycopyrrolate (0.1-0.2 mg) administered in the preanesthetic holding area. With the exception of ketamine, doses of sedatives are reduced in cases where decreasing SVR would increase right-to-left shunting. Cyanotic infants are usually polycythemic and may be prone to thromboses of vital organs if they are not adequately hydrated with IV fluids preoperatively.

3. **Monitoring and equipment.** In addition to the standard monitoring required for all patients, a precordial or esophageal stethoscope and three temperature probes (tympanic membrane, esophageal, and rectal) should be available. Intra-arterial pressure monitoring is usually necessary. Prior surgical procedures, such as Blalock-Taussig shunt construction or coarctation repair, may influence the choice of site for radial artery cannulation. **Central venous catheters** are typically inserted. A 4-French double-lumen catheter can be used for infants weighing less than 10 kg, and a 5-French triple-lumen catheter can be used for larger children. A warming blanket, radiant heating lamps, and a heated humidifier are useful perioperatively. TEE is an important diagnostic and intraoperative management tool.

4. **Resuscitation drugs** and infusions of inotropic medications appropriate for pediatric use must be available. Commonly used inotropes include dopamine (2-10 µg/kg/min), epinephrine (0.01-0.1 µg/kg/min), and dobutamine 2-10 µg/kg/min). **Air bubbles** must be meticulously removed from IV tubing and syringes. **Air filters** should be used whenever possible. Even in the absence of shunts, paradoxical air emboli may traverse a probe-patent foramen ovale (PFO).

5. **Induction.** The choice between an inhalational and IV induction is based primarily on ventricular function and the degree of patient cooperation. A slow, carefully titrated induction by either technique usually provides a safe and stable anesthetic. Theoretically, patients with right-to-left shunts may have a slower rate of induction with volatile anesthetics because blood is shunted past the lungs. Similarly, arterial concentrations of IV anesthetics may increase more rapidly in patients with a significant right-to-left shunt.

E. Cardiopulmonary bypass

1. **Pump prime volume** ranges between 150 and 1200 mL. Packed red blood cells are frequently added to the prime to yield an initial Hct of approximately 25% when on bypass. For smaller children, the red cells may be washed to remove potassium, lactic acid, and citrate-phosphate-dextrose-adenine preservative. Cells may be leukocyte depleted to decrease patient exposure to cytomegalovirus. Typical constituents of pump prime include sodium bicarbonate (to counteract acidosis), mannitol (to promote diuresis), heparin, and calcium (to offset the effects of the citrate in blood). Albumin solutions and FFP may be added to the prime for neonates.

2. **Infants and children** generally lack vasoocclusive disease. Consequently, blood flow during CPB is more important than arterial pressure. Flows as high as 150 mL/kg/min may be used in infants weighing less than 5 kg, while MAP as low as 30 mm Hg is well tolerated provided that SVC pressure is low (indicating that venous drainage is adequate).

3. **DHCA** is used extensively for infants weighing less than 10 kg. Up to 1 hour of circulatory arrest is tolerated without neurologic injury at a core and brain temperature of 15 °C to 20 °C. Where appropriate, low-flow CPB may offer advantages over circulatory arrest. Management points include adequate brain hypothermia (eg, packing the head with ice packs), hemodilution, acid-base balance, muscle relaxation, and blood glucose control.

F. **Procedures that do not require CPB** include PDA ligation, aortic coarctation repair, PA banding, and most procedures, which create shunts designed to increase pulmonary blood flow (eg, modified Blalock-Taussig shunt). Procedures such as pulmonary valvotomy, aortic valvotomy, and the creation of ASDs can be accomplished with percutaneous techniques.

G. **Management of specific CHD lesions** (Table 29.7)

1. **Cyanotic lesions** are secondary to **right-to-left shunting** either alone or in the presence of an obstruction to pulmonary blood flow. Typical conditions include tetralogy of Fallot, tricuspid atresia, pulmonary atresia, and pulmonary hypertension.

   a. **Management goals** are to decrease PVR, increase pulmonary blood flow, maintain SVR, and maintain central volume.

   b. **Ventilation management** include using modest hypocarbia, increasing inspired oxygen concentration, maintaining normal functional residual capacity, and avoiding acidosis.

   c. Patients with **tetralogy of Fallot** are prone to hypercyanotic spells (rapid desaturation usually in response to surgical or other stimulation). Management of these spells includes measures that reduce infundibular spasm and improve pulmonary blood flow (eg, β-blockers such as propranolol), volume loading (15-20 mL/kg), and use of α-agonists (eg, phenylephrine) to increase SVR. Alprostadil (prostaglandin E_1 0.05-0.1 µg/kg/min IV) may be used to maintain ductus arteriosus patency, decrease PVR, and increase pulmonary blood flow.

2. **Lesions with increased pulmonary blood flow** and left-to-right shunting include ASDs, VSDs, and PDA.

   a. **Management goals** are to avoid negative inotropes and excessive pulmonary blood flow.

   b. **Anesthetic maneuvers** include minimizing myocardial depressants (eg, volatile anesthetics) and increasing PVR and decrease pulmonary blood flow in favor of systemic blood flow through maintaining normocarbia to slight hypercarbia, limiting inspired oxygen concentration, and using PEEP.

3. **Balanced shunts** have the potential for a ventricle's output to be directed to the pulmonary or systemic circulation and include hypoplastic left heart syndrome, truncus arteriosus, double-outlet RV, and complete AV canal defect. The direction of blood flow is governed by the relative resistances of the pulmonary and systemic vasculatures (PVR/SVR ratio).

   a. **Management goals** are to manipulate pulmonary blood flow to maintain adequate systemic perfusion. Often both a low-normal blood pressure (eg, MAP of 40 mm Hg) and a low PaO_2 (eg, 40 mm Hg) must be tolerated.

   b. **Anesthetic maneuvers** depend on the balance of systemic versus pulmonary blood flow, which can be affected by altering $Paco_2$, inspired oxygen concentration, and PEEP.

TABLE 29.7	Specific Congenital Cardiac Lesions			
Lesion	**Anatomy**	**Pathophysiology**	**Surgical Correction**	**Anesthetic Considerations**
ASD	Three varieties: 1. Ostium secundum: defect in septum (most common) 2. Ostium primum: endocardial cushion defect 3. Sinus venosus: caval-atrial defect often with partial anomalous pulmonary venous return	Left-to-right shunt RV volume overload Potential for right-to-left shunting (eg, during Valsalva maneuver) with paradoxical embolus risk Minimal symptoms until later age, when CHF may develop	Suture or patch closure Percutaneous catheterization device closure	Inhalation or intravenous induction Potential extubation at end of procedure Avoid air bubbles
VSD	Supracristal, membranous canal, and muscular subtypes	Left-to-right shunt Increased pulmonary blood flow Pulmonary hypertension and reversal of shunt as a late effect (Eisenmenger syndrome)	Dacron patch closure of singular or multiple defects Muscular defects may be difficult to locate Selected defects may be amenable to percutaneous catheterization device closure	Hypocarbia and low FiO_2 to decrease pulmonary blood flow Avoid myocardial depressants Avoid air bubbles Potential for postoperative AV block and pacing requirement Potential need for postrepair inotropic support
Coarctation of the aorta	Narrowing usually distal to origin of left subclavian artery May be preductal or postductal in location Often associated with a VSD	Increased blood flow to upper extremities and head Systemic hypoperfusion Pressure overload of LV	Left thoracotomy approach Subclavian artery flap angioplasty or resection and end-to-end anastomosis	Non-CPB case Arterial line on right Suitable for regional anesthesia supplementation Potential for postrepair hypertension
PDA	PDA	Right-to-left shunt when PVR is high Left-to-right shunt as PVR decreases Necessary for survival with certain lesions (eg, hypoplastic left heart syndrome)	Left thoracotomy vs thoracoscopic approach Ligation and occasional division of PDA Potential for percutaneous catheterization coil embolization	Usually premature infants with concomitant pulmonary disease Avoid high FiO_2 (risk of retrolental fibroplasia) Risk of recurrent laryngeal nerve damage

Tetralogy of Fallot	1. VSD 2. Pulmonary outflow tract obstruction 3. RV hypertrophy Overriding aorta	Right-to-left shunting through VSD into overriding aorta Fixed (pulmonic stenosis) and dynamic (infundibular hypertrophy) RV outflow obstruction components Systemic desaturation ("Tet" spell)	Patch closure of VSD RV outflow tract reconstruction/augmentation Excision of infundibular muscle band (when appropriate)	Management of "Tet spell": augment intravascular volume, minimize PVR (increase FiO_2 and decrease $Paco_2$), increase SVR (knee-chest position and phenylephrine), and consider negative inotropes (halothane and β-blockade) Potential need for postoperative pacing
Transposition of the great arteries	Transposition of both the aorta to the RV and the PA to the LV resulting in isolation of pulmonary and systemic circulations	ASD, VSD, and/or PDA required for pulmonary and systemic blood mixing and, hence, survival	Atrial switch procedure (Mustard and Senning): rarely performed Arterial switch procedure (Jatene) When associated with a VSD and pulmonic stenosis, a Rastelli procedure (LV to aorta baffle closure via the VSD, and RV to PA allograft conduit)	Ductus/mixing lesion-dependent CHD lesion Prostaglandin E_1 to maintain ductus patency (when appropriate)
Truncus arteriosus	Single great artery that gives rise to the aorta, PA, and coronary arteries Associated VSD	Mixing of pulmonary and systemic blood Most commonly presents with pulmonary overcirculation Valvuloplasty of truncal valve	VSD closure RV to PA valved conduit	Increase PVR or decrease pulmonary blood flow precorrection (based on the degree of pulmonary overcirculation) Normalize PVR postcorrection Potential need for inotropic support postrepair

(continued)

TABLE 29.7 Specific Congenital Cardiac Lesions (Continued)

Lesion	Anatomy	Pathophysiology	Surgical Correction	Anesthetic Considerations
Atrioventricular canal defect	Common AV valve. Deficiency of atrial and ventricular septae	Mixing of blood at the atrial and ventricular levels Usually presents with pulmonary overcirculation	Closure of ASD and VSD Mitral/tricuspid valvuloplasty	Manipulate PVR to balance/optimize pulmonary systemic blood flow Anticipate need for inotropic support postrepair Associated with Down syndrome (potential airway issues)
Hypoplastic left heart syndrome	Atretic/hypoplastic mitral valve, aortic valve, LV, and ascending aorta	Left-to-right shunt (obligatory) at atrial or ventricular level for mixing Ductus arteriosus dependent for right-to-left (ie, systemic) perfusion	Palliative, staged repair: 1. Norwood I: atrial septectomy, reconstruction of aortic arch, PA plasty, and creation of systemic to pulmonary shunt 2. Bidirectional Glenn: takedown of systemic to pulmonary shunt, creation of SVC to PA (cavopulmonary) shunt 3. Modified Fontan procedure: creation of an IVC to PA anastomosis via an intra-atrial baffle; creates total cavopulmonary continuity Alternatively, cardiac transplantation is an option	Critically ill neonates. Preoperative intensive care unit (ICU) management will impact outcome. Prostaglandin E_1 to maintain ductal patency Inotropes often necessary prerepair and postrepair Avoid myocardial depressants Fentanyl >50 µg/kg prior to sternotomy. Manipulate PVR via adjustments in FiO_2 and Pco_2 to balance/optimize pulmonary vs systemic perfusion Target goal: MAP = 40, pH = 7.40, $Pao_2 = 40$, $Paco_2 = 40$

ASD, atrial septal defect; AV, atrioventricular; CHD, congenital heart disease; CHF, congestive heart failure; CPB, cardiopulmonary bypass; FiO_2, fraction of inspired oxygen; ICU, intensive care unit; IVC, inferior vena cava; LV, left ventricle; MAP, mean arterial pressure; PA, pulmonary artery; Pao_2, partial pressure of oxygen; $Paco_2$, partial pressure of carbon dioxide; PDA, patent ductus arteriosus; PVR, pulmonary vascular resistance; RV, right ventricle; SVC, superior vena cava; SVR, systemic vascular resistance; VSD, ventricular septal defect.

VII. OTHER CARDIAC PROCEDURES

A. Off-bypass CABG is performed to avoid the complications associated with CPB and to minimize aortic manipulation. Proximal grafts are performed using either a partial aortic cross-clamp technique or a specifically designed proximal anastomotic device that precludes aortic clamping. Distal grafts are performed using one of several heart stabilizing devices. Considerations for this procedure include the following:

1. Consider tailoring anesthetic management to allow possible **early extubation** after surgery (eg, fentanyl 5-10 µg/kg, volatile anesthetic followed by an infusion of propofol or dexmedetomidine).

2. **Heparin** is given to maintain ACT above 400 seconds. This allows the patient to be emergently initiated on CPB if necessary. Antifibrinolytic therapy is avoided. A small dose of protamine (50-100 mg) is given after the procedure.

3. **Hemodynamic instability** is common, particularly when the surgeon is performing the distal anastomoses. Grafts to vessels with less disease tend to be associated with more instability than those to vessels that are occluded. Increasing MAP to optimize coronary perfusion is critical for the ischemic heart during creation of the distal anastomosis. If hemodynamically intolerable ischemia results, coronary shunting may be indicated. Occasionally, repositioning of the heart is required to permit augmented right-sided filling when hemodynamic instability is due to obstruction of right heart inflow.

4. **Volume requirements** tend to be high. A full heart tends to tolerate physical manipulation better.

5. **Ventricular dysrhythmias** may be treated with an amiodarone 150 mg IV bolus and then followed with 1 mg/min infusion. Acid-base and electrolyte abnormalities should be corrected.

B. "Redo" cardiac surgery

1. **Mediastinal structures**, including the heart, major vessels, prior coronary bypass grafts, as well as the lungs may be adherent to the underside of the sternum. They can be lacerated during sternotomy. Usually, 2 to 4 units of blood must be in the OR before sternotomy begins. An additional 14 g IV catheter or a rapid infusion catheter should be placed to facilitate volume resuscitation. Because the patient may need to go on CPB emergently, heparin must be in a syringe ready to administer immediately. In emergency situations, venous return may be supplied from the pump suction line on the field ("sucker bypass").

2. Insertion of a PA catheter equipped with pacing capability is prudent as epicardial pacing may not be possible during chest opening. Transcutaneous defibrillation pads should be applied to treat malignant arrhythmias.

3. **Diffuse bleeding** from dissection of scar tissue may occur after CPB. Amicar is useful in standard doses.

4. **ECG monitoring** is imperative because manipulation of atheromatous grafts may send emboli to the coronary circulation. Because myocardial protection is more challenging in patients with previous coronary grafts, post-bypass myocardial dysfunction is more likely.

C. DHCA may be necessary for surgery on the distal ascending aorta or aortic arch (eg, for an aneurysm or aortic dissection). Circulatory arrest provides a bloodless field for distal aortic anastomosis. Hypothermia decreases the metabolic rate and minimizes the risk of cerebral and organ ischemia during circulatory arrest. Problems associated with DHCA include increased CBP time, coagulopathy, and end-organ dysfunction. The risk

of permanent neurologic injury after aortic arch surgery using DHCA is approximately 3% to 12%. Most patients tolerate 30 minutes of DHCA without significant neurologic dysfunction. Management issues include the following:

1. **Organ protection during DHCA**
   a. **Hypothermia.** Systemic cooling to 18 °C produces electrical silence on the EEG in most patients. There is no outcomes evidence to support topical cooling of the head in humans.
   b. **Antegrade cerebral perfusion (ACP)** via the right axillary artery or **retrograde cerebral perfusion (RCP)** via the SVC cannula can be used to extend the duration of safe circulatory arrest. ACP is thought to be superior to RCP for cerebral protection and avoid deep hypothermia.
2. **Glycemic control** is important. Glucose metabolism is impaired under DHCA. Blood glucose concentration should be maintained below 180 mg/dL to avoid worsening neurologic injury.
3. **Temperature monitoring.** It is commonly preferred to use more than one site for core body temperature monitoring. Nasopharyngeal temperature provides the closest assessment of brain temperature for adults.
4. **Acid-base management** depends on whether α-stat or pH-stat is used (see Section IV.C.2). The pediatric literature generally recommends the use of pH-stat management during DHCA for both cerebral and myocardial protection.

D. **Cardiac tamponade and constrictive pericarditis**
   1. Avoid decreases in myocardial contractility, peripheral vascular resistance, and heart rate. **Pericardiocentesis** prior to induction may be advisable in patients with tamponade unless the condition is secondary to aortic dissection.
   2. An arterial catheter, a large-bore IV catheter should be inserted. A central venous catheter or PA catheter may be used if the patient can tolerate insertion.
   3. Useful **induction agents** include etomidate and ketamine.
   4. A method for **backup atrial pacing** (transesophageal or transvenous) should be available.
   5. Patients should be prepped and draped for surgery prior to induction. In **severe cases**, awake intubation with maintenance of spontaneous ventilation should be considered.

E. **Cardiac transplantation**
   1. **Anesthetic management of the donor**
      a. Basic management of donor patients and organs is discussed in Chapter 21.
      b. Donor after cardiac death organ transplantation is an emerging technique with promising initial results that serves to increase the overall number of organ donations. In donor patients, after cardiac arrest has occurred and is deemed irreversible, both heart and lungs may be harvested and transported with various preservation techniques. Outcomes in transplant recipients of these organs have been comparable with recipients of organs from donor after brain death patients.
   2. **Anesthetic management of the recipient**
      a. **The key to patient survival** is minimizing the ischemic time of the donated heart. Consequently, expeditious preparation of the recipient and communication with the surgical team are essential.
      b. **Preoperative evaluation** of the recipient should determine whether the patient has had previous chest surgery, has an elevated PVR (>6

Wood units, transpulmonary gradient >12 mm Hg), has pulmonary hypertension responsive to venodilators, or is coagulopathic.

c. **Invasive monitoring** includes arterial and central lines. A PA catheter and TEE should be used. Internal cardiac defibrillator (ICD) should be turned off.

d. **Precautions for a full stomach** may be necessary during induction. If the patient is receiving inotropic infusions, consider increasing their doses before induction. If a ventricular assist device (VAD) is present, venous return must be maintained for the pump to maintain its flow rate.

e. **Right heart failure and coagulopathy** are common during the rewarming phase of bypass. Cellular blood products should be irradiated or leukocyte depleted to minimize foreign HLA antigen exposure.

f. The donor heart may be unresponsive to drugs whose actions are mediated by the recipient's cholinergic nervous system (eg, atropine and glycopyrrolate). Upon termination of CPB, the recipient's heart rate should be maintained between 80 and 110 beats/min. This can be accomplished with epicardial pacing or pharmacologically with a dopamine (2-10 μg/kg/min), epinephrine (0.01-01 μg/kg/min), or isoproterenol infusion (0.5-5 μg/min).

g. **Immunosuppressants** and steroid will be necessary and are administered in consultation with the surgeon and transplant cardiologist.

F. **Lung transplantation**

1. **Indications and surgical technique**: Lung transplantation is performed for end-stage nonmalignant lung disease. Common indications are severe emphysema, α1-antitrypsin deficiency, cystic fibrosis, pulmonary fibrosis, and pulmonary hypertension. Specific operations include living-related lobar lung transplant (LRLLTx), single-lung transplant (SLTx), double-lung transplant (DLTx), sequential SLTx, and combined heart-lung transplantation. The patient's position depends on the incision required for adequate surgical exposure (lateral decub/thoracotomy for SLTx and clamshell incision/supine for DLTx or LRLLTx). Patients will have undergone preoperative counseling, exercise and cardiac testing, and a conditioning program.

2. **Anesthetic management of the recipient**

a. **Invasive monitoring** with arterial line, central venous line, and PA catheter. A femoral arterial line and large bore femoral venous access are contemplated for patients who have a high likelihood of requiring extracorporeal membrane oxygenation (ECMO) or CPB. TEE is useful for assessing heart function and pulmonary blood flow after implantation.

b. **Medications** should be immediately available to treat bronchospasm, electrolyte disturbances, pulmonary hypertension, and right ventricular failure. Immunosuppressants, steroids, and antibiotics should also be administered. All blood products must be leukocyte depleted and transfused via a filter. Anticipation of a large transfusion requirement and maintenance of an ample supply of blood products are important.

c. **An epidural catheter** is typically placed for postoperative pain management unless the patient is already on ECMO or has other contraindications.

d. **Bypass or ECMO equipment** should be available if hypoxemia becomes a significant problem. Indications for full CPB include arterial oxygen saturation less than 90% after clamping of the PA, low cardiac index less than 2.0 L/min/m^2 despite therapy with dopamine and nitroglycerin, or a systolic blood pressure less than 90 mm Hg. Continuous cardiac output monitors may be used to assess cardiac function.

e. **Induction with a** technique that provides cardiovascular stability is appropriate. Most recipients are considered "full stomachs."

f. **Lung isolation** is best achieved with a left side DLT or large (>8 mm) single-lumen endotracheal tube with an endobronchial block. The DLT is exchanged for a single-lumen tube at the end of operation.

g. **Capnography** may be misleading because of severe mismatching of ventilation to perfusion. Frequent measurements of ABG tensions are warranted to assess ventilation. Worsening acidemia may also signal inadequate tissue perfusion from a variety of causes (hypovolemia, airtrapping, and decreased cardiac output).

h. **Postoperative management**

1. Pulmonary hypertension will cause increased hydrostatic pulmonary edema and worsening gas exchange and lung compliance. Serial ABGs are followed to document the function of the transplanted lung.

2. Acute rejection may manifest as decreasing pulmonary compliance with worsening arterial oxygenation.

3. Many patients will remain intubated until the transplanted lung begins to function well, and symptoms of reperfusion edema and acute rejection are controlled. The trachea is extubated only when the patient is hemodynamically stable and breathing comfortably, which is sometimes possible in the OR.

4. Observe for signs of toxicity from the immunosuppressive regimen, including acute renal failure.

5. Repeated bronchoscopies and biopsies of the transplanted lung are necessary after surgery and are often managed under local anesthesia with intravenous sedation.

G. **VADs** may be classified as extracorporeal, implantable, and percutaneously inserted. The extracorporeal employ a pump positioned outside of the body and have largely been replaced by smaller pumps implanted inside of the chest.

1. **Implantable devices** (eg, Novacor LVAS, HeartMate XVE/IP/VE, HeartMate Pneumatic, HeartMate II/III, Thoratec IVAD, Impella).

a. These devices are used as a bridge to cardiac transplantation, destination therapy, or recovery.

b. Except for the Thoratec LVAD, these devices are designed for LV support only. They consist of an inflow cannula, a pump, and an outflow cannula. The inflow cannula is inserted into the LV apex while the outflow cannula is inserted into the ascending aorta. A driveline is tunneled through the skin to connect the implanted pump to the external console. CPB is always necessary for placement.

c. The Novacor LVAS, HeartMate VXE, and HeartMate devices are electrically driven. A rechargeable power source fits into a backpack or holsters and allows the patient to leave the hospital.

d. **Axial flow devices** provide constant flow with reduction in pulsatile arterial perfusion.

1. The HeartMate II is smaller than other devices, making it appropriate for use in a wider range of patients and may be used as a bridge to transplant or to improve survival and quality of life as a long-term device in transplant-ineligible heart failure patients. It represents an improvement in survival over HeartMate XVE.

  2. The HeartMate III represents an improvement over the HeartMate
  II in rate of adverse events and battery life and is smaller, which
  may facilitate more minimally invasive techniques for placement.
  2. The Impella is a percutaneously inserted VAD that can be placed via retrograde approach across aortic valve using femoral or axillary artery
  access. It has been in patients with heart failure, cardiogenic shock
  (CS), and high-risk patients undergoing percutaneous intervention. It
  provides up to 6.2 L/min of cardiac output.
  3. Anesthetic considerations for VAD insertion
  a. Patients will have **marginal cardiac function.** Extreme care is required
  during induction to minimize decreases in contractility and preload.
  b. Large-bore IV access and anti-fibrinolytics are recommended.
  c. If the patient is receiving the device as a bridge to transplantation,
  transfuse with leukocyte-depleted cellular blood products to minimize HLA antigen exposure.
  d. **TEE is required to assess the position and flow of the cannula** in addition
  to facilitating air removal. It also evaluates the position of the interventricular septum to guide the pump output and evaluate ventricular functions and volume status.
  e. Patients receiving an LVAD frequently require RV support. Inotropes,
  inhaled prostaglandin or nitric oxide, and occasionally an RVAD are
  required.
  f. The flow of the device depends largely on the volume in the ventricle. Decreased venous return or hypovolemia will be signaled by a
  decreased pumping rate which is typically improved with volume
  repletion. Vasopressors such as norepinephrine and vasopressin are
  typically needed to ameliorate vasodilation.
H. ECMO is an alternative form of extracorporeal life support to VADs. ECMO
is indicated for the short-term management of severe but reversible CS
or respiratory failure that is refractory to conventional treatment. It is an
option for treatment of severe postcardiotomy ventricular dysfunction
with or without hypoxemia. It consists of an external pump that pushes
venous blood through a membrane allowing gas exchange before returning the blood to the circulation via a warmer.
  1. Venous drainage usually occurs from the internal jugular (IJ) vein or
  femoral vein. Blood is returned either to an artery (venoarterial ECMO)
  or a central vein (venovenous ECMO).
  2. Venoarterial (VA) ECMO bypasses the patient's heart and lungs with
  diversion of complete or partial flow through the ECMO circuit, providing both respiratory and hemodynamic support. It can be used for
  refractory postcardiotomy CS. The same cannulation setup during
  CPB can be used for ECMO. If considered subsequently, ECMO can
  be established from the femoral artery and vein. A condition called
  differential hypoxemia can occur in VA ECMO when a proportion of
  venous blood in a patient with some return of cardiac function is
  pumped into the diseased lungs, with subsequent ejection of hypoxic
  blood to the coronaries and great vessels. This may be revealed by a
  difference in oxygenation from sampling of left-sided and right-sided
  arterial lines.
  3. Venovenous (VV) ECMO provides gas exchange support in patients with
  good left cardiac function. Venous cannulae are usually placed in the
  right femoral vein for drainage and right IJ for infusion. A dual-lumen
  cannula (Avalon or Protek Duo) can be inserted into the IJ vein. The
  cannula drains blood from IVC and SVC or RA returns oxygenated
  blood into RA or PA.

4. **Aggressive medical support** is required to optimize the results of ECMO and facilitate weaning. Interventions may include the use of pulmonary vasodilators for pulmonary hypertension, lung-protective ventilation strategies; optimization of preload to provide pulmonary perfusion; and the use of renal replacement therapy. To avoid thrombus formation in the ECMO circuit, heparin is administered to maintain the ACT at 1.5 to 2.0 times normal.

5. **Continual assessment** of native cardiopulmonary function is essential. If the heart and lungs do not recover within the expected timeframe (1-2 weeks), the decision should be made to convert to long-term support such as a VAD or transplant. A discussion of the goals of care is important if the disease process is believed to be nonreversible.

I. **Transcatheter aortic valve replacement (TAVR)** is conducted for patients who are not surgical candidates for aortic replacement. An expanding bioprosthetic valve is placed over the native aortic valve. The procedure may be carried out using a transfemoral arterial or open transapical approach. The procedure is typically carried out in a hybrid OR or cardiac catheterization laboratory.

1. Anesthetic management

a. **General anesthesia** is required for proper positioning of the new valve with TEE. The procedure can be well tolerated under monitored anesthesia care or conscious sedation if fluoroscopy and TTE are used for valve deployment and evaluation.

b. **Rapid ventricular pacing** is required to minimize cardiac motion during valve deployment. A transvenous pacing lead is inserted into the right ventricle. A pacing rate of 140 to 200 beats/min frequently results in 1:1 ventricular capture and sufficiently lowers the pulse pressure and cardiac output. The rapid pacing periods must be minimized to avoid hemodynamic instability, especially in patients with depressed LV function and CAD.

c. **TEE** is particularly useful to assess adequate placement and function of the valve. It is crucial to ensure accurate positioning of the valve with TEE and fluoroscopy prior to deployment to avoid embolization of the valve or a large perivalvular leaks. TEE can assess stability, location, and function of the valve as well as the degree of perivalvular leak.

2. **Complications** include tamponade, cerebral vascular accident, aortic rupture or dissection, AI, conversion to emergent surgical aortic valve replacement, myocardial infarction, suboptimal valve deployment, and AV block.

J. **Percutaneous MV repair** is effective for both degenerative and functional MR in patients who are not suitable surgical candidates. The mechanical device (MitraClip, Abbott Vascular) is advanced through the IVC and delivered into the LA through transseptal access; it then grasps and approximates the valve leaflets. Short- and medium-term outcomes have been favorable in the randomized EVEREST II study. Compared to surgical repair, there is less reduction in MR with the percutaneous approach.

1. **General endotracheal anesthesia** with **TEE** and fluoroscopic guidance is required for the procedure. In some centers, the procedure is done under sedation and local anesthesia.

a. Right heart catheterization or PA catheter placement is often performed to monitor right- and left-sided hemodynamics before and after the procedure.

b. TEE guidance is crucial for the transseptal puncture and device positioning.

c. Brief periods of apnea may be required to allow precise placement of the device.

  d. Vasoactive agents and inotropes may be required to raise the blood pressure to adequately assess the severity of residual MR.

 2. Complications include tamponade, systemic embolization, worsening of MR, and arrhythmias (especially atrial fibrillation).

VIII. ANESTHESIA FOR "OFF-SITE" CARDIAC PROCEDURES

The goal of anesthesia is to provide sufficient sedation to allow the procedure to be completed without excessive movement while avoiding cardiopulmonary instability. The issues pertinent to anesthesia outside of the OR for noncardiac procedures apply to cardiac procedures as well.

A. The **IABP** is normally placed in the cardiac catheterization lab under sedation. It provides circulatory assistance for the failing or ischemic heart. Inflation of the intra-aortic balloon augments aortic diastolic pressure and thus coronary perfusion. The effect is most beneficial for the LV that receives most of its blood supply during diastole. Deflation of the balloon reduces the impedance to LV ejection, thereby reducing myocardial oxygen consumption.

 1. Preoperative indications for placement include unstable angina that is refractory to medical therapy; LV failure due to myocardial infarction, ruptured papillary muscle, or VSD; and prophylaxis for a high-risk patient with severe left main disease.

 2. Post-bypass indications include refractory LV failure preventing successful termination of CPB and refractory ST-segment elevation. The IABP is inserted through a femoral artery and advanced until the tip is 1 to 2 cm distal to the left subclavian artery in the descending thoracic aorta. It can be placed in a transthoracic manner if iliofemoral disease precludes the use of a femoral artery.

 3. Inflation of the IABP is synchronized with the patient's ECG, a pacemaker potential, or the arterial blood pressure trace. Balloon inflation occurs early in diastole either at the dicrotic notch of the arterial pressure waveform or following a time delay after the R wave on ECG.

 4. Balloon deflation occurs during isovolumic contraction. Intraoperative triggering directly from a pacemaker generator will eliminate interference otherwise caused by electrocautery or blood sampling from an arterial catheter.

 5. Relative contraindications include severe AI, aortic aneurysm, and severe peripheral vascular disease.

 6. Complications of the IABP include distal embolization, aortic dissection, aortic rupture, and lower extremity ischemia. **Anticoagulation** is indicated for extended IABP use. Heparin is usually used with a target ACT or aPTT that is 1.5 to 2 times the baseline.

 7. Percutaneous device closure of PFO or ASD. Following induction of general endotracheal anesthesia, right heart catheterization is performed, and a guidewire is threaded across the PFO or ASD. TEE is used to define the intracardiac anatomy and in guidance of device placement.

B. Aspiration thrombectomy with the AngioVac device (Vortex Medical) combines a venous suction cannula with VV bypass to achieve filtering of aspirated thrombus and other debris. This may be utilized to remove thrombi from the pulmonary vasculature, peripheral vasculature, or right atrium without the need for concomitant thrombolytic therapy.

 1. Anesthetic management is driven by the indication for the procedure. Complications associated with acute PE, RV dysfunction, cardiac arrhythmias, venous embolic event, or previous failed thrombolytic therapy should be anticipated. General anesthesia with TEE and arterial line for invasive BP monitoring are indicated, with consideration given to central venous access.

2. **VV bypass** is established for filtering of thrombotic material and other debris. Patients are heparinized to ACT of 250 to 300 seconds before initiation. Access site for VV bypass should be discussed with the proceduralist, as right IJ access may be limited if the need for more central venous access should arise.

C. **Implantable Cardioverter Defibrillator (ICD).** Modern ICDs consist of an endocardial lead system and a pectoral pulse generator. Older systems used epicardial lead systems and abdominal generators.

1. ICDs are used for primary prevention of sudden cardiac death in patients with systolic heart failure (EF < 35%) refractory to medical therapy or in those with high-risk conditions such as long QT syndrome, hypertrophic cardiomyopathy, Brugada syndrome, and arrhythmogenic right ventricular dysplasia. In addition to ICD placement, patients with dilated cardiomyopathy and a widened QRS have been shown to also benefit from cardiac resynchronization therapy.

2. Devices are placed under local anesthesia in the electrophysiology laboratory. A brief period of general anesthesia is necessary for testing of the device once it is implanted. A deep sedation anesthetic with propofol is suitable.

3. If intracardiac electrodes are inadequate, patients may require intraoperative epicardial electrode placement. These patients are often hemodynamically compromised. They should have an arterial catheter and catheter for vasoactive medication administration. Emergency drugs, including epinephrine, must be immediately available.

4. **Noninvasive programmed stimulation** is used to test the function of an ICD after it has been implanted. An ICD programmer is used to induce the irregular rhythm (ventricular fibrillation or tachycardia). The device is then checked for proper sensing and dysrhythmia termination.

D. **Cardioversion.** A short-acting sedative (eg, propofol or etomidate) can be administered for brief loss of consciousness. The combination of fentanyl and midazolam is an alternative but not ideal due to prolonged duration of action. Routine fasting guidelines should be followed for all elective cardioversions. Hemodynamically unstable patients often warrant immediate cardioversion, and a small dose of amnestic may be all that can be tolerated.

E. **Transcatheter ablation and electrophysiology** procedures take place in cardiac catheterization or electrophysiology labs. Common procedures include pulmonary vein isolation (PVI) for ablation of atrial fibrillation/flutter and supraventricular tachycardia (SVT).

1. **Anesthetic management** is determined by the type of procedure performed. PVI is performed under general anesthesia, as more durable response to therapy has been documented as compared to PVI under conscious sedation. However, SVT ablations are carried out under sedation, as to avoid suppression of arrhythmia by a general anesthetic.

Suggested Readings

American Society of Anesthesiologists and Society of Cardiovascular Anesthesiologists Task Force on Transesophageal Echocardiography. Practice guidelines for perioperative transesophageal echocardiography. An updated report by the American society of anesthesiologists and the society of cardiovascular anesthesiologists task force on transesophageal echocardiography. *Anesthesiology.* 2010;112:1084-1096.

Diaz LK, Andropoulos DB. New developments in pediatric cardiac anesthesia. *Anesthesiol Clin.* 2005;23:655-676.

El-Marghabel I. Ventricular assist devices and anesthesia. *Semin Cardiothorac Vasc Anesth.* 2005;9:241-249.

Feldman T, Foster E, Glower D, et al. Percutaneous repair or surgery for mitral regurgitation. *N Engl J Med.* 2011;364(15):1395-1406.

Ferraris VA, Ferraris SP, Saha SP, et al. Perioperative blood transfusion and blood conservation in cardiac surgery: the STS and SCA clinical practice guideline. *Ann Thorac Surg.* 2007;83:S27-S86.

Gilani FS, Farooqui S, Doddamani R, Gruberg L. Percutaneous mechanical support in cardiogenic shock: a review. *Clin Med Insights Cardiol.* 2015;9(suppl 2):23-28.

Gravlee GP, Davis RF, Kurusz M, et al, eds. *Cardiopulmonary Bypass.* 2nd ed. Lippincott Williams & Wilkins; 2000.

Gryka RJ, Buckley LF, Anderson SM. Vorapaxar: the current role and future directions of a novel protease-activated receptor antagonist for risk reduction in atherosclerotic disease. *Drugs R D.* 2017;17(1):65-72.

Han JJ, Acker MA, Atluri P. Left ventricular assist devices. *Circulation.* 2018;138(24): 2841-2851.

Hanke JS, Dogan G, Rojas SV, et al. First experiences with HeartMate 3 follow-up and adverse events. *J Thorac Cardiovasc Surg.* 2017;154(1):173-178.

Hensley FA, Martin DE, Gravlee GP, eds. *A Practical Approach to Cardiac Anesthesia.* 3rd ed. Lippincott Williams & Wilkins; 2002.

Karl TR. Neonatal cardiac surgery. Anatomic, physiologic, and technical considerations. *Clin Perinatol.* 2001;28:159-185.

Koenig-Oberhuber V, Filipovic M. New antiplatelet drugs and new oral anticoagulants. *Br J Anaesth.* 2016;117(suppl 2):ii74-ii84.

Konstadt S, Shernan S, Oka Y. *Clinical Transesophageal Echocardiography: A Problem-Oriented Approach.* 2nd ed. Lippincott Williams & Wilkins; 2003.

Kothandan H, Ho VK, Yeo KK, et al. Anesthesia management for MitraClip device implantation. *Ann Card Anaesth.* 2014;17(1):17-22.

MC Ashley E. Anaesthesia for electrophysiology procedures in the cardiac catheter laboratory. *Cont Educ Anaesth Crit Care Pain.* 2012;12(5):230-236.

Murkin JM, Arango M. Near-infrared spectroscopy as an index of brain and tissue oxygenation. *Br J Anaesth.* 2009;103(suppl 1):i3-i13.

Murkin JM. Perioperative multimodality neuromonitoring: an overview. *Semin CardioThorac Vasc Anesth.* 2004;8:167-171.

Myles PS, McIlroy D. Fast-track cardiac anesthesia: choice of anesthetic agents and techniques. *Semin Cardiothorac Vasc Anesth.* 2005;9:5-16.

Piquette D, Deschamps A, Belisle S, et al. Effect of intravenous nitroglycerin on cerebral saturation in high-risk cardiac surgery. *Can J Anaesth.* 2007;54:718-727.

Rajab TK, Singh SK. Donation after cardiac death heart transplantation in America is clinically necessary and ethically justified. *Circ Heart Fail.* 2018;11(3):e004884.

Ram H, Gerlach RM, Hernandez Conte A, Ramzy D, Jaramillo-Huff AR, Gerstein NS. The AngioVac device and its anesthetic implications. *J Cardiothorac Vasc Anesth.* 2017;31(3):1091-1102.

Reul H, Akdis M. Temporary or permanent support and replacement of cardiac function. *Expet Rev Med Dev.* 2004;1:215-227.

Riess FC. Anticoagulation management and cardiac surgery in patients with heparin-induced thrombocytopenia. *Semin Thorac Cardiovasc Surg.* 2005;17:85-96.

Roasio A, Lobreglio R, Santin A, et al. Fenoldopam reduces the incidence of renal replacement therapy after cardiac surgery. *J Cardiothorac Vasc Anesth.* 2008;22:23-26.

Sato K, Jones PM. Sedation versus general anesthesia for transcatheter aortic valve replacement. *J Thorac Dis.* 2018;10(suppl 30):S3588-S3594.

Serna DL, Thourani VH, Puskas JD. Antifibrinolytic agents in cardiac surgery: current controversies. *Semin Thorac Cardiovasc Surg.* 2005;17:52-58.

Speiss BD. *Perioperative Transfusion Medicine.* 2nd ed. Lippincott Williams & Wilkins; 2005.

Thys D. *Textbook of Cardiothoracic Anesthesiology.* McGraw-Hill; 2001.

Wan S, LeClerc JL, Vincent JL. Inflammatory response to cardiopulmonary bypass: mechanisms involved and possible therapeutic strategies. *Chest.* 1997;112:676-692.

Warkentin TE, Koster A. Bivalirudin: a review. *Expert Opin Pharmacother.* 2005;6:1349-1371.

Woo YJ. Cardiac surgery in patients on antiplatelet and antithrombotic agents. *Semin Thorac Cardiovasc Surg.* 2005;17:66-72.

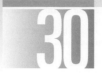

Anesthesia for Head and Neck Surgery

Nancy M. Wu and Jason M. Lewis

I. ANESTHESIA FOR OPHTHALMIC SURGERY

A. General considerations

1. **Intraocular pressure** (IOP; normal range 10-22 mm Hg) is principally determined by (1) aqueous volume (the rate of production of aqueous humor in relation to its rate of drainage) and (2) the blood volume within vessels of the eye. Owing to scleral inelasticity, small changes in volume result in large changes in IOP.

   a. **Factors that may increase IOP** include hypertension, hypercarbia, hypoxia, laryngoscopy and endotracheal intubation, venous congestion, vomiting, coughing, straining, bucking, external pressure on the eye, succinylcholine, and ketamine.

   b. **Factors that may decrease IOP** include hypocarbia, hypothermia, central nervous system (CNS) depressants, ganglionic blockers, most volatile and intravenous (IV) anesthetics, nondepolarizing neuromuscular blockade (NMB), mannitol, diuretics, acetazolamide, and head elevation.

2. **Glaucoma**

   a. **Open-angle glaucoma** usually arises from chronic obstruction of the aqueous humor drainage and is characterized by a progressive, insidious course that may *be painless*.

   b. **Closed-angle glaucoma** results from acute aqueous outflow obstruction due to a narrowing of the anterior chamber. This occurs as a result of pupillary dilation or lens edema and is *painful*.

3. **Oculocardiac reflex**

   a. The oculocardiac reflex (OCR) is mediated by afferent impulses via the ophthalmic branch (cranial nerve [CN] VI) of the trigeminal nerve and efferents from the vagus nerve (CN X). Increases in IOP, manipulation of the globe, or traction on the extrinsic eye muscles may result in bradycardia, atrioventricular block, ventricular ectopy, or asystole. Administration of ocular regional anesthesia may also elicit this response. OCR is common in patients undergoing strabismus surgery.

   b. The OCR should be promptly treated by cessation of the stimulus. Atropine (0.01-0.02 mg/kg IV) may be administered if bradyarrhythmias persist. The reflex fatigues quickly with repeated stimulation. However, if the reflex persists, infiltration of local anesthetic near the extrinsic eye muscles or placement of a peribulbar or retrobulbar block is effective. Alternatively, pretreatment with atropine or glycopyrrolate can be helpful in preventing the reflex.

4. **Commonly used drugs**

   a. **Topical.** Most ophthalmic medications are highly concentrated solutions that are administered topically and may produce systemic effects.

      1. **Mydriatics**

         a. **Phenylephrine** eye drops may cause hypertension and reflex bradycardia, especially when administered as a 10% solution.

For this reason, a 2.5% solution is commonly used. It dilates the pupil and constricts periocular blood vessels.

b. **Cyclopentolate, atropine, and scopolamine** are anticholinergic agents that can produce CNS toxicity (eg, confusion seizures), particularly in the elderly and young. Additional effects include flushing, thirst, dry skin, and tachycardia.

c. **Epinephrine** 2% topical solution reduces IOP in open-angle glaucoma by decreasing aqueous secretion while improving outflow. Complications can include hypertension, tachycardia, dysrhythmias, and syncope.

2. **Miotics.** Cholinergic drugs (eg, pilocarpine 0.25%-4% solution) may produce bradycardia, salivation, bronchorrhea, and diaphoresis.

3. **Drugs that decrease IOP**

a. β-**Adrenergic antagonists** (eg, timolol or betaxolol) may cause bradycardia, hypotension, congestive heart failure, and bronchospasm.

b. **Anticholinesterases**, such as echothiophate, depress plasma cholinesterase activity for 2 to 4 weeks and may prolong recovery from succinylcholine and mivacurium (not available in the United States).

c. **Apraclonidine**, an α_2-adrenergic agonist, is used to reduce IOP by decreasing aqueous production and improving outflow. Systemic side effects may include sedation and drowsiness. Rebound hypertension may result from acute withdrawal after chronic therapy.

b. **Systemic**

1. **Acetazolamide**, a carbonic anhydrase inhibitor, is administered systemically to decrease aqueous humor secretion, thus lowering IOP. Chronic use can lead to the development of hyponatremia, hypokalemia, and metabolic acidosis.

B. **Anesthetic management**

1. **Preoperative evaluation.** Patients undergoing eye surgery are often at the extremes of age, presenting with significant concomitant diseases that may require careful evaluation (eg, the formerly premature infant with bronchopulmonary dysplasia for retinal surgery or the elderly patient with cardiovascular disease for cataract excision). Preoperative testing should be dictated by medical comorbidities. However, recent evidence indicates that even patients with complex conditions undergoing low-risk eye surgery without routine testing have no increased risk of adverse events as compared with those who do undergo evaluation.

2. **Avoidance of coughing, sudden movement, or straining is essential.** Unexpected patient or eye movements during delicate microscopic intraocular surgery can lead to increased IOP, choroidal hemorrhage, expulsion of vitreous material, or loss of vision.

3. **Regional anesthesia**

a. **Ophthalmic procedures** such as cataract extraction, corneal transplant, anterior chamber irrigation, oculoplastic procedures, and even vitreoretinal procedures lasting 3 to 4 hours can be performed under regional anesthesia and light sedation.

b. Patient cooperation and lack of head motion are important for the success of this technique. Patients who are unable to participate owing to extremes of age, impaired hearing, psychiatric illness, language barrier, inability to tolerate supine position or maintain a relatively motionless position may not be candidates for regional anesthesia for delicate eye surgery.

c. Advantages of regional anesthesia include a lower incidence of coughing, straining, and emesis on emergence, reliable postoperative analgesia, lower perioperative morbidity, and earlier discharge compared with general anesthesia (GA).

d. **IV sedation** may be used perioperatively. Midazolam (0.25-1 mg IV), fentanyl (10-50 μg IV), remifentanil (0.25-1 μg/kg IV), or propofol (5-20 μg IV) can be administered just before the regional injection. Patients should have standard ASA monitors during regional block placement and receive supplemental oxygen if indicated.

e. **Technique.** Intraocular surgery requires adequate sensory and motor block of the eye and often the eyelids as well. Anesthesia of the eye is accomplished by injecting local anesthetic into the retrobulbar space, peribulbar space, or episcleral space, facilitating neural blockade of CNs II through VI.

f. **Retrobulbar block** is achieved by injecting 4 to 6 mL of a 50:50 mixture of 1% lidocaine and 0.375% bupivacaine (with 5 units hyaluronidase) within the muscle cone formed by the four recti muscles and the two oblique muscles. With the eye in a neutral position, a 23- or 25-gauge blunt Atkinson 1 ¼-inch needle is inserted through the lower lid or conjunctiva at the level of the inferior orbital rim in the inferotemporal quadrant. The needle is first advanced slightly inferiorly and temporally approximately 1.5 cm; once past the equator of the eye, the needle is then directed superiorly and nasally toward the apex of the orbit to a depth of approximately 3.5 cm, while feeling for a "pop" as the needle penetrates through the muscle cone (**Figure 30.1**).

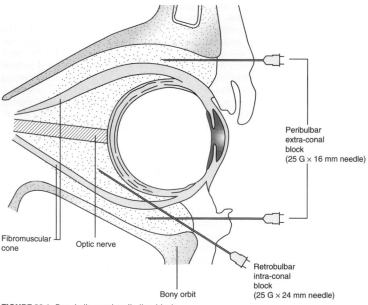

FIGURE 30.1 Retrobulbar and peribulbar blocks.

g. **Peribulbar block.** No attempt is made to enter the muscle cone. A 25-gauge ¾-inch Atkinson needle is advanced along the inferior orbital floor to a depth of approximately 2.5 cm. Between 8 and 10 mL of local anesthetic is required, and hyaluronidase (3.75-15 U/mL) is frequently added to help facilitate spread through the muscle cone. Careful aspiration before injection is required for both blocks, followed by gentle massage or orbital compression to promote the spread of the anesthetic (although orbital compression should be avoided in patients with glaucoma). If desired, the facial nerve can also be blocked by infiltrating 2 to 4 mL of additional local anesthetic along the inferior and superior orbital rim to help prevent squinting. The retrobulbar block provides faster, more reliable anesthesia and akinesia but has a higher complication rate as compared with the peribulbar block (**Figure 30.1**).

h. **Episcleral block (sub-Tenon block).** Local anesthetic is injected into the episcleral space via a needle or cannula. Needle entry is into the fornix at an angle tangential to the globe, between the conjunctival semilunaris fold and globe. Upon entry into the conjunctiva, the needle is shifted medially and advanced posteriorly until a "click" is felt. Local anesthetic is then injected, with volumes greater than 6 mL producing both globe analgesia and akinesia. Using the cannula technique, topicalization is performed and the bulbar conjunctiva lifted in the inferonasal quadrant with forceps. A small nick is made in the conjunctiva and Tenon capsule using blunt Westcott scissors, accessing the episcleral space. A specially designed blunt cannula is inserted, advanced into the episcleral space, and 3 to 4 mL of local anesthetic injected.

i. **Complications of regional anesthesia** are infrequent but include direct optic nerve trauma, transient globe compression with increased IOP, retrobulbar hemorrhage, globe perforation, and stimulation of the OCR. Hyaluronidase is toxic to the eye if injected into the globe. Intravascular injection of local anesthetic may cause seizures or myocardial depression. Rarely, the local anesthetic may dissect proximally along the neural sheath of the optic nerve and a total spinal can occur; treatment is supportive.

j. During the procedure, fresh air at a flow rate of 10 to 15 L/min is provided to the patient under the drapes using a large face mask. This helps to remove exhaled carbon dioxide and helps offset the sense of claustrophobia some patients may experience. Oxygen may be used if indicated, but the surgeon should be notified not to use electrocautery while oxygen is flowing. Capnography is frequently used since visual inspection of respiration may be difficult while patients are draped.

4. **General anesthesia**

a. Goals include (1) a smooth induction and maintenance of stable IOP, (2) avoidance and treatment of OCR, (3) maintenance of a motionless field with sufficient depth of anesthesia with or without NMB since the eye is highly innervated, (4) avoidance of postoperative nausea and vomiting (PONV), and (5) a smooth emergence.

b. **Smooth emergence and extubation** are particularly desirable after ophthalmic surgery. This may be facilitated by thorough posterior pharyngeal suctioning while the patient is still deeply anesthetized, administration of an opioid to reduce the cough reflex, and IV lidocaine or dexmedetomidine before planned extubation.

Deep extubation is also an option but does not guarantee a smooth emergence.

c. **Ketamine** can cause blepharospasm, nystagmus, and vomiting. It may increase arterial pressure and IOP. For these reasons, ketamine usually is a poor choice for most ophthalmic surgeries.

C. **Ophthalmic procedures**

1. **Open-eye injury.** Penetrating eye trauma may be a surgical emergency or needs to be addressed within 24 hours of injury to minimize the risk of infection. It requires a carefully conducted anesthetic designed to prevent aspiration and favorably affect IOP. A sudden increase in IOP can result in extrusion of ocular contents and cause permanent vision loss. Trauma to the eye and orbit, long-duration and complex surgery, and a crying patient with a full stomach usually mandate general endotracheal anesthesia.

   a. Succinylcholine causes an increase in IOP of approximately 6 to 12 mm Hg for 10 minutes before returning to baseline. This has not been shown to be clinically significant and succinylcholine often is the drug of choice during a rapid sequence induction (RSI) in the eye surgery patient with a full stomach. Alternatively, 1.2 mg/kg of rocuronium can be used during an RSI.

   b. An adequate depth of anesthesia and degree of NMB must be ensured before laryngoscopy and intubation to minimize increases in IOP (which may rise to 40-50 mm Hg) secondary to straining, coughing, and bucking.

   c. In children, if an IV cannot be placed, an inhalation induction along with cricoid pressure may be necessary.

2. **Strabismus repair** is a procedure to alter the lengths of the extraocular muscles.

   a. Surgical manipulation frequently elicits **the oculocardiac reflex** (see Section I.A.3).

   b. **PONV** is very common (40%-85% incidence in untreated patients). Strategies to reduce the incidence of PONV include minimizing opioids, multimodal analgesia, combination of antiemetics with different mechanisms of action (ondansetron, dexamethasone, haloperidol, etc.), gastric decompression using orogastric tube (OGT), ensuring adequate hydration, and possible total intravenous anesthetic (TIVA).

3. **Retinal surgery for detachment and vitreous hemorrhage** often is performed on patients in extremes of age and/or with multiple comorbidities. Meticulous attention to airway management, fluid status, normothermia, and postoperative transport is crucial. Premature infants, especially those less than 60 weeks postconceptional age, are at risk for postoperative central apnea. They should demonstrate a 12-hour apnea-free interval before discharge. Patients with diabetes or sickle cell anemia also may require retinal surgery (see Chapter 7, Section I.G and Chapter 37, Section X.C).

   a. **Regional anesthesia** is suitable for short procedures (<3 hours) in cooperative patients, although unexpected movement during the delicate retinal repair may result in vision loss.

   b. An **intravitreal gas bubble** containing an inert, high-molecular-weight, low-diffusivity gas such as sodium hexafluoride (SF_6), perfluoropropane (C_3F_8), octofluorocyclobutane (C_4F_8), or air, may be injected at the conclusion of surgery to reduce intravitreal bleeding. Nitrous **oxide should be avoided** in surgeries where an intravitreal gas bubble is injected as it will rapidly expand the bubble and increase IOP. Because these gas bubbles remain for various periods of time, administration of nitrous oxide should be avoided for 5 days after an air injection, 10 days after SF_6 injection, and 60 days after C_3F_8 injection. *Owing to pressure changes associated with air travel, patients should be instructed to avoid air travel for 3 to 4 weeks after intravitreal gas injection.*

II. ANESTHESIA FOR OTORHINOLARYNGOLOGIC PROCEDURES

A. General considerations

1. **Airway.** The airway during otorhinolaryngologic (ORL) procedures is often shared with the surgeon. Pathology, scarring from previous surgery or irradiation, congenital deformities, trauma, or manipulation can produce chronic or acute airway obstruction, bleeding, and a potentially difficult airway. Preoperative discussion with the surgeon and analysis of previous anesthetic records regarding perioperative airway management, endotracheal tube (ETT) size and position, patient positioning, and use of nitrous oxide and NMB are essential. The patient may require awake examination of the airway under sedation and topical anesthesia or an awake fiberoptic intubation (FOI) before induction of GA.

2. Patients presenting for ORL surgery may have a history of heavy smoking, alcohol abuse, obstructive sleep apnea (OSA), and chronic upper respiratory tract infections. Preoperative testing should be dictated by medical comorbidities.

3. In addition to standard monitors, intra-arterial blood pressure and urine output monitoring may be needed for major surgeries with significant anticipated blood loss.

4. **Extubation** after any upper airway surgery requires careful planning. Extubation is performed once the throat packs are removed, the pharynx is suctioned, and full protective laryngeal reflexes return. Excessive upper airway bleeding, edema, or pathology may preclude extubation in the operating room.

B. Ear surgery

1. Preoperative considerations
   a. Ear surgery often involves dissecting and preserving the **facial nerve (CN VII)**. Primary anesthetic concerns include patient positioning, facial nerve preservation, use of nitrous oxide, adequate hemostasis, smooth emergence, and prevention of PONV.
   b. The **middle ear** communicates with the oropharynx via the eustachian tube. If eustachian tube patency is compromised by trauma, edema, inflammation, or congenital deformity, normal venting of middle ear pressure cannot occur. In this situation, a high concentration of nitrous oxide can increase middle ear pressure to 300 to 400 mm Hg in 30 minutes. Conversely, acute cessation of nitrous oxide can result in rapid resorption and a net negative pressure in the middle ear. These changes may result in alteration of middle ear anatomy, rupture of tympanic membrane, disarticulation of artificial stapes, disruption of surgical grafts, and PONV.
   c. **Positioning.** During surgery, the patient's head often is elevated and turned to the side. Extremes of head position should be assessed preoperatively to determine limits of range of motion, especially in patients with arthritis or cerebrovascular disease. Furthermore, attention to adequate venous drainage is necessary with extremes of head position.

2. **Anesthetic technique.** Anesthesia is induced with a hypnotic and short-acting NMB or by inhalation and is maintained with a volatile anesthetic or TIVA. The use of nitrous oxide should be discussed with the surgeon or avoided; nitrous oxide should be discontinued at least 30 minutes before placement of a tympanic membrane graft.
   a. Delicate microsurgery of the ear requires adequate hemostasis. Volatile anesthetics, remifentanil, and α- or β-adrenergic antagonists work well to maintain mean arterial pressures of 60 to 70 mm Hg. Elevation of the head of the bed to approximately 15° to decrease venous congestion and local application of epinephrine for vasoconstriction usually improve operating conditions.
   b. Myringotomy with tube placement is one of the most frequently performed outpatient pediatric surgeries. These procedures are short and can usually be performed under mask anesthesia with or without an IV placement. Deep anesthesia using volatile anesthetics alone or in combination with remifentanil can be used. If the procedure is performed without an IV line, intranasal fentanyl (1-2 µg/kg) and preoperative oral acetaminophen (20-40 mg/kg) can be used for postoperative pain management.

C. Nasal surgery

1. **Anesthetic technique.** Nasal surgery is often performed under GA, although local anesthesia can be considered for minor procedures or high-risk patients. The surgeon may apply topical cocaine to the nasal mucosa with or without injection of lidocaine with epinephrine for vasoconstriction and hemostasis. These agents may cause tachycardia, hypertension, and arrhythmias. In a healthy adult, the cocaine dose should not exceed 1.5 mg/kg (each drop of a 4% solution contains about 3 mg of cocaine). Smaller doses should be used when administered with epinephrine or in patients with cardiovascular disease. GA may be needed to provide immobility, airway protection, or amnesia.

2. After **nasal cosmetic surgery**, the nose is unstable and application of a face mask is undesirable. Smooth emergence and extubation are important to decrease postoperative bleeding and to avoid laryngospasm and the need for positive-pressure ventilation by mask.

3. **Blood loss** during nasal surgery may be substantial and difficult to estimate. A throat pack may help decrease PONV by preventing passage of blood into the stomach. An OGT may be placed to evacuate the stomach of any swallowed blood.

4. Patients with **severe epistaxis** presenting for internal maxillary artery ligation or embolization often are anxious, hypertensive, tachycardic, and hypovolemic. They are assumed to have a full stomach containing blood, and induction of anesthesia and endotracheal intubation should be planned accordingly. Hypertension should be controlled to reduce blood loss. Posterior nasal packing, although helpful, can cause edema and hypoventilation. Because the extent of blood loss is difficult to assess, adequate IV access and blood for transfusion should be available. Removal of the posterior packing can be associated with substantial blood loss.

D. Upper airway surgery

1. **Tonsillectomy and adenoidectomy**
   a. **Preoperative evaluation** should seek a history of bleeding disorders, recent respiratory tract infection, and OSA. The STOPBANG questionnaire for OSA is a useful screening tool.
      1. Do you **snore** loudly at night?
      2. Do you feel **tired** during the day?

3. Has anyone **observed** apnea?
4. Do you have or are you being treated for high blood **pressure**?
5. Is your **BMI** greater than 35?
6. Is your **age** over 50?
7. Is your **neck** circumference over 17 inches (male) or 16 inches (female)?
8. Is your **gender** male?

A score of 5 or greater is strongly predictive of OSA. Patients with OSA may be difficult to ventilate and intubate. They are also at an increased risk of postoperative respiratory complications and should be considered for prolonged observation in the postanesthesia care unit (PACU) or overnight admission to monitor for respiratory compromise.

b. Most **children** receive an inhalation induction, followed by placement of an appropriately sized IV. Maintenance anesthetic with a volatile agent, supplemented with an opioid (eg, morphine 0.05-0.1 mg/kg IV), usually is performed. NMB facilitates intubation but is not mandatory. Inadvertent ETT obstruction, disconnection, or dislodgement can occur during head and mouth gag manipulation. ETT should be firmly secured at the midline of the mandible for surgical access.

c. **At the end of surgery**, the throat pack is removed, an OGT is placed to empty the stomach of swallowed blood, and the pharynx is suctioned thoroughly. Administration of antiemetic agents should be considered. Extubation may be performed under deep anesthesia or when the patient is awake with intact airway reflexes. The use of an oropharyngeal airway after surgery can cause surgical wound disruption and bleeding if not carefully placed in the midline. Nasal airways are useful alternatives.

d. Auscultate for unobstructed breathing before transport to the PACU and check for a dry pharynx before discharge.

2. Tonsillar rebleeding

a. **Rebleeding** after a pediatric tonsillectomy occurs in approximately 5% of cases. Primary bleeds occur within 24 hours after surgery. Secondary bleeding is common 7 to 10 days postoperatively as the eschar sloughs. Hematemesis, tachycardia, frequent swallowing, pallor, and airway obstruction may be seen. The extent of blood loss is often underestimated because the blood is swallowed.

b. **Post-tonsillectomy hemorrhage** is a surgical emergency, and induction of anesthesia in a bleeding, hypovolemic child can result in severe hypotension or cardiac arrest. Appropriate IV access is necessary, and the patient should be adequately resuscitated (with blood products if necessary) before reoperation. Hematocrit, coagulation studies, and availability of blood products should be ascertained. Doses of anesthetic agents may need to be reduced in the setting of hypovolemia.

c. Because the stomach is full of blood, a **rapid-sequence induction** should be performed. Two working suctions and an additional styletted ETT one size smaller than anticipated should be available. The surgeon should be present. Extubation is safest with the patient awake.

3. **A tonsillar or parapharyngeal abscess** may present with trismus, dysphagia, and a distorted, compromised airway. The surgeon may be able to decompress the abscess with needle aspiration before the induction of anesthesia. If needed, an awake FOI may be performed. Anesthetic

management and extubation procedures are similar to those for tonsillectomy (see Section II.D.1). In Ludwig angina, a cellulitis of the submandibular and sublingual spaces may extend to the anterior compartments of the neck. Trismus, airway edema, and distorted anatomy often make visualization by direct laryngoscopy of the glottic opening difficult. Asleep intubation is contraindicated if stridor occurs at rest. *Awake FOI is the safest approach in this scenario.* If awake FOI is not possible, consider tracheostomy under local anesthesia to secure the airway.

4. **Cleft lip and palate (CLP) repair**
   a. A detailed preoperative evaluation is necessary as patients may have associated anomalies including cardiac or airway deformities.
   b. GA is required for CLP repair. Oral RAEETT is used and may become kinked or dislodged during placement of a mouth gag.
   c. Prior to emergence, an OGT is used to evacuate the stomach of blood. The oropharynx is gently suctioned with soft tip catheter, while avoiding the newly repaired palate by advancing along the tongue.
   d. Given concern for postoperative airway obstruction, multimodal analgesia is used to minimize opioid requirement, and the patient is extubated when fully awake. The surgeon may place a tongue stitch to allow forward tongue displacement if patient obstructs. Postoperative monitoring in the pediatric intensive care unit is required.

5. **Direct laryngoscopy** is indicated for diagnostic (biopsy) or therapeutic (vocal cord polyp removal) purposes and may involve potentially compromised airways. Evaluation of imaging studies (magnetic resonance imaging or computed tomography) and laboratory studies (pulmonary flow-volume loops) may help identify airway abnormalities and potential perioperative problems. Many patients have a history of smoking and cardiopulmonary disease.
   a. **Anesthetic management** is described in Chapter 27, Section IV.
   b. **Postoperative airway edema** may develop. If anticipated, dexamethasone (4-10 mg IV) may be given. Additional treatment includes head elevation, humidified oxygen by mask, and nebulized racemic epinephrine. Occasionally, cessation of nebulized racemic epinephrine is associated with the return of airway edema.

6. **Laser use in ORL surgery. Laser** (**l**ight **a**mplification by **s**timulated **e**mission of **r**adiation) produces a high-energy, high-density beam of coherent light that generates focused heat on contact with tissue. The emission media used to produce the monochromatic light determines the wavelength.
   a. **Short-wavelength (1-µm) laser** (argon gas, ruby, neodymium:yttrium aluminum garnet [Nd:YAG]) emissions in the red-green visible part of the electromagnetic spectrum are poorly absorbed by water but well absorbed by pigmented tissues such as the retina and blood vessels.
   b. **Infrared (10-µm) carbon dioxide laser** emissions are well absorbed by water and superficial surface cells and are commonly used to treat laryngeal lesions. They cannot be transmitted through fiberoptics.
   c. **Eyes must be protected** from the laser beam. Operating room personnel must wear appropriate safety goggles (green tinted for argon, amber for Nd:YAG, and clear for carbon dioxide). The patient's eyes should be taped closed and covered with safety goggles.

d. **The most serious complication of laser airway surgery is airway fire.** The likelihood of fire depends on the gas environment of the airway, the energy level of the laser, the manner in which the laser is used, the presence of moisture, and the type of ETT used. Oxygen and nitrous oxide both support combustion. A safe gas mixture during laser upper airway surgery is oxygen/air or oxygen/helium to achieve a fraction of inspired oxygen of 21% to 30%.

e. **Safe laser use.** Lasers should be used intermittently, in the noncontinuous mode, and at moderate power (10-15 W). Surgeons should not use the laser as a cautery and should share responsibility for fire prevention by limiting the energy input, allowing time for heat dispersal, packing aside nontarget tissue and ETT cuffs with moist gauze, and maintaining moisture (as a heat sink) in the field.

f. **Airway options during laser surgery.** Specially designed, fire-resistant, impregnated, or shielded ETTs (eg, Xomed Laser-Shield II endotracheal tube) are used, and the cuff is filled with blue saline. For some procedures, intubation is not possible because the surgeon requires free access to the surgical field. Options include the following:

1. Jet-Venturi technique. This technique eliminates the need for an ETT, but airway fire may still occur owing to dry tissue igniting. All patients are at risk for barotrauma; pediatric patients and patients with chronic obstructive pulmonary disease are at the highest risk.

2. Ventilation and apneic oxygenation. The surgeon operates during periods of apnea and stops intermittently to allow the anesthesiologist to ventilate and oxygenate the patient.

g. **If an airway fire occurs**, immediately remove the ETT, stop flow of airway gases, remove any flammable material from the airway, and pour saline in the airway. Once the fire is out, reestablish ventilation while avoiding oxidizer-enriched environment, examine ETT for possible fragments left behind in the airway, and consider bronchoscopy. **Complications** include airway edema, inhalation injury, tracheal and laryngeal granulation tissue formation, and airway stenosis.

h. The **anesthetic technique** for laser surgery is similar to that described above (Section II.D.6.f) and in Chapter 27, Section IV. Goals include adequate surgical exposure, fire prevention, and return of protective airway reflexes before extubation. Clear communication with the surgical team is essential. Endotracheal intubation, jet ventilation, or intermittent mask ventilation may be used. TIVA is used to maintain GA for open airway procedures. Because airway edema may occur, the patient is given humidified oxygen postoperatively and is observed closely in the PACU. Corticosteroids or aerosolized racemic epinephrine may be necessary.

III. ANESTHESIA FOR PROCEDURES OF THE NECK

A. General considerations

The primary anesthetic concerns during neck surgery are establishing and maintaining a secure airway, tissue preservation, and nerve monitoring.

1. An **armored endotracheal tube** (eg, Tovell) may be necessary to prevent kinking.

2. An **elective tracheostomy** under local anesthesia may be performed before induction of GA for certain extensive procedures with anticipated difficult airway.

3. **Teflon injection of the vocal cords** must be performed during awake laryngoscopy to allow continuous assessment of voice quality. The procedure should be performed with adequate local anesthesia and light sedation.

B. **Radical neck dissection**

1. **Patient condition.** These patients are often elderly, chronically debilitated, and malnourished and frequently have a history of tobacco and alcohol use. The severity of comorbidities will determine the extent of preoperative evaluation and choice of perioperative monitoring. Radical neck dissection in previously irradiated patients may be associated with large blood loss and a difficult airway.

2. **Anesthetic technique.** Airway management is of primary concern in this patient population, particularly if mass lesions exist. Awake FOI, rigid fiberoptic scopes, video laryngoscope, or awake tracheostomy may be necessary in patients with compromised airways. Long-acting NMB is generally avoided to allow the surgeon to use a nerve stimulator. A 15° to 30° head-up tilt and mild hypotension (mean arterial pressure 60-70 mm Hg), facilitated by a volatile anesthetic, vasodilators, or remifentanil, may help reduce blood loss. However, prolonged, profound hypotension and anemia may increase the risk of end-organ damage.

3. Neck dissection often involves rotational flaps or free flaps. During dissection, traction or pressure on the carotid sinus can cause dysrhythmias such as bradycardia or asystole. Treatment is immediate cessation of the stimulus. If necessary, the surgeon can infiltrate local anesthetic near the sinus.

4. If airway compromise is anticipated postoperatively, the ETT is left in place or an elective tracheostomy is performed.

5. Maintenance of normothermia and adequate hydration and minimizing the use of vasoconstrictors are desirable during reconstructive flap transfer surgery. Intraoperative predictors of free flap compromise include significant medical comorbidity, administration of greater than 7 L of crystalloid, and prolonged operative time. Postoperatively, blood pressure should be adequate to maintain flap perfusion, but not so high that a hematoma develops.

C. **Thyroid and parathyroid surgery**

1. General endotracheal anesthesia is the most common technique. Approximately 40% of surgically associated recurrent laryngeal nerve (RLN) palsies are related to thyroid surgery. Use of a "nerve integrity monitor" endotracheal tube for intraoperative RLN monitoring may be considered. Succinylcholine is the agent of choice for intubation, and additional NMB should be avoided in the setting of RLN monitoring (**Figure 30.2**).

2. Injury to one RLN may cause unilateral vocal cord paralysis, leading to hoarseness, weak voice, and poor cough. Bilateral vocal cord paralysis usually leads to upper airway obstruction and stridor and requires reintubation and possible tracheostomy.

3. **Anesthetic technique.** Surgical manipulation near the trachea can be very stimulating, while postoperative pain may only be mild to moderate. Inhalational anesthetics, sometimes augmented with a remifentanil infusion, is commonly used to maintain an adequate plane of anesthesia and avoid the use of NMB.

4. **Bleeding** at the operative site after thyroid or parathyroid surgery may compress the trachea and cause acute airway obstruction. Opening the

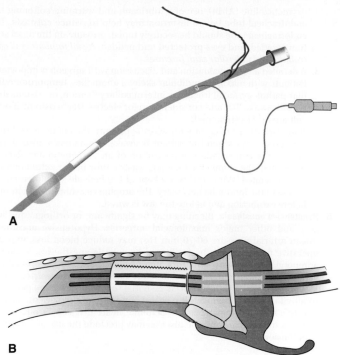

FIGURE 30.2 Intraoperative recurrent laryngeal nerve monitoring. A, Xomed NIM II endotracheal tube electrode (Medtronic Xomed). B, Proper intraluminal position of NIM II. NIM, nerve integrity monitor. (Redrawn from White WM, Randolph GW, Hartnick CJ, et al. Recurrent laryngeal nerve monitoring during thyroidectomy and related cervical procedures in the pediatric population. *Arch Otolaryngol Head Neck Surg.* 2009;135(1):88-94.)

wound by placing a sterile hemostat through the incision allows egress of trapped blood. If this maneuver fails, the obstruction may be secondary to acute lymphedema and may necessitate immediate reintubation.

IV. ANESTHESIA FOR DENTISTRY AND ORAL AND MAXILLOFACIAL SURGERY

A. Anesthetic technique. Most dental and oral surgery procedures can be done under local anesthesia with or without sedation in the outpatient setting, whereas most maxillofacial surgeries require GA.

1. Patients requiring GA for dentistry may be young children, adults with severe phobias, or the mentally or physically impaired; thus, they often require **premedication.** Oral or intranasal midazolam and intranasal dexmedetomidine can be given to cooperative patients. Intramuscular ketamine may be necessary for the agitated or uncooperative patient and can be combined with midazolam and glycopyrrolate to combat undesirable psychological reactions and sialorrhea, respectively.

2. **Nasal intubation** is usually preferred; care must be taken not to damage the turbinates or adenoids. Prior to intubation, identification of the more patent nasal passage, topicalization of the nasal mucosa with

oxymetazoline (Afrin), use of a lubricant, and warming/softening the endotracheal tube before insertion may help to reduce epistaxis. The endotracheal tube should be securely taped, pressure on the nasal septum avoided, and eyes protected and padded. *Nasal intubation is contraindicated in basilar skull fractures.*

3. A detailed airway evaluation and discussion with surgeon is important. Patients with maxillomandibular skeletal anomalies, temporomandibular pathology, facial fractures, intermaxillary fixation, or trismus may require awake FOI and consideration for elective tracheostomy if difficult airway is anticipated.

4. If intermaxillary fixation with wires is present, the endotracheal tube is removed only when the patient is awake, edema has subsided, and bleeding is controlled. Administration of an antiemetic and decompression of the stomach with a nasogastric tube before extubation are recommended. Wire cutters are kept at the bedside should emergent access to the mouth be necessary. The oropharynx should be suctioned before extubation and before the jaw is wired.

B. **Hypotensive anesthesia.** Bleeding may be significant for orthognathic surgery and other major maxillofacial surgeries. Hypotensive anesthesia (mean arterial pressure 60-70 mm Hg) may reduce blood loss, improve operative field, and can be facilitated by volatile anesthetics, α- and β-adrenergic blockers, vasodilators, potent opioid infusion, and head elevation. Meticulous monitoring (blood pressure with possible arterial line, E, blood loss, and urine output) is essential to ensure adequate perfusion to all vital organs. The overall medical condition of the patient, such as poorly controlled hypertension, ischemic heart disease, carotid artery stenosis, and hepatic or renal disease, may preclude the use of controlled hypotension.

Suggested Readings

Barak M, Yoav L, El-Naaj IA. Hypotensive anesthesia versus normotensive anesthesia during major maxillofacial surgery: a review of the literature. *ScientificWorldJournal.* 2015;2015:1-7.

Brimacombe J, Berry A. The laryngeal mask airway for dental surgery—a review. *Aust Dent J.* 1995;40:10-14.

Choi WS, Samman N. Risks and benefits of deliberate hypotension in anaesthesia: a systematic review. *Int J Oral Maxillofac Surg.* 2008;37:687-703.

Chung F, Subramanyam R, Liao P, et al. High STOP-Bang score indicates a high probability of obstructive sleep apnoea. *Br J Anaesth.* 2012;108:768-775.

Doyle DJ. Anesthesia for ear, nose, and throat surgery. In: Miller RD, ed. *Anesthesia.* 8th ed. Elsevier Saunders; 2015:2523-2549.

Feldman MA. Anesthesia for eye surgery. In: Miller RD, ed. *Anesthesia.* 8th ed. Elsevier Saunders; 2015:2512-2522.

Ghazal EA, Vadi MG, Coté CJ, et al. Preoperative evaluation, premedication, and induction of anesthesia. In: Coté CJ, Lerman J, Andereson BJ, et al, eds. *A Practice of Anesthesia for Infants and Children.* 6th ed. Elsevier; 2019:35-68.

Litman RS. Anesthesia for pediatric ophthalmologic surgery. In: Litman RS, ed. *Pediatric Anesthesia the Requisite in Anesthesiology.* Elsevier Mosby; 2004:267-274.

Litman RS, Samadi DS, Tobias JD. Anesthesia for pediatric ENT surgery. In: Litman RS, ed. *Pediatric Anesthesia the Requisite in Anesthesiology.* Elsevier Mosby; 2004:236-251.

McGoldrick KE, ed. *Anesthesia for Ophthalmic and Otolaryngologic Surgery.* WB Saunders; 1992.

Modest VE, Alfille PH. Anesthesia for laser surgery. In: Miller RD, ed. *Anesthesia.* 8th ed. Elsvier Saunders; 2015:2598-2611.

Pattani KM, Byrne P, Boahene K, et al. What makes a good flap go bad? A critical analysis of the literature of intraoperative factors related to free flap failure. *Laryngoscope.* 2010;120:717-723.

Philips MB, Bendel RE, Crook JE, et al. Global health implications of preanesthesia medical examination for ophthalmic surgery. *Anesthesiology*. 2013;118(5):1038-1045.

Raafat SH, Brown KA, Verghese ST. Otorhinolaryngologic procedures. In Coté CJ, Lerman J, Anderson BJ, ed. *A Practice of Anesthesia for Infants and Children*. 6th ed. Elsevier; 2019:754-789.

Ragab SM, Hassanin MZ. Optimizing the surgical field in pediatric functional endoscopic sinus surgery: a new evidence-based approach. *Otolaryngol Head Neck Surg*. 2010;142(1):48-54.

Somerville N, Fenlon S. Anaesthesia for cleft lip and palate surgery. *Cont Educ Anaesth Crit Care Pain*. 2005;5:76-79.

Supkis DE, Dougherty TB, Nguyen DT, et al. Anesthetic management of the patient undergoing head and neck cancer surgery. *Int Anesthesiol Clin*. 1998;36:21-29.

Tobin JR, Weaver RG. Ophthalmology. In Coté CJ, Lerman J, Anderson BJ, ed. *A Practice of Anesthesia for Infants and Children*. 6th ed. Elsevier; 2019:790-803.

Troll GF. Regional ophthalmic anesthesia: safe techniques and avoidance of complications. *J Clin Anesth*. 1995;7:163-172.

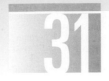

Anesthesia for Urologic Surgery

Jenny Zhao Cheng and Dan Ellis

I. ANESTHESIA FOR SPECIFIC UROLOGIC PROCEDURES

A. **Cystoscopy and ureteroscopy** are performed to diagnose and treat lesions of the lower (urethra, prostate, and bladder) and upper (ureter and kidney) urinary tracts.

1. Warmed irrigation fluids are used to improve visualization and to remove blood, tissue, and stone fragments.

a. **Electrolyte solutions** (normal saline and lactated Ringer) are isotonic and do not cause hemolysis upon intravascular absorption. Because of ionization, they cannot safely be used for procedures involving monopolar electrocautery. These solutions can be used with bipolar electrocautery.

b. **Sterile water** has optimal visibility and is nonconductive, but intravascular absorption can cause hemolysis and hyponatremia/hypoosmolality.

Nonelectrolyte solutions of glycine, sorbitol, and mannitol have good visibility and are nonconductive. Near-isotonicity minimizes hemolysis, although large volume absorption may cause hyponatremia (see section on TURP syndrome that follows).

2. Anesthesia

a. Depending on the patient and procedure, anesthesia for cystoscopy/ureteroscopy can range from topical lubrication to monitored anesthesia care (MAC), regional, and/or general anesthesia (GA). Placement of a rigid cystoscope (particularly in males) and distention of the bladder and ureters can be quite stimulating. Postoperative pain is minimal.

b. If regional anesthesia is used, a T6 level is required for upper tract instrumentation, whereas a T10 level is adequate for lower tract surgery.

c. GA can be effective with short-acting intravenous (IV) and inhaled anesthetics. Transient muscle relaxation may be required.

d. Lithotomy position is most common.

B. **Transurethral resection of the bladder (TURB)** is performed to diagnose and treat lesions of the bladder. Anesthetic considerations are similar to TURP (see below). Muscle relaxation should be considered as inadvertent simulation of the obturator nerve, deep to the lateral bladder wall, may result in leg adduction, and risk damage to the bladder. Additionally, chemotherapy instillation during TURB for bladder cancer may impact operating room cleaning and scheduling of anesthetists.

C. **Transurethral resection of the prostate (TURP)** is performed to relieve urinary obstruction from benign prostatic hypertrophy (BPH). This procedure uses a modified cystoscope (resectoscope) with a wire connected to an electrocautery unit for resection of tissue and coagulation of bleeding vessels. Alternatives to TURP include medical management

(α-blockers and hormonal therapies) and minimally invasive techniques such as laser ablation, microwave thermotherapy, and prostatic stents.

1. During surgery, large prostatic venous sinuses can be opened, allowing irrigant to be absorbed. The quantity of fluid absorbed depends on the following:

   a. Hydrostatic pressure related to the height of the irrigant above the patient.

   b. Surgical technique: duration of exposed sinuses, irrigation flow rate, and cystoscope size.

   c. Number and size of venous sinuses opened (influenced by prostate size).

   d. Peripheral venous pressure (lower pressure increases absorption).

2. Anesthesia

   a. If GA is used, it is essential to prevent coughing or movement that increases the risk of bleeding or bladder/prostatic capsule perforation. Positive-pressure ventilation may decrease irrigant absorption by raising venous pressure.

   b. Advantages of regional anesthesia may include an atonic bladder (improved surgical visualization) and elimination of bladder spasms (more rapid postoperative hemostasis). Awake patients may also report symptoms that allow earlier detection of TURP syndrome (see below) or bladder perforation.

   c. Spinal anesthesia can be achieved with an iso- or hyperbaric solution of local anesthetic with or without opioid. A T10 sensory level is recommended to counteract pain from bladder distention. Lower venous pressures associated with neuraxial blockade may reduce bleeding but increase irrigant absorption.

   d. Methods for monitoring fluid absorption intraoperatively may include volumetric fluid balance, gravimetric weighing, and measurement of exhaled ethanol when a known amount of ethanol is added to the irrigating fluid.

3. **Complications**

   a. **TURP syndrome** is a collection of neurologic and cardiovascular signs and symptoms caused by excessive irrigant absorption. It may appear early (direct intravascular absorption) or after several hours (absorption from retroperitoneal and perivesicular spaces).

      1. **Central nervous system** symptoms include nausea, agitation, confusion, visual changes, seizures, and coma. These symptoms are likely multifactorial and have been attributed to hyponatremia/hypoosmolality with accompanying cerebral edema, hyperglycinemia, and hyperammonemia (glycine is hepatically metabolized to ammonia).

      2. **Cardiovascular** symptoms include hypertension/hypotension, bradycardia, dysrhythmias, pulmonary edema, and cardiac arrest likely secondary to pronounced fluid shifts and associated electrolyte disturbances. Hypervolemia initially occurs with fluid absorption followed by rapid redistribution of the irrigant to the interstitium.

      3. **Treatment involves** notifying the surgeon, completing the procedure as quickly as possible, and maintaining hemodynamic stability. There is disagreement in the literature about the most appropriate therapy. Fluid restriction and diuresis with

furosemide have been advocated to treat volume overload, and hypertonic saline is reserved for severe symptoms or hyponatremia (serum sodium <120 mmol/L). Others suggest that the diuretic strategy may exacerbate intravascular volume depletion and hyponatremia and recommend early use of hypertonic saline (with slow correction of hyponatremia to minimize the risk of central pontine myelinolysis) and reserving diuresis for acute pulmonary edema. Any therapy should be guided by regular measurements of serum sodium and osmolality.

b. **Bladder perforation** is a serious complication. Muscle relaxation with an adequate level of anesthesia, neuromuscular blockade, or spinal anesthesia minimizes this risk.

1. Extraperitoneal perforation is more common and manifests as suprapubic fullness, abdominal spasm, or pain in the suprapubic, inguinal, or periumbilical regions.

2. Intraperitoneal perforation presents as upper abdominal pain or referred pain from the diaphragm to the shoulder. This may result in hypertension, tachycardia, and abdominal distention followed by hypotension and cardiovascular collapse.

c. **Bacteremia** may occur due to absorption of bacteria through prostatic venous sinuses and is commonly associated with indwelling urinary catheters or with subclinical/partially treated prostatitis.

d. **Blood loss and coagulopathy.** Assessing blood loss is extremely difficult during a TURP because of irrigant dilution. Continuous postoperative bleeding may result from surgical bleeding, dilutional thrombocytopenia, disseminated intravascular coagulation, or the release of fibrinolytic enzymes from the prostate. Hemodynamic responses to blood loss may be masked by hypervolemia from irrigant absorption.

D. **Laser resection of the prostate** is a clinical approach to treating BPH and has less perioperative morbidity. Hemostatic properties of a laser limit tissue penetration and create a practically bloodless field. This procedure is an alternative for seriously ill patients (TURP morbidity 18%) and patients on anticoagulants. Bladder irritation (transient), delayed gross hematuria, and transient dysuria are common complications. The procedure time is relatively short in duration. General anesthesia and regional anesthesia (subarachnoid or sacral canal block) may be safely performed.

1. The **holmium** (yttrium-aluminum-garnet = YAG) laser is a 60- to 80-W high-power pulse laser with a wavelength = 2140 nm. The high absorption of this laser by water limits tissue penetration. It is used to enucleate the prostate. Holmium laser preserves the histologic architecture of the prostate and facilitates prostate cancer detection.

2. The **KTP** (potassium titanyl phosphate) is a 60- to 80-W high-power laser through a crystal with a wavelength = 532 nm. It is highly absorbed by oxyhemoglobin, potentially creating a bloodless field, and is poorly absorbed by water. It is used for the enucleation of the prostate in a procedure known as "photoselective vaporization of prostate" (PVP). PVP is as effective as TURPs (2- to 4-year follow-up) for relief of BPH symptoms and has less perioperative morbidity, postoperative bladder irrigation, catheterization time, incidence of sexual dysfunction, and hospital stay. A disadvantage is that it alters prostatic histology samples. It is also important to have muscle relaxation with either an adequate level of anesthesia, neuromuscular blockade, or spinal anesthesia during PVPs.

E. Radical retropubic prostatectomy (RRP) is the operative procedure for the treatment of prostate cancer. Prostatectomy is rarely done for BPH.

1. Anesthesia

a. Open RRP may be performed safely using general, general/epidural, epidural, or spinal anesthesia. Several small-scale prospective randomized trials compared general with epidural techniques and found modest benefits of epidural anesthesia in reducing operative blood loss, reducing postoperative pain, and hastening recovery of bowel function. Regardless of these results, experienced surgeons routinely perform prostatectomies using GA with minimal blood loss, well-controlled intraoperative and postoperative pain, and short hospital stays. Currently, transverse abdominis plane (TAP) blocks and rectus sheath blocks are used in opioid-sparing techniques.

b. Laparoscopic prostatectomies (LRPs) are promoted for their minimal invasiveness and comparable clinical outcomes. Prospective, nonrandomized trials comparing LRP to RRP show no significant differences in postoperative pain score, amount of narcotics administered, length of hospital stay, readmission rates, or complication rates. Anesthetic considerations for LRP are similar to those for other laparoscopic procedures. Retroperitoneal insufflation of carbon dioxide may be associated with increased systemic absorption compared with intraperitoneal insufflation, although reports are conflicting.

c. Robotic-assisted retropubic prostatectomies (RARPs) have become increasingly more common for decreased transfusion rates, faster return of urinary continence, and decreased erectile dysfunction when compared to open and laparoscopic prostatectomies. The anesthetic plan for an RARP is similar to the anesthetic plan for an LRP. GA with standard intravenous induction and tracheal intubation is required. As the patient's arms will be tucked while he is in the lithotomy position, many anesthetists advocate two intravenous lines with a noninvasive blood pressure cuff on each of the patient's arms. These redundancies help compensate for difficulties assessing the patient arms measuring blood pressure intraoperatively. Notably, trocar advancement may unexpectedly invade large vessels or enter the stomach. Therefore, a preoperative blood bank sample and decompressing the stomach with an orogastric tube is recommended. Decompressing the stomach may also decrease ocular damage caused by gastric contents draining onto a patients' eyes. Neuromuscular blockade is extremely important because any movement by the patient while the robot is docked may lead to significant and serious complications. Patients are often placed in steep Trendelenburg position to facilitate surgical exposure of deep pelvic organs. Trendelenburg positioning increases intracranial and intraocular pressures and may also result in physical objects hitting the patient's face. Therefore, clinicians must monitor patients closely to prevent harm. Fluid management is also very important during robot prostatectomies. Too much fluid is associated with an increased risk of postoperative anastomotic leak as well as increased risk of glottic and periocular edema during Trendelenburg position. However, restrictive fluid management may cause acute tubular necrosis and compartment syndrome due to hypotension in the lower extremities.

    d. Diagnostic dyes may be used during the procedure to demonstrate the integrity of the reconstructed urinary tract.

        1. Methylene blue 1% (1 mL) bolus may impact blood pressure. It may also cause transient erroneous decreases in pulse oximetry readings (SaO_2) to as low as 65%, lasting 10 to 70 seconds.

        2. Indigo carmine 0.8% (5 mL) is an α-agonist and may cause hypertension.

    e. Complications generally relate to blood loss, including hypothermia, anemia, and coagulopathy. Large-bore IV access is suggested. Two intravenous lines and two blood pressure cuffs are recommended (see above section on RARP). Urine output measurements are interrupted during mobilization of the prostatic urethra. Venous sinuses can be exposed during surgery, which can increase blood loss and potentially lead to air emboli.

F. Nephrectomy is performed for neoplasm, transplantation, chronic infection, trauma, and severe cystic or calculous disease.

    1. Patients undergoing nephrectomy for renal cell carcinoma require preoperative staging. These tumors can be quite large. If the tumor extends into the inferior vena cava (IVC) or right atrium, then two potential complications must be considered:

        a. The tumor may partially or fully occlude the IVC with poor venous return and hypotension.

        b. Tumor fragments may embolize to the pulmonary circulation. Consequently, pulmonary artery catheterization and central venous access may be risky if catheter placement dislodges tumor into the IVC or right atrium. Transesophageal echocardiogram should be considered if there is high risk of tumor embolism. Cardiopulmonary bypass may be used to minimize the risk of pulmonary emboli intraoperatively.

    2. Patients undergoing nephrectomy for transitional cell carcinoma will likely undergo an associated complete ureteral resection.

    3. Anesthesia

        a. The patient is positioned supine for a transabdominal approach or in the lateral decubitus position for a retroperitoneal approach. In the lateral position, the kidney rest and table flexion are often used to improve exposure. Hypotension can be produced by the kidney rest position, likely due to IVC compression, or blood pooling in dependent extremities.

        b. A thoracoabdominal incision may be required for larger or upper pole tumors.

        c. Combined general/epidural anesthesia can maximize postoperative analgesia with an upper abdominal or thoracoabdominal incision. TAP block can also be considered for adequate pain control.

        d. Large-bore IV access with or without arterial line is appropriate as blood loss can be massive due to tumor size and vascularity.

G. Cystectomy

    1. Simple and partial cystectomy is the removal of all or part of the bladder. Adjacent organs and structures, including pelvic lymph nodes, are left intact.

    2. Radical cystectomy is performed for invasive bladder tumors. It frequently involves removal of other pelvic organs, such as the prostate or uterus. Patients with pelvic malignancies, neurogenic bladder dysfunction, chronic lower urinary tract obstruction, or postradiation bladder dysfunction may require an ileal or colonic urinary diverting procedure.

3. Anesthesia

    a. Large-bore IV access may be indicated as substantial blood loss may occur.

    b. Arterial or central venous access may be indicated as large volume shifts occur while the ureters are disconnected.

    c. GA with epidural anesthesia or TAP catheter is recommended.

H. Orchidopexy, orchiectomy, and urogenital plastic surgery procedures are performed to treat congenital deformities, neoplasms, and impotence. Patients with torsion of the testicle may require emergency reduction and orchidopexy to prevent ischemia.

I. Renal transplantation is performed for patients with end-stage renal disease. Recipients commonly have hypertension and/or diabetes mellitus and are at increased risk for coronary artery disease and congestive heart failure. Patients may present with electrolyte and acid-base abnormalities, anemia, and platelet dysfunction. Preoperative dialysis, if possible, can improve potassium and acid-base abnormalities. The anesthetist must also make sure that the patient receives the proper perioperative immunosuppressants.

1. Anesthesia

    a. IV access may be difficult, and IV placement in extremities with fistulas or shunts should be avoided. The benefits of additional invasive monitors (arterial or central venous lines) should be weighed against the risks of catheter-related complications in immunosuppressed patients.

    b. Patients may have delayed gastric emptying from diabetes, uremia, and preoperative opioids. Rapid sequence induction should be considered for patients receiving peritoneal dialysis or patients with autonomic neuropathy.

    c. Muscle relaxation is important and should be maintained until fascia is closed. Coughing may dislodge a transplanted kidney from its vascular anastomosis. Cisatracurium is the preferred neuromuscular blockade agent. Rocuronium has also been used. Sugammadex, however, has not yet been approved for patients with end-stage renal disease.

    d. Graft function depends on adequate intravascular volume before and after vascular anastomosis to maintain perfusion to the transplanted kidney. Intravascular volume expanders include crystalloid, albumin, and mannitol.

    e. Intraoperative hypotension may compromise renal perfusion and should be treated promptly by addressing mechanical factors such as IVC compression or treating hypovolemia with additional volume. If pharmacologic support is necessary, phenylephrine boluses, phenylephrine infusions, or dopamine infusions may be considered. α-Agonists such as phenylephrine were previously thought to decrease renal blood flow via vasoconstriction. However, α-agonists have been used successfully in these procedures. In cases of marked acidemia, sodium bicarbonate may improve hemodynamics.

    f. Urine output provides an immediate gauge of renal function, which may be affected by hypovolemia, acute rejection, or patency of the anastomoses. Both mannitol and furosemide may be requested by a surgeon to promote diuresis after anastomosis.

II. LITHOTRIPSY

    A. Treatment of kidney stones ranges from open surgical procedures to less invasive approaches such as cystoscopy/ureteroscopy with mechanical stone extraction and/or laser lithotripsy.

1. Anesthetic options include regional, MAC, and GA (laryngeal mask airway vs endotracheal tube), depending on both patient and surgical factors.

B. **Extracorporeal shockwave lithotripsy**, a noninvasive technique, focuses acoustic shock waves aimed at urinary stones. At interfaces between materials of differing density, such as between soft tissues and stones, reflections of these acoustic waves set up complex patterns of internal echoes resulting in stresses that cause stones to fracture. While early-generation lithotripters required patient immersion into water baths, current models allow positioning on an operating table, have smaller cutaneous "shock entry" zones, and are more precisely focused onto the stone with less energy dissipated on surrounding structures.

C. **Anesthesia**

1. The patient is generally positioned supine but may be prone depending on the precise location of the stone(s). Lithotomy position may be necessary for concurrent cystoscopy or stent placement.

2. MAC is usually adequate with newer lithotripters. Other strategies include neuraxial blockade and GA.

3. Adequate IV hydration may aid passage of stone fragments.

4. Absolute contraindications are pregnancy, untreated infections, bleeding diatheses, and abdominal pacemakers. Relative contraindications are pacemakers/implantable cardioverter defibrillator, abdominal aortic or renal artery aneurysms, orthopedic prostheses, and morbid obesity.

D. **Complications**

1. Ureteral colic soon after the procedure may manifest as nausea, vomiting, or bradycardia.

2. Hematuria is common and can be treated with hydration and diuretics.

3. Cardiac dysrhythmias such as bradycardia, premature atrial contractions, and premature ventricular contractions can occur intraoperatively secondary to mechanical (shock wave) strains on the cardiac conduction system. If premature ventricular contractions are frequent or symptomatic, they may be minimized by synchronization of the shock waves to the cardiac cycle.

4. Hypertension can reach extreme levels in patients who have autonomic dysreflexia.

5. Renal (subcapsular) hematoma may result from collateral damage to renal vasculature, especially in hypertensive patients.

6. Severe pulmonary or intestinal damage is rare and occurs if the shock waves are inadvertently applied to the lung or intestines, as may occur with a patient movement during treatment.

III. PATIENTS WITH SPINAL CORD PATHOLOGY

A. Spinal cord injury frequently causes urinary retention, which promotes urinary tract infections, nephrolithiasis, and vesicoureteric reflux.

B. **Autonomic dysreflexia** is manifested by an acute onset of sympathetic hyperreactivity to certain stimuli below the level of a spinal cord lesion, generally at or above the T6-T7 level. The syndrome may appear at any time from a few months to many years after the injury.

1. Common findings include hypertension (potentially severe), headache, diaphoresis, flushing or pallor, and bradycardia.

2. Precipitants include visceral stimulation, most commonly bladder distention, although urinary tract infection, fecal impaction, uterine contraction, bowel distention, and other intra-abdominal and cutaneous stimuli have been reported.

3. Pathophysiology is thought to involve disorganized connections between afferent neurons and sympathetic neurons below the level of the injury that lead to vasoconstriction and hypertension. The parasympathetic nervous system is unable to counteract this vasoconstriction resulting from the spinal cord injury.

4. Treatment of autonomic dysreflexia includes removal of the inciting stimulus, increasing anesthetic depth, and pharmacologic treatment of persistent hypertension with rapidly acting agents such as sublingual nifedipine, or IV nitroglycerin or nitroprusside. Neuraxial anesthesia blocks both limbs of the reflex arc and prevents dysreflexia. However, a preexisting complete sensory deficit impairs determining the level of anesthesia by cutaneous testing. For short procedures, spinal may be preferable to epidural anesthesia because of more reliable block without spared segments.

Suggested Readings

Biki B, Mascha E, Moriarty DC, Fitzpatrick JM, Sessler DI, Buggy DJ. Anesthetic technique for radical prostatectomy surgery affects cancer recurrence: a retrospective analysis. *Anesthesiology.* 2008;109(2):180-187.

Conacher ID, Soomro NA, Rix D. Anaesthesia for laparoscopic urological surgery. *Br J Anaesth.* 2004;93(6):859-864.

Domi R, Sula H, Ohri I, et al. Anesthetic challenges of patients with cardiac comorbidities undergoing major urologic surgery. *Int Arch Med* 2014;7:17. doi:10.1186/1755-7682-7-17

Ellis DB, Albrecht M. Anesthesia for robotic surgery. In: Gropper MA, ed. *Miller's Anesthesia.* 9th ed. Elsevier; 2020:2236-2250.

Gravenstein D. Extracorporeal shock wave lithotripsy and percutaneous nephrolithotomy. *Anesthesiol Clin North Am.* 2000;18(4):953-971.

Hahn RG. Fluid absorption in endoscopic surgery. *Br J Anaesth.* 2006;96(1):8-20.

Hambly PR, Martin B. Anaesthesia for chronic spinal cord lesions. *Anaesthesia.* 1998;53:273-289.

Hanson R, Zornow M, Coulin M, Brambrink AM. Laser resection of the prostate: implications for anesthesia. *Anesth Analg.* 2007;105(2):475-479.

Hsu RL, Kaye AD, Urman RD. Anesthetic challenges in robotic-assisted urologic surgery. *Rev Urol.* 2013;15(4):178-184.

O'Malley C, Frumento R, Hardy M, et al. A randomized, double-blind comparison of lactated Ringer's solution and 0.9% NaCl during renal transplantation. *Anesth Analg.* 2005;100:1518-1524.

Scavonetto F, Yeoh TY, Umbreit EC, et al. Association between neuraxial analgesia, cancer progression, and mortality after radical prostatectomy: a large, retrospective matched cohort study. *Br J Anaesth.* 2014;113(suppl 1):i95-i102.

Schmid S, Jungwirth B. Anaesthesia for renal transplant surgery: an update. *Eur J Anaesthesiol.* 2012;29(12):552-558.

Sprung J, Scavonetto F, Yeoh TY, et al. Outcomes after radical prostatectomy for cancer: a comparison between general anesthesia and epidural anesthesia with fentanyl analgesia. A matched cohort study. *Anesth Analg.* 2014;119(4):859-866.

Whalley DG. Anesthesia for radical prostatectomy, cystectomy, nephrectomy, pheochromocytoma, and laparoscopic procedures. *Anesthesiol Clin North Am.* 2000;18(4):899-917.

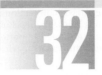

Anesthesia for Obstetrics and Gynecology

Hilary Gallin and Andrew N. Chalupka

I. MATERNAL PHYSIOLOGY IN PREGNANCY (TABLE 32.1)

A. Respiratory system

1. **Capillary engorgement of the mucosa** may occur throughout the respiratory tract, beginning early in the first trimester and increasing throughout pregnancy. Historically, a 6.0- to 6.5-mm (inner diameter) endotracheal tube has been recommended for intubation to decrease the possibility of airway trauma. However, the use of larger tubes may be possible in most patients should it be required. Fluid retention may lead to an enlarged tongue that may explain the increased prevalence of Mallampati class 3 and 4 airways in term parturients compared to the general population. Additionally, the airway examination may change during the course of labor resulting in a further increase in the airway class. Lastly, because of mucosal engorgement, nasotracheal intubation may cause epistaxis and is best avoided in pregnant women.

2. **Minute ventilation increases by 45%** to support the higher oxygen requirements of the mother and fetus and is driven by a proportional increase in tidal volume. Pulmonary resistance is decreased by 50% to accommodate these changes. As the pregnancy progresses, elevation of the diaphragm from the gravid uterus leads to 20% decrease in maternal **functional residual capacity** (FRC). The resultant decrease in oxygen reserve mandates adequate preoxygenation prior to induction of general anesthesia.

B. Cardiovascular system

1. **Cardiac output increases** progressively up to 50% from the end of the second trimester to term primarily due to increased stroke volume with a small contribution of increased heart rate. A grade II systolic ejection murmur at the left sternal border can be commonly heard because of cardiac enlargement due to increases in intravascular volume. During labor, contractions of the engorged uterus provide a 300- to 500-mL autotransfusion into the maternal circulation, further increasing cardiac output. Cardiac output becomes highest immediately postpartum and may increase 80% to 100% above prelabor values due to further autotransfusion and loss of inferior vena cava (IVC) compression by the fetus. Despite the significant increase in cardiac output, blood pressure is not elevated at term from prepregnancy levels due to decreased peripheral vascular resistance.

2. **Supine hypotension** usually occurs after 20 weeks of gestation when the gravid uterus compresses the aorta and IVC of the patient in the supine position. Aortocaval compression decreases venous return and results in maternal hypotension and decreased uteroplacental blood flow. Providing left uterine displacement of at least 15° when the patient is supine may mitigate this problem.

C. Hematology

1. **Blood volume increases** markedly throughout the course of pregnancy. Because the plasma volume increases (up to 50% by 34 weeks gestation) more than does red cell mass, a relative **dilutional anemia** occurs.

2. The pregnant patient is **hypercoagulable** throughout gestation. The concentration of most coagulation factors increases, with the exception of factors XI and XIII, in pregnancy as does platelet production, activation, and consumption. This hypercoagulable state helps to limit blood loss at delivery although it also increases the risk for thrombotic complications.

D. Nervous system
    1. The **minimum alveolar concentration** (MAC) for inhalational anesthetics is decreased up to 40% during pregnancy. The etiology is unclear but may be related to alterations of hormone and endorphin

System	Parameters	Changes
Respiratory	*Capacities/volume*	
	Total lung capacity	−5%
	Vital capacity	No change
	Functional residual capacity	−20%
	Inspiratory reserve volume	+5%
	Expiratory reserve volume	−20%
	Residual volume	−15
	Closing capacity	No change
	Tidal volume	+45%
	Mechanics	
	FEV_1	No change
	FEV_1/FVC	No change
	Minute ventilation	+45%
	Alveolar ventilation	+45%
	Blood gases	
	$Paco_2$	−10%
	Pao_2	+5%-10%
	pH	No change
	HCO_3	Decrease
	Oxygen consumption	+20%
	P50 at term	30 mm Hg
Cardiovascular	Cardiac output	+50%
	Stroke volume	+25%
	Heart rate	+20%-25%
	Systematic vascular resistance	−20%

Physiologic Changes Associated With Pregnancy

System	Parameters	Changes
Hematology	Blood volume	+45%
	Plasma volume	+55%
	Red blood cell volume	+25%
	Coagulation factors	
	Factors VII, VIII, IX, X, XII, fibrinogen	Increase
	Prothrombin	No change
	Factors XI, XIII	Decrease
	Platelet count	No change or decrease
	Total protein (albumin, globulin)	Decrease
Central nervous system	MAC	Decrease
	Local anesthetic requirement	Decrease
Gastrointestinal	*Gastric emptying*	
	First trimester	No change
	Second trimester	No change
	Third trimester	No change
	Labor	Decrease
	Postpartum (18 h)	No change
	Barrier pressure	
	First, second, third trimesters, labor	Decrease
Hepatic	AST, ALT, LDH, bilirubin	Increase
	Alkaline phosphatase	Increase
Renal	Glomerular filtration rate	+50%
	Renal plasma flow	+75%

TABLE 32.1 Physiologic Changes Associated With Pregnancy (Continued)

ALT, alanine aminotransferase; AST, aspartate aminotransferase; FEV_1, forced expiratory volume in one second; FVC, forced vital capacity; LDH, lactate dehydrogenase; MAC, minimum alveolar concentration.

concentrations during pregnancy, which result in an increased pain threshold or pregnancy-induced analgesia. However, this increased sensitivity to volatiles may not translate to enhanced effect in the brain; therefore low MAC should be used with caution to avoid an increase in the incidence of awareness under anesthesia. The speed of induction for intravenous agents is increased in pregnant women secondary to the increase in cardiac output in contrast to inhalational agents that act slower because of the increase in minute ventilation and decreased FRC.

2. The **local anesthetic** dose required for regional anesthesia is reduced in the parturient compared to the patient who is not pregnant. Reasons for this include the following:

a. **A decrease in cerebrospinal fluid (CSF) protein** results in a greater proportion of free and active drug.

b. **Elevated CSF pH** increases the un-ionized fraction of the local anesthetic.

c. **Distention of epidural veins** during pregnancy results in a decrease in lumbar CSF volume with enhancement of local anesthetic spread and reduction of the segmental dose requirement for **spinal anesthesia**.

3. **Sympathetic nervous system (SNS) activity increases** from as early as 6 weeks of gestation despite decreases in diastolic pressure and total peripheral resistance. The parturient is highly dependent on the SNS for hemodynamic control, which is reflected by the significant decrease in blood pressure seen after regional anesthesia. SNS activity may return to normal by 24 to 48 hours postpartum.

4. The apex of **lumbar lordosis is shifted cephalad** with reduced thoracic kyphosis in the supine position. This may contribute to the increased cephalad spread of spinal anesthesia during pregnancy.

E. **Gastrointestinal system.** Because of the **relaxation of the lower esophageal sphincter** and mechanical **displacement of the stomach** by the gravid uterus, gastric reflux and heartburn are present in 30% to 50% of pregnant patients. It is not clear when during the pregnancy the risk for aspiration increases, although the difference between intragastric pressure and lower esophageal sphincter tone is decreased as early as the first trimester. Gastric emptying is not delayed during pregnancy, but it is slowed during labor, particularly following the administration of opioids. When a general anesthetic is planned, a nonparticulate antacid should be given routinely; a histamine (H_2) blocker and metoclopramide should be considered. Patients in the second and third trimesters should have a rapid sequence induction for general anesthesia.

F. **Renal system.** Renal plasma flow and glomerular filtration increases by up to 50%, leading to increased creatinine clearance and decreased blood urea nitrogen and serum creatinine levels.

G. **Musculoskeletal system.** Increased lumbar lordosis and intra-abdominal pressure secondary to the enlarging uterus can stretch and compress the lateral femoral cutaneous nerve and produce a sensory loss over the anterolateral thigh ("meralgia paresthetica"). Carpal tunnel syndrome is common with a possible multifactorial etiology. Widening of the pubic symphysis is likely secondary to an increase in the hormone relaxin during pregnancy.

II. LABOR AND DELIVERY

A. **Labor** is defined as the onset of regular painful uterine contractions that lead to cervical change, and it may be divided into three stages.

1. The **first stage** begins with the onset of regular contractions and ends with full cervical dilation. It is divided into a slow latent phase and a rapidly progressive active phase characterized by accelerated cervical dilation. Patients with body mass index greater than 30 kg/m² and male fetuses may experience prolonged first stage of labor. Such factors highlight the limitations of widespread use of a single labor curve for all patients.

2. The **second stage** extends from full cervical dilation until delivery of the infant.

3. The **third stage** begins after delivery of the infant, ending with delivery of the placenta.

B. **Pain** during the early first part of labor is primarily caused by uterine contractions and cervical dilation. Pain during the first portion of labor is mediated by the T10 to L1 segments of the spinal cord. In the active phase of the first stage of labor and in early second-stage labor, there is an additional component of pain due to perineal stretching that travels via the pudendal nerve to enter the spinal cord between the S2 and S4 segments.

C. **Intrapartum fetal evaluation** is most commonly accomplished with **fetal heart rate (FHR) monitoring**—either continuous or intermittent. Continuous FHR monitoring is used in up to 85% of laboring patients in the United States. The normal FHR ranges from 110 to 160 beats per minute (bpm) over 10 minutes. Fetal tachycardia may signify fetal asphyxia, maternal fever, and/or chorioamnionitis or may be the result of maternally administered drugs. Persistent fetal bradycardia is most commonly due to hypoxia, but other etiologies include congenital heart block, maternally administered β-blockers, or hypothermia. FHR baseline variability is defined as the fluctuation in FHR of two cycles or greater per minute. Minimal variability refers to less than 5 bpm fluctuation, moderate ranges from 6 to 25 bpm, and marked greater than 25 bpm. It is modulated by fetal vagal tone and is a sign of underlying fetal health. Lack of variability may be associated with fetal hypoxia, neurogenic abnormalities, and resulting central nervous system (CNS) depression due to side effects from opioids or other medications given throughout labor and must be interpreted in the context of FHR decelerations (decreases in FHR of 15 seconds or more from baseline to nadir). Recurrent concerning decelerations (late or deep variables), especially in the setting of minimal or absent variability, should prompt further evaluation to detect fetal compromise. Decelerations have been categorized (**Figure 32.1**) as follows:

1. **Early decelerations** are gradual FHR decelerations (normally up to 20 bpm below baseline) that occur concomitantly with uterine contractions providing a mirror image of the uterine contraction, with the nadir of the deceleration occurring at the peak of the contraction. They are caused by an increase in fetal vagal tone, likely from mild hypoxia and compression of the fetal head, and do not require intervention.

2. By definition, **variable decelerations** are variable in both duration and appearance and can occur spontaneously. Variable decelerations are associated with umbilical cord compression and decreased umbilical blood flow or compression of the head of the fetus in the second stage of labor. They may indicate fetal compromise when severe and/ or repetitive. Amnioinfusion (the instillation of amniotic fluid through a transcervical catheter after rupture of the fetal membranes) has been demonstrated to decrease the need for emergent cesarean delivery by improving or eliminating them.

3. **Late decelerations** are gradual repetitive decelerations that begin 10 to 30 seconds after the onset of a uterine contraction with a return of the FHR to the baseline only after the contraction has ended. Late decelerations suggest impaired maternal-fetal oxygen exchange and are triggered in susceptible fetuses by the decrease in fetal reserve with resulting intolerance of transient hypoxia. Medical interventions are tailored to improve placental oxygen delivery, among them left uterine

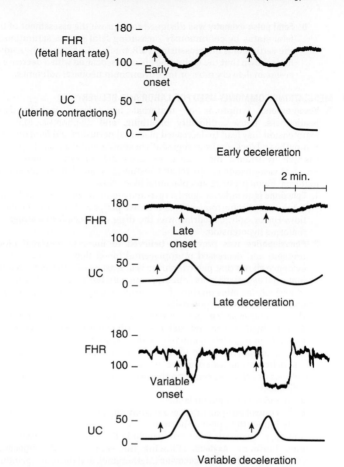

FIGURE 32.1 Patterns of periodic fetal heart rate (FHR) decelerations in relation to uterine contractions.

displacement, correction of maternal hypotension, reconsideration of oxytocin dosing, and oxygen by face mask to the mother. A persistent late deceleration pattern might require delivery of the fetus.

4. Electronic FHR monitoring has several significant limitations including a high rate of false positives and significant variability in its interpretation. Lastly, the use of electronic fetal monitoring has been associated with an increase in operative deliveries. While it has not resulted in a decrease in cerebral palsy rates, it has been associated with a lower rate of neonatal seizures. To minimize intervention based on false positives, additional ancillary tests may be considered:

   a. **Fetal scalp stimulation.** An FHR acceleration in response to digital or instrumental stimulation of the fetal head is associated with a healthy nonacidotic fetus and a pH of at least 7.19.

b. **Fetal pulse oximetry** was designed to improve the assessment of the fetal status by continuously measuring fetal oxygen saturation in the setting of a nonreassuring FHR tracing. Unfortunately, studies have shown that the technology is not associated with a decrease in cesarean delivery rates or improvement in neonatal outcomes.

III. MEDICATIONS COMMONLY USED FOR LABOR AND DELIVERY

A. **Vasopressors.** Symptoms of maternal hypotension include light-headedness, nausea, difficulty breathing, and diaphoresis. Maternal hypotension may lead to decreased placental perfusion and fetal distress. Sympathetic blockade from regional anesthesia and decreased systemic vascular resistance may cause symptomatic maternal hypotension. An ideal vasopressor for obstetric anesthesia is one that increases both maternal blood pressure and placental blood flow.

1. **Ephedrine** is an indirect agonist of α- and β-adrenergic receptors. Its inotropic and chronotropic effects increase peripheral and uterine blood flow. Historically, ephedrine was the drug of choice for treatment of maternal hypotension.

2. **Phenylephrine** was previously believed to increase maternal blood pressure and decreased uteroplacental blood flow, but more recent evidence shows that phenylephrine is at least as effective in correcting maternal hypotension as ephedrine but with less risk of fetal acidemia. Phenylephrine infusions have become increasingly common to prevent and treat maternal hypotension.

3. Dilute **norepinephrine** may be used to counteract spinal anesthesia-induced hypotension and increases cardiac output with a lower incidence of bradycardia compared with phenylephrine. Less commonly used than ephedrine and phenylephrine, norepinephrine use in labor and delivery is an area of active investigation.

B. **Uterotonics** or ecbolics are agents that stimulate uterine contractions.

1. **Indications**
   a. To induce or augment labor
   b. To control postpartum uterine atony and bleeding
   c. To induce therapeutic abortion

2. The most frequently used drugs include the synthetic posterior pituitary hormone, **oxytocin** (Pitocin); the ergot alkaloids, **ergonovine** (Ergotrate) and **methylergonovine** (Methergine); and the prostaglandins, **prostaglandin 15-methyl F$_2\alpha$** (carboprost; Hemabate) and **prostaglandin E$_1$** (misoprostol).

   a. **Oxytocin** acts on the uterine smooth muscle to stimulate the frequency and force of contractions. Cardiovascular side effects of oxytocin include vasodilation, hypotension, tachycardia, and arrhythmias. In high doses, oxytocin may have an antidiuretic effect and produce hyponatremia, cerebral edema, and subsequent seizures. With a half-life on the order of minutes, continuous intravenous infusion is required.

   b. **Ergot alkaloids** control postpartum bleeding following the third stage of labor by producing tetanic uterine contractions. Side effects include systemic vasoconstriction and hypertension, which may be amplified in the presence of vasopressors. IV injection has been associated with severe hypertension, seizures, stroke, myocardial infarction, and pulmonary edema. Intramuscular (IM) administration is therefore highly recommended. Ergot alkaloids should be used with caution or avoided in patients with peripheral vascular disease, preeclampsia, hypertension, or coronary artery disease.

c. **Prostaglandin 15-methyl F$_2\alpha$**, or **carboprost**, is a treatment for uterine atony. The usual dose is 250 µg IM or by intramyometrial injection, not more frequently than every 15 minutes, with a total maximum dose of 2 mg. Transient hypertension, severe bronchoconstriction, and increased pulmonary vascular resistance have been reported, contraindicating its use in patients with a history of asthma. Fever, nausea, vomiting, and diarrhea are additional side effects.

d. **Prostaglandin E$_1$** increases myometrial intracellular free calcium concentrations and improves uterine tone. It is available in 200-µg tablets that are placed rectally or vaginally for the treatment of postpartum hemorrhage. Side effects are less common but are similar to those of prostaglandin 15-methyl F$_2\alpha$.

C. **Tocolytics** are used to delay premature labor in patients with viable fetuses less than or equal to 34 weeks of gestation. Cervical dilation of less than 4 cm and cervical effacement of less than 80% are associated with a greater likelihood of success in terminating premature labor.

1. **Indications**
   a. To stop preterm contractions
   b. To slow or arrest labor while initiating other therapeutic measures (eg, betamethasone to accelerate fetal lung maturation)
   c. To allow transfer from a community hospital to a tertiary care center with a neonatal intensive care unit

2. **Contraindications**
   a. Chorioamnionitis
   b. Fetal distress
   c. Intrauterine fetal demise
   d. Severe hemorrhage

3. **Specific drugs**
   a. **β_2-Adrenergic agonists** such as **terbutaline** produce myometrial relaxation, maternal bronchodilation, vasodilation, and tachycardia. In addition, they cause hyperglycemia, hypokalemia, hyperinsulinemia, and metabolic acidosis. Pulmonary edema and chest pain are rare in the setting of less than 24 hours of therapy. Preexisting hyperglycemia should be corrected, and a baseline electrocardiogram should be considered for patients with preexisting cardiac disease.

   b. **Cyclooxygenase inhibitors** such as **indomethacin** inhibit arachidonic acid conversion to prostaglandins. Maternal side effects are uncommon but possible fetal side effects include premature closure of the ductus arteriosus and decreased fetal urine output. They should therefore be used with caution after 32 weeks of gestation and in oligohydramnios.

   c. **Calcium channel blockers** block the release of calcium from smooth muscle sarcoplasmic reticulum, thus inhibiting uterine contractions. Calcium channel blockers are effective tocolytic agents and are well tolerated. Hypotension is an expected side effect.

   d. **Magnesium sulfate** is no longer recommended for tocolysis due to ineffectiveness. It may be used for the prevention of eclamptic seizures in at-risk patients. It antagonizes intracellular calcium and inhibits myometrial contraction. Side effects include hyporeflexia, lethargy, and nausea; at higher serum concentrations, peripheral respiratory depression, electrocardiogram changes, and pulmonary edema are possible.

IV. PLACENTAL TRANSFER OF DRUGS

A. **Passive diffusion** is responsible for the placental transfer of the majority of drugs, although some facilitated and active transport occurs. Factors that promote rapid diffusion include the following:
   1. Low molecular weight
   2. High lipid solubility
   3. Low degree of ionization
   4. Low protein binding

B. Most of the **inhalational** and **intravenous anesthetics** readily cross the placenta because they have a low molecular weight, have high lipid solubility, are relatively nonionized, and are minimally protein bound.

C. **Opioids** cross the placenta readily and cause fetal neurologic and respiratory depression.

D. **Muscle relaxants** are water-soluble, ionized molecules, with high molecular weights, and therefore do not readily cross the placenta.

E. The transfer of **anticholinergic** drugs is variable: glycopyrrolate is poorly transferred while atropine is completely transferred. Small amounts of **acetylcholinesterase inhibitors** are transferred.

F. **Vasoactive medications**—antihypertensive, antiarrhythmic medications, and vasopressors (with the exception of phenylephrine)—cross the placenta and do exert some effect on the fetus.

G. **Local anesthetics** are weak bases with low degrees of ionization and therefore may cross the placenta when absorbed into the maternal bloodstream (eg, via epidural venous plexuses). Fetal acidosis, exacerbated in fetal distress, favors ionization and subsequent placental transfer and accumulation of basic drugs, in a process known as "ion trapping." However, in normal circumstances, these concentrations rarely result in clinical toxicity.

V. ANALGESIA FOR LABOR AND VAGINAL DELIVERY

A. **Natural childbirth.** Some women favor a delivery plan with minimal medical intervention. Nonetheless, it is important to evaluate each patient's medical history and physical findings to provide informed and expedient emergency care.

B. **Systemic analgesia**
   1. **Mixed opioid agonist-antagonists.** Nalbuphine or butorphanol are often the initial choice for systemic analgesia due to their efficacy combined with a ceiling effect on maternal ventilatory depression.
   2. **Opioids.** Meperidine, morphine, remifentanil, and fentanyl are commonly used opioids. Maternal side effects, including dose-dependent respiratory depression, sedation, and rapid placental diffusion, limit their use overall. These drugs may also contribute to neonatal respiratory depression and cause decreased FHR variability, a need for active neonatal resuscitation, and possible neurobehavioral effects in the neonate. Of note, remifentanil and fentanyl have the advantage of self-administration via PCA. Remifentanil is rapidly metabolized by the fetus and has a short maternal half-life. Fentanyl is preferred to meperidine due to lower rates of respiratory depression and nausea. Both drugs have favorable fetal outcomes.
   3. **Inhalational analgesia.** Nitrous oxide is used in different parts of the world, most commonly in a 50% mixture with oxygen. Its analgesic efficacy is limited. Environmental pollution is a concern, and hypoxemia is possible in combination with systemic opioids. Neonatal depression is rare.

C. Epidural provides the most effective labor analgesia and eases the transition to effective neuraxial anesthesia if a cesarean delivery becomes necessary. Existing evidence does not show an increased rate of cesarean delivery when compared to systemic analgesia. The duration of the second stage of labor is about 15 minutes longer, and the instrumental delivery rate is increased with epidurals.

1. **Technique**
   a. Initial IV access should be established. Prehydration with 500 mL of fluid may be routine among some anesthetists, but data from small studies have provided conflicting results regarding the effect on FHR.
   b. Vital signs and FHR should be monitored according to institutional protocol.
   c. It is customary to administer a dose of oral nonparticulate antacid.
   d. Specific physiologic and anatomic features of term pregnancy—for example, epidural venous distention, increased abdominal size, and intermittent uterine contractions—must be taken into account for positioning. A patient may be seated or in the lateral decubitus position.

2. **Advantages**
   a. Epidurals offer continuous analgesia for the duration of labor and cesarean section if necessary.
   b. Drug dose and delivery mode (eg, patient controlled analgesia) may be individualized.
   c. The hyper-/hypoventilation cycle and associated decrease in PaO_2 or O_2 saturation are favorably modified.
   d. Memory, alertness, and emotional perception are preserved.

3. **Disadvantages**
   a. Patient cooperation is necessary.
   b. Providers skilled in neuraxial technique in pregnant women are required.
   c. Vital signs must be regularly monitored and systemic hypotension corrected.
   d. Accidental dural puncture complicates approximately 1.5% of placements.

4. **Contraindications**
   a. Patient refusal or inability to cooperate during placement.
   b. Coagulation disorder or significant thrombocytopenia—either acquired or inherited.
   c. Infection at the site of catheter placement.
   d. Severe hypovolemia.
   e. Space-occupying lesion with increased intracranial pressure predisposing the patient to herniation after accidental dural puncture and CSF loss.

5. **Anesthetics**
   a. **A test dose** of 3 mL of 1.5% lidocaine (45 mg) with 1:200,000 epinephrine (15 μg) aids in detection of intrathecal or intravascular placement. The test dose should be given after the completion of a contraction if possible to isolate the potential cause of tachycardia or hypertension.
   b. The ideal analgesia in labor provides adequate pain relief and minimizes motor block. The combination of a local anesthetic and an opioid helps to achieve this goal. Our current practice is to administer an epidural mix of 0.08% (0.8 mg/mL) bupivacaine

with 2 µg/mL of fentanyl. Epidural administration is now preferred through programmed intermittent epidural bolus instead of continuous epidural infusion (CEI) with patient controlled epidural anesthesia. There is a greater spread of anesthetic with intermittent bolus compared to the continuous infusion that results in a local anesthetic sparing effect and less dense motor block while having greater patient satisfaction. Additional clinical boluses are typically between 5 and 10 mL. In the course of labor, it is not uncommon to administer concentrated local anesthetics—for example, 0.125% to 0.25% bupivacaine or 0.1% to 0.2% ropivacaine—to meet analgesic requirements. Malfunction and malposition of the epidural catheter must be considered when the observed analgesic effect is lower than expected.

c. Blood pressure monitoring must be more frequent at the onset of epidural analgesia and after local anesthetic boluses since hypotension may become symptomatic and cause impaired placental perfusion. The usual treatment of the hypotension is crystalloid volume expansion, ephedrine 5 to 10 mg, and/or phenylephrine 80 µg IV repeated as necessary.

d. **Continuous infusion for labor** is also possible but not common practice in our hospital.

6. **Complications**

a. Epidural failure—Epidural catheter replacement rates range between 5% and 13% due to inadequate analgesia.

b. **Dural penetration** complicates 1.5% of labor epidural placements. Increased depth of the epidural space and number of attempts correlate with increased frequency of this complication. Conversely, practitioners' skill and experience as well as loss of resistance to saline might decrease the incidence of inadvertent dural puncture. Accidental intrathecal catheters can be kept and dosed accordingly in particularly difficult epidural placements. Careful attention must be paid to label the catheter accordingly.

c. **Postdural puncture headache (PDPH).** Approximately 52% of inadvertent dural punctures with an epidural needle will cause frontal or occipital headache of variable intensity with possible radiation to the neck defined to be within 5 days post puncture. The headache is often orthostatic with symptoms that appear within seconds of being upright and resolve quickly after becoming horizontal. Risk factors for PDPH include young age (<40), female gender, low BMI, history of PDPH, use of a needle with a cutting bevel, and vaginal delivery. In mild PDPH, hydration, bed rest, analgesics, caffeine, and avoidance of heavy lifting may be helpful in treating symptoms, but studies have not shown efficacy in preventing PDPH. Severe PDPH may warrant an **epidural blood patch (EBP).** Immediate symptomatic relief occurs in up to 75% of cases. A second EBP might be considered in refractory cases. Rare complications include meningitis, subdural hematoma, diplopia, hearing loss, and cerebral venous thrombosis. These serious complications should be considered if the headache does not respond to conservative measures or the EBP described above.

d. **Intravascular injection.** Total dose and rate of intravascular injection are correlated with signs and symptoms of local anesthetic toxicity. When intravascular injection is suspected, infusion should be discontinued and appropriate therapy immediately instituted, including the administration of Intralipid. Cardiovascular collapse must be treated with cardiopulmonary resuscitation (CPR), left uterine displacement, and, potentially, perimortem cesarean delivery (PMCD).

   e. **Intrathecal injection.** Aspiration before each epidural dose helps to detect intrathecal catheters. Large epidural doses inadvertently injected into the intrathecal space may produce high or total spinal anesthesia. Nausea, hypotension, and loss of consciousness may precede cardiopulmonary arrest. Critical interventions include IV crystalloid, vasopressors, inotropes, left uterine displacement, and 100% oxygen administration. Cardiac and respiratory arrest associated with a total spinal must be emergently treated in accordance with the advanced cardiac life support (ACLS) principles.

D. Spinal anesthesia. A small single intrathecal dose of 0.25% bupivacaine (1-2.5 mg) provides prompt analgesia lasting up to 90 minutes. Single shot spinals are not preferred for laboring women due to the prolonged duration of labor and fixed duration of the spinal. They may be used if delivery is imminent due to their rapid onset. Morphine may be added to the spinal to prolong the duration of analgesia, but data are inconsistent.

E. Combined spinal-epidural analgesia (CSE) offers both a rapid onset (2-5 minutes) of sacral analgesia for advanced labor and the benefit of CEI. In a subset of patients for whom labor pain inhibits active participation in the epidural placement process, initiation of spinal analgesia may improve the success of a subsequent epidural placement. However, it prevents immediate verification of epidural function. Additionally, spread of the intrathecal anesthetic may be unpredictable on initiation of the epidural. Addition of a lipophilic opioid may decrease the dose of local anesthetic required, thereby limiting the motor blockade and significant hypotension associated with local anesthetics. This may be helpful in patients who are preload dependent. Despite the dura being punctured, there has not been an increase in PDPH noted when a small-gauge pencil point needle is used. The dural puncture may increase the risk of a neuraxial infection. Intrathecal opioid administration is associated with a higher incidence of pruritus compared to epidural administration.

F. Dural puncture epidural (DPE) is a technique in which the dura is punctured with a spinal needle, but unlike a CSE, no medication is injected into the intrathecal space. Studies have shown more frequent blockade of the sacral dermatomes compared to a lumbar epidural due to migration of local anesthetic into the intrathecal space. Data are conflicting, but some studies suggest DPE produces improved block quality compared with labor epidural and fewer side effects compared with CSE.

VI. ANESTHESIA FOR CESAREAN DELIVERY

The anesthetic technique for cesarean delivery must be planned according to the urgency of the delivery. Indications may be either maternal (eg, prior cesarean delivery, arrest of labor, failed induction, placental or uterine pathology) or fetal (eg, malpresentation, concern for fetal well-being).

A. Positioning, regardless of anesthetic technique, should include a **15-degree left table tilt** to relieve aortocaval compression and prevent maternal hypotension and uterine insufficiency.

B. Aspiration prophylaxis should be carried out with a nonparticulate antacid, H_2 receptor antagonist, and/or metoclopramide. In the case of elective cesarean delivery, clear liquids may be consumed until 2 hours prior to surgery. While laboring patients may be allowed moderate amounts of clear liquids throughout labor, those laboring patients with additional risk factors for aspiration (eg, morbid obesity) or at increased risk of operative delivery (eg, nonreassuring fetal heart tracing) should be subject to additional restrictions on oral intake.

C. **Anesthetic technique**

1. **Regional anesthesia** is more commonly employed and offers maternal and fetal benefits, including avoidance of airway manipulation, minimal fetal drug exposure, and decreased blood loss.

   a. **Spinal anesthesia** provides rapid onset of surgical anesthesia, but its duration is time-limited. T4 sensory for adequate coverage of abdominal viscera. The use of hyperbaric bupivacaine (0.75% in dextrose 8.25%) allows positional control over the cephalad spread of the local anesthetic. The ED_{95} for spinal bupivacaine in cesarean delivery is 11.2 mg. Common adjuvants include a lipophilic opioid (eg, fentanyl or sufentanil) for intraoperative pain control and a hydrophilic opioid (eg, morphine or hydromorphone) for longer term analgesia. Concomitant fluid load and prophylactic phenylephrine infusion may reduce sympathectomy-associated hypotension. Postoperatively, patients should be monitored and assessed for delayed respiratory depression and pruritus.

   b. **Epidural anesthesia** is most commonly used during cesarean delivery when a labor epidural is used to provide surgical anesthesia. In comparison with spinal anesthesia, epidural anesthesia is slower in onset, requires higher local anesthetic doses, and may be redosed as necessary. Commonly used local anesthetics include 2% lidocaine with epinephrine and 3% 2-chloroprocaine; the utility of bupivacaine is limited by the slow onset time. The addition of sodium bicarbonate to lidocaine or 2-chloroprocaine may speed their onset. Ongoing attention should be paid to the patient's sensory level and epidural should be redosed as necessary. Postoperative analgesia is improved by epidural administration of 2 to 3 mg of preservative-free morphine after delivery of the fetus. Monitoring for postoperative respiratory depression and pruritus is indicated.

   c. **CSE** combines the advantage of rapid anesthetic onset with the option to prolong its duration. Although the function of the epidural catheter is not tested at the start, recent literature has shown that positioning of the epidural catheter is usually correct with this technique.

2. **General anesthesia**

   a. Indications
      1. Failure of neuraxial technique
      2. Insufficient time to implement neuraxial anesthesia
      3. Maternal preference
      4. Medical contraindication to regional anesthesia

   b. The potential for a difficult airway and increased risk of aspiration in the pregnant patient mandate careful preparation and discussion of alternative airway plans and immediate availability of advanced airway equipment. Preoxygenation followed by rapid sequence intravenous induction with endotracheal intubation is the technique of choice.

   c. To minimize fetal exposure to anesthetics, the cesarean section should begin immediately upon securing the airway. Halogenated agents antagonize uterine contracture; therefore, it is customary to decrease their inhaled concentration to 0.75 to 0.5 MAC and increase the N_2O fraction immediately after delivery or transition to a propofol infusion. Risk of awareness is elevated in emergency cesarean delivery; consider administration of midazolam to reduce this risk.

d. Additional neuromuscular blockade following induction is not usually necessary.

e. Emergence and extubation represents a high-risk time, especially if difficult intubation or large fluid shifts occurred intraoperatively. Strict extubation criteria should be applied and delayed extubation may be considered.

f. In the absence of long-acting neuraxial opioid, adequate postoperative pain control may require regional block (eg, transversus abdominis plane block, assuming no contraindication) or initiation of intravenous opioid patient controlled analgesia.

VII. PREECLAMPSIA

Preeclampsia is a common diagnosis occurring in approximately 5% of pregnancies, particularly in nulliparous, diabetic, hypertensive patients or those with chronic disease. Although the etiology is incompletely understood, possible mechanisms of disease include a combination of factors including exaggerated maternal immune and inflammatory responses as well as chronic uteroplacental ischemia leading to upregulation of angiogenic factors.

A. Diagnosis

1. Persistent hypertension after 20 weeks of gestational age should prompt a diagnostic workup for preeclampsia.

2. The American College of Obstetricians and Gynecologists defines a diagnosis of preeclampsia as a single blood pressure measurement of >160/110 mm Hg or two measurements more than 4 hours apart of >140/90 mm Hg combined with *either* proteinuria or evidence of end-organ damage (thrombocytopenia, pulmonary edema, renal insufficiency, or impaired liver function).

3. Preeclampsia with severe features is defined as a blood pressure of >160/110 mm Hg on two occasions at least 4 hours apart in addition to visual disturbances, new-onset headache, or the end-organ sequelae listed above.

4. Two additional diagnoses, **HELLP syndrome** and **eclampsia,** are also part of this spectrum of disease.

   a. Eclampsia describes the new onset of seizures in a parturient with preeclampsia due to CNS involvement. It is observed in approximately 50% of maternal deaths associated with preeclampsia.

   b. HELLP syndrome (**h**emolysis, **e**levated **l**iver enzymes, and **l**ow **p**latelets) involves a constellation of laboratory abnormalities and is generally regarded as a subset of severe preeclampsia. The diagnosis of HELLP syndrome is also associated with an increased risk of adverse outcomes including placental abruption, renal failure, hepatic subcapsular hematoma formation and liver rupture, and fetal and maternal death.

B. Management

1. Obstetric management

   a. Expectant management and monitoring until 37 weeks' gestation is preferred for women with a preterm fetus and preeclampsia without severe features.

   b. Delivery is recommended for preeclampsia with severe features at 34 weeks' gestation or beyond. Delivery of the placenta is the accepted treatment for preeclampsia.

2. **Pharmacologic therapy**
   a. **Seizure prophylaxis** may be carried out with **magnesium sulfate**. Magnesium is administered during labor and delivery and for 24 to 48 hours postpartum via an IV loading dose of 4 g given over 30 minutes, followed by an infusion of 1 to 2 g/h. Due to its relaxant effect on smooth muscle, magnesium therapy may decrease maternal blood pressure and predispose the patient to postpartum uterine atony and hemorrhage.
   b. **Antihypertensive medications** such as **labetalol, hydralazine,** and **calcium channel blockers** are frequently administered for blood pressure control. The goal of therapy is not to normalize blood pressure but to prevent progression to hypertensive crisis, encephalopathy, or stroke. It is important to remember that the placenta has minimal ability to autoregulate flow. A sudden drop in maternal blood pressure may decrease placental perfusion and result in significant fetal compromise.
   c. **Fluid management.** Volume assessment is challenging. Intravascular depletion should be corrected with judicious administration of crystalloid, as preeclamptic patients are at increased risk for the development of pulmonary edema.
   d. **Coagulation abnormalities.** A platelet count less than 100,000/µL is the most common coagulation abnormality. The threshold for neuraxial placement for most providers is a platelet count greater than 75,000/µL. Vigilance for the risk of epidural hematoma and availability of neurosurgical consultation are essential. The coexistence of other hemostatic abnormalities (eg, prolonged prothrombin time or partial thromboplastin time, low fibrinogen) should be taken into account. Repeated coagulation testing at regular intervals may be advisable.
C. **Anesthesia**
   1. **Neuraxial** anesthesia.
      a. Neuraxial anesthesia is the preferred type of anesthesia for labor, vaginal delivery, or cesarean delivery.
      b. A platelet count of $<150,000 \times 10^9/L$ is present in about 20% of preeclamptic patients overall and up to 50% of patients with severe disease. Investigation of platelet count is advisable prior to any instrumentation of the neuraxis (including epidural catheter removal).
      c. **Epidural anesthesia.** Early epidural placement offers possible improved uteroplacental perfusion, reduction in circulating maternal catecholamines, and assessment of the function of the epidural catheter prior to the development of fetal intolerance to labor and urgent cesarean section
      d. **Spinal anesthesia.** Growing evidence in the literature shows that spinal anesthesia is not associated with more severe hypotension in preeclamptic patients, supporting the safe use of this technique.
   2. **General anesthesia** is usually reserved for emergent cesarean sections or for patients with coagulopathy or other contraindications to regional techniques. The disadvantages of general anesthesia include autonomic stimulation and hypertension that may occur with intubation and extubation. The hypertensive response to laryngoscopy can be blunted by the use of remifentanil on induction. Diffuse, severe interstitial edema of the airway may also increase the likelihood of a difficult intubation. The interaction of magnesium with nondepolarizing muscle relaxants might prolong their duration of action in preeclamptic patients.

VIII. PERIPARTUM HEMORRHAGE

Peripartum hemorrhage is the leading cause of maternal mortality worldwide, accounting for approximately 15% of deaths.

A. **Antepartum hemorrhage** threatens oxygen transfer to the fetus since it is most commonly due to hemorrhage originating along the uteroplacental interface.

1. **Placenta previa** occurs when the placenta implants in advance of the fetal presenting part. A placenta that covers the cervical os is considered a true placenta previa. If it is near the cervical os, it is classified as a low-lying placenta. The hallmark presentation is painless vaginal bleeding in the second or third trimester. The first hemorrhage is usually self-limiting and does not compromise the fetus. Patients with a previous cesarean section and placenta previa have a higher incidence of **placenta accreta** with a subsequent need for a gravid hysterectomy. A minimum distance of 1 cm from placental edge to the internal os is recommended to proceed with vaginal delivery. The amount and rate of blood loss and severity of associated signs and symptoms are the primary considerations in the anesthetic choice.

2. **Placental abruption** is the premature separation of part or all of a normally implanted placenta. Classically, an abruption is painful and associated with either vaginal bleeding or hemorrhage concealed behind the placenta. Hypertension, preeclampsia, advanced maternal age, and abdominal trauma are associated with an increased risk for abruption. Patients may deliver vaginally or via cesarean section depending on the degree of compromise. Anesthetic management is similar to the management of placenta previa. One-third of coagulopathies in pregnancy are a result of abruption, which increases the risk for disseminated intravascular coagulation (DIC).

3. **Vasa previa** is a condition in which the fetal vessels are in front of the presenting part of the fetus and are not protected by the umbilical cord. Trauma during vaginal examination, artificial rupture of membranes, or descent of the presenting part might tear the vessels causing fetal hemorrhage. Immediate cesarean section is warranted.

4. **Vaginal birth after cesarean (VBAC) section.** Patients with a singleton fetus in vertex presentation and a history of a single low transverse uterine incision might be candidates for a trial of labor and VBAC. Although induction with prostaglandins is contraindicated, oxytocin augmentation may be administered to patients attempting a VBAC. Uterine scar dehiscence occurs in 0.7% of VBAC and does not compromise the fetus nor cause excessive hemorrhage. Uterine rupture (0.65% of VBAC), however, may result in fetal compromise, maternal hemorrhage, or both, necessitating cesarean section or postpartum exploratory laparotomy. If uterine rupture occurs, the presence of a functioning epidural may provide a means for establishing a quick, safe anesthetic for cesarean section. If uterine rupture causes massive hemorrhage, anesthetic management is the same as for any actively bleeding patient.

B. **Postpartum hemorrhage:** Defined as >500 mL blood loss following vaginal delivery or >1000 mL following cesarean delivery.

1. **Uterine atony**, defined as the inadequate contractile response of the uterus after delivery, is the most common cause of postpartum hemorrhage. Risk factors include cesarean delivery, induced labor, hypertension, diabetes, prolonged labor, and advanced maternal age. Uterotonics, as discussed above, should be initiated. Oxytocin is

typically the first-line agent. Patients should receive adequate resuscitation with crystalloid, colloid, and blood products as clinically indicated. If conservative measures fail, surgical management or arterial embolization may be necessary.

2. **Retained placenta** occurs in up to ~3% of all vaginal deliveries and often requires manual exploration of the uterine cavity facilitated by epidural or spinal block. When additional uterine relaxation is needed, nitroglycerin in 50 to 100 μg IV boluses can be used. For analgesia, small doses of ketamine may be administered. Volatile anesthetic via facemask should be avoided due to the risks of a full stomach and unprotected airway. If there has been significant bleeding and the patient is hypovolemic, general endotracheal anesthesia with a volatile agent to help relax the uterus may be necessary. When the retained placenta has been removed, the volatile anesthetic must be discontinued to reverse uterine relaxation. Many patients require additional uterotonics to improve uterine tone.

3. **Retained products of conception** may cause significant postpartum bleeding. Uterine relaxation is usually not necessary for uterine curettage to remove remaining placental fragments. Anesthetic options are augmentation of an existing labor epidural, spinal, or general anesthesia.

4. **Laceration of the vagina, cervix, or perineum** is a common cause of postpartum hemorrhage. Bleeding may be insidious and difficult to estimate. Patients require adequate analgesia to facilitate repair that may involve augmentation or placement of regional blocks, infiltration of local anesthetics, or a general anesthetic.

5. **Uterine inversion** is a rare cause of postpartum hemorrhage (~1 in 3400) that represents a true obstetric emergency. Nitroglycerin in small IV boluses may produce adequate uterine relaxation and may avoid the need for general anesthesia. Atony commonly follows the replacement of the uterus after inversion, and uterotonic medications are indicated.

6. **Placenta accreta** refers to an abnormally adherent placenta with increasing incidence in patients with prior cesarean sections or placenta previa. The rising prevalence is directly related to the increase in cesarean delivery rate. The condition may be divided into three types: accreta vera (abnormal placental attachment to the myometrium), increta (invasion into the myometrium), and percreta (invasion through the myometrium into the serosa and adjacent organs). Placenta accreta generally necessitates peripartum hysterectomy with antenatal diagnosis improving the chance of favorable outcomes. Anesthetic management should include close interdisciplinary communication and planning as well as preparation for major hemorrhage.

IX. AMNIOTIC FLUID EMBOLISM

A. **Amniotic fluid embolism (AFE)** is a rare and catastrophic condition unique to pregnancy that should be considered in the differential diagnosis for any sudden cardiorespiratory collapse or seizure during this period. It commonly presents with hypotension, hypoxia, and coagulopathy. The true incidence of AFE is unknown since it is a diagnosis of exclusion, often made postmortem, but must include documentation of coagulopathy. US estimates range from 1.7 to 5.4 per 100,000 live births with mortality rates as high as 80%, usually occurring within the first hours of onset. Permanent neurologic dysfunction affects up to 85% of survivors. AFE is a diagnosis of exclusion. Myocardial infarction, pulmonary embolism, anaphylaxis, eclampsia, and sepsis should be considered on the differential as well.

B. Pathophysiology. The pathophysiology of AFE is poorly understood and likely does not arise from an embolic event in the classical sense. AFE seems to involve an initial breach in the barrier between the maternal and fetal compartments resulting in an abnormal maternal systemic response to the fetal tissue, activation of proinflammatory mediators, and a resulting syndrome similar to the systemic inflammatory response syndrome.

C. Clinical presentation. Risk factors include advanced maternal age, placental abruption, eclampsia, and induction of labor. The diagnosis is made based on clinical features of acute peripartum hypoxia and hypotension, with rapid deterioration to cardiovascular collapse, coagulopathy, and death. AFE remains a clinical diagnosis, and laboratory tests are not recommended to confirm or rule it out.

D. Manifestations. AFE affects multiple organ systems, and the presentation may vary.

1. **Cardiovascular.** Hypotension is a key feature of the disease, present in 100% of patients with severe disease. A biphasic model of shock has been proposed with an initial transient pulmonary hypertension—likely from the release of vasoactive substances—resulting in hypoxia and right-sided heart failure. The patients who survive the initial insult develop a left heart failure and pulmonary edema due to left ventricular ischemic injury or direct myocardial depression.

2. **Respiratory.** Hypoxia is an early manifestation of AFE, thought to arise from acute pulmonary hypertension, decreased cardiac output, and ventilation-perfusion mismatch. Later, pulmonary edema develops in association with left ventricular failure. Many patients will also manifest noncardiogenic pulmonary edema when the left ventricular function improves.

3. **Coagulation.** Disruption of the normal clotting cascade occurs in most patients resulting in DIC and hemorrhage in women who survive the initial cardiopulmonary instability.

E. Management of AFE involves aggressive resuscitation. Right heart failure from pulmonary artery hypertension can be treated with inotropes such as dobutamine and milrinone. Patients may respond to sildenafil, inhaled or IV prostacyclin, and inhaled nitric oxide to decrease pulmonary vascular resistance. To address abnormalities in coagulation, maintaining a platelet count >50,000 and a normal international normalized ratio are recommended. Uterine atony should be treated with oxytocin, ergot derivatives, and prostaglandins when indicated. Serious AFE will result in total cardiovascular collapse requiring intubation and CPR. Extracorporeal membrane oxygenation has recently the most immediately available rescue method. Intra-aortic balloon counterpulsation and cardiopulmonary bypass have also been used. The decision for immediate delivery of the fetus should be made by the obstetrician to maximize chances of fetal survival and aid maternal resuscitation, but is recommended after 23 weeks.

X. ANESTHESIA FOR NONOBSTETRIC SURGERY DURING PREGNANCY

A. Approximately 1% to 2% of women undergo nonobstetric surgery during pregnancy. Purely elective surgical procedures are relatively contraindicated in pregnancy and should be postponed until 6 weeks postpartum.

If a surgical procedure must be performed, the second trimester is the preferred time. The objectives in the anesthetic management include the following:

1. **Maternal safety.** Induction and emergence from general anesthesia are more rapid in pregnant patients due to the increase in minute ventilation and decrease in FRC. Uterine displacement to minimize aortocaval compression should be considered as early as the second trimester. During any anesthetic, oxygen transport to the placenta must be maintained.

2. **Teratogenicity.** In 2016, the U.S. Food and Drug administration released a Drug Safety Communication warning that "repeated or lengthy use of general anesthetic or sedation drugs during surgeries or procedures in children younger than 3 years or in pregnant women during their third trimester may affect the development of children's brains." However, no data from pregnant women were included among the clinical studies cited, and a series of subsequent studies showed no evidence of an effect on neurodevelopmental outcomes in young children exposed to anesthesia. Nitrous oxide may interfere with DNA synthesis and is often avoided by practitioners in the first and second trimesters.

3. **Fetal well-being.** Pregnant women who undergo surgery during their pregnancies have a higher rate of preterm labor. Laparoscopy is not associated with a higher rate of adverse pregnancy outcomes.

4. **Reversal of residual neuromuscular block.** The use of the combination of neostigmine and glycopyrrolate might expose the fetus to unopposed neostigmine and cause fetal bradycardia, as the placenta is more permeable to neostigmine than glycopyrrolate.

B. **Procedures directly related to pregnancy**

1. **Ruptured ectopic pregnancy** is the leading cause of maternal death in the first trimester. It is a surgical emergency requiring laparoscopy or laparotomy. Intra-abdominal hemorrhage is common, and it is prudent to have blood available in the room even without hemodynamic instability.

2. **Abortion or miscarriage.** Spontaneous abortion refers to the loss of pregnancy before 20 weeks or at a fetal weight of less than 500 g (**Table 32.2**). A dilatation and evacuation is often indicated for incomplete abortions and missed abortions.

TABLE 32.2	Spontaneous Abortion Classification			
Type	**Vaginal Bleeding**	**Cervix**	**Products of Conception**	**Management**
Threatened	Y	Closed	In utero	Observation
Inevitable	Y	Dilated	In utero	Await spontaneous passage or induce labor
Missed	N	Closed	In utero	Await spontaneous passage, induce labor, or D&C
Incomplete	Y	Dilated	Partial expulsion	Emergent D&C
Complete	Y	Dilated	Complete expulsion	Observation

D&C, dilation and curettage.

3. Monitored anesthesia care, spinal, epidural, or general anesthesia can be used after careful assessment of the patient to evaluate PO status, volume status, and presence of DIC or sepsis. Consideration to airway protection should be given in the second trimester and beyond.

4. **Incompetent cervix** might lead to early pregnancy loss and is treated with cerclage. Regional block is the preferred anesthetic choice for cerclage except when the myometrial relaxation associated with inhalational agents is necessary. A sensory block to T10 is necessary for to cover the cervix, vagina, and perineum.

5. **Anesthesia for postpartum sterilization.** Elective postpartum tubal ligation is performed through a small infraumbilical incision typically within the first 48 hours after delivery. The labor epidural may be appropriately dosed to achieve a T4 sensory level, although the function of the epidural becomes less likely the longer the interval after delivery. Alternatively, spinal anesthesia is a frequent choice. Our practice is to use an intrathecal dose of 15 mg of 0.75% hyperbaric bupivacaine with 10 to 15 μg fentanyl. General anesthesia is reserved for rescue of intraoperative neuraxial failure. All patients should receive aspiration prophylaxis.

6. **Cerclage placement:** A prophylactic cerclage is placed early in the second trimester to prevent preterm birth. A rescue cerclage placement may be complicated by prolapse of membranes and cervical dilation. A T10 sensory level is required for the ~30 minute procedure. A spinal anesthetic is recommended, but a catheter-based anesthetic may be more appropriate if the procedure is anticipated to be complex.

C. **Procedures incidental to pregnancy**
1. When a nonemergent procedure must be performed, the second trimester is the preferred time since organogenesis is complete and the risk of preterm labor is minimized.
2. The most common urgent/emergent procedures in pregnancy include appendicitis, cholecystitis, and bowel obstruction.
3. **Consultation with an obstetrician** preoperatively improves the assessment of risks and benefits to the patients and guides the choice of perioperative monitoring. Most commonly, FHR is measured before and after surgery. In select cases, continuous intraoperative FHR monitoring and uterine tocometry might be indicated.
4. **Use regional techniques when possible.**

XI. CPR DURING PREGNANCY

A. **Cardiac arrest during pregnancy** occurs in 1 per 12,000 admissions for delivery. CPR is more difficult than in individuals who are not pregnant, but survival to hospital discharge is as high as 58.9%. The American Heart Association recommends the following changes in the ACLS algorithm for cardiac arrest in pregnancy:

1. Standard **basic life support** and activation of the maternal cardiac arrest team (if present in the institution) should be initiated immediately upon discovery of a pregnant patient in cardiac arrest.
2. The patient should be placed **supine** for chest compressions. If the uterus is palpated at or above the umbilicus, or if the uterus cannot be assessed, **manual left uterine displacement** should be employed to relieve aortocaval compression. (Left lateral tilt is no longer recommended due to hindrance of effective chest compressions.)
3. **No change in the hand position** for chest compressions is recommended. (Prior guidelines to perform compressions higher on the sternum were not supported by evidence.)

4. When indicated, **defibrillation should not be delayed to allow for removal of invasive fetal monitors.** Defibrillation energy does not change in pregnancy. Anterolateral pad placement is the recommended default, with attention to the placement of the lateral pad underneath breast tissue.

5. **Rapid development of hypoxemia** should be anticipated in the pregnant patient due to lower oxygen reserve and higher metabolic demand. Difficult airway management should also be expected.

6. Intravenous or intraosseous **access** should be obtained **above the diaphragm** due to possibly impeded lower extremity venous return.

7. Resuscitation drugs should be administered as per ACLS guidelines without modification.

8. Evaluation of fetal well-being during maternal cardiac arrest should not be carried out due to the risk of interference with maternal resuscitation or monitoring.

9. **Perimortem cesarean delivery** (PMCD) should be completed **within 5 minutes** of maternal arrest with unsuccessful resuscitation in a woman with fundal height at or above the umbilicus. PMCD may facilitate maternal resuscitation while also limiting fetal anoxia. Delivery should be performed at the site of arrest; the patient should not be transported.

10. Causes of maternal cardiac arrest may be remembered with the mnemonics **BEAUCHOPS** (**b**leeding/DIC, **e**mbolism, **a**nesthetic complications, **u**terine atony, **c**ardiac disease, **h**ypertension, **o**ther [common etiologies as in standard ACLS guidelines], **p**lacenta previa or placental abruption, **s**epsis) or **ABCDEFGH** (**a**nesthetic complications or **a**ccidents/trauma, **b**leeding, **c**ardiovascular causes, **d**rugs, **e**mbolic phenomena, **f**ever, **g**eneral [Hs and Ts], **h**ypertension [preeclampsia/eclampsia/HELLP syndrome]).

XII. ANESTHESIA FOR GYNECOLOGIC SURGERY
A. Abdominal procedures

B. Pelvic surgery can be performed under regional anesthesia. Duration of the procedure, intraoperative blood loss, fluid shifts, and Trendelenburg positioning might require control of the airway and general anesthesia. Laparoscopic procedures are performed under general anesthesia. Rescue IV and radial artery access may be limited by draping and position of the patient.

C. Vaginal procedures

D. Vaginal and intrauterine surgeries may be performed using regional or general anesthesia. A T10 level is sufficient for these procedures, while a T4 to T6 level is necessary for vaginal hysterectomy.

XIII. ANESTHESIA FOR OOCYTE RETRIEVAL

A. Oocytes are retrieved with a transvaginal needle under ultrasound guidance. Immobility during the procedure minimizes risks and improves the quality of retrieval. **Monitored anesthesia care** with moderate-to-deep sedation is the most common anesthetic choice. Midazolam, fentanyl, remifentanil, and meperidine do not appear to affect fertility.

B. General anesthesia. There is no conclusive evidence that the commonly used inhalational anesthetics adversely affect pregnancy and live birth rates for in vitro fertilization procedures. However, nitrous oxide might be avoided due to its interference with DNA synthesis. Volatile halogenated anesthetics may interfere with DNA synthesis and mitosis. While propofol is found in follicular fluid, no DNA damage has been observed and fertility outcomes are comparable to regional anesthetic techniques.

C. Spinal anesthesia can provide excellent surgical conditions and provides the advantage of minimizing oocyte exposure to anesthetic agents. Postoperative recovery is often longer than with general anesthesia.

Suggested Readings

Chestnut D, Wong C, Tsen L, et al, eds. *Chestnut's Obstetric Anesthesia: Principles and Practice.* 6th ed. Elsevier; 2020.

Committee on Practice Bulletins – Obstetrics. ACOG Practice Bulletin No. 202: gestational hypertension and preeclampsia. *Obstet Gynecol.* 2019;133(1):e1-e25.

Devroe S, Bleeser T, Van de Velde M, et al. Anesthesia for non-obstetric surgery during pregnancy in a tertiary referral center: a 16-year retrospective, matched case-control, cohort study. *Int J Obstet Anesth.* 2019;39:74-81.

Jeejeebhoy FM, Zelop CM, Lipman S, et al. Cardiac arrest in pregnancy. *Circulation.* 2015;132(18):1747-1773.

Lim G, Facco FL, Nathan N, Waters JH, Wong CA, Eltzschig HK. A review of the impact of obstetric anesthesia on maternal and neonatal outcomes. *Anesthesiology.* 2018;129(1):192-215.

Lipman S, Cohen S, Einav S, et al. The Society for Obstetric Anesthesia and Perinatology consensus statement on the management of cardiac arrest in pregnancy. *Anesth Analg.* 2014;118:1003-1016.

Mhyre JM, Sultan P. General anesthesia for cesarean delivery: occasionally essential but best avoided. *Anesthesiology.* 2019;130(6):864-866.

Mushambi MC, Kinsella SM, Popat M, et al. Obstetric Anaesthetists' Association and Difficult Airway Society guidelines for the management of difficult and failed tracheal intubation in obstetrics. *Anaesthesia.* 2015;70(11):1286-1306.

Practice guidelines for obstetric anesthesia: an updated report by the American Society of Anesthesiologists Task Force on Obstetric Anesthesia and the Society for Obstetric Anesthesia and Perinatology. *Anesthesiology.* 2016;124:270.

Suresh M, Segal BS, Preston R, Fernando R, Mason CL, eds. *Shnider and Levinson's Anesthesia for Obstetrics.* 5th ed. Lippincott Williams & Wilkins; 2013.

U.S. Food and Drug Administration. *FDA Drug Safety Communication: FDA Review Results in New Warnings about Using General Anesthetics and Sedation Drugs in Young Children and Pregnant Women.* FDA; 2016.

Weiniger CF, Gerard W. Ostheimer lecture: what's new in obstetric anesthesia 2018. *Anesth Analg.* 2020;131:307-316.

Anesthesia for Pediatric Surgery and Care of the Neonate

Rupeng Li and Chang A. Liu

I. DEVELOPMENT

A. Organogenesis is virtually complete after the 12th gestational week.

B. Respiratory development

1. Anatomic

a. **The lungs** begin as a bud on the embryonic gut in the fourth week of gestation. Failure of separation of the lung bud from the gut later results in the formation of a **tracheoesophageal fistula (TEF)**.

b. **The diaphragm** forms during the 4th through 10th week of gestation, dividing the abdominal and thoracic cavities.

   1. If the diaphragm is not completely formed when the midgut reenters the abdomen from the umbilical pouch, the abdominal contents can enter the thorax.

   2. The presence of abdominal contents within the thorax is associated with arrested lung growth.

   3. The lungs from patients with **congenital diaphragmatic hernia** (CDH) have a decreased number of arterioles in the hypoplastic lung. In addition, the pulmonary arteries of both lungs are abnormally thick and reactive, resulting in increased pulmonary vascular resistance.

2. Physiologic

a. **Lung development** is generally insufficient for survival at less than the 23rd week of gestation, prior to the saccular stage of lung development when thinning of the pulmonary interstitium due to decreased collagen fiber deposition, increased cellular differentiation, and capillary development begins the capacity for gas exchange.

b. Secretion of **surfactant,** which reduces alveolar wall surface tension and promotes alveolar aeration, is often inadequate until the last month of gestation.

   1. Birth before 32 weeks of gestation is associated with **respiratory distress syndrome (RDS)**.

   2. Because glucose metabolism affects lung surfactant maturation, infants of diabetic mothers are at increased risk of RDS when prematurely born at later stages of gestation.

   3. Antenatal treatment with steroids is associated with a decrease in the incidence of RDS in prematurely born infants.

c. After birth, the onset of breathing is stimulated by hypoxemia, hypercarbia, tactile stimulation, and a decrease in plasma prostaglandin E_2. After aeration and distention of the lung, the pulmonary vascular resistance decreases, and pulmonary blood flow increases nearly 10-fold. Failure of the reduction of pulmonary vascular resistance after birth is associated with extrapulmonary shunting of blood and severe hypoxemia and is called **persistent pulmonary hypertension of the newborn (PPHN)**.

C. Cardiovascular development

1. Anatomic

a. The cardiovascular system is the first organ system to function in utero. Its formation consists of three developmental stages including tube formation, looping, and septation. Heart formation is complete by approximately 8 weeks of gestation.

b. The primitive **cardiac tube** consists of the sinoatrium, the ventricle, the bulbus cordis (primitive right ventricle), and the truncus (primitive main pulmonary artery). During the second month of gestation, a heart with two parallel pumping systems develops out of this initially tubular system. During this process, various structures divide and migrate. Failure of structural maturation at this stage of development causes numerous cardiac malformations. For example:

1. Failure of division of the sinoatrium into the two atria results in a single atrium. Improper closure results in an **atrial septal defect**.

2. Failure of migration of the ventricular septum and atrioventricular valve between the primitive ventricle and the bulbus cordis results in a **double-outlet left ventricle** (single ventricle). Minor migrational defects result in **ventriculoseptal defects**.

3. Failure of division of the truncus into the pulmonary artery and the aorta results in **truncus arteriosus**.

c. The aortic arch system initially consists of six pairs of arches.

1. The sixth arches produce the pulmonary arteries. The **ductus arteriosus** develops from the distal portion of the right sixth arch. Although the left proximal sixth arch usually degenerates, it can persist and form an aberrant left ductus arteriosus.

2. Failure of regression of various portions of the aorta and arch system also can result in aberrant vessels and vascular rings. For example, failure of regression causes a **double aortic arch**. Regression of the left-sided but not the right-sided arches can result in a right-sided aortic arch.

2. Physiologic

a. Fetal circulation: After the 12th week, the circulatory system is in its final form. Oxygenated blood from the placenta passes through the umbilical vein and the ductus venosus and returns to the heart. Subsequently, 85% to 95% of fetal cardiac output bypasses the pulmonary circulation by flowing right to left through the foramen ovale and the ductus arteriosus into the aorta.

b. At birth, umbilical placental circulation ceases with the clamping of the umbilical cord, and blood flow through the ductus venosus ceases. However, the ductus venosus often remains patent for up to a week. Also, the interruption of umbilical blood flow at birth reduces right atrial pressure and causes functional closure of the foramen ovale. Moreover, pulmonary resistance decreases as the lungs are distended and ventilated at birth, while systemic resistance increases with removal of the high-capacitance placental circulation. Constriction of the ductus arteriosus occurs with increasing Pao_2. Cessation of ductus arteriosus blood flow often occurs within several hours to days in term infants but may be delayed in prematurely born or sick infants.

D. Body composition

1. Extracellular fluid (ECF) and total body water decrease as the fetus grows, while intracellular fluid increases with gestational age. ECF is 90% of total body weight at 28 weeks, 80% at 36 weeks, and 75% at term.

2. After birth, a physiologic diuresis occurs, with the term infant losing 5% to 10% of ECF in the first few days of life. Premature infants may lose up to 15% of ECF.

3. Before 32 weeks of gestation, the **neonatal kidney is immature** and has a relatively low glomerular filtration rate and altered tubular function. This leads to difficulties in excreting water loads and diminished capacity to reabsorb sodium and water and thereby concentrate urine. In part, this is due to incomplete glomerular development, tubule insensitivity to vasopressin, loops of Henle that have not yet penetrated into the medulla, low osmolality in the medullary interstitium, and low serum urea levels. Renal tubular function increases with postnatal age, and the concentrating ability of the kidney reaches adult levels at 6 to 12 months postnatal age.

II. GENERAL ASSESSMENT
A. History
1. In collecting the neonatal patient's medical history, it is important to include information about antenatal events. Fetal growth and development are affected by **maternal disorders,** including hypertension, diabetes, lupus, and drug, cigarette, and alcohol use. Poly- or oligohydramnios, abnormal α-fetoprotein, maternal infections, and premature labor are often associated with neonatal problems.

2. **Perinatal history** also includes gestational age, time of onset of labor and rupture of membranes, use of tocolytics and fetal monitors, signs of fetal distress, type of anesthesia used and mode of delivery (spontaneous, forceps or vacuum assisted, or cesarean), condition of the infant at delivery, and immediate resuscitation steps required (eg, intubation for meconium, ventilatory assistance, surfactant administration, CPR, or medication administration). **The Apgar score** should be noted as it reflects the degree of intrapartum stress as well as the effectiveness of initial resuscitation (**Table 33.1**). Points are awarded for each of the five criteria, with the maximum score being 10. Although the Apgar score at 1 minute correlates with intrauterine conditions, the 5- and 10-minute Apgar scores correlate best with neonatal outcome. In addition, ensure that vitamin K and ocular antibiotic ointment were given after birth to prevent hemorrhagic disease of the newborn and ophthalmia neonatorum, respectively.

B. Physical examination
1. A complete, systematic evaluation is needed. No assumptions should be made about the development, location, or function of organ systems. An abnormality in one system may be associated with abnormalities in another.

TABLE 33.1	Normal Vital Signs	
Vital Sign	Term	Preterm
Pulse (beats/min)	80-120	120-160
Respiration (breaths/min)	30-40	50-70
Blood pressure (mm Hg)	60-90/40-60	40-60/20-40
Temperature (°C)	37.5 (rectal)	37.5

TABLE 33.2	Apgar Scores		
Sign	Score		
	0	1	2
Heart rate	Absent	<100/min	>100/min
Respiratory effort	Absent	Irregular	Good, crying
Muscle tone	Limp	Some flexion	Active motion
Reflex irritability	Absent	Grimace	Cough or sneeze
Color	Blue	Acrocyanosis	Completely pink

2. **Vital signs** provide a useful physiologic screen of organ function. If a cardiac abnormality is suspected, a chest x-ray (CXR), electrocardiogram (ECG), and four extremity blood pressure measurements are required. Postductal oxygen saturation should be greater than 94%. In addition, an echocardiogram and pediatric cardiology consultation should be considered. Normal vital signs are summarized in **Table 33.2**.

3. **Gestational age** influences care, management, and survival potential of the neonate. An infant is considered preterm if the gestational age is less than 37 weeks, term if it is 37 to 41 weeks, and postterm if the gestational age is more than 42 weeks. Although the date of conception and ultrasound examination can be used to predict gestational age, a physical examination to determine gestational age should be performed. **The Dubowitz-Ballard scoring system** involves evaluation of physical characteristics of the skin, external genitalia, ears, breasts, and neuromuscular behavior to assess gestational age.

4. **Weight determination.** Similar to gestational age, birth weight is an important prognostic factor for premature infants. By convention, low birth weight infants weigh less than 2500 g, very low birth weight infants less than 1500 g, and extremely low birth weight infants less than 1000 g. Intrauterine growth restriction (IUGR) is defined as a rate of growth less than a fetus' predetermined genetic potential. **Small for gestational age infants at birth are less than 10th percentile of the standard population–based weight.** This may be the result of chromosomal defects, maternal hypertension, chronic placental insufficiency, maternal cigarette or drug use, or congenital infection. These infants have a high incidence of hypoglycemia, hypocalcemia, and polycythemia. Infants who are **large for gestational age** (LGA) are greater than 90th percentile of standard population–based weight and may have mothers with diabetes. In the immediate postnatal period, LGA newborns should be evaluated for hypoglycemia and polycythemia. Infants of diabetic mothers and LGA infants are at risk of complications from fetal macrosomia, including shoulder dystocia and brachial plexus injuries.

5. **Respiratory.** Signs of respiratory distress include tachypnea, grunting, nasal flaring, intercostal and subcostal retractions, rales, rhonchi, asymmetry of breath sounds, and apnea. **Pulse oximetry** is used to screen the levels of systemic oxygenation in neonates. Blood gas tensions should be measured in patients with suspected cardiopulmonary abnormalities.

6. **Cardiovascular.** Central cyanosis and capillary refill should be assessed. Distal pulses should be palpated, noting whether they are bounding. A delay between brachial and femoral pulses is suggestive of **coarctation of the aorta**. Note the character and location of murmurs and splitting of the second heart sound. During the first 48 hours after birth, murmurs may appear as intracardiac pressure gradients change and disappear as the ductus arteriosus closes.

7. **Abdominal exam.** A scaphoid abdomen suggests **diaphragmatic hernia**. A normal umbilical cord has two arteries and one vein. In nearly 40% of cases, the existence of a single umbilical artery is associated with renal abnormalities. The size of the liver, spleen, and kidneys and the presence of hernias or abdominal masses should be determined by inspection and palpation. The location and patency of the anus should be assessed.

8. **Neurologic.** A thorough examination includes evaluation of motor activity, muscle strength and tone, and newborn reflexes (Moro, tonic neck, grasp, suck, and stepping reflexes). Full-term newborns should have an upgoing Babinski reflex and brisk deep tendon reflexes.

9. **Genitourinary.** The gonads may be differentiated or ambiguous, and in males, the testes should be palpable. The location of the urethra should be determined, remembering that hypospadias precludes a circumcision. A male infant with hypospadias and bilateral cryptorchidism must be evaluated for congenital adrenal hyperplasia.

10. **Musculoskeletal.** Any deformities, unusual posturing, or asymmetric limb movement should be noted, and the hips should be examined for possible dislocation with congenital hip dysplasia, particularly in breech infants. A clavicle or humerus may be fractured during a difficult delivery.

11. **Craniofacial.** One should determine head circumference, the location and size of the fontanelles, the presence of a cephalohematoma or caput, and ensure the palate is intact. Observing nasal gas flow despite occluding each naris or passage of a nasogastric tube will rule out choanal atresia.

C. **Laboratory studies.** Routine initial laboratory studies may include hematocrit and serum glucose. Additional studies should be guided by the individual problem. For example, blood type and Coombs determination may be indicated in infants at risk for hyperbilirubinemia such as those whose mothers who are blood type O. In addition, a CBC and blood culture should be checked and wide spectrum antibiotic therapy initiated if there is suspicion of neonatal sepsis or maternal chorioamnionitis.

D. **Fluids**

1. **The total fluid requirement** varies with birth weight.
   a. Less than 1.0 kg, use 100 mL/kg/d.
   b. 1.0 to 1.5 kg, use 80 to 90 mL/kg/d.
   c. 1.5 to 2.5 kg, use 80 mL/kg/d.
   d. Greater than 2.5 kg, use 60 mL/kg/d.

2. **Isosmolar solutions** should be used.
   a. **Electrolyte supplementation** is not required within the first day of life for maintenance fluids in full-term infants. For premature infants, check the electrolytes at 8 to 12 hours of life and consider adjusting the fluid infusion rate and/or adding electrolytes as indicated.
   b. **10% dextrose** in water is typically used as the initial intravenous (IV) fluid in preterm and term infants. Blood glucose concentrations should be monitored closely in high-risk infants and the dextrose concentration of IV fluids should be adjusted as required to maintain serum glucose levels described below.

3. Additional fluids may be required **for insensible water loss.**
   a. Fluid requirements increase with lower birth weight and gestational age, as well as with many neonatal interventions including phototherapy, radiant warmer use, and support of infant with respiratory distress.
   b. Insensible losses from pathologic causes (eg, omphalocele, gastroschisis, neural tube defect, bladder exstrophy) must similarly be taken into account and replaced. The electrolyte composition of the replacement fluid should match that of what is lost.
   c. Infants who are mechanically ventilated absorb free water through their respiratory system.
4. Several signs will determine the adequacy of fluid infusions.
   a. Urine output at least 1 mL/kg/h.
   b. Only a 1% loss in body weight per day for the first 10 days of life.
   c. Stable hemodynamics and good perfusion.

E. Electrolytes
1. The usual electrolyte requirements after the first 12 to 24 hours of life are as follows:
   a. Na^+, 2 to 4 mEq/kg/d.
   b. K^+, 1 to 2 mEq/kg/d.
   c. Ca^{+2}, 150 to 220 mEq/kg/d.
2. The frequency of laboratory tests for serum electrolyte levels will be determined by the rate of insensible loss.

F. Glucose. Supplemental glucose should be given after birth to keep blood glucose levels between 50 and 125 mg/dL.
1. In most infants, 10% D/W at maintenance fluid rates will provide adequate glucose. This infusion rate provides the 5 to 8 mg/kg/min of glucose that is required for basal metabolism.
2. Infants with hyperinsulinism, IUGR, or metabolic defects can require glucose infusion rates as high as 12 to 15 mg/kg/min.
3. In peripheral IV lines, up to 12.5% D/W may be infused. In central lines, 15% to 20% D/W may be infused.
4. **Hypoglycemia** (glucose <50 mg/dL) is treated with a bolus of glucose and increased glucose infusion rate.
   a. Glucose at 200 mg/kg IV is given over a minute (eg, 10% D/W at 2 mL/kg).
   b. The glucose infusion rate is increased from the current level or started at 8 mg/kg/min IV.
   c. Serial blood tests are necessary to determine the effectiveness of the increased glucose.

G. Nutrition. The gastrointestinal tract is functional after 28 weeks of gestation but is of limited capacity. Requirements vary with each neonate.
1. **Calories.** Requirements are 100 to 130 kcal/kg/d.
2. **Protein.** Requirements are 2 to 4 g/kg/d.
3. **Fat.** Initiate at 1 g/kg/d and increase gradually as tolerated up to 3 to 4 g/kg/d so that the fat provides 40% of the daily calories.
4. **Vitamins** A, B, D, E, C, and K should be provided.
5. **Iron.** Requirements are 2 to 4 mg/kg/d of elemental iron. The adequacy of iron supplementation can be assessed by measuring the hemoglobin or hematocrit and the reticulocyte count.
6. **Minerals.** Calcium, phosphate, magnesium, zinc, copper, manganese, selenium, and iron need to be replaced. Premature infants, in particular, have increased calcium and phosphate requirements in order to prevent metabolic bone disease of prematurity.

7. **Enteral feedings.** Feedings are usually initiated with breast milk or a formula contains the whey-to-casein ratio that is contained in breast milk. For infants that exhibit lactose intolerance, non- or low-lactose-containing formulas are available. Infants less than 32 weeks of gestation often have poor suck and swallow reflexes and require gavage feedings. For premature infants or ill full-term neonates, small volume enteral feedings are generally initiated once the baby is stable. Subsequently, the volumes of the feedings are gradually increased every 12 to 24 hours as they are tolerated. Once the desired goal volume of enteral feedings is reached, the breast milk or formula is supplemented with additional calories, as needed, to attain the desired weight gain.

8. **Parenteral feeding.** If enteral feeding is impossible, parenteral nutrition should be started as soon as possible to promote positive nitrogen balance and growth. The metabolic status of the infant should be assessed frequently so that the parenteral formulation can be adjusted to meet the infant's needs and to identify signs of toxicity from hyperalimentation. Usual studies include serum glucose, electrolytes, osmolality, liver function tests, blood urea nitrogen, creatinine, lipid levels, and platelet count.

H. **Thermoregulation.** It is critical to measure the newborn's body temperature and use active measures to maintain it in a euthermic range. Babies exhibit thermal instability because of decreased epidermal and dermal thickness, minimal subcutaneous fat, immature nervous system, and increased surface area to body weight ratio with a relatively large head size. Moreover, premature newborns are particularly susceptible to hypothermia because they lack thermogenic brown fat cells. Measures to maintain the newborn's body heat include using a warm incubator during transport to and from the nursery; keeping the ambient operating room (OR) temperature at 85 °F (30 °C); using warming blankets, radiant warmers, and a head cover; and prewarming IV fluids. Neonates with significant cold stress are particularly prone to hypoglycemia.

III. COMMON NEONATAL PROBLEMS PERTINENT TO ANESTHESIA
A. Preparation for surgery

1. Conditions that require emergent surgery in neonates are often accompanied with medical problems. As a result, the care for these critically ill newborns requires careful coordination of medical, surgical, and nursing management. In some cases, surgical procedures might occur at the bedside in the neonatal intensive care unit (NICU). In these instances, before the surgical procedure is initiated, it is important to identify and integrate the key resources and care measures provided by the NICU team into the anesthetic management of the surgical procedure.

2. Routine standard monitoring for neonates undergoing surgical procedures includes blood pressure monitoring and continuous electrocardiograph, temperature, pulse oximetry, and O_2 and CO_2 gas measurements. Specialized monitoring for surgical procedures detailed below may also include postductal pulse oximetry, chest piece stethoscopes, and continuous blood pressure monitoring and intermittent blood sampling through arterial and central lines. In infants with umbilical arterial and venous catheters, it is important to confirm the precise location of the tips of the lines and their suitability for fluid and drug infusions and blood sampling.

3. Nonrebreathing circuits are effective for ventilating and for delivering gaseous anesthetic agents to newborns and infants. The system must have provisions for humidification of the inspired gases to decrease

the insensible fluid losses and thereby help maintain the patient's thermostability. The specialized ventilators used in the NICU (eg, high-frequency oscillator ventilator) and continuous infusions of anesthetics and analgesics are often used for the patient during bedside surgery. A warm environment (85 °F), underbody heaters, radiant warmers, head wraps, and prewarmed IV and surgical fluids are also critical in helping the infant maintain thermoregulation.

4. A warm neonatal transport isolette complete with monitors, adequate oxygen supply, and emergency airway and drugs is required for moving neonatal patients to and from the intensive care unit and OR.

B. Respiratory disorders

1. **Differential diagnosis.** The following diseases present similarly as pulmonary parenchymal disease and should be considered when evaluating an infant with respiratory distress.

   a. **Airway obstruction.** Choanal atresia, vocal cord palsy, laryngomalacia, tracheal malacia or stenosis, and compression of the trachea by external masses (eg, cystic hygroma, hemangioma, and vascular ring).

   b. **Developmental anomalies.** TEF, CDH, congenital lobar emphysema, pulmonary sequestration, bronchogenic cysts and congenital pulmonary airway malformations/congenital cystic adenomatoid malformations.

   c. **Nonpulmonary.** Cyanotic heart disease, PPHN, congestive heart failure, and metabolic disturbances.

2. **Laboratory studies** for an infant in respiratory distress should include an arterial blood gas, pre- and postductal oxygen saturation (determined by pulse oximetry), hemoglobin or hematocrit, 12-lead ECG, and CXR. If these results are abnormal, potential cardiac disease should be evaluated by assessing blood gas tensions while the neonate breathes 100% O_2 (hyperoxia test). As indicated, cardiology consultation and an echocardiogram will help evaluate potential congenital heart disease.

3. **Apnea**

   a. **Etiology and treatments**

   1. **Central apnea** is due to immaturity or depression of the respiratory center (eg, narcotics). It is related to the degree of prematurity and is exacerbated by metabolic disturbances (eg, hypoglycemia, hypocalcemia, hypothermia, hyperthermia, and sepsis). Before 34 weeks of gestational age, central apnea is often treated with **methylxanthines** such as caffeine citrate.

   2. **Obstructive apnea** is caused by inconsistent maintenance of a patent airway. It can result from incomplete maturation and poor coordination of upper airway musculature. This form of apnea may respond to changes in head position, insertion of an oral or nasal airway, or placement of the infant in a prone position. Occasionally, administration of **continuous positive airway pressure** (CPAP) or a high-flow oxygen nasal cannula may be beneficial. These therapies especially may be effective in infants with a large tongue, such as with trisomy 21 or Beckwith-Wiedemann syndrome.

   3. **Mixed apnea** represents a combination of both central and obstructive apnea.

   b. **Postoperative apnea in the neonate**

   1. Apnea is associated with anesthesia in infants that are born prematurely. The etiology of postoperative apnea is multifactorial. Risk factors have been identified including postconceptual

age less than 60 weeks at time of surgery, anemia, LGA infants, hypothermia, and altered ventilatory response to hypoxemia and hypercarbia induced by general anesthesia.

2. If it is not possible to delay surgery until the patient is more mature, it is prudent to use **postoperative apnea monitoring** for 24 hours in neonates who undergo anesthesia at less than 60 weeks postconceptual age. In the previous meta-analysis done by Cotes CJ et al, it was demonstrated that the incidence of apnea following hernia repair remains above 5% until postconceptual age of 48 weeks and the incidence is reduced to less than 1% beyond postconceptual age of 56 weeks. Infants with a history of apnea is at increased risk for postoperative apnea and should be actively monitored.

4. **Respiratory distress syndrome (RDS)**
   a. **Pathophysiology.** RDS results from physiologic surfactant deficiency. This causes decreased lung compliance, alveolar instability, progressive atelectasis, and hypoxemia resulting from intrapulmonary shunting of deoxygenated blood.
   b. Prematurely born infants have an increased incidence of RDS. Newborns at risk for RDS can be identified prenatally by amniocentesis and evaluation of the amniotic fluid phospholipid profile. Lung surfactant maturity in the fetus is associated with a lecithin-to-sphingomyelin ratio greater than 2, saturated phosphatidylcholine level greater than 500 μg/dL, or presence of phosphatidylglycerol in the specimen.
   c. **Glucocorticoid (betamethasone) treatment** of the mother at least 48 hours prior to delivery decreases the incidence and severity of RDS. Only one full course of a glucocorticoid treatment regimen during a pregnancy is necessary. This is accomplished by giving one dose of glucocorticoid to the pregnant woman per day for 2 days.
   d. **Clinical features** of RDS include tachypnea, nasal flaring, grunting, and retractions. Cyanosis appears shortly after birth. Because of the intrapulmonary shunt across atelectatic lung units, infants with RDS remain hypoxemic despite breathing at high FIO_2.
   e. The **CXR** will show low lung volumes. A "ground-glass" pattern of the lung fields and air bronchograms may also be evident.
   f. **Initial treatment** includes warmed, humidified oxygen administered by hood or nasal cannula. The FIO_2 should be adjusted to maintain the PaO_2 between 50 and 80 mm Hg (SaO_2 between 88% and 92%). If an FIO_2 greater than 60% is required to keep the patient oxygenated, **nasal CPAP** should be administered. With more severe disease, or if the nasal CPAP is poorly tolerated, intubation and ventilation with positive end-expiratory pressure may be required. In intubated newborns with RDS, endotracheally administered exogenous **surfactant** decreases the morbidity and mortality of the disease. In babies with severe RDS, **high-frequency oscillatory ventilation** (HFOV) decreases the incidence of air leaks and chronic lung disease (CLD).
   g. **Broad-spectrum antibiotics** are often begun after appropriate cultures are obtained because the clinical signs and CXR of patients with RDS are indistinguishable from pneumonia.
   h. In more mature newborns, RDS may be self-limited. Clinical improvement often occurs after 2 to 3 days and is associated with a spontaneous diuresis. In extremely premature newborns, RDS may progress to CLD.

i. The **morbidity and mortality** of patients with RDS are directly related to the degree of prematurity, perinatal resuscitation, and the coexistence of other complications of prematurity (eg, patent ductus arteriosus [PDA], infection, intraventricular hemorrhage). **Pneumothoraces, pulmonary interstitial emphysema, and pulmonary hemorrhage** may complicate the recovery and can be associated with the evolution to CLD.

5. **Bronchopulmonary dysplasia (BPD)**

   a. **Etiology. BPD** is defined as the continued need for oxygen therapy or mechanical ventilation beyond 36 weeks postconceptual age. BPD is also referred to as CLD of prematurity and is associated with oxygen toxicity, chronic inflammation, and mechanical injury in the lung. BPD can be worsened by the presence of a PDA or infection. However, in some premature infants, BPD occurs in the absence of significant lung injury. Recent studies suggest that BPD is associated with excessive transforming growth factor-beta signaling in the injured developing lung. Preventive strategies include vitamin A or caffeine administration and early initiation of CPAP.

   b. **Clinical features** include retractions, rales, and areas of lung hyper- and hypoinflation. Because of nonhomogenous ventilation, an intrapulmonary shunt may produce hypoxemia and hypercarbia in patients with BPD. Hypoxia and hypercarbia may also be associated with bronchospasm in many patients with severe BPD. Many patients with severe BPD have growth failure and require high-caloric feeds.

   c. **Treatment** consists of supportive respiratory care, aggressive nutrition, and diuretic therapy. Because patients with BPD may have lung segments with long time constants, a ventilatory pattern with low respiratory rates and increased inspiratory and expiratory time may decrease gas trapping and improve gas exchange. Permissive hypercapnia is typically utilized to minimize further lung injury. In addition, **bronchodilator therapy** may be lifesaving in patients with BPD and bronchospasm. Systemic steroids sometimes are used to treat patients with CLD. However, because of adverse long-term neurodevelopmental outcomes observed in infants treated with systemic steroids, this therapy is typically reserved for the most severe cases. In some patients with severe BPD, pulmonary hypertension might be observed. In these cases, pulmonary vasodilators including inhaled NO and type 5 phosphodiesterate inhibitors have been used.

   d. **Prognosis** of BPD varies with the severity of the disease. Of severely affected infants, 20% die within the first year. Most infants are generally asymptomatic by 2 years of age, but additional morbidities include recurrent respiratory infections, increased pulmonary reactivity and asthma, repeated hospitalizations, pulmonary hypertension, and neurodevelopmental abnormalities.

6. **Pneumothorax**

   a. **Etiology.** Pneumothorax can occur in infants requiring positive pressure or mechanical ventilation. In addition, spontaneous pneumothorax can occur in 1% to 2% of otherwise healthy full-term infants who often remain asymptomatic or mildly symptomatic and require no intervention. The incidence increases up to 5% to 10% of full-term infants with meconium staining or prematurely born infants with RDS.

b. **Clinical features.** The diagnosis should be considered in any neonate with an acute deterioration in clinical condition (eg, sudden cyanosis and hypotension). Occasionally, asymmetric chest movement with ventilation and asymmetric breath sounds may be appreciated; however, endobronchial intubation should be ruled out.

c. **Laboratory studies.** Transillumination of the chest with a strong light usually will show a hyperlucent hemithorax. If the patient is stable, a CXR may be obtained to confirm the diagnosis.

d. **Treatment**

1. In otherwise stable and well-oxygenated term infants with minimal respiratory distress, a nitrogen washout by breathing a high concentration of oxygen has historically been used to assist with resolution of the pneumothorax. However, the data supporting this mode of therapy are minimal and should be weighed against newer ones, suggesting that hyperoxia is associated with end-organ injury.

2. In the **unstable infant,** immediate aspiration of the pleural space with an IV catheter should be performed. Reaccumulation of clinically significant air after aspiration warrants placement of a chest tube.

7. **Meconium aspiration syndrome**

a. **Meconium staining of amniotic fluid** occurs in 12% of all births and may be associated with fetal distress and perinatal depression.

b. To **decrease the effects of aspiration,** it is prudent to intubate and suction the airways of infants with meconium-stained fluid who are born with depressed respirations and poor tone.

c. **Meconium aspiration** may produce lung airspace disease by mechanical obstruction of the airways with fecal matter and chemical inflammation and surfactant inactivation causing pneumonitis. Complete obstruction of the airways by meconium results in distal atelectasis. Partial obstruction of the airways may produce overinflation of distal air spaces by a ball-valve effect, leading to pneumothorax. The bile in meconium may cause chemical pneumonitis and airway edema.

d. **Meconium aspiration syndrome** is also associated with PPHN (see Section III.C.5).

e. Chest radiographic findings can include diffuse, patchy intraparenchymal densities with areas of hyper- and hypoinflation.

f. **Respiratory support** for meconium aspiration is dependent on the etiology of the poor gas exchange. Obstruction of airways with meconium may require mechanical ventilation with long expiratory times to decrease gas trapping. Pneumothorax is treated by placement of a chest tube. Sometimes HFOV can recruit closed lung segments and improve gas exchange. Alkalosis and **inhaled nitric oxide (INO)** have been useful to decrease pulmonary vasoconstriction. Exogenous **surfactant** has also been observed to be beneficial as meconium inhibits endogenous surfactant activity.

8. **Congenital diaphragmatic hernia (CDH)**

a. **CDH** is a defect of the diaphragm allowing abdominal contents to herniate into the chest. CDH occurs in 1 in 5000 live births and has a high mortality, with 40% not surviving infancy.

b. **Clinical features.** CDH is usually detected during a prenatal ultrasound. Eighty-five percent of defects occur in the left posterior lateral region of the diaphragm through the foramen of Bochdalek. The neonate often has a scaphoid abdomen with absent breath sounds on the involved side. Rarely, bowel sounds are heard in the affected hemithorax. The clinical spectrum of CDH may vary and is probably related to the degree of lung hypoplasia and associated pulmonary hypertension and cardiac dysfunction.

c. The **diagnosis** is confirmed by CXR. The intestines and stomach are typically observed in the thorax. The liver, spleen, and/or kidneys may also be involved. Approximately 40% of infants with CDH have associated anomalies including cardiac, gastrointestinal, genitourinary, or renal anomalies that significantly increase the risk of mortality.

d. Treatment is geared toward decreasing pulmonary vascular resistance and facilitating CO_2 elimination prior to surgical correction. Insufflation of the stomach and intestines is minimized by intubating the patients while they are spontaneously breathing and may often take place in the delivery room. However, if necessary, ventilation with bag and mask should be accomplished with minimal airway pressures. Continuous gastric suction also decreases air insufflation. Conventional ventilation or HFOV is used. Ventilation with INO has been observed to decrease pulmonary vasoconstriction and cyanosis in some patients with CDH. The main causes of mortality are respiratory insufficiency and pulmonary hypertension. Pneumothorax in the unaffected lung can occur and is often the cause of death during resuscitation. Hypotension and shock are frequently seen secondary to prolonged systemic hypoxemia, cardiac impairment caused by shifting of the mediastinal contents by the hernia, and gastrointestinal fluid losses.

e. Surgical repair involves replacing the abdominal contents and repairing the diaphragm. Current evidence supports first stabilizing the patients with medical therapy and gentle ventilation, using **extracorporeal membrane oxygenation** (ECMO) as a last resort (see Section III.C.5.d.3). During the stabilization period, pulmonary artery pressures fall, and the patient is subsequently taken to the OR for repair.

f. Anesthetic considerations: Decompression of the gut with continuous nasogastric suction is helpful. An arterial catheter is indicated for the frequent assessment of acid-base balance, oxygenation, and ventilation. Sodium bicarbonate and hyperventilation are used to treat metabolic and respiratory acidosis, respectively. In addition, alkalosis and INO may decrease pulmonary vasoconstriction. Although spontaneous ventilation may prevent gastric inflation and lung compression, ventilator support is often needed. Using the lowest effective inflating pressures reduces the risk of pneumothorax and ventilator-induced lung injury. Nitrous oxide is avoided because it may distend the gut and compromise lung function. Muscle relaxation, narcotics, and oxygen therapy are often used during anesthesia.

g. Postoperative morbidities include feeding difficulty, gastroesophageal reflux, hearing loss, neurodevelopmental disability, and potential recurrence of the diaphragmatic hernia, particularly in those infants with a large defect requiring a patch repair.

C. Cardiovascular disorders

1. Congenital heart disease should be suspected in the setting of persistent cyanosis, hypotension, respiratory distress, murmur, hypoxemia, poor perfusion, or shock. Congenital heart disease occurs with an overall incidence of 8 per 1000 live births with 2 per 1000 presenting in the first year of life. The most common congenital heart disease lesions include ventricular septal defects, pulmonary stenosis with intact ventricular septum, tetralogy of Fallot, atrial septal defects, or transposition of the great arteries.

2. **Cyanosis**
    a. **Etiology.** There are many causes of cyanosis, including diffusion abnormalities in the lung, intracardiac and extracardiac shunts, and polycythemia. The pulmonary causes of cyanosis are described above.
    b. **Cardiac lesions** may cause systemic hypoxemia by decreasing pulmonary blood flow or by causing admixture of systemic and pulmonary venous blood via shunts.
    c. Several factors allow the majority of fetuses to tolerate congenital heart lesions in utero. Fetal oxygenation occurs via the placenta, rather than being dependent on pulmonary blood flow. Both the left and right ventricles contribute to systemic blood flow, and mixing occurs at atrial and ductal levels. Furthermore, the fetus has greater oxygen carrying capacity because of fetal hemoglobin and an elevated hemoglobin concentration.
    d. In the newborn, the **ductus arteriosus may initially permit pulmonary blood flow** in patients with transposition of the great arteries, pulmonic stenosis or atresia, tetralogy of Fallot, or ventricular hypoplasia. Most of these infants become symptomatic as the ductus arteriosus closes at 2 to 3 days of life. If a ductal-dependent cardiac lesion exists, prevention of ductal closure is critical to maintain pulmonary blood flow. This may be accomplished with a **prostaglandin E$_1$** infusion. Side effects of prostaglandin treatment include apnea, hypotension, and seizure activity.
    e. Many patients with **septal defects** are asymptomatic during the fetal and neonatal period. However, with increased pulmonary vascular resistance, right-to-left shunting of deoxygenated blood may produce systemic hypoxemia. Later in life, the normal decrease in pulmonary vascular resistance increases blood flow to the lung and potentially causes pulmonary vascular overcirculation and pulmonary hypertension.
    f. **Laboratory studies.** In the infant with signs and symptoms of cardiovascular disease, relevant studies include an arterial blood gas, pre- and postductal oxygen saturations, four extremity blood pressures, an ECG, CXR, hemoglobin or hematocrit, and determination of arterial blood gas tension during inhalation of pure oxygen ("**hyperoxia test**"). A Pao$_2$ that remains below 150 mm Hg while the infant breathes 100% oxygen is suggestive of an intracardiac shunt. Cardiology consultation is indicated, and echocardiography is frequently performed to detect potential structural heart lesions.

3. **Patent ductus arteriosus (PDA)**
    a. **Clinical features.** PDA is commonly encountered in the premature infant and is characterized by a murmur at the left sternal border radiating to the back, bounding pulses, widened pulse pressure, evidence of increased pulmonary blood flow by CXR, respiratory distress, and excessive weight gain. The PDA often can be confirmed by cardiac ultrasound. In some cases, cardiac dysfunction associated with a PDA may decrease systemic blood pressure, peripheral perfusion, and urine output and may be associated with metabolic acidosis.

b. Although **early treatment** of a PDA consists of fluid restriction and supportive care, it is important to maintain systemic perfusion. If the degree of shunt through the ductus arteriosus is significant, and renal and platelet function are adequate, pharmacologic closure of the ductus with **indomethacin** or **ibuprofen** may be attempted.

c. **Surgical closure** of a PDA is indicated in symptomatic infants for whom medical therapy has either failed, is contraindicated, such as those with decreased renal or platelet function, or thought not to be effective.

d. **Anesthetic considerations:** Often these infants are critically ill, requiring high levels of oxygen support, ventilator support, and vasopressor therapy. They may have renal dysfunction, because of decreased cardiac output caused by the PDA and fluid restriction, and platelet dysfunction because of medical therapies. Many PDA closures may take place in the NICU to avoid the risk of transporting the infant to the OR. In addition to a preductal pulse oximeter that is used to assess cerebral oxygen delivery, a postductal oximeter can be helpful during the surgical procedure for detecting inadvertent occlusion of the aorta during assessment of the anatomy of the central circulation. An opiate-based anesthetic (eg, fentanyl) with muscle relaxation is a common technique used for infants undergoing PDA ligation. Infants should be monitored closely in the postoperative period for complications including pneumothorax, hypotension, and oliguria.

4. **Dysrhythmias**

a. **Supraventricular tachycardia** (SVT) is the most frequent dysrhythmia seen in fetuses and neonates. The associated heart rate greater than 250 beats/min is often self-limited and well tolerated. However, if the SVT is associated with hypotension or hemoglobin oxygen desaturation, prompt treatment is required.

b. **SVT treatment** consists of vagal maneuvers such as nasopharyngeal stimulation or placement of a cold pack glove or ice-filled glove on the infant's face. Massage of the eye should be avoided, as this may lead to disruption of the lens in neonates. **Adenosine** and **esophageal pacing** are also useful for acute management of symptomatic SVT.

c. Synchronized electrocardioversion is indicated if the patient is hemodynamically unstable.

5. **Persistent pulmonary hypertension of the newborn (PPHN)**

a. **Pathophysiology.** PPHN, previously referred to as persistent fetal circulation, is manifested by an increase in lung vascular resistance with resulting pulmonary arterial hypertension, right-to-left shunting across the foramen ovale and the ductus arteriosus, and systemic hypoxemia.

b. **Etiology.** It is suspected that many newborns with PPHN have abnormal muscularization of the distal lung vascular bed and reactivity of the pulmonary arteries. Although PPHN is associated with perinatal depression, meconium aspiration, bacterial pneumonia, or sepsis, the exact role of these in the etiology of PPHN is unknown.

c. **Clinical features.** Typically, term or near-term newborns with PPHN have severe systemic hypoxemia unrelieved by breathing at high FIO_2. They may have shunt evidenced by higher oxygen saturations in the upper versus lower extremities. ECG may reveal right ventricular hypertrophy, and CXR may show decreased pulmonary vascular markings. Echocardiography may demonstrate shunting of blood at the level of the PDA and/or PFO.

    d. Treatment of PPHN

      1. Specific treatments include intubation and mechanical ventilation with high FIO_2, induced respiratory or metabolic alkalosis, and INO administration. In nearly 50% of cases, carefully administered inhaled NO gas rapidly vasodilates the pulmonary vasculature, decreases shunt, and increases systemic oxygenation. In babies breathing NO gas, the levels of methemoglobin and inhaled NO oxides need to be measured.

      2. Nonspecific and supportive treatments include aggressive blood pressure support, sedation with narcotics (eg, fentanyl), and occasionally muscle relaxants.

      3. ECMO may be lifesaving for some patients with PPHN refractory to ventilatory and medical therapy.

        a. The **ECMO circuit** consists of tubing, a reservoir, pump, membrane oxygenator, and heat exchanger. To prevent clotting, the patient is treated with heparin. Because of platelet consumption during ECMO, platelet infusions are often required.

        b. Access. General anesthesia is required for central vascular cannulation during the initiation of ECMO. In neonates with adequate cardiac function, **venovenous (VV)** ECMO is performed with a single double-lumen catheter placed in the right ventricle via the right internal jugular vein. In neonates with compromised cardiac function and/or congenital heart disease associated with the PPHN, **venoarterial (VA)** ECMO is facilitated by cannulation of the right common carotid artery and the right internal jugular vein or the femoral artery and vein.

        c. Potential morbidities are associated with ECMO. Heparin treatment can cause intracranial hemorrhage and bleeding from other sites. Right-sided cerebral injuries (focal left-sided seizures, left hemiparesis, and progressive right cerebral atrophy) are thought secondary to cannulation and ligation of the right internal carotid artery.

        d. Because of the potential risks of ECMO, it is reserved for term and late preterm (>34 weeks) infants with a birth weight generally greater than 1800 to 2000 g with severe systemic hypoxemia. Prior to ECMO cannulation, a screening head ultrasound, echocardiogram, and baseline laboratory evaluation should be performed. Most infants with significant intracranial hemorrhage are excluded because of the unacceptable risk of hemorrhage extension while being treated with heparin. Also excluded are infants with multiple congenital anomalies, severe neurologic impairment, or cyanotic congenital heart disease.

D. Hematologic disorders

  1. Hemolytic disease of the newborn (erythroblastosis fetalis)

    a. Isoimmune hemolytic anemia in the fetus is caused by transplacental passage of maternal IgG antibodies against fetal erythrocytes.

    b. Rh hemolytic disease is usually caused by anti-D antibodies but can also be caused by antibodies to minor antigens including Kell, Duffy, and Kidd. The absence of D antigen makes one Rh negative. A mother can be sensitized to fetal antigens by leakage of fetal blood into the maternal circulation during pregnancy, delivery, abortion, or amniocentesis. To prevent sensitization, an unsensitized Rh-negative mother is given **anti-D immune globulin (Rhogam)** during pregnancy at 28 weeks of gestation, after any invasive procedure (eg, amniocentesis), and at delivery. Once a mother is sensitized, immune prophylaxis is of no value. Even if treated with immune globulin, a mother can still be sensitized during pregnancy if a large fetomaternal transfusion occurs.

c. **ABO hemolytic disease** can occur without maternal sensitization, because a mother with group O blood has naturally occurring anti-A and anti-B antibodies in her circulation. Because these are usually IgM antibodies that cannot cross the placenta, ABO hemolytic disease tends to be milder than Rh disease, with little or no anemia, mild indirect hyperbilirubinemia, and rare need for exchange transfusion.

d. An **indirect Coombs test** on maternal blood can detect the presence of IgG antibodies.

e. A **direct Coombs test** on the infant's red blood cells can detect cells already coated with antibody, thus indicating a risk for hemolysis.

f. **Hemolysis** occurs when antibodies cross the placenta and attach to the corresponding antigens on fetal erythrocytes. Hepatosplenomegaly results from increased hematopoiesis triggered by hemolysis.

g. **Clinical features.** Physical examination may reveal hepatosplenomegaly, edema, pallor, scleral icterus, or jaundice.

h. **Laboratory studies** often reveal anemia, thrombocytopenia, a positive direct Coombs test, indirect hyperbilirubinemia, hypoglycemia, hypoalbuminemia, and an elevated reticulocyte count that increases proportionally with the severity of the disease. Serial hematocrit and indirect bilirubin levels should be followed.

i. **First-line treatment** consists of **phototherapy.** Intravenous immunoglobulin (IVIG) administration and/or an exchange transfusion may be required if the total indirect bilirubin level is very high or the rate of rise of bilirubin exceeds 1 mg/dL/h.

2. **Hydrops fetalis**

a. **Hydrops fetalis** is associated with excessive accumulation of fluid in at least two body compartments of the fetus and can range from mild peripheral edema to massive anasarca with pleural and/or pericardial effusions.

b. **Etiologies.** Hydrops fetalis is associated with anemia (eg, hemolytic disease, fetomaternal hemorrhage, donor twin-twin transfusion), cardiac arrhythmias (eg, complete heart block, SVT), congenital heart disease, vascular or lymphatic malformation (eg, hemangioma of the liver, cystic hygroma), and infection (eg, viral, toxoplasmosis, syphilis).

c. **Treatment.** The main goals of therapy include prevention of intrauterine or extrauterine death from anemia and hypoxia, restoration of intravascular volume, and avoidance of neurotoxicity from hyperbilirubinemia.

1. Survival of the unborn fetus may be improved by in utero transfusion via the umbilical vein.

2. Care of the live born infant with hydrops may include respiratory support with intubation and mechanical ventilation, paracentesis and/or thoracentesis, echocardiogram, placement of central lines, correction of hypovolemia and acidosis, and exchange transfusion. Some of these babies require aggressive and prolonged ventilator support because of pulmonary hypoplasia.

3. Late complications include anemia, mild graft-versus-host reactions, inspissated bile syndrome (characterized by persistent icterus with elevated direct and indirect bilirubin), and portal vein thrombosis (as a complication of umbilical vein catheterization).

E. Gastrointestinal disorders

1. Hyperbilirubinemia

a. **Pathophysiology.** Bilirubin is formed from the breakdown of hemoglobin. It is rapidly bound to albumin, transported to the liver (where it is conjugated with glucuronate), and delivered to the intestine in bile. In the intestine, it is either deconjugated by intestinal bacteria and reabsorbed or converted to excretory urobilinogen.

b. **Etiology.** Hyperbilirubinemia results from overproduction (eg, hemolysis, absorption of sequestered blood, polycythemia), underconjugation (eg, immature or damaged liver), or underexcretion (eg, biliary atresia). It is often seen in sepsis, asphyxia, and metabolic disorders (eg, hypothyroidism, hypoglycemia, galactosemia) as well as in healthy, typically breast-fed infants.

c. **Toxic effects.** Unconjugated (indirect) bilirubin is lipid soluble and is capable of crossing the blood-brain barrier and entering the central nervous system. Toxic levels of bilirubin result in damage of neurons. This process leads to **bilirubin encephalopathy** or **kernicterus** and may cause symptoms ranging from mild lethargy and fever to convulsions. Infants with prematurity, respiratory distress, sepsis, metabolic acidosis, hypoglycemia, hypoalbuminemia, or severe hemolytic disease are at risk for kernicterus. Later in life, kernicterus causes neurologic sequelae including diminished cognitive function, mental retardation, sensorineural hearing loss, dental dysplasia, and choreoathetoid cerebral palsy.

d. **Physiologic jaundice** results from increased red cell turnover and an immature hepatic conjugation system. It occurs in 60% of term newborns, and peak bilirubin levels occur by day 2 to day 4 of life. Premature infants have an increased incidence (80%) and later bilirubin peak (day 5-day 7 of life).

e. **Breast milk jaundice** develops gradually in the second or third week of life. In this disease, bilirubin levels peak at 15 to 25 mg/dL, and the elevated bilirubin levels may persist for 2 days to 3 months. Other causes of hyperbilirubinemia should be excluded before making this diagnosis. Interrupting nursing for a few days and supplementing with formula results in a marked decrease in serum levels, at which time nursing can be restarted. This is a benign type of jaundice without adverse sequelae.

f. **Laboratory studies** include total and direct bilirubin, blood type and direct Coombs test, hemoglobin or hematocrit, reticulocyte count, blood smear for red cell morphology, electrolytes, blood urea nitrogen, creatinine, and appropriate cultures if sepsis is suspected. Because hyperbilirubinemia may be the presenting sign of a urinary tract infection, urinalysis and urine cultures should be considered.

g. **Treatment**

1. An elevated bilirubin level in the first 24 hours of life is pathologic and always warrants further investigation.

2. Management of physiologic or mild hemolytic jaundice consists of monitoring serial bilirubin levels and starting early feeding to reduce enterohepatic cycling of bilirubin.

3. **Phototherapy** is used if moderate indirect bilirubin levels or an accelerated rate of rise is noted. Light therapy of 420- to 470-nm wavelength results in photoisomerization of bilirubin, making it water soluble. Eyes must be shielded during phototherapy to prevent retinal damage.

   4. For severe hyperbilirubinemia, IVIG administration and/or **exchange transfusion** are indicated (eg, indirect bilirubin >25 mg/ dL in a full-term infant).

2. **Esophageal atresia (EA) and tracheoesophageal fistula (TEF)**

   a. EA is usually associated with TEF. The location of the fistula in patients with TEF is variable, with the most common configuration consisting of a proximal esophageal pouch and a distal TEF. EA/TEF is often accompanied by other congenital abnormalities, particularly cardiac defects.

   b. Pathophysiology. The proximal esophageal pouch has a small capacity, resulting in overflow aspiration. Aspiration leads to the classic clinical triad of coughing, choking, and cyanosis in patients with EA. Occasionally, copious secretions with drooling requiring frequent suctioning may be the only early symptom.

   c. The **diagnosis** is confirmed by the inability to pass a nasogastric tube into the stomach. A CXR that includes the neck with air- or water-soluble contrast agent will confirm the existence of esophageal atresia.

   d. Medical treatment is directed at reducing aspiration. Neonates should be kept NPO. A nasogastric tube is placed on continuous low suction and the head of the bed is elevated. Aspiration pneumonia should be treated with antibiotics and oxygen as required. Endotracheal intubation and ventilation may be required for severe pneumonia. However, ventilation may be difficult when a TEF exists.

   e. Surgical treatment depends on the stability of the infant. In newborns with severe aspiration pneumonia, surgery may be delayed until the lungs improve. If gastric distention because of air transiting the TEF into the GI tract compromises pulmonary function, a gastrostomy tube may be placed under local anesthesia. After initial stabilization, definitive repair of the esophagus and fistula may occur.

   f. Anesthetic considerations: It is critical, and sometimes difficult, to establish an airway in patients with a TEF. Surgeons should be readily available during the induction should emergent decompression of the stomach be required. The patient should be fully monitored; a precordial chest piece should be placed over the left thorax to aid in the assessment of ventilation. If the patient has a gastrostomy tube, it should be placed to water seal. Spontaneous ventilation during induction, intubation until the time of surgical ligation of the fistula should be maintained. To facilitate placement of the endotracheal tube so that its tip resides between the fistula and the carina, the tube may be placed first into the right mainstem bronchus. The tube then may be withdrawn slowly until breath sounds are heard over the left thorax. Decreased breath sounds and insufflation of the stomach or gas exiting from the gastrostomy tube suggest that the end of the endotracheal tube is above the fistula and that it should be advanced. Once the tube is in a good location, it must be carefully secured and monitored for dislodgement during the surgical procedure.

3. **Duodenal atresia**

   a. Clinical features. Duodenal atresia usually presents with bile-stained emesis, abdominal distention, and increased volume of gastric aspirates. It is associated with trisomy 21 and may coexist with other intestinal malformations.

b. Prenatal ultrasound or a postnatal **abdominal x-ray** often reveals a **"double bubble,"** representing air in the stomach and proximal duodenum.

c. **Treatment** consists of avoiding oral feeds, use of nasogastric suction, ensuring adequate hydration, and managing electrolytes. Anesthesia consists of an awake or rapid sequence intubation, avoidance of nitrous oxide, and often the use of muscle relaxants.

4. **Pyloric stenosis**

a. **Clinical features:** Pyloric stenosis usually presents in the third to fifth week of life and is characterized by hypertrophy of the pylorus, which causes gastric outlet obstruction. The patient may present with persistent nonbilious emesis. Although the infant may exhibit hypochloremic, hypokalemic metabolic alkalosis from loss of hydrochloric acid, protracted vomiting may result in metabolic acidosis, intravascular volume depletion, and shock. An abdominal mass consisting of the hypertrophic pylorus or "olive" may be palpable.

b. An **abdominal x-ray** usually shows gastric dilatation. The diagnosis is confirmed by abdominal ultrasound. In the past, x-ray examinations with contrast were performed to confirm this disease.

c. **Treatment** consists of rehydration, correction of metabolic alkalosis, and nasogastric or orogastric drainage before surgical repair via pyloromyotomy.

d. **Anesthetic considerations:** It is critical to empty the stomach before anesthetic induction. Since the patient's nasogastric tube is often blocked with gastric secretions, it is best replaced just before induction and the patient suctioned while they are positioned supine, lateral, and prone. A rapid-sequence or awake intubation may then be performed. Inhalation anesthetics or muscle relaxants can be used as needed. Opioids often are not necessary, and the patient may be prone to respiratory depression from opioids due to cerebrospinal fluid (CSF) alkalosis. Rectal acetaminophen and local anesthetic infiltration of the surgical incision may be sufficient for analgesia. The neonate should be fully awake and breathing adequately before removing the endotracheal tube.

5. **Omphalocele and gastroschisis**

a. **Clinical features.** An **omphalocele** is caused by failure of the migration of the intestine into the abdomen and subsequent closure of the abdominal wall at 6 to 8 weeks of gestation. The viscera remain outside the abdominal cavity and are covered with intact peritoneum. Associated defects are present in 45% to 80% of patients with an omphalocele and can include genetic abnormalities (50%), cardiac defects (28%), exstrophy of the bladder and other genitourinary abnormalities (20%), craniofacial defects (20%), and CDH (12%). **Gastroschisis** occurs later in fetal life (12-18 weeks of gestation) from interruption of the omphalomesenteric artery. The resulting paraumbilical defect allows exposure of the bowel to the intrauterine environment without peritoneal coverage. Bowel loops are often edematous and covered with an inflammatory exudate. In contrast to omphalocele, gastroschisis is associated with other congenital abnormalities in only 10% to 20% of cases but may be complicated by intestinal atresia/stenosis or midgut volvulus in up to 16% of cases.

b. **Medical stabilization** includes nasogastric drainage, IV hydration, and protection of the viscera before surgical repair. If the peritoneal sac is intact, the omphalocele should be covered with sterile, warm, saline-soaked gauze to decrease heat and water loss and the risk of infection. If the sac has ruptured or if the infant has gastroschisis, warm saline-soaked gauze should be used to wrap the exposed viscera or the infant can be placed in a sterile plastic bag with careful ongoing monitoring of intestinal perfusion. The infant should then be wrapped in warm sterile towels before surgical repair.

c. **Anesthetic considerations.** In the OR, special measures are directed at compensating for the increased insensible water and heat loss associated with the abdominal surgery. After carefully emptying the stomach, a rapid-sequence induction is performed to minimize gaseous distention of the gastrointestinal tract. Muscle relaxation aids the surgeons in placing the organs into the abdominal wall or silo placement. Special attention is required to maintain ventilation and systemic blood flow after the organs are placed in the abdomen, which can be facilitated by measuring ventilatory pressures, urine output, and lower body blood pressure and oxygen saturation. These data aid in the decision of whether the lesion should be corrected in a single or staged procedure. It is essential to assess ventilation and oxygenation of the patient prior to extubation. The increased intra-abdominal pressures associated with the procedure can compromise the pulmonary function of the patient and perfusion of the abdominal contents.

6. **Necrotizing enterocolitis (NEC)**

   a. **NEC** is an acquired intestinal necrosis that appears in the absence of functional or anatomic lesions. It occurs predominantly in premature infants with an increased incidence at lower gestational ages. It usually develops during the first few weeks of life and almost always after the institution of enteral feedings. Mortality may be as high as 40%.

   b. **Pathogenesis** is unclear but involves critical stress of an immature gut by ischemic, infectious, or immunologic insults. Enteral feedings seem to potentiate mucosal injury, though feeding with breast milk may be protective.

   c. **Clinical features** include abdominal distention, feeding intolerance with gastric aspirates or emesis, ileus, abdominal wall erythema, and bloody stool. The infant may demonstrate temperature instability, lethargy, respiratory and circulatory instability, apnea, oliguria, and DIC.

   d. **Laboratory studies** should include an abdominal x-ray (which may show **pneumatosis intestinalis,** fixed loops of bowel, portal venous air, or free intraperitoneal air), CBC (revealing leukocytosis, leukopenia, thrombocytopenia), arterial blood gases (demonstrating acidosis), electrolytes (showing hyponatremia or acidosis), stool guaiac (often showing occult blood), and stool Clinitest (showing evidence of carbohydrate malabsorption). Because the differential diagnosis includes sepsis, cultures of blood and urine should also be obtained. If the patient is stable and disseminated intravascular coagulation is not evident, CSF should be obtained by lumbar puncture for Gram stain and culture.

   e. **Treatment.** When NEC is suspected, enteral feedings are discontinued, and the stomach is decompressed with a nasogastric tube. Oral feeds are withheld for at least 10 to 14 days, and the patient is supported with parenteral nutrition. Broad-spectrum antibiotics (ampicillin, an aminoglycoside and, if perforation is suspected, metronidazole or clindamycin) are administered empirically.

f. **Surgical consultation** is indicated, although laparotomy or abdominal drain placement is usually reserved for intestinal perforation, a fixed loop on serial abdominal x-rays, or persistent metabolic acidosis.

g. **Anesthetic concerns** include hemodynamic instability due to abdominal sepsis, increasing abdominal girth leading to ventilation challenges, and profound metabolic acidosis, which is associated with severe NEC. It is also important to prevent aspiration of gastric contents and maintaining organ perfusion in the presence of significant third-space fluid losses.

7. **Volvulus**

a. **Volvulus** may occur as a primary lesion or, more commonly, as the result of intestinal malrotation, which can rapidly compromise blood flow to the intestine causing ischemia. If present in utero, intestinal necrosis may be present at birth, and immediate resection is indicated.

b. **Clinical features** may include abdominal distention, bilious emesis, and signs of dehydration, acidosis, sepsis, or shock.

c. **The diagnosis** of malrotation is made by upper gastrointestinal and small bowel follow-through examination, which demonstrates an abnormally positioned ligament of Treitz.

d. **Treatment** involves volume resuscitation, placement of a nasogastric tube, cessation of feeding, antibiotic administration, and surgical repair.

e. **Anesthetic considerations:** After evacuation of the stomach, a rapid sequence induction should be performed and anesthesia maintained with inhalation or IV anesthetics as tolerated. Nitrous oxide should be avoided to prevent further distention of the bowel.

F. **Neurologic disorders**

1. **Seizures**

a. **Seizures** may be generalized, focal, or subclinical.

b. **Etiologies** include birth trauma, intracranial hemorrhage, hypoxic ischemic encephalopathy, metabolic disturbances (hypoglycemia or hypocalcemia), drug withdrawal, and infections.

c. **Laboratory evaluation**

1. Initial evaluation includes electrolytes, glucose, calcium, magnesium, and arterial blood gas and pH determination. If a metabolic disease is suspected, serum lactate and ammonia, serum/urine amino acids, and urine for organic acids should be obtained.

2. CBC with differential, platelet count, and the appropriate cultures, including blood and CSF.

3. To identify underlying causes of the seizures, neuroimaging is performed, which may include cranial ultrasound, computed tomography (CT) scan, and/or magnetic resonance imaging (MRI) sometimes with T2 diffusion-weighted imaging, and electroencephalograms may be obtained, sometimes during pyridoxine administration.

d. **Treatment** includes supportive care. It is critical to ensure that the patient maintains adequate oxygenation. In addition, it is important to correct potential underlying metabolic abnormalities that cause the seizures (eg, hypoglycemia, hypocalcemia). Anticonvulsants are started and, if indicated, a test dose of pyridoxine is administered. In newborns ≥36 weeks of gestational age, if a hypoxic-ischemic event at or near the time of birth is thought to be contributing to the brain injury, and clinical signs suggest that there is moderate-to-severe encephalopathy, then total body or head cooling to 33.5 °C to 34.5 °C is often initiated in the NICU within the first 6 hours of life and employed for 72 hours. In these cases, consultation with experts in neonatal neurology is often sought.

- **e. Anticonvulsants**
    1. Acute medical treatments include the following:
        - **a. Phenobarbital,** 20 mg/kg IV load over 10 minutes; maintenance dose of 2.5 mg/kg twice daily to maintain a serum level of 20 to 40 μg/mL.
        - **b. Benzodiazepine** (eg, lorazepam 0.1-0.3 mg/kg IV).
        - **c. Fosphenytoin,** 15 to 20 mg/kg IV load over 15 minutes; maintenance dose of 2.5 mg/kg twice daily to maintain a therapeutic level of 15 to 30 μg/mL.
    2. Chronic treatment for neonatal seizures is usually with phenobarbital or levetiracetam.
- **2. Intracranial hemorrhage**
    - **a. Intraventricular hemorrhage** occurs in more than 30% of infants with birth weights below 1000 g typically within the first 7 days of life. Subdural and subarachnoid hemorrhages are much less common.
    - **b. Clinical features.** Intraventricular hemorrhage is often asymptomatic, although it may present with unexplained lethargy, apnea, or seizures. On examination, the head circumference can be increased, and the fontanelle may be bulging.
    - **c. Laboratory studies.** Laboratory examination may show anemia and acidosis. Screening head ultrasounds are generally performed in infants under 32 weeks of gestational age.
    - **d. Grading of intraventricular hemorrhage**
        1. **Grade I.** Subependymal or choroid plexus bleeding only.
        2. **Grade II.** Intraventricular bleeding without dilatation of ventricles.
        3. **Grade III.** Intraventricular bleeding with dilatation of ventricles.
        4. **Grade IV.** Intraparenchymal bleeding.
    - **e.** The **major complication** of intraventricular hemorrhage is CSF obstruction resulting in **hydrocephalus.** This is followed by measuring daily head circumferences and by serial cranial ultrasounds. Serial lumbar punctures or intraventricular shunting is often required.
    - **f.** Hypertonic agents (eg, 25% dextrose in water) that had previously been advocated in the treatment of hypoglycemia have been implicated in the etiology of intraventricular hemorrhage and should be avoided.
- **3. Myelodysplasia**
    - **a.** Abnormal neurulation of the embryo can result in failed closure of the posterior neural tube by the fourth week of gestation. A **meningocele** is caused when the meninges herniate through a bony abnormality in the spine (spina bifida) and form a sac filled with CSF. The spinal cord and nerve roots are generally not involved. A **myelomeningocele** is the result of spinal cord and meninges herniating through a defect in the spinal canal. Eight percent of myelomeningoceles involve the lumbar spinal region. Hydrocephalus may affect as many as 90% of newborns with myelomeningocele because the cord lesion can displace the cerebellum and interfere with CSF flow.
    - **b.** Myelomeningoceles occur with an incidence of 4 to 10 per 10,000 live births. The incidence has significantly decreased with maternal folic acid supplementation. Women with diabetes or taking certain medications (eg, antiepileptics) are at increased risk of having a child with myelodysplasia.

    c. **Postnatal management** includes covering the defect with a warm, normal saline-soaked sterile dressing to prevent adhesion of the dressing to the defect. The infant should be kept prone, and latex exposure should be avoided. Preoperatively, the infant should undergo assessment for additional abnormalities (eg, scoliosis, hydrocephalus, Arnold-Chiari malformation), and neuroimaging is recommended. Early surgical repair significantly decreases the risk of infection. Postoperatively, infants must be monitored closely for seizures and hydrocephalus that may require shunt placement. Prognosis ultimately depends on the level of the lesion and the presence of other congenital anomalies.

    d. **Anesthetic considerations:** During intubation of the patient in a supine position, special care must be taken to pad the exposed neural tissue to prevent injury. In some cases, intubation of the patient in the left lateral decubitus position may be preferred to protect the lesion. Many patients with myelomeningocele may have a short trachea, creating an increased risk for endobronchial intubation. Blood loss tends to be minimal unless extensive subcutaneous tissue dissection is required to mobilize the skin so that it can cover a large lesion. If hydrocephalus is present, the neonate may have a diminished response to hypoxia causing an increased risk of apneic episodes in the postoperative period.

4. Retinopathy of prematurity (ROP)

    a. **Etiologies**

        1. **The risk of ROP** is increased in premature neonates requiring oxygen therapy. ROP is seen in infants with birth weights less than 1500 g and gestational age less than 30 weeks. There is an 80% incidence in infants weighing less than 1000 g. To decrease the incidence of ROP, **hyperoxia should be avoided.**

        2. Factors other than hyperoxic exposure and prematurity may produce ROP, as it has been demonstrated in full-term infants, infants with cyanotic heart disease, stillborn infants, and infants without hyperoxic exposure. Factors that may increase risk include anemia, infection, intracranial hemorrhage, acidosis, and PDA.

    b. **Pathophysiology.** ROP begins in the temporal peripheral retina, which is the last part of the retina to vascularize. An elevated ridge demarcating vascularized and nonvascularized retina is initially seen. **Fibrovascular proliferation** from this border extends posteriorly, and in 90% of patients, gradual resolution occurs from this stage. These patients may develop strabismus, amblyopia, myopia, or peripheral retinal detachment in later life.

    c. In 10% of patients, fibrovascularization extends into the vitreous, resulting in vitreous hemorrhage, peripheral retinal scarring, temporal dragging of the disk and macula, and partial retinal detachment. In severe disease, extensive fibrovascular proliferation can result in a retrolental white mass (leukocoria), complete retinal detachment, and loss of vision.

    d. **Infants ≤32 weeks of gestational age, birth weight ≤1500 g, or with additional risk factors should undergo** indirect ophthalmoscopy at 34 weeks of corrected gestational age. If ROP is identified, the infant is reexamined at 1- to 2-week intervals until spontaneous resolution occurs. New cases of ROP do not occur after 3 months of age.

    e. **Treatment** for severe manifestations of ROP has included photocoagulation, diathermy, cryotherapy, vitrectomy, and bevacizumab injection.

G. Infectious diseases

1. Environment

a. **Neonates are particularly vulnerable to infection.** They have decreased cellular and humoral immune defense systems and are at increased risk for colonization and nosocomial infection.

b. **Prevention.** Infectious transmission may be reduced by using separate equipment and isolettes for each infant, by hand washing before and after each contact, and by wearing cover gowns.

2. Risk factors for infection. Prolonged rupture of membranes is associated with a high incidence of chorioamnionitis and subsequent ascending bacterial and viral infection in the neonate. Maternal fever, maternal leukocytosis, prolonged rupture of membranes, and fetal tachycardia are also associated with neonatal infection.

3. Laboratory studies include complete blood count with differential and blood cultures. A lumbar puncture for culture and analysis of CSF may be indicated. If appropriate, viral cultures should be obtained.

4. Neonatal sepsis

a. Organisms responsible for infections soon after birth are usually acquired in utero or during birth. These can include group B β-hemolytic streptococcus, *Escherichia coli*, *Listeria monocytogenes*, and herpes simplex virus. Later-onset infections may be caused by *Staphylococcus aureus*, *Staphylococcus epidermidis*, *Enterobacter cloacae*, *Enterococcus*, and *Pseudomonas aeruginosa*.

b. **The clinical features of sepsis** include respiratory failure, seizures, and shock. Subtle signs, including respiratory distress, apnea, irritability, and poor feeding, are often seen first and warrant evaluation.

c. **Laboratory studies** should include blood, urine, and CSF cultures; CBC with differential; blood glucose; urinalysis; and CXR.

d. **Antibiotic coverage** with ampicillin and an aminoglycoside is begun and continued for 48 to 72 hours. If cultures are positive, treatment should continue as indicated by the severity and location of infection. Aminoglycoside serum levels should be monitored and dosages adjusted to prevent toxicity.

IV. ANATOMY AND PHYSIOLOGY

A. Upper airway

1. Neonates are obligate nose breathers due to weak oropharyngeal muscles and increased compliance of the pharynx, larynx, and bronchial tree. Their nares are relatively narrow, and a significant fraction of the work of breathing is needed to overcome nasal resistance. Occlusion of the nares by bilateral choanal atresia or tenacious secretions can cause complete airway obstruction; however, some infants will convert to mouth breathing. Placement of an oral airway, a laryngeal mask airway, or an endotracheal tube may be necessary to reestablish airway patency during sedation or anesthesia.

2. Infants have relatively large tongues, which can make mask ventilation and laryngoscopy challenging. A recent study called tongue size into question and found the tongue to be proportional in children aged 1 to 12. Clinically, the tongue can easily obstruct the airway if excessive submandibular pressure is applied during mask ventilation.

3. Infants and children have a more cephalad glottis (C3 vertebral level in premature infants, C4 in infants, and C5 in adults) and **a narrow, long, angulated epiglottis,** which can make laryngoscopy difficult.

4. In infants and young children, **the narrowest part of the airway is at the cricoid cartilage** (recent studies have questioned this; see suggested readings), rather than at the glottis (as in adults). An endotracheal tube that passes through the cords may still be too large distally.

5. **Deciduous teeth** erupt within the first year and are shed between ages 6 and 13 years. To avoid dislodging a loose tooth, it is safest to open the mandible directly, without introducing a finger or appliance into the oral cavity. Loose teeth should be documented on the preoperative evaluation. In some instances, unstable teeth should be removed before laryngoscopy. Parents and patients should be informed of this possibility in advance.

6. **Airway resistance** in infants and children can be increased dramatically by subtle changes in an already small-caliber system. Even a small amount of edema can significantly increase airway resistance and cause airway compromise.

B. Pulmonary system

1. Neonates have **higher metabolic rates,** resulting in an elevated oxygen consumption (6 mL/kg/min) when compared with adults (3 mL/kg/min).

2. **Neonatal lungs have high closing volumes,** which fall within the lower range of their normal tidal volume. Below closing volume, alveolar collapse and shunting occur.

3. To meet the higher oxygen demand, infants have a **higher respiratory rate and minute ventilation.** An infant's functional residual capacity (FRC) is nearly equivalent to that of an adult (FRC of an infant, 25 mL/kg; adult, 35 mL/kg). Their higher minute ventilation to FRC ratio results in rapid inhalational induction. The tidal volume for infants and adults is equivalent (6-7 mL/kg).

4. **Anatomic shunts** including PDA and patent foramen ovale may develop significant right-to-left flow with increases in pulmonary artery pressure (eg, hypoxia, acidosis, or high positive airway pressure). This may predispose to air emboli if care is not taken to remove it from the IV tubing.

5. The characteristics of the infant's pulmonary system contribute to **rapid desaturation during apnea.** Profound desaturation can occur when an infant coughs or strains and alveoli collapse. Treatment may require deepening anesthesia, using neuromuscular relaxants, as well as alveolar recruitment.

6. The **diaphragm** is the infant's major muscle of ventilation. Compared with the adult diaphragm, the newborn has only half the number of type I, slow-twitch, high-oxidative muscle fibers essential for sustained increased respiratory effort. Thus, the infant's diaphragm fatigues earlier than the adult's. By 2 years of age, the child's diaphragm would have attained mature levels of type I fibers.

7. The **pliable rib cage** (compliant chest wall) of an infant cannot maintain negative intrathoracic pressure easily. This diminishes the efficacy of the infant's attempts to increase ventilation.

8. An infant's **dead space** is 2 to 2.5 mL/kg, equivalent to an adult's.

9. Infants' high baseline minute ventilation limits their ability to increase their ventilatory effort further. End-tidal CO_2 concentrations should be followed if spontaneous ventilation is permitted under anesthesia; assisted or controlled ventilation may be necessary.

10. **Alveolar maturation** occurs by 8 to 10 years of age when alveoli number and size reach adult ranges.

11. **Retinopathy of prematurity** (see Chapter 30).
12. **Apnea and bradycardia** after general anesthesia occur with increased frequency in infants who are premature and in infants who have anemia, sepsis, hypothermia, central nervous system disease, hypoglycemia, hypothermia, or other metabolic derangements. These patients should have cardiorespiratory monitoring for a minimum of 24 hours postoperatively. Such infants are not candidates for ambulatory day surgery. The guidelines for discharge vary among institutions. Most hospitals agree that infants who are less than 45 to 60 weeks of postconceptual age are monitored postoperatively. Any full-term infant who displays apnea after general anesthesia should also be monitored.

C. **Cardiovascular system**
1. **Heart rate** and **blood pressure** vary with age and should be maintained at age-appropriate levels perioperatively (**Tables 33.3** and **33.4**).
2. **Cardiac output** is 180 to 240 mL/kg/min in newborns, which is two to three times that of adults. This higher cardiac output is necessary to meet the higher metabolic oxygen consumption demands.
3. The **ventricles** are less compliant and have a relatively smaller contractile muscle mass in newborns and infants. The ability to increase contractility is limited; increases in cardiac output occur by increasing heart rate rather than stroke volume. Bradycardia is the most deleterious dysrhythmia in infants, and hypoxemia is a frequent cause of bradycardia in infants and children.
4. Neonates have immature calcium signaling and handling in the sarcoplasmic reticulum and myocardium and are more dependent on ionized calcium concentrations for myocardial function.

D. **Fluid and electrolyte balance**
1. The **glomerular filtration rate** at birth is 15% to 30% of the normal adult value. Adult value is reached by 1 year of age. Renal clearance of drugs and their metabolites is diminished during the first year of life.

TABLE 33.3	Age Dependence of Typical Respiratory Parameters				
Variable	**Newborn**	**1 Y**	**3 Y**	**5 Y**	**Adult**
Respirations (breaths/min)	40-60	20-30	Gradual decrease to 18-25	18-25	12-20
Tidal volume (mL)	15	80	110	250	500
FRC (mL/kg)	25		35		40
Minute ventilation (L/min)	1	1.8	2.5	5.5	6.5
Hemoglobin (g/dL)	14-20	10-11	–	–	13-17
Hematocrit (%)	47-60	33-42			38-50
Arterial pH	7.30-7.40	7.35-7.45	–	–	–
Paco$_2$ (mm Hg)	30-35	30-40	–	–	–
Pao$_2$ (mm Hg)	60-90	80-100	–	–	–

FRC, functional residual capacity.

TABLE 33.4	Cardiovascular Variables		
Age	Blood Pressure (mm Hg)		
	Heart Rate (Beats/min)	Systolic	Diastolic
Preterm neonate	120-180	45-60	30
Term neonate	100-180	55-70	40
1 y	100-140	70-100	60
3 y	84-115	75-110	70
5 y	84-100	80-120	70

2. Neonates have an intact renin-angiotensin-aldosterone pathway, but the distal tubules resorb less sodium in response to aldosterone. Thus, newborns are "obligate sodium losers," and IV fluids should contain sodium.

3. The **total body water** in the preterm infant is 90% of body weight. In term infants, it is 80%; at 6 to 12 months, it is 60%. This increased percentage of total body water affects drug volumes of distribution. The dosages of some drugs (eg, propofol, succinylcholine, pancuronium, and rocuronium) are 20% to 30% greater than are the equally effective dose for adults.

E. **Hematologic system**

1. Normal values for hemoglobin and hematocrit are listed in **Table 33.3**. The nadir of physiologic anemia is at 3 months of age, and the hemoglobin may reach 10 to 11 g/dL in an otherwise healthy infant. Premature infants may demonstrate a decrease in hemoglobin concentration as early as 4 to 6 weeks of age.

2. At birth, **fetal hemoglobin** (HbF) predominates, but β-chain synthesis shifts to the adult type (HbA) by 3 to 4 months of age. HbF has a higher affinity for oxygen; that is, the oxyhemoglobin dissociation curve is shifted to the left, but debate exists regarding the clinical relevance.

3. See Section XII.B for calculations of blood volume and red cell mass.

F. **Hepatobiliary system**

1. **Liver enzyme systems,** particularly those involved in phase-II (conjugation) reactions, are immature in the infant. Drugs metabolized by the P-450 system may have prolonged elimination times.

2. **Jaundice** is common in neonates and can be physiologic or have pathologic causes.

3. **Hyperbilirubinemia** and displacement of bilirubin from albumin by drugs can result in kernicterus. Premature infants develop kernicterus at lower levels of bilirubin than do term infants.

4. **Plasma levels of albumin** are lower at birth and as a result, drugs that are protein bound may have a higher free fraction and higher effective concentration.

G. **Endocrine system**

1. **Newborns,** particularly premature babies and SGA infants, have decreased glycogen stores and are more susceptible to **hypoglycemia**. Infants of diabetic mothers have high insulin levels because of prolonged exposure to elevated maternal serum glucose levels and are prone to hypoglycemia. Infants who fall into these groups

may have dextrose requirements as high as 5 to 15 mg/kg/min. Normal glucose concentrations in the full-term infant are ≥45 mg/dL (2.5 mmol/L).

2. **Hypocalcemia** is common in infants who are premature, are SGA infants, have a history of asphyxia, are offspring of diabetic mothers, or have received transfusions with citrated blood or fresh-frozen plasma. Serum calcium concentration should be monitored in these patients and calcium administered if the ionized calcium is less than 4.0 mg/dL (1.0 mmol/L).

H. Temperature regulation

1. Compared with adults, infants and children have a greater surface area to body weight ratio, which increases loss of body heat.

2. Infants have significantly less muscle mass and cannot compensate for cold by shivering or adjusting their behavior to avoid the cold.

3. Infants respond to cold stress by increasing norepinephrine production, which enhances metabolism in brown fat. Norepinephrine also produces pulmonary and peripheral vasoconstriction, which can lead to right-to-left shunting, hypoxemia, and metabolic acidosis. Sick and preterm infants have limited stores of brown fat and therefore are more susceptible to cold. Strategies to prevent cold stress are discussed in Section IV.C.

V. THE PREANESTHETIC VISIT

General principles of the preanesthetic visit are discussed in Chapter 1. The preoperative visit is an excellent opportunity to address the concerns of the child and parents.

A. History should include the following:

1. Maternal health during gestation, including alcohol or drug use, smoking, diabetes, and viral infections.
2. Prenatal tests (eg, ultrasound and amniocentesis).
3. Gestational age and weight.
4. Events during labor and delivery, including Apgar scores and length of hospital stay.
5. Hospitalizations/emergency room visits.
6. Congenital, chromosomal, metabolic anomalies or syndromes.
7. Recent upper respiratory infections, tracheobronchitis, "croup," reactive airway disease (asthma), exposure to communicable diseases, cyanotic episodes, or history of snoring.
8. Sleeping position (prone, side, or supine).
9. Respiratory quality and pattern (ie, noisy breathing that increase with sleep; periods of apnea with sleep).
10. Growth history.
11. Vomiting and gastroesophageal reflux.
12. Siblings' health.
13. Parents who smoke.
14. Past surgical and anesthetic history.
15. Allergies (environmental, drugs, food, and latex).
16. Bleeding tendencies.

B. Physical examination should include the following:

1. General appearance, alertness, color, tone, congenital anomalies, head size and shape, activity level, and social interaction.
2. Vital signs, height, and weight.
3. Loose teeth, craniofacial anomalies, or large tonsils that could complicate airway management.

4. Respiratory pattern and quality. Signs of upper respiratory infection and/or reactive airways disease (excessive secretions may predispose patients to laryngospasm and bronchospasm during induction and emergence of anesthesia).

5. Cardiac exam including age-appropriate heart rate, rhythm, and heart murmurs (which may indicate flow through anatomic shunts).

6. Potential vascular access sites.

7. Strength, developmental milestones, activity level, and motor and verbal skills.

8. Additional exam(s) pertinent to specific anesthetic/surgical condition.

C. Laboratory data appropriate for the child's illness and proposed surgery should be obtained. Most centers agree that a "routine hemoglobin" is unnecessary for healthy children. If indicated, laboratory tests can often be obtained after induction of general anesthesia (eg, blood bank sample).

VI. PERIPROCEDURAL CONSIDERATIONS AND FASTING GUIDELINES
A. Periprocedural considerations

1. Children face multiple stressors in the perioperative period. They may not understand the specific disease; the concept of anesthesia, or the procedure itself. Honesty about the procedure(s), associated pain, and the sequence of events is essential in maintaining the trust of children regardless of their level of development.

a. Approaches to optimize the periprocedural experience include the use of nonpharmacologic techniques. Examples of these strategies include distraction, humor, sharing control (eg, would you like to sit up or lie down for induction?), and medical reinterpretation of equipment. The use of a child life specialist, tablet, and/or a teaching module may decrease the need for preprocedure pharmacologic therapy and improve a child's experience.

2. Infants less than 8 months old generally tolerate short periods of separation from parents and usually do not require premedication.

3. Children 8 months to 5 years of age likely have developed separation anxiety and may require sedation before the induction of anesthesia (see Section V.B).

4. Older children generally respond well to information and reassurance. Parental and patient anxiety may be reduced by having parents accompany their children to the OR. An especially anxious child may benefit from premedication.

5. Premedication with intramuscular (IM) **anticholinergics** generally is not recommended. If vagolytic drugs are indicated, they are usually administered IV at the time of induction of anesthesia.

6. In the presence of **gastroesophageal reflux, ranitidine** (2-4 mg/kg PO, 2 mg/kg IV) along with **metoclopramide** (0.1 mg/kg) can be administered 2 hours before surgery to increase gastric pH and reduce gastric volume.

7. Children receiving medications for medical problems such as reactive airways disease, seizures, or hypertension should continue to take these medications preoperatively.

B. Fasting guidelines

1. Milk, breast milk, formula, and solid foods should be restricted as outlined in **Table 33.5**.

2. The **last feeding** should consist of clear fluids or sugar water. Studies document that there is no increased risk of aspiration if clear fluids are offered up to 2 hours preoperatively. This policy minimizes preoperative

TABLE 33.5	Fasting Guidelines
Type of Food	**Fasting Guidelines (Hours)**
Clear fluids	2
Breast milk	4
Nonhuman milk	6
Solid food	8

dehydration and hypoglycemia and contributes to a smooth induction and stable operative course. We recommend that patients receive clear fluids until 2 hours before surgery is scheduled. Oral intake is then restricted (see **Table 33.5**).

3. If schedule delays occur, clear fluids may be given. Some patients may require IV placement for hydration and/or glucose administration.

VII. PREPARATION OF THE OR

A. Perioperative/procedure huddle is a useful meeting to confirm procedure details, anesthetic requirements, special concerns, patient-specific factors, and nonroutine steps.

B. **Anesthetic circuit**

1. The **semiclosed circuit** normally used in adults has some disadvantages if used in very small infants:

   a. The inspiratory and expiratory valves increase resistance during spontaneous ventilation: This can be overcome by closing the APL valve to 3 to 5 cm of water and providing adequate gas flow rates to maintain pressure, or the use of pressure support.

   b. The large volume of the absorber system acts as a reservoir for anesthetic agents.

   c. The breathing circuit tubing has a large compression volume; however, neonatal and pediatric tubing are available that help compensate for this, as well as decrease the circuit dead space volume.

2. The **nonrebreathing, open circuit (Mapleson D)** solves these problems (see Chapter 9). **Rebreathing** is prevented by using fresh gas flows 2.0 to 2.5 times the minute ventilation to wash out carbon dioxide. Capnography is essential in recognizing rebreathing (inspired $CO_2 > 0$) and avoiding excessive hyperventilation. This circuit is useful for very small infants who are allowed to breathe spontaneously and during transport.

3. A passive heat and moisture exchanger may be used with either circuit.

4. The **reservoir bag volume** should be at least as large as the child's vital capacity but small enough so that a comfortable squeeze does not overinflate the chest. General guidelines for bag volumes are as follows: newborns, 500-mL bag; 1 to 3 years, 1000-mL bag; and more than 3 years, 2000-mL bag.

5. For **most infants and children,** the semiclosed-circuit-absorber system can be used with a smaller reservoir bag and a pediatric breathing circuit with small-caliber tubing (ie, circle system).

C. **Airway equipment**

1. A **mask** with minimal dead space should be chosen. A clear plastic type is preferred because the lips (for color) and mouth (for secretions and vomitus) can be visualized.

2. The appropriate size of **oral airway** can be estimated by holding the airway in position next to the child's face. The tip of the oral airway should reach to the angle of the mandible with the base at the lips.

3. **Laryngoscopy**

   a. A **narrow handle** is often preferred because it has a more natural feel when using a smaller blade.

   b. **Straight blade** (Miller or Wis-Hipple) is recommended for children less than 2 years old. The smaller flange and long tapered tip of the straight blade provide better visualization of the larynx and manipulation of the epiglottis in the confined spaces of a small oral cavity (see Section IX.A).

   c. **Curved blades** are generally used for patients more than 5 years old.

   d. **Guidelines for laryngoscope blade sizes** (Table 33.6).

4. **Endotracheal tubes.** Traditionally, uncuffed tubes were used for children under 6 to 7 years of age (5.5-mm inner diameter endotracheal tube or smaller). However, the risk of tracheal stenosis is minimal with modern low-pressure cuffs, and cuffed tubes are more commonly used currently and provide additional benefit against aspiration in airway and abdominal surgeries. The size of the endotracheal tube is a significant factor for postoperative recovery in the pediatric patients. In our institute, we primarily use cuffed tubes. The size of cuffed endotracheal tube can be estimated with the equation: endotracheal tube size (mm internal diameter) = (age/4) + 3.5.

5. Care must be taken **not to overinflate** the cuff and to realize that N_2O can diffuse into the cuff which can increase cuff pressure. At the time of intubation, endotracheal tubes that are one size larger and smaller than the estimated size should be available. Special techniques of endotracheal intubation are discussed in Section IX. **Table 33.7** provides guidelines for endotracheal tube sizes.

TABLE 33.6	Guidelines for Choice of Laryngoscope Blades
Age	**Blade**
Premature and neonate	Miller 0
Infant up to 6-8 mo	Miller 0-1
9 mo-2 y	Miller 1
	Wis-Hipple 1.5
2-5 y	Macintosh 1
	Miller 1-1.5
	Wis-Hipple 1.5
Child over 5 y	Macintosh 2
	Miller 2
Adolescent to adult	Macintosh 3
	Miller 2

TABLE 33.7	Guidelines for Endotracheal Tube Sizes
Age	**Size (mm Internal Diameter)**
Premature newborn	2.5-3.0
Full-term newborn	3.0
6-12 mo	3.5
12-20 mo	4.0
2 y	4.5
Over 2 y	4 + (age [years]/4)
6 y	5.5
10 y	6.5

Tube length at mouth (cm) = (10 + age [years])/2.

D. Temperature control

1. The **OR should be warmed** to 80 °F to 90 °F before the child's arrival and an underbody warmer placed on the OR table. Infants should be kept covered with a blanket and a hat.
2. **A servocontrolled radiant warmer** will keep infants warm during the induction of anesthesia and positioning. Skin temperature should be measured and should not exceed 39 °C.
3. **Passive heat and moisture exchangers** can be used for most routine cases. Some practitioners prefer to actively heat and humidify inspired gases during prolonged surgery.
4. Fluids, blood products, and irrigation solutions should be warmed.

E. Monitoring

1. In addition to standard monitoring (Chapter 10), a **precordial or esophageal stethoscope** provides information about heart and respiratory function.
2. **Blood pressure**
   a. A blood pressure cuff should cover at least two-thirds of the upper arm but not encroach on the axilla or antecubital space.
   b. The cuff can be placed on the leg if the arms are inaccessible (eg, cast present).
   c. Several manufacturers of oscillometric blood pressure cuffs have different preset initial pressure settings and cycle durations, for neonate, pediatric, and adult sized cuffs. Care should be taken to choose the appropriate size/setting to avoid inadvertent injury.
3. **Pulse oximetry** is one of the best indicators for the early detection of desaturation. It can also provide plethysmographic data on perfusion and respiratory variation.
4. Observed **end-tidal carbon dioxide measurements** usually will be lower than expected when a nonrebreathing circuit is used, because exhaled gas will be diluted with high flows of fresh gases.
5. **Temperature** should routinely be monitored. In small infants, esophageal, rectal, or axillary probes are acceptable. Once the drapes are placed, the warming blanket and room temperature should be adjusted so that children (especially small infants) do not become hyperthermic.

6. **Urine output** can provide a good reflection of volume status in children. In newborns, 0.5 mL/kg/h is adequate; for infants over 1 month of age, 1.0 mL/kg/h usually indicates adequate renal perfusion.

7. **Noninvasive cardiac output monitoring** is a developing technology that may provide earlier identification of hemodynamic changes in the pediatric patient when compared to the current monitoring methods. When this monitor was compared with transthoracic echocardiography, it was shown to have variability with absolute cardiac output; however, it has been shown to accurately predict volume responsiveness.

8. **EEG** utilization and density spectral array data (see Chapter 11) to determine depth of anesthesia can be a useful tool(s) to monitor the cortical biorhythm in the pediatric patient and prevent anesthetic overdose. Caution is advised in children under 2 years of age due to developmental changes in the EEG signal.

F. **IV setup and supplies**

1. For children less than 10 kg, a control chamber (burette) should be used to prevent inadvertent fluid administration and to quantify the fluid volume given.

2. Extension tubing (low volume) used as a drug push-line connected proximally to the patient facilitates drug administered as close to the IV insertion site as possible and prevents excessive flush fluid administration.

3. For older children, a pediatric infusion set is used where 60 drops equal 1 mL.

4. Extra care should be taken to purge IV tubing of air because right to left shunting of blood (and possibly air) can occur in infants with a patent foramen ovale. An air filter should be used in infants and children with known or suspected intracardiac shunts (some drugs are not compatible with these filters; ie, propofol).

VIII. INDUCTION TECHNIQUES

A. **Infants less than 8 months old** can often be transported to the OR without premedication; anesthesia can then be induced by an inhalation technique (see Section VIII.C.3). The vessel-rich organs are proportionately larger, and the muscle and fat groups are smaller in neonates than in adults, affecting uptake and distribution of inhalation agents (see Chapter 11).

B. **Preoperative sedation options for children 8 months to 5 years old** (without established IV access) include the following:

1. Often children who are older than 5 to 6 years are able to proceed to the procedure without sedation (see Section VI); however, these techniques are useful in special circumstances where sedation in an older child is required (ie, developmental delay, extreme anxiety, etc.)

2. **Oral midazolam,** 0.5 to 0.75 mg/kg, dissolved in sweet syrup, usually produces sedation within 20 minutes, although the time to onset of action can be quite variable. Patients often remain awake but sedated, and, generally, they will have no recall of leaving their parents or of induction of anesthesia.

3. **Oral ketamine,** 5 mg/kg given orally, produces sedation within 10 to 15 minutes and is synergistic with oral midazolam. Emergence time may be prolonged.

4. **Intranasal dexmedetomidine** (0.5-2 µg/kg) is an effective sedative given 30 to 75 minutes prior to induction with relatively preserved respiratory function. It has also been used to reduce emergence delirium, an

adjunct to postoperative pain management, and opioid withdrawal. Side effects can include decreased sympathetic activity, including bradycardia and hypotension. Delayed emergence time should also be anticipated.

5. **Oral clonidine** (4 μg/kg) is an effective sedative medication given approximately 45 minutes prior to induction. Its mechanism is similar to that of dexmedetomidine (α_2-agonist) and has been shown to have good sedating qualities with relatively preserved respiratory function, with side effects including impaired insulin release, bradycardia, and possible hypotension. It has been used to reduce emergence delirium, an adjunct to postoperative pain, and has been added to regional and neuraxial anesthesia techniques for synergistic pain management.

6. **Chloral hydrate** (25-50 mg/kg orally or rectally) is a drug used by pediatricians and radiologists for sedation during procedures. It causes minimal respiratory depression but may need to be repeated.

7. **Pulse oximetry** is used routinely once a patient is sedated.

C. **Inhalation induction**

1. This is the most common approach for pediatric patients, except when a rapid sequence IV induction is indicated.

2. An **excitement stage or "stage two"** of anesthesia with disconjugate gaze, injected conjunctiva, increased airway obstruction, altered breathing pattern, increased risk for laryngospasm and bronchospasm, muscular jerkiness, as well as sympathetic discharge as reflected by elevated heart rate and blood pressure is often encountered during inhalation induction. This is the critical period during induction of anesthesia; therefore, noise and activity in the OR should be minimized during this stage. This stage should be explained to parents if they will be present during induction.

3. **Techniques**

a. **Children 8 months to 5 years old** may be anesthetized after premedication. The inhalational induction can begin with nitrous oxide initially (ie, 4 L/min O_2 and 6 L/min nitrous oxide). Once the effect of the nitrous oxide is apparent, characterized by loss of attention and lack of patient response, the concentration of sevoflurane can be gradually increased in 0.5% to 1% increments.

b. A **slow inhalation induction** may be used in cooperative toddlers and older children who have not received premedication. Children are shown how to breathe through a clear anesthetic mask. O_2 and N_2O are delivered via facemask, and sevoflurane is gradually added to the mixture. An engaging story incorporating breathing instructions can be very useful.

c. A **"single-breath induction"** may be accomplished with a mixture of a volatile anesthetic with nitrous oxide.

1. Loss of consciousness can be achieved with a single vital capacity breath of 8% sevoflurane and 70% N_2O in O_2. Desflurane and isoflurane are pungent volatile anesthetics that are not recommended for inhalation induction.

2. The circuit is primed with 70% N_2O–O_2 and 7% to 8% sevoflurane. The end of the circuit should be occluded with a plug or another reservoir bag. Care should be taken to avoid environmental exposure of anesthetic gas to personnel in the room.

3. Painting the mask with flavor extracts or flavored lip balm may increase acceptance by children.

4. The child is instructed to take a deep breath approaching vital capacity of room air, blow it all out as a forced expiration, and then hold his or her breath. At this point, the anesthetist gently places the mask on the patient's face. The child then takes a deep inspiration of the anesthetic mixture and again holds his or her breath. This sequence is repeated for four or five breaths.

5. Most children will be anesthetized with an adequate vital capacity single-breath sevoflurane inhalational induction within 60 seconds; a few children will need longer.

   d. Children can become frightened, uncooperative, and even combative during an inhalation induction. Should this occur, it is imperative to have a backup plan, such as an IM injection of a sedative or hypnotic medication.

D. Intramuscular induction. For the extremely uncooperative or developmentally delayed child, anesthesia may be induced with ketamine (4-8 mg/kg IM), which takes effect in 3 to 5 minutes. Atropine (0.02 mg/kg IM) or glycopyrrolate (0.01 mg/kg IM) should be mixed with the ketamine to prevent excessive salivation. Midazolam, 0.2 to 0.5 mg/kg IM, may also be given to reduce the chance of emergence delirium.

E. IV induction

  1. For children more than 8 years old: Often, older children may prefer an IV technique rather than a mask. Anesthesia can be induced with propofol (3-4 mg/kg). Ketamine (1-2 mg/kg) is a useful inductive agent in patients requiring hemodynamic stability upon induction. Etomidate (0.2-0.3 mg/kg) can be used in children with major trauma associated with hemodynamic instability or children with cardiomyopathy.

  2. IV induction at this age is often preferable to a mask induction because many older children do not like the smell of volatile anesthetics. Local anesthesia before IV placement can be achieved with subcutaneous injection of lidocaine 1%. Alternatively, **EMLA cream** (a eutectic mixture of 2.5% lidocaine and 2.5% prilocaine), **LMX cream** (lidocaine 4%), or Synera (a heated topical patch with a eutectic mixture of lidocaine and tetracaine) can be applied to the skin approximately 45 minutes before IV placement. EMLA cream is also useful to reduce the pain of accessing a Portacath. The use of the jet injection lidocaine applicator is another method for achieving analgesia for IV placement.

F. Children with "full stomachs"

  1. For **rapid sequence induction,** in general, the same principles apply to infants and children as for adults.

    a. Atropine (0.02 mg/kg) may be given IV to prevent bradycardia, especially if succinylcholine will be used.

    b. Children often require larger doses propofol (3-4 mg/kg) and succinylcholine (1-2.0 mg/kg) because of a larger volume of distribution for these drugs.

    c. Infants with gastric distention (eg, pyloric stenosis) should have their stomachs decompressed with an orogastric tube before induction of anesthesia. This gastric tube should be suctioned again before the trachea is extubated.

    d. Ranitidine (2-4 mg/kg) can be given to decrease gastric volume and increase gastric pH. **Ondansetron** (0.1 mg/kg) can be given for postoperative nausea and vomiting prophylaxis.

    e. Metoclopramide should not be given if gastric outlet or bowel obstruction is suspected.

2. **An awake laryngoscopy and intubation** is an option for the moribund infant or an infant with a grossly abnormal airway (eg, severe craniofacial anomaly) and a "full stomach."

3. **A cuffed endotracheal tube** should be considered for a child with a full stomach. This option minimizes the need for replacing an uncuffed tube that proves too small. The cuff volume can be adjusted to ensure an appropriate air leak.

IX. ENDOTRACHEAL INTUBATION

A. Oral approach

1. Older children are placed in the "sniffing" position using a blanket or shoulder roll. Infants and small children have large occiputs, and a small rolled towel placed under the scapulae can be helpful.

2. During laryngoscopy, the tip of the blade is used to elevate the epiglottis. If this technique does not provide a good view of the glottis, the laryngoscope blade can be placed in the vallecula even with a straight blade.

3. In a previous study done by Hochman and Zeitels et al, it was demonstrated that complete exposure of vocal cord can be achieved by positioning the patient in an alternative flexion-flexion position during intubation. This technique has been practiced in our institute under certain circumstances when clear view of vocal cord cannot be achieved with sniffing position.

4. The distance from the glottis to the carina is about 4 cm in a term neonate. Pediatric endotracheal tubes have a single black line located 2 cm from the tip and a double black line at 3 cm; these markings should be observed while the tube is passed beyond the vocal cords.

5. If resistance is met during intubation, a half-size smaller tube should be tried.

6. After intubation, the chest should be examined for bilateral equal expansion, end tidal CO_2, and the lungs auscultated for equal breath sounds. There should be a leak around an uncuffed tube when 15 to 20 cmH_2O positive pressure is applied. If the leak is present at less than 10 cmH_2O pressure, the endotracheal tube should be exchanged for the next larger size.

7. The chest should be auscultated after every change in head or body position to verify equal bilateral breath sounds. Extension of the head can result in extubation, while flexion can result in tube advancement into either mainstem bronchus.

8. Endotracheal tubes should be securely taped and the numerical marking on the tube closest to the gingiva noted; migration of the endotracheal tube will be apparent from any change in this relation.

B. Nasal approach

1. This method is generally similar to that for adults (see Chapter 14).

2. The cephalad position of the infant larynx makes unaided intubation difficult; Magill forceps or a fiberoptic scope is frequently needed to guide the tip of the tube through the vocal cords.

3. Nasal intubation should be performed only when specifically indicated (eg, oral surgery) because of the risk of epistaxis from enlarged adenoids.

C. Muscle relaxants

1. **Muscle relaxants** often are used to facilitate endotracheal intubation. Muscle relaxants may be contraindicated in infants and children with abnormal airway anatomy.

2. **Succinylcholine** can cause bradycardia and may be exaggerated with repeated doses. Atropine (0.02 mg/kg) may be given before administration of succinylcholine in infants or children with immature respiratory and autonomic nervous systems. The use of succinylcholine in children with occult myopathies may result in life-threatening hyperkalemia, manifesting as wide complex bradycardia, ventricular tachycardia, ventricular fibrillation, or asystole. A history of mild muscle weakness or failure to attain age-appropriate physical milestones may be absent, as the Duchenne and Becker types of muscular dystrophy may not be apparent until the child is 4 years of age. Any suspicion of muscle weakness, particularly in male infants, should warrant a preoperative creatine kinase level. The FDA "black box" warns that "succinylcholine in children should be reserved for emergency intubation or instances where immediate securing of the airway is necessary, for example, laryngospasm, difficult airway, full stomach." Succinylcholine should be avoided in children with a close family history of malignant hyperthermia (see Chapter 19).

3. **Rocuronium** (0.6-1.2 mg/kg) has a quick onset of action (40-90 seconds), and in most cases, this drug has replaced succinylcholine when a rapid sequence induction is mandated. Reduced dosing (0.25-0.5 mg/kg) is recommended in infants due to pharmacokinetic/dynamic properties.

4. Routine neuromuscular relaxation can be achieved with **cisatracurium** (0.1-0.2 mg/kg).

5. For very long cases (eg, craniotomy and cardiac surgery), **pancuronium** (0.1 mg/kg) is an option which has the wanted side-effect of supporting the heart rate in pediatric patients.

6. Reversal of neuromuscular blockade with **neostigmine** (0.05-0.06 mg/kg) and an anticholinergic drug (eg, atropine or glycopyrrolate) should occur if the twitch monitor (train of 4 ratio is less than 0.9) or clinical examination suggests weakness.

D. The **laryngeal mask airway** (see Chapter 14) has revolutionized pediatric anesthesia. It has replaced the mask airway for simple cases (eg, herniorrhaphy) and the endotracheal tube for many procedures (eg, MRI or CT scan).

X. ANALGESIA

Perioperative/periprocedural pediatric pain evaluation, treatment, and monitoring are essential to mitigate biologic and psychological stresses and improve long-term outcomes. Multiple methods are used for treatment of pediatric pain and include nonpharmacologic and pharmacologic techniques. These include neuraxial, regional, nonopioid, and opioid pharmacotherapy.

XI. PHARMACOTHERAPY

A. Nonopioid pharmacotherapeutic agents can be used as sole or adjuvant therapy for the treatment of pain. Common medications include the following:

1. **Acetaminophen** 10 to 15 mg/kg PO (IV administration is also 10-15 mg/kg) and 30 to 45 mg PR. Daily dosing should not exceed 75 mg/kg for children, 60 mg/kg for neonates, and 45 mg/kg for preterm infants.

2. **Ketorolac** given 0.5 mg/kg IV or 1 mg/kg IM (given q6h). Caution is used in patients less than 2 years old.

3. Additional agents include ketamine, gabapentin, dexmedetomidine, clonidine, and magnesium.

TABLE 33.8	Guidelines for Opioid Administration in Pediatric Patients		
Drug	**Starting IV Dose and Interval**	**Parenteral: Oral Dose Ratio**	**Starting Oral Dose and Interval**
Codeine	–	–	0.5-1 mg/kg q 3-4 h
Morphine	0.05-0.1 mg/kg q2-4 h	1:3	0.3 mg/kg q 3-4 h
Oxycodone	–	–	0.1-0.2 mg/kg every 3-4 h
Methadone	0.1 mg/kg every 4-8 h	1:2	0.1 mg/kg every 4-8 h
Fentanyl	0.5-1.0 µg/kg every 1-2 h Infusion: 0.5-2.0 µg/kg/h	–	–
Hydromorphone	0.02 mg/kg every 2-4 h	1:4	0.04-0.08 mg/kg every 3-4 h
Meperidine	0.8-1.0 mg/kg every 2-3 h	1:4	2-3 mg/kg every 3-4 h
Remifentanil	0.1-0.25 µg/kg 1-4 µg/kg for intubation Infusion 0.05-0.15 µg/kg/min	–	–

B. Opioid therapy is summarized in **Table 33.8.** There are multiple PO and IV agents to achieve analgesia. Codeine received a black box warning by the FDA in 2013 and warning in 2012 for tonsillectomy and adenoidectomy and caution in postsurgical pediatric for rare but adverse events (rapid metabolism to morphine), respectively. Controversy exists surrounding the use of remifentanil and the induction of rapid tolerance and hyperalgesia. It should also be noted that clearance is higher in neonatal patients. As previously discussed, remifentanil can be used to facilitate endotracheal intubation; caution should be taken due to the side effects of hypotension and bradycardia, especially with elevated dosing.

C. **Regional and neuraxial anesthesia** for pediatric patients has gained acceptance because of a better understanding of the pharmacokinetics and pharmacodynamics of local anesthetics in infants and children and the availability of specifically designed equipment. In addition, regional anesthesia has been demonstrated to be safe when performed during general anesthesia, and complication rates are comparable under general anesthesia versus sedated or awake children.

D. **Pharmacology of local anesthetics**
1. **Protein binding** of local anesthetics is decreased in neonates because of decreased levels of serum albumin. Free drug concentration may be increased, especially for bupivacaine.
2. **Plasma cholinesterase activity** may be decreased in infants less than 6 months old, which theoretically diminishes clearance of amino esters.
3. **Hepatic microsomal enzyme systems** are immature in the neonate, and this will decrease the clearance of amino amides.
4. **The increased volume of distribution** in the infant and child acts to decrease free local anesthetic concentrations in the blood.

5. **Systemic toxicity** is the most frequent complication of regional anesthetics, and doses should be carefully calculated on a weight basis. The risk of accumulation of free drug after repeated doses of local anesthetics is increased in infants and children.

E. **Brachial plexus block and additional regional blocks.**

F. **Brachial plexus blocks** (for upper extremity surgery), **penile blocks** (for circumcision), and **ilioinguinal blocks** (for inguinal herniorrhaphy) are particularly useful and common regional techniques in the pediatric population. In addition, regional techniques as performed in pediatric patients as in the adult population have yielded great postoperative analgesia and are discussed in Chapter 18.

G. **Spinal anesthesia**

1. **Indications**

   a. Premature infants less than 60 weeks postconceptual age and infants with a history of apnea and bradycardia, BPD, or need for long-term ventilatory support are at increased risk for apnea and cardiovascular instability after general anesthesia. Spinal anesthesia may decrease the likelihood of these postoperative anesthetic complications. The benefit of spinal anesthesia is beyond postoperative pain management. These techniques in infants can avoid airway instrumentation, decrease the risk of early postoperative apnea, and maintain hemodynamic stability. In the Cochrane review done by Jones LJ et al, it was demonstrated that moderate-quality evidence supports spinal anesthesia is preferred comparing to general anesthesia with possible risk of postoperative apnea reduced up to 47% in preterm infants. The number needed to treat is estimated at 4. In the recently published study done by Liu et al, it is demonstrated that infants that received spinal anesthesia for hernia repair have significantly lower r-FLACC score (the revised Face, Legs, Activity, Cry, and Consolability score) and less requirement for acetaminophen postoperatively in infants younger than 60 weeks postmenstrual age comparing to general anesthesia. These infants still require a minimum of 24 hours of cardiorespiratory monitoring postoperatively, regardless of the anesthetic technique. IV or inhalational medications during spinal anesthesia may negate the potential benefits of protection toward early postoperative apnea.

   b. Children at risk for malignant hyperthermia.

   c. Children with chronic airways disease such as reactive airway disease or cystic fibrosis.

   d. Cooperative older children and adolescents with full stomachs undergoing peripheral emergency surgery (eg, fractured ankle).

2. **Anatomy.** The spinal cord in an infant terminates at approximately L3 and does assume the adult L1-L2 termination until approximately 12 months.

3. **Technique**

   a. The procedure may be performed with the patient in the lateral decubitus or sitting position in the OR using a team approach. All infants undergoing spinal anesthesia had EMLA cream applied to the L4-L5 interspace and covered with a Tegaderm for 30 minutes before coming into operation room. An assistant is present for positioning the infant (refer to **Figure 33.1**). Premature infants and neonates are positioned in the sitting position to limit rostral spread of drug. The head is supported upright to prevent upper airway obstruction. A 22-gauge 1.5-inch spinal needle is used for infants, because CSF

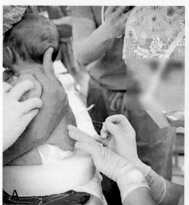 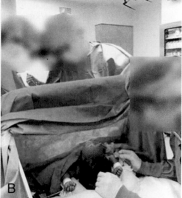

FIGURE 33.1 Demonstration of spinal anesthesia for infant surgeries. A, Optimized patient position for spinal anesthesia is achieved using a team approach. B, An ether screen was placed so that the awake patient could be monitored, soothed, and reached easily during surgery. It is crucial to position infants in a way so that they are ready for induction of general anesthesia and intubation at any time during the spinal.

flow can be very slow especially with a smaller needle. In children older than 2 years, a 25-gauge needle is acceptable. A timer is started as soon as the spinal is placed. We place IV catheter in one of the extremities following the placement of spinal anesthesia. Absence of infant response to attempted IV placement in the lower extremity or detection of lower extremity motor paralysis was used as an indication for successful onset of spinal anesthesia. If an IV was unable to be placed in the lower extremities, it was then attempted in the upper extremities. The surgeons are informed of the time since spinal placement at 30, 45, and 60 minutes to help track progression of the surgery.

b. Patient should be monitored throughout the procedure. Maintaining normothermia is essential, especially for premature infants and neonates. The infant should remain supine after placement of the spinal anesthetic; the Trendelenburg position and leg raising should be avoided because of possible cephalad migration in the subarachnoid space. Special attention should be paid to the tone of crying in the infants under spinal anesthesia. Muffled or weaken crying is a sign of high spinal in this population. Rarely, transient Horner syndrome has been reported in this population with no report for long-term effect so far.

4. **Drugs and dosage**
   a. Hyperbaric solutions of bupivacaine or tetracaine are used most frequently.
   b. The dosage requirements are increased, and the duration of action is decreased in infants.
   c. **Recommended dosages** for infants, for a T6 level of anesthesia.
      1. **Bupivacaine** 0.5% (isobaric solution): 0.5 to 1 mg/kg.
      2. **Bupivacaine** 0.75% in 8.25% dextrose: 0.5 to 1 mg/kg.

    3. **Tetracaine,** 1% in 5% dextrose: 0.8 to 1.0 mg/kg in an infant and 0.25 to 0.5 mg/kg in a child. This dose is large compared with adult dosage, but it is necessary in infants.

  d. **Duration of surgical anesthesia** averages 90 minutes with both tetracaine and bupivacaine. Multiple agents have been added to the local anesthetic in attempts to prolong the block. **Epinephrine** 2 to 5 µg/kg and **clonidine** 1 µg/kg have been shown to prolong duration of spinal block.

5. **Complications and contraindications**

  a. **The anesthetic level** recedes more quickly in children than in adults. If the block subsides, supplemental sedation must be used cautiously, especially in premature infants and neonates. If subarachnoid anesthesia is inadequate, it is best to initiate general anesthesia before positioning.

  b. **Hypotension** is rare in children less than 7 to 10 years old, perhaps because resting sympathetic vascular tone is lower than in adults. A high spinal anesthetic may be heralded only by mottled skin or apnea and bradycardia.

  c. **Contraindications** are similar to those in adults, with particular attention to congenital anatomic defects of the central nervous system and a history of intraventricular hemorrhage.

H. **Caudal and epidural anesthesia**

1. **Indications.** These techniques are useful in combination with general anesthesia for minor and major procedures of the thorax, abdomen, pelvis, bladder, and lower extremities, particularly when significant postoperative pain is anticipated (eg, orthopedic surgery).

2. **Anatomy** is outlined in Chapter 17. Note that the dural sac ends at the level of the S3 vertebra in the neonate; care is required to avoid dural puncture during placement of the caudal needle.

3. **Technique** is outlined in Chapter 17.

  a. Most caudal and lumbar epidural anesthetics are placed after induction of general anesthesia.

  b. **Caudal anesthesia** may be administered as a single injection of local anesthetic through a 1.5-inch, short-bevel styletted needle placed into the caudal epidural space. This technique is ideally suited for short procedures with mild-to-moderate postoperative pain such as inguinal herniorrhaphy, orchiopexy, and circumcision. For longer procedures or prolonged postoperative analgesia, a catheter may be advanced from the sacral epidural space. Intermittent boluses or a continuous infusion of local anesthetic with or without an opioid may be used. In infants, 22-gauge caudal catheters are placed through 20-gauge, 40- to 50-mm Tuohy needles; older children require 20-gauge catheters placed through 17- or 18-gauge, 90- to 100-mm Tuohy needles.

  c. **Caudal catheters** can be advanced to lumbar or thoracic levels in young children because the epidural space is not yet extensively vascularized. The recommended levels are T6-T9 vertebral level for thoracic surgery (eg, pectus excavatum repair), T10-T12 vertebral level for abdominal surgery (eg, Nissen fundoplication or bowel resections), and L3-L4 vertebral level for pelvic procedures. Usually, these catheters advance easily; resistance may indicate malpositioning. If necessary, confirmation of catheter placement can be done with contrast dye, stimulation, ECG, and fluoroscopy techniques. While easy to place when compared with a lumbar catheter, the caudal catheter has a greater potential to become contaminated from stool. Also, the catheter may become dislodged postoperatively.

d. **Epidural catheters** may be placed via lumbar or thoracic approaches. The distance from the skin to the epidural space is short (1-2 cm) in children, and, again, care must be taken to avoid dural puncture. Loss of resistance is usually accomplished with saline. In older children, 18-gauge Tuohy needles and 20-gauge catheters are used. Thoracic catheters are useful for petus excavation repair or thoracotomy.

4. **Drugs and doses**

   a. In **single-dose caudal anesthesia,** a long duration of sensory blockade with minimal motor blockade is desirable. Bupivacaine, 0.125% to 0.25% with epinephrine, is administered according to the formula of 0.06 mL of local anesthetic per kg per segment, where the number of segments is counted from the S5 spinal level to the desired level of analgesia. A simple alternative dosing scheme is to administer 0.125% bupivacaine with epinephrine at a dose of 1 to 1.25 mL/kg. Increasing the concentration of bupivacaine above 0.25% does not appear to improve analgesia. Dosages of bupivacaine 2.5 mg/kg without epinephrine and 3 mg/kg with epinephrine result in plasma levels in infants and children below the toxic range determined for adults. Ropivacaine 2% has been successfully used in caudal anesthesia at doses of 1 mL/kg for minor elective surgery. The addition of **clonidine** 0.5 to 2 μg/kg to bupivacaine prolongs the duration of analgesia by 2 to 3 hours. It may cause increased sedation postoperatively and should be avoided in babies at risk of apnea (neonates and ex-preterm infants).

   b. **Continuous infusion:** Bupivacaine 0.05% to 0.1% or ropivacaine 0.2% can be infused epidurally at a dose of 0.2 to 0.3 mg/kg/h in infants and 0.2 to 0.4 mg/kg/h in children. Opioids may be added in μg to the local anesthetic solution: fentanyl (1-3 μg/mL), infused at 0.3 to 1 μg/kg/h; morphine 5 to 10 μg/mL, infused at 1 to 5 μg/kg/h; or hydromorphone 3 to 7 μg/mL, infused at 1 to 2.5 μg/kg/h. Infants younger than 6 to 12 months generally do not receive opioids in the epidural infusion, unless they are in a closely monitored setting.

   c. **Postoperative analgesia** may be provided by infusion through the caudal or epidural catheter. Generally, an infusion of 0.1% bupivacaine with fentanyl, 1 to 3 μg/mL at 0.3 to 1 μg/kg/h, will provide good analgesia without motor blockade. However, some patients benefit from omission of local anesthetic from the infusion, and fentanyl, 0.5 to 1 μg/kg/h, can be used in these patients. Because of concern about postoperative respiratory depression, infants younger than 6 to 12 months generally do not receive epidural opioids unless they are in a closely monitored setting. These infants receive an infusion of 0.1% bupivacaine, 0.2 to 0.4 mL/kg/h.

5. **Contraindications** are the same as for spinal anesthesia (see Section XI.F.5).

   Chlorhexidine use in infants less than 2 months old or with skin breakdown is controversial due to systemic absorption and risk of burn injury.

6. **Complications** of epidural and caudal anesthesia are discussed in Chapter 17.

XII. FLUID MANAGEMENT

The following calculations may be used to estimate fluid requirements for infants and children. Other reflections of volume status, including clinical exam, blood pressure, heart rate, urine output, central venous pressure, pulse pressure variation, straight leg raise, noninvasive cardiac output monitoring, fluid challenge, and osmolarity, may guide further adjustments.

A. Maintenance fluid requirements

1. Administer 4 mL/kg/h for the first 10 kg of body weight (100 mL/kg/d), 2 mL/kg/h for the second 10 kg (50 mL/kg/d), and then add 1 mL/kg/h for more than 20 kg (25 mL/kg/d). For example, maintenance fluids for a 25-kg child would be ([4 mL/kg × 10 kg] + [2 mL/kg × 10 kg] + [1 mL/kg × 5 kg]) = 65 mL/h.

2. The usual solution for replacement of fluid deficits and ongoing losses in the healthy child is **lactated Ringer solution**. A second solution of 5% dextrose is frequently used in the perioperative period for premature infants, septic neonates, infants of diabetic mothers, and those receiving total parenteral nutrition. These patients should have their blood glucose levels measured periodically.

B. Estimated blood volume (EBV) and blood losses

1. **EBV** is 95 mL/kg in premature neonates, 80 to 90 mL/kg in full-term neonates, 75 to 80 mL/kg in infants up to 1 year old, and 70 mL/kg thereafter.

2. **Acceptable blood loss (ABL).** ABL can be estimated with a simple formula. This should be used with caution if fluid redistribution/equilibration has not occurred.

   $$ABL = EBV \times (Hct_{initial} - Hct_{acceptable})/Hct_{initial}$$

   General guidelines are as follows:

   a. If the amount of the blood loss is less than one-third of the ABL, it can be replaced with lactated Ringer solution.

   b. If the amount of blood loss is greater than ABL, replace with packed red blood cells (leukoreduced, CMV negative, and irradiated). Fresh frozen plasma and platelet transfusions should be guided by the results of coagulation tests, estimates of the present and anticipated blood losses, and adequacy of clot formation in the wound.

   c. For infants and young children, blood loss should be measured using small suction containers and by weighing sponges. Because it is sometimes difficult to measure small-volume blood losses precisely in young children, monitoring of hemoglobin and hematocrit will help avoid unnecessary transfusions and also alert the anesthetist to the need for blood transfusion.

   d. The **"acceptable hemoglobin and hematocrit"** is no longer considered to be 10 g/dL and 30%. Each patient is evaluated with regard to the need for red blood cell transfusion. A healthy child with normal cardiac function can compensate for acute anemia by increasing cardiac output. A premature infant, a debilitated child, a child with sepsis, a child receiving chemotherapy, or one facing massive surgery may require a higher hemoglobin.

C. Estimated fluid deficit = (maintenance fluid per hour) × hours since the last oral intake. The entire estimated fluid deficit replaced during all major cases; the first half is administered during the first hour, and the remaining deficit is infused over the next 1 to 2 hours.

D. Third-space losses may require up to an additional 10 mL/kg/h of lactated Ringer solution or normal saline if there is extensive exposure of the intestine or a significant ileus.

XIII. EMERGENCE AND POST-ANESTHESIA CARE
A. Extubation
1. **Laryngospasm** may occur during emergence, especially during the critical period of the excitement stage before consciousness returns.
2. In most cases, the trachea is extubated after emergence from anesthesia. Coughing is not a sign that the child is ready for extubation. Instead, children should demonstrate purposeful activity (eg, reaching for the endotracheal tube) or eye opening before extubation. In the infant, hip flexion, strong grimaces and purposeful movements are useful indications of awakening.
3. Alternatively, the trachea may be extubated while the patient is in a deep plane of anesthesia with spontaneous ventilation. This can be done in operations such as inguinal herniorrhaphy where coughing on emergence is undesirable or in patients with reactive airways disease. Extubation under deep anesthesia is not appropriate for the child with a full stomach; a child whose trachea was difficult to intubate or the child who had oral or laryngeal surgery. Clinical judgment is essential.
4. **Emergence delirium** is a relatively common post-anesthetic event and can be difficult to differentiate from pain. Common risk factors include age (1 to 5 years old), surgery type (ENT/ophthalmic procedures), preoperative anxiety, preoperative medication, rapid emergence, and pain. Treatment options after treating pain include early reunion with parents, fentanyl (1 μg/kg), propofol (1 mg/kg), and dexmedetomidine (0.5 μg/kg).
B. During transport to the post-anesthesia care unit (PACU), the child's color and ventilatory pattern should be continuously monitored. Supplemental oxygen may be administered if indicated (eg, the child with anemia or pulmonary disease).
C. In the PACU, early reunion of the child and parents is desirable. Discharge criteria often follow the Aldrete Scoring system (motor function, breathing, blood pressure, consciousness, and oxygenation) as well as pain control. In addition, extended postoperative/procedural monitoring of infants and children should be considered on a case-by-case basis (obstructive sleep apnea, prematurity, children less than 3 years who underwent airway surgery including tonsillectomy, etc.).

XIV. SPECIFIC PEDIATRIC ANESTHESIA PROBLEMS
A. The compromised airway
1. **Etiologies**
   a. Congenital abnormalities (eg, choanal atresia, Pierre Robin syndrome, tracheal stenosis, or laryngeal web).
   b. Inflammation (eg, tracheobronchitis or "croup," epiglottitis, and pharyngeal abscess).
   c. Foreign bodies (FBs) in the trachea or esophagus.
   d. Neoplasms (eg, congenital hemangioma, cystic hygroma, or thoracic lymphadenopathy).
   e. Trauma.
2. **Initial management**
   a. Administer 100% oxygen by face mask (continually assess oxygenation and ventilation).
   b. Keep the child as calm as possible. Evaluation should be efficient, because it may increase agitation and cause further airway compromise. Parents are invaluable in their ability to pacify their children and should remain with them as long as feasible.

c. An anesthetist must be present during transport to the OR. Oxygen, a resuscitation bag and mask, laryngoscope, atropine, succinylcholine, drugs suitable for sedation and hypnosis, appropriate endotracheal tubes and laryngeal mask airways, oral airways, and pulse oximetry must be available.

3. **Induction of anesthesia with a compromised airway**
    a. **Minimize manipulation of the patient.** A precordial stethoscope and pulse oximeter are adequate monitors during the initial induction of anesthesia.
    b. The child may remain in a **semisitting position,** with the parents present if indicated. A **gradual inhalation induction** with sevoflurane is the next step (see Section VIII.C.3). Airway obstruction and poor air exchange will prolong induction.
    c. Parents are asked to leave when the child becomes unconscious, and an IV is started. If indicated, atropine may be given at this time. Alternatively, a preinduction IV may be started if there is concern for acute decompensation and proceed with IV or inhalational induction.
    d. **Patients with croup** may benefit from gentle application of CPAP, but any positive pressure can cause acute airway obstruction in patients with epiglottitis or an FB.
    e. The **oral endotracheal tube** should have a stylet and be at least one size smaller than the predicted size. If postoperative ventilation is anticipated (eg, epiglottitis), a cuffed endotracheal tube may be indicated.
    f. At this point, patients usually are hypercarbic ($ETCO_2$ between 50 and 60 mm Hg), but generally, this is well tolerated. Bradycardia is an indication of hypoxemia and requires immediate establishment of a patent airway.
    g. Perform laryngoscopy only when the child is deeply anesthetized. The decision to give a muscle relaxant depends on the situation. A muscle relaxant facilitates intubation and obviates the need for deep anesthesia in certain circumstances. In other cases, muscle relaxation may further compromise the airway. In general, orotracheal intubation should be accomplished before any further airway procedures are attempted. **Bronchoscopy** is indicated before intubation in cases of large upper airway FBs or friable subglottic tumors (eg, hemangioma).
    h. **A nasal tube** may be more appropriate for illnesses that require several days of intubation (eg, epiglottitis). An orotracheal tube may be changed to a nasotracheal tube at the end of the procedure, provided the oral intubation was easily accomplished. Never jeopardize a secure oral endotracheal tube for the sake of changing it to a nasal endotracheal tube.
    i. Children should be sedated during transport to the intensive care unit. A combination of a narcotic and a benzodiazepine, propofol infusion, or dexmedetomidine infusion or bolus can be effective. Breathing may be spontaneous or assisted during the immediate postoperative period. Propofol is not approved by the FDA for sedation of pediatric intensive care patients due to the risk of propofol infusion syndrome and its associated metabolic derangements.

4. **Management of the inhaled foreign body (FB)**
    a. FB aspiration usually occurs between 7 months and 4 years of age. About 75% of FBs lodge in the proximal airway (larynx, trachea, and right/left mainstem bronchus). Most deaths occur at the time

of aspiration, and the mortality in most series is zero if the child reaches the hospital alive.

b. Choking and wheezing following a witnessed aspiration event is the most common **presentation**. The triad of coughing, wheezing, and reduced breath sounds is present in only 50% of cases. CXR may show radiopaque objects, postobstructive emphysema, or a localized pneumonia but has a false-negative rate of 40%.

c. **Management** is prompt rigid bronchoscopy regardless of CXR findings. It is vital to communicate with the bronchoscopist before and during the procedure. An emergency tracheotomy and thoracotomy kit should be prepared. There are two approaches to the anesthetic: spontaneous ventilation and controlled ventilation.

d. **Spontaneous ventilation:** After preoxygenation and IV atropine or glycopyrrolate, a sevoflurane/100% oxygen induction is performed. Sevoflurane is preferred for inhalational induction, and spontaneous ventilation is maintained. Once an adequate depth is achieved, the vocal cords and subglottic space are sprayed with topical lidocaine (2% for school age children and 1% for small infants). The trachea is then intubated with a ventilating bronchoscope. A sufficient depth of anesthesia is required to prevent moving and coughing. Consider a small dose of muscle relaxant just before removal of the FB through the vocal cords. The stomach is then suctioned, and the patient is allowed to emerge breathing through either a mask or an endotracheal tube placed after FB removal. Advantages of this technique are better air flow distribution and ventilation-perfusion matching, uninterrupted ventilation, and the ability to immediately assess ventilatory mechanics after FB removal. Disadvantages are the risks of patient movement, coughing, laryngospasm, and prolonged emergence.

e. **Controlled ventilation:** Anesthesia is commenced with a rapid sequence induction using propofol and a muscle relaxant. Maintenance anesthesia can be provided with propofol and remifentanil infusions and muscle relaxant. The trachea is intubated with a ventilating bronchoscope, and ventilation is performed in concert with the bronchoscopist's interventions. When the bronchoscope is in place, ventilation is achieved with high inspiratory pressures, and long expiratory times are necessary to prevent barotrauma. Emergence is achieved in a manner similar to the spontaneous ventilation technique. The advantages of controlled ventilation are rapid control of the airway, no patient movement, and lower anesthetic requirements. However, ventilation is intermittently interrupted, and there are risks of displacing the FB distally and causing barotrauma with ball-valve hyperinflation.

f. A large retrospective study showed that **ventilatory technique** did not affect the success of FB removal or influence adverse outcomes (hypoxia, hypercarbia, bradycardia, and hypotension).

g. Subglottic edema resulting in postextubation croup can be treated with humidified oxygen. If symptoms are severe, then racemic epinephrine (0.5 mL of a 2% solution in 2-4 mL of volume) can be given. In addition, dexamethasone (0.25-0.5 mg/kg up to 8 mg) should be considered.

B. Recent upper respiratory infection. Infants and children can have 6 to 10 upper respiratory infections each year. It is important to balance the severity of symptoms with the urgency of surgery. Wheezing, fever, and cough are signs of lower respiratory inflammation and are associated with an increased risk of perioperative airway complications. Conversely, myringotomy and ear tube placement may relieve the rhinorrhea associated with chronic otitis media.

C. **Intra-abdominal malformations** include pyloric stenosis, gastroschisis, omphalocele, atresia of the small intestine, and volvulus (see Chapter 30).

1. **Gastrointestinal emergencies** frequently produce marked dehydration and electrolyte abnormalities. Repair of pyloric stenosis should be delayed until intravascular volume is restored and the hypokalemic, hypochloremic, and metabolic alkalosis is corrected. The situation is more urgent with other diagnoses (eg, duodenal atresia), and rehydration can be continued intraoperatively.

2. **Abdominal distention** in infants and young children rapidly causes respiratory compromise, so nasogastric drainage is mandatory. Even so, a few moribund infants may require endotracheal intubation before the induction of anesthesia.

3. Children with less severe physiologic disturbances and only mild or moderate distention can undergo a rapid sequence induction of anesthesia.

4. A severely dehydrated and septic child may require additional monitoring (eg, arterial line, central venous line, and urinary catheter).

5. Volatile anesthetics are appropriate for the previously healthy infant undergoing a simple operation (such as pyloromyotomy). In the case of an extremely ill child (eg, perforated viscous), the anesthetic management should include an O_2-air mixture and drugs causing minimal myocardial depression. Opioids, benzodiazepines, and neuromuscular relaxants are usually better tolerated than volatile anesthetics. Nitrous oxide should be avoided because it may add to abdominal distention.

6. **Fluid and heat losses.** When the bowel is exposed and manipulated, third-space losses may be excessive, and remarkable fluid volumes may be necessary. Even when using all possible warming strategies, heat loss may be unavoidable.

7. Postoperative ventilatory support is often indicated until abdominal distention is diminished, hypothermia resolves, and fluid requirements decrease.

D. **Thoracic emergencies**
1. **Tracheoesophageal fistula.** See Chapter 30.
2. **Congenital diaphragmatic hernia.** See Chapter 30.

E. **Congenital heart disease.** See Chapters 2, 23, and 30.

F. **Head and neck procedures**
1. Strabismus repair. See Chapter 26.
2. Tonsillectomy, adenoidectomy, and emergency surgery in the child with bleeding tonsils. See Chapter 26.

G. **Potential for neurotoxicity of general anesthetics**
1. In vivo and in vitro animal models of neuronal cell death have been demonstrated with almost all of the commonly used anesthetic agents (ie, propofol, ketamine, desflurane, halothane, isoflurane, sevoflurane, xenon, diazepam, midazolam, chloral hydrate, pentobarbital). However, the long-term outcomes regarding neurodevelopmental effects and tests of memory and cognitive processing in animal studies are mixed and call into question the effects of anesthetic drugs. Furthermore, significant limitations in animal studies (ie, developmental equivalence, dosing/duration of exposure controlled for life span, study design, etc.) preclude extrapolation to our pediatric patient.

2. Due to the in vitro and animal evidence, there has been growing concern regarding the long-term developmental effects of general anesthesia on our pediatric patients. The data regarding the long-term outcomes of pediatric patients exposed to general anesthesia early in development are mixed and have several limitations (ie, study design, anesthetic used, surgical exposure, comorbidities, etc.). The first prospective randomized control trial (GAS; NCT00756600) investigating the effects of general versus regional anesthesia on neurodevelopmental outcomes in infants undergoing inguinal hernia repair has concluded in two publications, Davidson et al and McCann et al. The "GAS study" showed that in healthy children receiving a single sevoflurane exposure of slightly less than 1 hour in duration, there is no change in intelligence scores at 2-year and 5-year of age. The long-term developmental effects of longer exposure duration, multiple exposures, and in children who have comorbidities remain unclear.

3. In advising a parent or caregiver concerned about the neurodevelopmental effects of general anesthesia, it may be helpful to discuss several points below:

   a. Alternatives if possible to general anesthesia (ie, spinal anesthesia).
   b. Necessity of surgical/procedural intervention.
   c. Necessity of anesthesia if surgery is indicated.
   d. Not exceeding the required amount of anesthesia for the indicated procedure to accomplish procedural and patient comfort goals.
   e. Uncertainty regarding the human and animal data.

Suggested Readings

Anand KJS, Hickey PR. Pain and its effects in the human neonate and fetus. *N Engl J Med.* 1987;317:1321-1329.

Arant BSJ. Developmental patterns of renal functional maturation compared in the human neonate. *J Pediatr.* 1978;92:705-712.

Bahrami KR, Van Meurs KP. ECMO for neonatal respiratory failure. *Semin Perinatol.* 2005;29:15-23.

Bell EF, Warburton D, Stonestreet BS, et al. Effect of fluid administration on the development of symptomatic patent ductus arteriosus and congestive heart failure in premature infants. *N Engl J Med.* 1980;302:598-604.

Berde CB, Sethna NF. Analgesics for the treatment of pain in children. *N Engl J Med.* 2002;347(14):1094-1103.

Cloherty JP, Eichenwald EC, Hansen AR, Stark AR. *Manual of Neonatal Care.* 7th ed. Lippincott Williams & Wilkins; 2011.

Constant I, Sabourdin N. The EEG signal: a window on the cortical brain activity. *Paediatr Anaesth.* 2012;22(6):539-552.

Cote CJ, Lerman J, Anderson BJ. *A Practice of Anesthesia for Infants and Children, and Adolescents.* 5th ed. Saunders Elsevier; 2013.

Coté CJ, Sui J, Anderson TA, et al. Continuous noninvasive cardiac output in children: is this the next generation of operating room monitors? Initial experience in 402 pediatric patients. *Paediatr Anaesth.* 2015;25(2):150-159.

Coté CJ, Zaslavsky A, Downes JJ, et al. Postoperative apnea in former preterm infants after inguinal herniorrhaphy. A combined analysis. *Anesthesiology.* 1995;82: 809-822.

Dalal PG, Murray D, Messner AH, et al. Pediatric laryngeal dimensions: an age-based analysis. *Anesth Analg.* 2009;108(5):1475-1479.

Dalens B, Khandwala R. *Regional Anesthesia in Infants, Children, and Adolescents.* Williams & Wilkins; 1995.

Davidson AJ, Disma N, de Graaff JC, et al; GAS Consortium. Neurodevelopmental outcome at 2 years of age after general anaesthesia and awake-regional anaesthesia in infancy (GAS): an international multicentre, randomised controlled trial. *Lancet.* 2016;387(10015):239-250. doi:10.1016/S0140-6736(15)00608-X

Dorsch JA, Dorsch SE. *Understanding Anesthesia Equipment.* 5th ed. Wolters Kluwer Health, Lippincott Williams & Wilkins; 2008.

Duracher C1, Schmautz E, Martinon C, Faivre J, Carli P, Orliaguet G. Evaluation of cuffed tracheal tube size predicted using the Khine formula in children. *Paediatr Anaesth.* 2008;18(2):113-118. doi:10.1111/j.1460-9592.2007.02382.x

Fanaroff AA, Wald M, Gruber HS, et al. Insensible water loss in low birth weight infants. *Pediatrics.* 1972;50:236-245.

Fluge G. Clinical aspects of neonatal hypoglycaemia. *Acta Paediatr Scand.* 1974;63:826-832.

Gallagher TM, Crean PM. Spinal anaesthesia for infants born prematurely. *Anaesthesia.* 1989;44:434-436.

Gersony WM, Peckham GJ, Ellison RC, et al. Effects of indomethacin in premature infants with patent ductus arteriosus: results of a national collaborative study. *J Pediatr.* 1983;102:895-906.

Greeley WJ. *Pediatric Anesthesia.* Churchill Livingstone; 1999.

Gregory GA. *Pediatric Anesthesia.* 4th ed. Churchill Livingstone; 2001.

Hall BD. Choanal atresia and associated multiple anomalies. *J Pediatr.* 1979;95:395-398.

Hochman II, Zeitels SM, Heaton JT. Analysis of the forces and position required for direct laryngoscopic exposure of the anterior vocal folds. *Ann Otol Rhinol Laryngol.* 1999;108(8):715-724.

Johns Hopkins Hospital; Custer JW, Rau RE, Lee CK. *The Harriett Lane Handbook.* 18th ed. Elsevier Health Sciences; 2008.

Keith CG, Doyle LW. Retinopathy of prematurity in extremely low birth weight infants. *Pediatrics.* 1995;95:42-45.

Kliegman RM, Behrman RE, Jenson HB, et al. *Nelson Textbook of Pediatrics.* 18th ed. WB Saunders Elsevier; 2007.

Koehntop DE, Rodman JH, Brundage DM, et al. Pharmacokinetics of fentanyl in neonates. *Anesth Analg.* 1986;65:227-232.

Krane EJ, Haberkern CM, Jacobson LE. Postoperative apnea, bradycardia, and oxygen desaturation in formerly premature infants: prospective comparison of spinal and general anesthesia. *Anesth Analg.* 1995;80:7-13.

Kurth CD, Spitzer AR, Broennle AM, et al. Postoperative apnea in preterm infants. *Anesthesiology.* 1987;66:483-488.

Lin EP, Soriano SG, Loepke AW. Anesthetic neurotoxicity. *Anesthesiol Clin.* 2014;32(1): 133-155.

Marks KH, Devenyi AG, Bello ME, et al. Thermal head wrap for infants. *J Pediatr.* 1985;107:956-959.

McCann ME, de Graaff JC, Dorris L, et al. Neurodevelopmental outcome at 5 years of age after general anaesthesia or awake-regional anaesthesia in infancy (GAS): an international, multicentre, randomised, controlled equivalence trial. *Lancet.* 2019;393(10172):664-677. doi:10.1016/S0140-6736(18)32485-1

Miller RD, ed. *Anesthesia.* 8th ed. Elsevier-Churchill Livingstone; 2009.

Motoyama EK, Brinkmeyer SD, Mutich RL, et al. Reduced FRC in anesthetized infants: effect of low PEEP. *Anesthesiology.* 1982;57:A418.

Motoyama EK, Davis PJ. *Smith's Anesthesia for Infants and Children.* 8th ed. St. Elsevier Mosby-Saunders; 2007.

Moya FR, Lally KP. Evidence-based management of infants with congenital diaphragmatic hernia. *Semin Perinatol.* 2005;29:112-117.

O'Neill JA, Rowe MI, Grosfeld J, et al. *Pediatric Surgery.* 5th ed. Mosby-Year Book; 1998.

Philippart AI, Canty TG, Filler RM. Acute fluid volume requirements in infants with anterior abdominal wall defects. *J Pediatr Surg.* 1972;7:553-558.

Roberts JD Jr, Fineman JR, Morin FC III, et al. Inhaled nitric oxide and persistent pulmonary hypertension of the newborn. The Inhaled Nitric Oxide Study Group. *N Engl J Med.* 1997;336:605-610.

Roberts JD Jr, Polaner DM, Lang P, et al. Inhaled nitric oxide (NO): a selective pulmonary vasodilator for the treatment of persistent pulmonary hypertension of the newborn (PPHN). *Circulation.* 1991;84:A1279.

Roberts JD, Polaner DM, Lang P, et al. Inhaled nitric oxide in persistent pulmonary hypertension of the newborn. *Lancet.* 1992;340:818-821.

Sola A. Oxygen in neonatal anesthesia: friend or foe? *Curr Opin Anaesthesiol.* 2008;21:332-339.

Srinivasan G, Jain R, Pildes RS, et al. Glucose homeostasis during anesthesia and surgery in infants. *J Pediatr Surg.* 1986;21:718-721.

Touloukian RJ, Higgins E. The spectrum of serum electrolytes in hypertrophic pyloric stenosis. *J Pediatr Surg.* 1983;18:394-397.

Tyszczuk L, Meek J, Elwell C, et al. Cerebral blood flow is independent of mean arterial blood pressure in preterm infants undergoing intensive care. *Pediatrics.* 1998;102:337-341.

Taenzer AH, Walker BJ, Bosenberg AT, et al. Asleep versus awake. Does it matter? Pediatric regional block complications by patient state: a report from the Pediatric Regional Anesthesia Network. *Reg Anesth Pain Med.* 2014;39(4):279-283. doi:10.1097/AAP.0000000000000102

Vergnaud E, Vidal C, Montmayeur Verchere J, et al. Noninvasive cardiac output measurement using bioreactance in postoperative pediatric patients. *Paediatr Anaesth.* 2015;25(2):160-166.

Wessel DL, Keane JF, Parness I, et al. Outpatient closure of the patent ductus arteriosus. *Circulation.* 1988;77:1068-1071.

Wright TE, Orr RJ, Haberkern CM, et al. Complications during spinal anesthesia in infants: high spinal blockade. *Anesthesiology.* 1990;73:1290-1292.

Yaster M, Buck JR, Dudgeon DL, et al. Hemodynamic effects of primary closure of omphalocele/gastroschisis in human newborns. *Anesthesiology.* 1988;69:84-88.

Non-Operating Room Anesthesia

Stephanie L. Counihan and Rafael Vazquez

I. GENERAL CONSIDERATIONS

The number of non-operating room anesthesia (NORA) procedures continues to increase rapidly. Ongoing technological advancements and innovations in percutaneous image-guided procedures have continued to rapidly evolve. As a result, procedures have become more technically complex. This has been paired with innovations in anesthetic care for complex cases such as advanced ventilation techniques. NORA locations typically include the following suites: interventional radiology (IR), diagnostic radiology (magnetic resonance imaging [MRI] and computed tomography [CT]), electrophysiology, and endoscopy. Although the same principles and considerations apply to patients who have monitored anesthesia care (MAC) or general anesthesia (GA) outside of the main operating room, this increase in cases is accompanied by an increase of oversight in safety in these remote locations. Three distinctive features characterize NORA: location, operator, and distinctive novelty. Factors relating to ergonomics, lack of anesthesia resources and personnel, and lack of familiarity with the environment are perhaps the biggest and most underestimated considerations. Considering these factors, team communication is paramount as is having a plan for crisis management with appropriate anesthesia equipment to promote patient safety and procedural success.

A. Required equipment in remote locations

1. Ensure that all standards (equipment, safety, patient evaluation) are met prior to the initiation of the anesthetic.
2. Verify a **central supply of oxygen and suction** that is functioning along with **patient supply and scavenging system**. A full reserve tank of O_2 and nitrous should be available. **Adequate electrical outlets and lighting** that are connected and a power source are mandatory. A source of air tank is necessary but not mandatory.
3. **Functioning anesthesia machine** appropriate for the anesthetic. Extra-long gas supply hoses may be necessary; anesthesia breathing circuit tubing may require extensions to reach the patient.
4. **Resuscitation equipment** must be immediately available, such as defibrillator, bag/valve/mask, and emergency and pertinent medications (ie, sugammadex and/or lipid emulsion if doing regional anesthesia).
5. Have a **dedicated NORA anesthesia supply cart** or Omnicell that can dispense controlled substances.
6. Dedicated advanced emergency airway equipment such as video laryngoscope and/or airway cart with a fiberoptic scope.
7. A NORA-specific *cognitive aid* such as an emergency manual to serve as a resource during a crisis situation.

B. Ergonomics and patient access

1. Ensure adequate space to deliver a safe anesthetic with a plan to access the patient if the layout (eg, moving C-arm, CT gantry) is less than ideal.

2. Ensure a means to remotely monitor patient and vital signs (eg, visible anesthesia display in control room) during intraprocedural points where additional irradiation and scans warrants the team exiting the room.

3. Plan in advance for positioning on hard surfaces when anesthetizing in the CT scanner and MRI suite. For prolonged procedures have additional blankets, pillows, prone face foam, etc.

4. Imaging often requires that the patient be moved great lengths frequently in and out of the gantry. Prepare to have additional length on circuit/O_2 tubing, $ETCO_2$, intravenous (IV) tubing, and monitoring cables. A "test scan" of full excursion is helpful prior to starting procedure to ensure the equipment has sufficient slack.

C. **Radiation safety**

1. ALARA—"As low as reasonably achievable" is the main tenant of radiation safety. The goal is to minimize radiation doses to patients, practitioners, and the environment. Three principles aid in ALARA:
   a. Time
   b. Distance
   c. Shielding

2. Radiation exposure is proportional to the distance from the source by a factor of 4. X-ray sources produce scatter. Given that exposure is cumulative, standing as far away as possible from the source is recommended to limit exposure. Extension IV tubing can decrease the radiation exposure to anesthesia providers during medication administration.

3. The use of mobile lead shields and wrap-around lead with a properly fitting thyroid shield is strongly recommended. A personalized radiation dosimetry badge is required to monitor radiation exposure. Lead goggles can be used to decrease radiation to the cornea that may cause cataracts.

II. ANESTHESIA TECHNIQUES

A. **Procedural sedation.** Sedation and analgesia comprise a continuum of states ranging from minimal sedation (anxiolysis) through GA. Specially trained nurses provide sedation for the majority of procedures outside of the operating room for patients deemed ASA I and ASA II. Procedural sedation encompasses **moderate sedation/analgesia**, also known as **conscious sedation (CS)**, and **deep sedation. CS** is defined as "a drug-induced depression of consciousness during which patients respond purposefully to verbal commands, either alone or accompanied by light tactile stimulation. No interventions are required to maintain a patent airway, and spontaneous ventilation is adequate. Cardiovascular function is usually maintained" (American Society of Anesthesiologists. Continuum of depth of sedation definition of GA and levels of sedation/analgesia. October 23, 2019). Common medications include midazolam and fentanyl. **Deep sedation** occurs when a deeper level of consciousness is reached. Patients can be aroused with repeated painful stimuli. Airway manipulation may be needed, and unintended GA may occur. **Deep sedation** requires special privileges and providers in airway management. The American Society of Anesthesiologists (ASA) and Joint Commission on Accreditation of Healthcare Organizations and state agencies (licensing boards) have a set of guidelines for provisions of nonphysicians to deliver conscious and deep sedation.

B. **MAC** is physician-directed anesthesia service performed by a qualified anesthesia provider, for a diagnostic or therapeutic procedure. It does not describe the continuum of depth of sedation. It provides deeper levels of analgesia and sedation than moderate sedation and is beneficial for certain patients and procedures. Advantages include preservation of hemodynamics over GA. Ventilation may be affected, and rescue airway maneuvers may need to be performed. Inadvertent conversion to GA may occur, and equipment should be available. Although a "deep MAC" is appropriate for some patients, the risks/benefits have to be carefully weighed. Various elements factor into this decision including procedure, patient comorbidities, and clinical experience. MAC is associated with fewer hemodynamic perturbations and may be a better choice for a subset of patients with severely compromised cardiovascular function. For high-risk aspiration patients and/or procedures MAC can be performed after careful consideration. Anxiolytic and analgesic techniques if employed should focus on preserving airway reflexes.

C. **GA** is used when a secured airway is necessary, when there is a need for a patient to be still (eg, long complex procedures), and when the procedures involve painful portions. The cardiopulmonary risk/benefits of GA in high-risk patients undergoing minimally invasive procedures have to be carefully considered on a case-by-case basis.

D. **Ultrasound-guided peripheral nerve blocks (PNBs)** may be used as the primary anesthetic or as an adjunct for procedural and/or postprocedural analgesia.
   1. **Brachial plexus nerve blocks** are options for specific dysfunctional arteriovenous access procedures in patients with ESRD.
   2. **Paravertebral nerve block (PVB)** may be beneficial for procedures of the liver and kidney, specifically transhepatic biliary drains, liver ablations and embolizations, and renal ablations. Bilateral T7 to T10 PVB can be beneficial for liver lesions (as the liver is innervated bilaterally), whereas a single PVB suffices for renal procedures.

E. **High-frequency jet ventilation (HFJV)** may be utilized to achieve a quiescent field superior to GA for intrathoracic or peridiaphragmatic percutaneous procedures such a pulmonary vein isolation, basilar pulmonary ablations and embolizations, or ablations of liver dome lesions.

F. **Selective lung isolation** utilizing a double lumen tube or bronchial blockers has been used to achieve a static lung. In addition, these techniques are useful for lung protection of the nonaffected lung from hemorrhage for procedures such as bronchial artery embolizations of patients with hemoptysis and lung ablation of large tumors. A **bronchoscope should be available to verify positioning.**

G. **Enhanced recovery after procedure (ERAP)** is an extension of ERAS and applied in NORA for painful procedures. Application of evidence-based opioid-sparing techniques can decrease post-procedural pain and opioid requirements. Preprocedural analgesics such as acetaminophen, celecoxib, and gabapentin can be beneficial. Administration of high-dose dexamethasone and antiemetics to avoid post-procedure ablation/embolization phenomena. This is most beneficial in the interventional oncology patient population undergoing embolizations and ablations and endoscopic retrograde cholangiopancreatography (ERCP).

III. CONTRAST MEDIA
A. **Ionic and nonionic contrast media** are administered intravenously and intra-arterially to supplement imaging; complexed gadolinium may be administered for both MRI and x-ray–based imaging. Low-osmolality contrast media (hypo and iso osmolar) are preferred over high-osmolality contrast media as they are less nephrotoxic.

1. **Contrast-induced nephropathy (CIN)** is defined as a deterioration in kidney function as a result of intravascular contrast administration.

   a. Risk factors include preexisting renal insufficiency (eGFR < 30) as well as diabetes and HTN. Cardiac angiography procedures are associated with a higher incidence owing to the nature of contrast injection.

   b. Baseline serum creatinine should be obtained in patients considered at risk.

   c. Precontrast IV volume expansion with crystalloid is the mainstay of prophylaxis for CIN. The ideal infusion rate and volume are unknown. Oral hydration has demonstrated less effectiveness. Other therapies do not have strong evidence, such as N-acetylcysteine and sodium bicarbonate.

2. **Nephrogenic systemic fibrosis** is a sclerosing skin condition that occurs after gadolinium exposure in patients with advanced or end-stage renal disease, with or without dialysis. This typically occurs days or months following exposure.

B. **Acute contrast media reactions** to modern contrast agents are rare (0.6% for iodinated and 0.01%-0.22% for gadolinium based) and not dose dependent. They are considered to be anaphylactoid (idiosyncratic) reactions since they are not IgE mediated but possess features of anaphylactic reactions and are unpredictable. Ninety percent of adverse reactions are associated with direct release of histamine and other mediators from mast cells, circulating basophils, and eosinophils.

   1. Risk factors include history of previous adverse reaction, asthma, anxiety, use of β-blockers, and severe cardiac disease.

   2. Symptoms are diverse ranging from a feeling of warmth/flushing, nausea/vomiting to pruritus, urticaria, and more severe with angioedema, hypotension, loss of consciousness, and cardiovascular collapse. They may develop immediately or be delayed up to 30 minutes during the procedure.

   3. Treatment is supportive. Administer corticosteroids and H1 and H2 blockers immediately and transition to additional O_2 or to an endotracheal tube for laryngeal edema and bronchospasm. Beta agonists, epinephrine, and vasopressors may be necessary.

C. **Contrast premedication strategies** reduce the likelihood of a reaction in high-risk patients receiving low-osmolality iodinated contrast media. Effective protocols center on adequate time to achieve effect to decrease circulating basophils and eosinophils. Oral premedication is preferable to IV premedication owing to greater evidentiary support in the literature. Eight-hour protocols are ideal with oral methylprednisolone and diphenhydramine (no evidence for H_2 blocker). This should be initiated by the scheduling providers ahead of time. Accelerated protocols are less than ideal; however, under urgent and emergent circumstances they have to be administered. Accelerated IV premedication as recommended by the American College of Radiologist Manual on Contrast Media (in decreasing order of desirability):

   1. Methylprednisolone 40 mg IV or hydrocortisone 200 mg IV immediately, and then every 4 hours until contrast medium administration, plus diphenhydramine 50 mg IV 1 hour before contrast administration. This regimen is usually 4 to 5 hours in duration.

   2. Dexamethasone sodium 7.5 mg IV and then every 4 hours until contrast administration, plus diphenhydramine 50 mg IV 1 hour before contrast administration.

3. Methylprednisolone 40 mg IV or hydrocortisone 200 mg IV, plus diphenhydramine 50 mg IV, each 1 hour before contrast administration.

These regimens with a duration less than 4 to 5 hours have no evidence of efficacy and are considered in emergent situations when there are no alternatives.

IV. ANESTHESIA FOR DIAGNOSTIC RADIOLOGY

CT scans and MRI are usually performed without GA. Children and uncooperative adults (eg, patients with head injury, claustrophobia, and chronic back pain) may require sedation or GA to minimize motion artifacts.

A. CT

1. **Adults.** Small IV doses of benzodiazepines, narcotics, or short-acting hypnotics (eg, propofol or dexmedetomidine) are useful for sedation; continuous infusions should be titrated to effect.

2. **Infants and children** less than 3 months of age may not need sedation; most children, however, will require some level of sedation or GA. Children provide specific challenges to the anesthetist as outlined in Chapter 33.

   a. Sedation

   1. Small IV doses of benzodiazepines, narcotics, or short-acting hypnotics (eg, propofol) may be used for sedation as either bolus or continuous infusions titrated to effect.

   2. **Chloral hydrate** (30-50 mg/kg orally or per rectum [PR] administered 30-60 minutes before the procedure) is an adequate mild sedative for children.

   3. **Methohexital, PR** (25-30 mg/kg), has more rapid onset (5-10 minutes) than does chloral hydrate and lasts approximately 30 minutes. It is useful for the induction of GA; however, effects may vary because absorption is unpredictable. Because deep sedation or GA may occur, only an anesthetist should administer methohexital with appropriate monitoring and provisions to secure the airway. The drug is not appropriate in patients at risk of reflux of gastric contents.

   b. GA maintained with either IV or inhalational agents may be required. The airway may be maintained naturally, with laryngeal mask airway (LMA) or endotracheal intubation as necessary.

B. Magnetic resonance imaging

1. The physical environment of the MRI suite presents several challenges for anesthetizing patients.

   a. The long, narrow bore of the magnet in which the patient reclines does not allow ready access to or viewing of the patient during imaging. Scanners are located in shielded rooms that contain the magnetic field and shield against radiofrequency noise that would produce image artifacts.

   b. The static **magnetic field is present at all times** and exerts a force on all ferromagnetic materials (eg, steel gas tanks, batteries, and standard stethoscopes). **Ferromagnetic objects brought near the magnetic field can be forcibly pulled toward the magnet, potentially injuring people or equipment in their path.** The static field and magnetic gradients generated during scanning can interfere with mechanical components (solenoids) in automated noninvasive blood pressure monitors, ventilators, and infusion pumps; specialized compatible equipment is necessary. Only plastic stethoscopes and commercially available magnet-compatible laryngoscopes should be used in the magnet area. Credit cards, watches, and pagers must be left outside the scanning room.

c. **Radiofrequency signals** and **shifting magnetic fields** generated during scanning may lead to artifacts on the electrocardiogram (ECG) and pulse oximeter.

d. **Non–MRI-compatible metallic implants (eg, joint prostheses, aneurysm clips, and cochlear implants) or implanted devices (eg, pacemakers, implantable cardioverter defibrillators [ICDs], insulin infusion pumps, intrathecal pumps, or spinal cord stimulators)** may potentially be dislodged, dysfunction, or suffer permanent damage by the magnetic field, and scanning or heating may occur from radiofrequency signals generated during scanning. Some specific pacemakers, ICDs, or pulmonary artery catheters are considered "MRI safe," and scanning can proceed. Imaging of patients with these devices should not be considered routine, and individual cases should be carefully reviewed for medical necessity. Imaging may require that the pacemaker be turned off while the patient is in the magnetic field; the device is turned on after scanning. Cerebral aneurysm clips are not considered an absolute contraindication to MRI; it is important, however, to identify the type of clip present to determine MR compatibility. Each MRI site carries a list of medical devices designated MRI compatible by the US Food and Drug Administration (FDA). Because medical devices may be upgraded or altered by a manufacturer without notifying the FDA, MRI centers should, in addition, contact the manufacturer about specific devices.

2. **Monitors** must be safe for the patient, function within the magnetic field, and have a minimal effect on imaging. Specialized compatible monitoring equipment is available that can remain in the magnetic field and communicate to a "slave" monitor outside the shielded magnet area.

a. The standard ECG is subject to interference during scanning.

b. Scanning interferes with standard **pulse oximeters**, which may also interfere with image acquisition. Specialized "MRI-compatible" monitoring systems utilizing fiberoptic cables are available.

c. A large amount of noise can be generated during imaging.

d. Temperature probes are not used because of the potential for thermal burns.

e. Visualization of patients during scanning is imperative and may occur via a shielded window or closed circuit video.

f. Electrical currents induced in coiled cables during scanning can burn patients; cables should be kept as straight as possible to minimize this risk.

3. **General issues.** The duration of an MRI scan varies. Immobility is required only during the actual scanning, 3 to 12 minutes at a time. GA is necessary for most infants and children, usually utilizing an LMA or endotracheal tube. GA can be induced in the magnet area. Alternatively, induction can be performed in an area out of the static magnetic field and the anesthetized patient moved into the scanner. Maintenance of anesthesia is provided with specially modified anesthesia machines that contain only nonferrous metals. The patient *must* be removed from the magnetic field if cardiopulmonary resuscitation is required. Challenges arise in developmentally delayed adults. A special pathway that may include oral sedative premedication prior to arrival to the scanner and a special induction area can be beneficial for these patients. Coordination with the patient's primary care physician is important. Intramuscular medications may be needed in patients unable to tolerate oral sedative.

V. ANESTHESIA FOR CT-GUIDED THERMAL ABLATIONS

Microwave, radiofrequency, and cryoablation are procedural modalities that utilize extreme thermal energy to induce cell apoptosis. Applicators/probes are guided using CT to the tumor tissue and emit the energy to achieve locoregional tumor treatment of lesions of a certain size (<3.0 cm for liver). The heat modalities include radiofrequency ablation (RFA) and microwave ablation (MWA). RFA involves electrical conduction through tissue, which generates resistive heating to achieve effect via thermal diffusion. Its cost-effectiveness makes it very popular worldwide; however, it is limited by tissue and thermal conductivity. MWA involves dielectric heating. The use of electromagnetic waves at frequencies of 900 to 2450 MHz causes intracellular water molecules to oscillate and produce heat. MWA is not dependent on tissue properties and heats faster in a larger volume. During cryoablation, the rapid expansion of argon gas achieves temperatures as low as -160 °C to freeze and destroy the tumor cells. Each procedure consists of 1 to 3 cycles of freezing and thawing per lesion. An advantage is that the ablation zone can be visualized real time with CT during treatment. In addition, cryoablation preserves collagenous structures; however, there is no coagulation effect and bleeding occurs more readily. If the targeted lesions are adjacent to delicate tissue structures such as bowel or the diaphragm, separation can be created by fluid hydrodissection or pneumoperitoneum with CO_2. A physical distance is created between the zone of ablation and the neighboring tissue to prevent collateral damage.

A. **CT-guided thermal ablations of liver, renal, bone, and soft tissue**
   1. **GA or MAC may be performed and supplemented with regional anesthesia.**
      a. HFJV can be utilized for hepatic dome lesions.
      b. **ERAP** can be beneficial as postprocedural pain can result from large ablations.
      c. Ultrasound-guided bilateral PVB can be beneficial for hepatic and unilateral renal ablations. Short-acting PNB can be used for musculoskeletal procedures.
   2. Discuss positioning with the proceduralist. Pad bony prominences and support the arms in pillow or blankets to be in an extended position without exaggerated abduction. Below are the typical positions; however, communicate and confirm with the IR team.
      a. Liver: supine with arms above head on towel rolls. Take care to not overextend the arms and prevent exaggerated abduction.
      b. Renal: usually lateral decubitus with targeted lesion typically dependent side down. This positioning decreases kidney mobility secondary to respiratory motion. For deep lesions the patients are positioned prone.
      c. Bone and soft tissue: involve heterogeneous lesions in the body including abdomen, retroperitoneum, chest wall, bones of upper extremities, vertebrae, and lower extremity. Patient positioning and anesthetic are variable as is anesthetic technique. Some centers use neuromonitoring when ablations are in delicate areas such as vertebrae or next to nerves.
   3. **Post ablation syndrome** occurs in up to 30% of patients undergoing liver MWA or RFA. The syndrome consists of nausea, fever, malaise, and immediate and delayed postprocedural pain. There is some evidence that this can be mitigated with dexamethasone, analgesics, and hydration.

B. CT-guided lung biopsies and ablations
1. Percutaneous procedures of the lung are becoming more common. Biopsies and ablations are amenable for small tumor lesions in patients who are poor candidates for surgical intervention owing to underlying comorbidities or anatomical reasons, ie, previous chest surgery or location of small tumor. These present special considerations for the anesthesiologist as some procedures can benefit from a static lung field to facilitate ablation, whereas others can benefit from lung isolation to induce pneumothorax (PTX) to separate pleural lesions from the chest wall. Treatment modalities include both heat ablations and cryoablations. Irrespective of modality, hemoptysis is a real concern especially for large ablations.
   a. When anesthesia support is provided the cases can be done with either MAC or GA. Lung biopsy is a relatively painless procedure amenable to procedural sedation or MAC. The pleura is well innervated, and penetration with a needle may be painful.
   b. MAC techniques should focus on keeping the patient immobile during needle placement and breathing in a normal pattern. Rapid, shallow, or deep and slow breathing can make procedures challenging.
   c. Ablations require the use of large-bore probes and are more painful especially during the ablation. GA can be performed, but the effects of positive pressure can lead to higher risk of PTX or tension PTX. GA is requested for cases involving complex lesions for advanced airway support.
2. Positioning is dependent on the location of tumor and planned trajectory: supine, prone, or lateral depending on the laterality and lesion location. Patient positioning and comfort are of utmost importance. Under GA prone positioning in the CT scanner bed is challenging. Pillows and abdominal rolls can be used to elevate the body, to keep the abdomen free, and to allow the head and face to be supported with the neck midline and neutral.
3. **HFJV or a double-lumen tube** can be utilized as previously described.
   a. Initial HFJV settings include driving pressure 10 to 15 psi, inspiratory time 30%, frequency 100 to 120 bpm. Alarm settings include pause pressure 15 to 25 cmH_2O, PIP 20 to 30 cmH_2O, and humidity 2 to 3.
   b. For these procedures, if positive pressure is utilized, it is prudent to use low pressure and consider chest tube placement by the interventionalist either prophylactically or if there is evidence of PTX on CT.
4. Post procedure the probe is removed and the wound immediately covered to prevent a sucking chest wound and PTX. This necessitates turning the patient prone or supine, depending upon the insertion site, immediately after removal of the probe. Extubation considerations include hemoptysis (for large ablations), tension PTX, or hemothorax (if chest tube is not in place). **Have two suctions readily available.** Ensure the patient has recovered cough reflex to protect the airway prior to extubation. Reintubation for airway protection may be necessary.

VI. ANESTHESIA FOR NEUROINTERVENTIONS
Anesthetic management may be necessary for both diagnostic (angiography, balloon test, and occlusion) and therapeutic (embolization and cerebral vasospasm) procedures. Patient access after start of the procedure may be limited to the left arm and leg.

A. **Endovascular embolization** is performed to treat ruptured as well as unruptured cerebral aneurysms, to interrupt blood supply to intracranial and extracranial arteriovenous fistulas and malformations, vascular tumors, and bleeding vessels in the nose or pharynx.

1. **Embolization** requires access to the vascular tree, commonly via the femoral artery, and advancement of a small catheter into the aneurysm or blood vessels supplying the area of pathology. Once position is confirmed by angiography, the vascular occlusive material (detachable metal coils, glue, or small particles) is deployed via the catheter.

   a. **Anesthetic goals** include provision of a still field during placement of the microcatheter and deployment of the occlusive material, stable hemodynamics, and rapid recovery after the procedure to test neurologic function. This often necessitates GA to provide amnesia in addition to paralysis. Anesthesia can be accomplished with IV medications (propofol, muscle relaxant, and narcotics) and/or volatile anesthetics. Nitrous oxide is avoided to minimize consequences of inadvertent arterial air emboli. These procedures are relatively painless with little stimulation from the procedure.

      1. If hypertonic contrast agents are used, bladder catheterization and fluid replacement may be necessary as these agents may produce diuresis.

      2. Invasive arterial blood pressure monitoring via a radial artery is often necessary for control of hemodynamics; alternatively, blood pressure may be transduced from the femoral artery sheath placed during the procedure.

      3. **Hypertension** should be avoided, because it may increase the risk of hemorrhage or aneurysm rupture. Vasoactive drugs such as phenylephrine should be used with great caution in patients with unprotected cerebral aneurysms. β-Blockers, calcium channel blockers, hydralazine, nitroglycerin, and sodium nitroprusside may be useful to treat hypertension.

      4. Procedures may be lengthy and place the patient at risk for untoward embolic events. Patients often require **anticoagulation** (heparin or argatroban) during the procedure to minimize propagation of thrombus from the embolization coils or microcatheters; anticoagulation is monitored by activated clotting time. Platelet inhibitors such as eptifibatide (Integrilin) may be administered by bolus and/or continuous infusion to minimize platelet aggregation. For some procedures, patients may receive aspirin and/or clopidogrel before the procedure. Aspirin can be given by suppository during procedures if necessary.

      5. Intraprocedural complications include rupture of the aneurysm, arteriovenous fistula or malformation, dissection or rupture of a blood vessel, and inadvertent occlusion of a blood vessel. If intracranial hemorrhage is suspected, immediate placement of a ventriculostomy may be necessary to drain cerebrospinal fluid (CSF) emergently to reduce intracranial pressure (ICP). Unlike intraoperative aneurysm rupture in open procedures (Chapter 23), there is no significant blood loss because the cranium is closed. Elevation of ICP may require hyperventilation, diuresis, or barbiturate coma. Immediate CT scan may be necessary to determine the extent of hemorrhage and need for emergency surgery to decompress the brain and definitive treatment.

B. **Embolization for control of epistaxis and extracranial vascular lesions** presents potential problems of hemorrhage, hemodynamic instability, large amounts of blood in the airway, and aspiration. Typed and cross-matched blood should be available; large-bore IV access may be necessary if acute hemorrhage is a potential threat. Endotracheal intubation is optimal especially for urgent cases, although it could be difficult if the pathology involves the airway and/or face. The nose and nasal pharynx may be packed as temporizing treatments.

C. **Balloon test occlusion** of the carotid artery is performed to determine whether permanent obstruction of the vessel will lead to neurologic deficit. Occlusion is performed endovascularly by temporarily obstructing blood flow with inflation of a balloon in the vessel; if no deficit is apparent on neurologic examination, hypotension is induced and maintained for 20 to 30 minutes to elicit signs of ischemia. Often, cerebral blood flow is evaluated during the hypotensive period by IV injection of a positron emission tomography (PET) isotope; PET scan is obtained after the procedure after the vessel is open and blood pressure returns to normal. If there is any deterioration in neurologic function, the balloon is immediately deflated and blood pressure is returned to normal. Although sedation is appropriate during initial angiography and placement of the balloon, **a completely awake, nonsedated patient is necessary for neurologic testing during occlusion**; short-acting agents are preferred. **Hypotension is induced with rapidly reversible agents** (nitroprusside or nitroglycerine). These agents may cause tachycardia, which can be offset by administering β-blockers. Emergency airway management including endotracheal intubation may be required if seizures or loss of the airway occurs during test occlusion.

D. **Intracarotid sodium amobarbital procedure** or the **WADA test** is performed for planned epilepsy surgery or less commonly for tumor resection. Sodium amorbarbital, a short-acting barbiturate, is carefully injected to limit spread beyond the brain hemisphere of interest. This test is effective in lateralizing speech and memory, seizure onset, predicting postoperative seizure control, and predicting degree of verbal memory decline following left temporal lobectomy. Anesthetic considerations are similar to BTO for which **a completely awake, nonsedated patient is necessary** for the patient to participate in the battery of neurocognitive tests. Emergency airway management including endotracheal intubation may be required if seizures, drastic disinhibition, or loss of the airway occurs during the injection.

E. **Cerebral angiography and spinal angiography** are generally painless diagnostic procedures. Only children or uncooperative adults usually require GA for angiography, although they may receive GA for comfort because of the potentially long duration. Adult patients requiring GA for intracranial angiography may have depressed mental status because of elevated ICP, encephalopathy, recent stroke, or intracerebral hemorrhage; meticulous attention to hemodynamics may require invasive blood pressure monitoring. Spinal angiography requires several hours for each vessel supplying the spinal cord to be identified and the angiogram to be performed. The duration of the procedure may need to be limited because the upper limit of contrast agent dosing may be reached. Patients are anesthetized for their comfort; invasive hemodynamic monitoring is not necessary unless dictated by comorbidity.

F. **Carotid stenting** with an embolic-protection device can be performed in lieu of CEA in average-surgical-risk symptomatic patients. This can be performed with the patient under sedation with MAC or GA. Tight hemodynamic control is important; stroke is a risk. Bradycardia may occur during the procedure and can be preemptively treated with an anticholinergic.

G. **Vertebroplasty and kyphoplasty** are percutaneous procedures performed to treat painful acute and subacute vertebral compression fractures or sacral fractures refractory to medical therapy via injection of acrylic cement. **Vertebroplasty** involves introducing a trocar-cannula via a transpedicular approach into the desired vertebral body. The cement is then deposited under steady pressure utilizing fluoroscopy. Multiple levels can be performed at one sitting, and often trochars are placed bilaterally at each level. A **kyphoplasty** is similar; however, after vertebral body access a balloon is inflated utilizing a contrast agent in the vertebral body to restore vertebral height; cement is then deposited. The procedures are performed in the prone position. The procedure is amenable to either MAC or GA. The majority of patients presenting for these procedures include frail elderly patients with cardiopulmonary insufficiency and either metastatic cancer and chronic pain and hyperalgesia. Positioning can present challenges as patients can have limited neck and shoulder mobility. GA may impact cardiovascular performance, and the patient has to be carefully turned prone. Sedation has to center on titrating in the judicious doses of anxiolytic(s) and synchronizing analgesia for portions of the procedure that are stimulating (ie, introduction of trocar). Sedatives and analgesics should have minimal residual effects as postprocedural pain is minimal. Short-acting analgesic such as remifentanil can be utilized as a bolus or infusion for these procedures. Post procedure patients remain supine for several hours to permit the cement to harden.

H. **Thrombolysis of acute ischemic stroke (AIS)** is an emergency procedure performed to restore blood flow to cerebral vessels occluded by thrombus. Prompt IV fibrinolytic therapy with tissue plasminogen activator (tPA) is the gold standard as the benefit is heavily time dependent. It is recommended in patients for up to 4.5 hours after onset of *disabling* symptoms. Recent recommendations include an expanded time window of 4.5 hours in patients *waking* with an AIS or having unclear time of onset >4.5 hours from last baseline state **and** if a large intracranial bleed is ruled out by MRI.

1. **Endovascular therapies (EVTs)** are indicated for large vessel occlusion of the anterior cerebral circulation (internal carotid and MCA branches). They include **mechanical retrieval or aspiration** of thrombus. It is recommended in conjunction with tPA in patients presenting within 6 hours of symptoms. Recent recommendations have extended the time window for EVT alone to 6 to 24 hours of last known normal. The concern is that reperfusion and anticoagulation after prolonged ischemia may predispose to hemorrhage into the site of infarction. Angioplasty of atherosclerotic plaque or placement of an intra-arterial stent may be used to supplement thrombolytic therapy to maintain patency of the occluded vessel. **Intra-arterial fibrinolysis** therapy can be administered, but not as first-line therapy, instead as a salvage technical adjunct.

   a. Anesthetic management is guided by the individual assessment of the patient. Airway support and ventilatory support are recommended for decreased consciousness or dysfunction that compromises airway. The literature is mixed as there are no prospective randomized studies comparing anesthetic techniques. Some suggest no difference between GA and MAC/CS on functional outcome. Either method is reasonable as long as it does not delay EVT. MAC can be performed with a wide array of anxiolytics and analgesics including midazolam and fentanyl. Dexmedetomidine may be beneficial for these cases; however, the impact on hemodynamics has to be taken into account. The airway must be maintained. Invasive arterial hemodynamic, if needed, can be placed during the procedure. There is no benefit for brain protection strategies. If GA is planned it should be executed expeditiously.

1. Blood pressure must be maintained to assist cerebral perfusion. Hypotension is associated with poor outcomes.

2. Hypovolemia should be corrected.
   a. No benefit or harm has been observed between colloid or crystalloid resuscitation.

3. Blood pressure (BP) should be maintained at or below 185/110 to decrease the risk of intracranial hemorrhage in patients receiving tPA.

4. Hyperthermia (>38 °C) and hypoglycemia (<60 mg/dL) should be promptly treated.

5. Complications arising from tPA include:
   a. **Intracranial bleeding.** Management includes stopping tPA, administering cryoprecipitate and TXA, as well as performing supportive maneuvers to decrease ICP.
   b. **Angioedema.** This can lead to partial or severe airway obstruction. Partial airway obstruction can be managed medically with methylprednisolone and H1 and H2 blockers. Nebulized epinephrine may be administered with cognizance of the impact on hemodynamics. ACE should be withheld. Preparation for awake FOI should be made if the airway is severely obstructed.
   c. For severe cases icatibant, a selective bradykinin antagonist, or plasma-derived C1 esterase inhibitor can be administered.

I. **Cerebral vasospasm** is a common and potentially devastating late complication of subarachnoid hemorrhage. Patients may require angiography and local **intra-arterial infusion** of vasodilating drugs (**papavarine, nicardipine, or milrinone**) or even angioplasty to increase the diameter of segments of cerebral blood vessels that are critically constricted. Medical management includes **hypervolemia, hemodilution, and hypertension** to increase blood flow through stenotic segments of feeding vessels; patients are often on large doses of vasopressors (phenylephrine, norepinephrine, or vasopressin) to induce hypertension. ICP may be elevated from brain edema secondary to initial injury or evolving ischemic strokes.

1. **ICP monitoring** may be helpful during the procedure because intracranial hypertension is common, and ICP may increase with therapy. Intraventricular catheter is preferable because it permits drainage of CSF to treat increased ICP; "Camino" bolt is adequate for monitoring, but CSF cannot be withdrawn.

2. Anesthetic goals are to optimize cerebral perfusion by **maintaining systemic hypertension and intracranial normotension**, maintain a hyperdynamic cardiovascular state, and provide a rapidly reversible general anesthetic so that neurologic examination can be assessed immediately after intervention. Patients may require postprocedural mechanical ventilation for control of ICP. Paralysis and mechanical ventilation may be necessary to control partial pressure of carbon dioxide. If ICP is not increased, GA may be accomplished with a low concentration of volatile anesthetic supplemented by narcotics and paralysis. Alternatively, propofol infusion may be necessary to control ICP.

3. ICP may rise and blood pressure may fall dramatically with intra-arterial infusions of **papavarine, nicardipine**, or **milrinone**. High doses of vasopressors such as phenylephrine or norepinephrine may be necessary. Supplementation with cardiac inotropes may be required to maintain blood pressure.

4. Because hyperglycemia may worsen consequences of cerebral ischemia, patients may be receiving an insulin infusion in conjunction with 5% dextrose in normal saline to maintain tight control of glucose.

5. Patients are often febrile. Normothermia can be maintained with surface cooling; hyperthermia may worsen consequences of cerebral ischemia.

VII. ANESTHESIA FOR GASTROINTESTINAL/GENITOURINARY AND VASCULAR RADIOLOGY PROCEDURES

A. Embolization for gastrointestinal bleeding and hemoptysis. Arterial embolization can be used to treat acute nonvariceal gastrointestinal hemorrhages of the upper or lower GI tracts that are not amenable to endoscopic treatment. Bronchial artery embolization is an effective treatment for massive hemoptysis. Both procedures are performed under angiographic guidance, through arterial access that allows delivery of embolic agents, such as gelatin sponges, beads, microcoils, or glues, to selected arteries through microcatheters. These procedures are typically performed under GA with the patient intubated for airway control with lung isolation for patients with hemoptysis. Muscle relaxants are helpful to minimize motion artifacts if digital subtraction angiography is used.

B. Transjugular intrahepatic portosystemic shunt (TIPS) decompresses the portal system in patients with decompensated portal hypertension. Often, patients may have advanced liver disease, actively bleeding esophageal varices, massive recurrent ascites, severely compromised liver function, or hypoxemia. Oliguria from hepatorenal syndrome is common. Patients with liver failure are often hyperdynamic with low systemic vascular resistance owing to arteriovenous fistulas in the liver and lung. Preprocedural hypoxemia may be multifactorial from V/Q mismatch or hepatopulmonary syndrome with associated intrapulmonary vascular dilations. The patient with actively bleeding varices may be on an octreotide infusion to decrease mesenteric blood flow.

1. The liver is commonly accessed via cannulation of the right internal jugular. Access to the portal circulation is achieved by sequentially placing a guidewire, needle, and sheath into the hepatic vein and through the liver parenchyma. A conduit is created via a balloon catheter dilation with stent placement to allow for egress of portal blood flow into the systemic circulation. Portal pressures are transduced to assess portosystemic gradient with a target portosystemic gradient of <12 mm Hg.

2. Sedation under MAC can be performed for patients without complex anatomy. GA, however, may be preferred owing to the duration and discomfort.

a. For a concomitant large-volume paracentesis (LVP) prior to TIPS it is recommended that albumin be replenished 6 to 8 g/L exceeding 5L drain. This counters the postparacentesis circulatory dysfunction that occurs after LVP resulting from decreased circulating blood volume. At our institution the goal is to avoid concomitant LVP and TIPS owing to large fluid shifts.

b. Patients with bleeding or massive ascites are considered to have full stomachs and receive a rapid sequence induction. It is preferable to perform paracentesis to drain ascites before induction of GA, if possible to reduce intra-abdominal pressure.

3. Delayed complications can include encephalopathy and/or heart failure.

C. **Balloon-occluded retrograde transvenous obliteration (BRTO)** is a method to treat gastric varices in patients who are not candidates for the TIPS procedure. Balloon-occluded sclerotherapy of gastric varices is achieved through either a transjugular or transfemoral venous approach, using 3% sodium tetradecyl sulfate as the sclerosing agent. Although it is an effective treatment for gastric varices, BRTO can increase the risk of esophageal varices and ascites. This procedure can be performed under MAC or GA.

D. **Selective internal radiation therapy (SIRT) and transarterial chemoembolization (TACE)** are procedures performed in patients presenting with large hepatic tumors not amenable for surgical excision or percutaneous ablation. Treatment relies on taking advantage of the arterial hepatic blood flow tumors receive in contrast to normal tissue. SIRT involves guiding a microcatheter to the terminal arterial branches supplying the tumor with placement of radioactive isotope yttrium Y-90 microspheres or beads. The TACE procedure combines the local delivery of chemotherapy and embolization of the tumor to disrupt and cease the blood supply to the tumor. Access can be via the left radial or femoral artery.

1. These procedures are amenable to MAC as they are relatively painless; however, they can be long depending on anatomy and for some debilitated patients lying prone may be an issue.

2. TACE procedures can result in postprocedural pain secondary to ischemia of the hepatic tissues. These patients can benefit from **ERAP**.

E. **Transhepatic percutaneous biliary and nephrostomy drains** are performed when there is the need for diversion of biliary or urinary flow due to the presence of obstruction from anomalous anatomy, stones, malignancy, or infections of the biliary tree or renal collecting system. The procedures involve ultrasound guidance and fluoroscopy for access of the tract. Once access is obtained small flexible drain catheters are placed.

1. These patients can present under a wide variety of conditions ranging from nonurgent to emergent in the case of cholangitis or urosepsis.

2. Positioning for biliary drains is supine. Optimal positioning for nephrostomy drains is prone; however, lateral positioning is possible.

3. Anesthesia can be done with either MAC or GA, but it largely depends on the clinical context and patient condition. For complex anatomy and a deteriorating patient condition a secure airway may be prudent as well as invasive BP monitoring.

4. Elective primary placement of large biliary drains can be stimulating and painful post procedure. ERAP can be beneficial.

5. Catheter exchanges or upsizing is quick and can be amenable to MAC; however, large dilations and upsizes can be stimulating and deep sedation can be performed.

F. **Percutaneous gastrostomy and gastrojejunostomy (GJ) tube** placements are indicated in patients with dysphagia unable to meet nutritional requirements. A GJ tube is placed in cases where there is reflux of gastric tube feeds if an NG tube is in place or a preexisting gastrostomy tube (G tube) owing to an incompetent lower esophageal sphincter or inability to tolerate gastric tube feeds. The patient population consists of patients with depressed mental status secondary to a neurological insult, most commonly stroke, as well as **head and neck cancers undergoing radiation therapy** or **amyotrophic lateral sclerosis** (ALS). Patients with gastric outlet obstruction from abdominal malignancy may require a G tube as a vent for stomach contents and/or a jejunostomy tube for nutritional support; such patients must be treated with full stomach precautions. A G tube and

GJ tubes may be placed endoscopically with fluoroscopy or a gastroscope. Alternatively, in cases with altered anatomy the G tube may be placed under **CT guidance.**

1. Airway examination is particularly important in this patient population as tumors, prior surgeries, and radiation can make mask ventilation and intubation potentially difficult.

2. G tube placements can be performed under MAC or GA depending on the patient comorbidities, GI anatomy, and proceduralist.

3. Fluoroscopic and CT-guided procedures require gastric insufflation to expand the stomach below the inferior costal margin. This is achieved by placement of a 5-French nasogastric tube. Prior to insufflation glucagon is administered to prevent the gastric air from transiting through the small bowel. *Small amounts of contrast* are injected to verify stomach access.

4. After fluoroscopic identification of the stomach the feeding tubes are placed with care to avoid the liver edge and/or transverse colon. In certain circumstances a contrast enema is placed to identify the transverse colon.

5. For patients with severe neurodegenerative disease such as ALS care presents a challenge. These patients have extreme procedural anxiety. MAC with minimal sedation is ideal with avoidance of airway obstruction to avoid CO_2 narcosis due to their hypermetabolic state with high production of CO_2. The key is to establish rapport and set expectations. Succinylcholine is contraindicated owing to potential lethal hyperkalemia. At our institution we are able to perform these safely under MAC. The nasopharynx is anesthetized with 2% lidocaine jelly and in combination with judicious use of midazolam and fentanyl with or without glycopyrrolate for secretions.

G. **Anesthesia for vascular access procedures: Fistulograms/graftrograms, thrombectomies, and tunneled dialysis catheters (TDCs).** The majority of the patient population are those with ESRD and accompanying comorbidities. Often these patients require repeated interventions for maintenance of their dialysis access, which include arteriovenous fistula (AVF), AV graft (AVG), and TDCs. Vascular access dysfunction may be due to several etiologies such as failure of maturation of an AVF, stenosis at various sites along the AVF/AVG including perianastomic stenosis of the arterial inflow or venous outflow and/or central vein stenosis (cephalic arch). These manifest as excessive bleeding or increased pressures during hemodialysis (HD) runs. Clotted vascular access presents with absence of fistula thrill.

1. Patients require special attention to their electrolytes, in particular potassium, as HD runs are suboptimal. Hyperkalemia, especially with ECG changes, calls for immediate temporizing medical management and emergent HD via placement of a nontunneled dialysis catheter.

2. MAC is sufficient for most procedures; however, some patients may not be able to stay still or cooperate for a variety of reasons, including respiratory insufficiency or back pain. GA is the alternative with LMA or ETT. Angioplasty can vary in discomfort from minimal with angioplasty of central veins to very painful for angioplasty of stenotic regions located in the distal arm. Pain is proportional to the size and duration of the angioplasty. It is brief with no residual pain. Well-timed small propofol boluses can be administered to mitigate pain; however, patients may not be able to tolerate any decrease in SVR.

   a. RA techniques can be used for procedures *involving significant angioplasty* in the mid-distal arm, specifically for radiocephalic fistulas in patients with limited cardiopulmonary reserve. Short-acting local anesthetics should be used as procedures can last 1 to 3 hours. Extreme care must be taken to weigh risks and benefits as RA can impact pulmonary reserve.

3. **Thrombectomies (declotting)** are performed for clotted access. This procedure involves a combination of pharmacological and mechanical thrombolysis. Fibrinolysis is achieved with tPA, and mechanical thrombectomy includes embolectomy and/or aspiration devices. Prompt intervention is indicated. These patients need to be optimized and carefully assessed. A feared complication is pulmonary embolism with cardiogenic shock due to thrombus microemboli. Vulnerable populations include patients with large clot burden, compromised RV, or significant pulmonary hypertension with previous AV thrombectomies in a relatively short span. Anesthetic choice can be MAC or GA with invasive monitoring depending on patient comorbidities.

4. **TDCs** are indicated in situations where prolonged HD is anticipated, such as acute kidney injury and AV fistula maturation, or in patients with no other long-term vascular access. The catheter is commonly placed on the right IJ and tunneled under the skin overlying the scapula and proximal chest wall over the second or third intercostal space. Anesthetic approach can be with a variety of MAC sedation approaches or for uncooperative patients with GA and a secure airway.

VIII. ANESTHESIA FOR PROTON BEAM THERAPY AND RADIATION THERAPY

A. **Proton beam radiation therapy** is used to treat arteriovenous malformations, pituitary tumors, retinoblastomas, and an expanding number of other tumors. Irradiation is painless, but planning sessions and creation of molds may take many hours, whereas each individual therapy session is much shorter. During irradiation, the target area must remain in a fixed position using a stereotactic frame locked to a positioning device.

1. **In adults**, placement of small pins or screws in the skull can be performed under local anesthesia with 2% lidocaine with epinephrine. If "ear bars" are used, a satisfactory ear block can be performed by subcutaneous injection of 3 mL of 2% lidocaine with epinephrine in the outer ear canal. Sedation is usually not recommended because patient cooperation is required.

2. **For children**, a general anesthetic is usually administered. The procedure typically is performed daily for about 4 weeks; a propofol induction (2-4 mg/kg IV) and maintenance infusion ($\sim$75-300 µg/kg/min) through an implanted Broviac or Hickman catheter is a suitable technique. It is ideal to replicate the previous anesthetic in order to achieve similar conditions from session to session. Tachyphylaxis has been observed to propofol, and large doses are used. Spontaneous ventilation should be permitted whenever possible. The patient's head is placed in a sniffing position, and a plaster mold is formed that maintains the head in the correct position for treatment. Nasal prongs or a facemask can provide supplemental oxygen; a sidestream sampling line will provide qualitative assessment of ventilation. LMA is considered if a natural airway cannot be maintained. Standard monitoring is used, and patients are monitored and viewed via closed-circuit television because the anesthetist must leave the room during the brief period of radiation. Emergence delirium can occur and the anesthetist has to be prepared to treat it accordingly.

B. **Anesthesia for radiation therapy.** Children receiving radiation therapy often require GA.
   1. Typical treatment course is three or four times a week for 4 weeks. It is desirable to choose an anesthetic that allows rapid recovery with minimal risk of nausea and vomiting.
   2. The first radiation procedure may be time consuming (one to several hours) because measurements must be performed and molds made of the patient. Subsequent treatments are typically less than 30 minutes.
   3. Many patients have indwelling venous access for chemotherapy. An IV induction and maintenance with propofol infusion is a suitable technique. Intramuscular injection of a combination of midazolam, glycopyrrolate, and ketamine may be useful in children with difficult venous access.

IX. ANESTHESIA FOR ELECTROCONVULSIVE THERAPY

Electroconvulsive therapy (ECT) is used to treat major depression, catatonia, and mania along with other second-line indications such as in patients who have not responded to medications, are debilitated by serious side effects, or are acutely suicidal. Patients who suffer from delusions, hallucinations, or profound psychomotor retardation are less responsive to medication, and thus, early ECT is preferred for them as well. Usually, a series of 6 to 12 treatments over 2 to 4 weeks is required for a clinical response.

A. **Physiologic effects of ECT**
   1. The electrical stimulus produces a generalized tonic-clonic seizure consisting of a tonic phase lasting 10 to 15 seconds followed by a clonic phase lasting 30 to 50 seconds.
   2. An initial vagal discharge may result in severe bradycardia and mild hypotension. Subsequent sympathetic nervous system activation produces hypertension and tachycardia, which can persist for 5 to 10 minutes. ECG changes are common and may include pulse-rate interval prolongation, increased QT interval, T wave inversions, and atrial or ventricular arrhythmias.
   3. Increased cerebral blood flow and metabolic rate lead to increased ICP. Increased intraocular and intragastric pressure may occur.

B. **Anesthetic goals.** Provide amnesia and a rapid return to consciousness, prevent damage from tonic-clonic contractures (eg, long-bone fractures), control hemodynamic response, and avoid interference with initiation and duration of induced seizure.

C. The one absolute contraindication to ECT is **intracranial hypertension** (elevated ICP). **Relative contraindications** include presence of an intracranial mass lesion (with normal ICP), intracranial aneurysm, recent myocardial infarction, angina, congestive heart failure, untreated glaucoma, major bone fractures, thrombophlebitis, pregnancy, and retinal detachment. Patients on maintenance treatment with benzodiazepines or lithium should discontinue these treatments before ECT; benzodiazepines are anticonvulsants that may abolish or attenuate the seizure; lithium is associated with post-ECT confusion and delirium.

D. **Anesthetic management**
   1. Sedative premedication is not indicated and may prolong emergence. Anticholinergic drugs may be used to reduce secretions and to minimize bradycardia. Ondansetron may be useful in patients with a history of nausea and vomiting.
   2. A small-gauge IV cannula is placed for drug administration, and standard monitors are applied.

3. The patient is preoxygenated with 100% oxygen; anesthesia is induced with methohexital (1.5 mg/kg IV) or propofol (1 mg/kg IV) and succinylcholine (1.0 mg/kg IV). Patients are ventilated with 100% oxygen via mask and Ambu bag. Small doses of short-acting nondepolarizing muscle relaxant can be used in patients with contraindications to succinylcholine. Pretreatment with labetalol (10-50 mg IV) or esmolol (40-80 mg IV) blunts the hypertensive response and may be useful in patients with hypertension or coronary artery disease.

4. Ketorolac may decrease muscle pains after ECT.

5. Rolled gauze pads placed bilaterally as bite blocks protect gums and lips from biting from electrical stimulus and subsequent seizure.

6. The nature and duration of induced seizures can be monitored by electroencephalogram or by the "isolated arm" technique. With the latter, inflation of a blood pressure cuff interrupts blood supply to one arm before injecting muscle relaxant; seizure activity is apparent in the isolated arm.

7. Patients are ventilated with oxygen by facemask until spontaneous ventilation resumes. They are then placed in a lateral decubitus position and monitored in a recovery area until awake and alert. Agitated delirium from tardive seizures may occur after ECT and can be treated with small doses of propofol or benzodiazepine.

8. Patients with underlying medical conditions may require special attention:

   a. Patients with gastroesophageal reflux may require aspiration prophylaxis and rapid sequence intubation.

   b. Patients with severe cardiac dysfunction may require invasive monitoring.

   c. Patients with intracranial mass lesions may require invasive blood pressure monitoring for tight hemodynamic control; hyperventilation before inducing a seizure may reduce the ICP response.

   d. Pregnant patients may require endotracheal intubation, fetal monitoring, and left uterine displacement.

9. Rarely, an induced seizure will not spontaneously terminate. Ventilation with 100% oxygen is continued, and seizure is terminated within 3 minutes with propofol (20-50 mg IV) or benzodiazepines.

E. **Psychiatric drug interactions.** Patients requiring ECT may be treated with psychotropic drugs that have potent side effects and interactions with anesthetic drugs.

1. **Tricyclic antidepressants** (eg, amitriptyline, nortriptyline, desipramine, imipramine, and doxepin) potentiate effects of norepinephrine and serotonin by preventing reuptake. Untoward effects include postural hypotension, sedation, dry mouth, urinary retention, and tachycardia.

2. **Monoamine oxidase inhibitors (MAOIs)** (eg, phenelzine and isocarboxazid) increase availability of norepinephrine at postsynaptic receptors; orthostatic hypotension and severe hypertension may occur. Tyramine, present in certain foods, may produce a hypertensive crisis in patients taking MAOIs. Although it has been recommended previously that MAOI therapy be discontinued at least 10 days before elective surgery, the risk of severe depression outweighs the risks of discontinuing the drug. **Important interactions** between MAOIs and anesthetics include severe hypertension with indirectly acting vasopressors (ephedrine). Administration of **meperidine** (and meperidine derivatives) to patients receiving MAOIs has been associated with serotonin syndrome characterized by severe hemodynamic instability, respiratory depression, and malignant hyperpyrexia.

3. **Selective serotonin reuptake inhibitors** (eg, fluoxetine, sertraline, fluvoxamine, and paroxetine) are associated with mild adverse effects with no known significant interactions with anesthetic drugs.

X. ANESTHESIA FOR GASTROINTESTINAL PROCEDURES

These are the most common NORA procedures performed. Unique to these procedures is the ability to be performed bedside in the intensive care unit (ICU) or in the operating room for patients who are unstable or have medically complex conditions. The anesthetic approach is dictated by patient comorbidities, including body habitus, nature of procedure, and clinical context. This may be done with MAC and varying levels of sedation or GA.

A. **Esophagoduodenoscopy** permits assessment and treatment of esophageal, gastric, and duodenal structures. Indications include evaluation of dysphagia, abdominal pain, GERD, persistent nausea/vomiting, and upper GI bleeding. It is also used to clear foreign bodies including food impaction. Endoscopy is not painful, and stimulation is limited to insertion of the endoscope. It requires sharing the airway with the endoscopist.

1. **Esophageal banding** uses elastic bands to ligate large bleeding esophageal varices. Patients have portal hypertension often secondary to hepatic cirrhosis. Risks of the procedure include bleeding and esophageal perforation. The procedure can be very stimulating with high aspiration risk. The airway should be secured. If the patient is on octreotide, the infusion should be continued throughout the procedure.

B. **Endoscopic ultrasonography** is a diagnostic and therapeutic procedure for malignancies of the digestive tract including the esophagus, stomach, pancreas, colon, and rectum. It uses high-frequency sound waves emitted from the endoscope to produce detailed images. Using fine-needle aspiration (FNA) samples can be taken from tissue or fluid-filled cystic neoplasms. In addition, it can be used as a therapeutic tool for image-guided drainage of collections such as abscesses and infected necrosis of the upper and lower GI track including the pancreas. Specifically, for pancreatic tumors it has utility as an interventional tool for brachytherapy, fiducial placement, and fine needle injection of anti-tumor agents. It can also be used to perform celiac plexus blocks.

1. A deep MAC or GA may be employed with the goal to ensure the patient does not move during FNA, if planned. The GI tract may be irrigated with fluid to improve imaging. If this is planned a secured airway is prudent to prevent aspiration.

C. **Endoscopic retrograde cholangiopancreatography (ERCP)** is a procedure of the biliary tree, gallbladder, and pancreatic duct for diagnosis and treatment of malignancy and/or obstruction. These structures are accessed via the catheterization of the sphincter of Oddi through a side channel of the endoscope. A combination of contrast media and fluoroscopy is used to achieve calculi retrieval, stent placement(s), and/or sphincterotomy to facilitate drainage.

1. The vast majority of procedures are performed with the patient in the prone position.

2. MAC can be used if a relatively straightforward procedure is anticipated and the patient has low-risk aspiration with a favorable airway examination.

3. GA is performed if there is concern for aspiration and/or anticipated complex procedure.

D. **Colonoscopy** evaluates and treats pathologies of the large intestine and rectum such as polyps, cancer, inflammatory bowel disease, as well as other symptoms like abdominal pain and rectal bleeding. Successful procedure is predicated on an adequate bowel prep for visualization. It is performed in the lateral decubitus position.

1. MAC with a natural airway is a sufficient anesthetic choice in situations where there is not concern for aspiration. However, in situations of obstruction precautions should be taken to secure the airway.

2. Perforation of the colon is one of the most serious complications of a colonoscopy and is associated with a high rate of morbidity and mortality. The incidence ranges from 0.016% to 0.2% following diagnostic colonoscopies and could be up to 5% following some colonoscopic interventions. Patients present with persistent abdominal pain due to peritonitis. Prompt surgical evaluation and intervention is necessary.

3. **Flexible sigmoidoscopy** is a limited examination of the rectum and lower sigmoid colon. It is performed to rule out lower GI bleeding in situations where an adequate bowel prep is not possible. It can be done bedside or in the ICU. Anesthetic choice is dictated by the patient's hemodynamic status and clinical situation.

Suggested Readings

American College of Radiology. *ACR Manual on Contrast Media 2020 Version 10.3. ACR Committee on Drugs and Contrast Medial.* American College of Radiology; 2020. https://www.acr.org/-/media/ACR/files/clinical-resources/contrast_media.pdf

American Society of Anesthesiologists. *Continuum of Depth of Sedation. Definition of General Anesthesia and Levels of Sedation/Analgesia Committee of Origin: Quality Management and Departmental Administration* (Approved by the ASA House of Delegates on October 13, 1999, and last amended on October 23, 2019). ASA; 2019. https://www.asahq.org/-/media/sites/asahq/files/public/resources/standards-guidelines/continuum-of-depth-of-sedation-definition-of-general-anesthesia-and-levels-of-sedation-analgesia.pdf?la=en&hash=227C0F37B707290FDEB457AFC9FBDD914E1B3C2A

American Society of Anesthesiology. *Advisory on Granting Privileges for Deep Sedation to Non-anesthesiologist Physicians Committee of Origin: Quality Management and Departmental Administration* (Approved by the ASA House of Delegates on October 20, 2010 and last amended on October 25, 2017). ASA; 2017. https://www.asahq.org/-/media/sites/asahq/files/public/resources/standards-guidelines/advisory-on-granting-privileges-for-deep-sedation-to-non-anesthesiologist.pdf?la=en&hash=5FB478F0CBD0B8C248C5173D190FC5000AFBC514

American Society of Anesthesiology. Practice guidelines for moderate procedural sedation and analgesia 2018: A report by the American Society of Anesthesiologists Task Force on Moderate Procedural Sedation and Analgesia, the American Association of Oral and Maxillofacial Surgeons, American College of Radiology, American Dental Association, American Society of Dentist Anesthesiologists, and Society of Interventional Radiology. *Anesthesiology.* 1018;128:437-479.

American Society of Anesthesiology. *Statement on Nonoperating Room Anesthetizing Locations.* (Approved by the ASA House of Delegates on October 19, 1994, last amended on October 16, 2013, and reaffirmed on October 17, 2018). ASA; 2018. https://www.asahq.org/-/media/sites/asahq/files/public/resources/standards-guidelines/statement-on-nonoperating-room-anesthetizing-locations.pdf?la=en&hash=A01CBA489AC9FF4757081995827DF98B1406E54D

Amin A, Lane J, Cutter T. An anesthesiologist's view of tumor ablation in the radiology suite. *Anesthesiol Clin.* 2017;35:611-615.

Anastasian ZH, Strozyk D, Meyers PM, Wang S, Berman MF. Radiation exposure of the anesthesiologist in the neurointerventional suite. *Anesthesiology.* 2011;114(3):512-520.

Apfelbaummd JL, Singleton MA, Ehrenwerth J, et al. Practice advisory on anesthetic care for magnetic resonance imaging: an updated report by the American Society of Anesthesiologists Task Force on Anesthetic Care for Magnetic Resonance Imaging. *Anesthesiology.* 2015;122:495-520.

Bhagavatula SK, Lane J, Shyn P. A radiologist's view of tumor ablation in the radiology suite. *Anesthesiol Clin.* 2017;35:617-626.

Brott TG, Halperin JL, Abbara S, et al. ASA/ACCF/AHA/AANN/AANS/ACR/ASNR/ CNS/SAIP/SCAI/SIR/SNIS/SVM/SVS guideline on the management of patients with extracranial carotid and vertebral artery disease: executive summary. A report of the American College of Cardiology Foundation/American Heart Association Task Force on Practice guidelines, and the American Stroke Association, American Association of Neuroscience Nurses, American Association of Neurological Surgeons, American College of Radiology, American Society of Neuroradiology, Congress of Neurological Surgeons, Society of Atherosclerosis Imaging and Prevention, Society for Cardiovascular Angiography and Interventions, Society of Interventional Radiology, Society of NeuroInterventional Surgery, Society for Vascular Medicine, and Society for Vascular Surgery. *J Am Coll Cardiol.* 2011;57:1002-1044.

Chun JY, Morgan R, Belli AM. Radiological management of hemoptysis: a comprehensive review of diagnostic imaging and bronchial arterial embolization. *Cardiovasc Intervent Radiol.* 2010;33:240-250.

Chung M, Vazquez R. *Non-operating room Anesthesia.* In: *Miller's Anesthesia.* 9th ed. Elsevier; 2020:2284-2312.

Coté CJ. Anesthesia outside the operating room. In: Coté CJ, Lerman J, Anderson B, eds. *A Practice of Anesthesia for Infants and Children.* 6th ed. Elsevier; 2018:1077-1094.

Dougherty TB, Nguyen DT. Anesthetic management of the patient scheduled for head and neck cancer surgery. *J Clin Anesth.* 1994;6:74-82.

Friedberg SR, Lachter J. Endoscopic ultrasound: current roles and future directions. *World J Gastrointest Endosc.* 2017;9:499-505.

Joung KD, Yang HK, Shin WJ, et al. Anesthetic consideration for neurointerventional procedures. *Neurointervention.* 2014;9:72-77.

Lin OS, Weigel W. Nonoperating room anesthesia for gastrointestinal endoscopic procedures. *Curr Opin Anesthesiol.* 2018;31(4):486-491.

Powers WJ, Rabinstein AA, Ackerson T, et al. Guidelines for the early management of patients with acute ischemic stroke: 2019 update to the 2018 guidelines for the early management of acute ischemic stroke. A guideline for healthcare professionals from the American Heart Association/American Stroke Association. *Stroke.* 2019;50(12):e34 4-e418.

Prabhakar A, Owen CP, Kaye AD. Anesthetic management of the patient with amyotrophic lateral sclerosis. *J Anesth.* 2013;27:909-918.

Raiten J, Elkassabany N, Gao W, Mandel JE. Medical intelligence article: novel uses of high frequency ventilation outside the operating room. *Anesth Analg.* 2011;112(5):1110-1113.

Runyon BA; AASLD. Introduction to the revised American Association for the Study of Liver Diseases Practice Guideline management of adult patients with ascites due to cirrhosis 2012. *Hepatology.* 2013;57:1651-1653.

Uppal V, Doursish J, Macfarlance A. Anaesthesia for electroconvulsive therapy. *Contin Educ Anaesth Crit Care Pain.* 2010;10(6):192-196.

Vazquez R, Beermann SL, Fintelmann FJ, Mullen EM, Chitilian H. High-frequency jet ventilation in the prone position to facilitate cryoablation of a peridiaphragmatic pulmonary neoplasm. *A A Pract.* 2019;13(5):169-172.

Vazquez R. Peripheral nerve blocks. In: McCarthy CJ, Walker TG, Vazquez R, eds. *Specialty Imaging: Acute and Chronic Pain Intervention.* 1st ed. Elsevier; 2020:36-45.

Walker TG, Salazar GM, Waltman AC. Angiographic evaluation and management of acute gastrointestinal hemorrhage. *World J Gastroenterol.* 2012;18:1191-1201.

Anesthesia for Trauma and Burns

Evan Hodell, Stephanie Lankford, and Ilan Mizrahi

I. INITIAL EVALUATION OF THE TRAUMA PATIENT

Rapid assessment of injuries and institution of resuscitative measures are particularly important in trauma patients. Life-threatening injuries should be identified immediately based on **A**irway, **B**reathing, **C**irculation, **D**isability (neurologic evaluation) and **E**xposure (hypothermia, smoke inhalation, chemical substances). Treatment measures should be initiated simultaneously. Assume that all patients have a cervical spine injury, a full stomach, and hypovolemia until proven otherwise.

A. Airway

1. Airway assessment should include inspection for foreign bodies, facial and laryngeal fractures (palpable fracture and subcutaneous emphysema), and expanding cervical hematomas. Dyspnea, hemoptysis, dysphonia, stridor, and air leaking through the neck wound may also be signs of airway injury. Remove all secretions, blood, vomitus, and any existing foreign bodies (eg, dentures or teeth).

2. **Minimize movement of the cervical spine during airway manipulation.** If immobilizing devices must be removed temporarily, an assistant should keep the head in a neutral position with manual in-line stabilization.

3. **Establish** a definitive airway if there is any doubt about the patient's ability to maintain airway integrity. With blunt or penetrating injuries to the neck, endotracheal intubation may worsen a laryngeal or bronchial injury. Functional suction equipment should always be immediately available to prevent aspiration if the trauma patient with a full stomach vomits.

   a. **The awake patient.** Depending on the patient's injuries, the ability to cooperate, and cardiopulmonary stability, several options are available. Choice of technique for securing the airway should be individualized based on operator preference and level of experience, as well as patient circumstances.

      1. Intubation **after a rapid sequence induction** is the most common approach to the airway. Video laryngoscopy may be helpful in patients with suspected cervical spine injury.

      2. **Awake nasal or orotracheal intubation** with the use of a laryngoscope or fiberoptic bronchoscope is an alternative.

      3. **Blind nasal intubation** may be performed on the spontaneously breathing patient.

      4. **Awake cricothyroidotomy** or **tracheostomy** may be necessary for patients with severe facial trauma that might be contraindications to other methods of intubation.

   b. **The combative patient.** A rapid sequence orotracheal intubation is often the most expedient approach. Preoxygenation may be difficult, and any delay in securing the airway will cause progressive hypoxemia.

   c. **The unconscious patient.** Orotracheal intubation is usually the safest and most expeditious approach.

d. **The patient with a prehospital supraglottic airway.** If the patient arrives with a supraglottic airway, prioritize establishing a definitive airway with endotracheal intubation. Ventilating via a supraglottic airway may force air into the stomach, leading to gastric inflation and subsequent emesis. Common prehospital supraglottic airways include Laryngeal Mask Airways, King Laryngeal Tubes, and Combitubes.

e. **The intubated patient.** Verify the position of an endotracheal tube by auscultating for breath sounds bilaterally and by detecting end-tidal CO_2. Secure the endotracheal tube, and ensure adequate ventilation and oxygenation. If there are any problems with oxygenation, consider bronchoscopy to assess endotracheal tube placement and patency.

B. **Breathing.** Adequate function of the lungs, diaphragm, and chest wall should be evaluated rapidly. Supplemental oxygen should be provided to all trauma patients, either by mask or by endotracheal tube.

1. Assess the chest wall excursion. Auscultate the lungs to ensure adequate gas exchange. Visual inspection and palpation may rapidly detect injuries such as a pneumothorax.

2. Tension pneumothorax, massive hemothorax, and pulmonary contusion are three common conditions that may acutely impair ventilation and should always be identified.

   a. **Treatment of tension pneumothorax.** Perform needle decompression on the affected side with a large-bore 14-gauge, 3.25-inch/8-cm catheter in the fourth or fifth intercostal space, anterior axillary line. The second intercostal space at the mid-clavicular line is the primary site in children and secondary site in adults. Effective treatment will result in a normalization of physiologic parameters but rarely cause the classically taught "whoosh" of air.

3. Positive-pressure ventilation may worsen a tension pneumothorax and/or cardiac tamponade, which can rapidly lead to cardiovascular collapse.

4. **Lung protective ventilation.** Use tidal volumes of 6 to 8 mL/kg. In patients with metabolic acidosis or suspected traumatic brain injury, increase the respiratory rate to achieve a $Paco_2$ of 35 to 40 mm Hg. In patients with hemorrhagic shock, be wary that high levels of positive end-expiratory pressure (PEEP) and auto-PEEP will increase intrathoracic pressure and subsequently decrease venous return, cardiac output, and systemic blood pressure.

5. The trauma patient's breathing and gas exchange should continue to be periodically reevaluated after intubation or initiation of positive-pressure ventilation.

C. **Circulation**

1. In the severely injured trauma patient, rapid initiation of resuscitation measures is important to prevent and control the lethal triad: hypothermia, acidosis, and coagulopathy.

2. **Hemodynamics** are initially assessed by palpating pulses and measuring the blood pressure. Consider placing an intra-arterial catheter for continuous blood pressure measurement in unstable patients.

3. **Intravenous (IV) access.** Check IV lines already in place to ensure proper function. At least two large-bore catheters should be placed, preferably 16 gauge or larger. These lines should be placed above the level of the diaphragm in patients with injuries of the abdomen, where there is a potential for major venous disruption. IV access below the level of the diaphragm is helpful when obstruction or disruption of the superior vena cava, innominate, or subclavian vein is suspected.

4. **Peripheral venous cannulation failure.** In this event, percutaneous sub-clavian or femoral vein cannulation should be carried out. Although the internal and external jugular veins remain options, access to these structures is frequently hindered by immobilization of the head and neck for a suspected cervical spine injury. If these approaches prove unsuccessful, **surgical cutdowns** can be performed. The saphenous vein at the ankle and the antecubital venous system are acceptable options. When emergent access for vasoactive medications or fluid resuscitation is needed, intraosseous (IO) access to the vasculature is also an option for personnel trained in this technique.

   a. IO access locations: proximal tibia (most common), distal tibia, proximal humerus, iliac crest, and sternum.

   b. IO flowrates vary by site but are roughly 165 mL/min and can be optimized by initially flushing the line and then using a pressure bag. In awake patients, flushing the line under pressure is usually much more painful than initial placement.

   c. IO access can be used for blood and fluid resuscitation, as well as vasoactive medications.

5. **Volume resuscitation should be individualized.** The concept of "damage control" emphasizes multiple approaches to control and prevent tissue hypoperfusion, acidosis, coagulopathy, and hypothermia.

   a. **Damage control resuscitation (DCR)** refers to the strategy of limit-ing crystalloid use, early resuscitation with packed red blood cells and clotting factors, and maintenance of a systolic blood pressure at approximately 90 mm Hg or mean arterial pressure at 50 to 65 mm Hg. The disadvantages to crystalloid infusion include dilu-tion of coagulation factors, hemodilution, and clot disruption. Early administration of blood and clotting factors serves to treat trauma-induced coagulopathy that can occur early after injury. In a patient in whom hemorrhage has not been definitely controlled, elevation in blood pressure and cardiac output can cause dislodgement of a clot and further bleeding. DCR blood pressure parameters should not be used in certain subsets of patients, such as patients with head trauma. Avoiding hypotension is a priority in patients with moder-ate and severe traumatic brain injury. In this patient population, maintain a systolic blood pressure ≥100 mm Hg for patients 50 to 69 years old and ≥110 mm Hg for patients 15 to 49 or >70 years old.

   b. **Massive blood transfusion**, or the replacement of 50% of the total blood volume within 3 hours, is a response to massive and uncontrolled hemorrhage. In an emergency, type-specific uncross-matched blood or type O–negative blood may be given before cross-matched blood becomes available. A ratio of 1:1:1 or 2:1:1 (RBCs:plasma:platelets) is targeted for blood product administration. Although this ratio mir-rors the content of whole blood, superior clot formation is achieved with transfusion of whole blood compared with 1:1:1 component transfusion. Therefore, fresh whole blood has been used for combat injuries in the military. Some civilian institutions have now adopted its use in trauma. An intraoperative blood salvage system (cell saver) can also be used to help in the reduction of allogenic red blood cell administration. Aggressive resuscitation with blood products can lead to hypothermia, hyperkalemia, and hypocalcemia. Empiric treatment is often indicated as the laboratory results may lag behind the clinical scenario when massive transfusion resuscitation is undertaken.

   c. **Management of coagulopathy** is guided by point-of-care (POC) and stan-dard laboratory testing. POC tests, such as the thromboelastogram

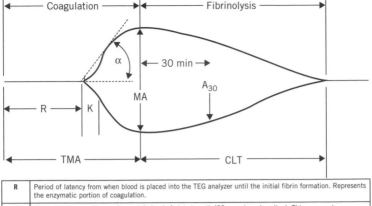

R	Period of latency from when blood is placed into the TEG analyzer until the initial fibrin formation. Represents the enzymatic portion of coagulation.
K	Measures the speed to reach a certain level of clot strength (20 mm above baseline). This represents clot kinetics.
α	Measures the rapidity of fibrin built up and cross-linking (clot strengthening). This represents fibrinogen level.
MA	Maximum amplitude, is a direct function of the maximum dynamic properties of the fibrin and platelet binding via GPIIb/IIIa and represents the ultimate strength of the fibrin clot. This represents platelet function/aggregation.
LY30	Measures the rate of amplitude reduction 30 min after MA. This represents clot lysis.

FIGURE 35.1 Overview of thromboelastogram parameters. (Reprinted with permission from Handa RR, Turnbull IR, Ismail O. Hemostasis, anticoagulation, and transfusions. In: Klingensmith ME, Wise PE, Courtney CM, et al, eds. *The Washington Manual of Surgery.* 8th ed. Wolters Kluwer; 2019. Figure 6.2.)

(**Figure 35.1**), provide rapid, near-real-time information regarding clot initiation, kinetics of clot formation, clot strength, and fibrinoloysis. Standard tests of hemoglobin levels, platelet counts, fibrinogen levels, prothrombin time, partial thromboplastin time, and international normalized ratio are useful but may lag behind rapidly evolving clinical situations. Utilizing dynamic parameters, such as transesophageal echocardiography (TEE) and the intra-arterial pressure waveform, can also assist in judicious blood and fluid administration.

    d. Severely injured trauma patients do not tolerate prolonged surgical procedures. **Damage control surgery** refers to the concept of employing initial short surgical procedures immediately after injury with the goals of controlling hemorrhage and preventing contamination (eg, due to GI tract injury) through temporary measures. Patients then undergo definitive corrective surgery at a later date after they have been stabilized.

6. Vasopressor infusions should not substitute for adequate volume replacement during initial resuscitation. Vasopressors may be necessary as a temporizing measure if perfusion pressure is clearly inadequate during ongoing volume resuscitation.

7. Antifibrinolytics, such as tranexamic acid (TXA), can reduce mortality in a bleeding trauma patient when started as soon as possible within 3 hours of injury. The safety of antifibrinolytics after 3 hours has yet to be fully elucidated. Immediate antifibrinolytic therapy is also associated with a decrease in mortality in patients presenting with traumatic brain injury. Administer 1 g of TXA over 10 minutes, followed by an intravenous infusion of 1 g over 8 hours.

TABLE 35.1	Glasgow Coma Score	
Eye Opening		**Score**
Spontaneous		4
To speech		3
To pain		2
No response		1
Best Verbal Response		
Oriented		5
Confused conversation		4
Inappropriate words		3
Incomprehensible sounds		2
None		1
Best Motor Response		
Obeys commands		6
Localizes pain		5
Normal flexion (withdrawal)		4
Abnormal flexion (decorticate)		3
Extension (decerebrate)		2
None (flaccid)		1

D. **Disability/neurologic evaluation.** A brief neurologic examination yields useful information in assessing cerebral perfusion or oxygenation and can provide a simple and quick means of predicting a patient's outcome.
  1. The level of consciousness can be described by the AVPU method (A, **a**lert; V, responds to **v**erbal stimuli; P, responds only to **p**ainful stimuli; and U, **u**nresponsive to all stimuli). A more detailed and quantitative assessment of neurologic function is with the Glasgow coma scale (**Table 35.1**) that is the sum of the best eye opening, verbal, and motor responses.
  2. An altered level of consciousness dictates immediate reevaluation of the patient's oxygenation and circulation, even though it can be of central nervous system origin (trauma or intoxication).
  3. Neurologic deterioration can rapidly occur in trauma patients and necessitates frequent neurologic reevaluation.

E. **Exposure.** Trauma patients are often hypothermic upon arrival at the hospital and require aggressive efforts to maintain normothermia (temperature ≥35.5 °C). Hypothermia can exacerbate coagulopathy.
  1. External warming devices should be applied, IV fluids and blood products warmed before infusion, and a warm environment maintained.
  2. If there is any suspicion of exposure to chemical agents, decontamination of the patient must be carried out before entrance into the hospital. This terminates exposure, protects the health care provider, and allows the hospital to function effectively.

F. Diagnostic studies

1. **Laboratory studies** include blood type and cross-match, complete blood count, platelet count, prothrombin time, activated partial thromboplastin time, electrolytes, glucose, blood urea nitrogen, creatinine, urinalysis, and, if indicated, toxicologic screening.

2. **Radiographic studies** should include a lateral cervical spine film, a chest radiograph (CXR), and an anteroposterior view of the pelvis on all patients with blunt trauma. At a minimum, a CXR is obtained in all patients with penetrating injuries of the trunk. Additional studies include thoracic, lumbar, and sacral spine films and chest and abdominal computed tomography (CT) studies.

    a. **Lateral radiographs of the cervical spine** must include the C7–T1 interface and must be of sufficient quality to delineate the structures of interest (ie, soft tissues and bones).

    b. If the patient's clinical condition allows time for additional studies, **open-mouth odontoid and anteroposterior views of the neck** (standard trauma cervical spine series) may be obtained.

    c. If the clinical evaluation demonstrates a patient with significant neck pain and tenderness but no evidence of fracture or dislocation on the plain radiographs, CT and magnetic resonance imaging may help delineate an occult injury.

3. A **12-lead electrocardiogram (ECG)** should be performed on all major trauma patients to help evaluate the presence of myocardial injury (eg, contusion, tamponade, ischemia, and arrhythmia).

4. Focused Assessment with Sonography in Trauma (**FAST, Figure 35.2**) is a rapid ultrasound examination evaluating for bleeding or free fluid around the heart or abdominal organs. The four areas that are examined are the perihepatic space (including Morison's pouch or hepatorenal recess), perisplenic space, pelvis, and pericardium. A negative FAST examination, however, cannot completely rule out significant intraperitoneal bleeding in patients with blunt abdominal trauma.

5. The extended FAST (eFAST) examination includes the ultrasound examination of a patient's bilateral lungs. It can be used to detect a pneumothorax with the absence of normal lung sliding.

G. Monitoring is dictated by the severity of the patient's injuries and preexisting medical problems.

1. **An arterial line** is useful in patients with hemodynamic instability or respiratory failure.

2. **A central venous catheter (CVC)** may be required to assess volume status via central venous pressure (CVP) measurements. Vasoactive medications can also be administered through a CVC.

3. A **pulmonary artery catheter** may be helpful in patients with ventricular dysfunction, severe coronary artery disease, valvular heart disease, multiple organ system involvement, or hemodynamics that seem disproportionate to their trauma burden. Placement is planned according to the time available and the clinical status of the patient.

II. SPECIFIC INJURIES

A. Intracranial and spinal cord trauma (see Chapter 23)

B. Facial trauma. Considerable force is required to produce facial fractures. Accordingly, these injuries often are associated with other injuries such as intracranial and spinal cord trauma, thoracic injury, myocardial contusion, and intra-abdominal bleeding. Brisk oral or nasal bleeding, limited mouth opening, broken teeth, vomitus, or tongue or pharyngeal injury

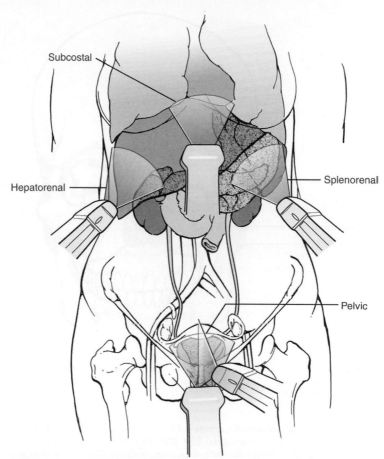

Subcostal

Hepatorenal

Splenorenal

Pelvic

FIGURE 35.2 FAST examination ultrasound locations. (Reprinted with permission from Berg SM, Bittner EA, Zhao KH. *Anesthesia Review: Blasting the Boards*. Wolters Kluwer; 2016. Figure 19.1.)

may occlude the airway, obscure visualization, and complicate airway management. Trismus may be associated with these injuries and should be assessed before the induction of anesthesia. Emergency cricothyroidotomy or tracheostomy done under local anesthesia may be lifesaving.

1. **Maxillary fractures** are grouped by the **LeFort classification** (**Figure 35.3**).
   a. **Type I (transverse or horizontal).** The body of the maxilla is separated from the base of the skull above the level of the palate and below the level of the zygomatic process.
   b. **Type II (pyramidal).** Vertical fractures through the facial aspects of the maxilla extend upward through the nasal and ethmoid bones.
   c. **Type III (craniofacial dysjunction).** Fractures extend through the frontozygomatic suture lines bilaterally, across the orbits, and through the base of the nose and the ethmoid region.

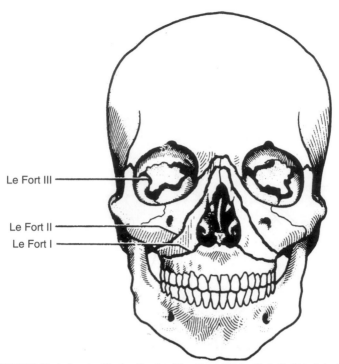

Le Fort III

Le Fort II
Le Fort I

FIGURE 35.3 The Le Fort classification. (Reprinted from Rosen P, Baker FJ, Barkin RM, et al, eds. *Emergency Medicine: Concepts and Clinical Practice.* 2nd ed. Mosby; 1988. Copyright © 1988 Elsevier. With permission.)

    d. Le Fort and related fractures are frequently associated with skull fractures and **cerebrospinal fluid (CSF) rhinorrhea.** Evaluation of radiographic images may help determine anatomic distortion and airway integrity. Nasotracheal intubation and placement of nasogastric tubes are relatively contraindicated under these circumstances. Elective nasal intubation (or tracheostomy) may be necessary, however, before operative repair. A fiberoptic bronchoscope may be used in these cases to guide an endotracheal tube into the trachea.

    e. In the presence of a CSF leak (rhinorrhea), positive-pressure mask ventilation can potentially cause pneumocephalus.

2. Mandibular fractures

    a. Malocclusion, limitation of mandibular movement, loose or missing teeth, sublingual hematoma, and swelling at the fracture site complicate airway management.

    b. Posterior displacement of the tongue producing airway obstruction is associated with bilateral condylar or parasymphyseal fractures of the mandible. Simple forward traction on the tongue often provides relief.

    c. Reestablishment of normal occlusion may necessitate intermaxillary fixation, which can also be combined with rigid fixation. Awake nasotracheal intubation is recommended if the nose has not been severely traumatized.

3. **Ocular trauma** usually requires general anesthesia for repair. Special considerations for open-eye injuries are discussed in Chapter 30.

4. **Anesthetic management.** Most displaced facial fractures require general anesthesia for repair. Although children usually require general anesthesia, many soft tissue injuries can be treated with local anesthesia. Maintenance of a patent airway is the principal concern, and induction may require awake nasotracheal intubation, fiberoptic laryngoscopy, or tracheostomy under local anesthesia.

C. **Neck trauma** may cause cervical spine injury, esophageal tears, major vascular injuries, and airway injuries. Airway injuries may present with obstruction, subcutaneous emphysema, hemoptysis, dysphonia, or hypoxemia.

1. The neck is divided into three anatomic zones when describing penetrating neck trauma (**Figure 35.4**). These zones guide surgical or conservative management:

   a. Zone 1: clavicles and sternal notch to cricoid cartilage. Greatest potential for injuries to intrathoracic great vessels. Important structures include the aortic arch, proximal common carotid arteries, vertebral arteries, subclavian vessels, innominate vessels, lung apices, esophagus, trachea, brachial plexus, and thoracic duct.

   b. Zone 2 (80% of injuries): cricoid cartilage to angle of mandible. Important structures include the common, internal and external carotid arteries, internal and external jugular veins, larynx, hypopharynx, and proximal esophagus.

   c. Zone 3: angle of mandible to base of skull. Important structures include internal carotid artery, vertebral artery, external carotid artery, jugular veins, prevertebral venous plexus, and facial nerve trunk.

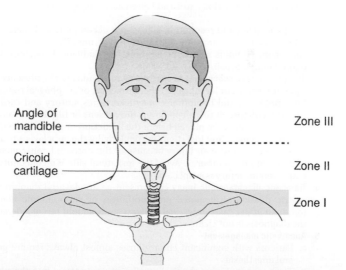

FIGURE 35.4 Zones of the neck. (Reprinted with permission from Fiser SM. *The ABSITE Review.* 3rd ed. Wolters Kluwer Health/Lippincott Williams & Wilkins; 2010. Figure 16.6.)

2. **"Clothesline"** injuries occur from direct trauma to the upper airway and can result in separation of the larynx from the trachea or separation between the cricoid cartilage and the first tracheal ring. These injuries do not always present with an open neck wound. Additional injuries include laryngotracheal transection, laryngeal fractures, and vascular injury.

3. Blunt injury over the carotid arteries may result in intimal disruption and dissection, even in the absence of initial symptoms. Angiography or ultrasonography may be required to exclude these injuries.

4. Initial management of **penetrating trauma** includes direct compression of involved vessels to control hemorrhage and prevent air embolism.

5. Associated **thoracic injuries,** such as pneumothorax and hemorrhage from injury to the great vessels, may occur with lower neck injuries.

6. **Anesthetic management**
   a. **Securing the airway** is the central issue in these patients. A coordinated approach among members of the trauma team is necessary. A surgical airway or direct intubation of an open airway defect can be lifesaving. Anesthesia induction via spontaneous ventilation of a potent inhalational agent can be useful in the presence of airway disruption with the caveat that the patient likely has a full stomach and is a high risk for aspiration. Preparations should be made for fiberoptic intubation, rigid bronchoscopy, and a surgical airway below the level of injury.
   b. **Great vessel injuries** in the neck may necessitate lower extremity IV access.

D. **Chest trauma** can involve injuries to the trachea or larynx, heart, great vessels, thoracic duct, esophagus, lung, or diaphragm.

   1. **Rib fractures** are a common feature of major thoracic trauma and mandate assessment for pneumothorax by CXR. First-rib fractures should alert the clinician to the potential for associated internal injuries due to severe forces needed to fracture the first rib. Multiple rib fractures most commonly involve ribs 7 to 10 and often accompany lacerations of the spleen or liver.

   2. The hypoxemia and respiratory failure that accompany **flail chest** and other major chest injuries are indicative of underlying pulmonary contusion. IV fluids should be administered judiciously because the injured lung is sensitive to fluid overload.

   3. The presence of **subcutaneous emphysema** may indicate the presence of a pneumothorax or laryngeal, tracheobronchial, or esophageal trauma. Pneumothorax and hemothorax may lead to respiratory and cardiovascular collapse. If these conditions are present or highly suspected, chest tubes should be placed before the induction of general anesthesia. Avoid central line insertion (particularly by the subclavian route) on the side opposite an injury because of the potential consequence of bilateral pneumothorax. Avoid the ipsilateral side if a concomitant major venous injury is suspected.

   4. **Traumatic diaphragmatic injury** can present as an elevated diaphragm, gastric dilatation, loculated pneumothorax, or subpulmonic hematoma. An upper gastrointestinal contrast study should be considered if the diagnosis is not clear.

   5. **Anesthetic management**
      a. Patients with significant chest injuries almost always require general anesthesia.
      b. The necessity for mechanical ventilation may extend into the postoperative period.

    c. Avoid nitrous oxide when a pneumothorax is suspected and a chest tube has not yet been placed. Airway pressures must be closely monitored during positive-pressure ventilation.

    d. Pulmonary hemorrhage into the main conducting airways calls for isolation of the uninjured side before it is flooded with blood. Double-lumen endotracheal tube placement, mainstem intubation, or endobronchial blockade may be needed to prevent blood from spilling into the noninjured side (see Chapter 27).

    e. Regional anesthesia (ie, intercostal nerve blockade, thoracic epidural anesthesia, or paravertebral blocks) may provide analgesia for multiple painful rib fractures. Adequate pain relief can reduce chest wall splinting, regional hypoventilation, and progressive hypoxemia.

E. Cardiac and major vascular trauma

  1. Blunt cardiac injury can result in myocardial muscle contusion, chamber rupture, valvular disruption, tamponade, or dysrhythmias.

  2. Cardiac trauma may be associated with a fractured sternum, hemothorax, pericardial tamponade, myocardial dysfunction, valvular dysfunction, and ECG changes (persistent sinus tachycardia, multiple premature ventricular contractions and other dysrhythmias, bundle branch block, nonspecific ST-segment and T-wave changes, and overt ischemia).

    a. Beck triad of distended neck veins, muffled heart sounds, and hypotension is present in only 30% of patients with pericardial tamponade, and pulsus paradoxus is even less reliable. The diagnostic test of choice is cardiac ultrasound.

    b. Pericardiocentesis may be used to stabilize the patient until surgical repair can be performed. A subxiphoid pericardial window is ideally performed in the operating room.

  3. A widened mediastinal profile, lack of clarity of the aortic knob, rightward tracheal shift, or widening of the left paraspinal line without associated fracture on the CXR mandate further workup to rule out traumatic aortic injury. CT is the diagnostic test of choice and is more sensitive than angiography. Potentially salvageable patients with aortic rupture often have an incomplete laceration near the ligamentum arteriosum. An intact adventitial layer or contained hematoma prevents immediate death. An arterial line should be placed in the right arm since the compromised aorta may not transmit a normal pulse distal to the left subclavian and the flow through the left subclavian may be occluded during the course of surgical repair.

  4. The subclavian artery is subject to injury with hyperextension of the neck and shoulder.

  5. Anesthetic management

    a. These patients are often **severely hypovolemic** and may have compromised cardiac function. Cardiopulmonary bypass may be required for certain repairs.

    b. Resuscitative endovascular balloon occlusion of the aorta (REBOA) is an option for patients presenting with noncompressible torso hemorrhage. REBOA does not provide definitive hemorrhage control. This temporary measure supports vital organ perfusion, decreases the amount of bleeding distal to the occluded site, and provides a window of opportunity for resuscitation and hemorrhage control.

    c. Monitors should include **intra-arterial catheter** placed in an upper extremity since lower-extremity arterial perfusion is lost during balloon inflation and occlusion of the aorta, CVC, and **TEE** to assess ventricular function, volume status, and position of the endovascular balloon.

d. Clear communication with the surgical team is essential in preparation for the physiologic changes of reperfusion following balloon deflation: hypoxemia, hypercarbia, acidosis, hyperkalemia, anemia, and disorders of hemostasis.

e. Etomidate and ketamine both provide hemodynamic stability for induction. However, ketamine use is cautioned in patients with concomitant head injury and those with cocaine abuse.

f. Cross-matched type-specific blood or O-negative blood should be available before induction. Inotropic and vasopressor agents should be immediately available to treat severe hypotension.

g. For refractory cardiogenic shock or acute respiratory distress syndrome, either venoarterial or venovenous extracorporeal membrane oxygenation, respectively, may be considered.

F. Peripheral vascular trauma

1. Check **peripheral pulses** in all extremities during the evaluation of trauma patients. Arteriography can be used to further define injuries.

2. **Anesthetic management** should focus on the recognition of hypovolemia secondary to uncontrolled hemorrhage. Regional anesthetic techniques may be considered in stable patients.

G. Abdominal trauma

1. In stable patients without peritonitis, **penetrating abdominal wounds** (with the exception of gunshot wounds) are initially evaluated by local wound exploration. If the exploration is equivocal, diagnostic peritoneal lavage, abdominal ultrasound, or an abdominal CT scan may be performed.

2. All patients with **gunshot wounds of the abdomen** are surgically explored.

3. With **impalement injuries** (eg, stab wounds or falls onto sharp objects), the penetrating object, if still present in the wound, will usually be removed in the operating room after anesthesia has been induced and the patient stabilized. Removal may result in exsanguination.

4. **Blunt trauma** may result in intra-abdominal or retroperitoneal bleeding.

a. The **spleen** is the most frequently injured abdominal organ in blunt trauma. Signs and symptoms include abdominal or referred shoulder pain, abdominal rigidity, a falling hematocrit, or hypotension. Minor splenic hematomas are often managed nonoperatively, but grade IV (active bleeding) and V (shattered/avulsed spleen) injuries require splenectomy.

b. The **liver** frequently fractures with blunt abdominal trauma. Minor injuries are managed nonoperatively unless other injuries mandate laparotomy. Thus, liver injuries that require operation are often complex with large blood loss and high mortality. Manual compression can temporarily control bleeding and allow time for volume resuscitation. Perihepatic packing (**"damage control surgery"**) with planned re-exploration is sometimes considered for patients with severe injuries.

5. **Abdominal compartment syndrome** (ACS) can occur in the setting of direct injury as well as after massive fluid resuscitation.

a. ACS often presents with a clinical triad of
   1. tense, distended abdomen.
   2. respiratory distress or high peak pressure if the patient is intubated.
   3. oliguria.

b. Intra-abdominal pressure greater than 12 mm Hg is indicative of abdominal hypertension. ACS is defined as a sustained intra-abdominal pressure >20 mm Hg that is associated with new organ dysfunction. ACS often warrants immediate decompression. Systemic hypotension is common because of a decrease in preload by compression of the inferior vena cava.

c. Retroperitoneal hematomas and aortic rupture may present with ACS. Bowel perforation can occur from ischemia, and peritonitis can lead to further tissue edema. Electrolyte disorders, myoglobinuria, and renal failure can occur.

d. Surgical decompression may be necessary. These patients are often **intravascularly depleted** and may **become severely hypotensive** after decompression owing to the newly uncompressed abdominal vasculature. Cross-matched type-specific blood or O-negative blood should be available before induction. Inotropic and vasopressor agents should be immediately available to treat severe hypotension.

H. Genitourinary trauma

1. All multiple trauma patients should have a **Foley catheter** placed. If pelvic or perineal injury has occurred, as evidenced by blood at the urethral meatus, a perineal hematoma, or a high-riding prostate, retrograde urethrography should be performed before urethral catheterization.

2. All patients with penetrating abdominal or back injuries and those with significant hematuria after blunt trauma should have a radiographic evaluation for damage to the kidneys, ureter, and bladder.

3. Eighty-five percent of renal injuries can be managed nonoperatively, but patients with refractory hypotension should go directly to the operating room for exploration.

   a. Ureteral laceration is managed by surgical intervention after locating the disruption by retrograde urography.

   b. Bladder contusions may be treated nonoperatively, but rupture usually requires exploration.

   c. The inability of the patient to void or clinical signs of injury indicate **injury to the urethra** (see Section II.H.1). Diagnostic urethrography should precede treatment with suprapubic cystostomy for urinary diversion and control of hemorrhage. Most disruptions can undergo delayed repair.

I. Orthopedic trauma

1. All **fractures or dislocations** that compromise nerve or vascular function may constitute surgical emergencies (eg, radial nerve injury with humeral shaft fractures and aseptic necrosis of the femoral head with hip dislocation) and must be reduced immediately. It is important to document the neurovascular examination immediately before anesthesia and upon awakening. Regional anesthesia may delay diagnosis of compartment syndrome and is relatively contraindicated if compartment syndrome is anticipated.

2. **Upper extremity**

   a. Severe **depression or hyperabduction of the shoulder girdle** can stretch or tear the brachial plexus. Horner syndrome may present with damaged cervical sympathetic chain.

   b. When the shoulder is struck hard from the side, the medial end of the clavicle may be dislocated upward or retrosternally. Pressure on the trachea in a retrosternal dislocation may cause life-threatening airway compromise.

   c. Dislocation of the glenohumeral joint can cause axillary nerve injury.

   d. Fractures of the humeral shaft, especially the middle or distal part, are frequently associated with radial nerve injury.

    e. Neurovascular compromise of the forearm can occur with **fracture or dislocation of the elbow.** Peripheral ischemia is often complicated by edema of the anterior compartment with risk for nerve and muscle necrosis. Fasciotomy may be indicated.

    f. Median nerve compression is possible with **fractures at the wrist** or with carpal dislocation and may require division of the transverse carpal ligament.

3. Pelvis

    a. Patients who have sustained pelvic injuries can be divided into three major categories:

        1. Exsanguinating hemorrhage from external bleeding in open fractures or from retroperitoneal hematoma in closed fractures (0.5%-1.0%). These patients almost always present with severe hypotension or cardiac arrest and rarely respond to resuscitative measures.

        2. Hemodynamically stable with a relatively uncomplicated course (75%). Urgent or elective surgery for repair of bony and ligamentous pelvic disruptions may be required.

        3. An **intermediate group** in critical condition with various degrees of overall injury, hemorrhage, and hemodynamic instability (25%).

    b. Initial management for these injuries may include the application of a compressive binder for "open-book" fractures, pelvic angiography (with or without therapeutic embolization to control hemorrhage), and external pelvic fixation.

    c. Pelvic fractures without major disruption, such as type I anterior-posterior compression (APC) injury or type I lateral compression injury, can be treated with bed rest and delayed open reduction and internal fixation (ORIF). More complex injuries such as APC II (widened sacroiliac joint with hemorrhagic and vascular consequences) require acute external fixation with delayed conversion to internal fixation, acute ORIF, or arterial embolization.

    d. Fat embolism can occur with pelvic and major long-bone fractures (see Chapters 17 and 22).

    e. Crush injuries may be associated with **myoglobinuria.** Aggressive and early hydration may help prevent acute renal failure.

4. Lower extremity

    a. Fractures of the **tibia and fibula,** the most common major skeletal injuries, can be associated with neurovascular trauma and attendant compartment syndrome.

    b. With a fracture of the **femur,** blood loss can be much greater than is evident from superficial inspection.

    c. Hip fractures are common in the elderly, whose clinical picture is often dominated by other complicating medical illnesses. Traction is used initially for pain relief, but most fractures require ORIF to ensure adequate healing and function and to avoid the complications of prolonged immobilization.

    d. Regional, general anesthesia, and combined techniques can be considered for patients with isolated lower-extremity injuries without concern for compartment syndrome.

5. Extremity reimplantation

    a. Indications. In general, these procedures are performed on the upper extremities and only in patients who are otherwise stable. An amputated arm, hand, or digit will not be reimplanted if it has sustained a severe crush injury or has been raggedly torn from major nerves and blood vessels. Reimplantations may be extremely lengthy procedures, occasionally in excess of 24 hours.

b. Anesthetic management

1. General anesthesia is usually chosen because of the long duration of these procedures. A combined technique will reduce anesthetic requirements and provide for postoperative analgesia (especially with catheter placements, rather than single-dose brachial plexus blocks). Regional anesthesia may improve blood flow via the induced sympathectomy.

2. During general anesthesia, the head and pressure points must be evaluated every 1 to 2 hours to avoid pressure-induced injury (eg, scalp ulceration and hair loss). Low-pressure mattresses and padded sponge blocks should be used to minimize pressure on susceptible peripheral nerves (eg, ulnar, sciatic, peroneal, or sural). The endotracheal tube cuff pressure should be periodically assessed because nitrous oxide will diffuse into the cuff and increase the pressure on the tracheal mucosa.

3. Patients should be kept warm and adequately hydrated. Avoid hyperventilation or the use of vasoconstrictors.

4. Consider invasive hemodynamic monitoring for optimization of the perfusion pressure and for prolonged cases. If a noninvasive blood pressure cuff is used, it should be rotated among multiple sites. The need for anticoagulation is determined intraoperatively.

5. Blood loss can be vastly underestimated. Blood samples should be sent periodically to assess hemoglobin levels.

III. THE PEDIATRIC TRAUMA PATIENT

A. General considerations

1. A clear understanding of the salient anatomic and physiologic differences among adults, children, and infants and a working knowledge of the specific anesthetic considerations for this patient population are required (see Chapter 33).

2. **Blunt trauma,** usually from falls or motor vehicle accidents, predominates in children. Multiple injuries are the rule rather than the exception, but diagnosis is often more difficult because of the child's inability to provide an accurate history.

B. Specific considerations

1. Although the pediatric trauma patient frequently presents with significant blood loss, initially, the **vital signs** may be minimally altered. **Reliance on vital signs alone may seriously underestimate the severity of the injury.**

2. Orotracheal intubation with protection of the cervical spine is the preferred method of obtaining airway control. Nasotracheal intubation is **not** recommended in children under the age of 12 years. **Surgical cricothyroidotomy** is rarely performed in an infant or a small child because of technical difficulties. If airway control and ventilation cannot be accomplished, needle cricothyroidotomy is an appropriate temporary approach for oxygenation.

3. **IO** is an acceptable procedure for critically injured pediatric patients in whom venous access cannot be established. An initial bolus of 20 mL/kg of crystalloid is recommended for initial resuscitation.

4. The small child who is **hypothermic** may be refractory to therapy for shock. During initial evaluation and management, overhead heaters or thermal blankets will be needed to maintain body temperature.

5. Avoidance of hypoxemia is pertinent in the pediatric population. Owing to high metabolic rate and oxygen consumption, desaturation can occur rapidly, followed by severe bradycardia. **Atropine IV 10 to 20 µg/ kg or IM 20 to 30 µg/kg** should be prepared to treat bradycardia.

IV. THE PREGNANT TRAUMA PATIENT
A. General considerations
1. Pregnancy must always be suspected in any female trauma patient of childbearing age (see Chapter 32 for management of the pregnant patient). All pregnant women greater than 24 weeks of gestation should have cardiotocographic monitoring for a minimum of 4 to 6 hours.
2. Kleihauer-Betke analysis helps in determining the amount of fetomaternal hemorrhage and should be performed. Volume replacement is preferable to vasopressor administration to support blood pressure. O-negative blood should be transfused in a Rh-negative pregnant patient until cross-matched blood becomes available. Fetomaternal hemorrhage in an Rh-negative patient warrants Rh immunoglobulin therapy.
3. Because the fetus depends on its mother for oxygen, an **uninterrupted supply of oxygenated blood** must be provided to the fetus at all times. The resuscitation of the fetus thus depends on the optimum resuscitation of the mother. The uterus remains an intrapelvic organ until the 12th week of gestation and reaches the umbilicus by 20 weeks. **Compression of the vena cava by the gravid uterus** after 20 weeks of gestation reduces venous return to the heart, thereby decreasing cardiac output and exacerbating shock. The pregnant patient should be transported and evaluated with **left uterine displacement**.
4. If intubation is necessary, a rapid sequence induction is recommended with a smaller-sized endotracheal tube and use of cricoid pressure. Advanced airway equipment (video laryngoscope, fiberoptic bronchoscope) should be readily available in anticipation of a difficult airway. Placement of a nasal or orogastric tube prior to induction of anesthesia should be considered to decompress the patient's stomach and reduce the risk of aspiration.
5. Although diagnostic irradiation poses a risk to the fetus, necessary radiographic studies should always be obtained. Consultation with a radiologist may be obtained for estimation of the total radiation dose to the fetus if multiple diagnostic imaging studies with ionizing radiation have been obtained.
6. If the amniotic fluid gains access to the intravascular space, it can be a source of amniotic fluid embolism and resultant disseminated intravascular coagulation.

B. Treatment
1. If the mother's condition is stable, the status of the fetus and the extent of uterine injury will determine further management. Consultation with the patient's obstetrician is advisable.
2. A potentially viable fetus at ≥24 weeks' gestation that shows no signs of distress should be monitored by external ultrasound. Premature labor is always a possibility in these patients, and tocolytic therapy should be initiated in consultation with the obstetrics team if premature labor develops.
3. When a viable fetus shows signs of distress despite successful resuscitative measures, a cesarean delivery must be performed expeditiously. A nonviable fetus may be managed conservatively *in utero* to optimize maternal oxygenation and circulation.
4. Primary repair of all maternal wounds should be attempted in a critically injured mother carrying a viable gestation, even at the expense of fetal distress.

5. Perimortem cesarean section/resuscitative hysterotomy is recommended for pregnant woman with fundus height at or above the umbilicus (20 weeks' gestation) or who are perimortem or after 4 minutes of advanced cardiac life support. If maternal viability is not possible (from fatal injury or pulselessness), it should be performed immediately.

V. MAJOR BURN INJURIES
A. Physical implications of burn injury
1. Thermal injury destroys skin, the body's barrier to the external environment. Skin plays a vital role in thermal regulation, fluid and electrolyte homeostasis, and protection against bacterial infection. Significant heat and protein loss, massive fluid shifts, and infections all commonly occur in patients with severe thermal injuries. Microvascular injury results from local damage by heat and from the release of vasoactive substances from the burned tissue.

B. Physiologic implications of burn injury
1. In major burns, circulating mediators trigger systemic inflammation, hypermetabolism, and immune suppression. There is also diffuse alteration in the permeability of cell membranes to sodium, resulting in generalized cellular swelling. Therefore, edema occurs in both burned and unburned tissues.

a. Cardiovascular effects
1. Alterations in microvascular permeability result in a transcapillary fluid flux and significant tissue edema 12 to 24 hours after a thermal injury. Large amounts of water, electrolytes, and proteins are lost into the extravascular space leading to intravascular fluid depletion and hypovolemic shock (burn shock).
2. Immediately after a burn injury, the cardiac output is frequently reduced owing to decreased preload and myocardial depression, possibly due to circulating humoral factors. Blood pressure may be normal owing to increased systemic vascular resistance (SVR). The magnitude of these pathophysiologic changes depends on the size and the depth of the burn injury.
3. The cardiovascular response 24 to 48 hours after successful resuscitation of a major burn is characterized by an *increase* in cardiac output and *reduced* SVR, consistent with the pathophysiology of the systemic inflammatory response syndrome.

b. Metabolic effects
1. "Ebb phase": During the first 2 days after severe, acute burns, a **hypo**metabolic state may be seen, accompanied by decreased oxygen consumption, cardiac output, and metabolic rate. This is also known as the "resuscitative phase" of the burn injury, where effective fluid resuscitation is guided by formulas targeted to achieve a urine output of 0.5 to 1 mL/kg/h.
2. "Flow phase": Starting days 2 to 5, there ensues a catecholamine, inflammatory, and hormonally mediated **hyper**metabolic-hyperdynamic state, which can persist for more than a year. It is frequently accompanied by high cardiac output, decreased SVR, increased oxygen consumption and carbon dioxide production, and protein wasting and catabolism. Treatment during the flow phase should be multifactorial and directed at the various physical and physiologic changes:
   a. Early skin grafting to aid thermal regulation, electrolyte homeostasis, and protect against bacterial infection.

     b. Strict temperature regulation with ambient temperature kept within the thermoneutral range to avoid shivering and a further increase in metabolic rate.

     c. Early nutrition with enteral feeding decreases muscle catabolism and may reduce bacterial translocation through the intestinal mucosa.

     d. Pharmacologic interventions, such as adrenergic blockade with propranolol, reduce resting energy expenditure, insulin resistance, and muscle-protein catabolism. Other pharmacologic interventions are areas of ongoing interest and research.

c. Capillary leakage results in **hemoconcentration** immediately after injury. Despite apparent adequate fluid resuscitation, the hematocrit level often remains increased during the first 48 hours after injury. Bleeding from wounds and a shortened erythrocyte half-life, however, can result in anemia.

d. Microaggregation of the platelets in the skin and smoke-damaged lung and aggressive volume resuscitation result in early **thrombocytopenia** after major burns. Thrombotic and fibrinolytic mechanisms are activated, and disseminated intravascular coagulation may complicate the course of a massive burn injury. A decrease in antithrombin III, protein C, and protein S levels can increase the thrombogenicity of these patients later in their clinical course and theoretically can cause venous thrombosis and pulmonary embolism.

e. **Acute renal failure** is not uncommon in patients with major burn injury and is associated with high mortality. Decreased renal blood flow secondary to hypovolemia and decreased cardiac output, as well as increased levels of catecholamines, aldosterone, and vasopressin, can contribute to renal failure. Other mechanisms include nephrotoxic effects of drugs, rhabdomyolysis, hemolysis, and sepsis (see Chapter 5).

f. **Gastrointestinal function** is diminished immediately after burn injury, secondary to the development of gastric and intestinal ileus. The stomach should be adequately vented with a nasogastric tube.

     1. **Curling ulcers (mucosal erosion)** will occur at variable times after major burns and may lead to gastric hemorrhage or perforation. These ulcers seem to be more common in children than in adults. Therapy consists of antacids, histamine (H_2) receptor antagonists, and proton pump inhibitors.

     2. **Other gastrointestinal complications of burns** include esophagitis, tracheoesophageal fistula (from prolonged intubation and the presence of a nasogastric tube), hepatic dysfunction, pancreatitis, acalculous cholecystitis, and mesenteric artery thrombosis.

g. **Infection** of burned areas delays healing and prevents successful skin grafting. Bacterial invasion of underlying tissue may result in septicemia. Common organisms involved are staphylococci, β-hemolytic streptococci, and gram-negative rods such as *Pseudomonas* and *Klebsiella* species. Local treatment with topical antimicrobials and early skin grafting are important measures to reduce risk of infection.

2. In **electrical burns,** current creates thermal energy that destroys tissue, particularly tissues with high resistance such as skin and bone. Exposure to high voltage can result in compartment syndromes, fractures of long bones and the axial spine, myocardial injury, and rhabdomyolysis with subsequent renal injury.

3. In **chemical burns,** the degree of injury depends on the chemical, its concentration, duration of contact, and the penetrability and resistance of the tissues involved. Some substances producing chemical burns, such as phosphorus, are absorbed systemically, producing significant and often life-threatening injury. Hydrofluoric acid exposure will cause severe hypocalcemia and requires close monitoring of serum calcium levels. Subeschar injection of calcium gluconate and emergent wound excision may be indicated. Many chemical agents can be safely and copiously irrigated with water. Chemicals that should *not* be irrigated include dry lime, elemental metals, and phenol. If the name of the offending chemical agent can be determined, websites, including OSHA, as well as Poison Control provide Safety Data Sheets (formerly known as Material Safety Data Sheets) that provide relevant chemical information and first aid care.

C. **Classification of burn injury**
   1. Burns are classified according to the total body surface area (TBSA) burned, depth of burn, and the presence or absence of inhalational injury. Superficial burns (first degree) should not be included in the TBSA assessment.
   2. **The extent of a burn** (TBSA) is calculated by using a Lund-Browder or other burn diagram.
      a. The **rule of nines** guides estimation (**Figure 35.5**).
         1. **Adults:** The head and each upper extremity each represent 9% TBSA. The anterior trunk, posterior trunk, and each lower extremity each represent 18% TBSA.
         2. **Infants and children:** Because of the different proportions of body surface area relative to patient age, reference must be made to the proper burn chart when calculating percent TBSA to avoid significant errors (**Figure 35.5**).
      b. Another practical method to estimate percent TBSA is that the area of the patient's hand will cover about 1% TBSA.
   3. The **depth of the burn** determines therapy (ie, conservative management vs excision and grafting). Burn depth is difficult to determine visually; however, there are some useful guidelines:
      a. The area under a **partial-thickness burn** should have normal or increased sensitivity to pain and temperature and should blanch with pressure.
      b. A **full-thickness burn** will be anesthetic and will not blanch with pressure. Commonly, the wound bed has varying depth of burn, so the presence of pain can still be common around areas of full-thickness burn where partial-thickness burns with surviving nerve tissue are also present.

D. **Initial evaluation of the burn patient**
   1. **Airway and breathing**
      a. Brief exposure of the epiglottis or larynx to either dry air at 300 °C or steam at 100 °C leads to massive edema and rapid airway obstruction. Chemical products of combustion such as ammonia, sulfur oxide, and chlorine dissolve in the tracheobronchial tree, forming acids and irritating the mucous membrane of the respiratory tract.
      b. When airway burns are suspected, early endotracheal intubation should be performed before airway edema occurs. Continued swelling and distortion of the soft tissues may progress at a rapid rate, rendering intubation difficult if not impossible. Upper airway edema usually resolves within the first week and can be reduced by avoiding excessive fluid administration and elevating the head of the bed.

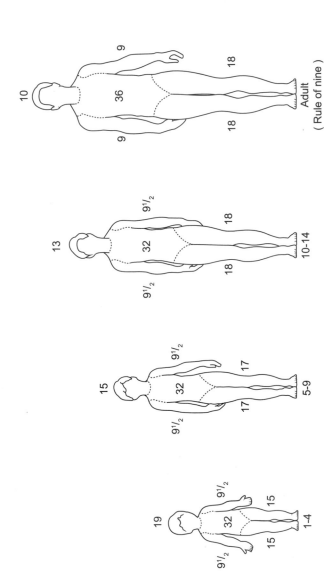

FIGURE 35.5 Rule of nines (Lung and Browder chart). (Modified from Ryan JF, Todres ID, Cote CJ, et al, eds. *A Practice of Anesthesia for Infants and Children*. WB Saunders; 1986:230. Copyright © 1986 Elsevier. With permission.)

c. **Circumferential full-thickness burns** of the thorax will decrease chest wall compliance, which can lead to hypoxemia and respiratory failure. Emergency escharotomies may be required.

d. **Ventilation strategies** involve avoidance of further respiratory compromise from barotrauma caused by increased alveolar distention and shearing forces. Low tidal volume ventilation is recommended. Bronchospasm is frequently present, and bronchodilator therapy with β_2-agonists is warranted. Intraoperatively, minimize retained secretions and cellular debris by attention to body positioning and frequent suctioning.

e. **Smoke inhalation injury** may occur during a fire within a closed space or when heated noxious vapors are inhaled.

1. An inhalation injury should be suspected in the presence of burns of the head or neck; singed nasal hairs; swelling of the mucosa of the nose, mouth, lips, or throat; a brassy cough; or carbonaceous sputum. Both the upper airway and pulmonary parenchyma may be affected.

2. **Chemical products** of combustion combine with water in the respiratory tract to form strong acids and alkali, causing bronchospasm, edema, and mucous membrane ulceration. Inhalation of gases such as phosgene and sulfuric acid can damage the alveolar membrane and cause partial or complete airway obstruction. Aldehydes such as acrolein impair ciliary function and damage mucosal surfaces.

3. Combustion of polyurethane-containing products (eg, insulation and wall paneling) releases **hydrogen cyanide,** which causes tissue asphyxia by inhibiting cytochrome oxidase activity. Patients may present with an anion gap metabolic acidosis and an elevated mixed venous PO_2. Plasma lactate levels correlate with the cyanide levels. Antidotal treatment of cyanide poisoning involves three strategies: binding of cyanide, induction of methemoglobinemia, and use of sulfur donors.

   a. Binding cyanide: Hydoxocobalamin/Cyanokit (dose 70 mg/kg IV, maximum dose 5 g) binds CN and forms cyanocobalamin, a less toxic substance.

   b. Induction of methemoglobinemia provides an alternative binding site for cyanide, rather than the cytochrome electron transport chain complex. Sodium nitrite is the drug of choice (300 mg IV over 5 minutes in 100 mL of 5% dextrose). Amyl nitrate (0.3 mL ampule, crushed and inhaled over 15-30 seconds, repeated every minute) is more technically challenging to administer and induces a much weaker methemoglobinemia, thus should be considered a second-line, temporizing agent. Treatment with amyl nitrite or sodium nitrite is **contraindicated** in cases of concurrent carbon monoxide toxicity.

   c. Sulfur donors aid the rhodanese enzyme in detoxifying cyanide and resulting in thiocyanate, which can be renally excreted. Usual dosing is sodium thiosulfate 12.5 g in a 50-mL solution.

4. **Carbon monoxide** binds hemoglobin, displacing oxygen and shifting the oxyhemoglobin curve to the left. Tissue hypoxia ensues.

   a. All burn-injured patients, especially those burned within a closed space, may have sustained some degree of CO exposure with their thermal injury. Oxygen administration should begin at the scene.

    b. Because oxyhemoglobin and carboxyhemoglobin absorb light at the same wavelength, conventional pulse oximetry cannot be used as an indicator of CO poisoning. Diagnosis is made on clinical suspicion and the level of arterial or venous carboxyhemoglobin, measured spectrophotometrically with a CO-oximeter.

    c. The half-life of CO is inversely related to the inspired oxygen concentration (FIO_2); it is 5 to 6 hours when breathing room air but 30 to 60 minutes when breathing 100% oxygen.

    d. Treatment is supportive and consists of supplemental oxygen until the carbon monoxide is eliminated. Hyperbaric oxygen should be considered in comatose patients and in those with severe carbon monoxide poisoning.

    e. **Indirect respiratory injury** and pulmonary edema may occur in burn patients without an inhalational injury. Mechanisms involved include the effect of burn wound mediators on the lung, decreased plasma oncotic pressure, and complications of burn therapy.

2. Cardiovascular resuscitation

    a. **Fluid replacement** consists of crystalloid, usually Ringer lactate, with or without the addition of colloid. Standard protocols for fluid replacement use body weight in kilograms and percent TBSA burned.

        1. **Parkland formula:** 4 mL of Ringer lactate per kg per % TBSA burn administered in the first 24 hours. Half of the fluid is given within the first 8 hours from the burn incident, and the remaining over the next 16 hours.

        2. **Brooke formula:** 1.5 mL of crystalloid per kg per % TBSA burn per 24 hours **plus** 0.5 mL of colloid per kg per % TBSA burn per 24 hours **plus** 2000 mL of 5% dextrose in water per 24 hours.

        3. **Rule of Tens:** 10 × % TBSA. The military Joint Trauma System Clinical Practice Guidelines use the Rule of Tens. It is simple to calculate and applies to most adults. The initial fluid rate is calculated as 10 mL × % TBSA, for patients between 40 and 80 kg. If over 80 kg, add 100 mL/h for every 10 kg > 80 kg.

    b. Half the calculated fluid deficit is administered during the first 8 hours postburn, and the remainder is administered over the next 16 hours. The patient's daily maintenance fluid requirements are given concurrently.

    c. The end points of fluid therapy are hemodynamic stability and maintenance of an adequate urine output. In extensive burns, fluid management is adjusted according to appropriate invasive monitors and laboratory studies.

E. Management of the burn wound

    1. **Early excision and grafting of burned areas** is a widely accepted procedure and appear to decrease mortality and hospital length of stay. Patients may be brought to the operating room in the acute phase of injury, with hemodynamic instability and respiratory dysfunction. Special emphasis should be placed on correcting acid-base and electrolyte disturbances, temperature normalization, and treatment of anemia and coagulopathy. Blood loss during wound excision and grafting can be massive. Adequate colloid and blood products should be ordered in advance. IV access should be adequate for resuscitation.

2. Topical agents are used to minimize the colonization of healing wounds. Burns should be kept moist, and many centers use petroleum-based agents with or without antibiotics (such as Bacitracin) and non-adherent, petroleum-impregnated dressings (such as Xeroform gauze). Other topical agents and their side effects include:

   a. **Silver nitrate** may cause hyponatremia or, rarely, methemoglobinemia.

   b. **Silver sulfadiazine** may cause leukopenia, which is reversible upon discontinuing the drug.

3. The incidence of **sepsis** may be reduced by using temporary biologic dressings, either allografts (cadaver skin or amnion) or xenografts (porcine). Artificial skin (eg, Integra) bioengineered from collagen and cultured epidermis can be used when a conventional autograft is not available.

4. The use of **systemic antibiotics** is limited to treatment of documented systemic infection (as opposed to colonization), and they are also used as prophylaxis before surgical procedures.

F. Anesthetic considerations

1. **Burn-injured patients may also suffer from nonthermal traumatic injuries** and should initially be assessed as a trauma patient (see Sections I.A to I.E). The patient's age, preexisting disease, and the extent of burn injury provide an index of the patient's likely physiologic condition. Altered pharmacokinetics, drug tolerance, difficult IV access, and anatomic derangements of the airway (neck scar or mouth contracture) are primary considerations.

2. **Airway.** Obtaining an adequate mask fit may be difficult because of edema in the early phases of burn injury or because of scars and contractures later on. The same processes can render endotracheal intubation extremely difficult in burn patients.

3. **Monitoring and IV access (Table 35.2)**

   a. Often IV access will still be in place from the initial resuscitation. Large-bore IVs are mandatory to allow for massive fluid replacement.

   b. In massive burns, ECG electrodes may be placed directly on debrided tissue. Alternatively, needle electrodes can be used.

TABLE 35.2	Intraoperative Monitoring Challenges in Patients With Major Burn Injury	
Monitor	Possible Challenges of Burn Injury	Possible Solutions
Electrocardiography (ECG)	ECG electrodes may not adhere	Consider needle electrodes or stapling of electrodes
Noninvasive blood pressure monitor	Edema or extensive burns in the extremities may limit use of cuff	Consider alternative location, use dressing or gauze under cuff Consider invasive monitoring
Invasive blood pressure monitor	Hypothermia, hypovolemia, initial decreased cardiac output, vasoconstriction	Consider alternative location, trend values, confirm with noninvasive blood pressure
Pulse oximetry	Extensive burn injury may limit placement Carboxyhemoglobin will falsely elevate oxygen saturation reading	Consider alternative location, trend values, assess partial pressure of oxygen by arterial blood gas (ABG)

   c. **Arterial lines** are indispensable for continuous blood pressure monitoring and frequent blood sampling. The cannulation site will depend on the availability of unburned areas. If all appropriate sites are burned, the line may have to be placed through the burn wound after the area has been prepared in a sterile fashion.

   d. **CVP lines** are useful both for monitoring central pressures and for central access for drug infusions.

   e. A **pulmonary artery catheter** may be required for management of patients with myocardial dysfunction, persistent oliguria or hypotension, or sepsis.

4. **Muscle relaxants. Extrajunctional nicotinic receptors** proliferate in muscle at the burn site and at sites distant from the burn injury. Succinylcholine is only safe in the immediate 24 hours after thermal injury. An increase in acetylcholine receptors is usually associated with resistance to nondepolarizing neuromuscular-blocking agents, increased sensitivity to depolarizing muscle relaxants, and life-threatening hyperkalemia when succinylcholine is used.

5. **Anesthetics**

   a. There is no single preferred agent or combination of agents; however, ketamine and etomidate may have advantages in patients with a tenuous hemodynamic status.

   b. These patients may have **greatly increased opioid requirements** owing to tolerance, hypermetabolic physiology, and an increase in the apparent volume of distribution for drugs. It is important to provide adequate analgesia, which may necessitate massive doses of opiates.

6. **Temperature regulation.** The most comfortable body temperature for a burn patient is about 100 °F (38 °C). In the burn intensive care unit, patients are cared for in warmed, humidified rooms. Every effort should be made to maintain normothermia during transport and surgery. The operating room, IV fluids, and blood products should be warmed and inspired gases heated and humidified. Pediatric patients should be placed under a radiant heat source and on a warming blanket whenever possible.

7. **Immunosuppression.** The immune system is suppressed for weeks to months after burn injury, and the wound itself serves as an excellent medium for bacterial growth. Every attempt should be made to practice aseptic technique when handling patients, suctioning airways, and inserting intravascular lines.

8. **Postanesthetic care.** It is important to maintain normothermia while transporting patients back to the intensive care unit because shivering results in vasoconstriction and could contribute to graft loss. Supplemental oxygen should be given until patients are fully recovered from anesthesia. Severe pain is common, and patient responses vary, necessitating individual titration of analgesics and frequent reassessment of the effect.

Suggested Readings

American College of Surgeons. *Advanced Trauma Life Support (ATLS) Student Manual.* 9th ed. American College of Surgeons; 2012.

Bickell WH, Wall MJ Jr, Pepe PE, et al. Immediate versus delayed fluid resuscitation for hypotensive patients with penetrating torso injuries. *N Engl J Med.* 1994;331:1105-1109.

Bittner EA, Shank E, Woodson L, Martyn JA. Acute and perioperative care of the burn-injured patient. *Anesthesiology.* 2015;122(2):448-464.

Bittner EA, Martyn JA, Sjöberg F. Chapter 87. Acute and anesthetic care of the burn-injured patient. In: Gropper M, ed. *Miller's Anesthesia.* Elsevier/Churchill Livingstone; 2020.

Bowen DK, Antevil JL, Gurney JM, et al. *Wartime Thoracic Injury. Joint Trauma System Clinical Practice Guidelines.* 2018. Accessed April 2, 2020. https://jts.amedd.army.mil/index.cfm/PI_CPGs/cpgs

Chung KK, Salinas J, Renz EM, et al. Simple derivation of the initial fluid rate for the resuscitation of severely burned adult combat casualties: in silico validation of the rule of 10. *J Trauma.* 2010;69(suppl 1):S49-S54.

Duchesne JC, Barbeau JM, Islam TM, et al. Damage control resuscitation: from emergency department to the operating room. *Am Surg.* 2011;77(2):201-206.

Driscoll IR, Mann-Salinas EA, Boyer NL, et al. Burn Care. Joint Trauma System Clinical Practice Guidelines. 2016. Accessed February 12, 2021. http://jts.amedd.army.mil/index.cfm/PI_CPGs/cpgs

Kaiser HE, Kim CM, Sharar SR, et al. Advances in perioperative and critical care of the burn patient. *Adv Anesth.* 2013;31(1):137-161.

Martyn JA, Richtsfeld M. Succinylcholine-induced hyperkalemia in acquired pathologic states: etiologic factors and molecular mechanisms. *Anesthesiology.* 2006;104:158-169.

Neschis DG, Scalea TM, Flinn WR, et al. Blunt aortic injury. *N Engl J Med.* 2008;359(16):1708-1716.

Roberts I, Shakur H, Ker K, et al. CRASH-2 Trial collaborators. Antifibrinolytic drugs for acute traumatic injury. *Cochrane Database Syst Rev.* 2012;12:CD004896.

Theusinger OM, Madjdpour C, Spahn DR. Resuscitation and transfusion management in trauma patients: emerging concepts. *Curr Opin Crit Care.* 2012;18(6):661-670.

Transfusion Therapy

Lukas H. Matern and Marvin G. Chang

I. THE DECISION TO TRANSFUSE

The decision to initiate transfusion is complex. There are many risks to transfusion (see Section VIII), and transfusion is ultimately indicated when the potential benefits outweigh these risks. In most civilian settings, transfusion therapy utilizes blood components rather than whole blood. The benefits of blood component transfusion stem from the correction of conditions that result in decreased production; increased utilization, destruction, or loss; or dysfunction of a specific blood component (usually red blood cells, platelets, or coagulation factors). Although many attempts at creating universal transfusion protocols have been introduced, few have successfully demonstrated definitive thresholds or clear superiority. The aim of this chapter is to provide the background to help clinicians make these decisions on an individual basis. A condensed summary of approaches to perioperative transfusion therapy and decision-making may be found in **Table 36.1.**

A. Assessing red cell mass and oxygen-carrying ability

1. **The decision to transfuse red blood cells** (also called erythrocytes, red cells, or RBCs). Most evidence suggests that higher red cell transfusion thresholds (eg, 10-12 g/dL) do not confer a mortality benefit and may even be harmful. Nonetheless, maintaining adequate red cell mass is essential for adequate oxygen-carrying capacity to the tissues, and it has been shown that perioperative anemia may increase the risk of acute kidney injury, acute coronary or cerebrovascular events, and prolonged postoperative hospital stays. The decision to transfuse, therefore, must be weighed carefully based on a variety of patient and situational factors rather than rigid guidelines.

2. **Patient factors.** The main reason for transfusing red cells is to maintain the oxygen-carrying capacity to the tissues, a primary determinant of which is the hemoglobin (Hb) level.

    a. **Healthy individuals** or **individuals with chronic anemia** can usually tolerate lower Hb levels of 6.5 to 8 g/dL, assuming normal intravascular volume. The use of a "restrictive" transfusion practice, aiming for Hb of 7 to 9 g/dL, is generally safe and may reduce the risk of death compared with transfusing toward a "liberal" Hb goal of 10 to 12 g/dL. The reasons for reduced mortality in the restrictively transfused group have not been clearly delineated, but the effects of allogeneic transfusion on diminished immune function have been substantiated in animal and human studies (see Section VIII.D).

    b. For **patients with coronary artery disease (CAD),** the risk of myocardial ischemia due to anemia has resulted in most practitioners transfusing to a higher (9-10 g/dL) Hb target. As the incidence of CAD rises substantially with age, many practitioners also opt to use a higher transfusion threshold in the elderly. Studies to support this practice, however, are lacking, and those that exist have produced

TABLE 36.1	Summary of Perioperative Transfusion Considerations

Preoperative Decision-Making

1. Evaluate indications for and contraindications to blood product transfusion, including patient history and comorbidities, surgical considerations, and allowable blood loss.
   a. Address preoperative anemia by administering iron, EPO, and blood products or adjuvants as appropriate.
   b. Hold nonessential anticoagulants and address preoperative coagulopathies.
   c. Consider preoperative autologous blood donation or acute normovolemic hemodilution strategies.
2. Perform a preoperative examination and review relevant laboratory tests to determine perioperative indications for blood products or adjuvants.
   a. Consider the need for a preoperative type and screen or crossmatch.
3. Discuss the risks and benefits of transfusion with the patient and obtain informed consent.
4. Prepare the operating room or anesthetizing location for blood product transfusion.
   a. Set up and prime an infusion circuit incorporating a fluid warmer and blood filter using calcium-free crystalloid, colloid, or blood components.
   b. Prepare rapid or pressure infusion devices as appropriate.
   c. Coordinate use of blood salvage and other devices with operating room staff.
5. Initiate discussion with the surgical team during a standardized huddle or time-out regarding how much blood loss is anticipated.

Intraoperative Decision-Making

1. Consider available blood-sparing measures, but do not withhold blood products when they may significantly improve patient outcomes.
   a. Administer adjuvant agents, particularly antifibrinolytics, to select patients when major blood loss is possible.
   b. Implement a controlled hypotension strategy if indicated.
   c. Replace simple fluid losses with non-blood product volume expanders (eg, crystalloid or colloid) prior to initiating transfusion.
   d. Consider recommending the use of hemostatic agents in the surgical field.
   e. Reinfuse perioperatively salvaged blood as appropriate.
2. Assess for clinical signs of adequate oxygen delivery and surgical blood loss using visual inspection and standard monitors.
   a. Consider additional hemodynamic monitoring techniques such as transesophageal echocardiography if substantial blood loss is present or expected.
3. Obtain point-of-care assessments of blood counts and coagulation (eg, TEG) to guide blood product and adjuvant administration.
4. Adhere to institutional and society-recommended transfusion thresholds and blood ordering protocols.
   a. Consider administration of leukoreduced red cells to patients at risk for CMV transmission and nonhemolytic transfusion reactions.
5. Monitor for and treat any early complications of transfusion therapy.

Postoperative Decision-Making

1. Maintain ongoing clinical and laboratory assessments of blood loss in the PACU or postoperative destination.
   a. Implement periodic evaluations of the operative site and drain outputs.
   b. Keep PACU phase I monitors applied until bleeding slows and vitals remain stable.
   c. Follow hemoglobin or hematocrit values serially if anemia is suspected.
2. Continue evaluation for and treatment of delayed complications of transfusion therapy.
3. Consider escalation of care or disposition to an intensive care setting if bleeding continues to be excessive, if the patient's status remains unstable, or if ongoing significant transfusion may be required.

contradictory results. For example, a study of medical patients with acute coronary syndromes also found a higher mortality rate attributable to red cell transfusion in otherwise stable patients with a hematocrit (Hct) greater than 25%.

3. **Situational factors**
   a. **Intraoperative red cell transfusion** depends on red cell loss. This can be roughly estimated by measuring blood in suction canisters, weighing sponges, and checking blood loss in the drapes. In the perioperative period, suspected or confirmed hemorrhage remains the most common indication for transfusion. During periods of ongoing blood loss, transfusion may be indicated even with a Hb > 10 g/dL if bleeding is brisk enough that the clinician expects a substantial drop in Hb without treatment.
   b. If a patient is anemic preoperatively, the etiology should be clarified. It may be secondary to decreased production (marrow suppression or nutritional deficiencies), increased loss (hemorrhage), or destruction (hemolysis). Such an assessment may then be used to guide perioperative therapy.

4. **Estimating blood volumes (BVs)**
   a. **Estimated allowable blood loss** (EABL) can be calculated as follows, using either Hcts (as shown) or Hbs:

$$EABL = \left[\left(Hct_{starting} - Hct_{allowable} \right) \times BV \right] \Big/ \left[\left(Hct_{starting} + Hct_{allowable} \right) \Big/ 2 \right]$$

   BV in an adult is approximately 7% of lean body mass. This may be calculated as approximately 70 mL/kg of body weight in an average adult man and approximately 65 mL/kg of body weight in an average adult woman (see Chapter 33 for pediatric considerations). Obese patients have a lower relative lean body mass and a lower relative BV; thus, the greater the degree of obesity, the lower the BV estimate relative to total body weight (TBW). For example, a patient with a body mass index (BMI) of 40 may have an estimated BV of 53 mL/kg TBW, whereas patients with a BMI of 70 may have an estimated BV of 40 mL/kg TBW.
   b. **The volume of blood to transfuse** can be calculated as follows:

$$\text{Volume to transfuse} = \left[\left(Hct_{desired} - Hct_{present} \right) \times BV \right] \Big/ Hct_{transfused\ blood}$$

   One unit of packed red blood cells (PRBCs) has a Hct of 70% to 85% when stored with the standard Adsol preservative.

B. **Thrombocytopenia** is due to either decreased bone marrow production (eg, chemotherapy, tumor infiltration, or alcoholism) or increased utilization or destruction (eg, trauma or surgery creating a large wound, hypersplenism, idiopathic thrombocytopenia purpura [ITP], disseminated intravascular coagulation [DIC], or drug effects). It also results from dilution and loss associated with massive transfusion (see Section IX.A.1). Spontaneous bleeding is unusual with platelet counts above 20,000/mm³. Platelet counts above 50,000/mm³ are preferable for surgical hemostasis. However, as in the case of red cell administration, the decision to transfuse must be made based upon clinical factors rather than platelet count alone. For example, patients with ITP have a high rate of platelet turnover and will often exhibit normal coagulation despite a low platelet count. In addition, as this form of thrombocytopenia is primarily due to platelet destruction, patients with ITP will not respond adequately to platelet transfusion.

Instead, treatments should be aimed at halting the underlying destructive process.

C. Coagulopathy. Bleeding associated with documented factor deficiencies or prolonged clotting studies (prothrombin time [PT] and partial thromboplastin time [PTT]) mandates replacement therapy to maintain normal coagulation function. See Sections II and IX for a discussion of coagulopathy.

II. COAGULATION STUDIES

The most important clues to a clinically significant bleeding disorder in an otherwise healthy patient may be obtained from a thorough history. In particular, a personal or family history of anemia requiring iron replacement or blood products may suggest a bleeding diathesis. Prior excessive surgical bleeding, gingival bleeding, easy bruising, epistaxis, or menorrhagia should raise concern. Many laboratory tests are available to assess the coagulation system. However, the clinician must remember that coagulation depends on a complex interplay of platelets and coagulation factors that may not be fully captured by any single test.

A. Activated partial thromboplastin time (aPTT or PTT) is measured by adding particulate matter such as silica or kaolin to a blood sample to activate the coagulation system. Normal values for the PTT are 22 to 34 seconds but vary according to the reagent and instruments used by the specific laboratory. The PTT assesses factors in the intrinsic (XI, XII, VIII, IX, and contact factors) and the common (II, V, X, and fibrinogen) coagulation pathways. The test is sensitive to decreased amounts of coagulation factors, and the value is elevated in patients on heparin therapy. The PTT will also be abnormally elevated in patients with hemophilia or a circulating anticoagulant (eg, lupus anticoagulant or antibodies to factor VIII). The clinician should remember that an abnormal PTT does not necessarily correlate with clinical bleeding severity. Therefore, aggressive correction of an abnormal PTT in surgical patients is not universally indicated unless the patient is actively bleeding.

B. PT is measured by adding tissue factor (thromboplastin) to a blood sample to activate coagulation. It serves as a measure of factors of the extrinsic (VII and tissue factor) and common (see above) coagulation pathways. Although both PT and PTT are affected by levels of factors V and X, prothrombin, and fibrinogen, the PT is specifically sensitive to deficiencies of factor VII. The PT is also normal in deficiencies of intrinsic pathway factors VIII, IX, XI, XII, prekallikrein, and high-molecular-weight kininogen. Normal values fall between 10 and 15 seconds, although the international normalized ratio (INR) (see below) is more commonly reported given the variability of PT results between laboratories.

C. The **INR** represents a means of standardizing PT values to allow reliable comparison among different laboratories. It is defined as the ratio of the patient's PT to the control PT value that would be obtained if international reference reagents had been used to perform the test. Oral warfarin anticoagulation therapy may therefore be guided by a target INR value that is independent of the laboratory variability of the PT. For example, an INR of 2.0 to 3.0 is recommended for prophylaxis against thromboembolism in atrial fibrillation. Higher INR values may be targeted in specific populations at increased risk for thromboembolic phenomena (eg, patients with mechanical mitral valves).

D. Activated clotting time (ACT) is a modified whole blood clotting time in which diatomaceous earth (celite) or clay (kaolin) is added to a blood sample to activate the intrinsic pathway. The ACT is the time until clot formation. A normal ACT is 90 to 130 seconds depending on the instrument used. Compared with the PTT, the ACT is a relatively easy and expedient test to perform and is useful in monitoring heparin therapy rapidly in the operating room (see Chapter 24). However, because the ACT is relatively insensitive to lower levels of heparin anticoagulation, it is typically reserved for settings that require higher doses of heparin, particularly cardiopulmonary bypass and extracorporeal membrane oxygenation.

E. **Platelet counts** can be measured to determine the risk of excessive bleeding due to platelet depletion. Commonly accepted normal values range between 150,000 and 450,000/mm^3, and a clinical threshold for perioperative platelet transfusion is often less than 50,000/mm^3. However, platelet counts do not provide a qualitative metric of platelet function and thus may not reliably reflect the risk of bleeding in certain populations.

F. **Platelet function tests** range from simple assessments of bleeding time to sophisticated optical aggregometry techniques. In circumstances involving elements of platelet dysfunction, including uremia and the use of antiplatelet agents, point-of-care tests of platelet activation and aggregation—such as that generated by the platelet function analyzer 100 (PFA-100) device—may provide insight into bleeding risk. However, these tests remain largely unvalidated for routine perioperative use. Thromboelastography may also allow for rapid assessment of platelet function.

G. **Fibrinogen** is the precursor protein that is activated to form fibrin and then cross-linked to strengthen clots. Assaying fibrinogen levels can be helpful when coagulopathy is present or suspected. Although the diagnostic specificity of the fibrinogen level is low, it can be helpful to guide further transfusion support (ie, the administration of fresh frozen plasma [FFP] or cryoprecipitate).

H. **Thromboelastography (TEG)** is available in some centers for clinical use, often as a point-of-care test. TEG is performed by placing a small aliquot of blood into a heated oscillating cup, into which a pin on a torsion wire is suspended. Clot formation in the oscillating cup generates torque on the pin, and the torque is measured and converted to an electrical signal. The signal is then recorded by a computer, creating a characteristic trace (**Figure 36.1**) that may be analyzed for abnormalities of clot formation. By measuring clot formation and viscoelastic clot strength, TEG provides information about the adequacy of clotting factors, fibrin levels, and platelets. In general, R time represents the activity of coagulation factors, the alpha angle and K time represent acceleration of fibrin formation, maximum amplitude represents platelet function, and percent lysis in 30 minutes (LY30) represents the rate of fibrinolysis. Thromboelastometry (TEM, previously ROTEM) uses similar technology with similarly measured parameters.

III. BLOOD TYPING AND CROSS-MATCHING

A. **Donor blood and recipient blood** are typed using the red cell surface **ABO and Rh systems** and screened for antibodies to other cell antigens. "Direct" cross-matching involves directly mixing the patient's plasma with the donor's red cells to establish that hemolysis does not occur from any undetected antibodies. An individual's red cells display A antigen, B antigen, both antigens (AB), or no surface antigens (O). If the patient's red cells do not display either surface antigen A or surface antigen B, then antibodies will be produced upon exposure to the absent antigen(s). Thus, a person

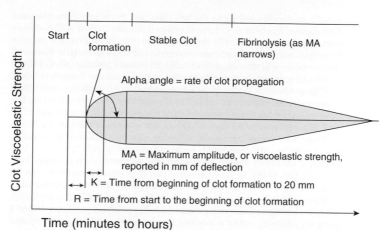

FIGURE 36.1 Thromboelastography.

who is type B may develop anti-A antibodies in the serum, and a type O individual may develop circulating anti-A and anti-B antibodies. A type AB individual will not produce antibodies to either A or B antigens and therefore can receive red cells from any donor blood type. People with type O blood display neither A nor B surface antigens and can donate blood cells to any other type (universal red cell donor; **Table 36.2**). The universal FFP donor, conversely, has type AB blood, which will contain neither anti-A nor anti-B antibodies to antigens on recipient RBCs. Whole blood donors and recipients must be exact ABO matches because whole blood contains both RBCs and serum. For example, a unit of type O whole blood will contain serum with anti-A and anti-B antibodies and therefore cannot be used to transfuse patients who are A, B, or AB blood types.

B. **Rh surface antigens** are either present (Rh positive) or absent (Rh negative). Individuals who are Rh negative will develop antibodies to the Rh factor when exposed to Rh-positive blood. Although this does not usually have clinical consequences at the time of the initial exposure, subsequent exposures to Rh-positive RBCs may cause circulating antibodies to produce hemolysis. This can pose a particular problem during pregnancy. Maternal

TABLE 36.2	Transfusion Compatibility	
Recipient Blood Type	**RBC Donor**	**FFP Donor**
AB	AB, A, B, or O	AB
A	A or O	A or AB
B	B or O	B or AB
O	O	A, B, AB, or O
Rh+	Rh+ or Rh+	Rh+ or Rh−
Rh−	Rh−	Rh+ or Rh−

anti-Rh antibodies belong to the IgG class and freely cross the placenta. Rh-negative mothers who have developed Rh antibodies will therefore transmit these antibodies to the fetus. If the fetus is Rh positive, massive hemolysis may occur (a phenomenon referred to as hemolytic disease of the newborn or erythroblastosis fetalis). **Rh immune globulin** (*RhoGAM*), an Rh-blocking antibody, prevents the Rh-negative patient from developing anti-Rh antibodies. It should be administered to Rh-negative individuals who receive Rh-positive blood and to Rh-negative mothers delivering Rh-positive babies (as some fetomaternal blood mixing often occurs at delivery). The recommended dose is 300 µg intramuscularly for every 15 mL of Rh-positive blood transfused, although administration of Rh-negative blood to Rh-negative mothers is preferred when available.

C. **Recipient antibodies against other donor RBC antigens** (such as those from the Kell, Kid, Duffy, or Lewis groups) can also cause hemolytic transfusion reactions. When a patient's blood sample is screened and found to contain antibodies against antigens found on donor RBCs, it complicates cross-matching and can delay the availability of blood products. When a patient's antibody screen is positive, it is advisable to discuss anticipated transfusion needs with the blood bank.

D. **If an emergency blood transfusion is needed,** type-specific (ABO) red cells can often be obtained within minutes at large centers if the patient's blood type is known. If type-specific blood is unavailable, type O Rh-negative red cells should be transfused (although type O–positive blood can be used emergently in males and postmenopausal women). Type-specific blood should be substituted as soon as possible to minimize the amount of type O plasma (containing anti-A and anti-B antibodies) transfused.

IV. BLOOD COMPONENT THERAPY
A. General considerations
1. One unit of **PRBCs**, which has a Hct of about 70% and a volume of about 250 mL, will usually increase the Hct by 2% to 3% or the Hb by 1 g/dL in the euvolemic adult once equilibration has taken place. In euvolemic children, PRBC volumes of 4 mL/kg will also increase the Hb by approximately 1 g/dL. PRBCs must be ABO compatible with the recipient.

2. One unit of **platelets** increases the platelet count by 5000 to 10,000/mm^3. A usual platelet transfusion is 1 unit per 10 kg of body weight. If thrombocytopenia is caused by a destructive or consumptive process or if platelets are dysfunctional, platelet transfusions will be less efficacious (see Section I.B). Transfusion of ABO-compatible platelets is not obligatory, although they may provide a better posttransfusion platelet count. Single-donor or HLA-matched platelets may be required for patients refractory to platelet transfusion. A unit of single-donor platelets provides the equivalent of approximately six random donor units of platelets. Owing to inactivation at low temperatures, **platelets should be stored at room temperature** and never placed in a cooler or refrigerator.

3. **FFP,** which is stored in volumes of about 250 to 300 mL/U and administered at doses of 10 to 15 mL/kg, should increase plasma coagulation factors to 30% of normal, the minimum necessary for hemostasis (except for fibrinogen, of which 50% of the normal 200-400 mg/dL concentration is required). Fibrinogen levels increase by 1 mg/dL per mL of plasma transfused. Acute reversal of warfarin is often achieved with only 5 to 8 mL/kg of FFP, although the PT may remain modestly prolonged. FFP transfusions must be ABO compatible, but Rh compatibility and cross-matching are not required (**Table 36.1**).

4. **Cryoprecipitate** is prepared via centrifugation of the plasma and contains concentrated factor VIII, factor XIII, fibrinogen, von Willebrand factor (vWF), and fibronectin. Indications for cryoprecipitate include hypofibrinogenemia, von Willebrand disease, hemophilia A (when recombinant factor VIII is unavailable), and preparation of fibrin glue. The usual dosage of 1 unit per 7 to 10 kg should raise the plasma fibrinogen by about 50 mg/dL in a patient without massive bleeding. ABO compatibility is not mandatory for cryoprecipitate transfusion.

B. **Technical considerations**

1. **Compatible infusions.** Blood products should not be infused with hypotonic (eg, 5% dextrose) solutions, as these may cause hemolysis. Recent studies have suggested that coinfusion with calcium-containing lactated Ringer's solution may not induce clot formation, but concern persists. Coadministration of blood products with Plasmalyte solutions is probably safe. Normal saline (0.9%) solution, albumin (5%), and FFP are compatible with RBCs and may be preferred in diluting blood products or priming blood delivery systems.

2. **Blood filters.** Standard blood filters (170-200 μm) remove debris and should be used for all blood components. However, manufacturer recommendations for specific bedside blood filters should be followed with respect to the component to be filtered and the number of units administered per filter.

   a. **Leukocyte reduction (leukoreduction)** is achieved by filtration, either in the blood bank or at the bedside. Microaggregate filters (20-50 μm), which should not be used for platelets, remove 70% to 90% of leukocytes. Third-generation or adhesion filters remove more than 99.9% of leukocytes via a combination of filtration and adhesion of white blood cells. These filters are recommended for use in patients with a history of febrile nonhemolytic transfusion reactions, for prevention of alloimmunization to foreign leukocyte antigens (eg, in the oncologic patient expected to require multiple platelet transfusions), or to prevent cytomegalovirus (CMV) transmission in organ transplant recipients. Other potential but unproven benefits of leukocyte reduction include a diminished immunomodulatory effect of allogeneic transfusion; reduced transmission of bacterial, viral, or prion diseases; prevention of transfusion-related acute lung injury (TRALI); and decreased incidence of graft-versus-host disease (GVHD). Several countries have implemented universal leukoreduction protocols for transfused cellular blood products. The proposed benefits and cost-efficiency of universal leukoreduction have generated significant controversy within transfusion medicine and are not mandatory in the United States at this time.

   b. **Hypotensive reactions** associated with the use of bedside leukocyte reduction filters have been reported. The pathophysiology may involve activation of bradykinin by the leukocyte filter, and the hypotensive effect may be exaggerated in patients taking ACE inhibitors. When this reaction occurs, the transfusion should be stopped and the blood pressure supported. These interventions usually result in rapid resolution of hypotension. Products that are leukoreduced in the blood bank may carry a lower risk of this hypotensive reaction, as bradykinin is rapidly metabolized in stored blood.

C. **Massive transfusion is traditionally defined as** transfusion of 10 or more units of PRBCs, or one BV, within a 24-hour period. When anticipating or initiating a large volume transfusion, coordination with the blood bank is crucial; therefore, many institutions have developed massive transfusion protocols to ensure availability and rapid mobilization of blood products when activated. The decision to activate a massive transfusion protocol may be complex but can be guided by validated clinical scoring systems such as the ABC score. Initial management should be aimed at correcting drivers of hemorrhage (eg, giving several units of FFP to correct a greatly elevated INR) prior to administering blood components according to any standard ratio. Some evidence suggests that transfusion of platelets, FFP, and PRBCs in a 1:1:1 ratio may be superior to a 1:1:2 ratio in promoting hemostasis and reducing mortality related to hemorrhage in the setting of trauma (see Chapter 35 for further discussion). Platelet counts may also be expected to fall by approximately 50% for each BV that is hemorrhaged; therefore, the early transfusion of platelets and consideration of antifibrinolytics may be beneficial.

D. **Blood substitutes.** Despite years of research intent upon finding a blood substitute capable of oxygen transport, none provides significant clinical usefulness at this time. Hemoglobin-based oxygen carriers trialed to date have been shown to scavenge nitric oxide, provoke inflammation, and produce other harms that outweigh their potential benefits. These products continue to be an area of research.

V. PLASMA SUBSTITUTES

Although various colloid products are available commercially, their use remains limited by cost, potential allergic reactions, adverse effects on coagulation, and a lack of clear benefits relative to crystalloids.

A. **Albumin** is available as either an isotonic 5% or a hypertonic 20% or 25% solution. Albumin has an intravascular half-life of 10 to 15 days. Although albumin is frequently used to avoid high volumes of crystalloid infusion and fluid creep, evidence supporting its routine use over crystalloids is lacking, and its cost is substantially higher than that of crystalloids. For these reasons, many authors argue against the routine use of albumin except in particular circumstances, which may include volume expansion for patients with substantial fluid third-spacing (eg, severe hepatic dysfunction) or replacement of rapid albumin losses (eg, after large-volume paracentesis).

B. **Hydroxyethyl starches** (hetastarch, Voluven [R]) are manufactured from amylopectin. Hetastarch's effects on coagulation include decreased fibrinogen, vWf, and factor VIII levels as well as impaired platelet function. It has also been shown to increase rates of renal failure and mortality in patients with severe sepsis and is now rarely used.

VI. PHARMACOLOGIC THERAPY

A. **Erythropoietin (EPO)** increases RBC mass by stimulating the proliferation and development of erythroid precursor cells. Recombinant EPO can be administered before elective surgery to increase RBC production. However, its role in the perioperative period is unclear, and its use may be associated with an increased incidence of hypertension and adverse thrombotic events.

B. **Desmopressin (DDAVP)** is a V2 receptor-selective analog of antidiuretic hormone (or vasopressin) that may be beneficial in patients with mild hemophilia A, von Willebrand disease (type 1), and uremic platelet dysfunction. DDAVP increases endothelial cell release (but not production) of vWF, factor VIII, and tissue plasminogen activator to promote coagulation. The standard dosage is 0.3 µg/kg diluted in normal saline and administered over 30 minutes. Tachyphylaxis is possible if doses are more frequent than every 48 hours. The intravenous (IV) dose should be administered slowly to avoid hypotension or hypertension, and hyponatremia may occur with excessive use.

C. **Lysine analogues** such as epsilon-aminocaproic acid (EACA) and tranexamic acid (TXA) inhibit fibrinolysis, the endogenous process by which fibrin clots are broken down. They act by displacing plasminogen from fibrin, inhibiting plasminogen conversion to plasmin, and preventing plasmin from binding to fibrinogen or fibrin monomers. Trials have shown that TXA may be useful in the early treatment of trauma victims to reduce bleeding and mortality as well as in modestly reducing bleeding-related mortality in women with postpartum hemorrhage (see Chapters 32 and 35). However, TXA has been associated with the development of perioperative tonic-clonic seizures, likely as a result of off-target GABA receptor inhibition, at therapeutic doses. Uses of EACA may include prophylaxis for dental surgery in hemophiliacs, reduction of bleeding in prostatic surgery, and reduction of hemorrhage in cases of excessive fibrinolysis. Because cardiopulmonary bypass has been shown to initiate fibrinolysis, EACA has been used during cardiac surgery to decrease postoperative chest tube drainage. However, the drug's efficacy in reducing blood transfusion requirements has been demonstrated only when the transfusion threshold is restrictive (Hb approximately 7 g/dL). Theoretical risks of thrombosis with EACA have not been demonstrated clinically; nevertheless, caution should be taken when administering these agents to treat DIC. The dosage of EACA in adults is a 5 g IV load over 1 hour followed by 1 to 2 g/h IV infusion, whereas the standard dosage of TXA is 1 g over 10 to 30 minutes. Dose reduction is commonly required in patients prone to drug accumulation, particularly those with renal insufficiency or failure.

D. **Serpins** (serine protease inhibitors) such as aprotinin function to directly inhibit the activity of plasmin and other proteases involved in fibrinolysis. Although these agents were previously used to reduce massive hemorrhage in cardiac surgery, they have been associated with increased mortality rates and have largely disappeared from use in the United States.

E. **Topical hemostatic agents** such as fibrin glue, thrombin gel, and oxidized regenerated cellulose (*Surgicel*) have been shown in trials to reduce perioperative transfusion requirements and time to hemostasis. Their use is now recommended for patients with potential or active excessive bleeding.

VII. CONSERVATION AND SALVAGE TECHNIQUES

A. **Autologous donation** usually begins 6 weeks before surgery and can greatly reduce the amount of homologous blood transfused. The length of the predonation period is limited by the length of time that blood can be stored, currently 42 days unless the blood is frozen. Current blood bank guidelines require a predonation Hb of at least 11 g/dL, donations no more frequently than every 3 days, and no donations in the 72 hours before surgery. Most patients tolerate autologous donation without complication. Patients with severe aortic stenosis or unstable angina are not candidates for autologous donation. Patients donating autologous blood should receive supplemental iron because depleted iron stores frequently limit RBC recovery. Recombinant EPO treatment (see Section VI.A) also may be considered. Because a risk of transfusion reactions due to clerical error still exists, autologous blood should not be transfused unless transfusion is clinically indicated.

B. **Acute normovolemic hemodilution (ANH)** entails removing one or more units of fresh whole blood from a patient while replacing the lost volume with either colloid or crystalloid. By implementing an ANH strategy in anticipation of intraoperative blood loss, fresh autologous blood is available for later reinfusion as surgical blood loss is complete. Any blood shed after hemodilution will also contain a smaller proportion of red cells relative to plasma, thus reducing the loss of hemoglobin and oxygen-carrying capacity. Hemodilution may be helpful in situations in which platelets are lost or altered intraoperatively (eg, cardiopulmonary bypass), as autologous blood retains normal platelet and clotting factor concentrations when reinfused. It should also be remembered that the autologous blood retains a Hct value similar to the patient's preoperative Hct (ie, approximately 40%-50% if normal); this is in contrast to a standard unit of PRBCs, which has a Hct of approximately 70%. Although ANH alone may not eliminate the need for allogeneic transfusion, it may decrease the need for allogeneic units when used in combination with preoperative autologous donation. In most cases, however, ANH will only modestly diminish the need for allogeneic transfusion unless the preoperative Hct is high, the patient can tolerate a low target Hct, and the expected blood loss is large.

C. **Intraoperative autotransfusion (cell salvage)** utilizes blood collected from the surgical field by a double-lumen suction device. As the shed blood is suctioned from the surgical field into one lumen, it is mixed with an anticoagulant (citrate-phosphate-dextrose or heparin) solution from the other lumen to prevent clotting of the blood in the filtered collecting reservoir. The blood then undergoes a series of steps including filtration, centrifugation, and washing; this process is designed to remove debris, plasma, free Hb, and anticoagulant factors. The final product is a collection bag of RBCs with a Hct of 50% to 70% that is ready for reinfusion after about 3 minutes of processing time. Although this technique remains highly useful, the clinician must note that blood collected via intraoperative salvage is deficient in plasma, clotting factors, and platelets. The technique is also generally restricted to procedures with clean surgical fields and nononcologic procedures because of the theoretical risks of reinfusing bacteria or tumor cells into the bloodstream.

D. **Controlled hypotension** (or induced hypotension) involves deliberate maintainence of a patient's blood pressure in a lower range than usual, often allowing a mean arterial pressure of 55 to 65 mm Hg or 30% less than the patient's baseline. This technique is most appropriate when performed in carefully selected patients for brief periods during specific procedures (eg, clipping of cerebral aneurysms). Short-acting, easily titratable vasodilator infusions are ideal for the maintenance of the hypotensive state. Although this technique may limit bleeding and potentially avoid the need for additional blood products, it has significant potential drawbacks including end-organ ischemia and thrombosis due to decreased forward blood flow. As these risks are amplified in states of preexisting cardiovascular disease and sensitivity to diminished perfusion, controlled hypotension is contraindicated in patients with severe atherosclerotic burdens in the coronary and cerebral circulations as well as those with increased intracranial pressure.

VIII. COMPLICATIONS OF BLOOD TRANSFUSION THERAPY
A. **Transfusion reactions**
1. **Acute hemolytic transfusion reactions** most commonly occur when ABO-incompatible blood is transfused, resulting in recipient anti-A and/or anti-B antibodies attaching to donor RBC antigens and forming

antigen-antibody complexes. These antigen-antibody complexes activate complement, precipitating intravascular hemolysis with the release of RBC stroma and free Hb. Immune system activation also results in endothelial and mast cell activation, stimulating the release of serotonin, histamine, and bradykinin; these mediators set off a cascade of widespread vasodilation, diffuse inflammation, and acute hypotension. The net results may include shock, kidney injury due to Hb precipitation in renal tubules, and DIC (see Section IX.B). Many signs and symptoms of an acute hemolytic transfusion reaction appear immediately and include fever, chest pain, anxiety, back pain, and dyspnea. Many are masked by general anesthesia, but intraoperative clues to the diagnosis include fever, hypotension, hemoglobinuria, unexplained bleeding, or failure of the Hct to increase after transfusion. **Table 36.3** outlines steps to take if a transfusion reaction is suspected. The incidence of fatal hemolytic transfusion reactions in the United States is approximately 1 in every 250,000 to 1,000,000 units transfused. Most reactions occur because of administrative errors, with the majority caused by improper identification of the blood unit or patient. The importance of adhering to strict policies of checking blood and matching to the correct patient in the operating room cannot be overemphasized.

2. **Delayed hemolytic transfusion reactions** occur because of antibodies targeting minor RBC antigens (eg, Kidd) and are characterized by extravascular hemolysis. Delayed hemolytic transfusions reactions are most common in patients with a history of multiple prior transfusions, especially those with chronic anemias or hemoglobinopathies. These reactions often present days to weeks after transfusion. Patients may experience minimal symptoms but may display signs of anemia and jaundice. Laboratory studies reveal a positive direct antiglobulin test, hyperbilirubinemia, decreased haptoglobin levels, and hemosiderin in the urine. Treatment is aimed at correcting the anemia.

3. **Febrile nonhemolytic transfusion reactions** (FNHTRs) are the most common transfusion reactions, occurring in approximately 1% of RBC transfusions and up to 30% of platelet transfusions. These may occur in response to cytokines in the stored product or may occur when anti-leukocyte or anti-HLA antibodies in the recipient react with donor white blood cells or platelets in the transfused blood product, thus producing pyrogen and proinflammatory cytokine release. Signs and symptoms include fever, chills, rigors, tachycardia, malaise, nausea, and vomiting. Approach to treatment involves first stopping the transfusion and excluding an acute hemolytic transfusion reaction or bacterial contamination of the donor unit. Acetaminophen and meperidine may diminish fever and rigors, respectively. Once the diagnosis of FNHTR has been made, future reactions may be avoided or diminished by administering leukoreduced blood products (see Section IV.B.2), premedicating at-risk patients with acetaminophen and hydrocortisone (50-100 mg IV), and administering the transfusion slowly.

4. **Allergic transfusion reactions** are common, occurring in 1% to 3% of transfusions. They arise from recipient IgE-mediated antibody responses to donor plasma proteins. Urticaria with pruritus and erythema is the most common manifestation, but bronchospasm or anaphylaxis may occur in rare instances. Many patients also develop fevers. Patients with IgA deficiency may be at an increased risk of allergic transfusion reactions and anaphylaxis because of the presence of anti-IgA antibodies

| TABLE 36.3 | Approach to Suspected Acute Hemolytic Transfusion Reaction |

1. Stop the transfusion.
2. Quickly check for error in patient identity or donor unit.
3. Send the donor unit and a newly obtained blood sample to blood bank for repeat cross-match.
4. Treat hypotension with fluids and vasopressors as necessary.
5. If ongoing transfusion is required, administer type O-negative PRBC and type AB FFP as necessary.
6. Insert a Foley catheter and support renal function with fluids to correct hypovolemia and, if needed, alkaline diuresis (sodium bicarbonate + furosemide ± mannitol) to maintain brisk urine output.
7. Monitor for signs of DIC clinically and with appropriate laboratory studies; treat supportively (see Section IX.B).
8. Send patient blood sample for direct antiglobulin (Coombs) test, free Hb, and haptoglobin; send urine for Hb.

DIC, disseminated intravascular coagulation; FFP, fresh frozen plasma; PRBC, packed red blood cells.

that react with transfused IgA; this is best prevented by administering plasma-free blood products (eg, washed PRBCs) to patients with known IgA deficiency. Treatment involves stopping the transfusion, excluding more severe reactions (see above), and administering antihistamines (eg, diphenhydramine 50 mg IV and ranitidine 50 mg IV). A significant reaction may warrant administration of a corticosteroid (methylprednisolone 80 mg IV). Bronchospasm and anaphylaxis should be treated as described in Chapter 17.

5. **TRALI** is a condition involving rapid-onset respiratory insufficiency following blood, FFP, cryoprecipitate, or platelet transfusion. Signs and symptoms include fevers, dyspnea, hypoxemia, hypotension, and low-pressure pulmonary edema developing within 4 hours of transfusion. TRALI is thought to occur when anti-HLA and anti-leukocyte antibodies present in donor plasma target recipient neutrophils, which damage the lung parenchyma. This mechanism also accounts for the transient leukopenia that may be observed in recipients who develop TRALI. TRALI may rapidly progress to hypoxemic respiratory failure and acute respiratory distress syndrome (ARDS) and is currently the leading cause of transfusion-related mortality in the United States. Most cases are traced to plasma-containing blood products from multiparous female donors who have developed anti-HLA antibodies; therefore, measures to prevent plasma donation by women who have been pregnant may reduce the incidence of TRALI-related episodes.

6. **Transfusion-associated circulatory overload (TACO)** is a condition of circulatory congestion secondary to the fluid volumes administered during massive transfusion. Symptoms often mimic those of decompensated congestive heart failure and include dyspnea, high-pressure pulmonary edema, tachycardia, and jugular venous distention. While TRALI usually produces pulmonary edema in the absence of overt hypervolemia, signs of hypervolemia and increased left ventricular filling pressures may be observed in TACO. TACO often affects

patients at risk for congestive heart failure and occurs in less than 1% of transfusions. If a patient is at risk for fluid overload with high-volume transfusion, diuretics or volume-reduced blood products may be administered prophylactically. However, as TACO is often traced to overly aggressive transfusion in patients with preexisting myocardial dysfunction, the clinician should also be judicious with respect to the volume transfused.

7. **GVHD** is a rare and serious complication of blood transfusion resulting from an attack of immunocompetent donor lymphocytes on the host's tissues. In a great majority of transfusions, donor lymphocytes are destroyed by the recipient's immune system, thus preventing GVHD. However, if the host is immunodeficient or if a specific type of partial donor-recipient HLA matching occurs, the risk of GVHD is increased. The condition often develops 4 to 30 days after transfusion, with patients typically presenting with fever and an erythematous rash that may become generalized. Other symptoms include anorexia, vomiting, abdominal pain, and cough. The diagnosis is made by skin biopsy and confirmed by demonstrating the presence of circulating lymphocytes with a different HLA phenotype, verifying their origin from the donor. GVHD is poorly responsive to most available treatments. Therefore, prevention is of utmost importance and is achieved by exposing lymphocyte-containing components to gamma radiation, thereby inactivating donor lymphocytes. In addition to immunocompromised recipients, patients receiving blood products from family donors or HLA-matched platelets are viable candidates for transfusion of irradiated blood components owing to an associated risk of partial HLA matching.

B. **Metabolic complications of blood transfusions**

1. **Hyperkalemia** is common with rapid blood transfusion but most often becomes clinically significant in cases involving massive transfusion or renal failure. During storage, red cells leak potassium into the extracellular environment, elevating potassium levels to greater than 20 mEq/U PRBCs after approximately 2 weeks. However, this state is rapidly corrected with transfusion and repletion of cellular energy stores.

2. **Hypocalcemia.** Citrate, which chelates calcium, is used as an anticoagulant in stored blood products. Consequently, rapid transfusion decreases ionized calcium levels in the recipient, potentially producing neuromuscular or cardiovascular complications. Although hypocalcemia is usually insignificant owing to efficient hepatic metabolism of the infused citrate, it may become problematic in small children, in patients with impaired liver function, in hypothermic or alkalemic patients, in patients with decreased hepatic blood flow, and during the anhepatic phase of liver transplantation. It is also more common with the transfusion of FFP, which contains higher concentrations of citrate. Ionized calcium levels should be followed, as total serum calcium includes inactive citrate-bound calcium and may not accurately reflect free serum calcium.

3. **Acid-base abnormalities.** Banked PRBCs become acidic because of accumulated red cell metabolites, with pH decreasing linearly to approximately 6.6 after 2 weeks in storage. However, the actual acid load delivered to the patient is minimal. Metabolic acidosis in the face of severe blood loss is more likely due to hypoperfusion and will typically improve with volume resuscitation. The development of a metabolic alkalosis is also common following massive blood transfusion because citrate is rapidly metabolized in the liver to bicarbonate.

4. **Hypothermia.** With the exception of platelets, blood products are typically refrigerated to a standard temperature of 4 °C. Rapid administration of a large volume of PRBCs and other cooled blood products may precipitate hypothermia, which may have adverse effects on immune function, wound healing, coagulation, myocardial function, and maintenance of electrolyte balance. Therefore, blood products other than platelets are best transfused through a primed warming device.

5. **Iron overload.** Repeated or high-volume transfusion of red cells has the potential to produce or worsen a state of hemochromatosis (systemic iron overload with consequent organ impairment). Although this is typically of little immediate concern in the setting of acute surgical or traumatic hemorrhage, patients with preexisting hereditary or transfusion-related hemochromatosis may exhibit progressive hepatic dysfunction, cardiomyopathy, and insulin resistance in addition to other endocrine abnormalities. As the body lacks a finely tuned mechanism for the elimination of excess iron, serial phlebotomy and iron chelation may be required as therapeutic measures. To minimize the buildup of excess iron in high-risk patients, perioperative blood-conserving approaches such as cell salvage and ANH may be appropriate (see Section VII).

6. **Derangements from blood storage.** It is known that stored red blood cells undergo progressive structural and functional alterations that decrease their functionality and viability following transfusion. For example, prolonged storage may diminish microvascular flow as red cells lose their deformability. A decrease in oxygen delivery also occurs secondary to depletion of 2,3-diphosphoglycerate, which results in a leftward shift of the oxyhemoglobin dissociation curve as well as increased adhesion and aggregation of red cells. In addition, there is an accumulation of proinflammatory substances and priming of the nicotinamide adenine dinucleotide phosphate ($NADP^+$) system with reduction in concentrations of nitric oxide (NO) and adenosine triphosphate (ATP). Some studies have suggested increased rates of complications and mortality following cardiac surgery in patients who received blood that was stored for more than 2 weeks, highlighting the potential clinical consequences of prolonged blood storage.

C. **Infectious complications of blood transfusions** have decreased with improved laboratory testing for transmissible diseases. Exposure to pooled products (eg, cryoprecipitate) increases the risk in proportion to the number of donors. See Chapter 8 for all infectious diseases transmitted by blood transfusion.

1. **Hepatitis B virus.** The risk of hepatitis B infection from a blood transfusion has decreased since testing donated blood for hepatitis B antigen became routine in 1971. The current risk is estimated to be 1:60,000 to 1:120,000 units transfused.

2. **Hepatitis C virus (HCV).** The institution of routine testing for antibodies to HCV in 1990 (and recently nucleic acid testing) has reduced the risk of transfusion-related HCV to approximately 1:800,000 to 1:1.6 million units transfused.

3. **Human immunodeficiency virus (HIV).** Because of improved screening and testing of patients and blood products, the risk of transfusion-associated HIV has been estimated to be about 1:1.4 to 1:2.4 million units transfused in the United States.

4. **Cytomegalovirus.** The prevalence of antibodies to CMV in the general adult population is approximately 70%. The incidence of

transfusion-associated CMV infection in previously noninfected patients is quite high, and CMV remains the most common infectious agent transmitted via blood product administration. Infection is typically asymptomatic; however, because immunosuppressed patients and neonates may develop severe disease, CMV-negative or leukoreduced blood products may be recommended.

5. **West Nile virus (WNV).** Following the 2002 epidemic of WNV in the United States, it was found that transfusion of red cells, platelets, and FFP can transmit WNV. With universal screening, the risk of WNV from transfusion has decreased to less than 1:1 million.

6. **Bacterial sepsis** caused by transfused blood products remains rare. Donors with evidence of infectious disease are excluded from transfusion, and the storage of PRBCs at 4 °C minimizes the risk of infection. Nonetheless, PRBCs may become contaminated, most frequently with *Yersinia enterocolitica*. Platelets, which are stored at room temperature, are more problematic, with an estimated infection rate of 1:1000 to 1:2000 units. The most common organisms associated with platelet contamination are *Staphylococcus* species (especially *S. aureus* and *S. epidermidis*) and diphtheroids. The risk of infection is directly related to the storage time of the product, with 15% to 25% of infected units causing severe sepsis in the recipient. Signs of infection usually become apparent during transfusion and should trigger immediate discontinuation of the transfusion and testing of the unit for contamination. Individual outcomes from transfusion-related sepsis depend on the size of the bacterial inoculum and the immunocompetence of the recipient, but overall mortality remains high at approximately 60%.

D. **Transfusion-related immunomodulation.** Transfusion of allogeneic blood is known to suppress the immune system. Although the exact mechanism is unknown, theories suggest that transfusion of donor leukocytes may induce an "immune-tolerant" state in the recipient. Thus, allogeneic blood transfusion has been used preoperatively and intraoperatively in renal transplant recipients to improve graft viability, although studies supporting this practice were largely performed prior to the advent of modern immunosuppressants such as cyclosporine. More controversial are the potential detrimental effects of intraoperative allogeneic blood transfusion on cancer recurrence rates, postoperative infections, activation of latent viral infections, and postoperative mortality. Some experts contend that many of the adverse immunomodulatory effects of allogeneic blood transfusion may be diminished by universal blood product leukoreduction, and promising research suggests that the use of leukoreduced blood products may improve survival in cardiac surgery. Universal leukoreduction protocols have therefore been increasingly adopted in various institutions.

IX. **PERIOPERATIVE COAGULOPATHY**
A. **Coagulopathy of massive transfusion** is unusual with transfusions less than 1 to 1.5 BVs, assuming the patient has a normal coagulation profile, platelet count, and platelet function initially.

1. **Thrombocytopenia.** Diffuse oozing and failure to form clots after massive transfusion may be precipitated in part by thrombocytopenia, which is typically due to the transfusion of platelet-poor blood products. However, clinically significant bleeding is unlikely with platelet counts above 50,000 cells/mm^3. If the loss of one BV or more is expected, platelets should be transfused to maintain a count of 50,000 cells/mm^3 or greater.

2. **Coagulation factor deficiencies.** The normal human body has tremendous reserves of clotting factors. In addition, the patient receives small amounts of the most stable clotting factors in the plasma of each unit of red cells. Bleeding from factor deficiency in the face of massive transfusion is therefore typically due to decreased levels of fibrinogen and labile factors with shorter storage half-lives (especially factors V, VIII, or IX). Bleeding from hypofibrinogenemia is unusual unless the fibrinogen level is below 75 mg/dL. In some patients, factor VIII levels increase with massive transfusion because of increased release from endothelial cells. Additional labile clotting factors are best repleted in the form of FFP. Six units of platelets contain coagulation factor levels equivalent to 1 unit of FFP. Cryoprecipitate may also provide a source of concentrated fibrinogen for the patient who cannot tolerate FFP owing to volume overload.

B. **DIC** refers to the abnormal, diffuse systemic activation of the clotting system. The pathophysiology involves excessive generation of thrombin (factor IIa), resulting in unrestrained fibrin cross-linking throughout the circulation accompanied by platelet activation, fibrinolysis, and coagulation factor consumption. The profound consumptive coagulopathy produced by DIC often results in hemorrhage.

1. **Causes** of DIC include infection, shock, trauma, burns, pancreatitis, and fat or cholesterol embolism. DIC is also common in extensive head injury and complications of pregnancy (eg, amniotic fluid embolism, placental abruption, or septic abortion) because of the high concentrations of tissue factor (thromboplastin) in brain and placental tissues, respectively. A chronic form of DIC may accompany cirrhotic liver disease, nephrotic syndromes, aortic dissection, and malignancy.

2. **Clinical features** include petechiae, ecchymoses, bleeding from venipuncture sites, and frank hemorrhage from operative incisions. Although the hemorrhagic manifestations of DIC are clinically most obvious, complications related to diffuse microvascular and macrovascular thromboses are more common, more difficult to treat, and more potentially life-threatening because of the resulting ischemia of vital organs. Systemic bradykinin release in DIC may also cause acute hypotension.

3. **Laboratory features** of DIC universally include an elevated D-dimer level and increased fibrin degradation products, although these abnormalities are nonspecific. The PT and PTT are typically prolonged, and serial measurements reveal decreased fibrinogen levels and platelet counts. After an initial PTT value is obtained, the waveform used to generate the PTT result can be reviewed for an early negative slope that is suggestive of DIC. Various TEG parameters, usually first indicating a hypercoagulable state followed by severe coagulation factor deficiencies, can also be followed as point-of-care assessments of a patient's coagulation profile.

4. **Treatment of DIC** involves addressing the precipitating cause and transfusing appropriate blood products (eg, FFP, platelets, and cryoprecipitate) to correct bleeding. It is now generally recommended that blood products not be withheld out of concern for "feeding the fire" of the consumptive coagulopathy, particularly if significant hemorrhage is present. However, inhibitors of fibrinolysis (eg, TXA) are contraindicated in DIC owing to the risk of exacerbating or precipitating further thrombotic complications.

C. **Chronic liver disease.** With the notable exceptions of factor VIII and vWF, which are produced by the endothelium, the liver synthesizes all coagulation factors. Assessment of serum factor VIII levels may thus be useful in distinguishing hepatic synthetic dysfunction from other coagulopathies. Patients with hepatic dysfunction may exhibit decreased production of inactive coagulation factors with decreased clearance of activated factors. If circulating levels of activated clotting factors are increased, patients may develop an ongoing consumptive coagulopathy similar to that seen in DIC. Because the liver is also instrumental in removing the by-products of fibrinolysis, levels of fibrin degradation products may be elevated. Note that, although the INR provides a reliable indicator of hepatic synthetic dysfunction, it does not correlate well with surgical bleeding risk in patients with significant liver disease.

D. **Vitamin K deficiency.** The fat-soluble vitamin K (phylloquinone) is required by the liver as a cofactor for the gamma-carboxylation of factors II, VII, IX, and X as well as anticoagulant proteins C and S. Because vitamin K cannot be synthesized endogenously, decreased vitamin K intake or malabsorption may cause a coagulopathy with a prolonged PT (see Chapter 6). In addition, because humans rely on gastrointestinal (GI) flora for some production of vitamin K, vitamin K deficiency is also commonly found in patients receiving broad-spectrum antibiotics, neonates who lack a mature GI microbiome, and patients with short bowel syndrome. Patients on warfarin therapy also exhibit a functional vitamin K deficiency (see Section IX.E.3). Patients with poor absorption or limited GI flora can be treated with subcutaneous vitamin K (eg, 10 mg daily for 3 days), whereas malnourished patients or those on warfarin may be given vitamin K orally. Intravenous administration of vitamin K (2.5-10 mg) may result in a faster correction of the PT but is accompanied by a greater risk of anaphylaxis. If used, IV vitamin K should be administered slowly. If faster correction of PT than by using vitamin K is required (as in active intracranial hemorrhage), FFP (5-8 mL/kg) or other blood products such as prothrombin complex concentrate (PCC or *Kcentra*) should be coadministered.

E. **Coagulopathy associated with cardiopulmonary bypass (CPB)** has long been recognized as a consequence of abnormal activation of the coagulation cascade and platelet dysfunction, which are likely precipitated by contact of blood with CPB circuit components. This increases the likelihood of bleeding in patients after cardiac surgery despite a lack of clear correlation with coagulation studies such as platelet counts. More recently, there has been an increased interest in the use of point-of-care platelet function assays as a metric of the risk of hemorrhagic complications associated with CPB.

F. **Pharmacologic interventions**

1. **Heparin** acts by accelerating the effects of antithrombin III, thus inhibiting both factors IIa (thrombin) and Xa. It prolongs the PTT and has a short half-life; therefore, its anticoagulant effect is usually reversed approximately 4 to 6 hours after discontinuation of the infusion. If faster reversal is required, protamine sulfate, a natural antagonist, may be administered.

2. **Low-molecular-weight heparins (LMWHs)** such as enoxaparin (*Lovenox*) are commercially prepared by fractionating heparin into molecules of 2000 to 10,000 Da. They exert their anticoagulant effect primarily by inhibiting factor Xa and usually do not require monitoring of the PTT. These drugs have longer half-lives than heparin and are incompletely reversed by protamine, yet protamine reversal may be indicated in the setting of a major bleeding episode. Faster reversal may require FFP transfusion.

3. **Warfarin (*Coumadin*)** is an oral vitamin K antagonist that inhibits vitamin K epoxide reductase. This produces a deficiency of activated vitamin K, preventing the hepatic gamma-carboxylation of factors II, VII, IX, and X and proteins C and S to their active forms. The PT and the INR are prolonged in patients taking warfarin. The onset and offset of warfarin's effects are slow due to the drug's half-life and the half-lives of vitamin K–dependent factors. If quick reversal of warfarin is required, vitamin K–dependent factors can be repleted in the form of FFP (5-15 mL/kg) or PCC. Vitamin K (2.5-10 mg by mouth, intravenously, or subcutaneously) can also be given to accelerate warfarin reversal.

4. **Platelet inhibitors** (or antiplatelet agents) target multiple pathways of platelet adhesion, activation, and aggregation. Irreversible inhibitors such as aspirin and clopidogrel generally impair the function of the platelets throughout their 7- to 10-day lifespan. Thus, immediate reversal of certain platelet inhibitors may require platelet transfusion and may not be effective if the inhibitor is still present in the plasma.

5. **Aspirin** and **nonsteroidal anti-inflammatory drugs (NSAIDs)** inhibit platelet aggregation by interfering with cyclooxygenase function. Non-aspirin NSAIDs reversibly inhibit the cyclooxygenase pathway, and their effects typically dissipate within 3 days of discontinuation.

6. **Ticlopidine**, **clopidogrel**, **prasugrel**, **ticagrelor**, and **cangrelor** are agents that inhibit ADP-mediated platelet aggregation by antagonizing the $P2Y_{12}$ receptor. Clopidogrel remains the most commonly coprescribed antiplatelet agent with aspirin in patients requiring dual antiplatelet therapy, although ticagrelor, a more potent reversible inhibitor, may have greater clinical efficacy in certain contexts. Ticlopidine is now rarely prescribed owing to the associated risk of neutropenia.

7. **Eptifibatide, abciximab,** and **tirofiban** are inhibitors of the platelet glycoprotein IIb/IIIa receptor. Abciximab, notably, is an IV monoclonal Fab antibody fragment directed against the receptor and thus also has the potential to produce thrombocytopenia. Although the drug's plasma half-life is short, impairment of platelet function may last for days, and reversal of its effects may require multiple platelet transfusions owing to ongoing adsorption of the antibody to donor platelets.

8. **Dipyridamole** and **cilostazol** are selective phosphodiesterase 3 inhibitors that increase platelet and endothelial cAMP levels, thereby inhibiting platelet aggregation and producing a degree of vasodilation. Cilostazol is commonly used in the management of symptomatic peripheral arterial disease.

9. **Thrombolytic agents** act by dissolving thrombi via direct conversion of plasminogen to plasmin, which lyses fibrin clots. They are intended to rapidly antagonize thrombosis and thus recanalize blood vessels occluded as a result of thrombotic phenomena (eg, thromboembolic stroke). Two thrombolytic agents, recombinant **tissue plasminogen activator** and **streptokinase,** are most commonly used in clinical practice. Each of these drugs results in a hypofibrinogenemic state and carries a substantial risk of bleeding. Therefore, they are generally contraindicated perioperatively, and the benefits of their administration should be carefully weighed against their considerable risks. If emergent surgery is required after thrombolytic therapy, the effect may be antagonized by administration of aminocaproic acid or TXA. Fibrinogen levels may also be restored by transfusion of cryoprecipitate or FFP.

10. **Direct thrombin inhibitors (DTIs)** such as **dabigatran, argatroban,** and **bivalirudin** inhibit thrombin (factor IIa). Dabigatran is an oral DTI often used for stroke prevention in atrial fibrillation and, unlike warfarin, does not require frequent INR monitoring. It also carries the advantage of an availability of a novel reversal agent called idarucizumab, a monoclonal antibody that targets and inactivates drug. Argatroban (often preferred in renal insufficiency) and bivalirudin are intravenous medications used for anticoagulation as alternatives to heparin in patients with heparin-induced thrombocytopenia. At this time, argatroban and bivalirudin lack specific reversal agents and can thus cause life-threatening bleeding if administered without due caution.

11. **Direct factor Xa inhibitors** such as **apixaban, edoxaban,** and **rivaroxaban** inhibit factor Xa. This mechanism lies in contrast to that of LMWHs and synthetic agents such as fondaparinux, which inhibit factor Xa indirectly via interaction with antithrombin III. Like dabigatran, these oral agents are also typically used for the prevention and treatment of thromboembolic events, and they have been demonstrated to be efficacious, safe, and convenient alternatives to warfarin therapy in patients with adequate renal function. Although direct factor Xa inhibitors were traditionally irreversible, a novel reversal agent called andexanet alfa (*Andexxa*), a recombinant derivative of factor Xa that acts as a decoy receptor for the anticoagulant drug, has gained US Food and Drug Administration (FDA) approval. Additional antidotes such as ciraparantag, a "universal" reversal agent potentially capable of counteracting a wide variety of anticoagulants, remain under investigation.

G. **Reversal of perioperative coagulopathy** can often be achieved with blood component therapies such as cryoprecipitate, platelets, and FFP, although the choice of therapy depends on the underlying cause of the coagulopathy. In addition, specific clotting factors are available for patients who require rapid reversal of coagulopathy and may not tolerate the large volumes or other risks associated with transfusion of conventional blood products.

1. **Recombinant factor VIIa (rFVIIa)** is FDA approved for the treatment of hemophiliacs with antibody inhibitors that prevent factor VIII or IX from normalizing their coagulation. Rather than replenishing factor VII levels directly, it produces direct and rapid platelet activation and can trigger the coagulation cascade with a "thrombin burst." The apparent efficacy of rFVIIa in massive surgical or traumatic bleeding, primarily shown in case studies, has generated interest in wider applications for the drug. A major trial of rFVIIa administration demonstrated reduced expansion of intracerebral hematoma in cases of nontraumatic hemorrhagic stroke, although a follow-up study showed no improvement in mortality or functional outcome. rFVIIa is expensive and has been associated with adverse thrombotic events.

2. **Prothrombin complex concentrates (PCCs)** are preparations of vitamin K–dependent factors II, VII, IX, X, and proteins C and S that are derived from FFP. They are useful for the urgent reversal of warfarin or other serious coagulopathies resulting from specific factor deficiencies. PCCs are expensive, and their use is currently restricted to particular clinical circumstances requiring immediate reversal of anticoagulation. Standard inactive PCC (*Kcentra*) is currently approved for the rapid reversal of warfarin anticoagulation in patients with severe acute bleeding or those requiring major surgery, whereas an activated form (factor eight inhibitor bypass activity or FEIBA) is primarily administered for uncontrolled

hemorrhage in patients with hemophilia A. Key adverse effects include thrombotic sequelae, especially with the use of activated PCC.

X. SPECIAL CONSIDERATIONS

A. **Hemophilias** are rare, mainly X-linked diseases affecting males almost exclusively. **Hemophilia A** is due to an abnormality or deficiency of factor VIII, whereas **hemophilia B (Christmas disease)** is due to an abnormality or deficiency of factor IX. The incidences in the United States are 1:10,000 males for hemophilia A and 1:100,000 males for hemophilia B. An even rarer autosomal recessive variant, hemophilia C (Rosenthal syndrome), is caused by a deficiency or dysfunction of factor XI.

1. **Clinical features.** Patients usually present early in childhood with deep bleeding manifestations such as hemarthroses and soft tissue (eg, skeletal muscle) hematomas after minor trauma. Such events may be painful and recurrent, potentially resulting in significant complications such as hemophilic arthropathy. Laboratory tests demonstrate a markedly prolonged PTT with a normal PT and platelet count.

2. **Treatment** with the appropriate factor (in the form of a recombinant or lyophilized concentrate) should be coordinated perioperatively with the patient's hematologist. Hemophilia A is treated with recombinant factor VIII to achieve preoperative activity levels of 25% to 100%, depending on the extent of the procedure. Some patients with mild hemophilia A may also respond to DDAVP therapy, which promotes release of factor VIII (with vWF) from the endothelium. If factor VIII is unavailable in an emergent situation, cryoprecipitate transfusion can provide the deficient factor, and antifibrinolytics such as TXA can reduce bleeding. Hemophilia B is treated with factor IX to achieve at least 30% to 50% activity before surgery.

B. **Von Willebrand disease** is caused by a deficiency or abnormality of vWF, a protein involved in anchoring platelets to injured endothelium and stabilizing factor VIII. It is the most common inherited bleeding disorder, affecting 1% to 2% of the population. It is inherited in an autosomal dominant pattern and affects both sexes equally. The disease is classified into three main phenotypes: type 1, characterized by mild to moderate quantitative deficiencies of vWF and factor VIII; type 2, characterized by a qualitative abnormality of vWF; and type 3, characterized by very low or undetectable levels of vWF in plasma with low but detectable levels of factor VIII.

1. **Clinical presentation.** The phenotypic expression is variable, and clinical manifestations may range from very mild to life-threatening hemorrhage. Usually, patients have a history of easy bruising and superficial bleeding from mucosal surfaces (eg, epistaxis or menorrhagia), but some patients are not diagnosed with a bleeding disorder until they suffer major trauma or undergo surgery complicated by abnormal bleeding. Laboratory tests may reveal a prolonged bleeding time without either PT or PTT elevation or thrombocytopenia.

2. **Treatment** of vWD depends on the subtype. Many patients respond to DDAVP treatment (type 1), but others (types 2 and 3) may require cryoprecipitate or a purified, lyophilized complex of vWF and factor VIII derived from pooled human plasma (*Humate-P*). There is evidence that administration of DDAVP in certain patients with vWD type 2 may precipitate paradoxical thrombosis or thrombocytopenia; therefore, empiric administration of DDAVP in patients with uncharacterized vWD is not recommended. Antifibrinolytics such as TXA also have

been used in some patients to reduce surgical bleeding. Preoperative consultation with the patient's hematologist is recommended.

C. Sickle cell disease (or sickle cell anemia) is an inherited hemoglobinopathy that is particularly prevalent in patients of African descent, affecting 1:600 African Americans. The disease is caused by the substitution of valine for glutamic acid at the sixth position (E6V) on the β-chain of Hb. Homozygotes for this substitution (as well as double heterozygotes for HbS and HbC or β-thalassemias) produce significant quantities of an abnormal sickle-type hemoglobin variant (HbS) and thus have clinical sickle cell disease. Patients who are heterozygous for the E6V substitution are said to have sickle cell trait, which is largely asymptomatic but may produce hyposthenuria or hematuria due to intermittent sickling in the relatively hypoxic and hypertonic renal medulla.

1. **Clinical features.** In sickle cell disease, abnormal HbS molecules polymerize and cause a sickling deformity of the red cell under certain conditions, notably hypoxia, hypothermia, acidosis, and dehydration. Sickled cells are poorly deformable and may become lodged in small vessels, producing microvascular occlusion with tissue ischemia and infarction. A sickle cell crisis typically presents with excruciating bone or abdominal pain, fever, tachycardia, leukocytosis, and hematuria. Particularly concerning is the development of acute chest syndrome, which manifests with dyspnea, hypoxia, chest pain, fevers, and new pulmonary infiltrates on chest radiography. However, many signs and symptoms may be masked by anesthesia. Sickled RBCs exhibit a shortened survival time of 12 days, leading to chronic anemia and extramedullary hematopoiesis.

2. **Anesthetic management** of patients with sickle cell disease includes avoiding conditions that promote sickling (especially hypoxia, hypovolemia, acidemia, and hypothermia). Conservative transfusion management to a preoperative Hct of approximately 30% prevents postoperative complications as effectively as the traditional "exchange transfusions" that sought to reduce the amount of HbS to 30% of total Hb. If acute chest syndrome is suspected perioperatively, the patient may require broad-spectrum antibiotics, ongoing respiratory support, and PRBC transfusions or exchange transfusion to rapidly reduce the proportion of sickled red cells.

D. Jehovah's Witness (JW) patients generally refuse to receive allogeneic as well as certain autologous blood products because of their religious beliefs, even if such refusal results in death. Special considerations apply if the patient is a minor, does not have the capacity to make healthcare-related decisions, or has responsibilities for dependents as well as in certain emergency circumstances (see also Chapter 1). However, under elective conditions, a physician is not required to agree to treat a patient who refuses a transfusion if doing so is contrary to the physician's ethical beliefs. Blood conservation measures are crucial in these patients (see Section VII). Jehovah's Witnesses may allow transfusion of intraoperatively phlebotomized blood (see Section VII.B) as long as the blood remains in continuity with the body (ie, the blood tubing must always remain connected to the patient). EPO is sometimes used to increase red cell mass perioperatively. A more conservative transfusion threshold (eg, transfusing only at a Hb of 6 g/dL) may sometimes be used intraoperatively to reduce the need for blood administration. However, the use of colloid instead of crystalloid has not been shown to help reduce the need for transfusions despite its theoretical benefit in expanding intravascular volume. In all major surgical procedures planned for a JW patient, it is crucial that the anesthesiologist fully discuss the patient's beliefs and decisions concerning transfusion and document these decisions clearly in the medical record as well as on operative consent forms.

XI. ACKNOWLEDGMENT

The authors would like to acknowledge Dr. Michael R. King and Dr. Jonathan E. Charnin for their work on prior editions.

Suggested Readings

American Society of Anesthesiologists Task Force on Perioperative Blood Management. *Practice Guidelines for Perioperative Blood Management.* Approved October 15, 2014. Accessed March 1, 2020. https://www.asahq.org/~/media/sites/asahq/files/public/resources/standards-guidelines/practice-guidelines-for-perioperative-blood-management.pdf

Carson JL, Stanworth SJ, Roubinian N, et al. Transfusion thresholds and other strategies for guiding allogeneic red blood cell transfusion. *Cochrane Database Syst Rev.* 2016;10:CD002042.

Cotton BA, Dossett LA, Haut ER, et al. Multicenter validation of a simplified score to predict massive transfusion in trauma. *J Trauma.* 2010;69(suppl 1):S33-S39.

Crash-2 Trial Collaborators. Effects of tranexamic acid on death, vascular occlusive events, and blood transfusion in patients with significant haemorrhage (CRASH-2): a randomised, placebo-controlled trial. *Lancet.* 2010;376:23-32.

Fergusson DA, Hebert PC, Mazer CD, et al. A comparison of aprotinin and lysine analogues in high-risk cardiac surgery. *N Engl J Med.* 2008;358:2319-2331.

Goodnough LT, Brecher ME, Kanter MH, et al. Transfusion medicine. I. Blood transfusion. *N Engl J Med.* 1999;340:438-447.

Goodnough LT, Brecher ME, Kanter MH, et al. Transfusion medicine: II. Blood conservation. *N Engl J Med.* 1999;340:525-533.

Goodnough LT. Risks of blood transfusion. *Crit Care Med.* 2003;31(12 suppl):S678-S686.

Hebert PC, Wells G, Blajchman MA, et al. A multicenter, randomized controlled clinical trial of transfusion requirements in critical care. *N Engl J Med.* 1999;340:409-417.

Holcomb JB, Tilley BC, Baraniuk S, et al. Transfusion of plasma, platelets, and red blood cells in a 1:1:1 vs a 1:1:2 ratio and mortality in patients with severe trauma: the PROPPR randomized clinical trial. *J Am Med Assoc.* 2015;313(5):471-482.

Kopko PM, Holland PV. Transfusion-related acute lung injury. *Br J Haematol.* 1999;105:322-329.

Lake CL, Moore RA, eds. *Blood: Hemostasis, Transfusion, and Alternatives in the Perioperative Period.* Raven Press; 1995.

O'Connell NM, Perry DJ, Hodgson AJ, et al. Recombinant FVIIa in the management of uncontrolled hemorrhage. *Transfusion.* 2003;43:1711-1716.

Rao SV, Jollis JG, Harrington RA, et al. Relationship of blood transfusion and clinical outcomes in patients with acute coronary syndromes. *J Am Med Assoc.* 2004;292:1555-1562.

Shaw AD, Stafford-Smith M, White WD, et al. The effect of aprotinin on outcome after coronary-artery bypass grafting. *N Engl J Med.* 2008;358:784-793.

Tanaka KA, Bader SO, Görlinger K. Novel approaches in management of perioperative coagulopathy. *Curr Opin Anaesthesiol.* 2014;27:72-80.

WOMAN Trial Collaborators. Effect of early tranexamic acid administration on mortality, hysterectomy, and other morbidities in women with post-partum haemorrhage (WOMAN): an international, randomised, double-blind, placebo-controlled trial. *Lancet.* 2017;389(10084):2105-2116.

37

The Post-anesthesia Care Unit

Jared R. B. Wortzman and Sheri M. Berg

I. GENERAL CONSIDERATIONS

For most patients, recovery from anesthesia is uneventful. Nevertheless, when postoperative complications occur, they may be sudden and life-threatening. The **post-anesthesia care unit (PACU)** is designed to provide close monitoring and care to patients recovering from anesthesia and sedation. This care covers the transition period from one-on-one monitoring in the operating room to a patient's disposition to either a hospital ward or independent function at home. The PACU is staffed by a dedicated team of anesthesiologists, nurses, and aides. Medical oversight may range from anesthesia providers near the PACU to a team consisting of intensivists, residents, and other clinicians with critical care experience. It is ideally located in immediate proximity to the operating room (OR), with access to radiology and the laboratory. Medications and equipment for routine care and advanced support must be readily available.

II. ADMISSION TO THE PACU

A. **Transport** from the OR should only be considered once a patent and stable airway is confirmed. The patient should be transported under direct supervision of the anesthetist, preferably with the head of the bed elevated or with the patient in the lateral decubitus position to maximize airway patency. Oxygen delivered via face mask is indicated in most patients to prevent hypoxemia due to hypoventilation or diffusion hypoxia (see Section VI.A). Unstable patients, such as those receiving vasoactive medications, usually require monitoring of oxygenation and hemodynamics during transport. The anesthetist may opt to bring rescue medications and airway management tools as the clinical situation dictates.

B. A complete **report** should be provided to the PACU team upon arrival. The anesthetist remains in charge of the care of the patient until the PACU team is prepared to assume responsibility.

C. As clinically indicated, the anesthetist may speak directly to the anesthesiologist in charge of the PACU, the surgeon, or a consultant about issues of particular importance for the patient. The report from the anesthetist to the PACU team is often the only formal account of the intraoperative events between the OR team and the personnel who will manage the immediate postoperative care. The report should include the following:

1. **Clinical history:** patient identification, age, surgical procedure, diagnosis, medical history (including hearing and visual impairments,

psychiatric conditions, and precautions for infection control), medications, allergies, preoperative vital signs, and language preference.

2. **Intravascular access:** location and size of catheters.

3. **Intraoperative pharmacology:** premedication, antibiotics, anesthesia induction and maintenance agents, opioids, muscle relaxants, reversal agents, vasoactive drugs, bronchodilators, and other clinically relevant agents administered.

4. **Surgical procedure:** exact nature of the surgery and relevant surgical issues (eg, adequacy of hemostasis, care of drains, restrictions on positioning); the surgeon may present these details to the PACU team.

5. **Anesthetic course:** emphasis on problems that may affect the immediate postoperative period including laboratory values, difficult intravenous (IV) access, airway management issues, intraoperative hemodynamic instability, and electrocardiographic (ECG) changes.

6. **Fluid balance:** amount, type, and reason for fluid replacement, urine output, and estimated fluid and blood losses.

III. MONITORING

Close observation of the patient's level of consciousness, breathing pattern, oxygen saturation, and hemodynamics is of utmost importance. The nurse-to-patient ratio for routine cases and postoperative care is one nurse to two or three patients and increases to single coverage for high-acuity patients, such as those with significant comorbidities, intraoperative complications, or particularly complex procedures. Vital signs are monitored and recorded at regular intervals according to clinical necessity. Standard monitoring includes **respiratory rate** measurement, continuous **electrocardiogram**, noninvasive **blood pressure**, and **pulse oximetry. Temperature** should be monitored and recorded.

A. Invasive monitoring such as arterial catheters, central venous catheters, and pulmonary artery catheters can be instituted if necessary. Arterial catheters provide continuous measurement of the systemic blood pressure and provide access for blood sampling. Central venous and pulmonary artery catheters should be considered when the etiology of hemodynamic instability is unclear (see Chapter 15) or when there is a requirement for vasopressors that can be administered only in the central venous system. Bedside transthoracic echocardiography may provide a less invasive alternative to assessing cardiac function and intravascular volume status. If monitoring and care requirements needed to appropriately care for the patient are escalating and a prolonged or complicated recovery is expected, plans should be made to transfer the patient to an intensive care unit (ICU).

IV. GENERAL COMPLICATIONS

The incidence of overall PACU complications has been found to be as high as 24%, although this number varies with specific patient populations and is likely dependent upon a patient's medical history as well as the anesthesia and procedure performed. The most frequent issues encountered in the PACU setting include the following:

A. **Respiratory and airway complications**

B. **Hemodynamic perturbations**

C. **Postoperative nausea and vomiting**

D. **Renal complications**

E. **Neurologic compromise**

V. EFFECTS OF ANESTHETICS AND SEDATIVES

General anesthesia (GA) affects the respiratory system by altering respiratory drive and mechanics via the following mechanisms:

A. **Reduction in respiratory drive.** Volatile anesthetics, sedatives, and opioids are respiratory depressants. They exert their effects by blunting central and peripheral chemoreceptor responsiveness to hypoxemia and hypercapnia, suppressing normal reflexive responses to negative upper airway pressure, and decreasing wakefulness.

1. **Opioids,** the most commonly prescribed analgesics for postoperative pain control, are potent inhibitors of the hypercapnic ventilatory drive. Respiratory failure secondary to postoperative opioid use peaks during the first 24 hours. Patients treated with opioids have a decreased respiratory rate and may become apneic if not stimulated. **Benzodiazepines** also inhibit ventilatory drive, but to a lesser extent than opioids. The effects of these drugs are dose dependent and influenced by age and comorbidities such as intracranial pathology, obstructive sleep apnea (OSA), or chronic obstructive pulmonary disease (COPD).

B. **Residual neuromuscular blockade** often persists despite reversal of muscle relaxants. The upper airway dilator muscles are particularly sensitive to the effects of muscle relaxants, increasing the risk of upper airway obstruction, aspiration, and reintubation when not fully reversed. Neuromuscular blocking agents should be avoided or administered judiciously in patients with neuromuscular disorders such as Guillain-Barré syndrome, myasthenia gravis, and muscular dystrophies.

C. **Modified respiratory mechanics.** GA alters lung and chest wall mechanics, causing reductions in lung volume and compliance, and chest wall compliance. Immediately after induction of GA functional residual capacity (FRC) decreases by as much as 20%, resulting in atelectasis in dependent regions of the lung. Atelectasis formation is further exacerbated by supine positioning of patients, as well as absorption of alveolar gas (absorption atelectasis) caused by high concentrations of oxygen. Reduced FRC and atelectasis cause ventilation perfusion mismatch, shunting, and hypoxemia.

D. **Intraoperative mechanical ventilation.** Ventilator-induced lung injury results from repetitive overdistention and collapse of dependent lung tissue. Lung protective ventilation with low tidal volumes, low plateau pressures, and the administration of positive end-expiratory pressure (PEEP) is the cornerstone of mechanical ventilation in ICU patients with ARDS. Patients undergoing surgery under GA may also benefit from low tidal volumes, low plateau pressures, higher levels of PEEP, and intraoperative recruitment maneuvers.

VI. RESPIRATORY AND AIRWAY COMPLICATIONS

Respiratory complications occur in 2% to 19% of postoperative patients, with atelectasis and alveolar hypoventilation being the most commons causes of these events. Additional causes of arterial hypoxemia include upper airway obstruction, laryngospasm, bronchospasm, and aspiration.

A. **Hypoxemia.** GA is associated with inhibition of hypoxic and hypercapnic ventilatory drive and a reduction in the lung's FRC. These changes may persist for a variable period of time postoperatively and predispose the patient to hypoventilation and hypoxemia. Supplemental oxygen can delay the detection of hypoventilation by pulse oximetry; however, it also reduces the incidence of hypoxia in the postoperative period. The decision to administer supplemental oxygen should be clinically determined for each patient but should generally be applied when transporting the patient from the OR to the PACU. Signs of hypoxemia include dyspnea, cyanosis, altered mental status, agitation, obtundation, tachycardia, hypertension, and arrhythmias. Hypoxemia should be diagnostically ruled out before undertaking specific treatment for these symptoms.

B. Causes of hypoxemia include the following:

1. **Atelectasis** is a predictable effect of the reduction in the FRC during GA and can lead to increased intrapulmonary shunting. Obese patients and those undergoing thoracic or upper abdominal procedures are more susceptible to atelectasis. Epidural anesthesia without GA is associated with little or no atelectasis formation. Deep breathing, intermittent positive-pressure breathing, and incentive spirometry are effective in rapidly reexpanding small areas of alveolar collapse, although their ability to reduce respiratory complications is uncertain. Noninvasive ventilation (NIV) has been shown to decrease atelectasis and improve oxygenation in postoperative patients. Occasionally, hypoxemia may persist, and a chest radiograph (CXR) may reveal a segmental or lobar collapse. Chest physiotherapy or fiberoptic bronchoscopy may help with reinflating the collapsed segment.

2. **Hypoventilation** causes hypoxemia by promoting alveolar collapse and increasing the partial pressure of CO_2 in the alveolar air.

3. **Diffusion hypoxia** may occur during washout of nitrous oxide upon emergence from GA. High-inspired O_2 fraction (FIO_2) by face mask can prevent hypoxemia.

4. **Upper airway obstruction** is most often caused by inadequate recovery of the airway reflexes and tone and is seen commonly in patients with obesity or preexisting OSA (see Section VI.D) or residual neuromuscular blockade (see Section VI.C.2.b).

5. **Bronchospasm** may cause hypoventilation, CO_2 retention, and hypoxemia.

6. **Aspiration of gastric contents** can lead to aspiration pneumonitis and pneumonia.

7. **Pulmonary edema** may occur from cardiac failure, increased pulmonary capillary permeability, or persistent exposure to negative pressure. Cardiogenic edema occurs mostly in individuals with preexisting cardiac disease and is characterized by hypoxemia, dyspnea, orthopnea, jugular venous distention, wheezing, and an S_3 gallop. It may be precipitated by fluid overload, dysrhythmias, and myocardial ischemia. A CXR, arterial blood gas, a 12-lead ECG, and troponin level should be obtained. Evaluation by a cardiologist may be indicated, particularly when aggressive management of conditions such as unstable angina or acute valvular disease is being considered. Inotropic agents, diuretics, and vasodilators are the mainstay of treatment. The use of NIV can obviate the need for intubation in patients with severe hypoxia, pending the response to the medical treatment. Noncardiogenic pulmonary edema secondary to sepsis, head injury, aspiration, transfusion reaction, anaphylaxis, negative pressure pulmonary edema, or upper airway obstruction is characterized by hypoxemia without the signs of left ventricular overload. Negative-pressure pulmonary edema (NPPE) can transpire secondary to persistent upper airway collapse such as laryngospasm, biting down on the endotracheal tube, or hypopharyngeal collapse, with continued diaphragmatic activity. Young, healthy, athletic patients with good muscle strength are at an increased risk for NPPE, which commonly develops immediately after airway obstruction is relieved.

It is characterized by hypoxemia, pink frothy sputum, and bilateral infiltrates on CXR that usually resolve within 24 to 48 hours. Treatment for pulmonary edema generally needs to be continued in an ICU.

8. **Pneumothorax** may cause hypoventilation, hypoxemia, and hemodynamic instability (see Section VI.C.2.e).

9. **Pulmonary embolism** seldom occurs in the immediate postoperative period. However, it must be considered in the differential diagnosis of hypoxemia in patients with deep venous thrombosis, cancer, multiple trauma, or extended periods of immobility.

C. **Hypoventilation** is characterized by inadequate minute ventilation resulting in hypercarbia and acute respiratory acidosis. When severe, hypoventilation can result in hypoxemia, mental status changes, and ultimately apnea. Supplemental oxygen may mask early detection of hypoventilation through pulse oximetry. Therefore, monitoring the ventilatory status of postoperative patients should not rely entirely on pulse oximetry. Etiologies of postoperative hypoventilation may be divided into two groups:

1. **Decreased ventilatory drive**

   a. All inhaled **halogenated agents** depress ventilatory drive (see Chapter 12) and may produce hypoventilation in the postoperative period. **Opioids** are also potent respiratory depressants. All μ-receptor agonists increase the apneic threshold. Narcotized patients typically appear pain-free, with a slow respiratory rate and a tendency to become apneic if left unstimulated. Large doses of **benzodiazepines** may also inhibit ventilatory drive. The safest treatment of anesthetic-related hypoventilation is to continue mechanical ventilation until breathing is adequate. Alternatively, pharmacologic reversal may be considered.

      1. Opioid-induced hypoventilation can be reversed by **naloxone**, an opioid antagonist with the greatest affinity for the μ-receptor. Doses of 40 to 80 μg IV are titrated to effect. Reversal occurs within 1 to 2 minutes and lasts for 30 to 60 minutes. Naloxone treatment may induce significant side effects such as pain, tachycardia, hypertension, and pulmonary edema. The respiratory depressant effects of the opioids may outlast a single dose of naloxone. Thus, the patient should be monitored for recurrence of opioid-induced hypoventilation. Naloxone should be used cautiously in patients with known or suspected history of chronic opioid use because it may precipitate acute withdrawal.

      2. Hypoventilation secondary to benzodiazepines can be reversed by **flumazenil** (increments of 0.2-1 mg IV over 5 minutes, up to a maximum of 5 mg). The onset of reversal occurs within 1 to 2 minutes with peak effect at 6 to 10 minutes. The patients should be followed closely after administration of flumazenil because resedation may occur owing to its short 7- to 15-minute half-life. Flumazenil should be used cautiously in patients with chronic benzodiazepine use because it may precipitate seizures.

   b. Less common, but potentially life-threatening, causes of decreased ventilatory drive include complications of **intracranial** and **carotid artery** surgery, **head injuries**, and intraoperative **stroke** (see Section IX).

2. **Pulmonary and respiratory muscle insufficiency**

   a. **Preexisting respiratory disease** is the most important risk factor for postoperative respiratory complications. COPD alters the match of ventilation and perfusion, resulting in hypoxemia and hypercapnia.

Impaired gas exchange and expiratory flow limitation cause a high ventilatory workload under normal circumstances. **Restrictive disease** (eg, pulmonary fibrosis, pleural effusions, obesity, scoliosis, massive ascites, and pregnancy) is associated with fewer complications than COPD, particularly when respiratory muscle strength is preserved and the restrictive defect is extrapulmonary. NIV can be beneficial in COPD and in restrictive pulmonary disease by decreasing the work of breathing, augmenting the ventilatory parameters, and avoiding intubation.

b. **Residual neuromuscular blockade** is defined as a train-of-four ratio less than 0.9 and suggested by the clinical observations of spasmodic twitching, generalized weakness, upper airway obstruction, or by more subtle signs such as hypoxemia or shallow breathing. Even with modern nondepolarizing neuromuscular blocking agents, approximately 30% of patients are admitted to the PACU with residual neuromuscular blockade. Adequacy of muscle strength can only be definitively assessed with the aid of a **quantitative neuromuscular transmission monitor** (see Chapter 14). If muscle weakness persists after adequate pharmacologic reversal (eg, **neostigmine** 20-60 μg/kg up to 5 mg, and **glycopyrrolate** 0.2 mg per 1 mg of neostigmine administered or **sugammadex** 2-4 mg/kg), it is best to institute or continue mechanical ventilation, administer adequate anxiolysis, and wait for the muscle strength to recover. At this point, special situations such as myasthenia gravis and myasthenic syndromes, pseudocholinesterase deficiency, succinylcholine-induced phase II block, hypothermia, acid-base and electrolyte imbalance, and anticholinesterase inhibitor–induced weakness should be considered.

c. **Inadequate analgesia** after thoracic or upper abdominal surgery may cause splinting and decreased minute ventilation, resulting in alveolar collapse, hypercapnia, and hypoxemia. This is preventable with early analgesia and encouragement of deep breathing and coughing. Compared with systemic opioids, epidural analgesia may reduce the incidence of respiratory complications (atelectasis, pulmonary infections, or hypoxia).

d. **Bronchospasm** is common in the pediatric population as well as patients with COPD, asthma, or a recent respiratory tract infection. It is often precipitated by manipulation of the airway, particularly tracheal intubation. Wheezing may also be heard upon chest examination of patients with pulmonary edema, endobronchial intubation, aspiration pneumonitis, and pneumothorax.

e. **Pneumothorax** may complicate certain procedures such as thoracotomy, mediastinoscopy, bronchoscopy, high retroperitoneal dissection for nephrectomy or adrenalectomy, laparoscopic surgery, and spinal fusion. Insertion of central venous lines and nerve blocks of the upper extremities are other possible iatrogenic etiologies. Diagnosis is made with a CXR in the upright position. In the presence of hemodynamic instability (tension pneumothorax), a needle decompression or tube thoracostomy must be performed emergently even without CXR diagnosis.

D. **Upper airway obstruction** may occur during recovery from anesthesia. Principal signs are the lack of adequate air movement, intercostal and suprasternal retractions, and paradoxical abdominal and chest wall motion during inspiration. Complete upper airway obstruction is silent. Partial obstruction is accompanied by either snoring (if the obstruction is above the larynx) or stridor (if perilaryngeal). Obstruction is more commonly seen in patients with OSA, obesity, tonsillar or adenoidal hypertrophy, or craniofacial abnormalities. Often times, airway obstruction may be relieved with a chin lift or jaw thrust. Patients with OSA may benefit from the use of continuous positive airway pressure. Common etiologies for upper airway obstruction include the following:

1. **Incomplete recovery** from GA and/or neuromuscular blockade (see Section VI.C.2.b). Decreased strength and coordination of the intrinsic and extrinsic airway musculature causes the tongue to fall backward and occlude the airway. Patency is reestablished by inserting a nasal or oral airway, by manually assisting ventilation, or by intubating the trachea.

2. **Laryngospasm is actually** a "protective reflex," which involves involuntary contraction of the vocal cords after stimulation of the superior laryngeal nerve by noxious stimuli such as blood and airway secretions, particularly while under light anesthesia. It is characterized by stridor or the absence of breath sounds and air movement. Children, smokers, and obese patients are at increased risk for laryngospasm.

3. **Airway edema** may be caused by laryngoscopy, bronchoscopy, nasogastric tube insertion, esophagoscopy, or surgery on the head and neck. It may also follow a traumatic intubation, allergic reaction, the administration of large amounts of IV fluids, or prolonged prone position. Children are particularly susceptible to airway obstruction from edema because of the small diameter of their upper airway. The cuff leak test is neither sensitive nor specific and should not be used as the sole determinant for extubation of a patient with suspected airway edema. Treatment of upper airway edema includes the following:
   a. Administration of warmed, humidified **100% O₂** by face mask.
   b. **Head elevation, fluid restriction**, and possible **diuresis**.
   c. Nebulization of racemic **epinephrine** 2.25% solution, 0.5 to 1.0 mL in normal saline, or L-epinephrine, 2 mL of a 1:1000 solution, which may be repeated in 20 minutes if needed.
   d. **Dexamethasone**, 4 to 8 mg IV every 6 hours for 24 hours.
   e. Administration of **Heliox** (helium:oxygen, 80:20) can dramatically improve gas exchange and the work of breathing by establishing laminar airflow and improving gas exchange at distal alveoli.
   f. **Reintubation** of the trachea must be considered early in the course of suspected airway obstruction as distortion of airway anatomy may occur rapidly, particularly in the setting of allergic reactions.

4. **Wound hematoma** caused by bleeding at the surgical site may complicate thyroid and parathyroid surgery, neck dissections, and carotid endarterectomy. The pressure caused by an expanding hematoma within the neck tissue planes causes obstruction of venous and lymphatic drainage and massive edema. Patients complain of local pain and pressure, dysphagia, and variable degrees of respiratory distress and may have drainage from the surgical site. Neck wound hematomas must be treated immediately by emergency reexploration and evacuation in the OR. The surgeon should be notified immediately and an OR prepared. The anesthesiologist must support the airway by mask ventilation with 100% O₂, followed by intubation of the trachea under direct vision. If tracheal intubation cannot be rapidly accomplished, opening the wound at the bedside can relieve soft tissue compression of the airway and improve airway patency.

5. **Vocal cord (VC) paralysis** may occur after thyroid, parathyroid, thoracic, tracheal, and neck surgery or a traumatic endotracheal intubation. VC paralysis may be transient, resulting from manipulation of

the recurrent laryngeal nerve, or permanent, from severing the nerve. Unilateral transient VC paralysis is relatively common, and the primary concern is potential aspiration of gastric contents. Permanent unilateral VC paralysis can occur without clinical symptoms as compensatory action of the contralateral VC minimizes the occurrence of aspiration. Bilateral VC paralysis can occur after radical surgery for thyroid or tracheal cancer when neoplastic infiltration makes identification of the recurrent laryngeal nerves difficult. Bilateral VC injury is a rare and serious complication that can lead to complete upper airway obstruction after extubation in the immediate postoperative period. It requires emergency endotracheal intubation (which may be more difficult owing to disrupted airway anatomy) and possibly a tracheostomy.

E. **The intubated patient** presents special considerations. The anesthesiologist in the PACU should establish a plan regarding weaning and extubation or, alternatively, transfer the patient to an ICU. Conditions that could delay the extubation at the end of the surgery include the following:

1. **Delayed emergence** from GA due to volatile or IV agents. Reversal may be facilitated pharmacologically for some agents, but generally it is prudent to support ventilation and allow the respiratory depression to resolve spontaneously. The presence of a full stomach mandates additional vigilance in ensuring the recovery of consciousness and pharyngeal reflexes before extubation.

2. **Deep intraoperative neuromuscular blockade** is not appropriate to pharmacologically reverse with **neostigmine and glycopyrrolate**. The steroidal neuromuscular blockers vecuronium and rocuronium can be reversed with appropriately dosed **sugammadex**. Absent the availability of sugammadex, the patient should remain intubated until the patient can be safely, and permanently, reversed. In addition, if muscle weakness persists after adequate pharmacologic reversal, the patient needs mechanical ventilation until full recovery is achieved.

3. **Inadequate O_2 and CO_2 exchange** often resolve as the effects of anesthesia, surgery, and positioning fade. While supporting ventilation, possible etiologies, discussed in Sections VI.A and VI.B, must be considered.

4. **Potential for airway obstruction** exists after any extubation but especially when the patient has had a head and neck procedure, drainage of pharyngeal abscesses, mandibular wiring, large fluid resuscitation, or a prolonged surgery in the prone position. These patients should not be extubated until fully awake.

5. **Hemodynamic instability**, when severe, may be associated with a variable degree of impaired gas exchange and/or consciousness that mandate continuation of mechanical ventilation. Transfer to an ICU should be arranged for patients who fail to improve.

6. **Hypothermia** has numerous adverse effects that may make extubation undesirable immediately after surgery (see Section XII.A).

F. **Guidelines for Extubation.** There is no single value or ventilatory parameter that will predict a successful extubation with certainty. The following criteria may be used when assessing the readiness to resume unassisted ventilation in a postoperative patient:

1. Adequate **arterial oxygen pressure** (PaO_2) or oxygen saturation (SpO_2) on minimal ventilatory support.

2. Adequate **breathing pattern.** Patients should be able to sustain spontaneous, unlabored breathing at a slow rate (<30 breaths/min) and adequate tidal volume (>6 mL/kg), as can be tested in a trial of unsupported breathing.

3. Adequate **level of consciousness** for cooperation and airway protection.
4. Full **recovery of muscle strength** that can be identified through neuro-muscular transmission monitoring.
5. Before proceeding with **extubation**, the PACU anesthesiologist should be aware of any preexisting airway problems in the event that reintubation is necessary. Supplemental O_2 is administered; the endotracheal tube, mouth, and pharynx are suctioned; and the tube is removed after a positive-pressure breath. Oxygen is then supplied by face mask as indicated, SpO_2 is monitored, and the patient is assessed for signs of airway obstruction or ventilatory insufficiency.

VII. HEMODYNAMIC AND CARDIOVASCULAR COMPLICATIONS

Hemodynamic and cardiovascular complications occur in approximately 5% of PACU admissions, with hypotension, arrhythmias, myocardial ischemia, and pulmonary edema being the most common complications recorded. Of interest, postoperative hypertension and tachycardia are associated with an increased risk of unplanned critical care admission and a higher mortality than hypotension and bradycardia.

A. **Hypotension** should prompt a review of the patient's history and the intra-operative management to generate a differential diagnosis. The anesthetist who performed the case can be contacted to help interpret the current events. Hemorrhage must remain a primary consideration in the evaluation of hypotension in the postoperative patient.

1. **Hypovolemia** is the most common cause of hypotension in the PACU, and administration of a fluid bolus during the initial assessment is generally appropriate. Ongoing hemorrhage, inadequate fluid replacement, osmotic polyuria, and fluid sequestration (eg, intestinal obstruction and ascites) are among the causes of hypovolemia in the PACU. Nonspecific signs include tachycardia, dry mucous membranes, oliguria, and thirst. A meaningful volume challenge (250-1000 mL of crystalloid or an equivalent volume of synthetic colloid, blood products, or both) should be considered for specific indications. Persistent hypotension after a seemingly adequate volume replacement mandates further assessment, starting with placement of a urinary catheter and consideration of ongoing surgical bleeding. Additional diagnostics may include transthoracic echocardiogram, a pulmonary artery catheter, or noninvasive cardiac output monitoring.

2. **Impaired venous return** occurs when mechanical forces decrease the venous return to the heart in the absence of a reduction of circulating blood volume. Common causes include **positive-pressure ventilation**, dynamic hyperinflation of the lungs resulting in **autopositive end-expiratory pressure**, **pneumothorax**, and **pericardial tamponade**. Signs of obstruction to venous return are similar to those of true hypovolemia except for the presence of jugular vein distention, an elevated central venous pressure, and possibly decreased breath sounds and heart tones. Volume administration is the mainstay of symptomatic therapy, but treatment of the underlying cause is the definitive intervention.

3. **Vasodilation** leading to hypotension can be caused by neuraxial anesthesia, residual inhalation agents, rewarming after hypothermia, transfusion reactions, adrenal insufficiency, anaphylaxis, systemic inflammation, sepsis, recent use of pharmacologic renin-angiotensin-aldosterone pathway modifiers, and the administration of vasodilating drugs. Hypovolemia accentuates the hypotension due to vasodilatation, but volume replacement alone cannot fully restore the blood

pressure. Pharmacologic treatment includes α–adrenergic receptor agonists such as **phenylephrine, norepinephrine**, and even **epinephrine**. Diagnosis and treatment of the specific etiology should be concurrent with symptomatic treatment.

4. **Decreased cardiac output** can be caused by myocardial ischemia and infarction, dysrhythmias, congestive heart failure, administration of negative inotropic drugs (anesthetics, β-adrenergic blockers, calcium channel blockers, and antidysrhythmics), sepsis, and hypothyroidism (see Chapters 3, 7, and 17). Symptoms include dyspnea, diaphoresis, cyanosis, jugular vein distention, oliguria, rhythm disturbances, wheezing, dependent crackles, and an S_3 gallop on auscultation. A CXR, 12-lead ECG, and basic laboratory tests may help with diagnosis. Invasive monitoring may be necessary to guide pharmacologic therapies, including:

   a. **Inotropic agents** such as dopamine, dobutamine, epinephrine, norepinephrine, and milrinone.

   b. **Afterload reduction** with nitrates and calcium channel blockers.

   c. **Diuresis** with loop diuretics for fluid overload.

   d. **Antiarrhythmics or electrical cardioversion** for arrhythmias.

B. **Hypertension** is most commonly observed in patients with preexisting hypertensive disease, particularly if antihypertensive medications were held preoperatively. Certain types of surgery such as carotid, vascular, endocrine, and intrathoracic procedures are more likely to be followed by hypertensive events. Other postoperative etiologies for hypertension may include pain, bladder distention, fluid overload, hypoxemia, hypercarbia, hypothermia, increased intracranial pressure (ICP), and administration of vasoconstrictive agents. Hypertension is usually asymptomatic, but patients with malignant hypertension may have headache, visual disturbances, dyspnea, restlessness, and even chest pain. In the initial assessment, one should verify the accuracy of blood pressure measurement by checking cuff size and placement, review the patient's history and operative course, and rule out correctable etiologies. The management of hypertension is aimed at restoring blood pressure close to the patient's baseline. Tight blood pressure control is extremely important after surgery for intracranial aneurysm, creation of vascularized muscular flaps, microvascular surgery, and in patients with severe vascular disease. If possible, resumption of chronic antihypertensive oral therapy is ideal. If needed, this can be supplemented or substituted with a fast-onset, short-acting IV medication.

   1. **β-Adrenergic blockers:** labetalol (an α-blocker and a β-blocker), 5 to 20-mg IV bolus or up to 2-mg/min IV infusion, and esmolol (β_1-blocker), 20- to 100-mg IV bolus or 25- to 300-µg/kg/min IV infusion, are first-line agents.

   2. **Calcium channel blockers:** nicardipine initiated at 5 to 15 mg/h or clevidipine 2 to 20 mg/h. Sublingual nifedipine is not recommended because it may cause an unpredictable, and at times severe, drop in blood pressure that may induce myocardial ischemia.

   3. **Hydralazine:** 5- to 20-mg IV bolus, vasodilator, and may induce reflex tachycardia.

   4. **Nitrates:** nitroglycerin, starting at 25 µg/min IV infusion, is preferentially a venodilator and useful for coexisting myocardial ischemia. Sodium nitroprusside, starting at 0.5 µg/kg/min IV infusion, is a potent arterial and venodilator and requires invasive blood pressure monitoring.

C. **Dysrhythmias** in the perioperative period can be caused by increased sympathetic outflow, hypoxemia, hypercarbia, electrolyte and acid-base imbalance, myocardial ischemia, increased ICP, drug toxicity, thyrotoxicosis, and malignant hyperthermia. Premature atrial contractions and unifocal premature ventricular contractions (PVCs) generally do not require treatment. In the presence of more worrisome rhythm disturbances, supplemental O_2 and supportive management should be administered while the etiology is investigated.

1. **Common supraventricular dysrhythmias**
    a. **Sinus tachycardia** may be secondary to pain, agitation, hypovolemia, fever, hyperthermia, hypoxemia, hypercarbia, congestive heart failure, and pulmonary embolism. Symptomatic treatment with β-blockers should be instituted only after its etiology is addressed, unless the patient is at risk of myocardial ischemia.
    b. **Sinus bradycardia** may result from a high neuraxial anesthetic block, opioid administration (with the exception of meperidine), vagal stimulation, β-adrenergic blockade, and increased ICP. Symptomatic treatment with anticholinergic muscarinic agents, **atropine**, 0.4 mg IV, or **glycopyrrolate**, 0.2 mg IV, is indicated when hypotension is present or for severe bradycardia (see Chapter 39).
    c. **Paroxysmal supraventricular tachydysrhythmias** occur with a higher incidence in patients over 70 years of age; after abdominal, thoracic, or major vascular procedures; and in patients with preoperative premature atrial contractions. They include paroxysmal atrial tachycardia, multifocal atrial tachycardia, junctional tachycardia, atrial fibrillation, and flutter. These rhythms may cause significant hypotension, and treatment may include the following:
        1. **Synchronized cardioversion** should be used if the patient is hemodynamically unstable, as per the ACLS protocol (see Chapter 39).
        2. **Adenosine:** 6 mg followed by 12 mg IV, administered rapidly, has a high success rate in converting paroxysmal atrial tachycardia to sinus rhythm.
        3. **Verapamil** (2.5- to 5-mg IV bolus) or **diltiazem** (5- to 20-mg IV bolus, or as an infusion with an initial 0.25- to 0.35-mg/kg IV bolus followed by an infusion rate of 5-15 mg/h IV) will slow the ventricular response.
        4. **Amiodarone** is the antiarrhythmic of choice for rate control of atrial dysrhythmias in the setting of a decreased myocardial function.
        5. **β-Blockers (metoprolol, esmolol, and atenolol)** also decrease the ventricular response to supraventricular tachydysrhythmias.
2. **Stable ventricular dysrhythmias** such as PVCs and stable nonsustained ventricular tachycardia generally do not require treatment; however, a search for reversible causes (hypoxemia, myocardial ischemia, acidosis, hypokalemia, hypomagnesemia, and irritation due to a central venous catheter) should be conducted. Stable sustained ventricular tachycardia can be treated with synchronized cardioversion or pharmacologic modalities. PVCs that are multifocal and occur in runs, or are close to the preceding T wave, should be treated, especially in patients with structural heart disease, owing to the risk of developing an unstable ventricular rhythm.
    a. **β-Blockers:** esmolol, 20- to 100-mg IV bolus, or 25- to 300-μg/kg/min IV infusion, metoprolol, 2.5 to 10 mg IV, and propranolol, 0.5- to 2.0-mg IV increments, may be used.
    b. **Amiodarone:** 150-mg IV bolus over 10 minutes followed by 1-mg/min IV infusion for 6 hours and then 0.5-mg/min IV infusion is indicated in patients with a decreased myocardial function.
3. Management for **unstable ventricular tachycardia** and **ventricular fibrillation** are described in the ACLS protocol (see Chapter 39).

D. Myocardial ischemia and infarction

1. **T-wave changes** (inversion, flattening, and pseudonormalization) may be associated with myocardial ischemia and infarction, electrolyte changes, hypothermia, surgical manipulation of the mediastinum, or incorrect lead placement. Isolated T-wave changes must be considered within the clinical context because they are common postoperatively and do not always indicate myocardial ischemia.

2. **ST segment changes** including depressions and elevations are generally indicative of myocardial ischemia and infarction, respectively. ST segment elevation can be a normal variant or can occur in other conditions such as left ventricular hypertrophy, left bundle branch block, and hyperkalemia. Unlike myocardial infarctions in the nonsurgical setting, in the postoperative period, most myocardial infarctions are associated with ST depression and have a non–Q-wave pattern. As supplemental O_2 is administered and a 12-lead ECG and cardiac enzymes are obtained, possible precipitating factors for the ST segment changes must be reviewed and corrected. Common etiologies include hypoxemia, anemia, tachycardia, hypotension, and hypertension. If ischemia is present, patients should be rate controlled with a *β*-blocker. Aspirin and statins may decrease the mortality of patients with acute coronary syndrome in the perioperative period. IV nitroglycerin is a good option for cases with ST segment elevations. Cardiology consultation and transfer to an ICU should be considered.

3. In patients at high risk for cardiac events (patients with a history of ischemic heart disease, congestive heart disease, cerebrovascular disease, renal insufficiency, and diabetes mellitus and patients undergoing intrathoracic, intraperitoneal, or suprainguinal vascular procedures), continuation, and in some settings initiation, of *β*-blockade may decrease the risk of adverse cardiac events perioperatively.

E. The patient with a permanent pacemaker (PPM) or an intracardiac defibrillator

(ICD) requires special care in the PACU. Information about the patient's pacemaker dependency state and the features of the device must be obtained from the OR team. Continuous ECG monitoring with special attention to the patient's rhythm, rate, and hemodynamic status is indicated. Electrocautery used during the surgery can potentially trigger arrhythmia responses in PPM and ICD. Modern devices are less likely to be affected by intraoperative electromagnetic interference. Placing a magnet over the PPM or ICD should not be standard practice without precise knowledge of its effects. Communication with the electrophysiology service before and after surgery is highly recommended for interrogation of the device. Interrogation and reprogramming of the device to the original parameters may be required in the PACU after the operation.

VIII. RENAL COMPLICATIONS

Acute renal failure in the postoperative period significantly increases the morbidity and mortality of the surgical patient. The physiology, diagnosis, and treatment of renal abnormalities are described in Chapter 4. Three common conditions encountered in the PACU that can indicate renal malfunction are discussed here.

A. Oliguria

is defined as a urine output of less than 0.5 mL/kg/h over 6 or more hours; however, reduced urine output in the PACU often precedes the official diagnosis. **Hypovolemia** is the most frequent cause of postoperative oliguria. Administration of a fluid bolus (250-500 mL of crystalloid or a synthetic colloid), even when other etiologies are not yet excluded, is acceptable, as well as placement of a urinary catheter. Further diagnostic tests (eg, plasma and urine electrolytes) and invasive monitoring should be considered when oliguria persists. **Diuretics** (see Chapter 4) should be used only when deemed necessary, such as in congestive heart failure and chronic renal insufficiency. Categorizing urinary pathology into prerenal, intrarenal, and postrenal is helpful in diagnosing the postoperative patient with oliguria.

1. **Prerenal** oliguria includes conditions that decrease renal perfusion pressure. Besides **hypovolemia**, other causes of decreased cardiac output must be considered (see Section VI.A.4). Abdominal compartment syndrome from high intra-abdominal pressures (ie, intraperitoneal hemorrhage and massive ascites) can also reduce renal perfusion. Analysis of urine electrolytes (see Chapter 5) will reveal a low fractional excretion of sodium (<1%).

2. **Intrarenal** causes of postoperative oliguria include acute tubular necrosis secondary to hypoperfusion (eg, hypotension, hypovolemia, and sepsis), toxins (eg, nephrotoxic drugs and myoglobinuria), and trauma. Urinalysis may show granular casts.

3. **Postrenal** causes include urinary catheter obstruction, trauma, and iatrogenic damage to the ureters.

B. **Polyuria**, defined as a urine output disproportionately high for a given fluid intake, occurs less frequently. Symptomatic treatment is based on volume replacement to maintain hemodynamic stability and adequate fluid balance. Electrolyte and acid-base equilibrium may be perturbed secondary to the etiology or to large volume loss. The differential diagnosis includes the following:

1. **Excessive volume** administration requiring simple observation in healthy subjects.

2. **Pharmacologic** diuresis.

3. **Osmotic diuresis** may be caused by hyperglycemia, hypercalcemia, alcohol intoxication, and administration of hypertonic saline, mannitol, or parenteral nutrition.

4. **Postobstructive diuresis** after resolution of urinary obstruction.

5. **Acute tubular necrosis** may cause transient polyuria owing to the loss of concentrating function of the tubules.

6. **Diabetes insipidus** secondary to the lack of antidiuretic hormone may follow head injury, infection, or hypothalamic-based intracranial surgery.

C. **Electrolyte disturbances** such as **hyperkalemia** and acidemia can develop within hours and need to be corrected emergently to avoid ventricular dysrhythmias and death (see Chapter 5). Polyuria may cause profound dehydration, with massive potassium losses and resulting alkalemia. **Hypokalemia**, often associated with **hypomagnesemia**, may also trigger atrial and ventricular dysrhythmias, although not as severe as those associated with hyperkalemia. Potassium should be replaced cautiously to avoid overdose. Magnesium replacement may effectively treat atrial and ventricular dysrhythmias, especially if the latter are in the form of torsade de pointes.

IX. NEUROLOGIC COMPLICATIONS

A. Delayed awakening

1. The most frequent cause of delayed awakening is **persistent effects of anesthetics** (see Section VI.B). Less common but possibly life-threatening causes include the organic cerebral events described below.

2. **Decreased cerebral perfusion** of sufficient duration, during or after surgery, may cause diffuse or localized cerebral damage responsible for

obtundation and delayed awakening. In patients with cerebrovascular disease, short periods of hypotension may cause a critical reduction of cerebral perfusion resulting in brain damage. If such an event is suspected, a neurologic consultation should be obtained as soon as possible, and specific tests (eg, computed tomography [CT], magnetic resonance imaging [MRI], or angiography) should be considered. If cerebral edema is suspected, treatment should be started immediately (see Chapter 29).

3. **Metabolic causes** of delayed awakening include hypothermia, sepsis, preexisting encephalopathies, hypoglycemia, and electrolyte or acid-base derangements.

B. **Neurologic damage** may be the result of a **stroke** or may be due to peripheral nerve injury (see Section IX.D). Strokes in the perioperative period have an incidence of 0.1% to 2.2% and may be ischemic or hemorrhagic. Early diagnosis of a stroke may be difficult because symptoms such as slurred speech, visual changes, dizziness, agitation, confusion, psychosis, numbness, muscular weakness, and paralysis may overlap with the manifestations of residual anesthetics. **Ischemic strokes** are more common in patients with cerebrovascular disease, hypercoagulable states, and atrial fibrillation, and they may be associated with intraoperative hypotension. Fat emboli secondary to long-bone fractures can also lead to strokes. **Hemorrhagic strokes** are more common in patients with coagulopathies, uncontrolled hypertension, cerebral aneurysms, arteriovenous malformations, and head trauma. Strokes are more frequent after intracranial surgery, carotid endarterectomy, cardiac surgery, and trauma. Neurologic consultation followed by brain CT or MRI is mandatory to guide immediate, and possibly brain-saving, treatment options.

C. **Emergence delirium** occurs in 5% to 20% of patients and is characterized by excitement alternating with lethargy, disorientation, and inappropriate behavior. Delirium may occur in any patient, but specific risk factors include age (<5 and >64 years old), preexisting anxiety or psychiatric diagnosis, type of surgery (breast, abdominal, ENT, and ophthalmic procedures), severe postoperative pain, and benzodiazepine premedication. Many drugs used perioperatively may precipitate delirium: ketamine, opioids, benzodiazepines, large doses of metoclopramide, and anticholinergics (atropine or scopolamine). Delirium may be a symptom of ongoing pathology such as hypoxemia, acidemia, hyponatremia, hypoglycemia, intracranial injury, sepsis, severe pain, and alcohol withdrawal. Along with addressing the underlying causes, treatment is symptomatic: supplemental O_2, fluid and electrolyte replacement, and adequate analgesia. Antipsychotic medications such as **haloperidol** (2.5- to 5-mg IV increments every 20-30 minutes) may be indicated. Benzodiazepines (**diazepam**, 2.5-5 mg IV, and **lorazepam**, 1-2 mg IV) may be added if agitation is severe; however, benzodiazepines carry an inherent independent risk of worsening delirium. **Physostigmine** (0.5-2.0 mg IV) may reverse delirium due to anticholinergic agents.

D. **Peripheral neurologic lesions** may follow improper intraoperative positioning or direct surgical damage or may be a complication of regional anesthetic techniques. In the American Society of Anesthesiologists (ASA) closed-claim analysis, ulnar nerve injury accounted for about one-third of the cases of nerve injury, followed by damage of the brachial plexus and the common fibular nerve. The risk factors for nerve injury after surgery include thin body habitus, previous history of neuropathy, smoking, and diabetes. Other sites of possible nerve damage are the wrist (median and ulnar nerve), internal aspect of the arm (radial nerve), and the points of emergence of the main branches of the VII cranial nerve, which can be compressed during mask-airway cases. Lithotomy position, especially when prolonged, may result in sciatic, femoral, common peroneal, and saphenous nerve injury. Improper positioning leads to compression or stretching of the nerve with demyelination. Remyelination often occurs in 6 to 8 weeks and results in complete recovery. Nevertheless, recovery may be more prolonged and, in some instances, the deficits are permanent. Early neurologic consultation for diagnosis and rehabilitation is crucial for a full recovery.

E. **Intraoperative awareness and recall** are rare complications of GA (0.13% in a large multicenter trial) that can be first detected in the PACU. These are often the consequences of light anesthetic techniques and occur especially after trauma, cardiac, and obstetric surgery. Risk factors include genetic or acquired (history of substance abuse or prescribed medications) resistance, ASA physical status III to V, and the use of muscular relaxants. The long-term effects of awareness under GA range from mild anxiety to overt posttraumatic stress disorder. A short interview (such as the modified Brice protocol) can be conducted in the PACU to identify patients with recall. Patients with recall should receive reassurance and close inpatient and outpatient follow-up. Referral for psychological counseling should be offered.

X. POSTOPERATIVE NAUSEA AND VOMITING

Postoperative nausea and vomiting (PONV) is a common complication of GA and less often of regional anesthesia. Patients should be stratified preoperatively with regard to their risk of PONV. The incidence of PONV is higher in women, nonsmokers, and patients with a history of PONV or motion sickness and when nitrous oxide and volatile anesthetics are used under GA. Certain types of surgery (cholecystectomy, laparoscopy, and gynecologic) may also increase the risk for PONV.

A. PONV prophylaxis is not recommended in individuals believed to be at low risk. If appropriate, patients with higher risk for PONV should be offered a regional anesthetic technique. If higher-risk patients undergo GA, they should receive antiemetic prophylaxis before or during the surgery. Monotherapy or a combination of two or three antiemetic drugs from different classes is recommended along with measures aimed to diminish the baseline risk factors for PONV: preoperative anxiolysis, use of propofol for induction and maintenance of anesthesia, total IV anesthesia, adequate hydration, and minimization of perioperative opioids. If PONV occurs in a patient who has not received prophylaxis, therapy should be initiated with a serotonin antagonist and supplemented, if necessary, with medications from other classes. In patients who have received prophylaxis, rescue therapy should consist of drugs from classes other than the ones already administered. Administration of drugs from the same class within the first 6 hours after surgery has not been found to be effective in treating PONV. Common antiemetic classes and agents include the following:

B. **Serotonin antagonists (ondansetron** 4-mg IV bolus) are well studied as prophylactic antiemetics when administered at the end of surgery, and rescue antiemetics when nausea and emesis have occurred postoperatively. However, if a serotonin antagonist has already been given prophylactically, there is no observed benefit of readministration as a rescue agent within 6 hours of the prophylactic dose.

C. **Corticosteroids** are commonly used for the prevention of PONV. **Dexamethasone** (4- to 8-mg IV bolus) is the best studied. It is most effective for prophylaxis if administered at induction of anesthesia and can be applied as a rescue drug for established PONV. Methylprednisolone (40-mg IV bolus) can also be used for PONV prevention.

D. **Butyrophenones** include haloperidol and droperidol. **Haloperidol** (0.5- to 2-mg IV bolus) is likely as effective as ondansetron (4-mg IV bolus) in preventing PONV. **Droperidol** (0.625- to 1.25-mg IV bolus) is no longer used as a first-line agent owing to a 2001 US Food and Drug Administration boxed warning associating it with QT segment prolongation and torsade de pointes. A normal QT segment should be documented before droperidol administration and continuous ECG monitoring for a few hours subsequent to the dose. Droperidol is still recommended as an alternative treatment for established PONV.

E. **Transdermal scopolamine** (1.5 mg) is effective in prophylaxis if applied 2 hours before the start of the surgery. It may cause visual changes and sedation.

F. **Phenothiazines** include **promethazine** (6.25- to 12.5-mg IV bolus) and **perphenazine** (2.5- to 5-mg IV bolus), which have been used for the prevention and treatment of PONV. Promethazine should be injected carefully as extravasation, or subcutaneous injection could result in tissue necrosis.

G. **Antihistamines** including **dimenhydrinate** (1-mg/kg IV bolus), and **meclizine** (50 mg by mouth [PO]) can be used for PONV prophylaxis. The major side effect is sedation.

H. **Propofol** (20-mg IV bolus) can be used as a rescue agent in the PACU.

I. **NK-1 receptor antagonists** are a newer class of antiemetic agents. The only one currently available for PONV prophylaxis is **aprepitant** (40-80 mg PO), and it should be taken within 3 hours prior to induction. Although there are limited clinical data, initial studies are promising.

XI. PRINCIPLES OF PAIN MANAGEMENT

Principles of pain management are described in Chapter 38. Adequate analgesia begins preoperatively and continues in the OR and in the PACU.

A. **Opioids** (IV or epidural) are the most common form of postoperative analgesia.

1. **Fentanyl,** a potent synthetic opioid with a rapid onset of action, is commonly limited to the operative setting. Occasionally, however, small IV doses (25- to 50-µg IV bolus) can be titrated postoperatively to establish rapid analgesia.

2. **Morphine** (2- to 4-mg IV bolus) may be repeated every 10 to 20 minutes until adequate analgesia is achieved. In children above 1 year of age, 15 to 20 µg/kg can be safely administered IV or intramuscularly at 30- to 60-minute intervals.

3. **Hydromorphone** (0.2- to 0.5-mg IV bolus) may also be repeated every 10 to 20 minutes until adequate analgesia is achieved. It is a synthetic opioid approximately eight times more potent than morphine and associated with significantly less histamine release.

4. **Meperidine** (25- to 50-mg IV bolus) is similarly effective. It lacks the vagotonic effect of other opiates and is frequently used to reduce post-anesthetic shivering. **Meperidine must be avoided in patients taking monoamine oxidase inhibitors** (serotonin syndrome) and must be administered cautiously in patients with renal insufficiency (toxic metabolite normeperidine is associated with seizures).

B. **Nonsteroidal anti-inflammatory drugs** (NSAIDs) and **acetaminophen** are effective complements to opioids. **Ketorolac** (15- to 30-mg IV bolus followed by 15-mg IV bolus every 6-8 hours in the perioperative period) provides potent postoperative analgesia. Other nonselective NSAIDs (**ibuprofen, naproxen,** and **indomethacin**) are also effective. Potential toxicities of all NSAIDs include decreased platelet aggregation resulting in increased bleeding risk and nephrotoxicity.

C. **Adjuvant analgesics** include spasmolytics (**cyclobenzaprine**) and small doses of benzodiazepines.

D. **Regional sensory blocks** can be very effective postoperatively (see Chapter 21).

E. **IV patient-controlled analgesia** has been shown to be superior in patient satisfaction compared with intermittent analgesia administered by the medical staff.

F. **Continuous epidural analgesia** should be continued postoperatively or promptly initiated in the PACU if not used in the OR.

XII. BODY TEMPERATURE CHANGES

A. Postoperative **hypothermia** causes vasoconstriction with secondary elevation of blood pressure, increased myocardial contractility, and tissue hypoperfusion; it impairs platelet function and clot formation and may increase the risk of bleeding. Changes in cardiac repolarization such as prolongation of the QT interval may induce dysrhythmias. In addition, the metabolism of various drugs is slowed and may result in prolonged recovery from the neuromuscular blockade. During rewarming, shivering significantly increases O_2 consumption and CO_2 production, which may be undesirable in patients with limited cardiopulmonary reserve. Hypothermia in the perioperative period can increase the length of stay in PACU, wound infection rates, and cardiac morbidity. Heated blankets, forced warm air blankets, and warm IV solutions should be used to correct hypothermia (see Chapter 17).

B. Etiologies of **hyperthermia** include infection, transfusion reaction, hyperthyroidism, **malignant hyperthermia**, serotonin syndrome, and neuroleptic malignant syndrome. Symptomatic treatment should be limited to situations in which hyperthermia is potentially dangerous, such as in young children or patients with compromised respiratory or cardiac reserve. **Acetaminophen** (suppositories 650-1300 mg or 10 mg/kg in children) and cooling blankets are commonly used. Hyperthermia can cause sinus tachycardia.

XIII. RECOVERY FROM REGIONAL AND NEURAXIAL ANESTHESIA

A. **Uncomplicated regional blocks** may not require recovery in the PACU. Postoperative monitoring is indicated when heavy sedation was administered, when a complication from the block occurred (eg, intravascular injection of a local anesthetic and pneumothorax), or when required by the nature of the surgery (eg, carotid endarterectomy).

B. **Recovery from spinal and epidural anesthesia** occurs gradually. Patients should show signs of regression of both sensory and motor blockade before discharge. If recovery seems delayed, a neurologic examination should be performed to investigate the possibility of epidural hematoma or nerve injury.

XIV. CRITERIA FOR DISCHARGE

At the Massachusetts General Hospital, all patients who undergo GA are observed until ready for discharge, with no mandatory minimum recovery time. At least 30 minutes of observation after the last dose of opioids (or other respiratory depressant medication) is required to ensure the adequacy of ventilation and oxygenation.

A. To be discharged from the PACU, patients must meet several criteria. They should be easily arousable and oriented, or at their baseline. Vital signs should be stable and within normal limits. Pain and nausea should be under control. The requirement for urination or ability to tolerate clear liquids before discharge may be required in select patients. There should be no obvious surgical complications (eg, active bleeding) present. Patients who have received neuraxial anesthesia should show signs of regression of both sensory and motor block before discharge. Effective communication with both the surgical team and the ward to which the patient is to be transferred can expedite the discharge of patients from the PACU. Outpatients should be discharged to a responsible adult with written instructions regarding postoperative diet, medications, etc, and with a phone number to call in case of emergency.

B. Fast-track recovery may be utilized for patients who meet certain criteria upon leaving the OR and are deemed ready to bypass the traditional PACU at the discretion of the anesthesia provider. These patients may be transferred directly to a second-stage recovery unit if they are ambulatory patients or to the floor if they are to be admitted as inpatients. Fast-track recovery criteria include the following:

1. The patient should be awake, alert, and oriented (or at the baseline state).

2. Vital signs should be stable (unlikely to require pharmacologic intervention).

3. Oxygen saturation should be 94% or higher on room air (3 minutes or longer) or at baseline.

4. If a muscular relaxant has been used, the patient should show no clinical signs of muscle weakness and/or the quantitative train-of-four monitoring should be greater than 0.9.

5. Nausea and pain should be minimal (unlikely to require parenteral medications).

6. There should be no active bleeding.

C. The intraoperative use of short-acting pharmacologic agents (midazolam, propofol, dexmedetomidine, remifentanil, succinylcholine, desflurane, and sevoflurane) and certain surgeries (orthopedic or simple gynecologic procedures) may make the fast-track recovery more likely.

XV. ENHANCED RECOVERY AFTER SURGERY

Enhanced Recovery After Surgery (ERAS) Society promotes a series of evidenced-based interventions and treatments encompassing the entire perioperative period. When these recommendations are applied, they lead to better clinical outcomes, including reduced mortality and shorter hospital lengths of stay. The foundational efforts were performed in patients who had elective colonic surgery, but additional guidelines have been presented for pancreaticoduodenectomies, rectal and pelvic surgeries, and radical cystectomies. In the PACU, specific attention can be given toward minimizing PONV, applying multimodal analgesia strategies, reducing opioid administration while maintaining adequate pain control, and judicious application of balanced crystalloids for resuscitation.

XVI. CONSIDERATIONS FOR PEDIATRIC RECOVERY

A. PONV is more common in the pediatric surgery population than in adults; however, children under the age of 2 years are exceptions and have a reduced incidence relative to adults. Certain operations (adenotonsillectomy, strabismus repair, hernia repair, orchidopexy, and penile surgery) are associated with increased incidence for PONV. Risk factors, as well as the general principles for prevention and treatment, are similar to those described in adults (see Section X). There is reasonable evidence to suggest **ondansetron** (100-μg/kg IV bolus for <6 months old; 150-μg/kg IV bolus >6 months old up to 4 mg) and **dexamethasone** (62.5-500 μg/kg up to 8 mg) are superior to other drugs in the prevention of PONV in children.

B. **Airway obstruction** results from similar etiologies and responds to similar treatments in children as in adults (Section VI.D). Active or recent upper respiratory infections increase the risk of postoperative laryngospasm, especially in children with a history of prematurity or reactive airway disease. Subglottic edema after extubation (postextubation croup) is associated with concurrent upper respiratory infections; traumatic, repeated, or prolonged intubations; tight-fitting endotracheal tubes; and surgeries of the head and neck. The treatment is outlined in Section VI.D. Placement of the children in the lateral decubitus position after emergence from anesthesia improves the patency of the upper airway and efficacy of chin lift and jaw thrust maneuvers, and it also minimizes the risk of aspiration of gastric contents should vomiting occur.

C. **Agitation** in children may be a normal response upon emergence from anesthesia in a strange, unfamiliar environment and in the absence of their parents. Intraoperative use of volatile anesthetics, ketamine, and atropine as well as inadequately treated pain may increase the incidence of agitation and anxiety. Other causes such as hypoxemia, hypercarbia, hypothermia, hypotension, metabolic disorders, and central nervous system pathology should be considered, investigated, and treated appropriately. Adequate pain control, reassurance, cuddling, and the presence of the parents at the bedside may mitigate the symptoms in most children.

XVII. CRITICAL CARE IN THE POST-ANESTHESIA RECOVERY UNIT

Increasingly, patients are admitted to the post-anesthesia recovery unit for short-term delivery of ICU level of care. Patients undergoing uncomplicated thoracic (eg, thoracotomies, lobectomies, and wedge resections) and vascular procedures (eg, infrarenal abdominal aortic aneurysm repairs, carotid endarterectomies), as well as other procedures involving large volume shifts, require a closer level of postoperative care. Care issues range from aggressive blood pressure management with IV medications to continued mechanical ventilation and hemodynamic resuscitation. It is important for the PACU care providers to establish a plan for continued monitoring and care. If longer-than-expected critical care needs arise, or respiratory and/or hemodynamic perturbations continue, transfer to the ICU should occur.

Suggested Readings

Apfelbaum JL, Walawander CA, Grasela TH, et al. Eliminating intensive postoperative care in same-day surgery patients using short-acting anesthetics. *Anesthesiology.* 2002;97:66-74.

Apfelbaum JL, Silverstein JH, Chung FF, et al. Practice guidelines for postanesthetic care: an updated report by the American Society of Anesthesiologists Task Force on postanesthetic care. *Anesthesiology.* 2013;118:291-307.

Bartels K, Karhausen J, Clambey ET, et al. Perioperative organ injury. *Anesthesiology.* 2013;119:1474-1489.

Brull S, Murphy G. Residual neuromuscular block. Lessons unlearned. Part II: methods to reduce the risk of residual weakness. *Anesth Analg.* 2010;111(1):129-140.

Chenitz KB, Lane-Fall MB. Decreased urine output and acute kidney injury in the postanesthesia care unit. *Anesthesiol Clin.* 2012;30:513-526.

Daley MD, Norman PH, Colmenares ME, Sandler ME. Hypoxaemia in adults in the postanesthesia care unit. *Can J Anaesth.* 1991;38(6):740-746.

Fu ES, Downs JB, Schweiger JW, et al. Supplemental oxygen impairs detection of hypoventilation by pulse oximetry. *Chest.* 2004;126:1552-1558.

Gan TJ, Diemunsch P, Habib AS, et al. Consensus guidelines for the management of postoperative nausea and vomiting. *Anesth Analg*. 2014;118(1):85-113.

Gustafsson UO, Scott MJ, Schwenk W, et al. Guidelines for perioperative care in elective colonic surgery: Enhanced Recovery After Surgery (ERAS) Society recommendations. *World J Surg*. 2013;37:259-284.

Hines R, Barash PG, Watrous G, O'Connor T. Complications occurring in the postanesthesia care unit: a survey. *Anesth Analg*. 1992;74(4):503-509.

Kluger MT, Bullock FM. Recovery room incidence: a review of 419 reports from the Anaesthetic Incident Monitoring Study (AIMS). *Anaesthesia*. 2002;57:1060-1066.

Lindenauer PK, Pekow P, Wang K. Perioperative beta-blocker therapy and mortality after major non cardiac surgery. *N Engl J Med*. 2005;353:349-361.

Mashour GA, Orser BA, Avidan MS. Intraoperative awareness: from neurobiology to clinical practice. *Anesthesiology*. 2011;114:1218-1233.

Munk L, Andersen LP, Gögenur I. Emergence delirium. *J Perioper Pract*. 2013;23(11):251-254.

Priebe HJ. Perioperative myocardial infarction-aetiology and prevention. *Br J Anaesth*. 2005;95:3-19.

Rose DK, Cohen MM, DeBoer DP. Cardiovascular events in the postanesthesia care unity: contribution of risk factors. *Anesthesiology*. 1996;84(4):772-781.

Sebel PS, Bowdle TA, Ghoneim MM, et al. The incidence of awareness during anesthesia: a multicenter United States study. *Anesth Analg*. 2004;99:833-839.

Thompson A, Balser JR. Perioperative cardiac arrhythmias. *Br J Anaesth*. 2004;93:86-94.

Wang K, Asinger RW, Marriott HJL. ST-segment elevations in conditions other than acute myocardial infarction. *N Engl J Med*. 2003;349:2128-2135.

Pain Management

Gloria Nadayil Berchmans and Peter Stefanovich

I. DEFINITION AND TERMINOLOGY

A. Pain is an unpleasant sensory and emotional experience associated with actual or potential tissue damage or described in terms of such damage (The International Association for the Study of Pain). Different categories of pain can be defined according to the duration, etiology, or perception of the painful experience.

1. **Acute pain** is caused by damage, ongoing inflammation, or physiological malfunction after a physical injury to body tissues and usually resolves as the wound heals. The intensity and duration of acute postoperative pain is a major risk factor in the development of chronic postsurgical pain. Improved control of acute pain following surgery has become a focus for practice improvement measures leading to a more timely and diversified approach to pain. Studies demonstrate that techniques that effectively reduce acute pain, including "prehabilitation," multimodal preventative analgesia, and the use of regional anesthetics are also associated with a lower incidence of subsequent chronic postsurgical pain and is a target as a primary prevention measure.

2. **Chronic pain** is pain that persists beyond the time of healing, often defined as pain persisting beyond 3 to 6 months. Common chronic pain conditions include chronic postsurgical pain, chronic low back pain, complex regional pain syndrome, postherpetic neuralgia, temporomandibular disorders, cancer pain, and myofascial pain. Current research suggests that mechanisms in the development of chronic pain involve signaling at both the site of tissue trauma and central sensitization at the level of the spinal cord and above.

3. **Neuropathic pain** results from pathologic function of the somatosensory system, either in peripheral elements (receptors or peripheral nerves) or in the central nervous system. The abnormal somatosensory function of neuropathic pain is a direct result of injury to the nervous system, and this type of pain persists even after tissue healing appears to be complete. It is most frequently described as burning, radiating, lancinating, or shooting in nature and can be accompanied by *allodynia*, or the perception of pain from a normally innocuous stimulus.

4. **Nociceptive pain** results from an injury that activates peripheral nociceptors, which can be somatic or visceral in origin, and is the pain associated with most acute injuries. Somatic pain typically reflects injury to the superficial structures of the musculoskeletal system and skin. Somatic pain is typically well localized in contrast to that of visceral pain, which arises from distention or injury to the viscera, owing to the less dense sensory innervation of the organs as compared with other tissues.

5. **Inflammatory pain** is categorized as nociceptive pain in the presence of acute inflammation, but chronic inflammatory states can play mechanistic roles in neuropathic pain states (Loeser & Treede, Kyoto). Inflammation resulting from tissue damage can lead to *hyperalgesia*, which is the exaggerated painful perception of a known noxious stimulus.

II. TREATMENT OF ACUTE PAIN IN THE PERIOPERATIVE SETTING
A. Pharmacologic treatment of pain

1. **Nonsteroidal anti-inflammatory drugs (NSAIDs, Table 38.1)** can effectively treat mild to moderate pain, particularly pain associated with inflammatory conditions. Drugs classified as NSAIDs have diverse chemical structures, but all share the ability to inhibit the enzyme cyclooxygenase (COX) and thereby inhibit the formation of prostaglandins from arachidonic acid. Combination therapy with the addition of NSAIDs to opioid during the perioperative period can often provide synergistic analgesia and reduce opioid-related side effects. Although it is important to avoid NSAIDs in patient populations at significant risk for toxicity, many patients having surgery can benefit from their addition.

   a. **Mechanism of action.** The apparent mechanism for analgesia produced by the NSAIDs is the prevention of neuronal sensitization by diminishing prostaglandin production. Type I cyclooxygenase (COX-1) is a constitutively expressed enzyme that is present in varying amounts in most cells at a fairly constant level. COX-1 serves a key role in cellular homeostasis and is the primary form of the enzyme present in platelets, the kidney, stomach, and vascular smooth muscle. COX-2 -selective inhibitors, developed with the goal to reduce side effects such as gastrointestinal (GI) bleeding associated with NSAIDs, have also been associated with a increase in the risk of adverse cardiovascular effects (eg, myocardial infarction and stroke). COX-2 inhibitors should be used with caution when cardiovascular risk factors are present and are contraindicated during coronary artery bypass graft surgery. Celecoxib is now the only available COX-2 inhibitor in the United States. For an overview of the NSAIDs according to their inhibition of COX and their selectivity for the COX-2 isoenzyme, see **Table 38.1**.

   b. **Toxicity** from NSAIDs impacts primarily the GI, renal, hematologic, and hepatic systems.

      1. GI system. Dyspepsia is the most common side effect, and nonselective NSAIDs lead to asymptomatic ulcers in 20% to 25% of users within 1 week of administration. Complicated ulcers, including perforated ulcers, upper GI bleeding, and obstruction

TABLE 38.1	Classification of Common NSAIDs Based on COX Inhibition and Selectivity
Aspirin	Irreversible inhibition of both COX-1 and COX-2
Ibuprofen, naproxen	Reversible, competitive inhibition of both COX-1 and COX-2
Ketorolac	Nonselective COX-1 and COX-2 inhibition
Indomethacin	Slower, time-dependent, but reversible inhibition of both COX-1 and COX-2
Celecoxib	Slow, time-dependent, and highly selective COX-2 inhibition

TABLE 38.2	Risk Factors That Increase the Risk of NSAID-Induced GI Toxicity

Age over 60 y

Prior history of peptic ulcer disease

Steroid use

Alcohol use

Use of multiple NSAIDs

The first 3 mo of use

occur in a significant number of long-term NSAID users. Factors that increase the risk of NSAID-induced GI toxicity are shown in **Table 38.2.**

2. Renal impairment occurs in some patients taking NSAIDs and results from reduction in renal perfusion due to inhibition of prostaglandin synthesis. In patients with contraction of their intravascular volume (eg, congestive heart failure, acute blood loss, and hepatic cirrhosis), renal perfusion is maintained through the vasodilatory effects of prostaglandins. Renal toxicity may manifest as acute interstitial nephritis or nephrotic syndrome. Acute renal failure occurs in as many as 5% of patients using NSAIDs; renal impairment typically resolves with the discontinuation of NSAID therapy but, rarely, progresses to end-stage renal disease. Factors that increase the risk of NSAID-induced renal toxicity are shown in **Table 38.3**.

3. Hematologic toxicity associated with NSAIDs takes the form of inhibition of normal platelet function. Platelet activation is blocked by the inhibitory effects of NSAIDs on cyclooxygenase and the secondary decrease of prostaglandin conversion to thromboxane A_2 (a platelet activator). Aspirin irreversibly acetylates cyclooxygenase, and thus, the platelet inhibition resulting from aspirin use persists for the 7 to 10 days required for new platelet formation. Nonaspirin NSAIDs induce reversible platelet inhibition that resolves when most of the drug has been eliminated. A recent metanalysis suggests that the effect of ketorolac on platelet function does not necessarily result in clinically appreciable postoperative bleeding.

TABLE 38.3	Factors That Increase the Risk of NSAID-Induced Renal Toxicity

Hypovolemia
- Acute blood loss
- Chronic diuretic use

Low cardiac output (congestive heart failure)

Hepatic cirrhosis

Preexisting renal insufficiency

4. Hepatic toxicity may also result from NSAID use. Minor elevations in hepatic enzyme levels appear in 1% to 3% of patients. The mechanism appears to be immunologic or metabolic-mediated direct hepatocellular injury, with dose-related toxicity occurring with both acetaminophen and aspirin. Periodic assessment of liver function is recommended in those on long-term NSAID therapy.

5. Inhibition of normal bone formation has been reported in both clinical and animal models. The clinical relevance to NSAID use in the immediate post–orthopedic surgery period and following acute fractures requires further study; despite the frequent use of NSAIDs to provide analgesia after orthopedic surgery and injury, there is little evidence that they dramatically affect healing.

c. **Clinical uses.** NSAIDs are used most widely to treat the pain and inflammation associated with rheumatic and degenerative arthritides. They also serve as a useful adjunct to opioids for providing control of acute pain, often reducing opioid requirements and opioid-related side effects in the postoperative period. Numerous agents are available for oral administration, and several are available without prescription. Thus, they are among the most common first-line analgesics.

d. **Available formulations.** Ketorolac and diclofenac are parenteral NSAIDs approved for clinical use in the United States. Both are potent analgesics and antipyretics, and several studies have demonstrated their usefulness in treating moderate postoperative pain. Ketorolac and diclofenac are nonselective NSAIDs, and despite a parenteral form, intravenous administration is still associated with GI toxicity similar to other orally administered NSAIDs. Familiarity with the dosing and administration of several oral NSAIDs as well as the parenteral formulations is an important tool for those treating acute pain. For a summary of comparative efficacy and dosages of commonly used nonopioid analgesics, see **Table 38.4**.

2. **Acetaminophen** is a para-aminophenol derivative with analgesic and antipyretic properties similar to NSAIDs. The exact mechanism by which acetaminophen exerts its effects has yet to be fully understood. Acetaminophen does not produce any significant peripheral inhibition of prostaglandin production. Acetaminophen causes no significant GI toxicity or platelet dysfunction, and there are few side effects within the normal dose range. Acetaminophen is entirely metabolized by the liver, and minor metabolites are responsible for the hepatotoxicity associated with overdose. The most common oral analgesics used to treat moderate to severe pain incorporate acetaminophen in combination with one of the opioids. Standing per os, per rectum, or IV dosing of 1 g of acetaminophen every 6 hours (<4 g/d) can be a very useful adjunct in the postoperative setting and can significantly improve pain and reduce opioid requirements.

3. **Ketamine** is an atypical dissociative anesthetic and potent analgesic that is an N-methyl-D-aspartate receptor (NMDA) receptor antagonist, which may play a role in decreasing central sensitization in the development of chronic pain. In contrast to opioids, spontaneous respiration and airway reflexes are relatively well maintained. Hypersalivation is a common side effect that can be eased by coadministration of an antisialagogue such as glycopyrrolate. Ketamine causes indirect stimulation of the sympathetic nervous system by inducing a catecholamine

TABLE 38.4 Selected Nonopioid Analgesics and Comparative Efficiency

Drug	Common Brand Names	Special Nonopioid Analgesic Dosage and Comparative Efficiency to Standards					
		Average Analgesic Dose (mg)	Dose Interval (h)	Maximum Daily Dose (mg)	Analgesic Efficacy Compared With Standards	Plasma Half-Life (h)	Comments
Acetaminophen	Tylenol numerous	500-1000 PO, PR, or IV	4-6	4000	Comparable to aspirin 650 mg	2-3	Use with caution in presence of alcoholism or liver disease Rectal suppository available
Aspirin (*Salicylate*)	Numerous	500-1000 PO	4-6	4000		0.25	Because of risk of Reye syndrome, do not use in children under 12 y with possible viral illness Rectal suppository available
Ibuprofen (*Propionic acid*)	Advil numerous	200-400 PO	4-6	2400	Superior at 200 mg to aspirin 650 mg	2-2.5	
Naproxen	Naprosyn	500 PO initial 250 PO	6-8	1250		12-15	

(*continued*)

TABLE 38.4 Selected Nonopioid Analgesics and Comparative Efficiency (Continued)

Drug	Common Brand Names	Average Analgesic Dose (mg)	Dose Interval (h)	Maximum Daily Dose (mg)	Analgesic Efficacy Compared With Standards	Plasma Half-Life (h)	Comments
			Special Nonopioid Analgesic Dosage and Comparative Efficiency to Standards				
Indomethacin	Indocin	25 PO	8-12	100	Comparable to aspirin 650 mg	2	Not routinely used because of high incidence of side effects
Ketorolac (*Pyrrolacetic acid*)	Toradol	15-30 IV or IM	6	150 first day, 120 thereafter	Comparable to 6-12 mg morphine	6	Do not take >5 d
Diclofenac (*Phenyl acetic acid*)	Dyloject	75-150 IV or IM	24	150 daily		1-2 h	Do not take >2 d
Celecoxib (*COX-2 inhibitor*)	Celebrex	100-200 PO	12	400			Not to be taken if allergic to sulfa

release. In high doses, ketamine causes a "dissociative" state and is associated with unpleasant side effects such as nightmares, which may be attenuated by concomitant administration of benzodiazepines. Use of ketamine as an adjuvant anesthetic has been shown to result in decreased opioid requirements in the immediate postoperative period in a majority of studies without significant increase in adverse outcomes and is especially useful in the management of perioperative pain in patients on chronic opioid therapy. Ketamine infusions (2.5-10 µg/kg/min) can be used as an intraoperative anesthetic adjunct for pain and has been shown to reduce opiate consumption in complex spine surgery up to 48 hours postoperatively. A Cochrane review of perioperative ketamine demonstrated both reduced pain and opioid consumption, increased time to first analgesic, and decreased postoperative nausea and vomiting, at the consequence of increased dysphoric side effects (hallucinations, unpleasant dreams, nystagmus). Ketamine bolus can also be used in the immediate postoperative period as a rescue analgesic, especially after opioid rescue has failed. Patients should be premedicated with a benzodiazepine to mitigate dysphoria and be monitored on telemetry (bolus 10-30 mg). A Cochrane review reported that 27 of 37 studies also demonstrated a significant reduction in postoperative pain with the use of ketamine.

4. **Opiates and opioids. Opiates** are among the most universally effective agents available for treating acute pain. Morphine, the prototypical opiate, is derived from the milk of the scored seed pod of the Oriental poppy, *Papaver somniferum*. Several other compounds can be derived directly through the chemical modification of morphine. Those drugs derived directly from morphine are termed the opiates. Other synthetic compounds have been produced that act via opiate receptors—all compounds that act via opiate receptors are termed the **opioids.** Although opioids form the cornerstone of effective acute pain management, they have significant side effects, and their long-term effectiveness is limited by tolerance, physical dependence, and the possibility of addiction. Common prescribing practices in the United States have led to an epidemic of prescription opioid misuse and abuse. Overdoses involving opioids killed nearly 47,000 people in 2018, and 32% of those deaths involved prescription opioids. Significant reform in physicians' prescribing patterns represents the first step in addressing this public health issue. Opioids are extremely useful for treating acute pain; although they are in widespread clinical use, their long-term effectiveness for treating chronic, noncancer pain is less clear.

a. **Metabolism.** Following injection, morphine rapidly undergoes hepatic conjugation with glucuronic acid; morphine remains largely in the ionized form at physiologic pH and is highly protein bound. The plasma concentration attained after an identical dose of morphine increases progressively with increasing age of patients. The plasma concentration of morphine correlates poorly with its pharmacologic effect. Analgesia and depressed ventilation correlate more closely with the cerebrospinal fluid (CSF) concentration. Of the metabolites morphine-3-glucuronide (M-3-G) and morphine-6-glucuronide (M-6-G), M-6-G, although produced in smaller amounts (a ratio of 1:9 in M-6-G:M-3-G), is pharmacologically active producing both analgesia and respiratory depression via interaction with μ-opioid receptors. As a result, prolonged respiratory depression can occur in patients with renal failure as M-6-G elimination is significantly impaired. Unlike fentanyl, histamine release follows IV morphine administration resulting in a decrease in systemic vascular resistance and blood pressure.

b. **Side effects** associated with opioid analgesics
   1. Respiratory depression. Opioids cause a dose-dependent reduction in the responsiveness of the brain stem respiratory centers to increases in arterial carbon dioxide tension ($Paco_2$) that manifests as a reduction in breathing rate and at high doses, apnea.
   2. Sedation. Mediated through the limbic system.
   3. Pupillary constriction. Excitatory action on the autonomic segment of the Edinger-Westphal nucleus of the occulomotor nerve.
   4. Nausea and vomiting. Direct stimulation of the chemoreceptor trigger zone within the area postrema in the medulla.
   5. Constipation. Reduction in the propulsive peristaltic contractions of the small and large intestines.
   6. Bradycardia. Central stimulation of the vagal nucleus within the medulla.

c. **Tolerance.** With continued use of substantial amounts of opioids, larger doses of the drug are required over time to produce the same physiologic effects. This phenomenon is called tolerance and is characteristic of the entire class of opioids.

d. **Physical dependence.** The precipitation of a distinct withdrawal (abstinence) syndrome when the opioid is discontinued. Manifestations of opioid withdrawal include diaphoresis, hypertension, tachycardia, abdominal cramping, and nausea and vomiting. Physical dependence occurs in any individual given sufficient doses of opioid for extended periods of time and is *not* synonymous with the complex disease that is addiction, although it can contribute to the neurobiological mechanisms driving compulsive opioid-seeking behaviors.

e. **Opioid-induced hyperalgesia (OIH).** This refers to a paradoxical increase in painful stimuli with opioid administration. This is thought to be secondary to the upregulation of compensatory pain pathways, of which the central glutaminergic system plays a central role. Discerning between OIH and tolerance is challenging, and as such, one must rule out an exacerbation of the patient's pain syndrome before considering OIH as a contributor. Strategies to address OIH once it occurs include opioid rotation and gradual dose reduction.

f. Forms of opioids
   1. **Oral opioids** are common agents used for the control of mild to moderate pain in those who are able to continue oral intake. Many agents are available as combination preparations containing an opioid along with acetaminophen. The duration of analgesic action for the orally administered opioids is similar and in the range of 3 to 4 hours. Commonly used oral opioids are listed in **Table 38.5.** In those with opioid tolerance or greater than average opioid requirements, oral opioid alone (without acetaminophen) should be used to avoid hepatic toxicity.
   2. **Intravenous (IV) opioids.** Control of moderate to severe pain or treatment of those who are unable to tolerate oral intake often requires the use of IV opioids. The pharmacokinetic profiles of opioid analgesics administered intramuscularly are similar but somewhat more erratic owing to variations in the muscle blood flow compared with that seen with IV administration; however, there is significant discomfort with intramuscular (IM) administration.

TABLE 38.5	Common Oral Opioid and Opioid/Acetaminophen Combinations Used to Treat Mild to Moderate Pain	
Drug	Equianalgesic Oral Dose (mg)	How Supplied
Acetaminophen	—	325-, 500-, 625-mg tabs; 500-mg/15-mL elixir
Codeine	60	15-, 30-, 60-mg tabs; 15-mg/5-mL elixir
Acetaminophen with codeine	—	300–15-, 300–30-, 300–60-mg tabs; 120–12/5-mL elixir
Hydrocodone	60	(Available only in combination with acetaminophen)
Acetaminophen with hydrocodone	—	500–2.5-, 500–5-, 500–7.5-, 660–10-mg tabs; 500–7.5/15-mL elixir
Oxycodone	10	5-mg tabs; 5-mg/5-mL elixir
Acetaminophen with oxycodone	—	325–5-, 500–5-mg tabs; 325–5/5-mL elixir
Morphine	10	15-, 30-mg tabs; 10-, 20-mg/5-mL elixir
Hydromorphone	2	2-, 4-, 8-mg tabs; 5-mg/5-mL elixir

There is no maximum dose for any of the pure opioid agonists (either orally or parenterally), and the dose can be increased until acceptable analgesia is produced or intolerable side effects ensue. Patients who require large doses of opioids should be closely monitored during initial dose titration as marked respiratory depression and apnea may occur unexpectedly.

5. **Muscle relaxants:** Medications used in the treatment of pain associated with musculoskeletal systems and spasms have varying mechanisms of action and unique safety and side-effect profiles. These include but are not limited to GABA-B agonists such as baclofen, α_2-agonists such as tizanidine, 5-HT2 antagonists such as cyclobenazeprine, and even benzodiazpenes such as diazepam. The mechanisms of action, side effects, and suggested dosing can be found in **Table 38.6**.

B. **Adjuncts used with opioids**

1. **Gabapentin:** Meta-analyses of preoperative use of gabapentin (250-500 mg) has shown decreased opioid use for 24 hours (by 35%), decreased pain at rest and with movement, decreased pruritus, nausea, and vomiting, but at the cost of increased dizziness and sedation.

2. **α_2-Agonists:** α_2-Agonists such as dexmedetomidine have been shown to decrease the risk of nausea and morphine consumption in the first 24 hours postoperatively without increased recovery times in abdominal surgery, and has also shown benefits in reducing pain scores and morphine consumption in the first 24 hours after cardiothoracic, breast, and bariatric surgery.

3. **Lidocaine (IV):** Meta-analyses of IV lidocaine infusion demonstrate decreased morphine consumption in both open and laparoscopic abdominal surgery. In addition, this review found moderate decreases

TABLE 38.6	Muscle Relaxants Used in the Management of Pain Related to Muscular Spasm		
Name	**Mechanism**	**Suggested Dose**	**Caution**
Baclofen	GABA-B receptor agonist	Starting dose: 5 mg PO up to 3 times daily Increase by 5 mg every 3 d, to max dose of 80 mg daily No hepatic or renal dose adjustments	Transient dizziness, withdrawal syndromes, interactions with CNS depressants
Tizanidine	Central α-2 receptor agonist	2-4 mg PO 3 times daily Increase as tolerated up to maximum dose of 36 mg daily Caution in renal or hepatic impairment; dose adjustments necessary	Hypotension, mild LFT elevation, and transient withdrawal syndrome with abrupt discontinuation
Diazepam	GABA-A receptor agonist	2 mg PO 2-3 times daily Contraindicated in hepatic impairment	Sedation, potential for dependence, withdrawal syndromes with abrupt discontinuation, interaction with CNS depressants
Cyclobenzaprine	Centrally acting 5HT2 receptor antagonist	5 mg PO 3 times daily Can be increased to 7.5 or 10 mg PO 3 times daily for up to 3 wk Use avoided in hepatic impairment, elderly patients. Long-term use not recommended	Anticholinergic effects including dizziness, dry mouth, visual disturbances, ocular hypertension, constipation, urinary retention, cardiac conduction disturbances

in pain at both rest and with movement, time to first flatus and bowel movement (7 and 12 hours, respectively), as well as hospital stay. Proposed mechanisms suggest that lidocaine exerts its effects not only through sodium channel blockade but also through interactions with inflammatory signaling cascades and inhibition of excitatory responses in wide dynamic range neurons. Additional studies have shown benefits in reducing opioid consumption in the ambulatory surgery setting and in thoracic surgery patients who are nonneuraxial candidates. Of note, although lidocaine did not show remarkable differences in opioid consumption in the perioperative setting in breast surgery, patients had a lower rate of chronic pain at 3 and 6 months, respectively. Similar studies in spine surgery show a decrease in postoperative pain 1 and 3 months after complex spine surgery. Lidocaine infusions can also be continued postoperatively for inpatient management of pain in conjunction with interdisciplinary support between pain service anesthesiologists, surgeons, and nursing staff, provided appropriate monitoring for signs of lidocaine toxicity as well as anesthesiology staff who can be available at all times to specifically address concerns relating to lidocaine infusion use is present. Intralipid emulsion should be readily available if lidocaine infusions are to be considered. At our institution, the acute pain service is routinely consulted on these patients, and nurses are given specific instructions on how to reach the service at any time.

C. **Specific pain treatment modalities used in the postoperative setting**

1. **Patient-controlled analgesia (PCA)** utilizes patient self-administration of opioid analgesia via a patient-activated infusion device. This method for delivering analgesics has evolved with the introduction of computer-controlled, programmable infusion pumps. The PCA paradigm holds that the timely administration of small intermittent doses of analgesics will allow maintenance of optimal plasma drug concentration while minimizing side effects and periods of poor analgesia associated with intermittent IV or IM administration. Typical PCA devices can be programmed to deliver a specified dose of opioid and then "lockout" further administration for a specified interval. Guidelines for PCA administration of common opioid analgesics are shown in **Table 38.7**. PCA provides superior analgesia in many settings where hospitalized patients experience acute pain. Patients are very accepting of this technology and are typically quite satisfied with the close degree of control of pain that PCA allows. The addition of a basal infusion to the PCA dosing regimen for opioid-tolerant patients is generally not recommended. Routinely including a basal infusion does not improve analgesia but increases the total opioid dose used and the frequency of opioid-related side effects.

   a. **Advantages** of PCA: PCA allows each patient to control their own pain relief, provides for rapid administration of analgesic immediately on patient request, has a high degree of patient acceptance and satisfaction, and reduces total opioid dose and related side effects.

   b. **Disadvantages** of PCA: PCA requires the patient's ability to understand and follow directions, requires enough mobility to utilize the PCA option, requires availability of specific infusion pumps, and is subject to programming errors that can cause overdosing or underdosing.

2. **Neuraxial analgesia.** The pharmacology and clinical use of intrathecal and epidural opioids and local anesthetics has been covered extensively in Chapter 20. In this section, we will focus on the practical aspects for using neuraxial techniques to provide postoperative analgesia. The combined use of thoracic epidural analgesia with general anesthesia (when compared with **general anesthesia** with IV opioids) has demonstrated

TABLE 38.7	Guidelines for Opioid Administration via IV PCA

Drug (Concentration)	Typical Demand Dose (Range)	Typical Lockout Interval (Range)
Morphine (1 mg/mL)	1 mg (0.5-3 mg)	10 min (5-12 min)
Meperidine[a] (10 mg/mL)	10 mg (5-30 mg)	10 min (5-12 min)
Fentanyl (10 μg/mL)	10 μg (10-20 μg)	10 min (5-10 min)
Hydromorphone (0.2 mg/mL)	0.2 mg (0.1-0.5 mg)	10 min (5-10 min)

[a]Use of meperidine has diminished, as this agent has an active metabolite, normeperidine, which can accumulate and lead to central nervous system excitation and seizures at very high doses.

many advantages for abdominal and thoracic surgery including decreased length of hospitalization, improved postoperative pain control with less sedation, improved respiratory function, accelerated recovery of bowel function, improved lower-extremity blood flow, and reduced stress response. In addition, the use of thoracic epidurals has shown to decrease mortality in elderly thoracic trauma patients as compared with parenteral medications in the setting of two or more rib fractures.

a. Intrathecal opioids can provide prolonged analgesia after a single injection. When a surgical procedure is to be carried out using spinal anesthesia, the addition of an opioid to the local anesthetic serves as a practical and effective means for improving postoperative analgesia. The technique is limited by the frequency of side effects at higher doses and the inability to provide complete analgesia for more extensive and painful procedures. There are two general classes of opioids used for spinal analgesia: those that are hydrophilic (eg, morphine) and those that are lipophilic (eg, fentanyl and sufentanil).

  1. Hydrophilic opioids are slower in onset (peak analgesic effect occurs between 20 and 60 minutes) but persist at significant levels within the CSF for prolonged periods of time. The prototypic hydrophilic agent is morphine. Although it produces prolonged analgesia, it has also been associated with a small incidence of delayed respiratory depression occurring as late as 18 to 20 hours after administration. This is believed to be due to the persistence of significant levels of the drug within the CSF for up to 24 hours and the rostral spread of drug within the CSF. Morphine 0.1 to 0.3 mg can provide analgesia for up to 8 to 24 hours; however, patients should remain hospitalized and observed periodically to detect and promptly treat delayed respiratory depression with this agent. The depression of ventilation can be difficult to detect because patients may demonstrate a relatively normal respiratory rate; however, hypoxemia detected by pulse oximetry, $PaCO_2$ (with bimodal peak of approximately 6 and 18 hours) detected by blood gas, and clinically depressed level of consciousness can point to undesired respiratory effects.

  2. Lipophilic opioids have a rapid onset (peak analgesic effect within 5-10 minutes), greater systemic absorption, and a short duration of analgesic action (2-4 hours). Delayed respiratory depression has not been observed with the lipophilic opioids. Fentanyl 10 to 25 µg or, less commonly, sufentanil 2.5 to 10 µg is often combined with small doses of local anesthetic to provide surgical anesthesia and postoperative analgesia for outpatient surgery.

b. Epidural opioids. Opioid analgesics also provide effective analgesia when administered into the epidural space. They can be administered as single-bolus injections, but it is far more common to place a catheter and administer combinations of opioid and low-dose local anesthetic to provide for continuous analgesia following surgery. It is imperative to understand the dermatomal extent of analgesia that can be expected from each agent and to place the injection at or near the midpoint of the dermatomal location of the surgical incision.

  1. Hydrophilic agents such as morphine or hydromorphone can be placed in the lumbar region and still provide analgesia for incisions that extend to the thoracic region, whereas fentanyl will not spread to the same extent.

  2. Local anesthetics provide analgesia only within the dermatomes adjacent to the site of injection. When administering combined opioid and local anesthetic infusions via an epidural catheter, we suggest an initial bolus to establish analgesia, prior to starting an infusion.

c. Continuous epidural infusion and patient-controlled epidural analgesia (PCEA). Continuous epidural infusions of opioids or opioid–local anesthetic combinations result in fewer fluctuations in the concentration of the analgesic drug and allows for patient-controlled supplementation via PCEA using programmable infusion pumps identical to those used for IV PCA. As discussed above, IV PCA relies on the patient-administered intermittent bolus doses to provide analgesia, and continuous infusions are seldom needed. In contrast, when using PCEA, the continuous infusion provides most of the analgesia, and small intermittent patient-administered doses are used to supplement its effect. There is evidence that patients can safely receive epidural opioids while on the regular hospital ward, provided that an anesthesiology-based acute pain service is responsible for all adjustments of analgesic and sedative medications.

d. Adverse effects associated with neuraxial opioid administration including sedation, pruritus, nausea, and vomiting, and urinary retention are common in patients receiving epidural or intrathecal opioids. Standing orders should be in place for addressing these common, minor side effects. Suggested standing orders for management of common side effects associated with neuraxial opioid administration are shown in **Table 38.8**.

e. Treatment of **inadequate analgesia** in patients receiving continuous epidural infusions requires a systematic approach. A member of the acute pain service should be immediately available to assess the patient and determine the cause for inadequate analgesia. A common algorithm for responding to inadequate analgesia in patients receiving epidural analgesia is shown in **Table 38.9**. Daily management of the patient receiving epidural analgesia requires a systematic approach aimed at assuring safe and effective pain treatment. A suggested daily checklist that will guide patient management is shown in **Table 38.10**.

TABLE 38.8	Pharmacologic Management of Common Side Effects Associated With Neuraxial Opioid Administration
Adverse Effect	**Standing Orders for Treatment**
Nausea	• Ondansetron 1-4 mg IV or dolasetron 12.5 mg IV • Nalbuphine 1-3 mg IV or butorphanol 0.25-0.5 mg IV every 4 h as needed
Pruritus	• Diphenhydramine 25-50 mg IV every 4 h as needed • Nalbuphine 1-3 mg IV or butorphanol 0.25-0.5 mg IV every 4 h as needed
Urinary retention	• Keep indwelling urinary catheter in place until discontinuation of the epidural analgesia
Sedation or respiratory depression	• Notify acute pain service immediately, for respiratory rate less than 6/min • Place supplemental oxygen 4 L/min via nasal cannula • Administer naloxone 0.4 mg IV

TABLE 38.9 Suggested Management of Inadequate Analgesia in Patients Receiving Continuous Epidural Analgesia

1. Assess the patient directly at the bedside to determine the cause for inadequate analgesia. If the patient is unable to respond in a timely fashion, consider alternate means for providing analgesia (eg, order a one-time IV dose of opioid by telephone; consider discontinuing epidural infusion and beginning IV PCA).
2. Examine the patient for signs of a unilateral block or a dislodged or disconnected epidural catheter.
3. Administer a bolus dose of the opioid or opioid–local anesthetic combination in use for continuous infusion. Choose the dose based on the severity of pain and use between ½ and 1 h worth of the medication (eg, 4- to 8-mL bolus of fentanyl 4 μg/mL/bupivacaine 0.0625% in a patient receiving 8 mL/h).
4. If there is no improvement in pain relief within 20-30 min, consider test dosing the epidural catheter with 10 mL of 2% lidocaine. *Do not* administer a test dose unless the patient can be attended continuously and monitored with blood pressure checks at least every 5 min for 20 min after the bolus is given. Means for treating hypotension must be readily available (IV access and ready availability of a vasopressor such as ephedrine or phenylephrine).
5. If no sensory or motor block appears within 20 min, replace or discontinue epidural catheter and begin an alternate means for providing analgesia (eg, IV PCA).
6. If a bilateral sensory or motor block develops, readminister an epidural bolus of the medication in use for continuous infusion and increase the epidural infusion rate. Be alert for causes of inadequate analgesia (eg, a lumbar epidural catheter in use for pain following thoracotomy). Consider changing the opioid in use if the catheter location is suboptimal or there is an extensive incision.

     f. Complications associated with epidural analgesia. Although the goal of epidural analgesia is to provide pain relief and minimize side effects, there are several serious complications associated with its use.
         1. Catheter migration into the intrathecal space can lead to increasing levels of sensory block and total spinal anesthesia.
         2. Indwelling epidural catheters can become infected directly at the skin entry site or through hematogenous seeding of the catheter

TABLE 38.10 Suggested Daily Checklist for Daily Management of Patients Receiving Epidural Analgesia

1. Examine the nursing record for adjustments and supplemental analgesics as well as medications for side effects. Check vital signs for evidence of persistent fever or hypotension.
2. Assess for adequate analgesia and side effects by directly questioning the patient. Be alert for sedation, pruritus, nausea and vomiting, and urinary retention.
3. Examine the patient to detect signs of unilateral block or excessive sensory or motor block.
4. Examine the epidural catheter site for signs of infection and the presence of an intact occlusive dressing.
5. Interrogate the infusion pump to assess the patient's use of supplemental doses, assure that it is properly programmed. Examine the infusion bag directly to be certain the medication ordered is what the patient is receiving.
6. Document your interaction in detail in the patient's chart and order any changes needed. Include when you anticipate changing or discontinuing therapy.

tip within the epidural space. Superficial site infection is common and rarely needs treatment beyond the removal of the catheter. Extension of a superficial infection or direct seeding of the catheter tip to produce an epidural abscess is rare.

3. Epidural hematoma formation is also uncommon but may follow epidural placement in a patient receiving systemic anticoagulants. Both epidural abscess and hematoma present with worsening back pain and neurologic deficit (urinary retention and sensory and motor loss in the lower extremities). The recognition and management of these complications are discussed in detail in Chapter 20.

3. **Continuous peripheral nerve blocks** using catheters are continuing to gain popularity in the inpatient as well as the ambulatory setting. The focus in this chapter is to outline a strategy for management of continuous nerve catheters in the postoperative period. For placement of peripheral nerve blocks, see Chapter 21. The availability of lightweight and sophisticated infusion pumps has greatly facilitated the use of continuous perineural infusions of local anesthetics. Ultrasound is now commonly used to guide catheter placement. Advances in technology and the emergence of the literature supporting continuous perineural infusions for improved postoperative analgesia and recovery have led to more widespread use of continuous perineural infusions of local anesthetics.

a. **Specific indications** for continuous peripheral nerve blocks vary in terms of surgical site. For example, femoral and **popliteal** fossa nerve catheters **are commonly used** following below-the-knee amputations. Similarly, brachial plexus blocks using continuous infusion have also proven effective for surgery on the shoulder and upper extremity.

b. **Choice of drug**, concentration, and infusion rate will depend on the target nerve or plexus, the surgical procedure, as well as the individual patient's response. Infusion rates can be fixed or variable including the possibility of a bolus (patient-controlled regional anesthesia). Continuous peripheral nerve blocks are carried out by infusing local anesthetic alone (for example, 0.1% bupivacaine or 0.2% ropivacaine) at a rate of 5 to 10 mL/h.

c. **Management of continuous peripheral nerve catheters.** Since the extremity will have decreased sensitivity for the duration of the block, care should be taken to prevent injury to exposed nerves. A properly fitted sling, brace, and thorough patient education are paramount to provide adequate protection. Given the high cumulative dose of local anesthetic, caution should be used in patients with renal failure and the drug should be avoided in those with hepatic failure. Daily follow-up of hospitalized patients with a perineural catheter should include close attention to specific aspects shown in **Table 38.11.**

d. **Use of perineural catheters in ambulatory patients.** Perineural catheters have been successfully employed in the ambulatory care setting. This requires careful patient selection, comprehensive patient education, and the implementation of a protocol for patient follow-up. Patient education should involve the patient's caregiver and include instructions on how to operate the pump, signs of catheter-related complications (such as infection, migration, and leak), and signs of local anesthetic toxicity. Patients should be aware of the expected time for resolution of the block and should understand the necessity to abstain from driving or operating machinery. A plan for

TABLE 38.11	Checklist for Daily Follow-Up of Patients With Perineural Catheters

1. Inspect the catheter insertion site to assess for signs of infection, leaks, and catheter dislocation.
2. Assure that ongoing analgesia is adequate.
3. Assess the patient for signs of excessive motor and/or sensory block.
4. Assess the patient for signs or symptoms of local anesthetic toxicity (local anesthetic toxicity is rare in the context of continuous perineural infusion, but the daily dose and any associated side effects should be assessed daily).

breakthrough pain management should be in place. Daily follow-up should be arranged, and provisions for immediate contact with an anesthesiologist should be available.

D. Acute pain management in patients with opioid tolerance or dependence.

  1. Patients with opioid tolerance or dependence represent a unique challenge to the anesthesiologist in the perioperative period. In contrast to the term addiction, dependence is defined by the World Health Organization as a cluster of physiological, behavioral, and cognitive phenomena in which the overwhelming desire and use of a substance, such as an opioid, takes on higher priority than other behaviors that once had value. Tolerance may or may not be present.

   a. **Perioperative management of patients with opioid tolerance or a history of opioid dependence.** Concepts to consider when managing patients who have been taking large doses of opioids for chronic pain and those with current or previous history of an opioid use disorder are shown in **Table 38.12.**

   b. **Managing acute pain in patients on buprenorphine maintenance therapy.** Buprenorphine, a semisynthetic, potent, and long-acting opioid, has been introduced for ambulatory treatment of patients with opioid dependence. It is a high-affinity partial agonist at the μ opioid receptor and antagonist at the $\hat{\kappa}$ opioid receptor that at higher doses exhibits a plateau effect in regards to euphoria and respiratory depression. When prescribed in the outpatient setting, buprenorphine is often mixed with naloxone (Suboxone) to be taken sublingually. Naloxone has poor bioavailability after oral and sublingual administration; however, if the drug combination is administered intravenously in an attempt for abuse, naloxone is present in high-enough concentrations to precipitate acute withdrawal symptoms in opioid-dependent patients. The addition of naloxone aims at limiting both abuse and diversion of the drug. Buprenorphine alone (Subutex) is used for initial testing prior to initiating a buprenorphine therapy–based maintenance regimen in the opioid-addicted patient. Subutex has also gained some popularity for use in the treatment of chronic pain, owing to its limited abuse potential and significant efficacy as an analgesic agent. There is a paucity of data for the management of patients receiving buprenorphine who present for surgery. In addition to the general principles for managing patients with opioid tolerance or addiction discussed above, specific considerations for the patient receiving buprenorphine are shown in **Table 38.13.**

   c. **Managing acute pain in patients on methadone maintenance therapy.** Methadone, a synthetic mixed μ-opioid and delta receptor

TABLE 38.12	Managing Patients With Opioid Tolerance or With Current or Previous Dependence

Consider use of regional anesthesia (spinal opioids and epidural infusions) to improve analgesia and minimize systemic opioid effects.

Use adjunctive analgesics whenever possible to reduce total opioid requirements (eg, NSAIDs, ketamine).

Administer opioids liberally to control pain in the immediate postoperative period. *Do not* attempt to limit opioid dose or wean opioid analgesics in the immediate postoperative period. Those with significant tolerance will probably require higher-than-average doses to control acute pain.

Use preoperative opioid doses as a baseline requirement and administer additional doses beyond this to control acute pain. This baseline requirement can be administered by continuing the preoperative long-acting opioid in addition to the use of a PCA.

Consider consultation with a substance abuse specialist during hospitalization for those with ongoing opioid abuse or a history of addiction.

Closely coordinate (communicate) the pain management with the patient's primary care provider before hospital discharge. Although acute escalation in the opioid requirement is often necessary in the perioperative period, a plan for weaning the opioids to their previous levels should be established *before* the patient is discharged from the hospital.

agonist, with NMDA receptor antagonist and serotonin norepinephrine reuptake inhibitor activity, has been used in the treatment of opioid-dependent patients for over 60 years and has found increasing applications in the treatment of cancer-related pain, neuropathic pain, and other chronic pain states. Its long half-life with a biphasic elimination profile exerts an effect both on pain control (8-12 hours) and on withdrawal (30-60 hours). However, variable oral bioavailability (40%-99%), variable hepatic elimination and the phenomena of incomplete cross tolerance, or lack of tolerance to the effects of opioids of other classes makes conversion from oral to IV formulations and calculating equianalgesic doses very challenging. Considering these attributes and its long half-life, titration to reach steady-state levels over days to weeks should only be done with assistance of a pain specialist owing to the risk of delayed respiratory depression. Furthermore, pretreatment EKG should be checked in any patient initiated or titrated on methadone, as QTC prolongation remains a significant concern. Patients who present for surgery should continue their baseline dose methadone on the morning of surgery, and pain should be managed proactively and aggressively in the perioperative period. The general principles for managing patients with opioid tolerance or addiction discussed above apply to these patients as well.

III. COMPLEMENTARY AND ALTERNATIVE MEDICINE IN PAIN MANAGEMENT

Complementary and alternative medicine (CAM) encompasses a broad range of therapeutic modalities that are often integrated into western medicine in the management of chronic conditions, including, but not limited to, pain.

A. Definitions of CAM

1. Practices that are not accepted as correct or in conformity with the beliefs of the dominant group of medical practitioners in a society.

TABLE 38.13 Perioperative Considerations for the Patient Receiving Long-Term Buprenorphine Treatment

For patients undergoing elective surgery, data from clinical studies suggest a possible synergistic and additive effect between buprenorphine at low to moderate analgesic doses (8-12 mg SL or less) and full μ-opioid receptor agonists. At doses less 12 mg SL studies suggest an at least 20% μ-opioid receptor availability for binding by full agonists. Furthermore, studies also suggest that 50%-60% receptor occupancy is what is needed to avoid withdrawal symptoms in patients managed on buprenorphine. Thus, our institutional policy is as follows: For surgeries in which postoperative pain is expected to be mild, home dose buprenorphine is recommended to be continued. For those in which moderate to severe pain is expected, the management depends on the buprenorphine dose. For those managed on 16 mg buprenorphine or less, it is recommended to continue the home dose until the day before surgery, and to continue patients on a regimen of 8 mg daily plus additional full opioid agonists and adjunctive pain medications as needed to manage pain postoperatively. Once postoperative pain subsides, patients can resume their home dose. For those managed on greater than 16 mg of buprenorphine, it is recommended that patients titrate down their therapy over time with the goal of 16 mg on the day before surgery with the assistance of the physician responsible for prescribing their opioid agonist therapy. Patients are then maintained on 8 mg daily plus full opioid agonists as needed until the period of acute pain resolves and the home regimen can be reinstated after full agonists are tapered off. Of note, some institutions recommend that buprenorphine therapy be completely discontinued and replaced with a full opioid agonist (eg, morphine and hydromorphone) 48-72 h prior to the scheduled surgery, with full opioid agonist dosages adjusted as needed to treat acute pain in the perioperative period. Buprenorphine maintenance therapy can then be reinstated using an induction protocol, coordinated with the physician primarily responsible for the opioid agonist therapy to ensure safety and supervision of the necessary changes in the therapeutic regimen after the period of acute pain resolves, as the initial dose of buprenorphine can precipitate withdrawal symptoms.

For patient requiring urgent or emergent surgery or when prior conversion to a full agonist is not feasible, a short-acting full agonist such as fentanyl can be titrated to effect. As is the case for patients maintained with other opioid agonists, higher-than-usual doses to achieve adequate analgesia are likely to be required. The appropriate dose of fentanyl in a patient taking buprenorphine might also be higher because of the strong affinity of buprenorphine for the μ receptor. After buprenorphine therapy is discontinued, the effects of a full agonist will become more pronounced; once the buprenorphine has been cleared from the body, the dose of the full agonist will need to be reduced over time. Close monitoring of the patient's response to therapy is required.

---

    2. Complementary practices are those that are used in conjunction with other medical practices, while alternative medicine is used in place of conventional medical practices.

  B. Categories of CAM practices. The National Center for Complementary and Integrative Health, a subdivision of the National Institutes of Health, has grouped CAM practices into several major subdivisions:

    1. Mind-body interventions use techniques to facilitate the mind's ability to affect bodily functions. Examples include hypnosis, mindfulness meditation, art therapy, and music medicine and therapy.

    2. Natural products refer to products such as herbs, botanicals, probiotics, and special diets designed to promote wellness and manage symptoms. Inquiry regarding the use of natural products is essential to the preoperative assessment described in Chapter 1.

3. **Alternative medicine** includes homeopathic medicine, Ayurvedic medicine, traditional Chinese medicine (acupuncture, massage, herbs), and other systems of belief typically used in place of conventional medicine.
4. **Manipulative therapies** include chiropractic manipulation, osteopathic manipulation, and massage.
5. **Energy-and biofield-based therapies** include qi gong and reiki, among other therapies that purport to direct healing by manipulating a body's perceived energy.

C. **Perioperative acupuncture**
   1. **Definition. Acupuncture** involves the insertion of fine needles into specific points on the body to produce therapeutic results. The analgesic effects of acupuncture have been attributed to the presynaptic release of enkephalins and dynorphin along the afferent fibers of the spinothalamic tract, the stimulation of norepinephrine and serotonin release in midbrain structures and in the periaqueductal gray matter to dampen nociceptive signaling, and the stimulation of the hypothalamus pituitary axis to effect systemic ACTH and endorphin release.
   2. **Preoperative use.** Numerous studies using preoperative acupuncture, including ear points, show significant relaxation. In two double-blinded studies, preoperative auricular acupuncture reduced anxiety up to 48 hours compared with sham acupuncture. This reduction in anxiety correlates with less pain and analgesic consumption postoperatively. Acupuncture may complement the use of preoperative anxiolytics and has also been shown in a few studies to reduce the incidence of postoperative nausea vomiting.
   3. **Intraoperative use.** Intraoperative acupuncture does not provide muscle relaxation, suppress autonomic reflexes, or provide unconsciousness. Available data show that acupuncture has little or no effect on anesthetic requirements—in some studies it slightly increased anesthetic requirements.
   4. **Postoperative use.** Studies regarding the effect of acupuncture on postoperative pain requirements remain conflicting and controversial, partially in part to variances in study design, patient population, practitioner experience level, and acupuncture methods. However, several studies do reveal substantial reduction in postoperative opioid consumption. In one study, acupuncture performed 20 minutes prior to induction reduced 24-hour morphine consumption by PCA after total abdominal hysterectomy. Other studies show similar opioid-reducing effects in abdominal surgery, in addition to significant decreases in serum plasma cortisol levels in the first 24 hours postoperatively.

D. **Hypnosis**
   1. **Definition.** Hypnosis involves the induction of a state of mind that allows for a heightened receptivity to suggestion. It is generally a state of relaxation in which critical thought is bypassed. The mechanism by which hypnosis can contribute to analgesia is thought to be mediated by a perceptual dissociation of the sensory and affective components of the pain experience.
   2. **Mechanism.** Hypnosis influences the affective (cognitive/evaluative) component of pain. Functional magnetic resonance imaging and positron emission tomography scans during hypnosis suggest that this affective processing of pain occurs in part in areas of the anterior cingulate gyrus, modulating pain unpleasantness without significant changes in perceived intensity encoded by activity in the primary and secondary somatosensory cortices.
   3. **Possible applications.** Many studies focus on the use of hypnosis to alleviate perioperative pain, anxiety, and nausea. Although findings vary,

the use of preoperative hypnotic suggestion has often been found to reduce emesis and narcotic requirements postoperatively. Children are often receptive to hypnosis-guided imagery. Hypnoanalgesia has emerged as a combination of hypnotic techniques with pharmacologic analgesics and sedation. In one study of 241 patients undergoing hypnosis as compared with standard IV conscious sedation and focused attention during percutaneous vascular and renal procedures, hypnosis showed the greatest reduction in intraoperative anxiety and the least pain over procedure time, as well as a lessened need for IV anxiolytics and opioid medications. It has been used effectively for dressing changes in burn patients, with the concurrent suggestions of improved appetite and nutrition. Positive suggestions to anesthetized patients may also promote fewer postoperative complications.

E. Mindfulness meditation

1. **Definition.** A "non-elaborative, non-judgmental awareness of the present moment experience," the recognition of such experiences as fleeting, and a resultant lack of emotional or cognitive reactions to such.

2. **Mechanism.** Although studies of the interplay between meditative practices and pain produced mixed results, they suggest that cognitive modulation reduces the influence of expectation and catastrophizing in the processing of painful stimuli in a manner that develops over time and experience. In one study, functional and structural MRI in experienced Zen meditation practitioners have exhibited increased activation in areas associated with sensory processing of pain, but reduced activity in the amygdala, caudate, and hippocampus suggesting decreased emotional reactivity to and appraisal of painful stimuli despite increased attention to such stimuli. Meditation's mechanism appears to not involve endogenous opioids in the perceived reduction of pain. In a randomized, double-blind study conducted in 2016 where 78 participants separated into mindfulness meditation and control groups were subjected to a noxious stimulus and given naloxone, mindfulness meditation produced significantly greater reductions in pain intensity and unpleasantness than the control groups in a manner that could not be reversed with naloxone, providing further support for the use of meditation as an adjunct to manage chronic pain.

3. **Preoperative use:** Studies are currently being conducted regarding the role of meditation in postoperative neurocognitive outcomes and pain as part of a "prehabilitation" program prior to cardiac surgery.

4. **Postoperative use:** Although a recent study examining postoperative pain scores in 52 patients receiving mindfulness meditation therapy via virtual reality headsets was underpowered to show any significance in narcotic utilization as compared with control, it highlights the potential for meditation to be utilized in postoperative period.

F. Music medicine and music therapy

1. **Definitions. Music medicine** is the practice of passive listening to prerecorded music; it is generally administered by physicians and nurses. **Music therapy** is the application of an individualized music intervention and therapeutic process based on music preferences administered by a trained music therapist.

2. **Preoperative use.** Music interventions offer a safe and inexpensive nonpharmacologic intervention for reduction of preoperative stress and anxiety that may complement the effect of other anxiolytics.

3. **Intraoperative use.** Several small studies show music interventions in patients undergoing neuraxial anesthesia for childbirth and for total knee replacement significantly decreased the need for intraoperative sedatives.

4. Postoperative use. Patients report increased satisfaction regarding their care and the postanesthesia care unit recovery period.

G. Virtual reality (VR)

    1. Definitions. Virtual reality is a fully immersive, engaging experience that incorporates a head-mounted display with an audio source and another device to allow for manipulation of a computer-generated environment, with applications in the attenuation and modulation of acute pain as well as procedural anxiety. The effectiveness of VR in reducing the intensity of perceived pain may stem from the engaging attention away from the painful stimulus using multisensory distraction, reflecting both gate control and multiple resources theories of pain perception.

    2. Perioperative use. It has been studied as a nonpharmacologic, noninvasive adjunct to pain medications in the management of acute burn patients, particularly in pediatric patients. Small studies have shown reductions in pain and anxiety scores during physiotherapy and wound dressing changes by various pain scales when used in conjunction with opioid pain medication as compared with medications alone. Other applications have included use of VR for unpleasant routine medical procedures such as phlebotomy, IV insertion, port access, and lumbar puncture as well as an adjunct to regional anesthesia and light sedation in orthopedic procedures.

Suggested Readings

Alford DP, Compton P, Samet JH. Acute pain management for patients receiving maintenance methadone or buprenorphine therapy. *Ann Intern Med.* 2006;144:127-134.

Amberger M, Stadelmann K, Alischer P, et al. Monitoring of neuromuscular blockade at the P6 acupuncture point reduces the incidence of postoperative nausea and vomiting. *Anesthesiology.* 2007;107(6):903-908.

Astin JA. Why patients use alternative medicine: results of a national study. *J Am Med Assoc.* 1998;279:1548-1553.

Benzon TB, Rathmell JP, Wu CL, et al. *Raj's Practical Management of Pain.* 4th ed. Mosby Elsevier; 2008.

Blaudszun G, Lysakowski C, Elia N, et al. Effect of perioperative systemic α2 agonists on postoperative morphine consumption and pain intensity: systematic review and meta-analysis of randomized controlled trials. *Anesthesiology.* 2012;116:1312-1322.

Boezaart AP. Perineural infusion of local anesthetics. *Anesthesiology.* 2006;104:872-880.

Chernyak GV, Sessler D. Perioperative acupuncture and related techniques. *Anesthesiology.* 2005;102(5):1031-1049.

Gobble RM, Hoang HL, Kachniarz B, Orgill DP. Ketorolac does not increase perioperative bleeding: a meta-analysis of randomized controlled trials. *Plast Reconstr Surg.* 2014;133(3):741-755.

Grant JA, Rainville P. Pain sensitivity and analgesic effects of mindful states in Zen meditators: a cross sectional study. *Psychosom Med.* 2009;71:106-114.

Haisley K, Straw O, Müller D, et al. Feasibility of implementing a virtual reality program as an adjuvant tool for peri-operative pain control: Results of a randomized controlled trial in minimally invasive foregut surgery. *Compl Ther Med.* 2020;49:102356.

Ilfeld BM, Enneking FK. Continuous peripheral nerve blocks at home: a review. *Anesth Analg.* 2005;100(6):1822-1833.

Jonas W, Levin J, eds. *Essentials of Complementary and Alternative Medicine.* Williams & Wilkins; 1999.

Joshi GP, Gertler R, Fricker R. Cardiovascular thromboembolic adverse effects associated with cyclooxygenase-2 selective inhibitors and nonselective antiinflammatory drugs. *Anesth Analg.* 2007;105:1793-1804.

Kaye AD, Kucera I, Sabar R. Perioperative anesthesia clinical considerations of alternative medicines. *Anesthesiol Clin North Am.* 2004;22:125-139.

Lang EV, Benotsch EG, Fick LJ, et al. Adjunctive non-pharmocological analgesia for invasive medical procedures: a randomized trial. *Lancet.* 2000;355:1486-1490.

Li A, Montano Z, Chen V, et al. Virtual reality and pain management: current trends and future directions. *Pain Manag.* 2011;1(2):147-157.

Manion SC, Brennan TJ. Thoracic epidural analgesia and acute pain management. *Anesthesiology.* 2011;115(1):181-188.

Martin S, Clark JD. Opioid-induced hyperalgesia: a qualitative systematic review. *Anesthesiology.* 2006;104(3):570-587.

Matsota P, Christodoulopoulou T, Smyrnioti ME, et al. Music's use for anesthesia and analgesia. *J Altern Complement Med.* 2013;19(4):298-307.

Micozzi M. *Fundamentals of Complementary and Alternative Medicine.* Saunders; 2010.

Mitra S, Sinatra RS. Perioperative management of acute pain in the opioid-dependent patient. *Anesthesiology.* 2004;101:212-227.

National Center for Complementary and Integrative Health. *The Use of Complementary and Alternative Medicine in the United States.* 2020. Accessed January 2020. http://www.nccam.nih.gov

Quaye AN, Zhang Y. Perioperative management of buprenorphine: solving the conundrum. *Pain Med.* 2019;20(7):1395-1408.

Rainville P, Duncan G, Price D, et al. Pain affect encoded in human anterior cingulate but not somatosensory cortex. *Science.* 1997;277:968-971.

Rathmell JP, Lair TR, Nauman B. The role of intrathecal drugs in the treatment of acute pain. *Anesth Analg.* 2005;101(5 suppl):S30-S43.

Rathmell JP, Neal JM, Viscomi CM. *Regional Anesthesia. The Requisites in Anesthesiology.* Elsevier Mosby; 2004.

Stewart JH. Hypnosis in contemporary medicine (review). *Mayo Clin Proc.* 2005;80(4):511-524.

Straube S, Derry S, Moore RA, et al. Single dose oral gabapentin for established acute postoperative pain in adults. *Cochrane Database Syst Rev.* 2010;5:CD008183.

Sun Y, Li T, Wang N, et al. Perioperative systemic lidocaine for postoperative analgesia and recovery after abdominal surgery: a meta-analysis of randomized controlled trials. *Dis Colon Rectum.* 2012;55:1183-1194.

Tsen LC, Segal S, Pothier M, et al. Alternative medicine use in presurgical patients. *Anesthesiology.* 2000;93:148-151.

Wobst AH. Hypnosis and surgery: past, present, and future. *Anesth Analg.* 2007;104(5):1199-1208.

Zeidan F, Adler-Neal AL, Wells RE, et al. Mindfulness-meditation-based pain relief is not mediated by endogenous opioids. *J Neurosci.* 2016;36(11):3391-3397. doi:10.1523/JNEUROSCI.4328-15.2016

Zeidan F, Grant JA, Brown CA, etal. Mindfulness meditation-related pain relief: evidence for unique brain mechanisms in the regulation of pain. *Neurosci Lett.* 2012;520(2):165-173.

Zhang Y, Peck K, Spalding M, et al. Discrepancy between patients' use of and health providers' familiarity with CAM. *Patient Educ Couns.* 2012;89(3):399-404.

Adult, Pediatric, and Newborn Resuscitation

John H. Nichols and Paul D. Guillod

I. OVERVIEW

Circulatory collapse and the need for cardiopulmonary resuscitation (CPR) is one of the more stressful crises that can occur in the operating room (OR). In such an emergency, it is the responsibility of the anesthesiologist to swiftly recognize and intervene to ensure recovery of spontaneous circulation (ROSC) without further injury. Success requires the necessary reflexive clinical skills, awareness of surrounding equipment, understanding of reversible etiologies, appropriate task delegation, and a composed demeanor. Fortunately, intraoperative cardiac arrest in noncardiac surgery is rare (1-7 cases per 10,000, ~40% 30-day survival) and an OR serves as an almost ideal location for such an event given its advanced monitoring, immediate medication availability, proximity to invasive line equipment, airway management tools, and pacemaking/defibrillation equipment. In addition, timely access to advanced imaging and treatment modalities such as transthoracic and transesophageal echocardiography, extracorporeal membrane oxygenation (ECMO), and cardiac catheterization (for example, emergent coronary stent, thrombectomy, intraaortic balloon pump) enhances the likelihood of a successful outcome.

In addition to the availability of physical resources, cognitive aids can help ensure successful resuscitation. The recent development of easily consulted emergency manuals within reach of the anesthesiologist has greatly facilitated accurate recall of critical resuscitation management steps during highly stressful situations. MGH includes an emergency manual adopted from the Stanford Cognitive Aid Working Group in all of its anesthetizing locations. In addition, simulation of intraoperative code events has become more integrated into the training curriculums of MGH and other institutions, which provides a structured, supportive environment to rehearse decision-making, enhance communication, and establish reflexive mental models. Together, simulation and easy access to emergency manuals promote a calm, quick adherence to optimal management protocols during otherwise difficult circumstances.

Essential to the swift return of spontaneous circulation after sudden cardiac arrest (SCA) are defibrillation for ventricular fibrillation (VF) or pulseless ventricular tachycardia (VT); prompt delivery of effective, minimally interrupted chest compressions to maintain cerebral and cardiac perfusion; and maintenance of effective oxygenation/ventilation. Effective compressions deliver oxygen and energy substrates to the myocardium and increase the likelihood that a perfusing rhythm will return after defibrillation. Appropriate oxygenation and ventilation are critical as hypoxemia inhibits oxygen delivery and hypo/hypercarbia can create decreased cerebral perfusion and unwanted sympathetic surges, respectively. Excessive tidal volumes can also reduce venous return, which inhibits cardiac output during CPR. CPR is more successful the earlier it is started; thus, prompt and clear communication with all team members about the emergency is essential.

T A B L E **39.1**	Classification System for Recommendation and Levels of Evidence		
Class of Recommendation		**Level of Evidence**	
I	Strongly recommended	A	High quality, 1+ RCT
IIa	Reasonable	B-R	Moderate quality from 1+ RCT
IIb	May be considered	B-NR	Moderate quality without RCT
III (NB)	No benefit	C-LD	Limited data
III (H)	Causes harm	C-EO	Expert opinion

Note that the recommendation class and quality of evidence are separate, independently determined factors. For instance, a class I recommendation may not have an A quality. RCT, randomized controlled trial.

In the OR, the patient is often poorly positioned for CPR (prone/lateral/elevated) and may have open surgical sites requiring rapid packing. Quick recognition and communication will facilitate optimal positioning and preparation for effective CPR.

There is a tendency after delivering defibrillating shocks to watch the monitors or check pulses for return in cardiac output, but CPR should be resumed immediately after defibrillation as the myocardium has been depleted of oxygen and metabolic substrates and is stunned. When possible, early consideration for patients with presumably reversible causes of cardiac arrest should include alerting the hospital ECMO and emergency echocardiography teams in accordance with institutional capabilities and policy.

The management and algorithms that follow are derived from evidence-based guidelines established through systematic reviews by the American Heart Association (AHA) in collaboration with the International Liaison Committee on Resuscitation, which has switched to a continuous review process since the last edition of this book. This section is current with respect to the 2015 *AHA Guidelines for Cardiopulmonary Resuscitation and Emergency Cardiovascular Care* and its yearly supplements up to 2019 for adult and pediatric management, which incorporates basic life support (BLS), advanced cardiac life support (ACLS), and pediatric advanced life support (PALS), which includes neonatal resuscitation.

Table 39.1 lists the AHA classifications used for the strength of recommendation and the quality of evidence used to support most of the protocol interventions presented in this chapter. Note that the recommendation class and quality of evidence are independently established. When helpful, the AHA recommendation class and quality will be provided next to suggestions in the form of *Class/Evidence*.

II. CARDIAC ARREST

    A. Diagnosis. The absence of a palpable pulse in a major peripheral artery (carotid, radial, or femoral), pulseless >10 seconds in an unconscious, unmonitored patient is diagnostic. Within the OR, monitoring equipment might show a precipitous drop in end-tidal CO_2, loss of pulse oximetry waveform, a low or nondetectable noninvasive blood pressure, or a flattening and drop in the arterial pressure waveform. Nonperfusing cardiac rhythms on EKG include tachyarrhythmias such as VF and VT as well as nontachyarrhythmias such as asystole, pulseless electrical activity (PEA), or severe bradycardia.

B. **Etiologies.** Common recognized causes of cardiac arrest, referred to using the mnemonic of the five "H's and T's" are:

1. **H**ypovolemia.
2. **H**ypoxemia.
3. **H**ydrogen ion/acid-base disturbances.
4. **H**yper/hypokalemia/electrolyte derangements (K, Ca, Mg).
5. **H**ypothermia.
6. **T**oxins (drug toxicity).
7. **T**amponade (cardiac).
8. **T**ension pneumothorax.
9. **T**hrombosis (pulmonary embolus).
10. **T**hrombosis (cardiac/myocardial infarction).
11. Hypoglycemia (not in the "5 H's and T's," but a critical assessment).

Within the OR, additional etiologies to consider are:

1. Local anesthetic systemic toxicity.
2. Neuraxial anesthesia causing severe sympathectomy.
3. Anaphylaxis (eg, paralytics, antibiotics).
4. Malignant hyperthermia.
5. Excessive vagal tone during surgical manipulation or laparoscopy.
6. Embolism of air, fat, amniotic fluid, or procedural cement.
7. Excessive anesthetic.
8. Coronary stent thrombosis (in setting of holding antiplatelet medication).
9. Postreperfusion syndrome in liver transplantation.

C. **Pathophysiology.** If CPR is not immediately started after cardiac arrest, the cessation of blood flow causes tissue hypoxia, anaerobic metabolism, accumulation of cellular wastes, depletion of ATP, and ion-gradient break-down (eg, uncontrolled calcium flow into cells that is excitotoxic and may trigger apoptosis). Widespread anaerobic metabolism leads to a sudden, severe acidemia with effects including systemic vasodilation, pulmonary vasoconstriction, and decreased response to catecholamines. Neurologic injury can become irreversible in as little as 4 to 6 minutes of absent cir-culation. After restoration of cardiac output, patients can have ischemia reperfusion injury with the generation of reactive oxygen species, mito-chondrial dysfunction, and an immune/inflammatory cascade for which targeted temperature management (formerly therapeutic hypothermia) may be beneficial. The cumulative effects of absent flow and reperfusion injury result in variable multiorgan damage and neurological disability.

D. **Epidemiology.** There are roughly 350,000 yearly out-of-hospital arrests in the United States, of which half are witnessed and only 1 in 10 survive to hospital discharge. Shockable rhythms (pVT/VF) represent around 20% of the initial observed rhythms.

III. ADULT RESUSCITATION

A. **BLS** refers to the core competency live-saving skill set of CPR, activation of the emergency response system, and expedient use of an automated external defibrillator (AED). BLS certification is offered to the public and is required for healthcare providers with variations in management sug-gestions based on level of training and comfort.

Any person found unresponsive or with absent or gasping/agonal breath sounds should be suspected to be in cardiac arrest (*IIa/C-LD*). Pulse checks by a healthcare provider in this setting should last at most 10 seconds (*II/C*). If the person cannot be aroused, the AHA guidelines for CPR and emergency cardiac care stress immediate activation of the emergency response system for out-of-hospital arrests and initiation of chest compressions to provide **C**irculation prior to **A**irway management and **B**reathing, or **C-A-B**. This was changed from **A-B-C** in 2010 to emphasize the initial focus on restoring circulation based on survival studies.

The C-A-B sequence emphasizes circulation first to minimize delays in chest compressions associated with establishing a patent airway. Beginning with chest compressions may also increase likelihood that bystanders will perform CPR on persons who have suffered from SCA as lay persons may find airway management challenging and hesitate to initiate CPR. In fact, the guidelines changed in 2017 to emphasize that untrained lay rescuers may provide compression only CPR (*I/C-LD*), and dispatchers should offer compression-only CPR instructions (*I/C-LD*). Lay persons trained in CPR should still add rescue breaths when trained or able.

For lone rescuers, the public is taught the "phone first/phone fast" rule. For adults, children aged 8 years and older, and all children known to be at high risk for arrhythmias, the emergency medical system (911; EMS) should be activated (phone first) before attempts at resuscitation by a lone rescuer. An initial resuscitation attempt followed by the activation of EMS ("phone fast") is indicated for children less than 8 years old and for all ages in cases of submersion or near drowning, arrest secondary to trauma, and drug overdose. Owing to the increased rate of unresponsiveness secondary to opioid overdose, family members are recommended to have naloxone available to administer in coordination with alerting EMS.

1. **Circulation (chest compressions).** It is estimated that chest compressions can provide up to one-third of the normal cardiac output. To ensure sufficient circulation, especially coronary and cerebral flow, compressions should occupy a minimum 60% of the arrest event time (*IIb/C-LD*) with a target of 80% and minimal pauses between shocks (*I/C-LD*). The patient should be on a firm surface, preferably a backboard when possible, and flat with their head at the level of the thorax. This is especially true in an OR where the soft surgical table padding/gel absorbs energy from compressions, which can decrease their effectiveness. For a prone, intubated patient in the OR who cannot be quickly turned supine for CPR, one member can place a clenched fist between the subxiphoid area and the OR table with compressions over the corresponding region of the back (*IIb/C*).

   Proper positioning involves placing the heel of your hand in the center of the patient's chest at the intermammary line with the heel of the other hand on top of the first so that the hands are overlapped and parallel (*IIa/B*). Shoulders can be positioned directly over the patient and elbows locked. The chest should depress to a minimum 2 inches in adults (*I/C-LD*) and at least one-third of the anterior-posterior chest diameter for pediatric patients (roughly 2 inches in children, 1.5 inches in infants) (*IIa/C-LD*). For children, single responders can use the heel of one or both hands (*IIb/C*). In infants, single responders should use a two-finger technique, whereas the two-thumb encircling hands technique is used with multiple responders (*IIb/C*).

   The chest compression rate should be at least 100/min, and allow for complete chest recoil by targeting equal compression and relaxation times (*IIb/C*). While rate and depth tend to err on the lower side, compressions quality can also suffer from being too deep or too fast, thus upper bounds of 2.4 inches for depth and 120 for rate were introduced. Given this notably small range of 2 to 2.4 inches (5-6 cm), compression feedback devices that optimize performance should be used when available (*IIb/B-R*).

The target compression-ventilation ratio is 30:2 for single responders with two breaths being delivered over less than 10 seconds (*IIa/C-LD*). With two or more people, the 30:2 ratio is preserved, and providers should switch every 2 minutes (five cycles) in less than 5 seconds (*IIa/B*). In children, the compression-ventilation ratio is 15:2 when there are two rescuers to reflect the more respiratory driven arrest incidence. If an advanced airway such as an endotracheal tube (ETT) or laryngeal mask airway (LMA) is in place during two-rescuer CPR, ventilations should be given at a rate of 10 breaths/min simultaneously with compressions without pauses.

Another described maneuver is the precordial "thump" whereby the rescuer slams the underside of their fist to the mid-sternum to depolarize the heart. This maneuver can be considered for monitored patients with unstable or pulseless VT if a defibrillator is not immediately available (*IIb/C*), although this method of triggering depolarization with swift mechanical impulses should not be used to "pace" the heart.

2. **Airway and breathing.** Although recent guideline changes have focused on circulation (all the way to compression-only CPR), maintaining a patent airway with adequate ventilation and oxygenation remains critical (*I/C*). It becomes more vital as arrest time increases owing to exhaustion of alveolar oxygen reserve and accumulation of carbon dioxide. Spontaneous ventilation is evaluated by observation and auscultation and aided by repositioning, most commonly through a head tilt-chin lift technique (*IIa/B*). If a cervical spine injury is suspected based on the scene or nature of injury, a jaw thrust without head extension should be attempted (*IIb/C*), although if unsuccessful at establishing airway patency, a head tilt should still be used (*I/C*). If ventilation remains impossible after these maneuvers and an advanced airway is not available, efforts to clear the airway of a suspected foreign body should be attempted. In primary foreign body obstruction, abdominal thrusts (Heimlich maneuver) should be attempted (*IIb/B*) and chest thrusts considered when unsuccessful (*IIb/B*). This differs for infants for whom back blows are delivered in succession with chest compressions for foreign body obstruction.

When an adult has spontaneous circulation by palpable pulses but ineffective breathing alone, rescue breaths should be provided 10 to 12 times per minute or every 5 to 6 seconds (*IIb/C*). Breaths should be delivered over 1 second with enough volume for visible chest rise, roughly 500 to 600 mL in adults (*IIa/C*). Rescue breaths during cardiac arrest should be similarly provided over 1 second with visible chest rise. In the absence of an advanced airway, compressions are briefly paused for breaths at the 30:2 ratio whether there are one or more providers. With an advanced airway in place, breaths should be given every 6 seconds (10/min) concurrent with compressions as mentioned above.

Hyperventilation (*III/B*) in any setting from excess respiratory rate or tidal volume should be avoided as it can cause gastric insufflation provoking aspiration and, more importantly, it can increase intrathoracic pressure, impair venous return, and lower cardiac output, which ultimately worsens outcomes.

3. **Defibrillation** in BLS refers to the use of AEDs, which should be retrieved as part of the initial activation of the emergency response system. Timely defibrillation and CPR are major determinants of a successful resuscitation. Defibrillation is the definitive management for pulseless VT and VF (*I/A*). When an arrest is witnessed and an AED is within

reach, the defibrillator should be used as soon as possible (*IIa/C-LD*). For unwitnessed arrests, CPR should be initiated while the AED is being retrieved (*IIa/B-R*).

Public access defibrillation programs have enabled public safety professionals (eg, fire personnel, police, security guards, and airline attendants) to employ readily accessible AEDs. The devices themselves are small and lightweight and use adhesive electrode pads for both sensing and delivering shocks. Visual and voice prompts are provided to assist the operators with the goal of making it usable by an untrained bystander. After analysis of the frequency, amplitude, and slope of the ECG signal, the AED *advises* either "shock indicated" or "no shock indicated." The AED is manually triggered and does not automatically defibrillate the patient as an automatic shock could injure someone touching the patient. AEDs are now also equipped with pediatric pad-cable systems that attenuate the adult dose to a smaller dose appropriate for children. The dose attenuators should be used in children less than 8 years of age and less than 25 kg in weight. For infants, manual defibrillation is recommended, but if unavailable, an AED with or without an attenuator can be used. There are efforts to make AED analysis more sophisticated such as incorporating artifact filtering so that compressions can be continued during rhythm analysis. At this point, these technologies are not reliable enough to promote (*IIb/C-EO*).

4. **Reassessment.** Although it is tempting to see if the defibrillation worked by checking for a pulse immediately after a shock, the heart still needs time to establish sufficient forward flow and compressions should be resumed immediately after shock delivery (*IIb/C-LD*) with a rhythm check after five cycles of CPR (2 minutes). For healthcare providers, if there is evidence of a perfusing rhythm, the pulse can be checked to determine if there is ROSC. If a nonshockable rhythm or no pulse is detected, CPR should be resumed with rhythm checks after every five cycles as before.

B. **ACLS** describes the definitive, medically exhaustive treatment for cardiac arrest taught exclusively to health professionals. It builds upon BLS skills and can be provided in the field by paramedics or in a hospital setting. As OR and intensive care unit (ICU) providers, anesthesiologists should keep themselves up to date with their certification and with changes to management protocols, which are amended yearly. Interventions described in ACLS include advanced airway management, manual defibrillation, synchronized cardioversion, pharmacologic management, and decisions toward more invasive mechanical circulatory support or withdrawal of care.

1. **Advanced airway.** Swift control of the airway optimizes oxygenation and the removal of carbon dioxide during resuscitation. Options are bag-mask ventilation or an advanced airway such as an ETT or LMA (*IIb/B-R*). The goal is to secure the airway via endotracheal intubation, which should be performed by the most experienced provider, often a trained anesthesiologist. Insertion of an oropharyngeal or nasopharyngeal airway can improve ventilation in an obstructed airway before intubation (*IIa/C*). Although cricoid pressure is sometimes used during bag-mask ventilation to decrease gastric insufflation, routine use is discouraged (*III/B*) as it tends to be performed incorrectly or in a manner that impairs ventilation.

Endotracheal intubation during an in-hospital arrest can be difficult given confined space, poor patient positioning, suboptimal visualization, and interference from chest compressions. Waveform capnography, which is often a component of modern defibrillators, is the most reliable method to confirm correct placement (*I/C-LD*), although a color-changing in-line CO_2 detector is frequently the most readily available. The ETT may be used to deliver certain lipophilic drugs like naloxone, atropine, vasopressin, epinephrine, or lidocaine (NAVEL, now known as LEAN with removal of vasopressin) if intravenous (IV) access has not been established. Higher doses of these drugs are needed (2-3 times as much) owing to lower peak blood concentrations and should be diluted in 10 mL of sterile saline.

2. **Defibrillation.** Pulseless VT and VF are shockable dysrhythmias associated with cardiac arrest (see **Figure 39.1**). As the duration of SCA increases, cardiac ischemia worsens, and it becomes more difficult to achieve ROSC. Rapid defibrillation is critical in this situation before the rhythm degenerates into PEA or asystole. It is the responsibility of the person operating the defibrillator to ensure that members of the resuscitation team are not in contact with the patient during defibrillation. Defibrillators deliver energy in a biphasic pulse that alternates current flow. The optimal dose to terminate VF is 150 to 200 J and is indicated on the front of the defibrillator. In children, an initial dose of 2 to 4 J/kg is advised (*IIa/C-LD*). The pediatric dose can be increased with successive

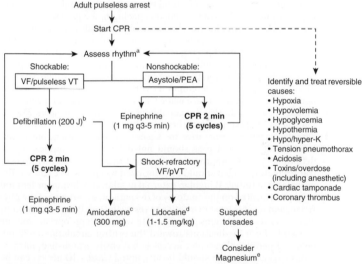

FIGURE 39.1 Algorithm for pulseless arrest. VF, ventricular fibrillation; VT, ventricular tachycardia. [a]When rhythm is unclear and could be VF, treat as shockable rhythm. [b]Biphasic. One cycle of CPR should follow any successful defibrillation. [c]Amiodarone bolus should be administered in 20 to 30 mL saline or D5W. This is followed by an infusion of 1 mg/min for 6 hours and then 0.5 mg/min thereafter. An additional dose of 150 mg IV can be readministered for recurrence of VF or VT. [d]Lidocaine can be bolused again at a dose of 0.5 to 0.75 mg/kg. [e]Magnesium sulfate 1 to 2 g can be considered for torsades (long-QT-associated polymorphic VT) but trials have not demonstrated an advantage. Vasopressin is no longer used in the ACLS protocol as its use had no added benefit relative to or in combination with epinephrine.

shocks but should not exceed 10 J/kg or the maximum adult dose (*IIb/C-LD*). The large adult pads/paddles (8-13 cm) are recommended in children above 1 year of age and at least 10 kg in weight. Infant pads/paddles (4.5 cm) are used in children less than 10 kg in weight. Pads are preferred to paddles, as they can aid in rhythm detection and pacing. The defibrillator should be charged while compressions continue, and once ready to discharge, the provider calls "clear" to alert everyone to remove their hands from the patient and the shock is delivered, and compressions are resumed.

a. **Cardioversion** using synchronized biphasic shocks are used for unstable tachyarrhythmias with pulses (rates generally >150 bpm) such as paroxysmal supraventricular tachycardia (PSVT), atrial fibrillation, re-entrant arrhythmias, or unstable VT. The recommended initial energy dose for synchronized cardioversion of atrial fibrillation is 120 to 200 J (*IIa/A*). Dosing can be increased in a stepwise fashion if the initial shock is ineffective. Hemodynamically stable VT can be cardioverted using 100 J as the starting point (*IIb/C*). The initial dose for cardioversion in children is 0.5 to 1 J/kg followed by subsequent doses of 2 J/kg. See **Figure 39.3** for management of tachyarrhythmias in adults.

3. **Pacing.** High-grade heart block with profound bradycardia is one etiology of cardiac arrest. Temporary pacing should be used when the bradyarrhythmia does not improve with medication (primarily atropine) and there are signs of instability (eg, altered mental status, severe hypotension) (*IIa/B*). Transcutaneous pacing is the easiest method to increase the ventricular rate but may require high currents for consistent capture, which can be very uncomfortable for awake patients. Transesophageal atrial pacing is efficacious for sinus bradycardia with maintained atrioventricular (AV) conduction and is useful intraoperatively for bradycardia-related hypotension in otherwise stable patients. Transvenous pacing via a temporary wire into the right heart is a third option to increase heart rate while CPR continues. Special pacing pulmonary artery catheters are capable of AV pacing. See **Figure 39.2** for management of symptomatic bradycardia.

4. **Vascular access** is imperative for successful resuscitation, but establishment of venous access should not delay chest compressions or defibrillation when appropriate. The most desirable route is into central circulation, which should be prioritized when possible (*IIb/C*). The insertion site (internal jugular, external jugular, subclavian, or femoral vein) is predicated on the anatomy of the patient, experience of the physician, and what is least disruptive to resuscitation. Peripheral IV catheters in antecubital veins are adequate when an appropriate volume is used to flush medications toward the central circulation (~20-mL bolus). If peripheral vascular access is not easily established, intraosseous (IO) cannulation should be attempted (*IIa/C*). IO access can be done in less than a minute in children. All drugs and fluids can be given through an IO route until good IV access is found.

Another form of vascular access to strongly consider is an arterial line, which is beneficial for sending arterial blood gases to aid in management and for evaluating compression quality (via pulsatile flow visualization) and return of spontaneous circulation.

5. **Drugs.** The drugs described below are used in ACLS protocols for the treatment of hemodynamic instability, myocardial ischemia/infarction, and arrhythmias. The doses of drugs used for PALS are in

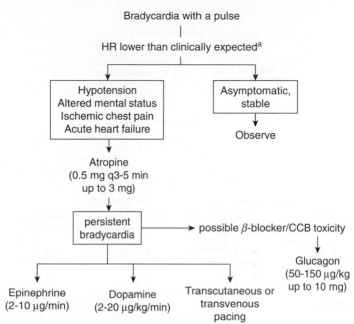

FIGURE 39.2 Algorithm for bradycardia. HR, heart rate; bpm, beats per minute; CCB, calcium channel blocker. ªNormal heart rate goal may be <60 bpm for patients receiving therapeutic nodal agents (eg, β-blocker). When IV access or medications are not immediately available, can jump to transcutaneous pacing.

parentheses following the adult doses. Drugs should be provided centrally whenever possible given the slow circulation times during CPR but can be given peripherally (IV or IO) or via ETT (LEAN medications as described previously).

a. **Adenosine** is an endogenous purine nucleoside with a half-life of 5 seconds. Adenosine slows or blocks anterograde AV node conduction and interrupts AV node reentry pathways to convert a stable PSVT to sinus rhythm. It can also slow the heart rate enough to identify an underlying rhythm that may be difficult to differentiate at elevated heart rates such as atrial fibrillation or atrial flutter. Adenosine can also be considered in the treatment of stable, regular, wide complex monomorphic VT. The initial dose is always a 6-mg rapid IV bolus immediately followed by a 20-mL saline flush (*I/B*). A brief asystole ensues, followed by P waves, flutter waves, or fibrillation waves that are initially without ventricular responses. The PSVT is sometimes converted to sinus rhythm by the initial dose, but a second injection of 12 mg may be required to terminate the PSVT if there is no effect of the first dose after 1 to 2 minutes. These doses are based on peripheral IV administration. If given via central access, the first and second doses are 3 and 6 mg, respectively.

Recurrent PSVT, AF, and atrial flutter will require longer-acting nodal agents for definitive treatment. The required dose of

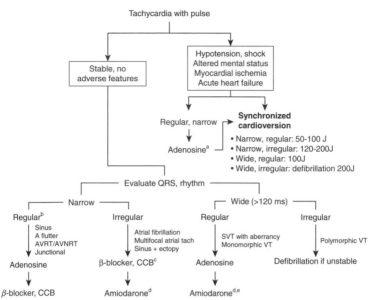

FIGURE 39.3 Algorithm for tachycardia with pulse. If there are signs of instability with hemodynamic compromise, the treatment of choice is immediate cardioversion. A useful estimate for peak heart rate is 220 − Age. When stable, EKG analysis and appropriate pharmacologic interventions should be attempted. [a]Adenosine should not be prioritized over cardioversion with unstable patients. It is given as a 6-mg IV push with a potential second dose of 12 mg (avoid with history or evidence of WPW). [b]Consider vagal stimulation before adenosine for stable, regular, narrow tachyarrhythmias. [c]Generally metoprolol, esmolol infusion, or diltiazem push. [d]Amiodarone given as 150 mg IV over 10 minutes followed by an infusion of 1 mg/min. [e]Alternatives to amiodarone for regular, wide complex include procainamide or sotalol.

adenosine may need to be increased in the presence of methylxanthines like theophylline owing to competitive inhibition and decreased if dipyridamole has been administered owing to potentiation via blockage of nucleoside transport (although such adjustments are usually made for infusions during stress tests to induce vasodilation and not in ACLS protocols) (PALS: 0.1 mg/kg; repeat dose 0.2 mg/kg; maximum dose 12 mg). Adenosine should not be used for irregularly irregular rhythms or pre-excitation syndromes like Wolff-Parkinson-White (WPW) as exclusive accessory tract conduction can precipitate VF (*III/C*).

b. **Amiodarone** is the most versatile drug in ACLS algorithms. It has the properties of all four classes of antiarrhythmics: lengthening of the action potential, sodium channel blockade at high frequencies of stimulation, noncompetitive antisynaptic actions, and negative chronotropism. Because of its high efficacy and low incidence of proarrhythmic effects, it is the preferred antiarrhythmic for patients with severely impaired cardiac function. For shock-refractory pulseless VT/VF, 300 mg diluted in 20 to 30 mL of saline or 5% dextrose in water (D5W) is administered as a bolus. To treat stable dysrhythmias (eg, hemodynamically stable AF, VT), 150 mg is administered over 10 minutes, followed by an infusion of 1 mg/min for 6 hours, and then 0.5 mg/min. The maximum daily dose is 2 g. Immediate side effects can be bradycardia and hypotension (PALS: loading dose 5 mg/kg; maximum dose 15 mg/kg/d). Amiodarone is indicated in the following situations:

1. Unstable VT (*IIb/C*).
2. VF or pulseless VT after failed electrical defibrillation and epinephrine treatment (*IIb/B-R*).
3. Attempted rate control during stable monomorphic VT, polymorphic VT (*IIb/B*), or AF.
4. Need for an adjunct to electrical cardioversion of refractory PSVT (*IIa*) or atrial tachycardia (*IIb*).

c. **Atropine** is an anticholinergic used as the first-line agent for hemodynamically significant bradycardia (*IIa/B*) or AV block occurring at the nodal level. It increases the rate of sinus node discharge and enhances AV node conduction by its vagolytic activity. It is not effective for Mobitz type II heart block, for complete heart block, or in transplanted hearts missing vagal innervation. It is also not indicated for asystole or PEA (*IIb/B*) but should be considered for treatment of profound bradycardia that may appear as asystole but with a preserved pulse. The dose of atropine for bradycardia or AV block is 0.5 mg repeated every 3 to 5 minutes to a total dose of 3 mg (PALS: 0.02 mg/kg; minimum dose, 0.1 mg; maximum single dose, 0.5 mg in child, maximum total dose for adolescent 3 mg).

d. **β-Adrenergic antagonists** (eg, atenolol, metoprolol, esmolol, propranolol) have established utility for patients with unstable angina or myocardial infarction. Their competitive inhibition of adrenergic receptors reduces heart rate, AV node conduction, blood pressure, and the effects of catecholamines. This action serves to reduce the rate of recurrent ischemia, nonfatal reinfarction, and postinfarction VF. In contrast to calcium channel blockers, β-blockers are not direct negative inotropes.

β-blockers are useful for the acute treatment of stable PSVT, AF, atrial flutter (I), and ectopic atrial tachycardia (IIb). Initial and subsequent IV doses, if tolerated, are atenolol, 5 mg over 5 minutes, repeated once at 10 minutes; metoprolol, three doses of 5 mg every 5 minutes; propranolol, 0.1 mg/kg divided into three doses given every 2 to 3 minutes; esmolol, 0.5 mg/kg over 1 minute followed by an infusion starting at 50 μg/min and titrated as needed up to 200 μg/min. Contraindications include second- or third-degree heart block, hypotension, and severe congestive heart failure. When a β-blocker might trigger bronchospasm in a patient with chronic lung disease, metoprolol with selective β1 blockade at therapeutic doses may be preferred.

e. **Calcium** is indicated during cardiac arrest only when hyperkalemia, hypermagnesemia, hypocalcemia, or toxicity from calcium channel blockers is suspected. Calcium chloride can be given as a dose of 8 to 16 mg/kg IV (usually 0.5-1g) and repeated as necessary (PALS: calcium chloride 10%: 20 mg/kg = 0.2 mL/kg). Although calcium plays a role in myocardial contraction, studies have not shown any benefit with routine use in cardiac arrest (*III/B*).

f. **Calcium channel blockers (nondihydropyridine)** such as verapamil and diltiazem depress AV nodal conduction and increase refractory time. These are used to treat hemodynamically stable, narrow complex

PSVT unresponsive to vagal maneuvers or adenosine (*IIa/B*). The initial verapamil dose is 2.5 to 5.0 mg IV, with subsequent doses of 5 to 10 mg IV administered every 15 to 30 minutes. Diltiazem is given as an initial bolus of 15 to 20 mg over 2 minutes. An additional dose of 20 to 25 mg and an infusion of 5 to 15 mg/h can be administered if needed. Their vasodilator and negative inotrope properties can cause hypotension, exacerbation of congestive heart failure, bradycardia, and enhancement of accessory conduction in patients with WPW syndrome. The hypotension can often be reversed with calcium chloride, 0.5 to 1.0 g IV. They are contraindicated for wide complex tachyarrhythmias (*III/B*).

g. **Dopamine** has dopaminergic (1-5 µg/kg/min), β-adrenergic (5-10 µg/kg/min), and α-adrenergic (>10 µg/kg/min) activity. Although those listed are "traditional" ranges for dose-dependent receptor agonism, the pharmacodynamics are not reliable (eg, tachycardia may occur with the lowest doses). Dopamine should be started at a low dose and titrated to the desired effect such as increased urine output, increased heart rate/inotropy, increased blood pressure or when undesired side effects limit further increases. It is the second-line agent to atropine for symptomatic bradyarrhythmias (*IIa/B*), alongside epinephrine and transcutaneous pacing. Infusions can range from 5 to 20 µg/kg/min.

h. **Epinephrine** continues to be the mainstay of pharmacologic therapy for all forms of cardiac arrest (*I/B-R*) given its demonstrated survival benefits. Its α-adrenergic vasoconstriction of noncerebral and noncoronary vascular beds produces compensatory shunting of blood toward the brain and heart. Its β1 and β2 agonism stimulates the heart and relaxes the bronchial tree. In normal circulation, its half-life is a few minutes. The recommended dose in SCA is 1 mg IV repeated every 3 to 5 minutes (*IIa,C-LD*). Epinephrine is second line to atropine for symptomatic bradycardia with a target dose range of 2 to 10 µg/min (*IIb/B*). It is the first-line agent, however, for bradycardia associated with neuraxial anesthesia (PALS: bradycardia with a pulse but poor perfusion, 0.01 mg/kg; pulseless arrest, 0.01 mg/kg). The optimal dose timing around defibrillation is not clear, but it is reasonable to give after the initial defibrillating shock fails (*IIb/C-LD*). In shock-refractory rhythms, epinephrine is combined with antiarrhythmics, including amiodarone or lidocaine. It is also commonly used in the OR in smaller, escalating doses for managing anaphylaxis and hypotension.

Studies have trialed high-dose epinephrine as high as 0.2 mg/kg but have not shown any advantage, and such doses are discouraged (*III/B-R*). High doses can contribute to myocardial dysfunction or even precipitate a stress cardiomyopathy.

i. **Isoproterenol** is a β_1 and β_2-adrenergic agent. It is another second-line drug used to treat hemodynamically significant bradycardia unresponsive to atropine and dobutamine in the event that a temporarily pacemaker is not available. It is not stocked in code carts. Its β_2 activity can cause hypotension. Isoproterenol is administered by IV infusion at 2 to 10 µg/min, titrated to achieve the desired heart rate.

j. **Lidocaine** acts on voltage-gated sodium channels and functions as both a local anesthetic and a class Ib antiarrhythmic. In the 2018 ACLS guidelines, lidocaine was added alongside amiodarone for VF/pVT unresponsive to defibrillation, especially for witnessed arrests

(*IIb/B-R*). It may be useful for the control (not prophylaxis) of ventricular ectopy during an acute myocardial infarction. The initial dose is 1 to 1.5 mg/kg IV and may be repeated as a 0.5- to 0.75-mg/kg bolus every 3 to 5 minutes to a total dose of 3 mg/kg followed by a continuous infusion at 2 to 4 mg/min. The lidocaine dose should be decreased for patients with reduced cardiac output, hepatic dysfunction, or advanced age (PALS: 1 mg/kg; infusion, 20-50 µg/kg/min).

k. **Magnesium** is a divalent cation with a myriad of regulatory roles such as being a cofactor in enzyme reactions including that of the Na^+, K^+-ATPase, decreasing nerve and muscle conduction, relaxing bronchial smooth muscle, acting as a vasodilator, and even effecting N-methyl-D-aspartate antagonism through competition at calcium-binding sites. That said, magnesium is not recommended for general use in cardiac arrest (*III/C-LD*) except in specific circumstances such as for preventing recurrent long QT associated polymorphic VT (torsades de pointes) (*IIb/C-LD*). The dose for emergent administration is 1 to 2 g in 10 mL D5W over 1 to 2 minutes. Hypotension and bradycardia are side effects of rapid administration (PALS: 25-50 mg/kg; maximum dose, 2 g).

l. **Oxygen** (100%) should be administered to all survivors of cardiac arrest by bag-valve-mask or advanced airway and to hemodynamically stable, breathing patients by unpressurized face mask. For neonates and infants not in cardiac arrest, high FIO_2 can be deleterious and is carefully titrated to preductal SpO_2.

m. **Procainamide** is a class Ia antiarrhythmic that can be used to convert atrial fibrillation/atrial flutter to sinus rhythm and control the ventricular response to supraventricular tachycardia secondary to accessory pathways and is useful during cardioversion of wide complex tachycardias of unknown origin. It has essentially been replaced by amiodarone. The loading dose is a continuous infusion of 20 to 30 mg/min that is terminated when the arrhythmia is suppressed, hypotension occurs, the QRS complex is widened by 50% of its original size, or a total dose of 17 mg/kg is reached. When the arrhythmia is suppressed, a maintenance infusion of 1 to 4 mg/min should be initiated, with a reduced dose considered in the presence of renal dysfunction. An ECG should be examined for QRS widening at least daily (PALS: 15 mg/kg over 30-60 minutes).

n. **Sodium bicarbonate** administration is detrimental in most cardiac arrests (*III/B*) because it creates a paradoxical intracellular acidosis. It can be considered when the standard ACLS protocol has failed in the presence of severe preexisting metabolic acidosis and for the treatment of hyperkalemia or tricyclic antidepressant overdose. The initial dose of bicarbonate is 1 mEq/kg IV, with subsequent doses of 0.5 mEq/kg given every 10 minutes (as guided by arterial blood pH and partial pressure of carbon dioxide [$PaCO_2$]) (PALS: 1 mEq/kg).

o. **Sotalol**, a type III antiarrhythmic and nonselective β-blocker can be considered alongside amiodarone and procainamide and is primarily used for atrial fibrillation/flutter and stable monomorphic VT (*IIb/B*). A dose of 1.5 mg/kg is given over 5 minutes for hemodynamically stable arrhythmias. Like procainamide, it should be avoided in patients with prolonged QT as it can precipitate torsade (*III/B*). Other side effects include bradycardia and hypotension.

p. **Vasopressin**, a hormone from the neurohypophysis, has pressor (V_1) and antidiuretic (V_2) activities. Endogenous levels of vasopressin are increased in patients undergoing CPR who eventually have ROSC. It is more effective than epinephrine in maintaining the coronary perfusion pressure, has a longer half-life of 10 to 20 minutes, and was conventionally substituted for either the first or second dose of epinephrine in the treatment of pulseless arrest at doses of 40 units IV. Although vasopressin may still be considered as a substitute or in combination with epinephrine (*IIb/C-LD*), it has not been shown to offer any clear advantage and is no longer part of the ACLS protocol (PALS: 0.4-1 U/kg bolus with a maximum dose of 40 units for cardiac arrest and 0.0002-0.002 U/kg/min for catecholamine-resistant hypotension).

6. **Specific ACLS protocols** are shown in **Figures 39.1-39.3**.
   a. Pulseless arrest (**Figure 39.1**).
   b. Bradycardia with pulse (**Figure 39.2**).
   c. Tachycardia with pulse (**Figure 39.3**).

7. **Open-chest direct cardiac compression** is an intervention used at institutions with appropriate resources to manage penetrating chest trauma, abdominal trauma with cardiac arrest, pericardial tamponade, hypothermia, or pulmonary embolism. Direct cardiac compressions also are indicated for individuals with anatomic deformities of the chest that prevent adequate closed-chest compression (*IIb/C*).

8. **ECMO** is a portable form of advanced mechanical cardiopulmonary support through invasive cannulation of large vessels. Recently, it has been referred to as extracorporeal cardiopulmonary resuscitation (eCPR). There are two forms of eCPR, venovenous (VV) and venoarterial (VA). Both provide respiratory support through external gas exchange, whereas VA provides additional circulatory (hemodynamic) support. eCPR is indicated when traditional CPR has failed, but it has many contraindications including, but not limited to, unwitnessed arrest, >30 minutes of traditional CPR without ROSC, severe bleeding, and the inability to tolerate systemic anticoagulation.

   Although eCPR can achieve normal cardiac output in situations where ROSC is not attainable through traditional CPR, it is not recommended as a routine intervention and should be reserved for patients who would likely recover (*I/C-EO*). Institutions that offer ECMO services should have a separate emergency consult team that screens, selects, and cannulates patients.

9. **Termination of CPR.** There are no absolute guidelines based on outcome studies to determine when to stop an unsuccessful resuscitation, but there is a very low probability of survival after 30 minutes. One objective measure is the failure to attain an end-tidal CO_2 of 10 mm Hg after 20 minutes of CPR (*IIb/C-LD*). It is at the discretion of the physician in charge to determine when the failure of the cardiovascular system to respond to adequately applied BLS and ACLS indicates that the patient has died. There should be meticulous documentation of the resuscitation, including the reasons for terminating the effort.

10. **Advanced directives**, such as "Do Not Resuscitate" (**DNR**), places the anesthesiologist in a key position with respect to intraoperative and postoperative care. It is often incorrectly *assumed* that a DNR order is suspended in the perioperative period. Each institution's written guidelines should be reviewed. In advance of a procedure, physicians and the patient with the DNR status or the patient's healthcare proxy should

clarify any resuscitative measures that would be compatible with the patient's wishes. For example, the use of a pressor to control hypotension following induction of general anesthesia might be permitted while defibrillation and CPR for spontaneous VF might be prohibited. When asked to perform an emergent intubation outside of the OR, the anesthesiologist should ask about the patient's code status and is ethically and legally bound to a known decision to limit treatment.

IV. PEDIATRIC RESUSCITATION

A. **Basic life support.** The need for CPR in the pediatric age group is rare after the neonatal period. Pediatric cardiac arrests usually result from hypoxemia linked to respiratory failure or airway obstruction. Initial efforts should be directed toward the establishment of a secure airway and adequate ventilation. The pediatric guidelines apply to infants between the ages of about 1 month and 1 year and to children more than 1 year of age. For newborns, see the next section. The definition of "children" for healthcare providers is patients between the ages of 1 year and the start of puberty; for the lay public, a child is defined as aged 1 to 8 years.

In contrast to the guideline of "phone first" for adult CPR, one should "phone fast" for infants and children. That is, the lone rescuer should perform five cycles (about 2 minutes) of CPR before phoning 911. The "phone fast" rule also applies to resuscitation from drowning, traumatic arrest, or drug overdose. Exceptions include witnessed and sudden arrests (eg, an athlete who collapses on the playing field) or situations in which a child is known to be at high risk for a sudden arrhythmia. Modifications to the rate and magnitude of compressions and ventilations, as well as to the hand positions for compressions are necessary because of anatomic and physiologic differences (**Table 39.2**). Differences between pediatric and adult resuscitation techniques are detailed below.

Airway and breathing. Maneuvers to establish an airway are the same as in the adult, with a few caveats. For children less than 1 year of age, abdominal thrusts are not used in the setting of airway foreign body obstruction since the gastrointestinal tract can be damaged easily. Hyperextension of an infant's neck for the head tilt-chin lift may lead to airway obstruction because of the small diameter and ease of compression of the

TABLE 39.2	Adult and Pediatric Cardiopulmonary Resuscitation			
Age	**Ventilations/ Minute**	**Compressions/ Minute**	**Ventilation:Compression Ratio**	**Depth of Compressions**
Neonate	30	90	3:1[a,b]	1/3 depth of chest
Infant (<1 y)	12-20	100	30:2[a]/15:2[b]	1/3-1/2 depth of chest
Child (1-8 y)	12-20	100	30:2[a]/15:2[b]	1/3-1/2 depth of chest
Adult and child >8 y	10-12	100	30:2[a,b]	1.5-2 inches

[a]One-person rescue.
[b]Two-person rescue.

immature airway. Submental compression while performing the chin lift can also lead to airway obstruction by pushing the tongue into the pharynx. Ventilations should be given slowly and with low airway pressures to avoid gastric distention and should be of sufficient volume to cause visible chest rise and fall.

B. Circulation. The brachial or femoral artery is used for pulse assessment in infants (<1 year old) because the carotid artery is difficult to palpate. Upon determination that a pulse is absent, chest compressions should be initiated. Chest compressions in infants are delivered using two fingertips applied to the sternum or by encircling the chest with both hands and using the thumbs to depress the sternum one fingerbreadth below the intermammary line (*IIb/C*). In older children, the correct hand position is determined as for adults, but with only one hand depressing the sternum. The chest should be compressed at least one-third of the anterior-posterior depth, roughly 1.5 in (4 cm) in infants and 2 in (5 cm) in children (*IIa/C-LD*). The compression-ventilation ratio is 30:2 for one-rescuer CPR of infants and children and 15:2 when two rescuers are available. If an advanced airway is in place during two-person CPR, there is no need to synchronize breaths between compressions. Ventilations should be given at a rate of approximately 10 breaths/min, and chest compressions should be given at a rate of 100 to 120/min without pauses for ventilation.

1. Pediatric advanced life support (PALS). Most pediatric cardiac arrests present as asystole and bradycardia, rather than ventricular arrhythmias, as they primarily occur secondary to respiratory failure or shock. In infants less than 1 year old, respiratory and idiopathic (sudden infant death syndrome) etiologies predominate. Anatomic and physiologic differences from the adult require weight-based defibrillator settings and drug dosing.

a. Intubation. Low-pressure high-volume cuffed ETT have mostly replaced uncuffed ones as the ETT of choice in children. Achieving an appropriate airway seal with an uncuffed ETT often requires multiple intubation attempts, which may predispose a child to iatrogenic airway edema. Whether using an uncuffed or cuffed ETT, a correctly sized tube should have an air leak at a driving pressure between 15 and 30 cm of water. For a cuffed ETT, this leak should be tested with the cuff deflated. Once the appropriately sized cuffed ETT has been selected, the cuff can be inflated and maintained at a pressure (as measured with a manometer) between 20 and 30 cm of water.

The internal diameter (ID) of an ETT required in children less than 1 year of age is 3.5 mm uncuffed or 3 mm cuffed and 1 to 2 years of age, the size is 4 mm uncuffed or 3.5 mm cuffed. The formula for the size of ETT (ID in millimeters) in children above 2 years of age is as follows: age in years/4 + 4 for uncuffed tubes and age in years/4 + 3.5 for cuffed tubes. Appropriate oral ETT depth (centimeters at teeth) can be calculated by the formulas: inner diameter × 3 for infants and neonates and age (in years)/2 + 12 for children >1 year. Correct ETT positioning should be confirmed with capnography, auscultation, and radiographic confirmation when available. If an intubated patient's condition deteriorates, the provider must rule out displacement or obstruction of the ETT, pneumothorax, or equipment failure (mnemonic DOPE).

b. Defibrillation. Defibrillator pads/paddles used for infants are 4.5 cm in diameter, and those used for older children (>8 years, <25 kg) are 8 cm in diameter (adult size). In an emergency and if no pediatric sizes are available, adult pads on the chest and back will suffice. The energy level is 2 J/kg for the initial biphasic shock and 4 J/kg or the lowest level that was previously successful for any subsequent shocks (*IIa/C-LD*). Hypoxemia, acidosis, or hypothermia should be considered as treatable causes of an arrest if the defibrillation attempts are unsuccessful. For synchronized cardioversion, the starting energy is 0.5 to 1 J/kg, which can be increased up to 2 J/kg (*IIb/C*). The configuration for pediatric pads/paddles varies among defibrillators.

c. **IV access.** During resuscitation, peripheral IV access is preferred over central venous access as central IV line placement may require an interruption in chest compressions. If central IV access is in place, it is the preferred route for delivery of drugs and fluids. All drugs by peripheral route should be flushed with saline to ensure delivery to the central circulation. IO access can be used in all age groups if needed.

d. **Medications.** Many of the drugs described in the adult ACLS section apply to PALS, with doses adjusted to the child's weight. Weight estimations can be obtained using body length tape with precalculated weights (Broselow tape) or formulas like the European pediatric life support formula [(age in years + 4) × 2 kg].

e. Specific PALS algorithms are shown in **Figures 39.4-39.6**.
   1. Pediatric cardiac arrest (**Figure 39.4**).
   2. Pediatric bradycardia with pulse (**Figure 39.5**).
   3. Pediatric tachycardia with pulse (**Figure 39.6**).

f. **Family presence.** Family presence during pediatric resuscitation is common in most institutions. Studies have shown that this is beneficial to family members, and parents should be offered the opportunity to observe the resuscitative efforts (*I/B*). One person should be assigned to stay with the family to explain the ongoing efforts, answer questions, and provide comfort and support. Parents can be requested to leave if they are disruptive (*IIa/C*). The resuscitation team should be aware of the presence of a family member.

V. NEONATAL RESUSCITATION

The neonatal period refers to the time from when a child is born and adjusting from intrauterine environment/physiology through the first month of life. About 10% of newborns require brief resuscitation at birth such as assistance with respiration, whereas 1% require more extensive interventions. At least one person who is skilled in the resuscitation of newborns should be present at every delivery. Rapid assessment of term gestation, respiration/crying, and good muscle tone ("yes" to all three predicts good outcome) helps identify babies who may require ongoing resuscitation from those who can stay with the mother. Resuscitation is often needed during an emergent cesarean section for fetal distress. In the event that the anesthesiologist is the only provider available to treat the newborn, the neonatal warmer should be brought to the head of the OR table to facilitate the treatment and monitoring of both the mother and child until a second provider (pediatrician) arrives (**Figure 39.7**).

A. **Assessment.** Immediate neonatal resuscitation is crucial, since profound hypoxemia can occur rapidly and may lead to persistence of the fetal circulation and resulting right-to-left shunting, which will exacerbate the hypoxemia. A neonate who requires resuscitation will likely have a significant right-to-left shunt.

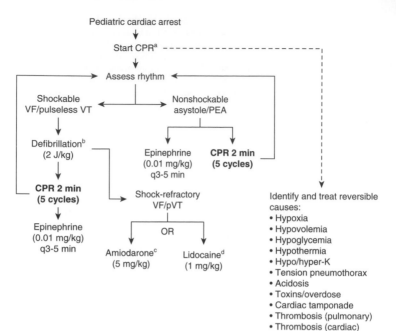

FIGURE 39.4 Algorithm for pediatric cardiac arrest. CPR, cardiopulmonary resuscitation; VF, ventricular fibrillation; VT, ventricular tachycardia. [a]Provide oxygen, establish intravenous or intraosseous access. [b]First shock, 2 J/kg; second shock, 4 J/kg; subsequent shocks ≥4 up to 10 J/kg or adult dose (200 J). [c]May repeat up to two times for VF or refractory VT. [d]Lidocaine can be used alternatively to amiodarone and following the bolus a maintenance of 20 to 50 µg/kg/min infusion may be used.

The **Apgar score** is an objective assessment of the physiologic well-being of the child as it relates to heart rate, respiration, tone, reflexes, and color and is taken at 1 and 5 minutes after birth.

B. An Apgar score of 0 to 2 mandates immediate CPR. Neonates with scores of 3 to 4 will need bag-mask ventilation and may require more extensive resuscitation. Supplemental oxygen and stimulation are normally sufficient for newborns with Apgar scores of 5 to 7. Respiratory activity should be evaluated by watching chest excursions and by auscultation. The heart rate is assessed by auscultation or by palpation of the umbilical pulse.

C. If rapid assessment at birth regarding term gestation, crying/breathing, and good muscle tone is "yes," then in most cases what is required is drying the baby and providing warmth (mother/wrapping). If the answer is "no," the following four categories should be followed in sequence.

   1. Initial steps in stabilization (dry, provide warmth, position, clear airway, stimulate to breathe).
   2. Ventilation.
   3. Chest Compressions.
   4. Medications/volume expansion.

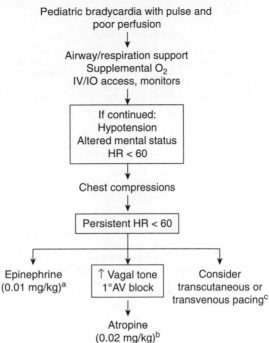

FIGURE 39.5 Algorithm for pediatric bradycardia. HR, heart rate; AV, atrioventricular. [a]May repeat every 3 to 5 minutes. If vascular access is not available, may give 0.1 mg/kg via endotracheal tube. [b]May repeat once. Minimum atropine dose is 0.1 mg; maximum 0.5 mg. If vascular access is not available, may give 0.04 to 0.06 mg/kg atropine via ETT. [c]Transcutaneous pacing is effective for bradycardia secondary to complete heart block or sinus dysfunction associated with a congenital heart disease but is not useful for asystole or hypoxic bradycardia. If pulse is lost, proceed to pulseless arrest PALS algorithm (**Figure 39.4**).

  D. Resuscitation. The first 60 seconds is referred to as the "Golden Minute" and is the time allotted for the initial steps and evaluation to decide if the baby requires ventilation. The decision to progress depends on the simultaneous assessment of two vital characteristics: appropriate respiration and heart rate. Once ventilation is required owing to inappropriate respiration or heart rate, ongoing assessment is based on three vital characteristics: heart rate, respiration, and oxygenation (pulse oximetry is used to avoid hyperoxia, and hence color is not recommended). An increase in heart rate with each intervention is the most valuable and sensitive indicator to a successful response.
  1. Initial steps. The cold-intolerant neonate should be dried thoroughly after birth and warmth provided by placing the baby under a radiant heat source. Temperature on admission to a neonatal ICU is a strong mortality predictor (*I/B-NR*) and should be maintained between 36.5 °C and 37.5 °C (*I/C-LD*). Risks of hypothermia include intraventricular hemorrhage, hypoglycemia, or delayed recognition of sepsis. Hyperthermia should also be avoided (*III/C-EO*). In the OR, a thermal mattress or

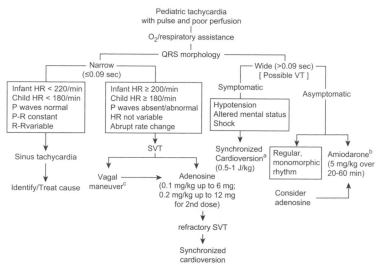

FIGURE 39.6 Algorithm for pediatric tachycardia with pulse and poor perfusion. HR, heart rate; SVT, supraventricular tachycardia; VT, ventricular tachycardia. [a]If not effective, increase to 2 J/kg. [b]Alternative to amiodarone is procainamide, 15 mg/kg over 30 to 60 minutes, but should not be given together and given with caution as can precipitate torsades. [c]Vagal stimulation should be attempted unless hemodynamically unstable or if it would delay medical or electrical cardioversion. Can be performed with ice applied to the face of infants/young children or carotid massage/Valsalva in older children.

warmed gases can be used in addition to the radiant warmer (*IIb/B-R*). It is unclear if there are risks with rapid rewarming (>0.5 °C/h) for newborns (*IIb, C-LD*).

Placement in the lateral Trendelenburg position with the head in a "sniffing" position helps to open the airway and allow secretions to drain. Routine suctioning of the oro/nasopharyngeal area is not recommended (meconium-stained *or* clear amniotic fluid) and should be reserved for babies with clear airway obstruction or who need positive-pressure ventilation (*IIB/C*). Suctioning the nasopharynx can induce bradycardia, reduce cerebral blow flow, and worsen pulmonary compliance. When necessary, clear the airway with a bulb syringe or suction catheter and use supplementary oxygen or bag-mask ventilation as needed. Drying and suctioning, however, usually provide adequate respiratory stimulation. Infants with meconium-stained amniotic fluid (vigorous or nonvigorous) are no longer routinely intubated for tracheal suctioning unless there are other reasons for intubation such as severe airway obstruction, slow heart rate or compromised breathing (*IIb/C-LD*).

Pulse oximetry is recommended during resuscitation to avoid hyperoxia, which has proved to be detrimental. Pulse oximetry (SpO_2) and heart rate are reliably measured 90 seconds after birth with a neonatal probe. Preductal values (right upper limb) are higher than postductal.

Oximetry should be used in conjunction with and not replace clinical assessment of heart rate.

2. **Ventilation.** Positive-pressure ventilation is initiated if the baby is apneic/gasping and if the heart rate is less than 100 beats/min with shorter or longer inspiratory times. The initial peak inspiratory pressure required for chest movement and increase in heart rate is variable. If airway pressure is monitored, an initial peak pressure of 20 cm of water may be required in preterm babies and higher pressures of 30 to 40 cm of water may be required in term babies (*IIb/C*). If airway pressures are not monitored, the minimal pressure required for heart rate response (increase) and chest rise should be used. In a preterm baby, excessive chest expansion could create lung injury. Assisted ventilation should be delivered at 40 to 60 breaths/min for a goal heart rate of above 100 (*IIb/C*).

PEEP at 5 cmH$_2$O has been shown to be beneficial and should be used if proper equipment is available for its delivery (*IIb/B-R*). Continuous positive airway pressure is recommended for preterm babies breathing spontaneously with difficulty, thus avoiding intubation (*IIb/B-R*). Endotracheal intubation is indicated in prolonged or ineffective bag-mask ventilation, during chest compression, and in special circumstances like a diaphragmatic hernia. Exhaled CO$_2$ monitoring should be used for confirmation of correct ETT placement including in very-low-birth weight neonates (*IIa/B*). An LMA can be considered as an alternative to an ETT (*IIb/B-R*) and is suggested for infants greater than 34 weeks gestation when ETT placement is unsuccessful (*I/C-EO*), although their efficacy during chest compressions is unclear.

Based on studies comparing air (21% O$_2$) and 100% oxygen for newborn resuscitation, air has been shown to have a higher survival rate and similar neurocognitive outcomes. Therefore, in term and late-preterm newborns air is most reasonable (*IIa/B-R*) and 100% O$_2$ should be avoided (*III/B-R*). From there, the F$_{IO_2}$ can be titrated to achieve the targeted range of preductal oxygen saturation (target SpO$_2$ table in **Figure 39.7**). If blended oxygen is unavailable, resuscitation should be started with air and if there is no improvement in 90 seconds, 100% oxygen should be used.

3. **Chest compressions** are indicated if the heart rate is **less than 60 beats/min** in spite of adequate ventilation with oxygen for 30 seconds. They should be delivered on the lower third of the sternum, and the chest should be compressed approximately one-third of its anterior-posterior depth (*IIb/C-LD*). Compressions and ventilations should be alternated and delivered while alternating at a 3:1 ratio, with 90 compressions and 30 breaths for approximately 120 events/min (*IIa/C-LD*). This 3:1 ratio reflects the predominant cardiopulmonary collapse secondary to poor gas exchange in infants, although if the arrest has a clear cardiac origin, a higher ratio such as 15:2 can be used (*IIb/C-EO*). There are two techniques, two thumb encircling hands and the two-finger with second hand on the back. The two thumb encircling hands is recommended as it generates higher pressures and is less exhausting to the provider (*IIb/C-LD*).

Frequent interruption of compressions should be avoided. Periodic assessment of ventilation, heart rate, and oxygenation should be done, and compressions are stopped when the spontaneous heart rate is greater than 60 beats/min. Whenever chest compressions are

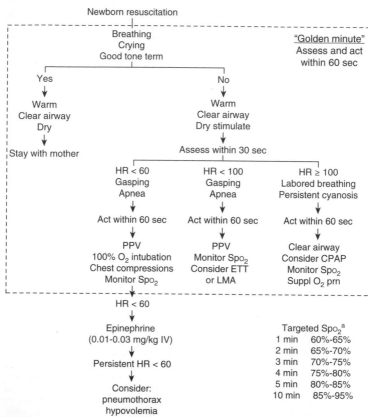

FIGURE 39.7 Algorithm for newborn resuscitation. HR, heart rate; PPV, positive pressure ventilation. [a]Target Spo$_2$ refers to preductal saturation (eg, right arm) as opposed to postductal (eg, feet). For access can place IV/IO but can consider umbilical venous catheter (UVC) placement as well.

provided, 100% O$_2$ is suggested (*IIa/C-EO*) but reduced as soon as possible (*I/C-LD*). CPR is continued until the heart rate is greater than 60 (*IIb/C*).

4. **Delivery of resuscitation drugs and fluids.** Resuscitation drugs should be administered when the heart rate remains below 60 beats/min despite adequate ventilation with 100% oxygen and chest compressions. The umbilical vein, the largest and thinnest of the three umbilical vessels, provides the best vascular access for resuscitation of the newborn. It is cannulated with a 3.5- to 5.0-French umbilical catheter after the umbilical cord stump has been prepped with an antiseptic and trimmed. Sterile umbilical tape placed at the base of the cord will prevent bleeding. The catheter should be placed below the skin level with blood aspirated freely, and care must be taken not to permit air into the system. If vascular access is unavailable, the ETT or IO access can be used to administer drugs.

5. **Medications and volume expansion**
   a. **Epinephrine.** The β-adrenergic effect of epinephrine increases the intrinsic heart rate during neonatal resuscitation. Epinephrine should be used for asystole and for heart rates less than 60 despite adequate oxygenation and chest compressions. The dose of 0.01 to 0.03 mg/kg per dose of a 1:10,000 solution is recommended intravenously (*IIb/C*). Higher IV doses are not recommended. If the drug is given via the endotracheal route, a dose of 0.05 to 0.1 mg/kg of 1:10,000 (0.1 mg/mL) should be considered.
   b. **Naloxone** is a specific opiate antagonist used for neonatal respiratory depression secondary to narcotics administered to the mother. The initial dose is 0.1 mg/kg. Naloxone is not recommended as part of the initial resuscitative efforts in newborns. Depressed respiration due to narcotics should be treated with assisted ventilation. Studies have shown misuse of naloxone in newborn and association of seizures following administration.
   c. **Sodium bicarbonate** is not recommended for newborn resuscitation unless specifically considered during prolonged arrests in an attempt to relieve depression of myocardial function and reduced action of catecholamines induced by marked acidemia. Intraventricular hemorrhage in premature infants has been associated with the osmotic load occurring with bicarbonate administration. A neonatal preparation of sodium bicarbonate (4.2% or 0.5 mEq/mL) should be used to prevent this from occurring. The initial dose is 1 mEq/kg IV given over 2 minutes. Subsequent doses of 0.5 mEq/kg may be given every 10 minutes and should be guided by arterial blood pH and $Paco_2$.
   d. **Atropine, calcium, and glucose** are not recommended for use in neonatal resuscitation unless specifically indicated.
   e. **Fluids.** Hypovolemia should be considered in the setting of peripartum hemorrhage, hypotension, weak pulses, and persistent pallor, despite adequate oxygenation and chest compressions. The fluid of choice for volume expansion in the delivery room is an isotonic crystalloid or blood (*IIb/C*). The volume infused should be 10 mL/kg and repeated as necessary. The administration of volume expanders too rapidly to premature infants has been associated with intraventricular hemorrhage (*IIa/C*).

6. **Post-resuscitation care.** After resuscitation, the baby should be in an environment where continuous monitoring and anticipatory care are provided. Maintenance of normothermia and normoglycemia is important in preventing any further injury to the brain. Therapeutic hypothermia should be offered to near-term babies with evolving moderate to severe hypoxic-ischemic encephalopathy. It should be conducted and initiated under clearly defined protocols in centers with facilities and capabilities of a multidisciplinary team.

7. **Guidelines for withholding and discontinuing resuscitation**
   a. It is considered reasonable to withhold resuscitative efforts when the conditions are known to be associated with high mortality and poor outcome especially with parental consent.
   b. The following guidelines should be interpreted according to current regional outcomes.
      1. Gestation (<23 weeks), birth weight (<400 g), and congenital anomalies (anencephaly, trisomy 13) associated with high mortality (*IIb/C*). Resuscitation is not generally indicated.

   2. High rate of survival and acceptable morbidity. Resuscitation is usually indicated. Includes gestational age >25 weeks and most congenital malformations (*IIb/C*).

   3. In conditions with an uncertain prognosis, borderline survival, high morbidity, and anticipated large burden to child, parental desires concerning initiation of resuscitation should be supported (*IIb/C*).

   E. Discontinuation of resuscitation is appropriate if no heart beat is detectable after 10 minutes of efficient resuscitation. The decision to continue after 10 minutes is influenced by presumed etiology of arrest, gestational age, potential reversibility of the situation, and parents' request.

Suggested Readings

Duff Jonathan P, Topjian Alexis A, Berg Marc D, et al. 2019 American Heart Association focused update on pediatric advanced life support: an update to the American Heart Association Guidelines for Cardiopulmonary Resuscitation and Emergency Cardiovascular Care. *Circulation.* 2019;140(24):e904-e914. doi:10.1161/CIR.0000000000000731

Panchal Ashish R, Berg Katherine M, Hirsch Karen G, et al. 2019 American Heart Association focused update on advanced cardiovascular life support: use of advanced airways, vasopressors, and extracorporeal cardiopulmonary resuscitation during cardiac arrest. An update to the American Heart Association guidelines for cardiopulmonary resuscitation and emergency cardiovascular care. *Circulation.* 2019;140(24):e881-e894. doi:10.1161/CIR.0000000000000732

Soar J, Maconochie I, Wyckoff MH, et al. 2019 International consensus on cardiopulmonary resuscitation and emergency cardiovascular care science with treatment recommendations. *Resuscitation.* 2019;145:95-150. doi:10.1016/j.resuscitation.2019.10.016

Vascular Access

Omar Hyder

I. OVERVIEW

Vascular access is necessary and tailored to the needs of the patient, procedure, and clinical setting. This chapter focuses on ultrasound guidance for peripheral intravenous (IV) and arterial access in short axis. Procedures for central venous and peripheral arterial access are discussed in Chapter 15—Monitoring.

II. APPLIED VASCULAR ANATOMY

A. Peripheral venous system

Preferred sites for ultrasound-guided IV placement in order of preference are the cephalic vein in the mid-to-distal forearm and the basilic vein in the upper arm. The cephalic vein runs a relatively consistent, linear, and superficial course through the anterolateral aspect of the forearm (**Figure 40.1**).

The basilic vein in the upper arm is a large and consistent vein. Risk of complications is higher because of its proximity to the brachial artery and nerves and undetected extravasation in deep tissues of the arm can occur.

Veins in antecubital fossa are ideal as a starting point for venous mapping but less preferable for cannulation because of venous confluences/branching, turns, changes in depth, and risk of inadvertent brachial arterial injury.

B. Peripheral arterial system

Distal radial, femoral, and axillary arterial cannulation can be performed for arterial line placement. Brachial artery has no collaterals and should be cannulated as last resort.

III. VASCULAR ACCESS DEVICES

A. Structure

Vascular access devices in anesthesia and critical care are typically a combination of needles, catheters, wires, and dilators.

B. IV catheters

The flow rate through an IV catheter depends on its diameter (Gauge; G) and length. They are available in sizes ranging from 26G to 14G and multiple lengths.

Sheath introducers and rapid infusion catheters (RICs) are large-bore intravenous access catheters placed percutaneously. They can be used for high flow fluid resuscitation. Hemodialysis catheters (Quinton) allow high flow rates and can be used for resuscitation in an emergency.

Table 40.1 shows the flow rates of commonly used sizes and lengths of IV catheters and access devices. Users are advised to review the device's packaging for flow rates.

IV. PRINCIPLES OF IMAGE-GUIDED VASCULAR ACCESS

A. Ultrasound basics relevant to vascular access

1. **Linear array probe:** High-frequency probes are ideal for imaging superficial structures such as veins and arteries in extremities. Use presets for vascular access on silicon-chip–based whole-body ultrasound systems (Butterfly IQ, Butterfly Network, Inc, Guilford, CT).

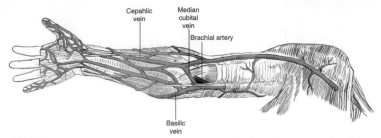

FIGURE 40.1 Venous anatomy of the upper extremity. Area highlighted in green is preferred site for ultrasound-guided IV placement. (Courtesy of Osman Hyder, MFA and redrawn from Lewis WH. *Anatomy of the Human Body.* 20th ed. Lea and Fabiger; 1918.)

2. **Depth setting:** Adjust depth setting to place the vessel of interest in the middle of the screen.
3. **Gain:** Use higher gain to distinguish between dark lumen and lighter walls of the vein and surrounding structures (blood is hypoechoic).
4. **Imaging the bevel:** Flat solid structures held perpendicular to ultrasound beam will reflect acoustic beams directly back at the probe and show brightest (hyperechoic) compared to surrounding structures. Bevel of the needle is the only relatively flat structure in cross section; therefore, it is the ideal target to guide vascular access.

TABLE 40.1 Maximal Flow Rates of Common Venous Access Catheters

Size	Length (mm)	Flow Rate (mL/min)
26G*	14	14
24G†	19	22
22G†	25	35
20G†	32	60
18G†	45	100
16G†	50	210
14G†	50	345
7-Fr triple lumen distal 16G port‡	160	56
MAC proximal 12G (no catheter)‡	100	216
Dual lumen dialysis line (12 Fr)§	200	400
9-Fr PSI/MAC distal lumen (no catheter)‡	100	550
8.5-Fr RIC‖	64	600

MAC, multi-lumen access catheter; PSI, percutaneous sheath introducer; RIC, rapid infusion catheter.
List not exhaustive. Consult manufacturer's information specific to the device.
Data from Manufacturer's product information (*ICU Medical Inc, San Clemente, CA; †B. Braun Medical Inc, Allentown, PA; ‡Arrow International Inc, Reading, PA; §Covidien LLC, Mansfield, MA). ‖ASA 2008 abstract A1484.

5. Further discussion showcases real-time ultrasound-guided peripheral IV placement with a focus on the bevel. Similar concepts apply to ultrasound guidance for arterial and central lines.

B. Explanation of procedure

1. Scanning technique

Apply tourniquet on upper arm. Sterile probe cover is recommended. Apply sterile gel to probe. Quickly map ventral forearm venous anatomy starting from the antecubital fossa and scanning down toward the wrist. Keep the vessel in the middle of the screen. Veins are easily compressible without pulsation.

2. Evaluation of vessel structure and choice of puncture site

Larger, thin walled, superficial vessels with a straighter course are easier to cannulate than smaller, thick-walled ones with turns and branching. Identify a 5-cm or longer linear segment.

Preferred location for ultrasound-guided IV is cephalic vein in the middle half of the forearm (**Figure 40.1**). IVs placed close to joints are more likely to be "positional."

3. Setup

Skin disinfectant, syringe of local anesthetic with a 27G or 30G needle, IV in the plastic sheath, gauze, securement materials. Clean off ultrasound gel; vigorously disinfect skin at and around the planned needle entry site.

4. Local infiltration

Vessels accessed with ultrasound guidance may be deep—local anesthetic infiltration is highly recommended. Place the probe over the planned vein entry site. Enter the skin in-line with center marker, 5 to 10 mm away from the probe if using a linear probe, directly under the probe if using a whole-body probe (wider footprint). Use an approximate middle of the probe if there is no center marker. Infiltrate down to the vein.

5. Insertion steps (⊙ Video 40.1)

a. Hold needle hub between thumb and index finger. Insert IV needle at infiltration site with bevel facing up. The shaft should be at angle of 15° to 30° with skin—deeper veins require a steeper angle.

b. Stop advancing as soon as the whole bevel disappears below the skin.

c. Tilt the probe away from the catheter entry site to make the beam approximately perpendicular to the plane of the bevel, slide toward the IV, and sonographically locate the bevel under the skin (**Figure 40.2** left panel).

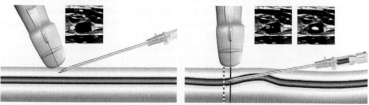

FIGURE 40.2 Technical considerations in positioning the probe and needle and representative ultrasound images. Left panel: Tilting the ultrasound probe to visualize the bevel (solid red arrow) above the cephalic vein (yellow arrow). Right panel: Sliding the ultrasound probe to visualize the bevel (solid red arrow) and tip of the needle (interrupted red arrow).

d. Smallest observable part of the bevel is the tip when probe is slid away from the IV. Ensure the bevel is above the center of the vessel. If not, adjust location of the tip with sideways movements of the hub.

e. When in correct position, advance the angiocath needle forward by 1 to 2 mm. Find the tip again using ultrasound. Keep the probe perpendicular to the angle of the bevel. Repeat this process until the tip of the bevel is directly over the top of the vein. Introduce it into the lumen with a short "jabbing" motion. Slow, gentle attempts at advancement through the vessel wall can redirect the tip off center—IV needles are dull by design to avoid back-walling during blind placement.

f. Stop advancing the apparatus as soon as the tip of the bevel is recognized within the vessel lumen.

g. Position the ultrasound probe upright, perpendicular to the skin to ensure visualization of the vessel lumen in perfect cross section. The body of the bevel is seen as a bright white object in the lumen against a dark background.

h. With the tip in real-time view on the ultrasound screen, adjust the angle of the shaft. Manipulate the hub to ensure that tip of the bevel is just cephalad to the center of the vessel.

i. Advance the IV about 2 mm until the body of the bevel is visualized as an enlarging, bright dot. Stop where it is brightest. Locate the tip of the bevel by sliding the probe away from the IV. Position the tip in the optimal position. Advance the IV apparatus in the vessel lumen until full view of bevel is obtained. Repeat the process until at least one-half to three-fourths of the catheter is inside the vein (**Figure 40.2** right panel).

j. For deployment, hold the hub between the thumb and the middle finger, visualize and center the tip in the vessel lumen, pull back slightly (~2-3 mm) on the needle hub to pull the sharp bevel inside the catheter. Advance the catheter fully into the vein. Pull needle out. Attach IV tubing and flush to verify free flow.

k. Thoroughly clean ultrasound contact gel from around the IV site. Apply occlusive dressing.

6. **Arterial line placement using the 4-Fr Micropuncture kit**

a. Radial artery is a small ultrasound target: ~2.4 mm in diameter with lumen as small as 0.5 to 1 mm.

b. For difficult arterial lines, Seldinger technique using real-time ultrasound guidance is recommended. A commonly used 4-Fr kit (Micropuncture Access Kit, Cook Medical, Bloomington, IN) has a 21G thin-wall needle that provides two points of confirmation of intra-arterial presence of its tip (ultrasound visualization of bevel and uninterrupted blood flow back from the hub). The platinum- or palladium-tipped wire is specialized for vascular access.

c. The procedure for real-time ultrasound guidance for needle puncture is like that described for ultrasound IV placement. After initially obtaining blood flow back, the tip should be advanced in the lumen by about 2 to 3 mm under real-time ultrasound guidance to anchor the thin-wall needle inside the artery; wire is threaded through the needle, which is then removed over the wire; 4-Fr catheter preloaded over dilator is threaded over wire into the vessel; the dilator is unscrewed from the catheter; both dilator and wire are removed together.

d. Radial arteries may contain clot or dissection flaps after repeated punctures. Compress along the whole sonographically visible length to ensure there is no clot at or proximal to intended puncture site.

e. Occasionally, upon first entry into the vessel lumen, the needle tip is clearly identified in the center of the vessel but no blood flows back through the hollow bore needle. This is likely because the bevel is dissecting subintimally. Advance the needle with meticulous attention to keeping the tip in the middle of the vessel with real-time ultrasound guidance until blood flow back is observed. This indicates location in the true lumen of the vessel.

V. COMMON ISSUES AND TROUBLESHOOTING

A. Site selection

Vessels deeper than 1.6 cm may be more challenging to cannulate because of difficulty in accurately visualizing the tip with increasing depth.

B. Catheter size

Novice operators should use 18G and larger catheters that are at least 1.5 inches long. Large bevels are easier to visualize. Longer length provides a margin of safety against an inadequate length of catheter in the vein.

C. Verifying IV location in vein

Inject agitated saline and observe it passing through the basilic system on ultrasound.

D. No reasonable venous targets in the forearm

Scan contralateral forearm. Use basilic or median cubital vein as a backup site. An experienced operator is preferred if upper arm basilic vein is being accessed.

Ultrasound-guided saphenous vein IV placement is complicated by superficial location and proximity to the bony prominence of medial malleolus, which limits "working space." External jugular vein can also be cannulated with real-time ultrasound guidance.

E. "Chasing" the vein

Insufficient length of catheter in vein occurs when the vessel lumen is entered far from skin entry site. These IVs are prone to displacement and extravasation with patient movement and arm manipulation that can result in compartment syndrome. Use the longest available IV catheters and abandon the attempt if vein entry does not occur within <15 mm from skin entry.

F. "Arterialized" veins

Veins with the visual appearance of an artery—small diameter, completely round, thick walled—spasm, extravasate quickly, and become obscured (isoechoic). They are associated with difficult ultrasound-guided IV placement. Meticulous attention to visualizing the bevel usually leads to first pass success.

G. "Wiring" IVs into peripheral veins

Use of wires should be restricted to arterial and central line placements. Most wires can easily tunnel subintimally and create a false passage in a small peripheral vein. This practice carries significant risk of unrecognized infiltration.

Suggested Readings

Blanco P. Ultrasound-guided peripheral venous cannulation in critically ill patients: a practical guideline. *Ultrasound J.* 2019;11:27.

Gottlieb M, Sundaram T, Holladay D, Nakitende D. Ultrasound-guided peripheral line placement: a narrative review of evidence based best practices. *West J Emerg Med.* 2017;18:1047-1054.

Drugs With Narrow Therapeutic Ranges and Potential for Harm

Richard M. Pino

Anesthetists frequently administer intravenous (IV) medications with narrow therapeutic windows and the potential for critical events. The drugs described in this section list agents that are not routinely administered by anesthetists but may be requested by others. It does not include agents that fall within the scope of the training and practice of anesthetists, for example, neuromuscular blockers.

A. Abciximab (ReoPro): Glycoprotein IIb/IIIa inhibitor preventing platelet adhesion and aggregation.

    1. Indications: Prevent thrombus formation peri–percutaneous transluminal coronary angioplasty (PTCA) and poststent placement.

    2. Administration guidelines

        a. Standard concentration: 9 mg/250 mL 0.9% sodium chloride.

        b. The IV tubing must have a filter on it (0.2- or 0.22-μm low–protein-binding filter) and no other medications should be piggybacked through this line.

        c. Loading dose (straight drug): 0.25 mg/kg administered 10 to 60 minutes prior to percutaneous coronary intervention (PCI). Withdraw through the 0.2- or 0.22-μm low–protein-binding filter the appropriate amount of abciximab for the patient's weight. Hypotension may occur with bolus dose.

        d. Maintenance at a rate of 0.125 μg/kg/min to a maximum of 10 μg/min (17 mL/h) for 12 hours. To prepare, withdraw 4.5 mL (9 mg) of abciximab through 0.2- or 0.22-μm low–protein-binding filter and inject into a 250-mL bag of 0.9% sodium chloride.

B. Alprostadil (prostaglandin E1 [PGE_1]): Vasodilator; decreases peripheral resistance, which causes reflexive increase in cardiac output and heart rate.

    1. Indications:

        a. Primary nonfunctional liver transplant characterized by rising transaminases, minimal bile production, and coagulopathy within 4 to 34 hours after transplantation.

        b. Pulmonary hypertension.

        c. Distal ischemia (limb or digit) refractory to conventional revascularization or drug therapy.

        d. Vasospastic disorders (Raynaud disease), vasculitis, Buerger disease, atheroembolic diseases.

        e. Protection against tacrolimus nephrotoxicity.

    2. Administration guidelines:

        a. Standard concentration: 500 μg of alprostadil in 1,000 mL NS (1 μg = 1,000 ng).

        b. Infusion rates should be titrated to patient response.

        1. Remove rings/tight-fitting jewelry during the infusion since most patients experience extremity swelling. Patients often experience a "flushing" feeling during the initiation that is not necessarily an indication to stop the infusion, unless there is a drop in blood pressure (BP).

    2. Start the infusion at 1 ng/kg/min. If the patient becomes hypotensive, wean back to the previous dose. A starting dose of 0.4 ng/kg/min is recommended for patient with borderline low BP and/or poor left ventricular (LV) function.

    3. The infusion rate (dose) may be doubled every 30 minutes as tolerated to a peak dose of 16 ng/kg/min.

C. Alteplase (Activase): Tissue plasminogen activator (tPA)

  1. Indications:

    a. Acute myocardial infarction.

    b. Pulmonary embolism.

    c. Peripheral arterial or venous thrombosis.

    d. Catheter occlusion.

  2. Administration guidelines:

    a. Acute myocardial infarction

      1. Standard concentration: 100 mg/100 mL.

      2. Patient weight less than 67 kg: 15-mg bolus; then 0.75 mg/kg (maximum 50 mg) over 30 minutes. Initiate **heparin** therapy with a bolus; then 0.5 mg/kg (maximum 35 mg) over the next hour.

      3. Patient weight greater than 67 kg: 15-mg bolus; then 50 mg over the next 30 minutes. Institute heparin therapy with a bolus. Infuse remaining 35 mg of tPA over the next hour (total dose of tPA = 100 mg).

    b. Pulmonary embolus:

      1. Standard concentration: 100 mg/100 mL.

      2. Maintenance infusion: 100 mg continuous infusion over 2 hours.

    c. Peripheral arterial or venous thrombosis

      1. Standard concentration: 50 mg/500 mL, 25 mg/250 mL.

      2. Loading dose: none.

      3. Maintenance infusion: 0.5 to 4 mg/h for 24 hours (recommended maximum 50 mg/24 h). Heparin (no loading dose) should be started after alteplase infusion is completed to maintain activated partial thromboplastin time (aPTT) in a therapeutic range.

    d. Venous and arterial thrombosis catheter-directed thrombolysis

      1. Standard concentration: 50 mg/500 mL, 25 mg/250 mL.

      2. Loading dose: 4 to 10 mg.

      3. Maintenance infusion: 0.5 to 4 mg/h for 4 to 24 hours IV. Recommended cumulative maximum of 50 mg (load plus infusion). Heparin should be used at a low non–weight-adjusted dose (eg, 250 units/h) keeping aPTT less than 1.5 times baseline during alteplase infusion.

D. Argatroban: Direct thrombin inhibitor

  1. Indications:

    a. Anticoagulation in patients with suspected or confirmed heparin-induced thrombocytopenia (HIT type II).

    b. Anticoagulation during and immediately following PCIs.

  2. Administration guidelines

    a. Standard concentration (1 mg/mL): 50 mg/50 mL premixed vial in NaCl for large volume infusion pump.

    b. Low concentration (0.05 mg/mL): 2.5 mg/50 mL bag.

    c. Microinfusion: 2.5 mg/50 mL syringe.

    d. Bolus: None.

    e. Maintenance:

      1. Start 0.5 to 2 μg/kg/min as a continuous infusion.

      2. Reduce initial dose to 0.5 μg/kg/min for hepatic and/or renal dysfunction, and critically ill.

    3. Check the partial thromboplastin time (PTT) 2 hours after the start of the infusion and after any rate change until stable (ie, two consecutive values within the goal range). Goal: aPTT 1.5 to 3× baseline not to exceed a PTT of 100 seconds.

    4. When activated clotting time (ACT) is greater than 450 seconds, reduce maintenance to 15 µg/kg/min and recheck in 5 to 10 minutes.

E. Bivalirudin (Angiomax): Direct thrombin inhibitor

    1. Indication: Anticoagulation in patients with strongly suspected or confirmed HIT (type II).

    2. Administration guidelines

      a. Standard concentration (5 mg/mL): 250 mg/50 mL bag.

      b. Low concentration (1 mg/mL): 100 mg/100 mL bag (low concentration).

      c. Microinfusion: 250 mg/50 mL syringe.

      d. Bolus: None.

      e. Maintenance

      1. Starting dose: 0.15 mg/kg/h (CrCl > 60 mL/min).

      2. If CrCl 30 to 60 mL/min: 0.05 mg/kg/h.

      3. If CrCl less than 30 mL/min or renal replacement therapy: 0.025 mg/kg/h.

      4. Goal aPTT: 1.5 to 2.5 times baseline. Check the PTT 2 hours after the start of the infusion and after any rate change until two consecutive PTT values are within the goal range.

F. Cangrelor: Antiplatelet agent. It is a direct $P2Y_{12}$ platelet-receptor inhibitor that blocks adenosine diphosphate (ADP)–induced platelet activation and aggregation.

    1. Indication: Use in PCI to reduce risk of myocardial infarction (MI), repeat coronary revascularization, and stent thrombosis for patients not previously treated with $P2Y_{12}$ inhibitor or glycoprotein IIb/IIIa inhibitor.

    2. Administration guidelines

      a. Bolus: 30 µg/kg. Administer over 1 min (<100 kg); 2 min (100-200 kg); or 3 min (>300 kg)

      b. Starting rate: 4 µg/kg/min

G. Epoprostenol sodium (Flolan): Potent vasodilator that also inhibits platelet aggregation.

    1. Indication: Pulmonary hypertension.

    2. Administration guidelines

      a. Do not give with other parenteral medications or carriers.

      b. A dedicated central venous catheter is required for administration with an air-eliminating filter.

      c. Do not flush catheter with epoprostenol in-line.

      d. Bolus: None.

      e. Maintenance infusion:

      1. Initial dose: 1 to 2 ng/kg/min IV.

      2. Titrate in 1 to 2 ng/kg/min increments every 15 to 30 minutes.

      f. If catheter needs to be flushed, withdraw 3 mL of fluid/blood from the catheter into a syringe and discard. The line should be primed with epoprostenol-specific diluent only.

      g. Avoid abrupt withdrawal that may cause rebound pulmonary artery hypertension.

      h. Syringe is only stable for 8 hours at room temperature.

H. Eptifibatide (Integrilin)

    1. Indication: Prevention of thrombus formation after PCI.

    2. Dosage: Bolus (180 µg/kg); then 2 µg/kg/min continuous infusion.

3. **Effect:** Inhibits glycoprotein IIb/IIIa; prevents platelet adhesion and aggregation.
4. **Comments:** Bleeding complications and thrombocytopenia are common side effects.

I. **Insulin, regular (human):** Humulin R, Novolin R
   1. **Indications:** Hyperglycemia, hyperkalemia, diabetic ketoacidosis.
   2. **Administration guidelines:**
      a. Regular insulin is the only insulin that can be administered intravenously.
      b. Insert infusion into y-site below any inline filters.
      c. Standard concentration for microinfusion: 50 units/50 mL normal saline.
      d. Loading dose: 5 to 20 units intravenous push (IVP) or bolus (usually given prior to starting maintenance).
      e. Maintenance infusion: 2 to 25 units/h IV titrated according to blood glucose level.
      f. Once under control, blood glucose should be monitored at a minimum of every 2 hours and more often as needed.

J. **Potassium chloride (KCl)**
   1. **Indication:** Correction of hypokalemia.
      a. **Caution: Hypokalemia is not usually treated in the operating room (OR).**
      b. The decision to administer KCl requires **anesthesia attending approval** in advance of administration.
   2. **Administration guidelines:**
      a. **Bolus dose: None. May cause cardiac arrest.**
      b. Peripheral concentration: 80 mEq/1,000 mL.
      c. Central concentration: 20 mEq/100 mL; 40 mEq/100 mL.
      d. Rate: Not to exceed 20 mEq/h.

Commonly Used Drugs

The drugs listed in this section are those that are commonly used or encountered by anesthetists during perioperative patient care. Anesthetics and muscle relaxants are not included and are covered in respective chapters.

I. ABCIXIMAB (REOPRO) (SEE APPENDIX I)

II. ADENOSINE
A. **Indications**: Paroxysmal supraventricular tachycardia.
B. **Dosage**: Adult: 6- to 12-mg peripheral intravenous (IV) bolus followed by rapid 20-mL saline IV flush. Central line: initial dose, 3 mg. Pediatric: 50 μg/kg IV.
C. **Effect**: Slows or temporarily blocks atrioventricular (AV) node conduction and conduction through reentrant pathways (especially those involving the AV node).
D. **Comments**:
1. Contraindicated in patients with second- or third-degree heart block or sick sinus syndrome.
2. Not effective in terminating atrial flutter or fibrillation but may aid in diagnosis by slowing ventricular response.
3. Asystole for 3 to 6 seconds after administration is common and resolves spontaneously.
4. May cause bronchospasm or hypotension.
5. Use with caution in patients with preexcitation syndromes (eg, Wolff-Parkinson-White).

III. ALBUTEROL
A. **Indications**: Bronchospasm.
B. **Dosage**: Aerosolized: 2.5 mg in 3 mL saline via nebulizer; 180 or 200 μg (two puffs) via metered dose inhaler (MDI). By mouth (PO): 2.5 mg. Pediatric: 0.1 mg/kg (syrup 2 mg/5 mL).
C. **Effect**: β_2-Receptor agonist, causing bronchial smooth muscle relaxation.
D. **Comments**: Possible β-adrenergic overload, tachydysrhythmias. Increased dose required when using MDI for intubated patients (four to six puffs).

IV. ALPROSTADIL (SEE APPENDIX I)

V. ALTEPLASE (SEE APPENDIX I)

VI. AMINOCAPROIC ACID (AMICAR)
A. **Indications**: Prevention of bleeding due to fibrinolysis.
B. **Dosage**: 5 g/100 to 250 mL of normal saline (NS) IV to load, followed by 1 g/h infusion.
C. **Effect**: Stabilizes the formed clot by inhibiting plasminogen activators and plasmin.
D. **Comments**: Contraindicated in disseminated intravascular coagulation.

VII. AMIODARONE

A. Indications: Refractory or recurrent atrial and ventricular tachydysrhythmias.

B. Dosage: 150 mg for Advanced Cardiac Life Support algorithm (ACLS 300 mg) intravenous push (IVP), then 1 mg/min for 6 hours (360 mg), then 0.5 mg/min for 18 hours (540 mg).

C. Effect: Depresses the sinoatrial node and prolongs the PR, QRS, and QT intervals; produces α- and β-adrenergic blockade.

D. Comments:

1. May cause severe sinus bradycardia, ventricular arrhythmias, AV block, liver and thyroid function test abnormalities, hepatitis, and cirrhosis.

2. Pulmonary fibrosis can result from long-term use.

3. Increases serum levels of digoxin, oral anticoagulants, diltiazem, quinidine, procainamide, and phenytoin.

VIII. ARGATROBAN (SEE APPENDIX I)

IX. ATENOLOL

A. Indications: Hypertension, angina, and postmyocardial infarction (post-MI).

B. Dosage: Oral (PO) 50 to 100 mg/d. IV: 5 mg as needed (prn).

C. Effect: β_1-Selective adrenergic receptor blockade.

D. Comments:

1. Relatively contraindicated in acute congestive heart failure and heart block.

2. Caution in patients on calcium channel blockers and other agents prolonging AV conduction.

X. ATROPINE

A. Indications: Antisialagogue; bradycardia; cardiac arrest (ACLS protocol).

B. Dosage:

1. Antisialagogue, adult, 0.2 to 0.4 mg IV; 0.4 to 1.0 mg IV; pediatric, 0.01 mg/kg/dose IV/intramuscular (IM) (<0.4 mg).

2. Bradycardia, adult, 0.2 to 0.4 mg IV; pediatric, 0.02 mg/kg/dose IV (<0.4 mg).

3. Cardiac arrest, adult, 1 mg IV; pediatric, 0.01 to 0.02 mg/kg/dose IV.

C. Effect: Competitive blockade of acetylcholine at muscarinic receptors.

D. Comments:

1. Low doses may cause paradoxical bradycardia.

2. May cause tachydysrhythmias, AV dissociation, premature ventricular contractions, dry mouth, or urinary retention.

3. Central nervous system (CNS) effects occur at high doses.

XI. BICARBONATE, SODIUM (NAHCO$_3$)

A. Indications: Metabolic acidosis; urinary alkalinization.

B. Dosage: IV dose in mEq $NaHCO_3$ = (base deficit × weight [kg] × 0.3) (subsequent doses titrated against patient's pH).

C. Effect: H^+ neutralization.

D. Comments:

1. Not compatible with many IV medications.

2. May cause metabolic alkalosis, hypercarbia, and hyperosmolality.

3. In neonates, can cause intraventricular hemorrhage.

4. Crosses placenta.
5. An 8.4% solution is approximately 1.0 mEq/mL; a 4.2% solution is approximately 0.5 mEq/mL.

XII. BIVALIRUDIN (SEE APPENDIX I)

XIII. CALCIUM CHLORIDE; CALCIUM GLUCONATE
A. **Indications:** hypocalcemia, hyperkalemia, and hypermagnesemia.
B. **Dosage:**
   1. Calcium chloride: 5 to 10 mg/kg IV prn (10% $CaCl_2$ = 1.36 mEq Ca^{2+}/mL).
   2. Calcium gluconate: 15 to 30 mg/kg IV prn (10% calcium gluconate = 0.45 mEq Ca^{2+}/mL).
C. **Effect:** Maintains cell membrane integrity, muscular excitation-contraction coupling, glandular stimulation-secretion coupling, and enzyme function. Increases blood pressure.
D. **Comments:**
   1. May cause bradycardia or arrhythmia (especially with digitalis).
   2. Irritating to veins. Ca^{2+} less available with calcium gluconate than with calcium chloride owing to binding of gluconate.
   3. Rapid infusion may cause coronary vasoconstriction.

XIV. CARBOPROST (PROSTAGLANDIN F_{2a}; HEMABATE)
A. **Indications:** Refractory postpartum hemorrhage.
B. **Dosage:** 250 μg IM; may repeat every (q)15-90 min, maximum total dose 2 mg.
C. **Effect:** Causes uterine muscle contraction.
D. **Comments:** May cause significant bronchospasm, especially in patients with reactive airways, or hypertension.

XV. CLEVIDIPINE (CLEVIPREX)
A. **Indications:** Treatment of acute hypertension when oral therapy is undesirable/unavailable.
B. **Dosage:** IV infusion: 1 to 2 mg/h; double the dose q90 seconds until approaching goal, then adjust q5-10 minutes. Maximum dose 32 mg/h.
C. **Effect:**
   1. Dihydropyridine calcium channel blocker; causes blood pressure reduction ± reflex tachycardia via decreased systemic vascular resistance.
   2. May have negative inotropic effects. Does not affect preload.
   3. No dose adjustments for hepatic/renal dysfunction.
D. **Effect:** Lasts 5 to 15 minutes after discontinuation.
E. **Comments:**
   1. Rapidly titratable. In lipid emulsion.
   2. Discard unused portion after 4 hours.
   3. Contraindicated in soy/egg allergic patients, defective lipid metabolism, or severe aortic stenosis.
   4. Risk of rebound hypertension with prolonged infusion; risk of atrial fibrillation.

XVI. CLOPIDOGREL (PLAVIX)
A. **Indications:** Antiplatelet agent.
   1. Acute coronary syndrome.
   2. Percutaneous coronary intervention (PCI).

3. Recent myocardial infarction (MI), recent thromboembolic stroke, or established arterial disease.
4. Coronary stent stenosis prophylaxis.

B. **Dosage:** Load, 300 to 600 mg PO; maintenance, 75 mg every day (qd).

C. **Effect:** Irreversible platelet ADP receptor blockade.

D. **Comments:**
1. Major side effect is bleeding.
2. Reduce dose in hepatic insufficiency.
3. Proton pump inhibitors may reduce clopidogrel efficacy.
4. Recommend discontinuing 7 days prior to neuraxial anesthesia.

XVII. DALTEPARIN (FRAGMIN)

A. **Indications:** Prophylaxis of acute coronary syndromes (ACSs), deep venous thrombosis (DVT).

B. **Dosage:**
1. DVT prophylaxis, 2500 to 5000 units subcutaneously (SC) qd.
2. ACS, 120 units/kg (maximum dose 10,000 units) SC q12h × 5 to 8 days with concurrent aspirin therapy.
3. DVT, 100 units/kg SC twice a day (bid) or 200 units/kg SC qd.

C. **Effect:** Anticoagulant; inhibits both factor Xa and factor IIa. See Heparin.

D. **Comments:**
1. Reduce dose for Cr clearance less than 30 mL/min.
2. Equally effective as unfractionated heparin; more predictable dose-response characteristics.
3. Spinal and epidural hematomas have been associated with spinals/lumbar punctures, or epidural catheter placement or removal. Use with caution when placing or removing neuraxial blockade in patients on Fragmin.
4. Only partially reversed by protamine.

XVIII. DANTROLENE

A. **Indications:** Malignant hyperthermia (MH); neuroleptic malignant syndrome.

B. **Dosage:** Mix 20 mg in 60 mL of sterile water. At first signs of MH, 2.5-mg/kg IV bolus; repeat dose, up to 10 mg/kg. Prophylactic IV treatment is not recommended.

C. **Effect:** Reduces Ca^{2+} release from sarcoplasmic reticulum; relaxes skeletal muscles.

D. **Comments:** Dissolves slowly into solution. Avoid extravasation as it is a tissue irritant.

XIX. DESMOPRESSIN ACETATE (DDAVP)

A. **Indications:**
1. Treatment of coagulopathy in von Willebrand disease, hemophilia A (but contraindicated if factor VIII > 5% activity), renal failure.
2. Central diabetes insipidus.

B. **Dosage:** Coagulopathy, 0.3 µg/kg IV (diluted 50 mL NS), infused over 15 to 30 minutes. Central DI, 5 to 20 µg intranasally qd/bid.

C. **Effect:** Increases plasma levels of factor VIII activity by causing release of von Willebrand factor from endothelial cells; increases renal water reabsorption (antidiuretic hormone [ADH] effect).

D. **Comments:** Chlorpropamide, carbamazepine, and clofibrate potentiate the antidiuretic effect. Repeat doses q12-24h will have diminished effect compared with initial dose. Has no vasopressor effect.

XX. DEXAMETHASONE (DECADRON)
- **A. Indications:** Cerebral edema; airway edema; prophylaxis of postoperative nausea and vomiting.
- **B. Dosage:**
    1. Edema: 10 mg IV, 4 mg IV q6h (tapered over 6 days).
    2. N/V: 4 mg IV.
- **C. Effect:** See Hydrocortisone. Has 20 to 25 times the glucocorticoid potency of hydrocortisone. Minimal mineralocorticoid effect.
- **D. Comments:** See Hydrocortisone.

XXI. DEXTRAN 40 (RHEOMACRODEX)
- **A. Indications:** Inhibition of platelet aggregation and improvement of blood flow in low-flow states (eg, vascular surgery).
- **B. Dosage:** 15 to 30 mL/h IV (10% solution); a load of 30 to 50 mL IV over 30 minutes is optional.
- **C. Effect:** Immediate, short-lived (1.5 hours) plasma volume expansion; decreases platelet adhesion.
- **D. Comments:** May cause volume overload, anaphylaxis, bleeding tendency, thrombocytopenia, interference with blood cross-matching, or false elevation of blood sugar.

XXII. DILTIAZEM (CARDIZEM)
- **A. Indications:** Angina pectoris, variant angina from coronary artery spasm, atrial fibrillation/flutter, paroxysmal supraventricular tachycardia, hypertension.
- **B. Dosage:** 20-mg IV bolus then 10-mg/h infusion; PO 30 to 60 mg q6h.
- **C. Effect:** Calcium channel antagonist that slows conduction through sinoatrial and AV nodes, dilates coronary and peripheral arterioles, and reduces myocardial contractility.
- **D. Comments:**
    1. May cause bradycardia and heart block.
    2. Possible impairment of contractility by interaction with β-blockers and digoxin.
    3. Causes transiently elevated liver function tests.
    4. Avoid use in patients with accessory conduction tracts, AV block, IV β-blockers, or ventricular tachycardia.

XXIII. DOBUTAMINE
- **A. Indications:** Inotropy for heart failure.
- **B. Dosage:** Begin infusion at 2 µg/kg/min and titrate to effect.
- **C. Effect:** β_1-Adrenergic agonist.
- **D. Comments:** May cause hypotension, arrhythmias, or myocardial ischemia. Can increase ventricular rate in atrial fibrillation.

XXIV. DOPAMINE
- **A. Indications:** Hypotension, heart failure.
- **B. Dosage:** 5 to 20 µg/kg/min IV titrate to effect.
- **C. Effect:** dopaminergic; α- and β-adrenergic agonist.
- **D. Comments:**
    1. May cause hypertension, dysrhythmias, or myocardial ischemia.
    2. Primarily dopaminergic effects (increased renal blood flow) at 1 to 5 µg/kg/min.
    3. Primarily α- and β-adrenergic effects at greater than or equal to 10 µg/kg/min.

XXV. ENOXAPARIN (LOVENOX)
A. Indications:
1. Prophylaxis of DVT.
2. Treatment of DVT.
3. Acute coronary syndromes.
B. Dosage:
1. DVT prophylaxis, 30 mg SC bid or 40 mg SC qd.
2. DVT treatment, 1 mg/kg SC q12h or 1.5 mg/kg SC qd.
3. ACS, 1 mg/kg SC bid for a minimum of 2 days, in conjunction with aspirin therapy.
C. Effect: Anticoagulant; inhibits both factor Xa and factor IIa. See Heparin.
D. Comments:
1. Equally effective as unfractionated heparin with more predictable dose-response characteristics.
2. Spinal and epidural hematomas have been associated with spinals/lumbar punctures, or epidural catheter placement or removal.
3. Only partially reversed by protamine.

XXVI. EPHEDRINE
A. Indication: Treatment of hypotension.
B. Dosage: 5 to 10 mg IV.
C. Effect: α- and β-adrenergic stimulation; norepinephrine release at sympathetic nerve endings.
D. Comments:
1. May cause hypertension, dysrhythmias, myocardial ischemia, CNS stimulation, decrease in uterine activity, and mild bronchodilation.
2. Minimal effect on uterine blood flow. Crosses the placenta.
3. Avoid in patients taking monoamine oxidase inhibitors (MAOI).
4. Tachyphylaxis with repeated dosing.

XXVII. EPINEPHRINE
A. Indications:
1. Heart failure.
2. Cardiac arrest (ACLS).
3. Bronchospasm, anaphylaxis.
4. Airway edema.
B. Dosage:
1. Heart failure, 1 to 12 µg/min titrated to effect.
2. ACLS, 0.1 to 1 mg IV or 1 mg intratracheal q5min prn. Pediatric, 0.01 mg/kg IV up to 0.5 mg. 0.01 mg/kg SC q15min × 2 doses up to 1 mg/dose.
3. Bronchospasm, anaphylaxis, 0.1 to 0.5 mg SC, 0.1 to 0.25 mg IV, or 0.25 to 1.5 µg/min IV infusion.
4. Airway edema, nebulized: 0.5 mL of 2.25% solution in 2.5 to 3.5 mL of NS q1-4h prn.
C. Effect: α- and β-adrenergic agonist.
D. Comments: May cause hypertension, arrhythmias, or myocardial ischemia. Topical or local injection (1:80,000-1:500,000) causes vasoconstriction. Crosses the placenta.

XXVIII. EPOPROSTENOL (FLOLAN) (SEE APPENDIX I)

XXIX. EPTIFIBATIDE (INTEGRILIN) (SEE APPENDIX I)

XXX. ERGONOVINE (ERGOTRATE) (SEE ALSO METHYLERGONOVINE)

A. Indication: Postpartum hemorrhage due to uterine atony.

B. Dosage: For postpartum hemorrhage: IV (emergency only), 0.2 mg in 5 mL of NS greater than or equal to 1 minute; IM, 0.2 mg q2-4h prn for less than or equal to 5 doses, then PO, 0.2 to 0.4 mg q6-12h for 2 days or prn.

C. Effect: Constriction of uterine and vascular smooth muscle.

D. Comments: May cause hypertension from systemic vasoconstriction (especially in eclampsia and hypertension), dysrhythmias, coronary spasm, uterine tetany, or gastrointestinal (GI) upset. Overdosage may cause convulsions or stroke.

XXXI. ESMOLOL (BREVIBLOC)

A. Indications: Supraventricular tachydysrhythmias and myocardial ischemia.

B. Dosage: Start with 5- to 10-mg IV bolus and increase q3min prn to total 100 to 300 mg; infusion 1 to 15 mg/min.

C. Effect: Selective β_1-adrenergic blockade.

D. Comments: May cause bradycardia, AV conduction delay, hypotension, congestive heart failure; β_2 activity at high doses.

XXXII. FENOLDOPAM

A. Indications: Hypertension.

B. Dosage: 0.03 to 0.1 µg/kg/min (most common dose); increase to 0.05 to 0.1 µg/kg/min every 15 minutes.

C. Effect: Selective postsynaptic dopamine-1 receptor agonist.

D. Comments:
1. Evidence does not indicate that it will prevent contrast-induced nephropathy.
2. May cause hyperkalemia.
3. Tachycardia possible at higher doses.
4. May increase intraocular pressure.

XXXIII. FLUMAZENIL (MAZICON)

A. Indications: Reversal of benzodiazepine overdose.

B. Dosage: 3 to 5 mg IV at 0.5 mg/min.

C. Effect: Competitive antagonism of CNS benzodiazepine receptor.

D. Comments:
1. Duration of action shorter than midazolam and other agonists.
2. May induce CNS excitation including seizures, acute withdrawal, nausea, dizziness, and agitation.
3. Only partial reversal of midazolam-induced ventilatory depression.

XXXIV. FOSPHENYTOIN

A. Indication: Seizure prophylaxis, treatment of seizures (see Phenytoin).

B. Dosage:
1. It is a prodrug; active metabolite is phenytoin.
2. 1.5 mg fosphenytoin is equivalent to 1 mg phenytoin and is referred to as 1 mg phenytoin equivalent (PE).
3. Dilute fosphenytoin in 5% dextrose or 0.9% saline solution for injection to a concentration ranging from 1.5 to 25 mg PE/mL.
4. The loading dose of fosphenytoin is 10 to 20 mg PE/kg given IV.
5. Maximum rate, 150 mg PE/min.

C. Effect: Anticonvulsant.

D. **Comments:**
1. Intravenous bolus may cause bradycardia, hypotension, respiratory arrest, cardiac arrest, or CNS depression.
2. Determination of unbound phenytoin levels may be helpful in patients with renal failure or hypoalbuminemia 2 hours after infusion has been completed.
3. Multiple drug interactions that may change the effective concentration of phenytoin.

XXXV. FUROSEMIDE (LASIX)
A. **Indications:** Edema, hypertension, intracranial hypertension, renal failure, and hypercalcemia.
B. **Dosage:** 2 to 40 mg IV (initial dose, dosage individualized).
C. **Effect:** Increases excretion of Na^+, Cl^-, K^+, PO_4^{3-}, Ca^{2+}, and H_2O by inhibiting reabsorption in loop of Henle.
D. **Comments:** May cause electrolyte imbalance, dehydration, transient hypotension, deafness, hyperglycemia, or hyperuricemia. Sulfa-allergic patients may exhibit hypersensitivity to furosemide.

XXXVI. GLUCAGON
A. **Indications:**
1. Duodenal or choledochal relaxation.
2. Refractory β-adrenergic blocker toxicity.
B. **Dosage:**
1. GI effects, 0.25 to 0.5 mg IV q20min prn.
2. β-Blocker toxicity, 5-mg IV bolus, with 1 to 10 mg/h titrated to patient response.
C. **Effect:** Catecholamine release. Positive inotrope and chronotrope.
D. **Comments:**
1. May cause anaphylaxis, nausea, vomiting, hyperglycemia, or positive inotropic chronotropic effects.
2. High doses potentiate oral anticoagulants.
3. Use with caution in the presence of insulinoma or pheochromocytoma.

XXXVII. GLYCOPYRROLATE
A. **Indications:** Decrease GI motility, antisialagogue. Bradycardia.
B. **Dosage:** 0.1 to 0.2 mg IV/IM/SC
C. **Effect:** Competitive blockade of acetylcholine at muscarinic receptors.
D. **Comments:** Longer duration, possibly less chronotropic effect than atropine. Does not cross the blood-brain barrier or placenta.

XXXVIII. HALOPERIDOL (HALDOL)
A. **Indications:** Psychosis, delirium, agitation, and postoperative nausea and vomiting.
B. **Dosage:** 0.5 to 10 mg IM/IV prn (dosage individualized); antiemetic, 1 mg IV.
C. **Effect:** Antipsychotic effects due to dopamine (D_2) receptor antagonism. CNS depression.
D. **Comments:**
1. May cause mild α-adrenergic antagonism.
2. Can prolong QT interval and produce ventricular arrhythmias, notably torsade de pointes, and lower seizure threshold.
3. May precipitate neuroleptic malignant syndrome.
4. Contraindicated in Parkinson disease.

XXXIX. HEPARIN—UNFRACTIONATED

A. **Indications**: Anticoagulation for:
1. Thrombosis, thromboembolism.
2. Cardiopulmonary bypass.
3. Disseminated intravascular coagulation.
4. Thromboembolism prophylaxis.

B. **Dosage:**
1. Thrombosis, load: 50 to 150 units/kg IV; maintenance: 15 to 25 units/ kg/h IV; titrate dosage with activated partial thromboplastin time.
2. CPBP, load: 300 units/kg IV; maintenance: 100 units/kg/h IV; titrate with activated clotting time (ACT).
3. Disseminated intravascular coagulopathy (DIC), load: 50 to 100 units/kg IV; maintenance: 15 to 25 units/kg/h IV; titrate with coagulation tests.
4. DVT prophylaxis, 5000 units q8-12h SC.

C. **Effect**: Potentiates action of antithrombin III; blocks conversion of prothrombin and activation of other coagulation factors.

D. **Comments:**
1. May cause thrombocytopenia, allergic reactions.
2. Half-life increased in renal failure and decreased in thromboembolism and liver disease.
3. Does not cross the placenta.
4. Reversed by protamine.
5. Spinal and epidural hematomas have been associated with neuraxial anesthesia (single-shot, or catheter placement or removal) and lumbar punctures in patients on heparin infusions.

XL. HYDRALAZINE

A. **Indication**: Hypertension.

B. **Dosage**: 2.5 to 5 mg IV. Repeat as needed up to total dose of 20 mg.

C. **Effect**: Reduces arterial smooth muscle tone; diastolic more effected than systolic.

D. **Comments**: May cause reflex tachycardia, systemic lupus erythematosus syndrome. Increases coronary, splanchnic, cerebral, and renal blood flows.

XLI. HYDROCORTISONE (SOLU-CORTEF)

A. **Indications:**
1. Adrenal insufficiency.
2. Inflammation and allergic reaction.
3. Cerebral edema from CNS tumors.
4. Asthma.

B. **Dosage**: 10 to 100 mg IV q8h. Physiologic replacement: IV: 0.25 to 0.35 mg/kg/d; PO: 0.5 to 0.75 mg/kg/d.

C. **Effect:**
1. Anti-inflammatory.
2. Mineralocorticoid effect.
3. Stimulates gluconeogenesis.
4. Inhibits peripheral protein synthesis.
5. Has membrane stabilizing effect.

D. **Comments:**
1. May cause adrenocortical insufficiency (Addisonian crisis) with abrupt withdrawal.
2. Delayed wound healing.
3. CNS disturbances, osteoporosis, or electrolyte disturbances.

XLII. INDIGO CARMINE

A. **Indications:** Evaluation of urine output. Localization of ureteral orifices during cystoscopy.

B. **Dosage:** 40 mg IV slowly (5 mL of 0.8% solution).

C. **Effect:** Rapid glomerular filtration produces blue urine.

D. **Comments:** Hypertension from α-adrenergic stimulation with rapid administration, lasts 15 to 30 minutes after IV dose. Dye color may interfere with pulse oximetry.

XLIII. ISOPROTERENOL

A. **Indications:** Heart failure; bradycardia.

B. **Dosage:** 2 µg/min titrated up to 20 µg/min.

C. **Effect:** β-Adrenergic agonist; positive chronotrope and inotrope.

D. **Comments:** May cause dysrhythmias, myocardial ischemia, hypertension, or CNS excitation.

XLIV. KETOROLAC (TORADOL)

A. **Indications:** Nonsteroidal anti-inflammatory drug (NSAID) for moderate pain. Useful adjunct for severe pain when used with parenteral or epidural opioids.

B. **Dosage:** 30 to 60 mg, then 15 to 30 mg q6h.

C. **Effect:** Limits prostaglandin synthesis by cyclooxygenase inhibition.

D. **Comments:**

1. Adverse effects are similar to those with other NSAIDs: peptic ulceration, bleeding, decreased renal blood flow.
2. Duration of treatment not to exceed 5 days.
3. Caution when used in the elderly or in patients with preexisting renal dysfunction or significant hypovolemia.

XLV. LABETALOL

A. **Indications:** Hypertension, controlled hypotension.

B. **Dosage:** 5 to 10 mg IV increments at 5-minute intervals, to 40 to 80 mg/ dose. Infusion: titrate to desired response, 10 to 180 mg/h.

C. **Effect:** Selective α_1-adrenergic blockade with nonselective β-adrenergic blockade. Ratio of α/β-blockade = 1:7.

D. **Comments:** May cause bradycardia, AV conduction delays, and postural hypotension. Crosses the placenta.

XLVI. LEVETIRACETAM (KEPPRA)

A. **Indication:** Seizure prophylaxis; treatment of seizures.

B. **Dosage:** 500 to 1000 mg IV.

C. **Effect:** Suppression of seizure activity.

D. **Comments:** Adjustment for renal insufficiency.

XLVII. LIDOCAINE (XYLOCAINE)

A. **Indications:**

1. Ventricular dysrhythmias.
2. Cough suppression.
3. Local anesthesia.

B. **Dosage:**

1. Dysrhythmias, 1 mg/kg IV × 2 (second dose 20 to 30 minutes after first dose) followed by 15 to 50 µg/kg/min IV (1 to 4 mg/min).
2. Cough 1 mg/kg IV.

C. **Effect:** Decreases conductance of sodium channels. Antiarrhythmic effect, sedation, neural blockade.

D. **Comments:**
1. May cause dizziness, seizures, disorientation, heart block (with myocardial conduction defect), or hypotension.
2. Crosses the placenta.
3. Caution in patients with Wolff-Parkinson-White syndrome.

XLVIII. LOW-MOLECULAR-WEIGHT HEPARIN
Please see individual entries for dalteparin (Fragmin) and enoxaparin (Lovenox).

XLIX. MAGNESIUM SULFATE
A. **Indications:**
1. Preeclampsia/eclampsia.
2. Hypomagnesemia.
3. Polymorphic ventricular tachycardia (torsade de pointes).
B. **Dosage:**
1. Obstetrics, 1 to 8 g IV, then 1 to 4 g/h.
2. Hypomagnesemia, 1 to 2 g q6-8h, prn.
3. VT, 1 to 2 g in 10 mL D5W over 1 to 2 minutes; 5 to 10 g may be administered for refractory arrhythmias.
C. **Effect:** Treatment and prevention of hypomagnesemia; prevents and treats seizures or hyperreflexia associated with preeclampsia/eclampsia.
D. **Comments:**
1. Potentiates neuromuscular blockade.
2. Potentiates CNS effects of anesthetics, hypnotics, and opioids.
3. Toxicity occurs with serum concentration greater than or equal to 10 mEq/L.
4. May alter cardiac conduction in digitalized patients. Avoid in patients with heart block.
5. Caution in patients with renal failure.

L. MANNITOL
A. **Indications:**
1. Increased intracranial pressure.
2. Oliguria or anuria associated with acute renal injury.
B. **Dosage:**
1. ICP, 0.25 to 1.0 g/kg IV as 20% solution over 30 to 60 minutes (in acute situation, can give bolus of 1.25 to 25.0 g over 5 to 10 minutes).
2. Renal, 0.2 g/kg test dose over 3 to 5 minutes, then 50 to 100 g IV over 30 minutes if adequate response.
C. **Effect:** Increases serum osmolality, which reduces cerebral edema and lowers intracranial and intraocular pressure; also causes osmotic diuresis and transient expansion of intravascular volume.
D. **Comments:**
1. Rapid administration may cause vasodilation and hypotension.
2. May worsen or cause pulmonary edema, intracranial hemorrhage, systemic hypertension, or rebound intracranial hypertension.

LI. METHYLENE BLUE
A. **Indications:**
1. Surgical marker for genitourinary surgery.
2. Methemoglobinemia.
3. Vasoplegic syndrome.

B. **Dosage:**
1. Genitourinary, 100 mg (10 mL of 1% solution) IV.
2. Methemoglobinemia, 1 to 2 mg/kg IV of 1% solution over 10 minutes; repeat q1h, prn.
3. Vasoplegia, 2 mg/kg IV.
C. **Effect:** Low dose promotes conversion of methemoglobin to hemoglobin. High dose promotes conversion of hemoglobin to methemoglobin.
D. **Comments:**
1. May cause red blood cell destruction (prolonged use), hypertension, bladder irritation, nausea, diaphoresis.
2. May inhibit nitrate-induced coronary artery relaxation.
3. Interferes with pulse oximetry for 1 to 2 minutes.
4. Can cause hemolysis in patients with glucose-6-phosphate dehydrogenase deficiency.

LII. METHYLERGONOVINE (METHERGINE)
A. **Indication:** Postpartum hemorrhage due to uterine atony.
B. **Dosage:**
1. IV (*emergency only*, after delivery of placenta): 0.2 mg in 5 mL of NS, dose over greater than or equal to 1 minute.
2. IM: 0.2 mg q2-4h, prn (<5 doses).
C. **Comments:** See Ergonovine. Caution in patients with hypertension, although the hypertensive response is less marked than with ergonovine.

LIII. METHYLPREDNISOLONE (SOLU-MEDROL)
A. **Indications:** See Hydrocortisone. Spinal cord injury; status asthmaticus.
B. **Dosage:**
1. 40 to 60 mg IV q6h. Higher doses in transplant patients.
2. Status asthmaticus, 2 mg/kg; then 0.5 to 1 mg/kg q6h.
3. Spinal cord injury, 30 mg/kg IV over 15 minutes; after 45 minutes begin 5.4 mg/kg/h × 23 or 47 hours.
C. **Effect:** See Hydrocortisone; has five times the glucocorticoid potency of hydrocortisone with almost no mineralocorticoid activity.
D. **Comments:** See Hydrocortisone.

LIV. METOCLOPRAMIDE (REGLAN)
A. **Indications:** Gastroesophageal reflux, diabetic gastroparesis, pulmonary aspiration prophylaxis, and antiemetic.
B. **Dosage:** 10 mg IV q6-8h.
C. **Effect:**
1. Facilitates gastric emptying by increasing gastric motility; relaxes pyloric sphincter and increases peristalsis in the duodenum and jejunum.
2. Increases resting tone of the lower esophageal sphincter.
3. Weak antiemetic effects appear secondary to antagonism of central and peripheral dopamine receptors.
4. Case causes neuroleptic malignant syndrome.
D. **Comments:**
1. Avoid in patients with GI obstruction, pheochromocytoma, or Parkinson disease.
2. Extrapyramidal reactions occur in 0.2% to 1% of patients.

LV. METOPROLOL (LOPRESSOR)
A. **Indications:** Hypertension, angina pectoris, dysrhythmia, hypertrophic cardiomyopathy, MI, and pheochromocytoma.

B. Dosage: 2.5 to 5 mg IV q2min, prn, up to 15 mg.
C. Effect: β_1-Adrenergic blockade (β_2-adrenergic antagonism at high doses).
D. Comments:
1. May cause symptomatic bradycardia.
2. Can increase the risk of heart block.

LVI. MILRINONE
A. Indication: Myocardial depressing requiring inotropy.
B. Dosage: 50 µg/kg IV over 10 minutes, then titrate 0.375 to 0.75 µg/kg/min to effect.
C. Effect: Phosphodiesterase inhibition causing positive inotropy and vasodilation.
D. Comments:
1. May increase ventricular ectopy.
2. Possible worsening of outflow tract obstruction in hypertrophic obstructive cardiomyopathy (HOCM).
3. Hypotension is common.

LVII. NALOXONE (NARCAN)
A. Indication: Reversal of systemic opioid effects.
B. Dosage: Adult: 0.04- to 0.4-mg doses IV, titrated q2-3min. Pediatric: 1 to 10 µg/kg IV (in increments) q2-3min (up to 0.4 mg).
C. Effect: Antagonizes effects of opioids by competitive inhibition.
D. Comments:
1. May cause hypertension, dysrhythmias, rare pulmonary edema, and delirium usually if given in high doses.
2. Reversal of analgesia.
3. Withdrawal syndrome in opioid-dependent patients.
4. Renarcotization may occur because antagonist has shorter duration than opiates.

LVIII. NICARDIPINE (CARDINE)
A. Indication: Hypertension.
B. Dosage: 2.5-5 mg/h
C. Effect: IV antihypertensive calcium channel blocker.
D. Comments:
1. Steady state achieved in 3 to 5 hours.
2. Maximum dose limit: 15 mg/h.
3. My cause hypoxemia secondary to inhibition of hypoxic pulmonary vasoconstriction.

LIX. NITROGLYCERIN
A. Indications:
1. Angina, myocardial ischemia, or infarction.
2. Hypertension.
3. Congestive heart failure.
4. Controlled hypotension.
5. Esophageal spasm.
B. Dosage:
1. Initial IV infusion at 50 µg/min, then titrate to effect.
2. Sublingual (SL): 0.15 to 0.6 mg/dose.
3. Topical: 2% ointment, 0.5 to 2.5 in q6-8h.
C. Effect:
1. Produces smooth muscle relaxation by enzymatic release of NO, causing systemic, coronary, and pulmonary vasodilatation (veins more than arteries).
2. Bronchodilation, biliary, GI, and genitourinary tract relaxation.

D. **Comments:**
1. May cause reflex tachycardia, hypotension, or headache.
2. Tolerance with chronic use may be avoided with a 10- to 12-hour nitrate-free period.
3. May be adsorbed by plastic in IV tubing.

LX. NITROPRUSSIDE (NIPRIDE)

A. **Indications:** Hypertension, controlled hypotension, and congestive heart failure.
B. **Dosage:** IV infusion initially at 0.1 µg/kg/min, then titrated to patient response to maximum 10 µg/kg/min.
C. **Effect:** Direct NO donor causing smooth muscle relaxation in both arterioles and veins.
D. **Comments:**
1. May cause excessive hypotension if not titrated slowly.
2. Reflex tachycardia.
3. Accumulation of cyanide with liver dysfunction; thiocyanate with kidney dysfunction. Cyanide/thiocyanate buildup with prolonged infusion.
4. Avoid with Leber hereditary optic atrophy, hypothyroidism, or vitamin B_{12} deficiency.
5. Solution and powder are light-sensitive and must be wrapped in opaque material.

LXI. NOREPINEPHRINE (LEVOPHED)

A. **Indication:** Hypotension, myocardial depression.
B. **Dosage:**
1. 1 to 30 µg/min IV, titrated to desired effect.
2. Administered through central venous catheter.
C. **Effect:** Both α- and β-adrenergic activity, with α-adrenergic activity predominating.
D. **Comments:**
1. May cause tachycardia and dysrhythmias in some patients.
2. Increased uterine contractility.
3. Constricted microcirculation.

LXII. OCTREOTIDE (SANDOSTATIN)

A. **Indications:**
1. Upper GI tract bleeding and acute variceal hemorrhage.
2. Treatment of symptomatic carcinoid.
B. **Dosage:** 25- to 50-µg IV bolus followed by continuous IV infusion of 25 to 50 µg/h.
C. **Effect:** Somatostatin analogue that suppresses the release of serotonin, gastrin, vasoactive intestinal peptide, insulin, glucagon, and secretin.
D. **Comments:** May cause nausea, decreased GI motility, and transient hyperglycemia.

LXIII. ONDANSETRON (ZOFRAN)

A. **Indications:** Prophylaxis and treatment of perioperative nausea and vomiting.
B. **Dosage:** Adult: 4 mg IV over greater than 30 seconds or 8 mg PO. Pediatric: 4 mg PO.
C. **Effect:** Selective 5-HT_3 receptor antagonist.
D. **Comments:** Used in much higher doses for chemotherapy-induced nausea. Mild side effects include headache and reversible transaminase elevation.

LXIV. OXYTOCIN (PITOCIN)

A. **Indications:** Postpartum hemorrhage, uterine atony, and augmentation of labor.

B. **Dosage:**
1. Hemorrhage, 10 units IM or 10 to 40 units in 1000 mL of crystalloid-infused IV at rate necessary to control atony (eg, 0.02 to 0.04 units/min).
2. Labor induction: 0.0005 to 0.002 units/min, increasing until contraction pattern established or maximum dose of 20 milliunits/min reached.

C. **Effect:** Reduces postpartum blood loss by contraction of uterine smooth muscle. Renal, coronary, and cerebral vasodilation.

D. **Comments:**
1. May cause uterine tetany and rupture, fetal distress, or anaphylaxis.
2. Intravenous bolus can cause hypotension, tachycardia, and dysrhythmia.

LXV. PHENOBARBITAL

A. **Indication:** Seizure suppression.

B. **Dosage:** 10 to 20 mg/kg IV, additional 5 mg/kg doses q15-30min for control of status epilepticus, then 3 to 5 mg/kg/d PO or IV in divided doses.

C. **Comments:**
1. May cause hypotension.
2. Multiple drug interactions through induction of hepatic enzyme systems.
3. Therapeutic anticonvulsant concentration 15 to 40 μg/mL at trough (just before next dose).

LXVI. PHENOXYBENZAMINE

A. **Indication:** Preoperative preparation for pheochromocytoma resection.

B. **Dosage:** 10 to 40 mg/d PO (start at 10 mg/d and increase dosage by 10 mg/d every 4 days prn).

C. **Effect:** Nonselective and noncompetitive α-adrenergic antagonist.

D. **Comments:** May cause orthostatic hypotension (which may be refractory to norepinephrine) and reflex tachycardia.

LXVII. PHENYLEPHRINE

A. **Indication:** Hypotension.

B. **Dosage:** 10 μg/min IV initially, then titrated to response; IV bolus 40 to 100 μg/dose. Customary mix: 10 to 30 mg in 250 mL of D5W or NS.

C. **Effect:** α_1-Adrenergic agonist.

D. **Clearance:** Hepatic metabolism; renal elimination.

E. **Comments:** May cause hypertension, reflex bradycardia, microcirculatory constriction, uterine contraction, or uterine vasoconstriction.

LXVIII. PHENYTOIN (DILANTIN)

A. **Indications:** Seizure prophylaxis, treatment of seizures.

B. **Dosage:** 10 to 15 mg/kg IV at less than 50 mg/min (up to 1000 mg cautiously, with ECG monitoring); for neurosurgical prophylaxis, then 100 to 200 mg IV q4h (at <50 mg/min).

C. **Effect:**
1. Anticonvulsant effect via membrane stabilization.
2. Antidysrhythmic effect similar to those of quinidine or procainamide.

D. **Comments:**
1. Intravenous bolus may cause bradycardia, hypotension, respiratory arrest, cardiac arrest, or CNS depression.

2. Nystagmus, diplopia, ataxia, drowsiness, gingival hyperplasia, GI upset, hyperglycemia, or hepatic microsomal enzyme induction.
3. Crosses the placenta.
4. Significant interpatient variation in dose needed to achieve therapeutic concentration of 7.5 to 20.0 μg/mL.
5. Determination of unbound phenytoin levels may be helpful in patients with renal failure or hypoalbuminemia.

LXIX. PHOSPHORUS (SODIUM PHOSPHATE)
A. **Indications:**
1. Treatment and prevention of hypophosphatemia.
B. **Dosage:** 0.15 to 0.25 mmol/kg IV over 6 to 12 hours.
C. **Effect:** Electrolyte replacement.
D. **Comments:**
1. Infuse doses of IV phosphate over a 4- to 6-hour period since risks of rapid IV infusion include hypocalcemia, hypotension, muscular irritability, calcium deposition, renal function deterioration, and hyperkalemia.
2. Use with caution in patients with cardiac disease and renal insufficiency.

LXX. PHYSOSTIGMINE (ANTILIRIUM)
A. **Indications:** Postoperative delirium, tricyclic antidepressant overdose, and reversal of CNS effects of anticholinergic drugs.
B. **Dosage:** 0.5 to 2.0 mg IV q15min prn.
C. **Effect:** Central and peripheral cholinergic effects; inhibits cholinesterase.
D. **Comments:** Rarely may cause bradycardia, tremor, convulsions, hallucinations, CNS depression, mild ganglionic blockade, or cholinergic crisis.

LXXI. POTASSIUM (KCl) (SEE APPENDIX I)

LXXII. PROCHLORPERAZINE (COMPAZINE)
A. **Indications:** Nausea and vomiting.
B. **Dosage:** 5 to 10 mg IV (≤40 mg/d); 5 to 10 mg IM q2-4h prn; 25 mg PR q12h prn.
C. **Effect:** Central dopamine (D_2) antagonist with neuroleptic and antiemetic effects with antimuscarinic and antihistaminic (H_1) actions.
D. **Comments:** May cause hypotension (especially when given IV), extrapyramidal reactions, neuroleptic malignant syndrome, leukopenia, and cholestatic jaundice.

LXXIII. PROMETHAZINE (PHENERGAN)
A. **Indications:** Nausea and vomiting.
B. **Dosage:** Adult: 12.5 to 25 mg IV q4-6h prn. Pediatric: 0.1 to 1 mg/kg IV, IM, PO, PR (per rectum) q4-6h prn.
C. **Effect:** Antagonist of H_1 and muscarinic receptors.
D. **Comments:** Lower doses (3-6 mg) may be effective in the immediate postoperative period for nausea and vomiting. May cause mild hypotension or mild anticholinergic effects.

LXXIV. PROPRANOLOL (INDERAL)
A. **Indications:**
1. Hypertension, atrial and ventricular dysrhythmias, myocardial ischemia, or infarction.

    2. Junctional rhythm.

    3. Hypertrophic cardiomyopathy.

    4. Thyrotoxicosis.

    5. Migraine headache.

B. Dosage: 0.5 to 1 mg IV, then titrate to effect; 0.5 mg IV for junctional rhythm.

C. Effect: Nonspecific β-adrenergic blockade.

D. Comments: May cause bradycardia, AV dissociation.

LXXV. PROSTAGLANDIN E₁ (ALPROSTADIL) (SEE APPENDIX I)

LXXVI. PROTAMINE

A. Indication: Reversal of the effects of heparin.

B. Dosage: 1 mg/100 units of heparin activity IV at less than or equal to 5 mg/min.

C. Effect: Polybasic compound forms complex with polyacidic heparin.

D. Comments:

    1. May cause myocardial depression and peripheral vasodilation with sudden hypotension or bradycardia.

    2. May cause severe pulmonary hypertension, particularly in the setting of cardiopulmonary bypass.

    3. Concern for allergic reaction/anaphylaxis for patients taking NPH insulin.

    4. Transient reversal of heparin may be followed by rebound heparinization.

    5. Monitor response with a partial thromboplastin time or ACT.

LXXVII. SCOPOLAMINE

A. Indications: Sedation, nausea/vomiting, motion sickness, amnesia.

B. Dosage: 0.3 to 0.6 mg IV/IM, 1.5-mg transdermal patch.

C. Effect: Peripheral and central cholinergic (muscarinic) antagonism.

D. Comments:

    1. Excessive CNS depression can be reversed by physostigmine.

    2. May cause excitement, delirium, transient tachycardia, hyperthermia, or urinary retention.

    3. Care when handling patch because contact with eyes may cause long-lasting mydriasis and cycloplegia.

    4. Crosses the blood-brain barrier and placenta.

LXXVIII. TRANEXAMIC ACID

A. Indications: Prevention of bleeding due to fibrinolysis.

B. Dosage: Intermittent IV infusion: 1000 mg over 10 minutes not to exceed 100 mg/min. Continuous IV infusion: 1 to 16 mg/kg/h not to exceed 100 mg/min.

C. Effect: Stabilizes the formed clot by inhibiting plasminogen activators and plasmin.

D. Comments:

    1. May cause hypotension with rapid administration.

    2. Commonly used for trauma, epistaxis, spine surgery, and joint arthroplasty.

    3. Used for management of postpartum hemorrhage.

    4. Cleared by the kidneys. It is contraindicated for patients with renal insufficiency since is may cause seizures.

    5. Contraindications for any prothrombotic state: previous DVT, PE, stroke, recent cardiac, vascular stent.

LXXIX. VASOPRESSIN (ANTIDIURETIC HORMONE, PITRESSIN)
A. Indications:
1. Diabetes insipidus.
2. Upper gastrointestinal (GI) hemorrhage.
3. Pulseless ventricular tachycardia or ventricular fibrillation.
4. Shock refractory to fluid and vasopressor therapy.

B. Dosage:
1. Diabetes insipidus (DI), 5 to 10 units IM/SC q8-12h.
2. GI, 0.1 to 0.4 units/min IV infusion.
3. ACLS, 40 units IV bolus (single dose).
4. Shock, 0.04 units/min IV infusion titrated as required.

C. Effect:
1. Increases urine osmolality and decreases urine volume.
2. Smooth muscle constriction; vasoconstriction of splanchnic, coronary, muscular, and cutaneous vasculature.

D. Comments:
1. May cause oliguria, water intoxication, pulmonary edema; hypertension, arrhythmias, myocardial ischemia; abdominal cramps (from increased peristalsis); contraction of gallbladder, urinary bladder, or uterus; vertigo or nausea.
2. Patients with coronary artery disease are often treated with concurrent nitroglycerin.
3. Useful in shock states as the effect of drug is not pH-dependent.

LXXX. VERAPAMIL
A. Indications: Supraventricular tachycardia, atrial fibrillation or flutter, Wolff-Parkinson-White syndrome.
B. Dosage: 2.5 to 10 mg IV over ≥2 minutes, repeat once if no response in 30 minutes.
C. Effect: Blocks slow calcium channels in the heart. Prolongs PR interval. Negative inotrope and chronotrope; systemic and coronary vasodilator.
D. Comments:
1. May cause severe bradycardia, AV block (especially with concomitant β-adrenergic blockade), excessive hypotension, or congestive heart failure.
2. May increase ventricular response to atrial fibrillation or flutter in patients with accessory tracts.
3. Active metabolite has 20% of the antihypertensive effect of the parent compound.

LXXXI. VITAMIN K
A. Indications: Deficiency of vitamin K–dependent clotting factors, reversal of warfarin anticoagulation.
B. Dosage: 2.5 to 10 mg IM/SC/PO or 1 to 10 mg IV at less than or equal to 1 mg/min (with caution). If prothrombin time is not improved 8 hours after initial dose, repeat prn.
C. Effect: Increases the levels of clotting factors II, VII, IX, and X by regeneration of vitamin K–dependent epoxide reductase blocked by warfarin.
D. Comments:
1. Excessive doses can make patient refractory to further oral anticoagulation.
2. Rapid IV bolus can cause profound hypotension, fever, diaphoresis, bronchospasm, anaphylaxis, and pain at the injection site.

LXXXII. WARFARIN (COUMADIN)

A. Indication: Anticoagulation.

B. Dosage: 5 mg PO × 2 to 5 days, then 2 to 10 mg PO, titrated to INR (international normalized ratio should be 2 to 3, based on indication).

C. Effect: Inhibits vitamin K epoxide reductase effectively lowering vitamin K levels to inhibit synthesis of factors II, VII, IX, and X and proteins C, S, and Z.

D. Comments:

1. May be potentiated by ethanol, antibiotics, dextran, thyroxine, diazoxide, ethacrynic acid, glucagon, methyldopa, monoamine oxidase inhibitors, phenytoin, prolonged use of narcotics, quinidine, sulfonamides, congestive heart failure, hyperthermia, liver disease, and malabsorption.

2. May be antagonized by barbiturates, chlordiazepoxide, haloperidol, oral contraceptives, hypothyroidism, and hyperlipidemia.

Common Intravenous Antibiotics

The antibiotics listed in this appendix are those usually given in the perioperative period. Doses marked by (+) are those that are recommended by the Massachusetts General Hospital (MGH) Infectious Disease service for standard surgical procedure antibiotic prophylaxis. These should be administered within 1 hour of incision unless indicated.

Drug	Dose: ≤80 kg	Dose: >80 kg	Dosing Interval (h)[a]	Comments
Ampicillin-sulbactam (Unasyn) (+)	3 g	3 g	q2h × 3 doses, then q6h	Not effective against *Pseudomonas* spp.
Aztreonam (+)	2g	2 g	q4h	
Cefoxitin	2 g	2 g	q2h	All cephalosporins require adjustment for renal function to prevent seizures in high concentrations.
Cefazolin (Ancef) (+)	2 g	2g 3 g if > 120 kg	q4h	5%-10% of penicillin-allergic patients will react to cephalosporins.
Ceftazidime	2 g	2 g	q4h	Preferred for *Pseudomonas aeruginosa* infections and neutropenic patients with fever.
Ceftriaxone (+)	2 g	2 g		Preferred for empiric coverage for bacterial meningitis.
Cefuroxime (+)	1.5 g	1.5 g	q4h	Preferred for community-acquired pneumonia.
Ciprofloxacin (+)	400 g	400 g	q6h	Administer within 2 h of incision.
Clindamycin (+)	900 g	900 g	q6h	Associated with *Clostridium difficile* colitis. May prolong neuro-muscular blockade.

(*continued*)

Drug	Dose: ≤80 kg	Dose: >80 kg	Dosing Interval (h)[a]	Comments
Doxycycline	100 g	100 g		
Fluconazole	200-400 mg	200-400 mg	q24h	
Gentamicin (+)	5 mg/kg	5 mg/kg	q24	Use adjusted body weight for high BMI. Initial dose unchanged for renal failure. Renal toxicity and ototoxicity. Precipitates with heparin. May prolong neuro-muscular blockade.
Imipenem-cilastatin	500 mg	500 mg	q2h × 3 doses, then q6h	Preferred for multiple-drug resistant gram-negative bacterial infections. Renal adjustment to prevent seizures.
Levofloxacin	500 mg	500 mg	qd	
Linezolid	600 mg	600 mg	q12h	Treatment of VRE. >7-10 d use may cause myelosuppression. **Do not give with meperidine or meth-ylene blue. MAO inhibition will cause serotonin syndrome.**
Meropenem	0.5-1 g	0.5-1 g	q2h × 3 doses, then q6h	Adjust for renal insuf-ficiency to prevent seizures.
Metronidazole (Flagyl) (+)	500 mg	500 mg	q12 h	
Nafcillin	1-2	1-2 g	q2h × 3 doses, then q6h	Preferred for antistaph-ylococcal coverage.
Penicillin G	500,000-2,000,000 U	500,000-2,000,000 U	q4h	Hypersensitivity is common. May induce seizures at high doses and induce interstitial nephritis.

Drug	Dose: ≤80 kg	Dose: >80 kg	Dosing Interval (h)[a]	Comments
Piperacillin-tazobactam (Zosyn)	3.375 g	3.375 g	q2h × 3 doses, then q6h	Tazobactam expands the activity of piperacillin to include β-lactamase–producing strains of *Staphylococcus aureus, Haemophilus influenzae, Enterobacteriaceae, Pseudomonas, Klebsiella, Citrobacter, Serratia, Bacteroides,* and other gram-negative anaerobes.
Vancomycin (+)	1 g over 30-60 min	2 g over 30-60 min	q24h	Preferred for MRSA patients. Increase dose interval in renal disease. Histamine release ("red man syndrome"). May precipitate with other medications.

BMI, body mass index; MAO, monoamine oxidase; MRSA, methicillin-resistant *Staphylococcus aureus*; VRE, vancomycin-resistant enterococci.

[a]Consider more frequent dosing during procedures with rapid blood loss.

Note: Page numbers followed by "f" indicate figures and "t" indicate tables.

CCS0521